Julien's
Primer of Drug Action

Julien's
Primer of Drug Action

A Comprehensive Guide to the Actions, Uses, and Side Effects of Psychoactive Drugs

Fourteenth Edition

Claire D. Advokat, Ph.D.
Louisiana State University

Joseph E. Comaty, Ph.D., M.P.
Baton Rouge, Louisiana

Robert M. Julien, M.D., Ph.D.
Portland, Oregon

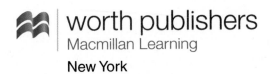

worth publishers
Macmillan Learning
New York

resident, Social Science and High School: Charles Linsmeier
tor of Content and Assessment, Social Sciences: Shani Fisher
tor Associate Editor: Sarah Berger
sistant Editor: Melissa Rostek
Marketing Manager: Clay Bolton
Marketing Assistant: Chelsea Simens
Director of Media Editorial: Noel Hohnstine
Associate Media Editor: Nik Toner
Media Project Manager: Joe Tomasso
Director, Content Management Enhancement: Tracey Kuehn
Senior Managing Editor: Lisa Kinne
Senior Project Manager: Matt Gervais, Lumina Datamatics, Inc.
Senior Project Manager: Andrea Stefanowicz, Lumina Datamatics, Inc.
Senior Workflow Project Manager: Paul Rohloff
Permissions Manager: Jennifer MacMillan
Director of Design, Content Management: Diana Blume
Senior Design Manager: Blake Logan
Art Manager: Matthew McAdams
Composition: Lumina Datamatics, Inc.
Printing and Binding: LSC Communications
Cover Photo: Greg Dunn

Library of Congress Control Number: 2018938114
ISBN-13: 978-1-319-01585-5
ISBN-10: 1-319-01585-9

Printed in the United States of America
1   2   3   4   5   6   23   22   21   20   19   18

Worth Publishers
One New York Plaza
Suite 4500
New York, NY 10004-1562
www.macmillanlearning.com

Claire Advokat received her Ph.D. in physiological psychology from Rutgers University, following which she completed an NIH Postdoctoral Fellowship at the College of Physicians and Surgeons of Columbia University in New York City. She then served on the faculty of the Department of Pharmacology at the University of Illinois Health Sciences Center in Chicago. In 1989, she joined the Department of Psychology at Louisiana State University, retiring in 2012 as an emerita professor. Her area of expertise is the neurobiology of psychoactive drugs, including substances of abuse as well as medications developed for the treatment of mental disorders.

Joseph E. Comaty received his M.S. in experimental psychology from Villanova University, his Ph.D. in psychology with a specialization in clinical neuropsychology from the Rosalind Franklin University of Medicine and Science in Illinois, and his postdoctoral Master's Degree in clinical psychopharmacology from Alliant University/CSPP in California. He retired from his position as chief psychologist, HIPAA privacy officer, and director of the Division of Quality Management of the Louisiana State Office of Behavioral Health, Louisiana Department of Health, in Baton Rouge. He currently serves as a consultant to that agency, conducts forensic fitness for duty evaluations, and has also held an adjunct faculty appointment in the Department of Psychology, Louisiana State University. Dr. Comaty is a clinical and medical psychologist, licensed to prescribe psychotherapeutic drugs in the state of Louisiana.

Robert M. Julien, M.D., received his M.S. and Ph.D. in pharmacology from the University of Washington and his medical degree from the University of California at Irvine. His many research articles focus on the psychopharmacology of sedative and antiepileptic drugs. Formerly an associate professor of pharmacology and anesthesiology at the Oregon Health Sciences University, Dr. Julien retired as staff anesthesiologist at St. Vincent Hospital and Medical Center in Portland, Oregon. For over three decades, Dr. Julien single-handedly accomplished the herculean task of revising each edition and maintaining a succinct yet comprehensive and clear review of the most up-to-date advances in psychopharmacology. He is also an active consultant and lecturer on pharmacology and anesthesiology.

CONTENTS

Preface   xi

PART 1

Introduction to Psychopharmacology   1

Biological Basis of Drug Action

1 Pharmacokinetics: How Drugs Are Handled by the Body   3

Drug Absorption / Drug Distribution / Termination of Drug Action /
Time Course of Drug Distribution and Elimination: The Concept of
Drug Half-Life / Drug Half-Life, Accumulation, and Steady State / Therapeutic
Drug Monitoring / Drug Tolerance and Dependence

2 The Neuron, Synaptic Transmission, and Neurotransmitters   39

Overall Organization of the Brain / Overview of Synaptic Transmission / Specific
Neurotransmitters / Monoaminergic Neurotransmitters

3 Pharmacodynamics: How Drugs Act   69

Receptors for Drug Action / Dose–Response Relationships / Variability in Drug
Responsiveness—The Therapeutic Index

PART 2

Pharmacology of Drugs of Abuse   101

Therapeutic Potential for Drugs of Abuse

4 Epidemiology and Neurobiology of Addiction   105

Extent of the Drug Problem / Nosology and Psychopathology of Substance
Abuse / Neurobiology of Addiction / Pharmacotherapy of Substance Use
Disorders / New Directions

5 Ethyl Alcohol and the Inhalants of Abuse   **135**

ETHYL ALCOHOL
Pharmacokinetics of Alcohol / Pharmacodynamics / Pharmacological
Effects / Psychological Effects / Tolerance, Dependence, and Withdrawal /
Toxicity / Teratogenic Effects / Alcoholism and Its Pharmacological Treatment
INHALANTS OF ABUSE
Why Inhalants Are Abused and Who Abuses Them / Consequences of Acute Use
of Inhalants / Long-Term Consequences of Chronic Inhalant Abuse
Chapter 5 Appendix: What is a Drink? How Much Alcohol is in Your Drink?

6 Caffeine and Nicotine   **177**

CAFFEINE
Pharmacokinetics / Pharmacological Effects / Mechanism of
Action / Reproductive Effects / Tolerance and Dependence
NICOTINE
Epidemiology and Public Policy / Pharmacokinetics / Mechanism of
Action / Pharmacological Effects / Tolerance and Dependence / Toxicity /
Effects of Passive Smoke / Effects During Pregnancy / Pharmacological
Approaches to Nicotine Dependence

7 Cocaine, the Amphetamines, and Other Psychostimulants   **217**

COCAINE
History / Forms of Cocaine / Pharmacokinetics / Mechanism of Action /
Pharmacological Effects in Human Beings / Comorbidity / Cocaine and Pregnancy
AMPHETAMINES
History / Pharmacokinetics of Amphetamine Compared with Cocaine /
Mechanism of Action / Pharmacological Effects / Methamphetamine /
Tolerance and Dependence
NONAMPHETAMINE BEHAVIORAL STIMULANTS
Synthetic Cathinones (Bath Salts) / Flakka (α-pyrrolidinovalerophenone) /
Pharmacological Treatment of Stimulant Dependency

8 Psychedelic Drugs   **257**

Scopolamine: The Prototype Anticholinergic (ACh) Psychedelic /
Monoaminergic Psychedelics / Catecholaminergic Psychedelics / Serotonergic
Psychedelics / Glutaminergic NMDA Receptor Antagonists / Salvinorin A

9 Cannabis: A New Look at an Ancient Plant   **291**

Epidemiology / History / What Is Cannabis? / Mechanism of Action:
Cannabinoid Receptors / Endocannabinoids / Pharmacokinetics /
Pharmacological Effects of Cannabis / Synthetic Cannabinoid
Agonists of Abuse / Cannabis Tolerance, Withdrawal, Addiction, and
Dependence / Treatment Issues

10 Opioid Analgesics   333

Opioid Misuse and Abuse / Opioid Terminology / History / Pain Signaling /
Opioid Receptors / Major Pharmacological Effects of Opiates / Genetic Opioid
Metabolic Defects / Tolerance and Dependence / Full Opioid Agonists / Partial
Agonists / Mixed Agonist-Antagonist Opioids / Pure Opioid Antagonists / Novel
Opioid-Based Compounds Under Development / Future Pharmacotherapy of
Opioid Dependence / Illicit Opioids of Abuse

PART 3

Psychotherapeutic Drugs   379

11 Antipsychotic Drugs   381

Schizophrenia / Historical Background and Classification of
Antipsychotic Drugs / First-Generation Antipsychotics /
Second-Generation Antipsychotics / Prominent Side Effects of Second-
Generation Antipsychotics / CATIE and CUtLASS Studies / In the
Pipeline / Recommendations for the Treatment of Schizophrenia / Additional
Applications for Second-Generation Antipsychotics

12 Antidepressant Drugs   433

Depression / First-Generation Antidepressants / Heterocyclic Antidepressants /
Selective Serotonin Reuptake Inhibitors / Serotonin + Norepinephrine
Reuptake Inhibitors / Serotonin-2 Antagonists/Reuptake Inhibitors (SARIs) /
Noradrenergic/Specific Serotonergic Antidepressant (NaSSA) / Atypical
Antidepressant Drugs or SSRI + Drugs / STAR*D Study / Additional, Alternative,
and Future Approaches to Treatment / Ketamine and Other Glutaminergic
Antagonists / Experimental Agents / In the Pipeline

13 Anxiolytics, Sedative Hypnotics, Anesthetics, and Anticonvulsants   489

Clinical Indications / Historical Background / Sites and Mechanisms of Action /
Sedative-Induced Brain Dysfunction / Barbiturates / Nonbarbiturate Sedative-
Hypnotic Drugs / Benzodiazepines / Flumazenil: A Benzodiazepine Receptor
Antagonist / New Approaches for the Treatment of Anxiety / Drugs Intended for the
Treatment of Insomnia / General Anesthetics / Antiepileptic Drugs

14 Drugs Used to Treat Bipolar Disorder   531

Bipolar Disorder / Diagnostic and Treatment Issues / STEP-BD Study /
Mood Stabilizers: Lithium / Mood Stabilizers: Antiepileptic Drugs / Atypical
Antipsychotics for Bipolar Disorder / In the Pipeline / Psychotherapeutic and
Psychosocial Treatments

PART 4

Special Populations and Integration   571

15 Child and Adolescent Psychopharmacology   573

Pregnancy and Psychotropic Drugs / Drugs of Abuse in Children and
Adolescents / Antidepressants in Childhood and Adolescence / Antipsychotics
in Children and Adolescents / Anxiolytics in Children and Adolescents /
Medications for the Treatment of Bipolar Disorder / Medications for Treating
Autism Spectrum Disorders / Medications for Treating Behavioral or Aggressive
Disorders / Analgesics in Childhood and Adolescence / Attention Deficit/
Hyperactivity Disorder

16 Geriatric Psychopharmacology   627

Inappropriate Drug Use in the Elderly / Control of Agitated and Aggressive
Behaviors in the Elderly / Undertreatment of the Elderly: Focus on
Depression / Parkinson's Disease / Alzheimer's Disease

17 Challenging Times for Mental Health   667

Epidemiology of Mental Illness

Appendix A: Quick Reference to Psychotropic Medication   681

Appendix B: Introduction to Epigenetics   689

Glossary   696

Index   709

The fourteenth edition of *Julien's Primer of Drug Action* marks over 40 years of continuous publication of this now classic textbook, which has as its goal the documentation of current understanding and advances in the psychopharmacological treatment of mental illness and substance abuse.

Historical discoveries that certain chemical compounds could help people who suffer from psychosis, depression, anxiety, mania, and other neurological and psychological conditions led to the development of medications that greatly improved the treatment of these devastating disorders. And similarly, during this time, there has been a corresponding explosion in our knowledge of the neurological substrates, the receptors, and enzymes that are affected by these drugs (discussed in Chapter 3), and an appreciation that they can be most effective when integrated with appropriate behavioral therapy. Unfortunately, progress in the basic science of psychopharmacology has not yet produced corresponding clinical improvements.

As with each of the prior editions, we strive in the fourteenth edition to present the information in a clear, concise, and timely manner, describing the general principles of each class of psychoactive drugs, as well as providing specific information about the individual agents. Each chapter includes an overview of the current models of the disorders, background and mechanisms of action of the drugs, and rationales for drug treatment. Chapters on drugs of abuse provide historical context and epidemiological updates, discussions of the classic agents, and descriptions of the most recent drugs of concern, as well as the latest developments in regard to pharmacological treatments of these disorders.

As in earlier editions, each chapter of the fourteenth edition has been revised to reflect the latest developments in the field. A broad overview of these changes since the last edition suggests the following prominent themes.

First, there has been continued expansion of the clinical indications for the major therapeutic drug classes. These ongoing changes reflect efforts on the part of the pharmaceutical companies to expand the use of their products to a broader array of behavioral health conditions.

Second, the rate of drug development for the treatment of behavioral health disorders has slowed. Although a few new agents have been brought to market since the last edition of this book, most of these agents are so-called "me too" drugs that are similar to those already on the market. In addition, the newer medications, referred to as "second generation" or even "third generation," have not been shown to produce better outcomes compared to what are referred to as "first generation" drugs originally marketed in the mid to late 1950s. The differences among these drugs are more a reflection of differing side effect profiles. This understanding has revived interest in the original agents and in comparisons of therapeutic effectiveness, not only among psychiatric medications, but also between pharmacological and nonpharmacological treatments. Accordingly, the discussion of antipsychotic drugs (Chapter 11) has been completely revised and updated to reflect current concepts of psychopharmacological mechanisms of action.

Third, one practical effect of this pessimistic view is a decrease in current pharmaceutical investment into research and development of new psychotropic medications—but with two exceptions. The first is the ongoing research, so far unsuccessful, for treatments of Alzheimer's disease (Chapter 16). The second major area of current psychiatric drug research involves an old drug, ketamine. This anesthetic agent has recently been shown to be a rapid-acting and effective antidepressant drug. Due to safety concerns and its short duration of action, ketamine itself cannot yet be used for routine clinical applications. Nevertheless, this finding has generated new interest in developing agents that have the same efficacy without the attendant risks (Chapter 12).

Fourth, although drug development may be undergoing a hiatus, there has been continuing interest in understanding the genetic basis of the disorders, drug effects, and interactions. Increased knowledge of how the environment interacts with our genetic substrate is having a profound effect on all aspects of medicine and in our context, especially on theories of addiction and how genetic susceptibility is involved in the etiology of substance abuse. In this edition, we have expanded the section on epigenetics with a summary of the CRISPR-Cas9 gene editing tool (Appendix B).

Fifth, there is increasing overlap between the therapeutic and addictive effects of drugs. Many therapeutic drugs, such as the stimulants (Chapters 6 and 7) and especially the opiates (Chapter 10), are involved in the ongoing epidemic of abuse and overdose deaths. Extraordinary efforts are being made to develop products that are resistant to misuse and diversion. At the same time, research on substances primarily considered to be drugs of abuse, such as hallucinogens (Chapter 8) and cannabis (Chapter 9), is revealing new therapeutic possibilities. As always, we are optimistic that scientific investigation will result in new insights into the etiology of mental illness and addiction and that the future will bring more effective treatments for these devastating disorders.

It is unrealistic to expect practitioners to read and analyze the field critically. Prescribers rely on sources of information that can be presented in compact formats or review articles that provide an informed, comprehensive summary of the important topics. Such resources include publications such as the *Carlat Psychiatry Report*, which does not accept any advertisements or drug company money, studies funded by government agencies such as the National Institute of Mental Health (NIMH), reviews of information by the Agency for Healthcare Research and Quality (AHRQ), and the Cochrane Library reviews. None of the authors of this book have financial ties with the pharmaceutical industry and we strive to ensure that the information we provide is as objective and unbiased as possible.

Finally, we appreciate that keeping current with medical literature is a daunting task. Even the most dedicated authors of textbooks on psychopharmacology too often miss some important developments. We also acknowledge that in order to be as succinct as possible, while remaining comprehensive, clinical data receive greater attention than preclinical results. We made this decision because it is difficult to predict whether or which preclinical outcomes will produce clinical breakthroughs. We accept the risk that by doing so, we may miss some important subsequent developments.

We are indebted to our colleagues, who review each edition and offer valuable criticism and suggestions for improvement. Their input is very much appreciated and we have attempted to incorporate their recommendations as much as possible. While making every effort to accommodate many of their proposals, we acknowledge and regret that we may have fallen short in some instances.

Dedication

Robert M. Julien, MD, Ph.D., was solely responsible for originally authoring and regularly updating this well-known book for over 30 years, beginning with the first edition in 1975. Dr. Julien's unique achievement was to author a text that has served for decades to make the immense amount of information accessible and timely to all those interested in understanding this important area of study. It is a testament to his expertise and dedication that the *Primer of Drug Action* has through the years attained and maintained its reputation as a resource that is always relevant, accurate, and remarkably up to date. Beginning with the eleventh edition, published in 2008, we have been honored to have been selected by Bob to join him in contributing to this stellar work. Only by being involved as authors over the last three editions and now the current one have we fully appreciated what a tremendous accomplishment it is for one person to have done what Bob has accomplished. And on top of his immense scholarship, integrity, and generosity, Bob is a wonderful person who is a delight to work with and who we are grateful to call our friend and colleague. So, it is a great honor to dedicate this fourteenth edition of *Julien's Primer of Drug Action* to Dr. Robert Julien on the occasion of his seventy-fifth birthday. Happy Birthday, Bob!

Claire D. Advokat, Ph.D.
Joseph E. Comaty, Ph.D., M.P.

PART 1

Introduction to Psychopharmacology

BIOLOGICAL BASIS OF DRUG ACTION

Pharmacology is the science of how drugs affect the body. *Psychopharmacology*, a subdivision of pharmacology, is the study of how drugs specifically affect the brain and behavior. To understand the actions, behavioral uses, therapeutic uses, and abuse potentials of psychoactive drugs, we need to know how the body responds when we take such drugs. This understanding involves some knowledge of brain anatomy, the basic principles of drug absorption, distribution, metabolism, and excretion (collectively termed *pharmacokinetics*), as well as the interactions of a drug with its "receptor," or the structure with which the drug interacts to produce its effects (the area of study termed *pharmacodynamics*).

This book specifically concerns drugs that affect the brain and behavior. It is an introduction to psychopharmacology, presenting not only drugs useful in treating psychological disorders, but also drugs prone to compulsive use and abuse. The book begins with three chapters devoted to the fundamentals of drug action.

Chapter 1 explores the area of *pharmacokinetics*, the movement of drug molecules into, through, and out of the body. It addresses such questions as: What are the ways by which drugs get into the body and how does that relate to their actions? Once in the body, how do drugs get to the sites at which they produce their effects? Once a drug exerts its effect, how is that action terminated? Finally, how does the body eventually get rid of the drug?

For readers without a background in neuroscience, Chapter 2 introduces the structure and function of the nervous system and the neuron, because this is where psychoactive drugs produce their effects. We focus on the connection between two different neurons, the *synapse*, and the chemical substances through which neurons communicate, the *neurotransmitters*. By studying the process of synaptic transmission, we begin to understand the mode of action of psychoactive drugs. The phenomenon of synaptic transmission is not static; rather, neurons have the ability to remodel themselves continually, a process called *synaptic plasticity*, which mediates learning and memory as well as such disorders as anxiety, depression, and addiction. A healthy, functioning brain is one that through this process of synaptic plasticity is continually remodeling itself in response to the environment. Healthy neurons continually form new synaptic contacts, maintaining the beautiful architecture that exists through normal interactions with millions of other neurons.

Chapter 3 explores the area of *pharmacodynamics*. It examines the interaction between drugs and the receptors to which the drugs attach and through which they produce their effects. Receptors are described both structurally and functionally, and how drugs alter receptor structure and function is discussed. Finally, we summarize the ways in which such actions underlie the therapeutic effects and the side effects of drugs. These three chapters provide the basic foundation for understanding more specific information in subsequent chapters.

CHAPTER 1

Pharmacokinetics:
How Drugs Are Handled by the Body

When we have a headache, we take it for granted that after taking some aspirin our headache will probably disappear within 15 to 30 minutes. We also take it for granted that, unless we take more aspirin later, the headache may recur within 3 or 4 hours. This familiar scenario illustrates four basic processes in the branch of pharmacology called *pharmacokinetics*. Using the aspirin example, the four processes are as follows:

1. *Absorption* of the aspirin into the body from the swallowed tablet
2. *Distribution* of the aspirin throughout the body, including into a fetus if a female is pregnant at the time the drug is taken
3. *Metabolism* (detoxification or breakdown) of the drug as the aspirin that has exerted its analgesic effect is broken down into metabolites (by-products or waste products) that no longer exert any effect
4. *Elimination* of the metabolic waste products, usually in the urine

These four processes are sometimes abbreviated as *ADME*. In concert, they determine the *bioavailability* of a drug, that is, how much of the drug that is administered actually reaches its target.[1]

The goal of this chapter is to introduce these pharmacokinetic processes. Because many drugs need to be taken chronically and for various periods of time, the chapter also explores the steady-state maintenance of therapeutic blood levels of drugs in the body and the usefulness of therapeutic drug monitoring. Finally, the chapter introduces the concepts of drug *tolerance* and drug *dependence*.

---

[1]An additional term may occasionally be encountered, the *liberation phase*, which extends from the time of drug administration to the point where the drug is dissolved in body fluids and ready for absorption.

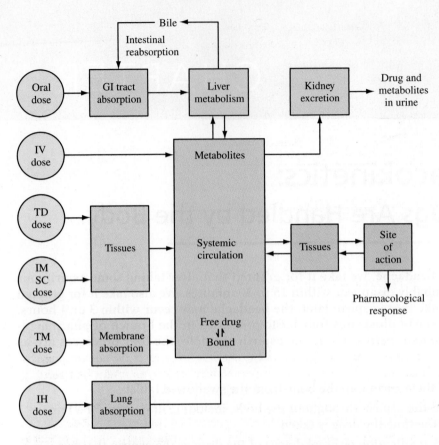

FIGURE 1.1 Schematic representation of the fate of a drug in the body. IM = intramuscular; IV = intravenous; TM = transmembrane; SC = subcutaneous; TD = transdermal; IH = inhalational.

In its simplest form, pharmacokinetics describes the time course of a particular drug's actions—the time to onset and the duration of effect. Usually, the time course simply reflects the amount of *time* required for the rise and fall of the drug's concentration at the target site. Figure 1.1 summarizes drug movement through the body and its equilibrium at its site of action.

The root *kinetics* in the word *pharmacokinetics* implies movement and time. Knowledge of movement and time offers significant insight into the action of a drug. At the very least, it helps distinguish a particular drug from other related drugs. For example, the main difference between the two benzodiazepines (see Chapter 13) *lorazepam* (Ativan) and *triazolam* (Halcion) is in their pharmacokinetics. Both these drugs depress the functioning of the brain, causing sedative and antianxiety effects. Lorazepam, however, persists for at least 24 hours in the body, while triazolam persists for only about 6 to 8 hours. If lorazepam is administered at bedtime for treatment of

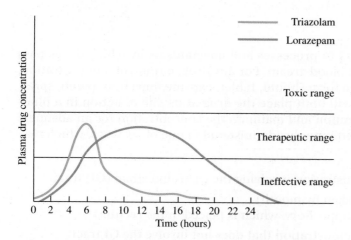

FIGURE 1.2   Theoretical blood levels of triazolam (a short-acting benzodiazepine) and lorazepam (a longer-acting benzodiazepine) over time following oral administration. Approximations for ineffective, therapeutic, and toxic blood levels are shown.

insomnia, daytime sedation the next day can be a problem, because lorazepam persists in the body through the next day. But for a longer, steady action, as might be useful in treating anxiety, lorazepam would be the superior agent to use.[2]

The kinetic differences between lorazepam and triazolam are illustrated in Figure 1.2, which shows three ranges in the blood plasma: an ineffective range (where not enough drug is present to produce either sedative or antianxiety effect), a therapeutic range, and a toxic range (where sedation becomes excessive). Triazolam reaches peak blood level rapidly and is of short duration. Lorazepam, on the other hand, reaches peak blood level later and persists longer in the therapeutic range. In essence, pharmacokinetic differences account for these results and allow two similar drugs to be used to achieve different therapeutic goals.

---

[2] Most drugs used in medicine are known by two or even three names. The most detailed name for a drug is its *structural name,* which accurately describes its chemical structure in words. In this book, such chemical names for drugs are not used. The second name for a drug is its *generic name,* often an abbreviated form derived from the structural name, given to the drug by its discoverer or manufacturer. After a drug's patent protection runs out (usually 17 years after the date of its patent registration by the manufacturer), any other generic drug manufacturer may legitimately sell the drug under this name. The third name is the drug's *trade name,* a unique name given to the drug by its original patent holder. Only that manufacturer can ever sell the drug under that name, even after the patent runs out and others sell the drug under its generic name. For example, many companies sell aspirin, a generic name for acetylsalicylic acid, the structural name. But only Bayer Pharmaceuticals, the original company that patented acetylsalicylic acid, can call it "Bayer Aspirin." In this book, when a drug is introduced, the generic name is given first and is not capitalized. The trade name follows in parentheses, is capitalized, and usually is not given again.

DRUG ABSORPTION

The term *drug absorption* refers to processes and mechanisms by which drugs pass from the external world into the bloodstream. For any drug, a route of administration, a dose of the drug, and a dosage form (liquid, tablet, capsule, injection, patch, spray, or gum) must be selected that will both place the drug at its site of action in a pharmacologically effective concentration and maintain the concentration for an adequate period of time. Drugs are most commonly administered in one of six ways, which may be divided into two categories:

1. *Enteral* routes refer to administration involving the gastrointestinal (GI) tract:
    a. Orally (swallowed when taken by mouth)
    b. Rectally (embedded in a suppository, which is placed in the rectum)
2. *Parenteral* routes refer to administration that does not involve the GI tract:
    a. Injected (given in liquid form with a needle and syringe)
    b. Inhaled through the lungs as gases, as vapors, or as particles carried in smoke or in an aerosol
    c. Absorbed through the skin (usually as a drug-containing skin patch)
    d. Absorbed through mucous membranes (from "snorting," or sniffing, the drug, with the drug depositing on the oral or nasal mucosa; termed *insufflation*)

Oral Administration

To be effective when administered orally, a drug must be soluble (able to dissolve) and stable in stomach fluid (not destroyed by gastric acids), enter the intestine, penetrate the lining of the stomach or intestine, and pass into the bloodstream. Because they are already in solution, drugs that are administered in liquid form tend to be absorbed more rapidly than those given in tablet or capsule form. When a drug is taken in solid form, both the rate at which it dissolves and its chemistry limit the rate of absorption. Food in the stomach may either increase or decrease the rate of absorption; carbonation may speed up absorption. As an example, absorption of the antipsychotic drug *ziprasidone* (Geodon) is cut in half if taken without food (Carlat, 2011). In some cases, rather than the active drug itself, the oral formulation contains a precursor (forerunner) of a drug, called a *prodrug*. A prodrug must undergo chemical conversion by metabolic processes before becoming an active pharmacological agent. An example of this type of medication is the drug *lisdexamfetamine* (Vyvanse), approved for the treatment of attention deficit/hyperactivity disorder (ADHD; see Chapter 15).

After a tablet dissolves, the drug molecules contained within it are carried into the upper intestine, where they are absorbed across the intestinal mucosa by a process of *passive diffusion*, passing from an area of high concentration into an area of lower concentration. This process necessitates that the drug molecules, at least to some degree, be soluble in fat (be *lipid soluble*). In reality, even a small amount of lipid solubility allows for absorption after oral administration; the most lipid-soluble drugs are merely absorbed faster than less lipid-soluble drugs. In general, most psychoactive drugs have good solubility in the lipid linings of the stomach and intestine; therefore, about 75 percent (or more) of the amount of an orally administered psychoactive drug is absorbed into the bloodstream within about 1 to 3 hours after its administration.

As illustrated in Figure 1.3, the digested nutrients from the small intestine (and most of the colon—the large intestine) flow into veins, which collect into the hepatic portal vein. Through the hepatic portal vein, nutrients and other products involved in digestion are transported to the liver as a first stop before going to other organs. This occurs *before general circulation of the blood to the rest of the body*. As described later in this chapter, a significant amount of drug metabolism takes place in the liver during this process, which is accordingly termed *first-pass metabolism*.

There are some exceptions to this general rule. One involves the antidepressant/antianxiety drug *buspirone* (BuSpar; see Chapter 13). This drug has limited clinical efficacy, primarily because most of it is rapidly metabolized by an enzyme located

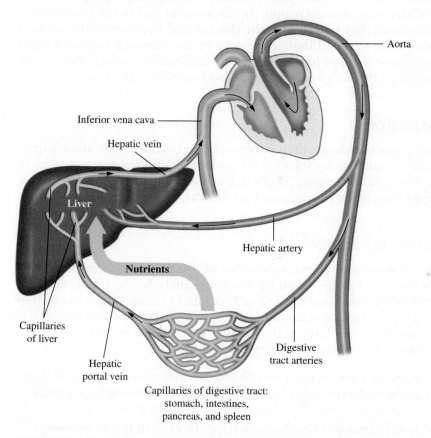

FIGURE 1.3 The hepatic portal connection between the gastrointestinal tract and the liver, illustrating the phenomenon of first-pass metabolism.

in the walls of the stomach lining. This enzyme (called CYP-3A4, discussed later) reduces the oral absorption of buspirone by over 90 percent. Should buspirone be taken with grapefruit juice, however, a component in the juice (furanocoumarin) inhibits the buspirone-metabolizing enzyme, allowing the drug to be more completely absorbed and increasing its therapeutic utility (Paine et al., 2006). It has recently been recognized that this interaction affects many more drugs than previously thought. In their review, Bailey et al. (2012) found that more than 85 drugs undergo this reaction with grapefruit juice and 43 have potentially serious consequences. This list includes drugs from many different categories, not just those that affect the brain. In general, these drugs are usually taken orally and it may take as little as 200 to 250 milliliters of grapefruit juice to produce an adverse reaction such as GI bleeding, urinary retention, dizziness, respiratory depression, and several others.

Although oral administration of drugs is common, it does have disadvantages. First, it may occasionally lead to vomiting and stomach distress. Second, although the amount of a drug that is put into a tablet or capsule can be calculated, how much of it will be absorbed into the bloodstream cannot always be accurately predicted because of genetic differences among people (in the amount and in the composition of the enzymes they have that metabolize the drugs) and because of differences in the manufacture of the drugs. Finally, the acid in the stomach destroys some orally administered drugs, such as local anesthetics and insulin, before they can be absorbed. To be effective, those drugs must be administered by injection.

Rectal Administration

Although the primary route of drug administration is oral, some drugs are administered rectally (usually in suppository form) if the patient is vomiting, unconscious, or unable to swallow. Absorption, however, is often irregular, unpredictable, and incomplete, and many drugs irritate the membranes that line the rectum.

Administration by Inhalation

In recreational drug misuse and abuse, inhalation of drugs is a popular method of administration. Examples of drugs taken by this route include nicotine in tobacco cigarettes and tetrahydrocannabinol (THC; see Chapter 9) in marijuana, as well as smoked heroin, crack cocaine, ice methamphetamine, and the various inhalants of abuse, all of which are discussed later in the book. The popularity of inhalation as a route of administration follows from two observations:

1. Lung tissues have a large surface area through which large amounts of blood flow, allowing for rapid absorption of drugs from the lungs into the blood (often within seconds).
2. Drugs absorbed into pulmonary (lung) capillaries are carried in the pulmonary veins directly to the left (arterial) side of the heart (Figure 1.4) and from

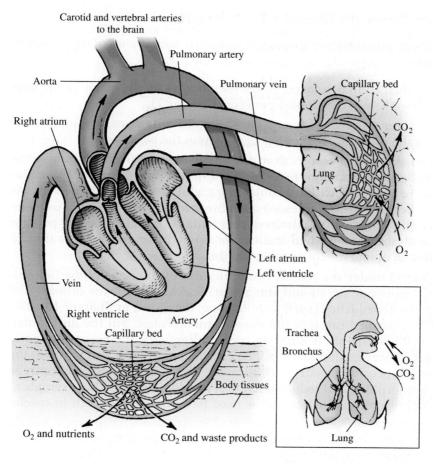

Carotid and vertebral arteries to the brain

Pulmonary artery

Aorta

Pulmonary vein

Capillary bed

Right atrium

CO_2

Lung

O_2

Left atrium

Left ventricle

Vein

Right ventricle

Artery

Capillary bed

Trachea

Bronchus

O_2

CO_2

Body tissues

Lung

O_2 and nutrients

CO_2 and waste products

FIGURE 1.4   Heart and circulatory system. Blood returning from the systemic venous circulation to the heart enters the right atrium and flows into the right ventricle. With contraction of the heart, this blood is pumped into the pulmonary arteries leading to the lungs. Once in the pulmonary capillaries, carbon dioxide (CO_2) is lost and replaced by oxygen. The oxygenated blood returns to the heart in the pulmonary veins, which empty into the left atrium. With heart contraction, the oxygenated blood is pumped from the left ventricle into the aorta and is carried to the body tissues and brain, where oxygen and nutrients are exchanged in the systemic capillary beds. Oxygen and nutrients are supplied to the body tissues through the walls of the capillaries; CO_2 and other waste products are returned to the blood. The CO_2 is eliminated through the lungs and the other waste products are metabolized in the liver and excreted in the urine.

there directly into the aorta and the arteries carrying blood to the brain. As a result, drugs administered by inhalation may have an even faster onset of effect than drugs administered intravenously. If drugs administered in this fashion are reinforcing, the rapid onset of effect can be intense and may promote compulsive use.

Administration Through Mucous Membranes

Occasionally, drugs are administered through the mucous membranes of the mouth or nose. A few examples:

• Cocaine powder, when sniffed, adheres to the membranes on the inside of the nose and is absorbed directly into the bloodstream (see Chapter 7).

• Nicotine (see Chapter 6) in snuff, nasal spray, or chewing-gum formulations is absorbed through the mucosal membranes directly into the bloodstream.

• For use before and after surgery on children, the opioid narcotic *fentanyl* (Sublimaze; see Chapter 10) became available in 1998 in lollipop form, allowing this pain-relieving drug to be provided without subjecting a child to a painful injection. As the lollipop is sucked, the drug is released and absorbed through the mucous membranes of the mouth. This form of administering fentanyl has also become popular for patients with disabling pain when orally administered pain relievers are insufficient and injection of opioid narcotics is too painful.

• A sublingual (placed under the tongue) combination of buprenorphine (an opioid narcotic) and naloxone (an opioid antagonist) is available for the office-based treatment of opioid dependency (such as Suboxone, discussed in Chapter 10). The buprenorphine is absorbed through the mucous membranes, but the antagonist, naloxone, is not. When the pill is administered sublingually, the desired narcotic effect is achieved. However, should the pill be crushed, dissolved, and injected, the antagonist naloxone precipitates drug withdrawal. This effect tends to discourage abuse of the buprenorphine and reduce illicit use, providing yet another example of how knowledge of pharmacokinetics can be used to therapeutic benefit in special circumstances.

Administration Through the Skin

Over the past several years, several medications have been incorporated into *transdermal patches* that adhere to the skin. A transdermal patch is a unique bandagelike therapeutic system that provides continuous, controlled release of a drug from a reservoir through a semipermeable membrane. The drug is slowly absorbed into the bloodstream at the area of contact. Examples of drug-containing patches include:

• Nicotine (used to deter smoking behaviors)
• Fentanyl (used to treat chronic pain)
• Clonidine (used to treat hypertension)
• Estrogen or other hormones (used to replace reduced hormones in postmenopausal women or for contraception)
• Scopolamine (used to prevent motion sickness)
• *Selegiline* (Emsam, used to treat depression)
• *Methylphenidate* (Daytrana, a 9-hour patch used to treat attention deficit/hyperactivity disorder in children)

All these transdermal skin patches allow for slow, continuous absorption of the drug over hours or even days, potentially minimizing side effects associated with rapid rises and falls in plasma concentrations of the drug contained in the patch.

Administration by Injection

Administration of drugs by injection can be *intravenous* (directly into a vein), *intramuscular* (directly into a muscle), *subcutaneous* (just under the skin), or *spinally* (*epidural* or *intrathecal*, that is, directly onto the spinal cord). Each of these routes of administration has its advantages and disadvantages (Table 1.1), but all share some features. In general, administration by injection produces a more rapid response than does oral administration because absorption is faster. Also, injection permits a more accurate dose because the unpredictable processes of absorption through the stomach and intestine are bypassed.

TABLE 1.1 Some characteristics of drug administration by injection

Route	Absorption pattern	Special utility	Limitations and precautions
Intravenous	Absorption circumvented Potentially immediate effects	Valuable for emergency use Permits titration of dosage Can administer large volumes and irritating substances when diluted	Increased risk of adverse effects Must inject solutions slowly as a rule Not suitable for oily solutions or insoluble substances
Intramuscular	Prompt action from aqueous solution Slow and sustained action from repository preparations	Suitable for moderate volumes, oily vehicles, and some irritating substances	Precluded during anticoagulant medication May interfere with interpretation of certain diagnostic tests (for example, creatine phosphokinase)
Subcutaneous	Prompt action from aqueous solution Slow and sustained action from repository (depot) preparations	Suitable for some insoluble suspensions and for implantation of solid pellets	Not suitable for large volumes Possible pain or necrosis from irritating substance
Epidural	Prompt action	Limited exposure of brain (localized effect)	Dural puncture or nerve damage, bleeding, or infection

Administration of drugs by injection, however, has several drawbacks. First, the rapid rate of absorption leaves little time to respond to an unexpected drug reaction or accidental overdose. Second, administration by injection requires the use of sterile techniques. Hepatitis and AIDS are examples of diseases that can be transmitted as a drastic consequence of unsterile injection techniques. Third, once a drug is administered by injection, it cannot be recalled.

Intravenous Administration

In an intravenous injection, a drug is introduced directly into the bloodstream. This technique avoids all the variables related to oral absorption. Intravenous injection can be done slowly and it can be stopped instantaneously if untoward effects develop. In addition, the dosage can be extremely precise, and the practitioner can dilute and administer in large volumes drugs that at higher concentrations would be irritants to the muscles or blood vessels.

The intravenous route is one of the most dangerous of all routes of administration because of the rapid onset of pharmacological action. Too-rapid injection can be catastrophic, producing life-threatening reactions (such as collapse of respiration or of heart function). Also, allergic reactions, should they occur, may be extremely severe. Finally, drugs that are not completely solubilized before injection usually cannot be given intravenously because of the danger of blood clots or emboli forming. Infection and transmission of infectious diseases are an ever-present danger when sterile techniques are not employed.

Intramuscular Administration

Drugs that are injected into skeletal muscle (usually in the arm, thigh, or buttock) are generally absorbed fairly rapidly. Absorption of a drug from muscle is more rapid than absorption of the same drug from the stomach but slower than intravenous absorption. The absolute rate of absorption of a drug from muscle varies, depending on the rate of blood flow to the muscle, the solubility of the drug, the volume of the injection, and the solution in which the drug is dissolved and injected.

Intramuscular injections are of two types: (1) fairly rapid onset and short duration of action and (2) slow onset and prolonged action (*depot* administration). In the former situation, the drug is dissolved in an aqueous (water) solution. Following injection, the water and dissolved drug are quite rapidly absorbed, with complete absorption occurring over a few hours. In the latter, depot type of administration, the drug has been classically suspended in an oily solution. The oil and dissolved drug solution is only slowly absorbed and complete absorption can take days or weeks. Modern manufacturing techniques have allowed the drug to be placed in bioabsorbable polymer microspheres, which release a constant amount of drug each day for a period of a week or more (such as with the antipsychotic Risperdal Consta; see Chapter 11). Similarly, the opioid narcotic antagonist naltrexone suspended in injected microcapsules releases a constant amount of drug into blood over a period of several weeks. This product is marketed under the trade name Vivitrol and is indicated in the treatment of opioid-dependent patients (see Chapter 10). Long-term absorption increases compliance, because the doses are given less frequently. Slow release means that the drug effect is not easily reversible.

Subcutaneous Administration

Absorption of drugs that have been injected under the skin (subcutaneously) is rapid. The exact rate depends mainly on how easy it is for the drug to penetrate the blood vessel and the rate of blood flow through the skin. Irritating drugs should not be injected subcutaneously because they may cause severe pain and damage to local tissue. The usual precautions to maintain sterility should be applied.

Spinal Administration

Protected by the bony vertebrae, the spinal cord consists of a large group of nerves that is located in the center of the spine and which carry messages between the brain and the rest of the body. Both the spinal cord and brain are protected by three layers of tissue or membranes called *meninges* (Figure 1.5). The outermost layer is called the *dura mater*. Between the dura mater and the surrounding bones of the vertebra is a space called the *epidural space*. Injections into this space are called *epidural injections*. The middle protective layer is called the *arachnoid mater*, because this tissue has a spiderweblike appearance due to the network of capillary blood vessels. The space between the arachnoid and the third and last membrane, the *pia mater*, is called the subarachnoid space. The pia mater is the innermost protective layer, tightly associated with the surface of the spinal cord. The subarachnoid space contains cerebrospinal fluid (CSF). The medical procedure known as a lumbar puncture (or "spinal tap") involves the use of a needle to withdraw cerebrospinal fluid from the subarachnoid space, usually from the lumbar region of the spine. Injections into this space are called *intrathecal injections*.

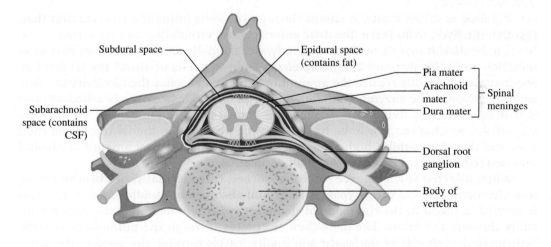

FIGURE 1.5 Cross section of spinal cord and vertebra, illustrating the meninges and accompanying spaces.

DRUG DISTRIBUTION

Once absorbed into the bloodstream, a drug is distributed throughout the body by the circulating blood, passing across various barriers to reach its target, that is, its site of action (its receptors). At any given time, only a very small portion of the total amount of a drug that is in the body is actually in contact with its receptors. For example, in the case of a psychoactive drug, most of the drug circulates outside the brain and therefore does not contribute directly to its pharmacological effect. This wide distribution often accounts for many of the side effects of a drug. *Side effects* are results that are different from the primary, or therapeutic, effect for which a drug is taken.

Bloodstream

Every minute, in an average-size adult, the heart pumps a volume of blood that is roughly equal to the total amount of blood in the circulatory system. That is, the entire blood volume circulates in the body about once every minute. Once absorbed into the bloodstream, a drug is rapidly (usually within the 1-minute circulation time) distributed throughout the circulatory system.

As seen in the schematic diagram of the circulatory system (Figure 1.4), blood returning to the heart through the veins is first pumped into the pulmonary (lung) circulation system, where carbon dioxide is removed and replaced by oxygen. The oxygenated blood then returns to the heart and is pumped into the great artery (the aorta). From there, blood flows into the smaller arteries and finally into the capillaries, where nutrients (and drugs) are exchanged between the blood and the cells of the body. After blood passes through the capillaries, it is collected by the veins and returned to the heart to circulate again. Psychoactive drugs quite quickly become evenly distributed throughout the bloodstream, diluted not only by blood but also by the total amount of water in the body.

If a drug is taken orally, it passes through the cells lining the GI tract and then through the liver; from there, the drug enters central circulation and is carried to the heart to be distributed throughout the body. Occasionally, in the process of first-pass metabolism (p. 7), drug-metabolizing enzymes in the cells of either the GI tract or the liver can markedly reduce the amount of drug that reaches the bloodstream. One example involves the enzyme that metabolizes alcohol. This enzyme is called *alcohol dehydrogenase*. It is found in the cells lining the GI tract and in cells of the liver. As we will see in Chapter 5, women have less of this enzyme in the GI tract cells than men and therefore exhibit higher blood alcohol levels for a given amount of alcohol ingested (corrected for body weight) than do men.

When injected (by whatever route), absorbed transdermally, or absorbed from mucous membranes, a drug bypasses intestinal absorption, rapidly enters veins, and is carried in blood to the right side of the heart (with minimal amounts passing initially through the liver). The drug then circulates through the pulmonary vessels, returns to the left side of the heart, and finally travels through the aorta to the brain and the body.

Cerebrospinal Fluid (CSF)

Cerebrospinal fluid (CSF) is a clear, colorless, bodily fluid that fills the subarachnoid space (between the arachnoid mater and the pia mater) and the *ventricular system* around and inside the brain and spinal cord (Figure 1.6). As seen in the figure, the ventricular system of the brain consists of *two lateral ventricles* (one on each side of the brain), which combine to produce a *third ventricle* that descends as the *aqueduct of Sylvius*, then expands near the base of the brain into the *fourth ventricle* and then becomes the spinal canal. Most of the CSF is produced by the *choroid plexus* (lining) of the lateral, third, and fourth ventricles and circulates through the subarachnoid space (between the arachnoid mater and the pia mater) and around the brain, and is absorbed into the superior sagittal sinus of the peripheral bloodstream across the arachnoid villi.

The human brain contains approximately 140 milliliters of CSF distributed among the four ventricles (20 milliliters), spinal subarachnoid space (30 milliliters), and the cranial subarachnoid space (90 milliliters). Because the brain floats in the CSF, its net weight is reduced from 1400 grams to about 50 grams, which not only reduces pressure at the base of the brain but also provides a protective buffer or cushion against physical impacts. The CSF circulates nutrients and chemical substances filtered from the blood, removes waste products from the brain, and transports hormones to the various brain structures. In the human brain, the entire CSF volume is produced and excreted into the blood every 4 to 5 hours or 4 to 5 times per day. Movement of a drug into the CSF is a function of drug transport across the choroid plexus, which forms

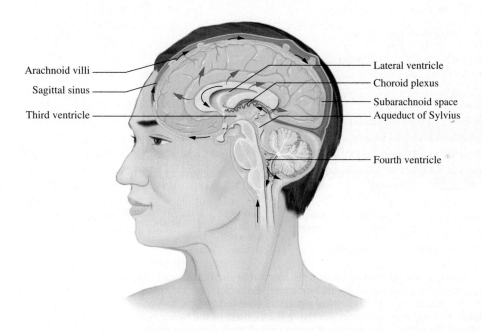

FIGURE 1.6 Circulation of cerebrospinal fluid (CSF) around the brain.

the blood–CSF barrier, and is not due to drug transport across the *blood–brain barrier* (see below). A drug injected into CSF undergoes rapid outflow to the blood compartment via bulk flow (Pardridge, 2016). Our understanding of the relationships between CSF, blood, and drug distribution in the central nervous system is currently undergoing reexamination and revision, which may ultimately lead to better ways of administering medicine to the brain (Brinker et al., 2014; Pardridge, 2011, 2016).

Body Membranes That Affect Drug Distribution

Four types of membranes in the body affect drug distribution: (1) cell membranes, (2) walls of the capillary vessels in the circulatory system, (3) the blood–brain barrier, and (4) the placental barrier.

Cell Membranes

The structure and properties of cell membranes determine their permeability to drugs. In Figure 1.7, the two layers of ovals represent the water-soluble head groups of complex lipid molecules called *phospholipids*. The phospholipid heads form a rather continuous layer on both the inside and the outside of the cell membrane. The wavy lines that extend from the heads into the membrane are the lipid chains of the phospholipid molecules. Therefore, for our present purposes, the interior of the cell membrane can be considered to consist of a sea of lipid in which large proteins are suspended.

Cell membranes provide a physical barrier that is permeable to small, lipid-soluble drug molecules but is impermeable to large, lipid-insoluble drug molecules. As a

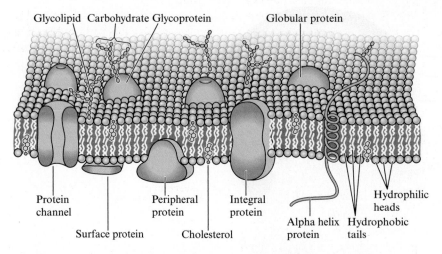

FIGURE 1.7 Diagrammatic representation of a cell membrane, a phospholipid bilayer in which cholesterol and protein molecules are embedded. Both globular and helical kinds of protein traverse the bilayer. Cholesterol molecules tend to keep the tails of the phospholipids relatively fixed and orderly in the regions closest to the hydrophilic phospholipid heads; the parts of the tails closer to the core of the membrane move about freely.

barrier, they are important for the passage of drugs (1) from the stomach and intestine into the bloodstream, (2) from the fluid that closely surrounds tissue cells into the interior of cells, (3) from the interior of cells back into the body water, and (4) from the kidneys back into the bloodstream.

Capillaries

Within a minute or so of entering the bloodstream, a drug is distributed fairly evenly throughout the entire blood volume. From there, drugs leave the bloodstream and are exchanged (in equilibrium) between blood capillaries and body tissues. Figure 1.8 shows a cross-sectional diagram and a schematic of a capillary. Capillaries are tiny, cylindrical blood vessels with walls that are formed by a single thin layer of cells packed tightly together. Between the cells are small pores (clefts or fenestra) that allow passage of small molecules between blood and the body tissues. The diameter of these pores is between 90 and 150 angstroms (Å), which is larger than most drug molecules. Thus, most drugs freely leave the blood through these pores in the capillary membranes, moving along their concentration gradient until equilibrium is established between the concentrations of drug in the blood, body tissues, and water.

The transport of drug molecules between plasma and body tissues is independent of lipid solubility because the membrane pores are large enough for even fat-insoluble drug molecules to penetrate. The pores in the capillary membrane, however, are not large enough to permit the red blood cells and the plasma proteins to leave the bloodstream. Thus, the only drugs that do not readily penetrate capillary pores are drugs that bind to plasma proteins. The rate at which drug molecules enter specific body tissues depends on two factors: the rate of blood flow through the tissue and the ease with which drug molecules pass through the capillary membranes.

Because blood flow is greatest to the brain and much less to the bones, joints, and fat deposits, drug distribution generally follows a similar pattern. For example, when marijuana is smoked, the active drug, tetrahydrocannabinol (THC; see Chapter 9), achieves

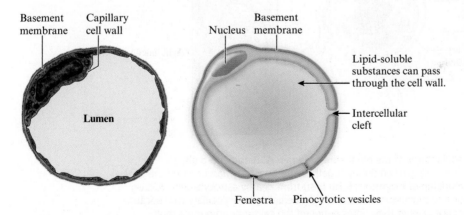

FIGURE 1.8 Cross section of a typical capillary (left) and the schematic (right), showing the pores (*fenestra*) and indicating that lipid-soluble substances can pass through the cell wall.

plasma concentrations of about 10 to 20 nanograms of drug per milliliter (ng/mL) of plasma soon after initiation of smoking. Within about 30 minutes, it achieves levels of about 50 to 100 ng/mL, which fall off within 1 hour to less than 5 to 10 ng/mL because the drug is rapidly taken up into body fat. From there, it slowly returns to plasma and is metabolized to an inactive metabolite (carboxy-THC) that is excreted in the urine.

Blood–Brain Barrier

The brain requires a protected environment to function normally and a specialized structural barrier, called the *blood–brain barrier* (BBB), plays a key role in maintaining this environment (Figure 1.9). In contrast to capillaries in most of the body, the capillary walls in the brain do not have pores. The endothelial cells that make up the

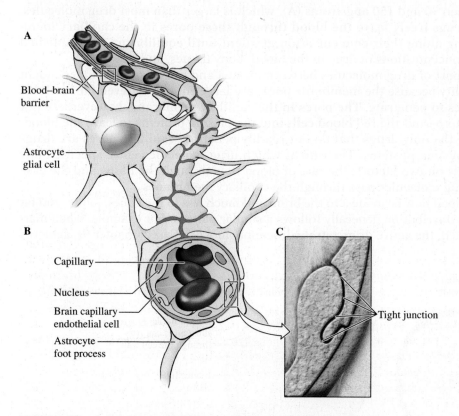

FIGURE 1.9 Cellular basis of the blood–brain barrier. **A.** Blood and brain are separated by capillary cells packed tightly together and by a fatty barrier called the *glial sheath*, which is made up of extensions (glial feet) from nearby astrocyte cells. A drug diffusing from blood to brain must move through the cells of the capillary wall because there are tight junctions rather than pores between the cells; the drug must then move through the fatty glial sheath. **B.** Cross section of a brain capillary. **C.** Electron micrograph of the section in the box from part B. Lines point to the tight junctions between the endothelial cells.

capillary walls are tightly joined together and covered on the outside by a fatty barrier called the *glial sheath,* which arises from nearby astrocyte cells.

Thus, to reach the neurons, a drug leaving the capillaries in the brain has to traverse both the wall of the capillary itself (because there are no pores to pass through) and the membranes of the astrocytes. Therefore, the rate of passage of a drug into the brain is generally determined by two factors: (1) the size of the drug molecule and (2) its lipid (fat) solubility. Large drugs penetrate poorly, while small, fat-soluble drugs penetrate rapidly. Oxygen is small enough and most psychoactive drugs are both small enough and sufficiently lipid soluble to cross the blood–brain barrier. Drugs that cannot cross the blood–brain barrier are restricted to structures outside the central nervous system (CNS). Penicillin is an example of such a drug. It does not cross the blood–brain barrier and its effectiveness as an antibiotic is restricted to infections located outside the brain.

Unfortunately, some other lipid-soluble drugs, such as steroids and beta blockers, are also unable to pass through capillary walls because they are detected as foreign and expelled by cellular export pumps, transporters (of which at least 15 are known) that protect the brain from toxins. Called *P-glycoproteins*, these are members of a larger group of transporters, called the ATP-binding cassette family. It is now known that these transporters are also found in the gut, gonads, and other organs as well as the brain, where they move substances either into or out of the tissue. Some prescription and over-the-counter drugs, foods, and substances made by the body may either inhibit or induce these transporters.

Larger molecules, such as glucose, amino acids, and vitamins, reach the brain because they are carried by special transport systems out of the capillaries. Even larger substances such as iron and insulin can be transported across the capillary wall by a process called *transcytosis*. In this situation, the substances attach to a receptor that is located in the cell wall membrane. A small segment of this membrane then forms a vesicle, which crosses over to and fuses with the membrane on the opposite side of the capillary wall, after which the receptor releases the substance into the brain.

Regardless of whether the drug crosses the blood–brain barrier, all drugs can enter the CSF from the blood. That a drug penetrates into the CSF, however, does not mean that the drug crosses the blood–brain barrier (Pardridge, 2011). Many serious brain disorders do not respond to the conventional lipid-soluble small-molecule model, including Alzheimer's disease, stroke, brain and spinal cord injury, brain cancer, HIV infections of the brain, various ataxia-producing disorders, amyotrophic lateral sclerosis, multiple sclerosis, Huntington's disease, and childhood inborn genetic errors of the brain. Researchers are trying to develop ways in which to "trick" the blood–brain barrier and "sneak" therapeutic drugs into the brain. Efforts are being made to inhibit specific export pumps or to devise lipid vesicles that could carry drug molecules inside their hollow cores and slide through the capillary walls. Perhaps someday we might be able to overcome the constraints of the blood–brain barrier and deliver medications for all types of brain disorders.

Placental Barrier

Among all the membrane systems of the body, the placental membranes are unique, separating two distinct human beings with differing genetic compositions and differing sensitivities to drugs. The fetus obtains essential nutrients and eliminates metabolic waste products through the placenta without depending on its own organs, many of which are not yet functioning. The dependence of the fetus on the mother places the fetus at the mercy of the placenta when foreign substances (such as drugs or toxins) appear in the mother's blood. In general, the mature placenta consists of a network of vessels and pools of maternal blood into which protrude treelike or fingerlike villi (projections) that contain the fetal blood capillaries. Oxygen and nutrients travel from the mother's blood to that of the fetus, while carbon dioxide and other waste products travel from the blood of the fetus to the mother's blood.

The membranes that separate fetal blood from maternal blood in the intervillous space resemble, in their general permeability, the cell membranes that are found elsewhere in the body. In other words, drugs cross the placenta primarily by passive diffusion. Fat-soluble substances (including all psychoactive drugs) diffuse readily, rapidly, and without limitation. The view that the placenta is a barrier to drugs is inaccurate. As a general rule, all psychoactive drugs (and all those discussed in this book) will be present in the fetus at concentrations quite similar to that in the mother's bloodstream. The presence of the drug in the fetus, however, is not necessarily detrimental to the fetus. Some drugs certainly are detrimental and their use should be avoided in women who are or might become pregnant. Ethyl alcohol is an obvious example. Many psychoactive medicines have been shown to be relatively safe to fetal growth and development when taken by a pregnant female. The effects of specific psychoactive drugs on the fetus are discussed in Chapter 15.

TERMINATION OF DRUG ACTION

Routes through which drugs can leave the body include (1) the kidneys, (2) the lungs, (3) the bile, and (4) the skin. Excretion through the lungs occurs only with highly volatile or gaseous agents, such as the general anesthetics and, in small amounts, alcohol "alcohol breath." Drugs that are passed through the bile and into the intestine are usually reabsorbed into the bloodstream from the intestine. Also, small amounts of a few drugs can pass through the skin and be excreted in sweat (perhaps 10 to 15 percent of the total amount of the drugs). Most drugs, however, leave the body in urine, either as the unchanged molecule or as a broken-down *metabolite* of the original drug. More correctly, *the major route of drug elimination from the body is renal (urinary) excretion of drug metabolites produced by the hepatic (liver) biodegradation of the drug.*[3]

Biotransformation (Drug Metabolism)

Biotransformation is what happens to drugs after they have entered the bloodstream and before they leave the body. Psychoactive drugs are usually too lipid soluble to be excreted passively with the excretion of urine. They have to be transformed into

---

[3]When evaluating urine for the presence of drugs of abuse, it is the inactive drug metabolites, rather than the active drug, which are in the urine. It is often unclear whether there is a correlation between the presence of the metabolite in urine and active drug in plasma *at the time the urine sample was taken.*

metabolites that are more water soluble, bulkier, less lipid soluble, and (usually) less biologically active (even inactive) when compared with the parent molecule (the molecule that was originally ingested and absorbed).[4] Thus, for a lipid-soluble drug to be eliminated, it must be metabolically transformed (by enzymes located in the liver) into a form that can be excreted rapidly and reliably. As a general, although not absolute, rule, most metabolites excreted in urine are either inactive or much less active than the parent drug. Examples of inactive metabolites include carboxy-THC (metabolite of THC) and benzoylecognine (metabolite of cocaine).

Biotransformation consists of two phases:

1. Phase I reactions (involving cytochrome P450 enzymes, described below)
2. Phase II reactions, or conjugation (primarily involving glucuronidation)

Phase I Reactions: The P450 System

The enzymes required for biotransformation are located in liver cells (*hepatocytes*) on membranes called the *smooth endoplasmic reticulum*. There are several categories, or families, of these enzymes; as a group they are called the *cytochrome P450 enzymes*, *P450 enzymes*, or *microsomal enzymes* (which relates to the component of the liver cell in which they are found). The main function of P450 enzymes is to turn lipophilic fat-soluble drugs into more water-soluble compounds. This process involves changing the drug molecule into a "polar" compound, a substance that is positively charged on one end and negatively charged on the other. Polar molecules are attracted to water, because water is also polar. Our kidneys are designed to excrete polar compounds and to reabsorb, and thus conserve, lipophilic compounds.

Three primary chemical reactions are catalyzed by P450 enzymes: oxidation, reduction, and hydrolysis. Oxidation means removing (negative) electrons, causing the compound to have a net positive charge. Most psychotropic medications are biotransformed through oxidation. A few are biotransformed by reduction (adding electrons by adding a hydrogen atom) and still others are biotransformed by hydrolysis (adding H_2O, that is, water, which causes a molecule to split up into two polar molecules).

Phase II Reactions: Conjugation

Conjugation means combining a drug with another molecule. "Phase II" means those reactions that usually occur after the Phase I reactions, when Phase I does not make the drug sufficiently hydrophilic to get eliminated. The most common conjugation

---

[4]Some drugs are exceptions: an administered drug may be metabolized into an "active" metabolite, which is at least as active, possibly more active, and may have a longer duration of action than the parent drug. Examples in psychopharmacology include *diazepam* (Valium; see Chapter 13), which is metabolized to nordiazepam, and *fluoxetine* (Prozac; see Chapter 12), which is metabolized to norfluoxetine. In both cases, the parent drug has an effect that lasts for two or three days, while the metabolite is active for over a week until it is eventually biotransformed to an inactive compound that can be excreted.

reaction is *glucuronidation*, in which glucuronic acid ($C_6H_{10}O_7$) is bound to the drug. Glucuronidation is common partly because glucuronic acid is made from glucose, which is plentiful in the body. Many psychotropic drugs are metabolized mainly by glucuronidation, including benzodiazepines, such as *lorazepam* (Ativan) and *temazepam* (Restoril), and drugs used to treat bipolar disorder (Chapter 14), such as *lamotrigine* (Lamictal) and *valproate* (Depakote). Carlat explains why this is important:

> Since both Lamictal and Depakote are metabolized by glucuronidation, there's a drug interaction between them. As it turns out, Depakote latches onto the glucuronidation enzyme more strongly than Lamictal, shoving Lamictal aside, preventing it from being metabolized, and thereby increasing its levels to about double what they are otherwise. Thus, when a patient is on Depakote, you have to start Lamictal at 12.5 mg QD rather than 25 mg QD, and you titrate the dose in smaller increments than usual. (Carlat, 2015, 51)

The *cytochrome P450 enzyme family*, physically located in hepatocytes (with a few located in the cells lining the GI tract), is the major system involved in drug metabolism. This gene family originated more than 3.5 billion years ago and has diversified to accomplish the metabolism (detoxification) of environmental chemicals, food toxins, and drugs. Thus, the cytochrome P450 enzyme system (about 50 of which are functionally active in humans) can detoxify a chemically diverse group of substances. Several P450 enzyme families can be found within any given hepatocyte.

A few of these enzyme families, particularly cytochrome families 1, 2, and 3 (designated *CYP-1*, *CYP-2*, and *CYP-3*), include enzymes involved in most drug biotransformations. By definition, because these three families promote the breakdown of numerous drugs and toxins, enzyme specificity is low (the enzymes are nonspecific in action). Thus, the body is enzymatically capable of metabolizing many different drugs. CYP-3A4 (a subfamily of CYP-3) catalyzes about 50 percent of drug biotransformations (Figure 1.10); this variant is found not only in the liver but also in the GI tract, as we saw with the metabolism of buspirone. CYP-2D6 catalyzes about 20 percent of drugs and CYP-2C variants catalyze an additional 20 percent. Other CYP enzyme variants are responsible for metabolizing the remaining 10 percent of drugs. Even though this may seem like a small proportion, the metabolic effects can be significant, especially considering the various different versions or *polymorphisms* of the enzymes that can occur genetically.

Factors Affecting Drug Biotransformation

Several different factors can alter the rate at which drugs are metabolized, either increasing or decreasing the rate of drug elimination from the body. In general, *genetic*, *environmental*, *cultural*, and *physiological factors* are the most relevant.

First, it is now becoming apparent that genetic variations may affect how different people respond to medications. Genetic DNA testing can now identify how a person may metabolize several drugs of different therapeutic classes, including antidepressants, analgesics, and antipsychotics. In general, DNA testing using a simple mouth swab can identify whether a person is a normal, slow, or fast metabolizer of

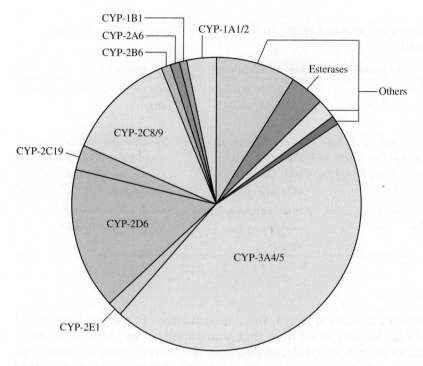

CYP-1B1
CYP-2A6
CYP-2B6
CYP-1A1/2
Esterases
Others
CYP-2C8/9
CYP-2C19
CYP-2D6
CYP-3A4/5
CYP-2E1

FIGURE 1.10   The approximate proportion of drugs metabolized by the major hepatic CYP enzymes. The relative size of each pie section indicates the estimated percentage of metabolism that each enzyme contributes to the metabolism of drugs.

a specific drug. Results provide a scientific basis for understanding why a person might have an unexpectedly toxic reaction after therapeutic doses of a drug or, on the other hand, might fail to respond to what was thought to be a therapeutic dose (Table 1.2).

Second, if more than one drug is present in the body, the drugs may interact with one another, either in a therapeutically beneficial way or in a way that can adversely affect the patient. Beneficially, two drugs can have additive therapeutic effects; for example, improving antidepressant or antianxiety treatment. In the liver, however, one drug can either increase or reduce the rate of metabolism of a second drug, reducing or increasing the blood level of the second drug. For example, *carbamazepine* (Tegretol; see Chapter 14) is particularly effective in stimulating the production of the drug-metabolizing enzyme CYP-3A3/4 in the liver (a process called *enzyme induction*), inducing an apparent *metabolic tolerance* to other drugs metabolized by CYP-3A3/4. In essence, in the presence of carbamazepine, the rate at which all drugs are metabolized by the CYP-3A3/4 enzymes increases. Therefore, metabolic drug *tolerance* develops as the blood level of drug falls more rapidly than would be expected if tolerance had not developed. Thus, increasing doses of a drug must be administered to maintain the same level of drug in the plasma and to produce the same effect

TABLE 1.2 Significance of genetic testing in the determination of drug dosage for an antidepressant

	Normal metabolizer	Slow metabolizer	Fast metabolizer
Genetic variation	Your genes produce a typical amount of enzyme.	Your genes produce too little enzyme.	Your genes produce too much enzyme.
Effects on you	The antidepressant helps your depression and causes few side effects.	The antidepressant builds up in your body, causing intolerable side effects.	The antidepressant is eliminated too quickly, providing little or no improvement in depression.
Treatment options	Follow the recommended dosage.	Switch antidepressants or reduce your dosage.	Switch antidepressants or increase your dosage.

as previously administered smaller doses. One consequence of this development of *metabolic tolerance* is that any other drug that is metabolized by the same enzyme will also be broken down more rapidly. In essence, the second drug becomes less effective because it is metabolized more rapidly as a result of the increased amount of metabolic enzyme. As a result, those drugs will also exert less of an effect, a phenomenon termed *cross-tolerance*.

In contrast to carbamazepine (which increases the rate of metabolism of other drugs), some psychoactive drugs *depress* the activity of the CYP enzyme that metabolizes other drugs metabolized by the same enzyme. This process *increases* the blood level of the other drugs and unexpectedly increases their toxicity. For example, antidepressants that are selective serotonin reuptake inhibitors (SSRIs), such as *fluoxetine* (Prozac; see Chapter 12), inhibit several metabolic enzymes, increasing the toxicity of several other types of antidepressants and certain antipsychotic drugs. This can happen when a person with schizophrenia who is taking the antipsychotic drug clozapine is also given an SSRI to treat obsessive-compulsive symptoms. By inhibiting the enzymes that metabolize clozapine, the blood level of clozapine may rise, increasing the risk of seizures and other adverse effects (Andrade, 2012b). As an interesting aside, the pain-relieving drug codeine (see Chapter 10) needs to be metabolized by CYP-2D6 into morphine, which is codeine's active metabolite responsible for its analgesic effect. Some SSRIs (for example, fluoxetine and paroxetine) block this metabolic conversion of codeine to morphine, so for patients taking SSRIs, codeine is ineffective as a pain-relieving agent.

The vast increase in the number of new drugs, both psychotropic and other medications, during the last two decades has increased the number of combinations and the likelihood of drug–drug interactions. Computer programs are now available to help detect and prevent dangerous combinations. Fortunately, not all interactions are common, clinically significant, or dangerous. One interaction that might be worth noting

Did You Know?

Microbiome

Even if you have not eaten in a long time, your gut is not empty! The average gastrointestinal tract is home to an estimated 100 trillion bacteria (and other genetic fragments), believed to include about 500 species on average. This population, known as the gut *microbiome*, is exceptionally diverse. While individual humans are ~99.9 percent identical to one another's genomes, they can be 80 to 90 percent different in terms of their individual microbiomes.

Although the term was coined by Joshua Lederberg in 2001, the existence of the microbiome was recognized in the 1680s by Antonie van Leeuwenhoek, who compared his oral and fecal material and noted the striking differences between them, and also between samples of healthy and sick individuals. But developments have since moved more quickly; in 2007, scientists announced plans for a Human Microbiome Project to catalog the microorganisms living in our body and several new terms have been derived. The relationship between the microbiota and the brain is referred to as the *brain–gut–microbiota axis* (BGM or GBM). The organisms are called *commensal* bacteria. An imbalance in the microbiota environment may be called *gut dysbiosis,* while neuroactive substances which affect the microbiome are called *psychobiotics*. Strains of good bacteria are called *probiotics* and carbohydrates that serve as food for those bacteria are called *prebiotics*.

What is the function of the microbiome? We give these organisms a home and food. In return, they help with digestion, provide vitamins, inhibit some pathogens, and affect intestinal motility. The consequence of this is that they may influence phenomena such as obesity, inflammatory bowel disease, and the toxic side effects of prescription drugs. In turn, they are affected by infections, antibiotics, and stress, especially during prenatal and early life.

Our current view is that there are several ways in which gut microbes and the brain interact. One method involves digestive products of the microbes that can cross into the blood and ultimately affect behavior by acting on various brain structures. Immune cells, after being programmed in the gut, might represent an additional method of communication, as they also eventually circulate to the brain. Finally, the vagus nerve provides a direct line, as it is a physical link between the gut nerves and the brain (Rogers et al., 2016).

Interestingly, several of the neurotransmitters produced and released by our neurons are also synthesized and secreted by the gut microbiota. These include serotonin, dopamine, and gamma-aminobutyric acid (GABA). Since nearly half of the dopamine and most of the serotonin comes from the intestinal biota, it is understandable that they would be involved in various digestive processes, such as appetite and satiation. Furthermore, it would not be surprising if they also contribute to gastrointestinal problems that accompany emotional disorders such as anxiety and depression (Smith, 2015).

Currently, the most dramatic effects of gut–brain interactions have been seen in nonhuman animal studies, specifically, germ-free mice. The most common findings are that various types of environmental stress, such as maternal separation and long-lasting restraint, produce more intense reactions (especially hormonal responses) in germ-free mice compared with normal mice. Replacing the microbiota (that is, by administering

(Continued)

feces from normal mice) corrects the imbalance, suggesting that early exposure to microbes is necessary for the normal development of physiological regulation of stress reactivity.

Although less dramatic, human studies have found that healthy persons given probiotics for weeks reported less psychological distress on questionnaires, less attention to "negative" stimuli on computer tests, or less cortisol (a stress hormone) on waking than persons not taking the substances.

A procedure known as *fecal microbiota transplant* (FMT) is currently the most successful available method of altering the microbiome. This procedure may be of benefit in many disorders, such as irritable bowel disease, Crohn's disease, and ulcerative colitis. But FMT was initially developed as a treatment for the infection of *Clostridium difficile* (*C. diff.*). This disorder produces debilitating diarrhea that can be fatal and has been implicated in the deaths of up to 14,000 people yearly just in the United States. The infection occurs when good bacteria in the colon is reduced or killed, commonly by antibiotic therapy. The loss of good bacteria causes an overpopulation of bad bacteria, which is corrected by the FMT replacement of healthy bacterial organisms. FMT involves inserting fecal matter from tested donors into a *C. diff.* patient by enema, colonoscopy, endoscopy, or sigmoidoscopy. Since June 2013, the FDA has permitted trained physicians to perform FMT for chronic *C. diff.* with the patient's consent (Fecal Transplant Foundation, 2017).

is that between lithium and nonsteroidal anti-inflammatory drugs (NSAIDs). NSAIDs cause a decrease in the renal elimination of lithium and may produce a dangerous increase in lithium blood levels and toxicity. In addition to prescription drugs, combinations of drugs with herbs and dietary supplements (HDS) can also increase the risk of adverse reactions. It has been estimated that more than 50 percent of patients with chronic disorders use HDS and that nearly 20 percent of patients take these products together with prescription medications (see Tsai et al., 2012).

Not all psychoactive medications are metabolized by the CYP liver enzymes. Several newer psychotropic medications are not. Moreover, some drugs may have active metabolites that are not further metabolized by this system. Such drugs may be useful in situations in which the normal metabolic enzyme systems are compromised. Examples of this are patients who have liver disease, are rapid metabolizers, or have induced enzymes (such as heavy cigarette smokers). A list of common psychotropic drugs that are not (or are minimally) metabolized by the CYP liver enzymes is shown in Table 1.3 (Andrade, 2012a).

Role of the Kidneys in Drug Elimination

Physiologically, our kidneys perform two major functions. First, they excrete most of the metabolic products; second, they closely regulate the levels of most of the substances found in body fluids. The kidneys are a pair of bean-shaped organs that lie at the rear of the abdominal cavity at the level of the lower ribs. The outer portion of the kidney

TABLE 1.3 Some neuropsychopharmacologic agents that are not metabolized or are minimally metabolized by CYP enzymes in the liver

Anxiolytics
  Pregabalin
  Lorazepam

Antidepressants
  Milnacipran
  Desvenlafaxine
  Low doses of amisulpride, sulpiride, and levosulpiride

Antipsychotics
  Paliperidone
  High doses of amisulpride, sulpiride, and levosulpiride

Anticonvulsants and mood stabilizers
  Gabapentin
  Levetiracetam
  Lithium
  Lamotrigine

Dementia treatment
  Memantine

SOURCE: C. Andrade, "Drugs That Escape Hepatic Metabolism," *Journal of Clinical Psychiatry* 73 (2012): e889–e890. Copyright © 2012, Physicians Postgraduate Press. Reprinted by permission.

is made up of more than a million functional units, called *nephrons* (Figure 1.11). Each nephron consists of a knot of capillaries (the *glomerulus*), through which blood flows from the renal artery to the renal vein. The glomerulus is surrounded by the opening of the nephron (*Bowman's capsule*), into which fluid flows as it filters out of the capillaries. Pressure of the blood in the glomerulus causes fluid to leave the capillaries and flow into the Bowman's capsule, from which it flows through the tubules of the nephrons into a duct that collects fluid from several nephrons. The fluid from the collecting ducts is eventually passed through the ureters and into the urinary bladder, which is emptied periodically.

In an adult, about 1 liter (1000 cubic centimeters) of plasma is filtered into the nephrons of the kidneys each minute. Left behind in the bloodstream are blood cells, plasma proteins, and the remaining plasma. As the filtered fluid (water) flows through the nephrons, most of it is reabsorbed into the plasma. By the time fluid reaches the collecting ducts and bladder, only 0.1 percent remains to be excreted. Because about 1 cubic centimeter per minute of urine is formed, 99.9 percent of filtered fluid is therefore reabsorbed.

Lipid-soluble drugs can easily cross the membranes of renal tubular cells and they are reabsorbed along with the 99.9 percent of reabsorbed water. Drug reabsorption occurs passively, along a developing concentration gradient—the drug becomes concentrated inside the nephrons (as a result of water reabsorption) and the drugs are

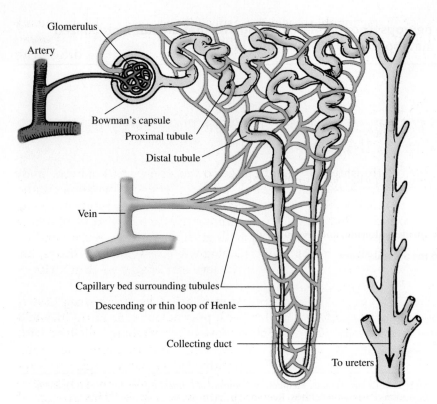

FIGURE 1.11 Nephron within a kidney. Note the complexity of the structure and the intimate relation between the blood supply and the nephron. Each kidney is composed of more than a million nephrons.

themselves reabsorbed with water back into plasma. Thus, the kidneys alone are not capable of eliminating most psychoactive drugs from the body; some other mechanism must overcome this process of passive renal reabsorption of the drug.

Role of the Liver in Drug Metabolism

The reabsorbed drug is eventually picked up by liver cells (*hepatocytes*) and enzymatically biotransformed (by enzymes located in these hepatocytes) into metabolites that are usually less fat soluble, less capable of being reabsorbed, and therefore capable of being excreted in urine. As the drug is carried to the liver (by blood flowing in the hepatic artery and portal vein), a portion is cleared from blood by the hepatocytes and metabolized to by-products that are then returned to the bloodstream. The metabolites are then carried in the bloodstream to the kidneys, filtered into the renal tubules, and poorly reabsorbed, remaining in the urine for excretion. Mechanisms involved in drug metabolism by hepatocytes are complex, but they have gained increased importance in psychopharmacology, especially because of the increasing number of prescription medications, OTC substances, and supplements being taken by consumers, which can potentially cause many complications from drug–drug interactions.

TIME COURSE OF DRUG DISTRIBUTION AND ELIMINATION: THE CONCEPT OF DRUG HALF-LIFE

Knowledge about the relationship between the time course of drug action in the body and its pharmacological effects is essential for (1) predicting the optimal dosages and dose intervals needed to reach a therapeutic effect; (2) maintaining a therapeutic drug level for the desired period of time; and (3) determining the time needed to eliminate the drug. The relationship between the pharmacological response to a drug and its concentration in blood is fundamental to pharmacology. With psychoactive drugs, the level of drug in the blood closely approximates the level of drug at the drug's site of action in the brain.

Figure 1.12 illustrates the time–concentration relationship for a drug that is injected intravenously and therefore reaches peak plasma concentration immediately. For our purposes, intravenous injection removes the variability involved with oral absorption and slow attainment of peak blood levels. Note that after the immediate peak in the plasma concentration, the concentration appears to fall very rapidly, followed by a slower decline in concentration. The rapid fall reflects the rapid *redistribution* of the drug out of the bloodstream into body tissues.[5] This process of redistribution takes only minutes to spread a drug nearly equally throughout the major tissues of the body. The upper left portion of the curve in Figure 1.12 represents this rapid distribution phase, which lasts only a few minutes. The shallower part of the curve represents the slower, prolonged decrease in the level of drug in the blood required for the body to detoxify the drug by hepatic metabolism. (The plasma concentration of the drug metabolites is not illustrated.) The calculated elimination half-life is a measure of this process and it allows the time course of drug action to be determined.

Figure 1.12 shows that the elimination half-life of the drug (the time for the blood level to fall from 4 to 2 micrograms per milliliter [µg/mL]) is about 4 hours. The 4-hour

---

[5]The movement of drug from more perfused organs to less perfused organs is known as *redistribution* of drugs. Initially the heart, liver, kidneys, brain, and other highly perfused organs (which may be referred to as the *Central Compartment*) receive most of the drug during the first few minutes after absorption. Other tissues (which may be referred to as the *Peripheral Compartment*) equilibrate with drugs less rapidly. Examples are skeletal muscle and adipose (fat) tissue. The result of compartmental drug redistribution is to alter the duration of effect at the target tissue. One example is the barbiturate thiopental, which produces anesthesia within seconds because of its high lipid solubility and rapid blood–brain equilibration. However, while rapidly induced, the duration of anesthesia is brief (even though the metabolism of thiopental is slow) because the agent is redistributed and stored in the adipose tissue that acts as a reservoir (Graziano, 2004).

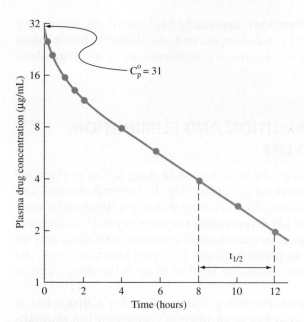

FIGURE 1.12 Plasma concentration–time curve following intravenous injection of a drug. In this example, drug concentrations are measured in plasma every 30 minutes for the first 2 hours following drug injection and then every 2 hours until 12 hours after injection. Over the first 2 hours, redistribution occurs as the drug leaves plasma, enters body tissues, and equilibrates with those tissues. After redistribution, the fall in plasma level is linear, exhibiting a metabolic half-life of 4 hours, regardless of the plasma concentration of the drug.

half-life then remains constant over time. In other words, it takes the same amount of time for the blood level to fall from 8 to 4 micrograms per milliliter as it does to fall from 4 to 2 micrograms per milliliter or from 2 to 1 micrograms per milliliter. Thus, although a different absolute amount of drug is metabolized within each half-life, the time interval remains constant.

The knowledge of a drug's half-life is important because it tells us how long a drug remains in the body. As shown in Table 1.4, it takes four half-lives for 94 percent of a drug to be eliminated by the body and six half-lives for 98 percent of the drug to be eliminated. At that point, a person is, for most practical purposes, drug-free. It is important to remember that even though the blood level of the drug is reduced by 75 percent after two half-lives, the drug persists in the body at low levels for at least six half-lives. The so-called drug hangover is a result.

Throughout this book, drug half-lives are cited to describe the duration of action of psychoactive drugs in the body and allow comparisons between drugs with similar actions but differing half-lives. Most drug half-lives are measured in hours; others are measured in days; and recovery from the drug may take a week or more. For example, the elimination half-life of *diazepam* (Valium; see Chapter 13) is about 30 hours in a

TABLE 1.4 Half-life calculations

Number of half-lives	Amount of drug in the body	
	Percent eliminated	Percent remaining
0	0	100
1	50	50
2	75	25
3	87.5	12.5
4	93.8	6.2
5	96.9	3.1
6	98.4	1.6

healthy young adult, much longer in the elderly. The half-life of its active metabolite is even longer, on the order of several days to a week. The elderly exhibit even more prolongation of the half-lives of both diazepam and nordiazepam; the duration of action can be four weeks or even longer.

Note that drug half-life is the *time* for the plasma level of drug to fall by 50 percent. Thus, half-life is independent of the absolute level of drug in blood: the level falls by 50 percent every half-life, regardless of how many molecules of drug were actually metabolized during that time. In such cases, called *first-order elimination* (or *kinetics*), the metabolism rate of the drug is a constant fraction of the drug remaining in the body, rather than a constant amount of drug per hour. Therefore, a varying amount of drug is metabolized with each half-life (fewer actual molecules are metabolized per half-life as the plasma level of drug falls).

One of the rare exceptions to this concept is the metabolism of ethyl alcohol by the enzyme alcohol dehydrogenase. In that case, a constant amount of alcohol is metabolized per hour, usually about 10 cubic centimeters (cc) of absolute alcohol regardless of the absolute amount of alcohol present in blood, and the blood level falls in a straight line. (The metabolism of alcohol is discussed in Chapter 5.) This type of metabolism is called *zero-order elimination* (or *kinetics*).

DRUG HALF-LIFE, ACCUMULATION, AND STEADY STATE

The biological half-life of a drug is not only the time required for the drug concentration in blood to fall by one-half; it also determines the length of time necessary to reach a plateau, or *steady-state concentration* (Figure 1.13). If a second full dose of drug is administered before the body has eliminated the first dose, the total amount of drug in the body and the peak level of the drug in the blood will be greater than the total amount and peak level produced by the first dose. For example, if 100 milligrams of a drug with a 4-hour half-life were administered at 12 noon, 50 milligrams

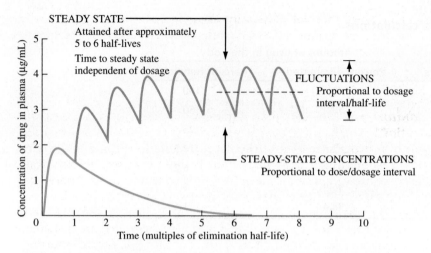

FIGURE 1.13 Plasma drug concentrations during repeated oral administration of a drug at intervals equal to its elimination half-life. The bottom curve illustrates elimination if only a single dose is given. Because only 50 percent of each dose is eliminated before the next dose is given, the drug accumulates, reaching steady-state concentration in five to six half-lives. The sinusoidal curve shows the maximal and minimal drug concentrations at the beginning and end of each dosage interval, respectively. The light dashed line illustrates the average concentration achieved at steady state.

of drug would remain in the body at 4 P.M. If an additional 100 milligrams of the drug were then taken at 4 P.M., 75 milligrams of drug would remain in the body at 8 P.M. (25 milligrams of the first dose and 50 milligrams of the second). If this administration schedule were continued, the amount of drug in the body would continue to increase until a plateau (steady-state) concentration was reached.

In general, the time to reach *steady-state concentration* (the level of drug achieved in the blood with repeated, regular-interval dosing) is about six times the drug's elimination half-life and is independent of the actual dosage of the drug. In one half-life, a drug reaches 50 percent of the concentration that will eventually be achieved. After two half-lives, the drug achieves 75 percent concentration; at three half-lives, the drug achieves the initial 50 percent of the third dose, the next 25 percent from the second dose plus half of the remaining 25 percent from the first dose. At 98.4 percent (the concentration achieved after six half-lives), the drug concentration is essentially at steady state. This is the rationale behind the general rule. The steady-state concentration is achieved when the amount administered per unit time equals the amount eliminated per unit time. The interdependent variables that determine the ultimate concentration (or steady-state blood level of drug) are the dose (which determines the blood level but not the time to steady state), the dose interval, the half-life of the drug, and other more complex factors that can affect drug elimination.

In summary, steady, regular-interval dosing leads to a predictable accumulation with a steady-state concentration reached after about six half-lives, which is proportional to dose and dosage interval. Clinically, these factors guide drug therapy when blood levels of the drug are monitored and correlated with therapeutic results.

THERAPEUTIC DRUG MONITORING

Therapeutic drug monitoring (TDM) can aid a clinician in making critical decisions in therapeutic applications. The basic principle underlying TDM is that a threshold plasma concentration of a drug is needed at the receptor site to initiate and maintain a pharmacological response. Critically important is that plasma concentrations of psychoactive drugs correlate well with tissue or receptor concentrations. Therefore, TDM is an indirect, although usually quite accurate, measurement of drug concentration at the receptor site. To make the correlation between TDM, dosage, and therapeutic response, large-scale clinical trials are performed and blood samples are drawn at several time periods during both acute (short-term) and chronic (long-term) therapy. Statistical correlation is made between the level of drug in plasma and the degree of therapeutic response. A dosage regimen can then be designed to achieve the appropriate blood level of a drug. A well-defined range of blood levels associated with optimal clinical response is called the *therapeutic window*. The important point is that levels either below *or above* that range are associated with a poor response. Figure 1.14A illustrates the concept of the therapeutic window and Figure 1.14B shows an example of the effective blood level range for the decrease in symptoms of the antipsychotic haloperidol.

One goal of TDM is to assess whether a patient is taking medication as prescribed; if plasma levels of the drug are below the therapeutic level because the patient has not been taking the required medication, therapeutic results will be poor. Another goal is to avoid toxicity; if plasma levels of the drug are above the therapeutic level, the dosage can be lowered, effectiveness maintained, and toxicity minimized. A third goal is to enhance therapeutic response by focusing not on the amount of drug taken, but on the measured amount of drug in the plasma. Other goals include possible reductions in the cost of therapy (since a patient's illness is better controlled) and the substantiation of the need for unusually high doses in patients who require a higher than normal intake of prescribed medication to maintain a therapeutic blood level of a drug.

An example of a drug that is routinely monitored is lithium (prescribed for bipolar disorder), because blood levels must be maintained within a narrow therapeutic range (see Chapter 14): too little and the medication will not be effective; too much and symptoms associated with lithium toxicity may develop. Author C.A. recalls an undergraduate student who had to miss several classes when he contracted a bad cold and became dehydrated. The loss of fluid caused his blood lithium concentrations to increase too much, requiring an adjustment. Other medications that show a correlation between blood levels and therapeutic effect include the antiepileptic valproate (also used to treat bipolar disorder); some antidepressants, such as imipramine, amitriptyline, nortriptyline, doxepin, and desipramine; caffeine (used as a bronchodilator); and sometimes other antiepileptics or mood stabilizers, such as carbamazepine.

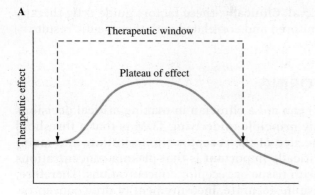

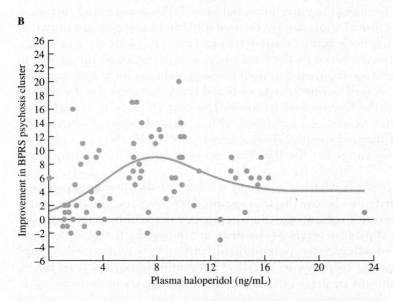

FIGURE 1.14 **A.** Schematic representation of the therapeutic window. The relationship between the therapeutic effect and the drug dose is in the shape of an inverted U. That is, after the therapeutic effect reaches a plateau, an increase in dose does not produce further improvement, but may actually decrease the drug's effectiveness. **B.** Example of the therapeutic window, showing improvement (of psychotic symptoms) as the plasma level of the antipsychotic drug haloperidol increases, followed by a decrease if the concentration continues to rise. [Data from Van Putten et al., 1991.]

DRUG TOLERANCE AND DEPENDENCE

Drug tolerance is defined as a state of progressively decreasing responsiveness to the same dose of a drug. A person who develops tolerance requires a larger dose of the drug to achieve the effect originally obtained by a smaller dose. At least three mechanisms are involved in the development of drug tolerance. Two are pharmacological mechanisms; one is a behavioral mechanism.

In *metabolic tolerance,* the first of the two types of pharmacological tolerance, more enzyme is available to metabolize a drug as a result of *enzyme induction.* This means that more drug must be administered to maintain the same concentration in the body and the same therapeutic response. *Cellular-adaptive,* or *pharmacodynamic, tolerance* is the second type of pharmacological tolerance. In this case, neurons adapt to excess drug either by reducing the number of receptors available to the drug or by reducing their sensitivity to the drug. Such reduction in numbers or sensitivity is termed *downregulation* and higher levels of drug are necessary to maintain the same biological effect (see Chapter 3).

Pharmacodynamic tolerance may be further divided into *acute* and *chronic* types. *Acute tolerance,* also known as *tachyphylaxis,* refers to the decrease in drug effect during a single exposure or within a short period of time. For example, the effect of nicotine may wane from the first cigarette of the day to subsequent cigarettes. Similarly, a single dose of most hallucinogens causes a reduced effect if the drug is taken again and even if a different type of hallucinogen is taken. For LSD-25, psilocybin, and other hallucinogens, it may take a week to regain full sensitivity to the drug. *Chronic tolerance* occurs after long-term, or several sessions of, exposure, covering at least several days. This phenomenon occurs during the development of drug addiction and abuse and is associated with an increase in drug dose to maintain the initial subjective reward.

Behavioral conditioning processes mediate the third type of drug tolerance. Neither enzyme induction nor receptor downregulation can account for the substantial degree of tolerance that many people acquire to opioids, ethyl alcohol, and other drugs. Instead, such tolerance develops when a drug is consistently administered in the context of predictable predrug cues and not in the context of alternative cues. In such situations, environmental cues routinely paired with drug administration will become conditioned stimuli and will elicit a conditioned response that is opposite in direction to, or compensates for, the direct effects of the drug. Over conditioning trials, the compensatory conditioned response grows in magnitude and counteracts the direct drug effects; that is, tolerance develops.

Instead of tolerance, a reverse phenomenon may occur to some drugs. *Sensitization,* or *reverse tolerance,* is an amplified, or potentiated, response to a drug after repeated exposure. That is, it is the opposite of tolerance. Cocaine and MDMA ("ecstasy") are examples of drugs that often produce sensitization.

Physical dependence is an entirely different phenomenon from tolerance, even though the two are often associated temporally. A person who is physically dependent needs the drug to avoid the withdrawal symptoms that occur if the drug is not taken. The state is revealed by withdrawing the drug and noting the occurrence of physical reactions and/or psychological changes (withdrawal symptoms). These changes are referred to as an *abstinence syndrome.* Readministering the drug can relieve the symptoms of withdrawal.

Because physical dependence is often seen after abstinence from drugs of abuse such as alcohol and heroin, the term has been linked with "addiction," implying that withdrawal signs are "bad" and observed only with drugs of abuse. This conclusion is incorrect; withdrawal signs can follow cessation of such therapeutic drugs as the SSRI type of clinical antidepressants (see Chapter 12).[6] In this situation, the phenomenon is more accurately referred to as a *discontinuation syndrome*. The occurrence of withdrawal signs after drug removal is not necessarily a sign of the drug "addiction" that is usually associated with "bad" drugs, such as heroin. Rather, physical dependence is an indication that brain and body functions were altered by the presence of a drug and that a different homeostatic state must be initiated when drug use is discontinued. It takes time (from a few days to about two weeks) for the brain and the body to adapt to the new state of equilibrium without the drug.

STUDY QUESTIONS

1. What is meant by the term *pharmacokinetics*?

2. Why must a psychoactive drug be altered metabolically in the body before it can be excreted?

3. Discuss the advantages and disadvantages of the various methods of administering drugs.

4. Discuss the blood–brain barrier as a limitation to drug transport.

5. Describe the basic characteristics of the cerebrospinal fluid system in the brain.

6. Describe the role of the liver and the hepatic enzyme system in drug metabolism.

7. Define *half-life*. How does *half-life* apply to steady state? If a drug has an elimination half-life of 6 hours, how long does it take for the drug to be essentially eliminated from the body after administration of a single dose?

8. What is meant by the terms *therapeutic drug monitoring* and *therapeutic window*? In what instances might they be useful?

9. What is drug tolerance and why does it occur?

REFERENCES

Andrade, C. (2012a). "Drugs That Escape Hepatic Metabolism." *Journal of Clinical Psychiatry* 73: e889–e890.

Andrade, C. (2012b). "Serotonin Reuptake Inhibitor Treatment of Obsessive-Compulsive Symptoms in Clozapine-Medicated Schizophrenia." *Journal of Clinical Psychiatry* 73: e1362–e1364.

---

[6]Discontinuation of SSRI-type antidepressants is followed in many patients by reactions that can be organized into five symptom categories: (1) disequilibrium (dizziness, vertigo, ataxia); (2) GI symptoms (nausea, vomiting); (3) flulike symptoms (fatigue, lethargy, myalgias, chills); (4) sensory disturbances (paresthesias, sensation of electric shocks); and (5) sleep disturbances (insomnia, vivid dreams).

Bailey, D. G., et al. (2012). "Grapefruit-Medication Interactions: Forbidden Fruit or Avoidable Consequences?" *Canadian Medical Association Journal* 185: 309–316. doi: 10.1503/cmaj.120951.

Brinker, T., et al. (2014). "A New Look at Cerebrospinal Fluid Circulation." *Fluids and Barriers of the CNS* 11: 10. doi: 10.1186/2045-8118-11-10.

Carlat, D. (2015). *Drug Metabolism in Psychiatry: A Clinical Guide*, 3rd ed. Newburyport, MA: Carlat Publishing, LLC.

Fecal Transplant Foundation. (2017). "What Is FMT?" http://thefecaltransplantfoundation.org/what-is-fecal-transplant/.

Graziano, J. (2004). "Drug Absorption, Distribution and Elimination." Columbia University. http://www.columbia.edu/itc/gsas/g9600/2004/GrazianoReadings/Drugabs.pdf.

Paine, M. F., et al. (2006). "A Furanocoumarin-Free Grapefruit Juice Establishes Furanocoumarins as the Mediators of the Grapefruit Juice-Felodipine Interaction." *American Journal of Clinical Nutrition* 84: 1097–1105.

Pardridge, W. M. (2011). "Drug Transport in Brain via the Cerebrospinal Fluid." *Fluids and Barriers of the CNS* 8: 7. doi: 10.1186/2045-8118-8-7.

Pardridge, W. M. (2016). "CSF, Blood-Brain Barrier, and Brain Drug Delivery." *Expert Opinion Drug Delivery* 13: 963–375. doi: 10.1517/17425247.2016.1171315.

Rogers, G. B., et al. (2016). "From Gut Dysbiosis to Altered Brain Function and Mental Illness: Mechanisms and Pathways." *Molecular Psychiatry* 21: 738–748.

Smith, P. (2015). "Can the Bacteria in Your Gut Explain Your Mood?" *New York Times*, September 23, 2015.

Tsai, H.-H., et al. (2012). "Evaluation of Documented Drug Interactions and Contraindications Associated with Herbs and Dietary Supplements." *International Journal of Clinical Practice* 66: 1056–1078.

Van Putten, T., et al. (1991). "Neuroleptic Plasma Levels." *Schizophrenia Bulletin* 17: 197–216.

CHAPTER 2

The Neuron, Synaptic Transmission, and Neurotransmitters

All our thoughts, actions, memories, and behaviors result from biochemical interactions that take place in and between *neurons*. Drugs that affect these processes are called *psychoactive drugs*. In essence, psychoactive drugs are chemicals that alter (mimic, potentiate, disrupt, or inhibit) the normal processes associated with neuronal function or communication between neurons. Therefore, to understand the actions of psychoactive drugs, it is necessary to have some idea of how the brain is organized, what a neuron is, and how neurons interact with each other.

OVERALL ORGANIZATION OF THE BRAIN

The human nervous system consists of two divisions, the *central nervous system* (CNS) and the *peripheral nervous system* (PNS). The CNS includes the brain and the spinal cord; the PNS includes the nerves that originate in the spinal cord and that connect the spinal cord to the organs of the body. The drugs discussed in this book exert their primary actions and some of their side effects by acting in the brain. Many of their side effects, however, are produced by their actions in the PNS, that is, at various organ systems, such as the digestive system and the cardiovascular system, as described in subsequent chapters.

The human brain consists of perhaps 90 billion individual neurons located in the skull and the spinal cord. A flow chart of the brain is shown in Figure 2.1A with the three major divisions indicated: the *hindbrain*, the *midbrain*, and the *forebrain*. The hindbrain and forebrain are further divided into two subdivisions each, which results in five major sections. Figure 2.1B shows the anatomical arrangement of these structures.

The *spinal cord* is essentially the "information highway of the body" through which messages are sent back and forth between the brain and the rest of the body. This information includes touch, temperature, pain, joint position, and signals telling muscles to move.

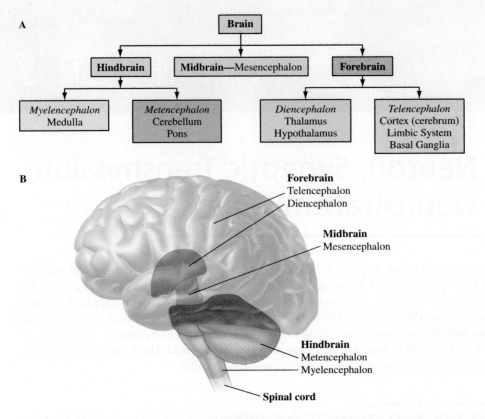

FIGURE 2.1 A. Flowchart of the brain and its major divisions. **B.** Outline of the human brain and its primary divisions.

Extending from the bottom of the brain (the medulla) to the sacrum (the bone in the lower part of the spine that forms the back of the pelvis), the spinal cord is made up of neurons and fiber tracts that

- Carry sensory information from the skin, muscles, joints, and internal body organs to the brain
- Modulate sensory input (including pain impulses)
- Organize and modulate the motor outflow to the muscles (to produce coordinated movement)
- Provide autonomic (involuntary) control of vital body functions

The part of the brain that is attached to the top of the spinal cord is the *brain stem* (Figure 2.2). It is divided into three parts: the *medulla* (its full name is the *medulla oblongata*), the *pons*, and the *midbrain*. All impulses that are conducted in either direction between the spinal cord and the brain pass through the brain stem, which is also important in the regulation of vital body functions, such as respiration (breathing), blood pressure, heart rate, gastrointestinal functioning, and the states of sleep

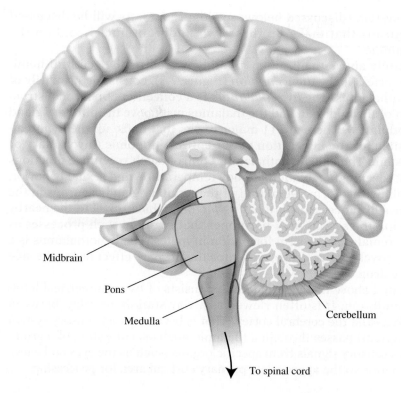

FIGURE 2.2   The brain stem is the portion of the brain consisting of the medulla, pons, and midbrain, which connects the spinal cord to the forebrain.

and wakefulness. The brain stem is also involved in behavioral alerting, attention, and arousal responses. Depressant drugs, such as the barbiturates, depress the brain-stem activating system, which probably underlies much of their hypnotic action.

Behind the brain stem is a large, bulbous structure—the *cerebellum*. A highly convoluted structure, the cerebellum is connected to the brain stem by large nerve tracts. The cerebellum is necessary for the proper integration of movement and posture. The staggering gait that is associated with drunkenness, termed *ataxia* (loss of coordination and balance), is caused largely by an alcohol-induced depression of cerebellar function.

An important part of the brain stem, even though it is only about 2 centimeters long, is the midbrain, which sits between the forebrain and the hindbrain. The upper half (*tectum*, or "roof") contains pathways that carry sensory information, while the bottom half (*tegmentum*, or "floor") contains two important nuclei, which are connected, respectively, to two other systems, whose primary structures are located in the forebrain. The first of these nuclei, the *substantia nigra*, is associated with the neuroanatomical system called the basal ganglia (discussed below; see Figure 2.4), which is responsible for coordination of movement and integration of motor control. Next to the substantia nigra is a more diffuse group of neurons called the *ventral tegmental area* (VTA), which is part of the neuroanatomical system called the *reward circuit*, located in the limbic system (discussed below; see Figure 2.5). As will be discussed later, most of the neurons that make up these two midbrain nuclei contain the neurotransmitter dopamine.

The area immediately above the brain stem and covered by the cerebral hemispheres (cerebrum or cortex) is the *diencephalon* (Figure 2.3), consisting primarily of the thalamus and hypothalamus. The *hypothalamus* is a collection of neuronal structures near the junction of the midbrain and the thalamus just above the pituitary gland (whose function it modulates). There are 11 major nuclei that make up the hypothalamus and are responsible for the integration of our entire autonomic (involuntary or vegetative) nervous system. Thus, the hypothalamus controls such vegetative functions as eating and drinking, sleeping, regulation of body temperature, and sexual behavior, in large part by controlling the hormonal output of the pituitary gland. Neurons in the hypothalamus produce substances called *releasing factors,* which travel to the nearby pituitary gland, inducing the secretion of hormones that regulate such processes as the menstrual cycle in females and sperm formation in males. The hypothalamus is a site of action for many psychoactive drugs, either for the primary effect or for the side effects produced by the drug.

The thalamus, located above the hypothalamus, consists of two symmetrical lobes on either side of the midbrain. It is often viewed as a way station, or relay, between multiple subcortical areas and the cerebral cortex. That is because every sensory system (except the olfactory system) passes through a thalamic nucleus, consisting of a group of neurons that receives sensory signals from specific organs (such as the eyes and ears), which sends the information to the appropriate primary cortical area for processing.

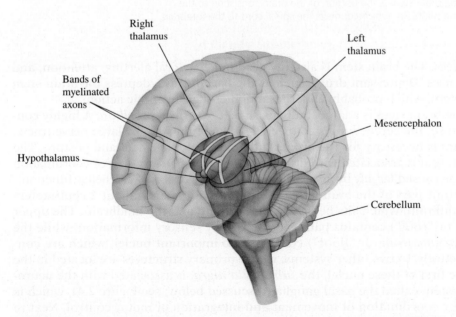

FIGURE 2.3   The diencephalon and its relationship to the mesencephalon (midbrain), cerebellum, and pons.

The last major division of the brain, the telencephalon, includes two important subdivisions, the *basal ganglia* and the *limbic system*. The major structures of the basal ganglia (Figure 2.4A and B) are the caudate nucleus and putamen (together, often referred to as the striatum) and the globus pallidus, which consists of two parts, the lateral (or external) and the medial (or internal) (see Figure 2.4B). Sometimes all three structures are referred to as the corpus striatum, because of their striated (striped) appearance when the tissue is stained so that it can be studied microscopically.

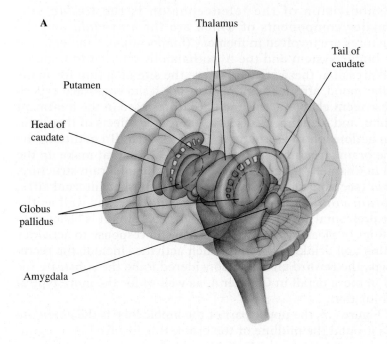

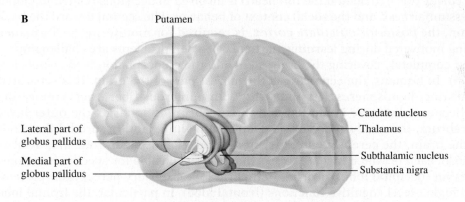

FIGURE 2.4   **A.** The basal ganglia (caudate, putamen, and globus pallidus). **B.** The relationship between the basal ganglia and two important associated structures, the subthalamic nucleus and substantia nigra.

In addition to these primary nuclei, the basal ganglia are associated with two additional structures, the subthalamic nucleus and the substantia nigra (see Figure 2.4B; located in the midbrain as noted above).

One major function of the basal ganglia is the integration of movement. Depending on which part of the system is impaired, disorders of the basal ganglia can cause the gradual loss of the ability to initiate movement, such as in Parkinson's disease, or conversely, an inability to prevent parts of the body from moving unintentionally, as in Huntington's disease.

The second major subdivision of the telencephalon is the *limbic system* (Figure 2.5A), the major components of which are the *amygdala* and the *hippocampus.* These structures are involved in memory (hippocampus) and emotion (amygdala). Because the limbic system and the hypothalamus interact to regulate emotion and emotional expression, these structures are the site of action for many psychoactive drugs that alter mood, affect, emotion, or responses to emotional experiences. As discussed in subsequent chapters, this includes drugs used in the treatment of schizophrenia, depression, and Alzheimer's disease. Many side effects of therapeutic drugs also result from actions on the structures in this system. In addition, the limbic system includes the brain structures, shown in Figure 2.5B, that make up the *reward circuit* (discussed in Chapter 4). This circuit includes the midbrain structure, the *ventral tegmental area* (see above), which is connected to other internal sites, such as the *medial forebrain bundle* and the *nucleus accumbens*, as well as the amygdala, septum and the prefrontal cortex (see Figure 2.6). This circuit is believed to be responsible for the feelings of pleasure that we experience in response to activities that we enjoy, such as eating and drinking. Because such activities include the recreational use of abused drugs, the reward circuit is considered to be the substrate for drug addiction, discussed in more detail in Chapter 4, as well as for the more typical sources of pleasurable stimulation.

As shown in Part A of Figure 2.5, the upper part of the limbic lobe is the *cingulate cortex*, located in the area around the midline of the brain. It is involved in integrating sensory, motor, visceral, motivational, and emotional information. The *anterior cingulate cortex* (located behind the forehead) is involved in decisions related to empathy, fairness/unfairness, and the social context of behavior. The section toward the back of the brain, the *posterior cingulate cortex*, is required for monitoring performance and keeping motivated during learning, particularly when problems are challenging.

Almost completely covering the brain stem and the diencephalon is the *cerebrum* (Figure 2.6). In humans, the cerebrum is the largest part of the brain. It is separated into two distinct hemispheres, left and right, with numerous fiber tracts connecting the two. Because skull size is limited and the cerebrum is so large, the outer layer of the cerebrum, the *cerebral cortex,* is deeply convoluted and fissured. Like other parts of the brain, the cerebral cortex is subdivided; it consists of four major lobes (Figure 2.6A), each of which includes areas that are responsible for specific functions, such as vision (occipital lobe), hearing (temporal lobe), sensory perception (parietal lobe), and higher-level cognitive functions (frontal lobe). In particular, the frontal lobe is further subdivided into more specific functional loci, as indicated in Figure 2.6B. The orbital prefrontal cortex modifies behavior depending on anticipated outcomes; that is, it mediates behavioral choice. The dorsal-lateral prefrontal cortex mediates

A

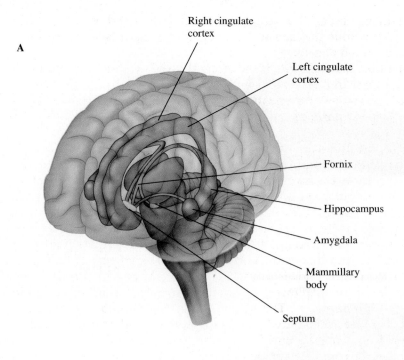

Right cingulate
cortex

Left cingulate
cortex

Fornix

Hippocampus

Amygdala

Mammillary
body

Septum

B

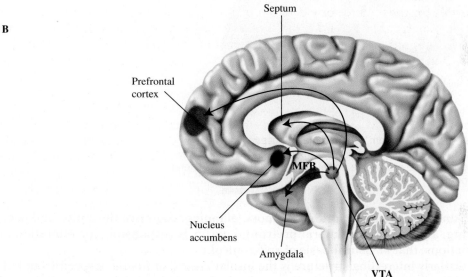

Septum

Prefrontal
cortex

MFB

Nucleus
accumbens

Amygdala

VTA

FIGURE 2.5   The limbic system. **A.** The major limbic structures. **B.** The structures that make up the reward system of the brain.

A

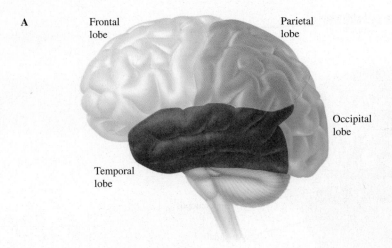

Frontal
lobe

Parietal
lobe

Occipital
lobe

Temporal
lobe

B

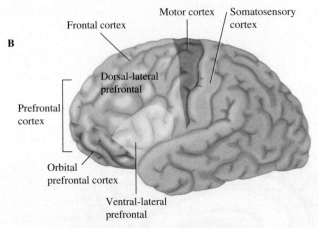

Motor cortex   Somatosensory
cortex

Frontal cortex

Dorsal-lateral
prefrontal

Prefrontal
cortex

Orbital
prefrontal cortex

Ventral-lateral
prefrontal

FIGURE 2.6 **A.** The cerebrum. The four major lobes of the human brain. **B.** Subdivisions of the frontal lobe, including the prefrontal cortex and its components: the orbital, the dorsal-lateral, and the ventral-lateral prefrontal cortex.

executive functions, such as working memory, planning, cognitive flexibility, and decision making, and the ventral-lateral prefrontal cortex is responsible for inhibition of motor functions, that is, neural basis of self-control.

A particularly interesting structure is the insular cortex, or *insula*, a specific but hidden lobe of the brain located within the cerebral cortex, behind the temporal lobe and beneath the frontal and parietal lobes (Figure 2.7). It receives information about the physiological state of the body and integrates it into a broader context. For example, unpleasant smells or tastes may be reimagined as a sensation of disgust. In 2007, it was reported that some people with damage to the insula were able to give up cigarettes instantly.

There is a special cell type in the insula, the Von Economo neurons, names for the neuroscientist who discovered them in 1925. For this reason, they are known as

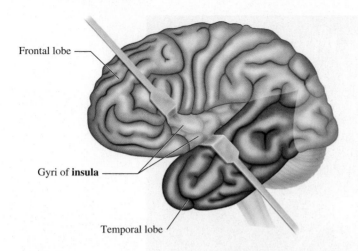

Frontal lobe

Gyri of **insula**

Temporal lobe

FIGURE 2.7 The Insula.

VENs. In addition to the frontal insula, these unusually large, cigar-shaped cells are also located in the anterior cingulate cortex. Aside from humans, only whales, great apes, and elephants are known to have them (Blakeslee, 2007).

In the last few years, there have been some remarkable technological developments in the neuroscience of the brain, especially in regard to understanding the neural basis of behavior. One significant international initiative is the Human Connectome Project (HCP). With start-up funding of $40 million, this collaboration began in 2010 with the goal of determining how neurons are connected across numerous brain sites. The first dataset was released in April 2015. This result consisted of connectomes obtained from about 460 people, 22 to 35 years old. In addition to the anatomical results, the outcome included information about personality variables, various intelligence assessments, social and economic conditions, and history of drug use, as well as age. The eventual goal is to collect data from 1200 adults in order to determine which systems across the brain are functioning while the brain is quiet. The connectomes are thought to indicate those neuronal associations that remain active to keep the brain ready to perform certain functions (Figure 2.8) (Reardon, 2015).

In July 2016, progress made by the HCP was made public with the publication of a new map of the brain, which contained nearly 100 previously unknown regions (Zimmer, 2016). The map was created by applying complex computer analyses to the large amount of data collected from the test subjects. Each participant had their brain mapped while they underwent hours of memory, language, and other neuropsychological tests. This update is the first large-scale revision of the cortex since 1907, when an atlas of 52 brain regions was published by Korbinian Brodman. According to one of the investigators, there were 112 different types of information used to construct the new map, including anatomical data, such as the amount of myelin, as well as the neuropsychological test results. (You can see the latest developments at www.humanconnectomeproject.org.)

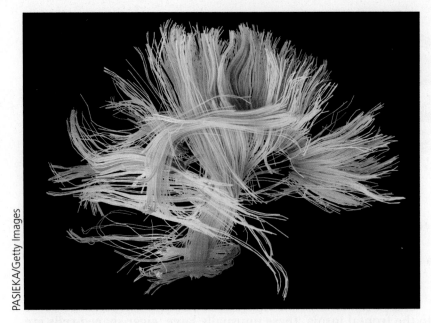

PASIEKA/Getty Images

FIGURE 2.8   A connectome of the brain shows active connections between neurons.

OVERVIEW OF SYNAPTIC TRANSMISSION

The central nervous system (CNS) is made up of two types of cells: neurons and a variety of nonneural cells, collectively called *glia* (from the Greek word meaning "glue"). It had long been thought that glia are more abundant than neurons and that there were from 10 to 50 times more glia than neurons in the CNS. There is recent evidence, however, that the 10:1 glia to neuron ratio is a myth and that the ratio in human and other primate brains is much closer to 1:1. It turns out to be more difficult to determine the ratio of glia to neurons than you might think. For example, some parts of the human brain have a higher ratio than others, and the ratio of other species differs from that of humans (Yuhas and Jabr, 2012).

The neuron is the basic functional unit, while glia provide support and protection. The main types of glial cells in the CNS are oligodendrocytes, astrocytes, and ependymal and microglial cells. Although glia may turn out to be less numerous than previously thought, they may in fact be more important than previously believed. Oligodendrocytes form the myelin sheath around axons. Astrocytes provide neurons with nutrients and structural support. They maintain the extracellular environment of neurons by regulating their ionic surroundings, modulating the rate of signal transmission and the reuptake of neurotransmitters. Astrocytes play a crucial role in synapse formation and they affect (by promoting or preventing) recovery after neural injury. Microglia are involved in cleaning up damaged cells and debris and pruning neurons.

Recent research suggests that they may be involved in disorders such as schizophrenia and Alzheimer's because of extensive pruning leading to massive synaptic loss (Hong et al., 2016).

A typical neuron has a *soma* (cell body), which contains the nucleus (including the genetic material of the cell) and several other structures, or *organelles*, that perform vital functions (Figure 2.9A). For example, mitochondria produce energy from nutrients, while Golgi bodies package substances (such as neurotransmitters) into vesicles for storage.

Extending from the soma in one direction are many short fibers, called *dendrites*, which receive input from other neurons through *receptors* located on the dendritic membrane (see Figure 2.9B). When a signal arrives from another cell, a message is generated and travels down the dendrite to the soma. Extending in another direction from the soma is a single process called an *axon*, which can vary in length from a few millimeters up to a meter (such as those that run from the motor neurons of the spinal cord out to the muscles that they stimulate). The axon transmits the signal through an electrochemical process (the *action potential*) from the soma to other neurons or to muscles, organs, or glands of the body. Longer axons are usually covered with a *myelin sheath*, produced by specialized types of glia, which increases the speed of the signal.

Information flows from the axon to the next neuron or cell by way of a specialized structure called a *synapse*. According to Thompson (1993), a "given neuron in the brain may receive ... thousand(s) of connections from other neurons" and the "number of possible different combinations of synaptic connections among the neurons in a single human brain is larger than the total number of atomic particles that make up the known universe. Hence the diversity of the interconnections in a human brain seems almost without limit" (2–3).

It was once thought that the brain has the maximal number of neurons at birth and that once a neuron dies, it is not replaced. This concept has been revised because we now realize that new neurons form every day (a process called *neurogenesis*) (Kempermann et al., 2004; Schaffer and Gage, 2004). Synaptic contacts between neurons are continually being reshaped, with axon terminals and dendrites re-forming new synaptic connections while eliminating old ones. This remodeling probably begins even before birth and continues throughout our lives.

A synapse consists of the presynaptic membrane (typically the axon terminal) of one neuron, the postsynaptic membrane of the receiving neuron (which might be a dendrite, the soma, or the axon terminal of another neuron), and a minute space (the *synaptic cleft*) between them (Figure 2.10). Among the numerous structural elements of the presynaptic side (for our purposes) are the synaptic vesicles, each of which contains several thousand neurotransmitter molecules that transmit information from one neuron to another. These vesicles serve two functions. They store the transmitter and protect it from being destroyed by metabolic enzymes so that it is available for release. When the action potential reaches the axon terminal, it triggers a series of biochemical actions, which cause the vesicles to fuse with the presynaptic membrane and release the transmitter, a process called *exocytosis*. The transmitter molecules diffuse across the synaptic cleft and attach to various types

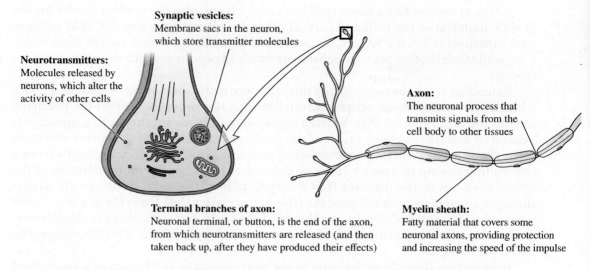

Synaptic vesicles:
Membrane sacs in the neuron, which store transmitter molecules

Neurotransmitters:
Molecules released by neurons, which alter the activity of other cells

Axon:
The neuronal process that transmits signals from the cell body to other tissues

Terminal branches of axon:
Neuronal terminal, or button, is the end of the axon, from which neurotransmitters are released (and then taken back up, after they have produced their effects)

Myelin sheath:
Fatty material that covers some neuronal axons, providing protection and increasing the speed of the impulse

FIGURE 2.9 Major parts of a neuron. Within the cell body is the nucleus, which contains the genetic code, DNA. The cell body is filled with a gelatinous substance, the cytoplasm. Within the cytoplasm are various organelles, which perform specific functions. The endoplasmic reticulum is a network of flattened sacs and branching tubules that extends throughout the cytoplasm, which provides a platform for ribosomes and a mechanism of transportation for movement of cellular products. Ribosomes synthesize proteins, mitochondria produce energy for cell functions, and the Golgi complex combines simple molecules into more complex structures and packages them into vesicles. Dendrites and axons are processes that receive incoming signals and send outgoing messages, respectively. Some axons are protected by myelin, a fatty sheath. The axons end in terminals, which contain membrane sacs filled with transmitter molecules.

of structures, called *receptors*, on both the presynaptic terminal and the postsynaptic membrane of the next neuron (see Chapter 3). The neurons do not physically touch each other; synaptic transmission is a chemical rather than an electrical process. Recently, however, it has been reported that, in at least some synapses, special proteins are arranged on the pre- and postsynaptic membranes such that the neurotransmitter molecules are aligned opposite their receptor sites. These structures, termed *nanocolumns*, appear to connect regions of neurotransmitter molecule release and activation (Tang et al., 2016).

Synaptic transmission is remarkably fast; the entire process may occur over a time span as short as a millisecond for transmitter release (from presynaptic vesicles), diffusion (across the cleft), receptor attachment, and activation. The nature of the response produced by synaptic transmission depends on the characteristics of the receptor that is activated (see Chapter 3). Receptors may respond quickly, within milliseconds, or they may produce responses that last hundreds of milliseconds. The ultimate outcome of receptor activation is a function of the organ or tissue in which it is located. In summary, the arrival of an action potential at the axon terminal induces

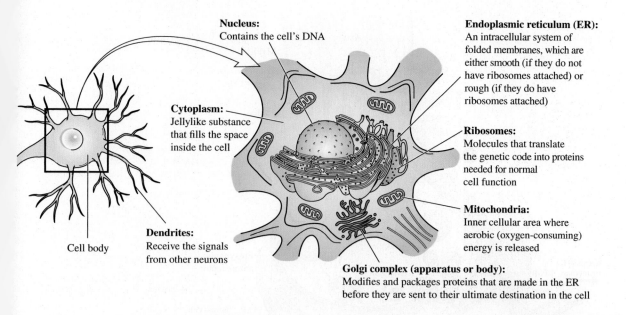

Nucleus:
Contains the cell's DNA

Cytoplasm:
Jellylike substance
that fills the space
inside the cell

Dendrites:
Receive the signals
from other neurons

Cell body

Endoplasmic reticulum (ER):
An intracellular system of
folded membranes, which are
either smooth (if they do not
have ribosomes attached) or
rough (if they do have
ribosomes attached)

Ribosomes:
Molecules that translate
the genetic code into proteins
needed for normal
cell function

Mitochondria:
Inner cellular area where
aerobic (oxygen-consuming)
energy is released

Golgi complex (apparatus or body):
Modifies and packages proteins that are made in the ER
before they are sent to their ultimate destination in the cell

release of a neurotransmitter into the synaptic cleft and the transmitter then activates its receptors.

The release of neurotransmitter may be modulated by presynaptic receptors, termed *autoreceptors* (see Figure 2.10). An autoreceptor is a presynaptic site on a neuron that binds the neurotransmitter *released by that neuron*. These receptors regulate the neuron's activity. Autoreceptors serve as negative feedback mechanisms. When stimulated by transmitter or by certain drugs, these receptors *reduce* the synthesis and further release of transmitter. Thus, when large amounts of transmitter are present in the synaptic cleft, excess transmitter molecules act on the autoreceptors to decrease further production and release. Conversely, if an antagonist blocks an autoreceptor, synthesis and release of transmitter is increased.

Once release has occurred, there must be a way to get rid of neurotransmitter; otherwise, transmitter would stay in the synaptic cleft and continually bind to and activate receptors. In most cases, transmitter removal occurs through one of two general types of mechanisms (see Figure 2.10; with some variations as described below for specific transmitters):

1. An enzyme present in the synaptic cleft breaks down any neurotransmitter remaining in the synapse. The metabolites are then taken back up into the presynaptic neuron to be resynthesized and repackaged for release. This is how the effect of the neurotransmitter acetylcholine is terminated. Drugs used in the treatment of Alzheimer's disease act by blocking this process, thereby increasing the amount of acetylcholine in the synapse, which may delay the progression of the dementia (see Chapter 16).

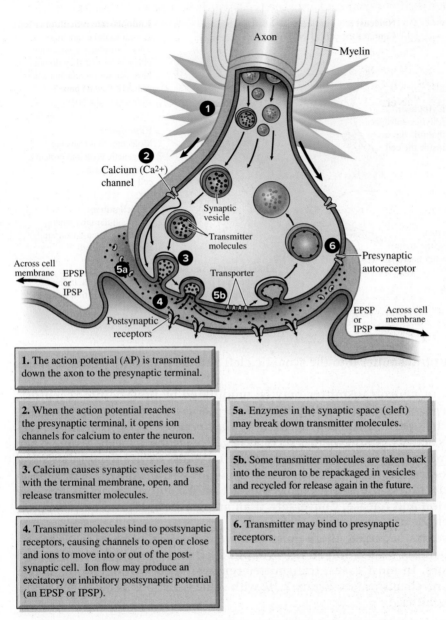

FIGURE 2.10   Structure and function of a generic synapse. Neurotransmitter is produced (synthesized) and stored in vesicles within the axon terminal. When an action potential reaches the terminal, it causes channels to open so that calcium can enter and initiate *exocytosis* (release of transmitter molecules) into the synaptic cleft. After release, neurotransmitter molecules bind to and activate receptors on the pre- and postsynaptic membrane. Transmitter effects are terminated either by breakdown of transmitter within the synaptic cleft or by reuptake back into the axon terminal to be recycled.

2. The transmitter itself is taken back into the presynaptic neuron and repackaged. The action of the neurotransmitters dopamine, norepinephrine, and serotonin is terminated by this mechanism. Drugs that block this reuptake process represent one class of antidepressant medication. In an alternative version of this process, transmitter is taken up into an adjacent glial cell and metabolized. The metabolites are then recycled back to the neuron where they are resynthesized into neurotransmitter and repackaged for release. The effect of the transmitter glutamate is terminated by this method.

Did You Know?

Optogenetics

In the last 10 years, neuroscience has been transformed by *optogenetics*, a remarkable new technology first described in 2005. Optogenetics is extraordinary because it permits scientists to actually control—activate or inactivate—specific neurons to see what happens. Optogenetics began in 2000, with neuroscientists Karl Deisseroth and Edward Boyden; in 2004, Deisseroth successfully inserted the gene for a molecule, an *opsin* (a light-sensitive protein found in the photoreceptors of the eye), into mammalian neurons in vitro. When these genes were ultimately inserted into living animals, flashes of light were used to stimulate regions deep inside the brain through a fiber optic wire attached to a laser diode. With this technique, researchers have identified new pathways that control anxiety in mice and used it to turn depression on and off in rats and mice as well as create false memories in laboratory animals (Colapinto, 2015; Deisseroth, 2015). Most recently, scientists have found that low-pressure ultrasound can be used as a noninvasive trigger to activate specific sensitized neurons in the nematode. In late February 2016, a blind woman in Texas became the first person to receive treatment developed from optogenetic therapy. The patient suffers from retinitis pigmentosa, a degenerative disease of the eye in which the rods and cones deteriorate. To try to recover some of her lost vision, DNA from light-sensitive algae was incorporated into viruses and injected into her eye. If the methodology is effective, these cells will become responsive to light and she will recover some vision. During 2017, the patient will be monitored to determine if the procedure is successful (Bourzac, 2016).

SPECIFIC NEUROTRANSMITTERS

Neurons release specific chemical substances from their presynaptic nerve terminals, and it is the interaction between psychoactive drugs and the receptors on which the natural transmitters act that underlies the actions of the drugs. Table 2.1 lists a few of the commonly recognized neurotransmitter families with some of the specific transmitters within each category. The earliest chemicals identified as CNS neurotransmitters were acetylcholine and norepinephrine, largely because of their established roles in the peripheral nervous system. In the 1960s, serotonin, epinephrine, and dopamine were recognized. In the 1970s, gamma aminobutyric acid (GABA), glycine, glutamate, and certain neuropeptides (such as the endorphins) were identified. In the late 1980s, the lipid amide anandamide was identified as the endogenous transmitter for the tetrahydrocannabinol (THC) receptor, followed by several other candidates after 2000.

TABLE 2.1 Classification of the major neurotransmitter families with selected neurotransmitters

	Specific neurotransmitters
Family and subfamily	**Transmitters**
AMINES	
Quaternary amine	Acetylcholine (ACh)
Monoamines	*Catecholamines:* Norepinephrine (NE), epinephrine (adrenaline), dopamine (DA)
	Indoleamines: Serotonin (5-hydroxytryptamine: 5-HT)
AMINO ACIDS	Gamma-aminobutyric acid (GABA), glutamate, glycine
NEUROPEPTIDES	
Opioid peptides	*Enkephalins:* Met-enkephalin, leu-enkephalin
	Endorphins: β-endorphin
	Dynorphins: Dynorphin A
PEPTIDES	Oxytocin, substance P, cholecystokinin (CCK), vasopressin, hypothalamic-releasing hormones
PURINES	Adenosine
LIPIDS	*Endocannabinoids:* arachidonoylethanolamine (anandamide or AEA), 2-arachidonoylglycerol (2-AG), 2-arachidonyl glyceryl ether (noladin ether), *N*-arachidonoyl dopamine (NADA), virodhamine (OAE), lysophosphatidylinositol (LPI)
GASES	Nitric oxide, carbon monoxide

Acetylcholine

Acetylcholine (ACh) was identified as a transmitter chemical first in the peripheral nervous system and later in brain tissue. Deficiencies in acetylcholine-secreting neurons have classically been associated with the dysfunctions seen in Alzheimer's disease. Certainly drugs that either potentiate or inhibit the central action of acetylcholine exert profound effects on memory. For example, scopolamine is a psychedelic drug that blocks central cholinergic receptors and as a result produces amnesia. Conversely, drugs that increase the amount of acetylcholine in the brain appear to improve memory function and are used to delay the progression of Alzheimer's disease.

Acetylcholine is synthesized in a one-step reaction from two precursors (choline and acetyl coenzyme A) and then stored within synaptic vesicles for later release (Figure 2.11). Like other neurotransmitters, acetylcholine is released into the synaptic cleft, rapidly diffuses across the cleft, and reversibly binds to postsynaptic receptors. Once acetylcholine has exerted its effect on postsynaptic receptors, its action is terminated by the enzyme *acetylcholinesterase* (AChE), which is located in the postsynaptic side of the synaptic cleft.

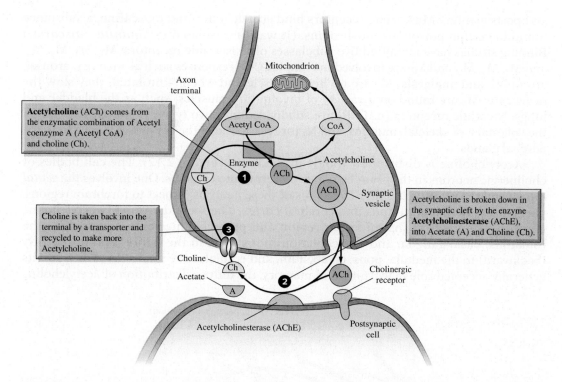

FIGURE 2.11 Schematic of an acetylcholine (ACh) synapse. Acetylcholine is made in the axon terminal from acetyl coenzyme A (acetyl CoA) and choline and stored in vesicles for release. After release, acetylcholine binds to its receptors and is immediately broken down at the receptors by acetylcholinesterase (AChE) into choline and acetate.

The enzymatic reaction that degrades acetylcholine is important not only in the treatment of Alzheimer's disease, but also in agriculture and the military. Drugs that block the action of acetylcholinesterase, referred to as *AChE inhibitors,* include both "reversible" and "irreversible" compounds. *Irreversible AChE inhibitors* form a permanent covalent bond with the enzyme and totally inhibit enzyme function. They are usually administered in "toxic" doses and the result is usually fatal. Some of these toxic drugs (such as *malathion* and *parathion*) have been exploited in gardening and agriculture as insecticides because they kill insects on contact. Other irreversible AChE inhibitors (such as *sarin* and *soman*) have been used in the military as lethal nerve gases.

Less toxic and shorter acting are the *reversible AChE inhibitors.* They are used clinically as putative cognitive enhancers to delay memory decline in patients with Alzheimer's disease. Individual agents are discussed in Chapter 16.

Cholinergic receptors are subclassified into two categories, nicotinic and muscarinic, named for substances that specifically stimulate each category. Muscarinic receptors are the "slow" type (metabotropic), while nicotinic receptors are the "fast" type (or ionotropic; see Chapter 3). They can be found on both sides of the synaptic cleft (presynaptic and postsynaptic). Muscarinic receptors bind acetylcholine and muscarine, a substance found in certain poisonous mushrooms. (It was first isolated in *Amanita muscaria.*) Binding studies have identified five subclasses of muscarinic receptors: M_1, M_2, M_3, M_4, and M_5. M_1, M_4, and M_5 are involved in complex CNS responses such as memory, arousal, attention, and analgesia. M_2 are on heart muscle and when stimulated, they slow the heart rate; M_3 are found on a variety of involuntary muscles, such as the bladder and lungs. Nicotinic receptors (nAChR) are subdivided into two types: N_1 (or N_M), found on the voluntary, or skeletal, muscles, and N_2 (or N_N), found in the nervous system and in the adrenal glands.

Acetylcholine is distributed widely in the brain (Figure 2.12). The cell bodies of cholinergic neurons in the brain lie in two closely related regions. One involves the *septal nuclei* and the *nucleus basalis.* The axons of these neurons project to forebrain regions, particularly the hippocampus and cerebral cortex. The second group of acetylcholine neurons originates in the midbrain region and projects anteriorly (forward) to the thalamus, basal ganglia, and diencephalon (not shown in the figure) and posteriorly (backward) to the medulla, pons, cerebellum, and cranial nerve nuclei. In addition to its generally accepted role in learning and memory, the diffuse distribution of acetylcholine

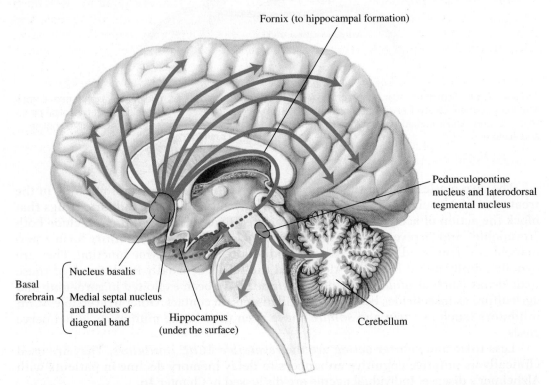

FIGURE 2.12 The two major cholinergic systems in the human brain. The basal forebrain cholinergic complex composed of neurons in the medial septal nucleus and nucleus basalis, which projects to the telencephalon; the pontomesencephalotegmental cholinergic complex, composed of cells in the pedunculopontine and laterodorsal tegmental nuclei, which ascend to the thalamus and other diencephalic loci (not shown) and descend to the pons, medulla, cerebellum, and cranial nerve nuclei.

is consistent with suggestions that acetylcholine is involved in circuits that modulate sensory reception; in mechanisms related to behavioral arousal, attention, energy conservation, and mood; and in REM (rapid eye movement) activity during sleep (dreaming).

MONOAMINERGIC NEUROTRANSMITTERS

Catecholamine Transmitters: Dopamine and Norepinephrine

The term *catecholamine* refers to compounds that contain a catechol nucleus (a benzene ring with two attached hydroxyl groups) to which is attached an amine group (Figure 2.13). In the CNS, the term usually refers to the transmitters *dopamine* (DA) and *norepinephrine* (NE). In the peripheral nervous system, *epinephrine* (adrenaline) is a third catecholamine transmitter. In the brain, a large number of psychoactive drugs (both licit and illicit, therapeutic and abused) exert their effects by altering the synaptic action of norepinephrine and dopamine.

The chemical synthesis of the catecholamines is illustrated in Figure 2.13. Biosynthesis of the catecholamines begins with the amino acid tyrosine (found in foods such as egg whites, cottage cheese, soy products, meat, fish, poultry, mustard greens, and spinach) and involves several steps controlled by specific enzymes. Following synthesis, these transmitters are stored in vesicles for release into the synaptic space. After release, norepinephrine and dopamine attach to pre- and postsynaptic receptors and initiate responses in the receiving cell or neuron. As noted earlier, inactivation occurs primarily by reuptake of the transmitter from the synaptic cleft into the presynaptic nerve terminal. Within the nerve terminal, catecholamines may be inactivated by enzymes such as *monoamine oxidase* (MAO). The class of antidepressants referred to as MAO inhibitors (MAOIs; see Chapter 12) acts by blocking monoamine oxidase, thereby increasing the amounts of dopamine and norepinephrine available for synaptic release.

Catecholamine Receptors

Each catecholamine transmitter exerts effects on a number of different receptors. Norepinephrine and epinephrine act on two primary types of receptors (alpha and beta), each of which has at least two subtypes. Dopamine exerts postsynaptic effects on at least six receptors, divided into two families (D_1 type and D_2 type). The D_1 receptor family consists of two subtypes—D_1 and D_5—and the D_2 receptor family consists of four subtypes—D_{2A}, D_{2B}, D_3, and D_4. Postsynaptic dopamine receptors of the D_2 family are responsible for at least part of the antipsychotic activity and side effects of the drugs discussed in Chapter 11. Alterations in dopamine receptor function have been implicated in numerous diseases and behavioral states, including schizophrenia, parkinsonism, affective disorders, sexual activity, addiction, and attention deficit/hyperactivity disorder.

Norepinephrine Pathways

The cell bodies of norepinephrine neurons are located in the brain stem, mainly in a structure in the pons called the *locus coeruleus* (Figure 2.14). From there, axons project widely throughout the brain to nerve terminals in the cerebral cortex, the limbic

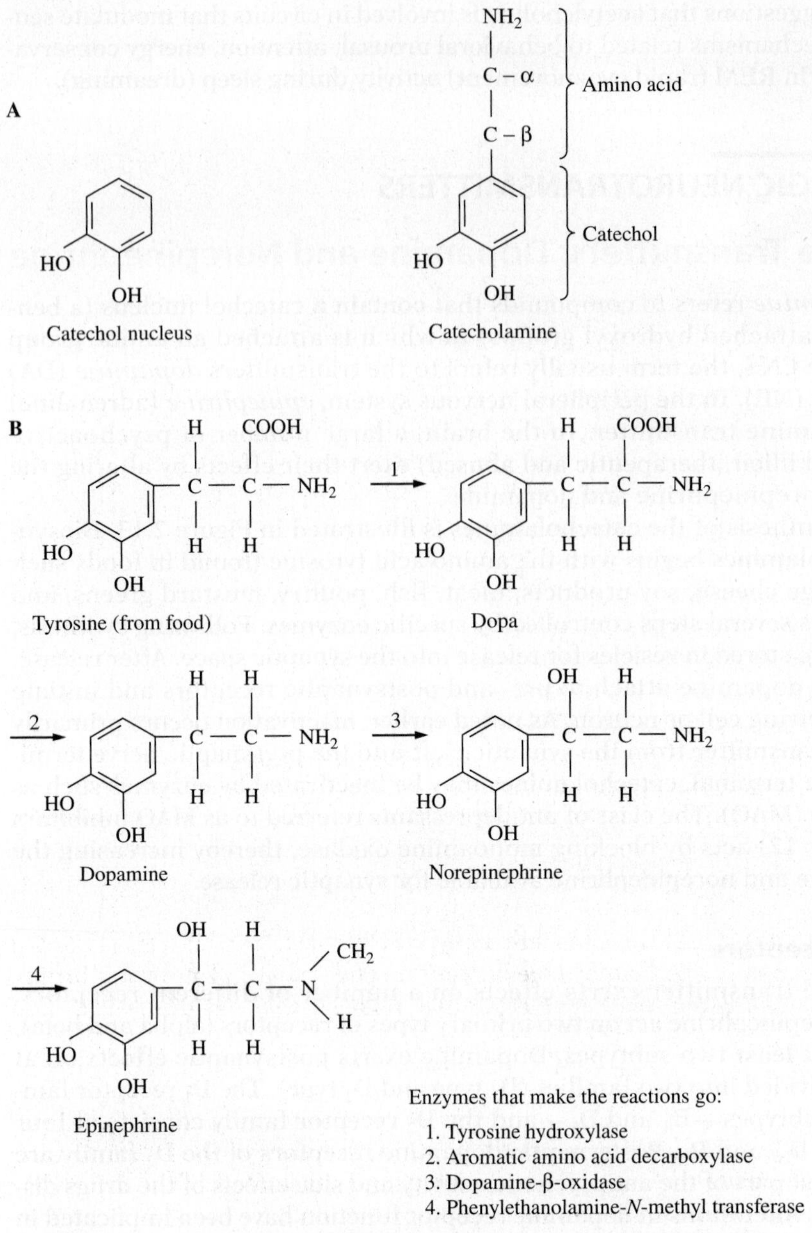

A

Catechol nucleus

Catecholamine

NH₂ — C–α, C–β (Amino acid)
Catechol

B

Tyrosine (from food)

Dopa

Dopamine

Norepinephrine

Epinephrine

Enzymes that make the reactions go:

1. Tyrosine hydroxylase
2. Aromatic amino acid decarboxylase
3. Dopamine-β-oxidase
4. Phenylethanolamine-N-methyl transferase

FIGURE 2.13 **A.** Catechol and catecholamine structure. All catecholamines share the catechol nucleus, a benzene ring with two adjacent hydroxyl (OH) groups. **B.** Structures and synthesis of the catecholamines. Tyrosine, an amino acid found in foods, is converted into dopa, then into dopamine, next into norepinephrine, and finally (in the peripheral nervous system) into epinephrine, depending on which enzymes (one to four) are present in the cell.

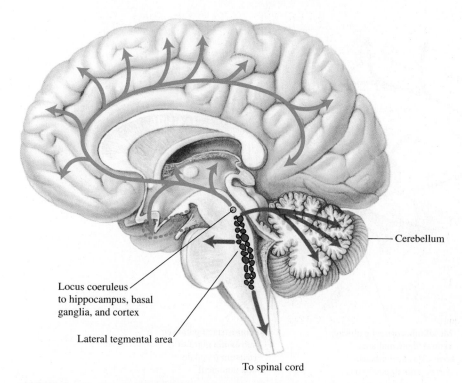

Cerebellum

Locus coeruleus
to hippocampus, basal
ganglia, and cortex

Lateral tegmental area

To spinal cord

FIGURE 2.14 Noradrenergic projection systems in the human brain. The cell bodies are in the locus coeruleus and adjacent regions of the brain stem and project widely to the forebrain and cerebellum and to the brain stem and spinal cord.

system, the hypothalamus, and the cerebellum. Axonal projections also travel down the spinal cord, where they exert an analgesic action. The release of norepinephrine produces an alerting, focusing, orienting response, positive feelings of reward, and analgesia.

Dopamine Pathways

Dopamine pathways also originate in the brain stem, sending axons both rostral (forward) to the brain and caudal (backward) to the spinal cord (Figure 2.15). Three dopamine circuits are most relevant for our discussions:

1. Neurons in the hypothalamus send short axons to the pituitary gland (not shown in Figure 2.15). These neurons regulate certain hormones. Alterations in hormone function are commonly seen in people with schizophrenia who are taking various antipsychotics, which block these dopamine receptors (see Chapter 11).

2. Neurons in the substantia nigra (see Figure 2.15) that project to the basal ganglia (see Figure 2.4) play a major role in the regulation of movement. As noted earlier, parkinsonism (see Chapter 16) and parkinsonian side effects produced by

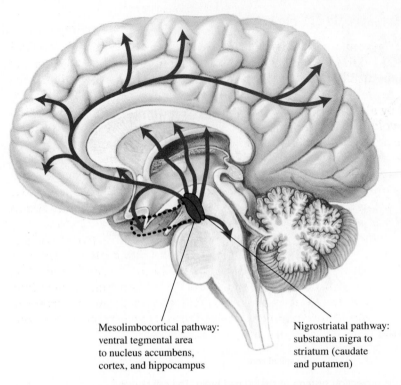

Mesolimbocortical pathway:
ventral tegmental area
to nucleus accumbens,
cortex, and hippocampus

Nigrostriatal pathway:
substantia nigra to
striatum (caudate
and putamen)

FIGURE 2.15 There are three major dopamine systems in the brain. One is a local circuit in the hypothalamus (not shown); another, the nigrostriatal pathway, projects from the substantia nigra to the caudate nucleus of the basal ganglia and is involved in motor functions and Parkinson's disease; the third consists of cell bodies next to the substantia nigra in the midbrain that project widely to the cerebral cortex and forebrain limbic system.

antipsychotic drugs (which block these receptors) (see Chapter 11) all involve this pathway.

3. Cell bodies of the VTA in the midbrain are located next to the substantia nigra (see Figure 2.15). Dopamine neurons of this nucleus extend forward and separate into two pathways. One branch, called the *mesocortical*, projects to the frontal cortex, and a second branch, called the *mesolimbic*, projects to the limbic system. These two dopaminergic pathways are extremely important in psychopharmacology. First, alterations in the development of these pathways may be involved in the pathogenesis of schizophrenia and its amelioration by antipsychotic drugs. That is because, as discussed in Chapter 11, drugs used in the treatment of schizophrenia all share the common action of blocking dopamine receptors in this pathway. Second, these dopaminergic pathways also include structures that are activated by drugs (and other stimuli) that produce sensations of pleasure. This group of structures constitutes our "central reward circuit," which is involved in addiction to most drugs of abuse (discussed in Chapter 4).

The Indolamine Transmitter: Serotonin

Serotonin (5-hydroxytryptamine, abbreviated as 5-HT) was first investigated as a CNS neurotransmitter in the 1950s when lysergic acid diethylamide (LSD) was found to resemble serotonin structurally and block the contractile effect of serotonin on the gastrointestinal tract. At that time, it was hypothesized that LSD-induced hallucinations might be caused by alterations in the functioning of serotonin neurons and that serotonin might be involved in abnormal behavioral functioning. Today, drugs that potentiate the synaptic actions of serotonin are widely used as antidepressants and as antianxiety agents (specifically, the serotonergic agents known as *selective serotonin reuptake inhibitors*, or SSRIs; see Chapter 12). Serotonin plays a role in depression, anxiety and obsessive-compulsive disorder, panic, phobias, sleep, sex, cardiovascular function, and the regulation of body temperature; use of an SSRI to treat depression can be associated with such side effects as insomnia, anxiety, and loss of libido.

Significant amounts of serotonin are found in the upper brain stem, particularly in the pons and the medulla, in structures collectively called the *raphe nuclei*. Anterior projections from the brain stem terminate diffusely throughout the cerebral cortex, hippocampus, hypothalamus, and limbic system (Figure 2.16). Serotonin projections largely parallel those of DA, although they are not as widespread. Axons of serotonin neurons descending to the spinal cord from cell bodies located in the raphe nuclei may be involved in the modulation of both pain and spinal reflexes.

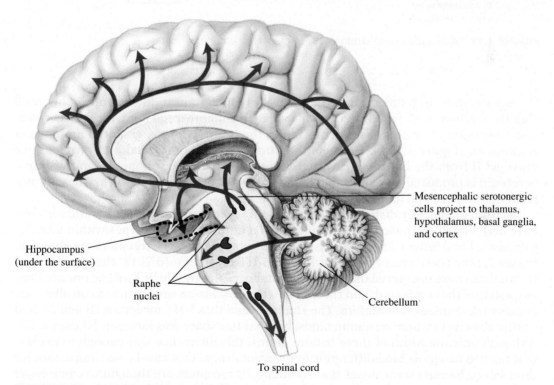

Mesencephalic serotonergic cells project to thalamus, hypothalamus, basal ganglia, and cortex

Hippocampus (under the surface)

Raphe nuclei

Cerebellum

To spinal cord

FIGURE 2.16 Serotonin pathways in the human brain.

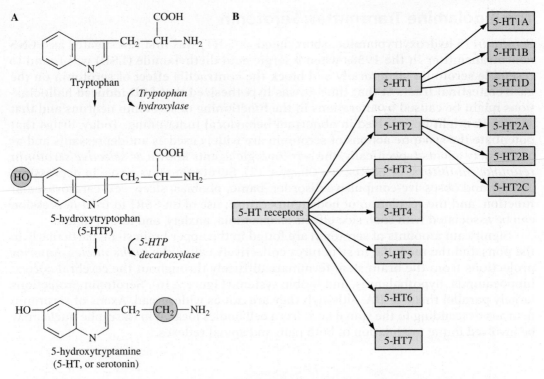

FIGURE 2.17 **A.** Biosynthesis of serotonin. **B.** Serotonin receptor nomenclature.

Serotonin is an indoleamine. Indoleamines all contain indole groups, a benzene ring (six-carbon ring) fused to a pyrrole ring (five-membered ring with four carbons and a nitrogen). Serotonin is synthesized in the brain from the essential amino acid tryptophan (Figure 2.17A). Because the human body cannot make tryptophan, we must get it from the foods we eat, such as poultry, bananas, tomatoes, and walnuts. Serotonin is produced by a short metabolic pathway consisting of two enzymes: trypto-phan hydroxylase and amino acid decarboxylase.

Several chemically distinct serotonin (5-HT) receptors have been identified. They have been classified in families (designated by a number) and subtypes within a family (designated by a letter). The main families and subtypes of 5-HT receptors are shown in Figure 2.17B. There are 14 different known 5-HT receptors. In 2013, the structures of two of these were uncovered using X-ray crystallography, by which X-ray beams are fired at crystals of the compound, and the way in which the beams are scattered can allow sci-entists to determine the structure. The studies found that 5-HT receptors 1B and 2B had similar structures where serotonin binds, but that this space was larger in 1B than in 2B. Although only the width of three helium atoms, this difference was enough to explain why the two receptors bind differently to different drugs. This may be very important for drug safety: because some drugs that stimulate 2B receptors are thought to cause heart problems, it has been nicknamed the "death receptor" (Wang et al., 2013).

Amino Acid Neurotransmitters

There are two amino acid neurotransmitters that are widely distributed in the brain. The first, *glutamic acid* (or *glutamate*), is the major universally excitatory neurotransmitter; the second is *gamma aminobutyric acid* (GABA), which is the major inhibitory neurotransmitter. Most other amino acids in the brain do not serve as neurotransmitters (with the exception of aspartate and glycine), but function as precursor molecules for the biosynthesis of other transmitters (for example, tyrosine for catecholamines and tryptophan for serotonin).

Both glutamate and GABA function to modulate a number of receptors, maintaining a balance between excitation and inhibition in the brain. The following sections focus on glutamate and GABA, because they are involved in the actions of several psychoactive drugs, ranging from the benzodiazepine antianxiety agents (see Chapter 13) to the mood stabilizers (see Chapter 14).

Glutamate

Glutamate is the major excitatory neurotransmitter in the brain and is also the precursor for the major inhibitory neurotransmitter GABA. GABA is formed from glutamate under control of the enzyme *glutamic acid decarboxylase.*

Glutamate is a nonessential amino acid, meaning that it is easily synthesized in the body and is not required in the diet. It does not readily penetrate the blood–brain barrier and is produced locally by specialized neuronal mechanisms. It can be synthesized by a number of different chemical reactions, among which is the normal breakdown of glucose. A second reaction, which might be the more important for neuronal glutamate, involves a glutamine cycle in which synaptically inactive glutamine serves as a reservoir of glutamate (Figure 2.18). In this process, after glutamate is released from a neuron and exerts its excitatory effect, it is transported into astrocytes and converted to glutamine. Eventually, the glutamine diffuses out of the astrocytes and enters the presynaptic nerve terminals, where it is converted to glutamate, the active neurotransmitter.

Glutamate receptors consist of two families, the *ionotropic* receptors (which respond quickly) that include NMDA and non-NMDA receptors (AMPA and kainate receptors) and *metabotropic receptors* (which respond more slowly). Metabotropic glutamate receptors (abbreviated as mGluRs) consist of eight members arranged into three groups (receptor classification is discussed more fully in Chapter 3). In the adult human brain, NMDA and AMPA receptors are colocalized in about 70 percent of their synapses. These receptors mediate rapid excitation of postsynaptic neurons, with especially high concentrations in the cerebral cortex, hippocampus, basal ganglia, septum, and amygdala.

NMDA receptors (Figure 2.19) have some unusual characteristics. First, in addition to glutamate, another amino acid, either glycine or serine, also needs to be present for the receptor to be activated. Second, in order for NMDA receptors to be activated, they not only need to be stimulated by glutamate, but they also need to be sufficiently stimulated electrically. The reason for this is that the NMDA ion channel is normally blocked by magnesium ions (Mg^{2+}). Glutamate alone is not able to activate the receptor because of this block. However, when the neuronal membrane is also electrically

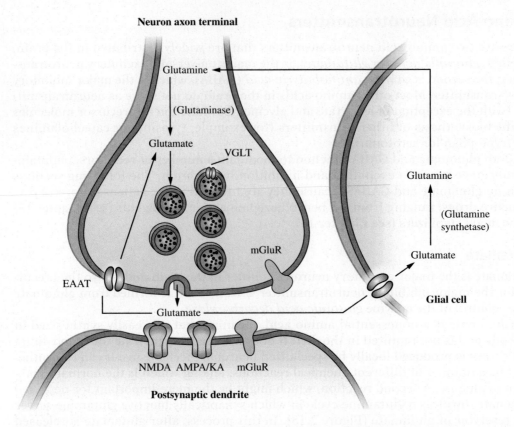

Neuron axon terminal

Glutamine

(Glutaminase)

Glutamate

VGLT

mGluR

Glutamine

(Glutamine synthetase)

Glutamate

EAAT

Glial cell

Glutamate

Glutamate

NMDA AMPA/KA   mGluR

Postsynaptic dendrite

FIGURE 2.18   Schematic of the glutamate synapse. Glutamate (Glu) is released into the synapse and recaptured by excitatory amino acid transporters (EAATs) located on the presynaptic terminal and on adjacent glial cells. Within the glial cells, glutamate is converted to glutamine by the enzyme *glutamine synthetase*. Glutamine diffuses back into neuronal terminals to replenish the Glu after conversion by the enzyme *glutaminase* and storage by vesicular glutamate transporters (VGLT). The "fast" (ionotropic) receptors, NMDA, AMPA, and kainate, are shown on the postsynaptic membrane; the "slow" (metabotropic, mGluR) receptors are shown on both the pre- and postsynaptic membranes.

stimulated, that is, depolarized (by the activation of AMPA or kainate receptors on the same postsynaptic neuron), the Mg^{2+} blockade of the ion channel is relieved. Then the NMDA receptor channel opens and permits the entry of both sodium and calcium ions, which further increases neuronal excitation. The NMDA receptor ion channel also has a binding site for phencyclidine (PCP) and ketamine (two psychedelic drugs discussed in Chapter 8). These two drugs also block the NMDA receptor (see Chapter 3) and therefore prevent glutamate-induced neuronal activation.

NMDA receptors play a critical role in regulating synaptic plasticity. Activation of these receptors is responsible for basal excitatory synaptic transmission and many forms of neurophysiological mechanisms that are thought to underlie learning and memory.

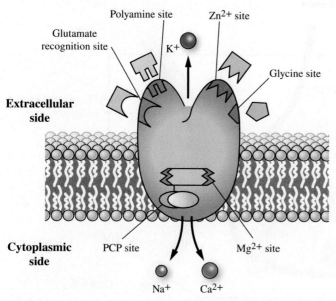

FIGURE 2.19 Schematic drawing of the NMDA (*N*-methyl-D-aspartate) receptor (PCP is discussed in Chapter 8).

Because these receptors are involved in cognitive processes, they are potential targets for therapies for Alzheimer's and other dementias. In 2004, memantine, the first anti-Alzheimer's drug that acts through a glutamatergic mechanism, became available for clinical use (see Chapter 16).

Although a normal amount of NMDA activity plays an important role in neuronal "health," excessive glutamatergic signaling is also involved in neuronal toxicity, a phenomenon by which nerve cells are damaged. Too much glutamate can lead to neuronal destruction through overactivity of NMDA receptors, which allows high amounts of calcium ions to enter the neuron (see Figure 2.19). Excess calcium activates enzymes, which then cause damage to cell structures and to DNA. For example, ethanol (see Chapter 5) reduces glutamate activity and alcohol withdrawal markedly increases glutamate release from neurons. Traumatic head injury also results in massive release of glutamate and attempts to provide "brain protection" after head injury is aimed at preventing glutamatergic overactivity. Anoxia (oxygen deficiency), hypoglycemia, and epilepsy are other glutamate-releasing events that can lead to neuronal damage. Research is also focusing on the possibility of glutamate dysfunction in the pathogenesis of schizophrenia, especially the negative symptoms and the cognitive dysfunction associated with the disorder (see Chapter 11).

Gamma Aminobutyric Acid

Gamma aminobutyric acid (GABA), the universal inhibitory transmitter, is found in high concentrations in the brain and spinal cord. Two different types of GABA receptors are categorized as GABA$_A$ and GABA$_B$ (Figure 2.20). *GABA$_A$ receptors* are fast

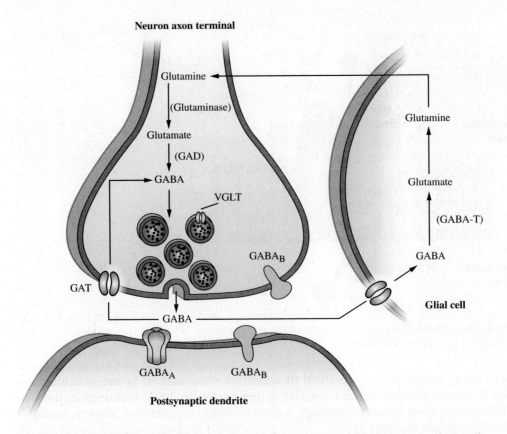

FIGURE 2.20 Schematic of the GABA synapse. GABA$_A$ receptors are fast (ionotropic; Chapter 3) receptors and found on the postsynaptic membrane. GABA$_B$ receptors are metabotropic and found on both pre- and postsynaptic membranes. GAT is the GABA transporter; GAD is glutamic acid decarboxylase, which converts L-glutamic acid to GABA; GABA-T is the enzyme transaminase, which metabolizes GABA.

receptors. Activation of this receptor by GABA opens an ion channel and leads to an influx of chloride into the cell, hyperpolarizing the cell and reducing its excitability. Barbiturate and benzodiazepine binding to this receptor facilitates the action of GABA (see Chapter 13), which is responsible for the anxiolytic, amnestic, and anesthetic effects of these sedative drugs. GABA$_A$ receptors are found in high density in the cerebral cortex, hippocampus, and cerebellum.

Numerous sub-subtypes of the GABA$_A$ receptor occur, allowing for the development of a variety of agonists and antagonists (see Chapter 13). Such drugs might be novel antianxiety agents, anticonvulsants, or cognitive enhancers.

GABA$_B$ receptors are slow-response receptors. Activation of GABA$_B$ receptors in the amygdala is associated with the membrane-stabilizing, antiaggressive properties of valproic acid, a drug widely used to treat bipolar disorder (see Chapter 14).

Peptide Neurotransmitters

Many newly identified neurotransmitters are peptides, which are small proteins (chains of amino acid molecules attached in a specific order). Peptide transmitters can be classified into several groups, including the hypothalamic-releasing hormones, the pituitary hormones, and the so-called "gut-brain peptides." In this book, one peptide transmitter of interest is the type involved in the actions of the opiates, such as morphine. *Opioid peptides* include the *endorphins* (about 16 to 30 amino acids in length) and the shorter-chain *enkephalins* (5 amino acids in length). These substances are formed from a larger protein produced elsewhere in the body. The endorphins may be involved in a wide variety of emotional states, including pain perception, reward, emotional stability, and energy "highs," as well as in acupuncture. Opiates such as morphine, codeine, and heroin activate receptors for endorphins and enkephalins (see Chapter 10). Opioid receptors are termed *mu, kappa,* and *delta*; the mu receptor mediates the analgesic and reinforcing properties of morphine and other opiates.

Another peptide transmitter of interest in this book is *substance P*, a *gut-brain peptide* (11 amino acids in length) that plays an important role as a sensory transmitter, especially for pain impulses that enter the spinal cord and brain from a peripheral site of tissue injury. Opioids, serotonin agonists, and norepinephrine agonists exert much of their analgesic effect by acting on substance P nerve terminals to limit the release of this pain-inducing peptide.

From Table 2.1, it can be seen that there are some additional transmitter substances that have not been mentioned here. The neuromodulator *adenosine* has several functions; the most relevant in this context is its role in promoting sleep. The effect of caffeine in maintaining wakefulness is due to the fact that it is an adenosine antagonist (discussed in Chapter 6). The endocannabinoids are the endogenous substances that stimulate the receptors on which cannabis (marijuana) acts. They are discussed in Chapter 9. The neurotransmitter gases that have also not been described do not play a major role in the action of the drugs described in this text.

Until recently, it was believed that only a single neurotransmitter could be produced, stored, and released at each synapse. But it is now clear that this situation is the exception rather than the rule. The "co-release" of more than one neurotransmitter is now a well-established phenomenon.

STUDY QUESTIONS

1. What are the major divisions of the central nervous system?

2. Summarize the major structures of the basal ganglia and the limbic system and their respective functions.

3. Describe the main parts of a neuron, including the components of the synapse.

4. Summarize the processes involved in synaptic transmission. How is synaptic transmitter action terminated? Give examples.

5. What are the six classical neurotransmitters and their major receptor types?

6. Which major brain structures are associated with the neural pathways that release norepinephrine, dopamine, and serotonin?

7. Which diseases and drugs of abuse are associated with each of the major neurotransmitters?

REFERENCES

Blakeslee, S. (2007). "A Small Part of the Brain, and Its Profound Effects." *New York Times.* February 16. http://www.nytimes.com/2007/02/06/health/psychology/06brain.html.

Bourzac, K. (2016). "Texas Woman Is the First Person to Undergo Optogenetic Therapy." *MIT Technology Review.* March 18. https://www.technologyreview.com/s/601067/texas-woman-is-the-first-person-to-undergo-optogenetic-therapy/.

Colapinto, J. (2015). "Lighting the Brain." *The New Yorker.* May 18. http://www.newyorker.com/magazine/2015/05/18/lighting-the-brain.

Deisseroth, K. (2015). "Optogenetics: 10 Years of Microbial Opsins in Neuroscience." *Nature Neuroscience* 18: 1213–1225. doi:10.1038/nn.4091.

Hong, S., et al. (2016). "Complement and Microglia Mediate Early Synapse Loss in Alzheimer Mouse Models." *Science.* March 31. doi: 10.1126/science.aad8373.

Kempermann, G., et al. (2004). "Functional Significance of Adult Neurogenesis." *Current Opinions in Neurobiology* 14: 186–191.

Reardon, S. (2015). "'Wiring Diagrams' Link Lifestyle to Brain Function." *Nature News.* September 28. doi:10.1038/nature.2015.18442.

Schaffer, D. V., and Gage, F. H. (2004). "Neurogenesis and Neuroadaptation." *Neuromolecular Medicine* 5: 1–9.

Tang, A.-H., et al. (2016). "A Trans-Synaptic Nanocolumn Aligns Neurotransmitter Release to Receptors." *Nature* 536: 210–214. doi: 10.1038/nature19058.

Thompson, R. F. (1993). *The Brain: A Neuroscience Primer,* 2nd ed. New York: Freeman.

Wang, C., et al. (2013). "Structural Basis for Molecular Recognition at Serotonin Receptors." *Science* 340: 610–614.

Yuhas, D., and Jabr, F. (2012). "Know Your Neurons: What Is the Ratio of Glia to Neurons in the Brain?" *Scientific American* June 3. https://blogs.scientificamerican.com/brainwaves/know-your-neurons-what-is-the-ratio-of-glia-to-neurons-in-the-brain/.

Zimmer, C. (2016). "Updated Brain Map Identifies Nearly 100 New Regions." *New York Times.* July 20. http://nyti.ms/2a9aU2a.

CHAPTER 3

Pharmacodynamics
How Drugs Act

While the body is in the process of ridding itself of an ingested psychoactive drug, the drug is exerting effects by attaching to *receptors* in cells in both the brain and the body. As a result of such interactions, the body experiences effects that are characteristic for the drug. *It is a basic principle of pharmacology that the pharmacological, physiological, or behavioral effects induced by a drug follow from their interaction with receptors.*

The study of these interactions, termed *pharmacodynamics,* involves exploring the mechanisms of drug action that occur at the cellular level. While *pharmacokinetics* is the study of what the body does to a drug, *pharmacodynamics* is the study of what the drug does to the body.

To produce an effect, a drug must bind to and interact with specific receptors which, in the case of psychoactive drugs, are usually located on the surface of neurons in the brain. The occupation of a receptor by a drug (termed *drug–receptor binding*) leads to a change in the functional properties of the neuron, resulting in the drug's characteristic pharmacological response. In most instances, drug–receptor binding is both *ionic* and *reversible* in nature, with positive and negative charges on various portions of the drug molecule and the receptor protein attracting one to the other. The strength of ionic attachment is determined by the fit of the three-dimensional structure of the drug to the three-dimensional site on the receptor,[1] the so-called "lock–and–key" relationship.

RECEPTORS FOR DRUG ACTION

A *receptor* is a fairly large molecule (usually a protein[2]) at which endogenous transmitters or modulators produce their biological effects. Literally hundreds of different types of receptors are known to have the ability to recognize one specific

---

[1]Reversible ionic binding is contrasted with the formation of a permanent, irreversible, covalent bond between a drug and receptor. One of the rare instances in psychopharmacology where an irreversible covalent bond forms is between certain antidepressant drugs and the enzyme monoamine oxidase (see Chapter 12).

[2]A protein is a complex chain of various amino acids that function, among other things, as metabolic enzymes and receptors.

neurotransmitter; that is, only one neurotransmitter might be specific enough to fit or bind to a specific receptor protein. For example, if only serotonin binds to a specific receptor, that protein is called a *serotonin receptor*. But although the receptor is specific for serotonin, serotonin, as a neurotransmitter, also binds to other, structurally different *receptor subtypes*.

To date, at least 11 (and perhaps 13 or 14) different serotonin receptor proteins have been identified (see Chapter 2).[3] This diversity makes it possible to develop closely related drugs, each with a slightly different degree of *affinity* (strength of attachment) for the different serotonin receptors. For example, a specific drug might have affinity for a serotonin 1 receptor, but not for any other serotonin receptor.

A given drug may even be more specific for a given set of receptors than the endogenous neurotransmitter. Serotonin, for example, must necessarily attach to all its receptors. However, a given drug might attach to only one receptor. For example, *buspirone* (BuSpar) attaches to one type of serotonin receptor, the 5-HT$_{1A}$ receptor, which results in antianxiety actions. It has no affinity for other serotonin receptors.

It is also a general rule of psychopharmacology that drugs do not create any unique effects; they merely modulate normal neuronal functioning, mimicking or antagonizing the actions of a specific neurotransmitter. Drug binding may mimic or facilitate neurotransmitter action, or drug occupation of a receptor might block access of the neurotransmitter to that receptor and prevent endogenous molecules from attaching, activating, and producing an effect at these sites.

Receptor Structure

What does a receptor look like? Although there are several different configurations of proteins that may serve a receptor function, the following is a brief summary of the major types most relevant to the action of drugs.

Ion Channel Receptors

Ion channel receptors (also called *ionotropic receptors*) are cell membrane-spanning receptors that form an *ion channel*. That is, the center of the receptor crosses the membrane of the neuron and forms a pore, which enlarges when either an endogenous neurotransmitter or exogenous drug attaches to the receptor-binding site. The attachment of the transmitter or drug molecule allows flow of a specific *ion* (such as chloride ions) through the enlarged pore (see Figure 3.1A). (It should be noted that, in some cases, the pore is normally open and the attachment of a drug or transmitter will close it. Although such situations are beyond the scope of this text, the general phenomenon is the same.)

As shown in Figure 3.1B, the ionotropic receptor is composed of five sections, or *subunits*, each of which crosses the cell membrane. Each of these sections is labeled, usually with a Greek letter. (If they are very similar in composition, two subunits may be given the same Greek letter.) Each of these subunits is, in turn, made up of four helical coils, which are also labeled, usually M$_1$ through M$_4$. It is the arrangement of

---

[3]Each receptor protein that binds serotonin, for example, has a slightly different amino acid composition; nevertheless, their three-dimensional structures are similar enough that serotonin, for example, still fits a "slot" (like a lock-and-key arrangement) and ionically binds to the protein.

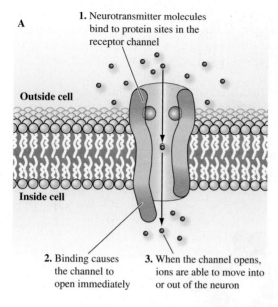

A

1. Neurotransmitter molecules bind to protein sites in the receptor channel

Outside cell

Inside cell

2. Binding causes the channel to open immediately

3. When the channel opens, ions are able to move into or out of the neuron

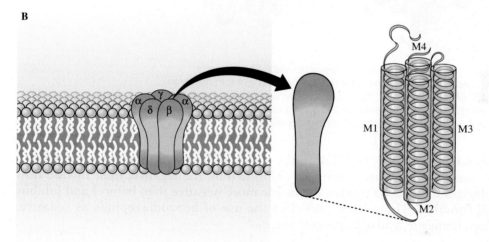

B

FIGURE 3.1 **A.** Schematic of neurotransmitter activation of an ionotropic receptor that contains an ion channel. **B.** Detailed schematic representation of the individual subunits of an ion channel (ionotropic) receptor, showing the helical coils of which they are composed.

these five transmembrane subunits that forms the channel of the ionotropic receptor, as seen in Figure 3.2.

Figures 3.2 and 3.3 illustrate how the neurotransmitter gamma aminobutyric acid (GABA) and various drugs (benzodiazepines, barbiturates) bind to the ionotropic GABA$_A$ receptor and affect the inward flow of chloride ions. Benzodiazepines (see Chapter 13) serve as *allosteric agonists* (discussed below) by binding to a site near the

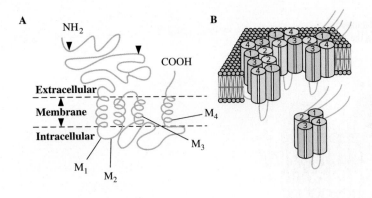

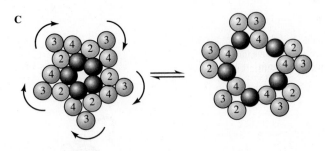

FIGURE 3.2   Hypothesized topology of the ionotropic GABA$_A$ receptor.
A. Single subunit with its large extracellular terminal part and four transmembrane
helical coils. **B.** Arrangement of the transmembrane domains of five subunits to
form a central channel. **C.** Transmembrane domain in a transverse section through
the membrane when the channel is closed (*left*) and open (*right*).

GABA-binding site and by facilitating the action of GABA in increasing the flow of
chloride ions into the neuron. Because chloride ions are negative, their inward flow
hyperpolarizes the neuron (makes the inside more negative than before) and inhibits
neuronal function. This action underlies the use of benzodiazepines as sedative,
antianxiety, amnestic, and antiepileptic agents.[4]

G-Protein-Coupled Receptors

The second type of membrane-spanning receptor protein is called a *G-protein-
coupled receptor* (GPCR). These receptors are also called *metabotropic* receptors (see
Figure 3.4). The activation of these receptors induces the release of an attached intracellular protein (a *G protein*) that in turn, controls enzymatic functions within the
postsynaptic neuron.

---

[4]Several other substances, such as barbiturates, also have binding sites on the GABA receptor complex, shown in Figure 3.3. Barbiturates (see Chapter 13) act like benzodiazepines in increasing the
effect of GABA on the chloride channel within the GABA receptor. Thus, with a site and mechanism
of action similar to that exerted by benzodiazepines, the two classes of drugs might be expected to
demonstrate similar clinical and behavioral effects. In general, they do.

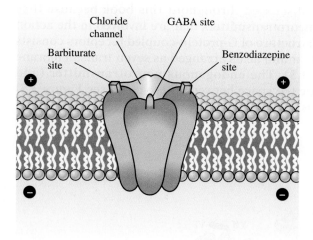

FIGURE 3.3 Schematic of the GABA$_A$ receptor, with its binding sites for GABA, benzodiazepines, and barbiturates.

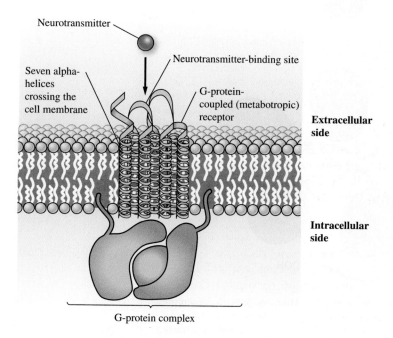

FIGURE 3.4 Schematic of a G-protein-coupled (metabotropic) receptor (GPCR), showing the seven helical, membrane-spanning coils.

G-protein-coupled receptors are discussed throughout this book because they mediate the synaptic effects of many neurotransmitters that are involved in the action of psychoactive drugs. The molecular structure of G-protein-coupled receptors consists of a single protein chain of 400 to 500 amino acids arranged as seven transmembrane alpha helices (see Figures 3.4 and 3.5). The endogenous neurotransmitter (and presumably drugs also) attaches inside the space between these coils (see Figure 3.5) and is held in place by ionic attractions.

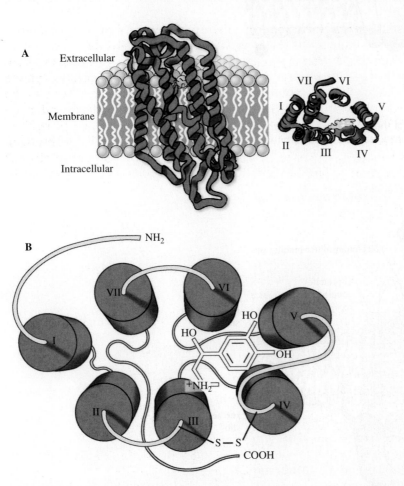

FIGURE 3.5 Schematic representation of a G-protein-coupled transmembrane receptor, with a molecule of neurotransmitter (norepinephrine) lying in its binding site. Note the arrangement of the seven transmembrane helical coils (numbered with roman numerals) and the site of the transmitter attachment deep within the structure. The ionic interactions between the transmitter and particular amino acid side chains are not illustrated. **A.** The membrane and continuous coils. **B.** The helical coils are represented as cylinders with the molecule of norepinephrine interacting with four of the coils.

G-protein-coupled receptors constitute a large and diverse family of proteins whose primary function is to change extracellular stimuli (transmitters and drugs) into intracellular signals. Unlike ionotropic receptors, metabotropic receptors do not form a membrane-spanning pore that can allow the direct passage of ions. Instead, when a neurotransmitter associates with the extracellular recognition (binding) site, the G protein is activated and either *directly* (see Figure 3.6) or *indirectly* (see Figure 3.7), through a series of enzymatic reactions, *opens or closes ion channels or alters other processes located at other places on the cell membrane or in the cell nucleus.* Because the effect of metabotropic receptors is not as immediate as that of ionotropic receptors, their action is slower.

The process starts when a hormone, neurotransmitter, or drug attaches to a receptor. This changes the shape of the receptor, which then activates the G protein on the inside of the cell membrane. One component of the G protein is released and then either *directly* activates an ion channel, as shown in Figure 3.6, or the G protein moves along the membrane until it finds and then *indirectly* activates an enzyme, such as the enzyme adenylyl cyclase, shown in Figure 3.8. In this example, the activated adenylyl cyclase then produces lots of cyclic AMP (cAMP), which spreads the signal through the cell. The cyclic AMP is called the *second messenger* (the first being the neurotransmitter). The ultimate cellular response produced by this process may be the opening of ion channels, the alteration of enzyme activities, or changes in gene activation in

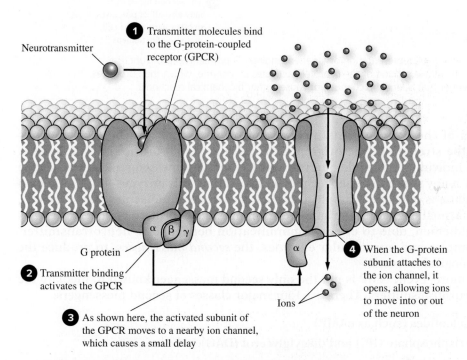

FIGURE 3.6 Schematic representation of G-protein-receptor function. In this situation, the ion channel is directly opened by the alpha subunit of the activated G protein.

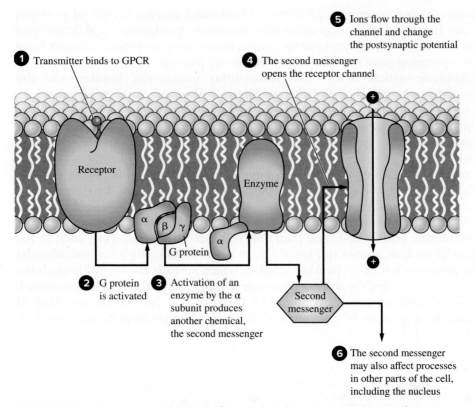

FIGURE 3.7 Schematic representation of a generic indirect G-protein-receptor function. In this situation, the alpha subunit of the G protein activates an enzyme, which then produces a second messenger that opens the channel, or causes other biochemical reactions.

the nucleus of the neuron. This mechanism provides the significant benefit of increasing the strength of the original extracellular signal of the first messenger. That is, the individual molecule of a transmitter, the first messenger, can trigger the synthesis of many second messenger molecules. Adding this enzyme "link," of which adenylyl cyclase is only one example, can elicit a cascade of molecules inside the cell, initiated by a small signal that originated from outside. G-protein-coupled receptors are the middlemen, able to effect communication between the neurotransmitter-receptor complex and intracellular enzymes, the *second messengers,* to produce the ultimate biological response.

Furthermore, cyclic AMP is not the only second messenger known to mediate the effects of neurotransmitters. There are four major classes of second messengers:

1. Cyclic nucleotides (such as cAMP)
2. Inositol trisphosphate (IP_3) and diacylglycerol (DAG)
3. Calcium ions (Ca^{2+})
4. Nitric oxide/carbon monoxide

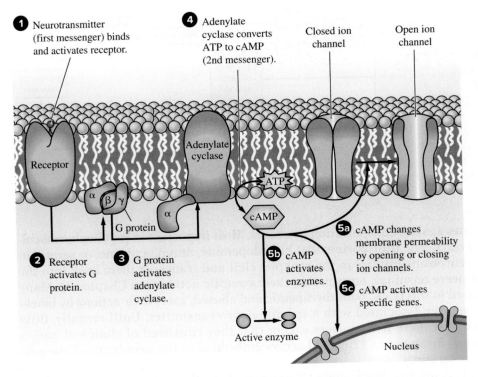

1 Neurotransmitter (first messenger) binds and activates receptor.

4 Adenylate cyclase converts ATP to cAMP (2nd messenger).

Closed ion channel

Open ion channel

Receptor

Adenylate cyclase

ATP

α β γ

cAMP

G protein

α

2 Receptor activates G protein.

3 G protein activates adenylate cyclase.

5b cAMP activates enzymes.

5a cAMP changes membrane permeability by opening or closing ion channels.

5c cAMP activates specific genes.

Active enzyme

Nucleus

FIGURE 3.8 Schematic representation of an indirect G-protein-receptor function, illustrating the specific activation of the cyclic amp second messenger system.

Figure 3.9 summarizes a general model of transmitter–receptor interactions and the resulting cascade of effects produced by second and, in some cases, third messengers (not shown here). Cyclic AMP is shown, associated with its enzyme, adenylyl cyclase, as well as another pair of second messengers, inositol triphosphate and diacylglycerol.

Ionotropic and (direct and indirect) metabotropic receptors are not the only receptor types important for understanding drug action. For example, the metabotropic glutamate (mGlu) and GABA receptors are atypical GPCRs, with more complicated biochemical characteristics than the basic structures described in this text (see Pin and Bettler, 2016 and Xu et al., 2014). Furthermore, there are additional receptors that mediate the effect of hormones (steroids) and neurotrophic substances (a generic term for any of a family of substances with roles in the maintenance and survival of neurons). Two other types of proteins are also crucial to understanding psychoactive drug mechanisms.

Transporter (Carrier) Proteins

The third type of membrane-spanning protein is a *carrier* (or *transport*) *protein*. This type of receptor transports small organic molecules (such as neurotransmitters) across

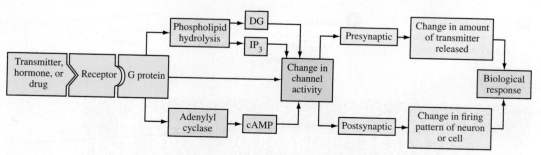

FIGURE 3.9 Major pathways for modulation of synaptic transmission. cAMP = cyclic adenosine monophosphate; IP_3 = inositol triphosphate; DG = diacylglycerol (all three substances are second messengers).

cell membranes against concentration gradients. Most important in psychopharmacology are the *presynaptic* transporters that bind dopamine, norepinephrine, or serotonin (and other neurotransmitters) in the synaptic cleft and transport them back into the presynaptic nerve terminal, terminating their synaptic action (see Chapter 2). Many drugs discussed in this book, both therapeutic and abused, exert their actions by blocking the transporter associated with a specific neurotransmitter. Until recently, little was known about these transporters except that they consisted of chains of amino acids (proteins) arranged as 12 helical arrays embedded in the membrane of the presynaptic nerve terminal.

Work by Gouaux and MacKinnon (2005) as well as others (Armstrong et al., 2006; Yernool et al., 2004) has added considerably to our knowledge of these transporters. To carry molecules of neurotransmitter across presynaptic membranes against a concentration gradient, the transporters are hypothesized to exist in at least three ionic states: open to the synapse, occluded with the transmitter "trapped" inside, and open to the cytoplasm of the presynaptic neuron (see Figure 3.10A). The transporter has been conceived as a bowl-shaped structure with a fluid-filled basin (open to the synaptic cleft) extending halfway across the membrane of the presynaptic nerve terminal (see Figure 3.10B). At the bottom of the basin are three binding sites for the neurotransmitter, each cradled by two helical "hairpins" reaching from opposite sides of the membrane. In the resting state, the bowl is open to the synaptic cleft. It traps one or more molecules of released transmitter per "cycle," allowing floods of molecules to move from the synaptic cleft into the presynaptic terminal and become available for rerelease. It is proposed that the transport of transmitter is achieved by movements of the hairpins that allow alternating access to either side of the membrane (for example, the outer layer closes, trapping the transmitter, and then the inner layer opens, ejecting the transmitter into the cytoplasm of the presynaptic terminal). Even more detailed biochemical descriptions of both serotonin transporters (Coleman et al., 2016) and the dopamine transporter (Wang et al., 2015) have recently been elucidated.

It should be appreciated that this is only a summary of neurotransporters and that there are many phenomena in this area that can be noted only briefly. One important concept is that there are several different versions, rather than a single type, of transporter for the various transmitters. Each neurotransmitter is associated with several forms of its respective transporter. A second important concept is that transporters are

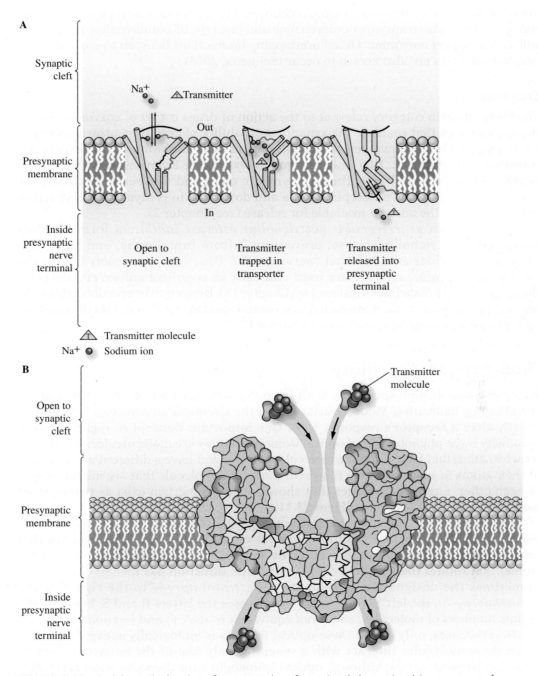

Na⁺ ○ Sodium ion

FIGURE 3.10 **A.** Schematic drawing of a proposed conformational change involving transport of transmitter and sodium ions across the membrane of the presynaptic nerve terminal. *Left:* Transporter open to the synaptic cleft. *Center:* Transmitter "trapped" inside the transporter. *Right:* Inward-facing state with transmitter "released" into the cytoplasm of the neuron. **B.** Schematic drawing of the proposed movement of neurotransmitter molecules through a transporter protein and into the presynaptic nerve terminal. The drawing illustrates the total movement and summarizes the three-step outline in Figure 3.10A. The deep aqueous basin reaches halfway across the membrane.

not completely selective to a single transmitter. For example, one type of dopamine transporter will also transport noradrenaline and one type of noradrenaline transporter will also transport dopamine. Other, overlapping interactions between transporters and neurotransmitters are also known to occur (Scimemi, 2014).

Enzymes

The fourth protein category relevant to the action of drugs is that of enzymes—in particular, enzymes that regulate the synaptic availability of certain neurotransmitters. These enzymes break down neurotransmitters and their inhibition by drugs increases transmitter availability. Two examples are *acetylcholine esterase*, the enzyme that breaks down acetylcholine within the synaptic cleft, and *monoamine oxidase*, the enzyme that breaks down norepinephrine and dopamine in presynaptic nerve terminals, controlling the amount available for release (see Chapter 2).

Drugs known as *irreversible acetylcholine esterase inhibitors* form covalent bonds with acetylcholinesterase, preventing it from functioning, and have been used as insecticides and as lethal "nerve gases." Drugs that *reversibly* inhibit the enzyme *acetylcholine esterase* are used clinically as cognitive enhancers, delaying the progression of Alzheimer's disease (see Chapter 16). Drugs that irreversibly inhibit the enzyme *monoamine oxidase* are called monoamine oxidase inhibitors (MAOIs) and are used primarily as antidepressants (see Chapter 12).

Drug–Receptor Specificity

Receptors exhibit high specificity both for one particular neurotransmitter and for certain drug molecules. Modest variations in the chemical structure of a drug may greatly alter a receptor's response to it. One important concept in regard to drug specificity is the phenomenon of optical isomers. *Isomers* are molecules formed around a carbon atom that have the same molecular formula but have a different arrangement of their atoms in space. Isomers represent forms of a molecule that are mirror images of each other. Simple substances that show optical isomerism exist as two or more isomers known as *enantiomers* (Figure 3.11).

The difference in the spatial arrangement of the two molecules means that they rotate a beam of polarized light in equal but opposite directions. The isomer that rotates the light in a clockwise direction is designated as the (+) isomer; conversely, the isomer that rotates the light in a counterclockwise direction has the (−) designation. Sometimes the designation is made as D (*dextrorotatory*—"to the right") and L (*levorotatory*—"to the left"). Yet another system uses the letters R and S, based on the atomic numbers of molecules, and is not equivalent to the (+) and (−) nomenclatures.

In most cases, only one of these optical isomers is biologically active. Therefore, when these molecules interact with a receptor, only one of the isomers would be effective. In other words, although optical isomers behave the same way chemically, they do not act in the same way biologically.

When drugs are made in the laboratory and eventually become medications, they are often produced as a 50/50 mixture of their two enantiomers. In the laboratory, it takes more work to separate the two, so it is the mixture (50 percent active and

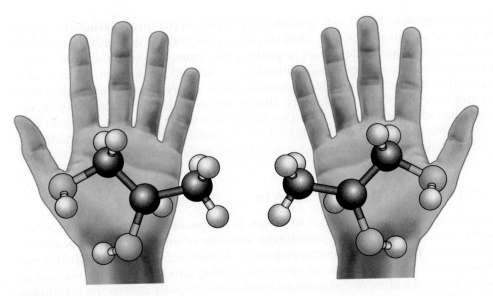

FIGURE 3.11 Illustration depicting the concept of enantiomers.

50 percent inactive) that is marketed, although only the (−) half of the medicine will be biologically active in the body. This is known as a *racemic mixture* or *racemate*. Most medicines are manufactured as racemates. However, sometimes an isomer is also produced. An example is the antidepressant citalopram. This is the racemate version, marketed as the antidepressant Celexa. When the patent on the racemate expired, the active isomer was separated out and is marketed as escitalopram, or Lexapro. As a result, escitalopram doses are approximately half of the clinically comparable citalopram doses (see Chapter 12).[5]

As a consequence of a drug binding to a receptor, cellular function is altered, resulting in changes in physiological or psychological functioning. The total effect of the drug in the body results from drug actions either (1) on one specific type of receptor or (2) at different types of receptors. However, whether the drug is used for therapeutic or recreational purposes, the total action will include additional responses, called *side effects.*

As an example of the side effects produced by the first mechanism, blockade of presynaptic serotonin reuptake, produced by the antidepressant class of selective

---

[5] Other drugs discussed in this book that have isomeric formulations include amphetamine and methylphenidate, stimulant drugs used in the treatment of ADHD (see Chapter 15), and modafinil, used in the treatment of narcolepsy (see Chapters 7 and 13). Both isomers of amphetamine are active; the D-isomer is familiar as Dexedrine. The L-isomer of methylphenidate is metabolized much faster than the D-isomer, which is marketed separately as Focalin. The racemic mixture of modafinil is marketed as Provigil; the R-isomer is marketed as Nuvigil, which is more soluble in water.

serotonergic reuptake inhibitors (SSRIs), increases serotonin availability at all postsynaptic serotonin receptors. This single action results not only in relief of depression but also in such side effects as anxiety, insomnia, and sexual dysfunction.

As an example of the side effects produced by the second mechanism, certain other antidepressants (the tricyclic antidepressants) reduce depression by increasing both serotonin and norepinephrine availability. But in addition, they produce sedation, dry mouth, and blurred vision because they also block cholinergic receptors. The goal is to find an acceptable balance between desirable therapeutic effects and undesirable side effects, and an important reason for understanding receptors is to achieve this outcome.

Acute and Chronic Receptor Effects

When a psychoactive drug binds to a receptor, it produces an immediate response. For example, smoking a cigarette containing nicotine or smoking illicit cocaine or methamphetamine releases the neurotransmitter dopamine; dopamine activates our reward system and a stimulant or pleasurable feeling can follow. With respect to medications, ingestion of *methylphenidate* (Ritalin) can rapidly relieve the symptoms of attention deficit/hyperactivity disorder (ADHD), potent opioid analgesics can rapidly relieve severe pain, and certain sedatives can rapidly induce drowsiness and be used in the treatment of insomnia. Similarly, many of the side effects of drugs (such as dry mouth, unwanted sedation, blurred vision, and so on) follow from acute actions at other receptors, often distinct from those responsible for the desired drug action.

But when the drug is given over a longer period of time, it produces long-term changes in the properties of the receptors. Here, the drug is in contact with its receptors for days to months. As a result, neurons "adapt" to the presence of a drug, resulting in long-term changes in neuronal functioning. There are two types of such adaptations, shown in Figure 3.12. The left panel of the figure shows the normal effect of transmission on receptors. Under normal physiological conditions, neurotransmitter molecules are released intermittently, only when the presynaptic neuron is activated. Therefore, the receptors for that transmitter are only transiently stimulated; the signal is received and then the transmitter molecules are removed.

However, if excessive numbers of transmitter molecules (or molecules of a drug that mimics a transmitter) are available to the receptor over a period of time, changes occur. In the presence of chronic stimulation, the number of receptor sites decreases[6] and the sensitivity of the receptors decreases. As indicated in the middle panel, this is called *downregulation* or *desensitization*. This may account for some types of tolerance, for example, when heroin consistently occupies the opioid–binding sites. Over time, often in a few weeks of continuous exposure, the postsynaptic neuron will no longer respond to average amounts of heroin and increased amounts are required to obtain the opioid effect.

When the reverse occurs, that is, when the number of transmitter molecules available at postsynaptic receptors is decreased, often because they are blocked by an antagonist drug, the opposite result may occur. That is, an *upregulation* or *supersensitivity* may develop, as shown in the right panel of Figure 3.12. In this case, the number of receptors

---

[6]Receptor number refers to the total number of receptors, expressed in terms of unit area of membrane, or per cell, or per unit mass of protein.

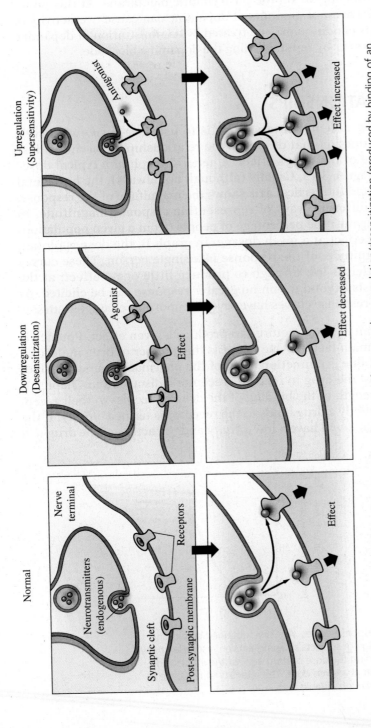

FIGURE 3.12 Schematic diagram depicting the phenomena of receptor downregulation/desensitization (produced by binding of an agonist drug) and upregulation/supersensitivity (produced by binding of an antagonist drug).

increases and the sensitivity of the receptors increase. For example, antipsychotic medications block dopamine receptors, which causes their upregulation. As a result, additional dopamine receptors appear on the postsynaptic membrane. At this point, if the blockade is ended, even average amounts of dopamine can cause overactivity of certain motor responses. This condition may be treated by administration of dopamine agonists (to decrease receptors) or by re-establishing the dopamine blockade.

DOSE–RESPONSE RELATIONSHIPS

One way of quantifying drug–receptor interactions is to use *dose–response curves*. A dose–response curve is a function that describes the relationship between the dose of a drug and the magnitude of the drug's effect. A generic graph of a typical dose–response curve is shown in Figure 3.13. Usually (although not always), the horizontal axis indicates the drug dose and the vertical axis shows the magnitude of the response. Figure 3.13 illustrates two different ways of representing response magnitude. In graph A, the dose is plotted against the percentage of people (from a given population) who exhibit a characteristic effect at a given dosage. In graph B, the dose is plotted against the intensity, or magnitude, of the response in a single person. These curves indicate that a dose exists that is low enough to produce little or no effect; at the opposite extreme, a dose exists beyond which no greater response can be elicited. As indicated in the figure, dose–response curves have several important characteristics:

• *Potency* refers to the amount of drug required to produce a given effect. Potency is largely determined by two main factors. One factor is the number of drug molecules at the receptor sites. This value is a function of all of the pharmacokinetic variables that influenced the ability of the drug to reach its receptors, discussed in Chapter 1. The second factor is the strength of the binding of the drug molecules to their receptors. The measure of how tightly a drug binds to the receptor is termed *affinity*. If the drug does not bind well, then it will have a low *affinity* and the action of the drug will

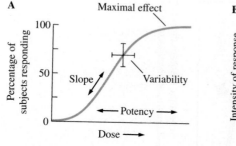
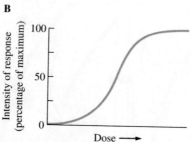

FIGURE 3.13 Two types of dose–response curves. **A.** Curve obtained by plotting the dose of drug against the percentage of subjects showing a given response at any given dose. **B.** Curve obtained by plotting the dose of drug against the intensity of response observed in any single person at a given dose. The intensity of response is plotted as a percentage of the maximum obtainable response.

be weaker. Therefore, if the respective doses of two drugs produce the same number of molecules at the receptor, then the drug with the greatest affinity will be more potent and produce a greater effect.

In addition to receptor affinity, the total duration of the ligand–receptor interaction, termed *residence time*, can also have a crucial impact on the drug response. Residence time describes how long the molecule is bound to its target. This is the interval between the time that the drug attaches to, or *associates* with, and detaches, or *dissociates* from, the receptor. A drug with a short residence time is said to have a *fast dissociation rate*. This phenomenon can significantly influence drug action. For example, a fast dissociation time might reduce the toxic effect of a drug because the drug molecules only act at the receptor for a short period of time (Pan et al., 2013). A clinical example is that of antipsychotic drugs used in the treatment of schizophrenia (Chapter 11). These drugs have a common action of blocking (antagonizing; see below) the D_2 dopamine receptor. Most members of the first group of antipsychotics that were discovered, such as haloperidol and chlorpromazine, are high-affinity antagonists of the D_2 dopamine receptor, with residence times greater than 30 minutes. In addition to their therapeutic benefit, these drugs elicit a number of adverse side effects. D_2 receptor antagonists with much shorter residence times (16 to 30 seconds), such as clozapine and quetiapine, have been developed, and this appears to have been an important mechanism for reducing the undesirable side effects of these drugs (Tummino and Copeland, 2008).

The location of the dose–response curve along the horizontal axis reflects the potency of the drug. If two drugs produce an equal degree of stimulation, but one exerts this action at half the dose level of the other, the first drug is considered to be *twice as potent* as the second drug. This concept is illustrated in Figure 3.14, which shows the dose–response curves for three different stimulant drugs—methamphetamine, D-amphetamine (see Chapter 7), and caffeine (see Chapter 6). The first two are powerful psychostimulants. Although their chemical structures are very close, they differ by the simple addition of a methyl (—CH₃) group to D-amphetamine, forming

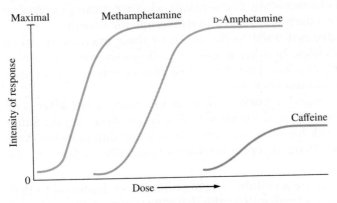

FIGURE 3.14 Theoretical dose–response curves for three psychostimulants illustrates equal efficacy of methamphetamine and dextroamphetamine, increased potency of methamphetamine, and reduced potency and efficacy of caffeine.

methamphetamine. Both drugs attach to the same receptors in the brain, but meth-amphetamine exerts a much more powerful action on them, at least in milligrams. In pharmacological terms, methamphetamine is more *potent* than D-amphetamine because a lower absolute dose achieves the same level of response as a higher dose of D-amphetamine. However, potency may be relatively unimportant because it makes little difference whether the effective dose of a drug is 1.0 milligram or 100 milligrams as long as the drug can be administered in an appropriate dose with no undue toxicity.

• *Variability* refers to individual differences in drug–response; some patients respond at very low doses and some require much more drug. As described in Chapter 1, differences in genetic makeup of metabolic enzymes are an important reason for the wide range in response magnitude.

• *Slope* refers to the relationship between the dose of a drug and its effect, as measured within the more or less linear (straight) central portion of the dose–response curve (see Figure 3.13). A flat, or shallow, slope suggests that large increases in dose do not produce big changes in effect. A steep slope on a dose–response curve indicates that there is only a small difference between the dose that produces a barely discernible effect and the dose that causes a maximal effect. This can be good because it may mean that there is little biological variation in the response to the drug. Conversely, it may be a disadvantage if it indicates that even a small increase in dose will produce a toxic reaction.

• *Efficacy* (at the level of the cell, this is often termed *intrinsic activity*) refers to the ability to produce a desired effect. The dose that exerts the maximum effect obtainable has 100 percent efficacy because it is not possible to produce a greater response. The *peak* of the dose–response curve indicates the maximum effect, or efficacy, that can be produced by a drug, regardless of further increases in dose. Not all psychoactive drugs can exert the same level of effect. For example, caffeine, even in massive doses, cannot exert the same intensity of central nervous system (CNS) stimulation as amphetamine (see Figure 3.14). Therefore, caffeine is less efficacious in regard to that reaction. Similarly, aspirin can never achieve the greater analgesic effect of morphine. Thus, the maximum effect is an inherent property of a drug and is one measure of a drug's efficacy. This pharmacological characteristic is essentially what we mean in everyday usage when we ask how *effective* a drug is in regard to its therapeutic benefit.

Most psychoactive drugs are not used to the point of their maximum effect because of side effects and toxicities. In other words, sometimes the usefulness of a compound is limited by side effects, even though the drug may be inherently capable of producing a greater or more intense response.

These parameters of dose–response curves allow us to compare the effects of drugs in a variety of different systems and the effects of different drugs on the same system. They provide a framework for understanding the relationship between drug binding and biological response. Drug–receptor interactions usually produce one of the following outcomes:

• Binding to a receptor site can initiate a cellular response similar or identical to that exerted by the natural, endogenous transmitter; the drug thus mimics the action of the transmitter. This is called an *agonistic action* and the drug is termed an *agonist* for that transmitter. Agonists are substances that have both affinity and efficacy. They must bind to their receptors and once bound to its receptor, must be capable of producing the targeted effect. If a drug is capable of eliciting the maximum

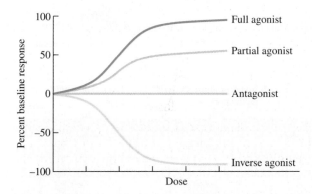

FIGURE 3.15 Dose–response functions produced by different types of drugs. A full agonist can produce the maximum possible effect; a partial agonist is not able to elicit the maximum effect at any dose; an antagonist does not produce an overt effect; an inverse agonist produces an effect opposite to that of an agonist.

response from a receptor system, then it is referred to as a *full agonist*. A *partial agonist*, therefore, is an agonist that is unable to induce maximal activation of a receptor population, regardless of the amount of drug applied (see Figure 3.15). Examples of drugs that act as partial agonists include the nicotine replacement medication varenicline (Chantix), discussed in Chapter 6 (Figure 6.4), and the opioid medications tramadol and buprenorphine (Suboxone), discussed in Chapter 10.

• Binding to a site other than the binding site for the endogenous transmitter can indirectly influence transmitter binding. This phenomenon makes it necessary to distinguish between the binding of the endogenous transmitter and the attachment of another substance. The binding site for the endogenous ligand on a receptor is called the *orthosteric* site. A binding site on a receptor that is at a different locus, which is distinct from the orthosteric site, is called an *allosteric* site. A ligand that binds to an allosteric site and modulates the binding and/or effect of an orthosteric ligand is called an *allosteric modulator* and the effect produced is termed an *allosteric action*. An allosteric drug may not produce an effect by itself, but in the presence of the natural transmitter, it may increase (*positive allosteric effect*) or decrease (*inhibitory or negative allosteric effect*) the response of the transmitter.

These processes are shown schematically in Figure 3.16. The first part of the figure illustrates orthosteric agonistic binding to the G-protein-coupled receptor (GPCR), which produces the standard effect. In the second part, a positive allosteric modulator binds to a site separate from that of the orthosteric agonist and enhances the *affinity* (indicated by the symbol α) and/or *efficacy* (indicated by the symbol β) of the orthosteric agonist. This increases the neural signal. The third segment represents a negative allosteric modulator, which decreases the affinity (indicated by the symbol α) and/or efficacy (indicated by the symbol β) of the orthosteric agonist, thereby decreasing the signal. The last segment shows allosteric ligands that have no effect on the affinity and/or efficacy mediated by the orthosteric agonist, which are termed neutral allosteric ligands (Wooten et al, 2013).

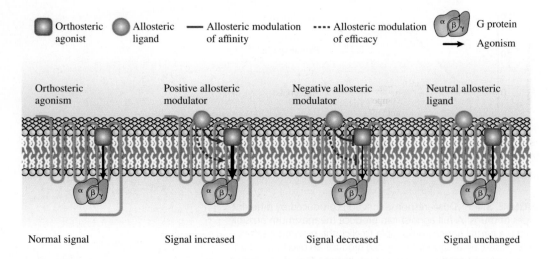

FIGURE 3.16 Schematic of allosteric influence on orthosteric function. See the text for discussion.

Examples of allosteric drugs are the benzodiazepines (such as diazepam), which do not, by themselves, affect the receptor's function but increase the activity of GABA at the receptor (see Chapter 13).

- Binding of a drug to a receptor site may block access of the transmitter to the site. This will prevent the normal effect of the transmitter or will cause transmitter molecules to be displaced from the site and inhibit its normal physiological action. This is called an *antagonistic action* and the drug is termed an *antagonist* for that neurotransmitter or receptor site (see Figure 3.15).

- Binding of a drug to a receptor site normally occupied by the endogenous neurotransmitter may produce the *opposite* pharmacological effect of an agonist. This type of drug is called an *inverse agonist*. According to Lambert (2004), the "actions of both the agonist and inverse agonist can be reversed by a competitive antagonist [described below]. The clinical significance of inverse agonism remains to be explored, but inverse agonism has been reported for several systems [relevant to this text], including benzodiazepine and cannabinoid receptors."

The hypothetical composite graph of Figure 3.15 indicates the shapes of DRCs for drugs that are full agonists, partial agonists, or inverse agonists. *It also illustrates the point that an antagonist drug by itself produces no response: that is, the effect of the drug on the baseline response level is not different from zero.* Therefore, in order to determine if a drug is in fact an antagonist as opposed to a substance that truly has no effect, it must be given in combination with an agonist. Only in the presence of a measurable response is it possible to determine if a drug has an antagonistic action by seeing if it *reduces the effect of the agonist*.

There are two primary categories of antagonistic drugs (see Figure 3.17). One type is called a *competitive antagonist*. These are drugs that bind to the receptor in a reversible way. They attach to the receptor, yet do not stimulate the effector system for that receptor. In this situation, both the agonist and antagonist bind to the same site on

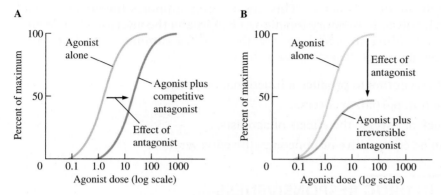

FIGURE 3.17   Agonist dose–response curves in the presence of competitive (Part A) and noncompetitive/irreversible (Part B) antagonists. The effect of a competitive antagonist is to shift the dose–response curve to the right. The noncompetitive/irreversible antagonist shifts the agonist curve down.

the receptor, hence the term "competitive." According to Lambert (2004), the "action of a competitive antagonist can be overcome by increasing the dose of the agonist (the block is surmountable)." In other words, if more molecules of agonist are added, then they "compete" with the antagonist for the receptor sites and eventually cause the antagonist to move off the receptor. The effect on the DRC of increasing the dose of agonist to overcome this type of block is to shift it to the right, making the agonist seem less "potent." Therefore, in the presence of a competitive antagonist, the dose–response curve is shifted to higher doses (horizontally to the right on the dose axis), but the same maximal effect is reached (see Figure 3.17A). An example of a competitive antagonist is the drug naloxone, which blocks the opiate receptor responsible for pain relief and for the euphoric effects of opiate drugs. If an overdose of an opiate drug has been taken, such as the analgesic OxyContin, then administration of naloxone will compete with OxyContin for the opiate receptor sites and prevent the overdose from being lethal. To regain the analgesic effect, more of the opiate drug would need to be taken.

In contrast, an *irreversible,* or *noncompetitive, antagonist* causes a downward shift of the maximum, with no shift of the curve on the dose axis (with some exceptions in more complex situations). (See Figure 3.17B.) As the name implies, the action of a noncompetitive antagonist differs from that of a competitive antagonist in that it does not attach at the same site as the agonist. Because of this difference in binding sites, the antagonist will not be displaced by the molecules of agonist. Thus the effect of the noncompetitive antagonist cannot be overcome by adding more of the agonist. Irreversible antagonists have actions comparable to those of noncompetitive antagonists (and the graphic depiction is the same), but for a different reason. In the case of the irreversible antagonist, the site of attachment may be the same as that of the agonist but, usually because of a chemical bond, the blocking molecule cannot be displaced and the antagonism cannot be overridden (Lambert, 2004). An example of a noncompetitive antagonist is the recreational drug PCP. PCP attaches to a site on the NMDA receptor for glutamate, but not at the same place as glutamate itself. Nevertheless, PCP prevents glutamate from performing its normal action. (One characteristic of PCP intoxication is memory loss—amnesia—for at least some of the time during which the drug is active. This observation supports the general belief that glutamate is involved in memory functions.) Eventually the antagonist molecules detach from their binding sites and are metabolized. In summary, the important concepts regarding pharmacodynamics are as follows:

- Agonists bind to receptors to produce a functional response.
- Agonists can be full, partial, or inverse.
- Antagonists block or reverse the effects of agonists.
- Antagonists can be competitive or noncompetitive/irreversible.

VARIABILITY IN DRUG RESPONSIVENESS— THE THERAPEUTIC INDEX

The dose of a drug that produces a specific response varies considerably among patients. Variability among patients can result from differences in rates of drug absorption and metabolism; previous experience with drug use; various physical, psychological, and emotional states; and so on. Despite the cause of the variability, any population will have a few subjects who are remarkably sensitive to the effects (and side effects) of a drug and a few who will exhibit remarkable drug tolerance, requiring quite large doses to produce therapeutic results. The variability, however, usually follows a predictable pattern, resembling a Gaussian distribution (also known as a "normal" distribution, sometimes called a "bell-shaped curve"; see Figure 3.18). In a few instances, however, a specific population will show a unique pattern of responsiveness, usually due to genetic alterations in drug metabolism.

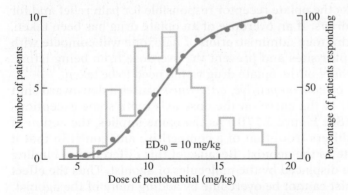

FIGURE 3.18 This figure is a theoretical, schematic, illustration of biological variation. Histogram (*left ordinate*) and cumulative frequency histogram (*right ordinate*) following intravenous administration of pentobarbital used to cause drowsiness in hospitalized patients. An ED_{50} of about 10 milligrams per kilogram (mg/kg) of body weight is shown. Note, however, that some patients exhibited sedation at about 4 milligrams per kilogram, while others required a dose of about 18 milligrams per kilogram. The stair-step bars illustrate the data behind the dose–response curve.

From Figure 3.18, it is obvious that although the average dose required to elicit a given response can be calculated easily, some people respond at very much lower doses than the average and others respond only at very much higher doses. The dose of a drug that produces the desired effect in 50 percent of the subjects is called the ED_{50} and the lethal dose for 50 percent of the subjects is called the LD_{50}. The LD_{50} is calculated in exactly the same way as the ED_{50}, except that the dose of the drug is plotted against the number of experimental animals that die after being administered various doses of the compound. Both the ED_{50} and the LD_{50} are determined in several species of animals to prevent accidental drug-induced toxicity in humans. The ratio of the LD_{50} to the ED_{50} is used as an index of the relative safety of the drug and is called the *therapeutic index* (TI) or *margin of safety*. A more precise definition is: the ratio of the highest amount of drug that does not produce toxicity/amount of drug required to produce the desired pharmacological response. Before giving the drug to patients, safety and efficacy data are obtained in nonhuman animals and exposure levels are studied in humans, taking into account species differences. Sometimes humans need more of the drug than expected from animal data and this can reduce the calculated safety margin. As stated by Muller and Milton (2012), in animal studies, the highest level of drug exposure that does not lead to toxicity, called the **no observable adverse effect level** (abbreviated as NOAEL), is usually the value used for the safety endpoint. This is a more conservative value than the lowest level of drug exposure that leads to toxicity, which is known as the **lowest observed adverse effect level** (LOAEL).

To illustrate, two dose–response curves are shown in Figure 3.19. The curve on the left represents the dose of drug necessary to induce sleep in a population of mice and the one on the right shows the dose of drug necessary to kill a similar population. In this example, the LD_{50}:ED_{50} ratio is seen to be 100:10, or 10. Although the response in this case is death, a therapeutic index can be determined for any drug effect.

The therapeutic index of 10 in this example may seem like a rather large margin, but note that at a dose of 50 milligrams, 95 percent of the mice sleep while 5 percent of the mice die. This overlap demonstrates both the difficulty in assessing the relative safety of drugs for use in large populations and the biological variation in individual responses to drugs. With this particular compound, a dose cannot be administered that will guarantee

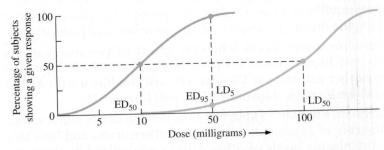

FIGURE 3.19 Illustration of therapeutic index. *Left*: Dose of drug required to induce a given response. *Right*: Lethal dose of the compound. See the text for discussion.

that 100 percent of the mice will sleep and none will die. Thus, a more useful indication of the margin of safety is a ratio of the lethal dose for 1 percent of the population to the effective dose for 99 percent of the population ($LD_1:ED_{99}$). A sedative drug with an $LD_1:ED_{99}$ of 1 would be a safer compound than the drug shown in Figure 3.18. The FDA defines a prescription drug as having a narrow therapeutic index (NTI) if very small changes in dose could cause toxic results in patients. Among these drugs is the class of lithium products (with a therapeutic index of 2 or 3) and some anticonvulsant drugs used in the treatment of bipolar disorder (see Chapter 14). Usually, although not always, the more selective that a drug is at its site of action, the better its therapeutic index.

This is a very simple and basic summary of the therapeutic index concept. In actual practice, it is more complicated. After all, even if a new medicine works, it will not be useful if it is not safe; therefore, the accuracy of this calculation is very important. The sooner during drug development that a therapeutic index can be determined, the sooner any problems can be addressed. It is certainly not desirable to expose human participants to unsafe drugs in the conduct of clinical trials. The expense of developing new medications also argues for early detection of side effects. Unfortunately, rare or idiosyncratic reactions usually will not appear at this stage; they may not be discernible until a large population of patients takes the drug after it is on the market.

Drug Interactions

Combining medications to improve therapeutic outcome, a practice termed *polypharmacy*, is common in psychiatric treatment. As noted by Zigman and Blier (2012), polypharmacy usually occurs because so few patients achieve remission of their illness from current medicines. Unfortunately, prescribing multiple medications may not be desirable because the combinations could be redundant, not useful, or even damaging. Zigman and Blier (2012) propose several principles to reduce the likelihood of what they call such inappropriate, or "irrational," polypharmacy:

- *Pharmacodynamic redundancy*, in which two drugs have the same or overlapping mechanism of action. For example, alcohol taken after ingesting a benzodiazepine tranquilizer or smoking marijuana increases sedation and loss of coordination. This action may have little consequence if the doses of each drug are low, but higher doses of either or both drugs can be dangerous both to the user and to others. The concurrent use of tranquilizers or marijuana may profoundly impair driving performance, endangering the driver, passengers, other motorists, and pedestrians.
- *Pharmacodynamic interactions* may occur when the effect of two medications oppose each other. This may happen when antipsychotics, which block dopamine type 2 receptors (among other actions; see Chapter 11), are combined with ADHD stimulant medications, which increase dopamine levels (see Chapter 15).
- *Pharmacokinetic interactions.* Chapter 1 explained how certain drugs might either increase or decrease the rate of hepatic metabolism of other drugs and how this interaction can affect the plasma levels of other drugs metabolized by the same enzymes. For example, carbamazepine increases the rate of metabolism of certain other medicines, reducing the blood concentration and effectiveness of the second drug. Conversely, valproic acid can inhibit the metabolism of other drugs, such

as lamotrigine, increasing its blood concentrations and potentially increasing its toxicity or side effects.

- *Inadequate dosing* may be a cause of irrational polypharmacy. Sometimes doses are too low because of side effects or concern about possible side effects. Sometimes the medication is given at a dose that is sufficient for one action, but not high enough for a second pharmacological action to be effective. For example, the dose at which the antidepressant venlafaxine blocks the reuptake of dopamine is lower than the dose at which it blocks the reuptake of norepinephrine.

- *Clinical evaluation and oversight* should be ongoing. Drugs started during exacerbation of an illness might need to be reassessed after the patient has restabilized. The natural history of a disorder might produce spontaneous remission, allowing dose reduction or elimination. The appearance of new symptoms might be a result of long-term drug exposure (tolerance or development of a side effect), which would be better treated by reassessment of the medication instead of adding a new agent.

Consideration of these possibilities can reduce unnecessary exposure to combinations that may be more harmful than helpful.

One of the most common types of adverse drug reaction is the phenomenon known as the *serotonin syndrome.* This is a rare but potentially serious untoward response caused by excess serotonergic action at 5-HT$_{2A}$ and 5-HT$_{1A}$ receptors in the central and peripheral nervous systems. Symptoms may develop relatively quickly, within hours of exposure. The syndrome may include altered mental states, such as delirium, clonus, tremor, hyperthermia, tachycardia, and akathisia,[7] among other reactions. As noted in Chapter 12, many antidepressant drugs are often involved in this adverse reaction because they inhibit serotonin reuptake. However, other drug classes that may promote this syndrome include drugs that increase 5-HT release, such as stimulants (see Chapter 7) and hallucinogens (see Chapter 8), drugs that are direct agonists, particularly the triptan category of migraine medications (sumatriptan, rizatriptan, naratriptan, and others), and drugs that decrease 5-HT metabolism, such as the MAOI category of antidepressants. It is not known why some people can tolerate the combination of serotonergic drugs while others do not. Patients are reminded to communicate with their prescribers and practitioners are advised to be aware of which drugs are associated with the syndrome, which drugs their patients are taking that might cause the condition, and to check the available resources, which are now accessible electronically, to be familiar with the risky combinations (Bishop and Bishop, 2011; for a recent update, see Werneke et al., 2016). An illustrative case study was presented in the *New York Times Magazine* (Sanders, 2013).

Drug Toxicity

All drugs can produce harmful effects as well as beneficial ones. It is important to categorize harmful effects of drugs in terms of their severity and to distinguish between

---

[7]Akathisia is a movement disorder. It consists of a subjective sensation of internal restlessness, which produces a persistent need to move, and elicits repetitive behaviors such as pacing, rocking, or marching in an effort to counteract the internal agitation. It most commonly occurs as a side effect of antipsychotics (see Chapter 11).

effects that cause temporary inconvenience or discomfort and effects that can lead to organ damage, permanent disability, or even death.

To achieve the desired therapeutic effect or effects, some side effects must often be tolerated; if they are serious, they may be a limiting factor in the use of the drug. The distinction between therapeutic effects and side effects is relative and depends on the purpose for which the drug is administered: one person's side effect may be another person's therapeutic effect. For example, in one patient receiving morphine for analgesia, the constipation that morphine induces may be an undesirable side effect that must be tolerated. For a second patient, however, morphine may be used to treat severe diarrhea, in which case the constipation induced is the desired therapeutic effect and relief of pain is a side effect. In addition to side effects that are merely irritating, some drugs may cause reactions that are very serious, including serious allergies, blood disorders, liver or kidney toxicity, or abnormalities in fetal development. Damage to the liver and kidneys results from the role of these organs in concentrating, metabolizing, and excreting toxic drugs.

Allergies to drugs may take many forms, from mild skin rashes to fatal shock. Allergies differ from normal side effects, which can often be eliminated or at least made tolerable by a simple reduction in dosage. However, a reduction in the dose of a drug may have no effect on a drug allergy because exposure to any amount of the drug can be hazardous and possibly catastrophic for the patient.

Placebos

Placebos have a long history in medicine. The first recorded clinical use was in 1772 (Schedlowski et al., 2015) and the word appeared in the first medical dictionary in 1785 (Lemoine, 2015). Translated from the Latin, the word means "I will please," and, in fact, the first modern definition, appearing in 1811, described placebos as "any medicine adopted more to please than to benefit the patient" (Scheindlin, 2009, 108). Since then, the role of the placebo in medicine has received increasing research interest, primarily for two reasons. First, during the course of drug development, placebo effects need to be minimized so that pharmacological effects can be separated from other influences on disease prognosis. Second, in clinical practice, it would be useful to maximize placebo effects to improve treatment outcomes and truly benefit the patient (see Holmes et al., 2016; Peciña and Zubieta, 2015; Schedlowski et al., 2015; Wager and Atlas, 2015, for current reviews).

Among the first to study the placebo response scientifically were Louis Lasagna and colleagues, who attempted to determine experimentally whether certain subgroups of patients were more likely to be placebo responders and, if so, whether they could be differentiated from nonresponders (Lasagna et al., 1954). Using a measure of postoperative pain, the researchers recorded the consistency of the placebo response and conducted thorough psychological evaluations of the patients. They concluded that their subjects could be divided into three groups: those who sometimes responded to placebo treatment (55 percent), those who always responded (16 percent), and those who never responded (29 percent). A colleague of Lasagna's, Henry Beecher, after further analyzing the data from 15 studies, reported that placebo reactions generally occurred in 30 to 40 percent of all patients (Beecher, 1955). Although placebo responders occurred in both sexes and across all ages, there was no clearly defined set of traits that differentiated them from nonresponders, a result that is supported by current research.

The neuroscientist Jon Levine is credited with initiating the modern era of the scientific study of placebos. In 1978, he infused patients with intravenous saline as they recovered from dental surgery, but told them that the solution could be morphine. A substantial decrease in pain was subsequently noted by about 30 percent of the patients. After the administration of placebo, naloxone, a drug that blocks the analgesia produced by opiates such as morphine or codeine, was secretly included in the infusion, the pain returned in the 30 percent of patients who experienced a pain reduction in response to the placebo. These results were extraordinary because they showed that the analgesia produced by placebos was not simply imagined or made up by the patients but could be biochemically antagonized (Marchant, 2016; Levine, 1978).

According to Schedlowski et al. (2015), in their extensive review of placebo mechanisms, three types of effects contribute to the placebo phenomenon: those relating to the interaction between the practitioner and the patient, those produced by the expectations of the patient, and those processes arising from conditioned drug actions. These effects can be elicited across a variety of disorders, including but not limited to pain conditions (diabetes, dental, migraine, fibromyalgia, and others), Parkinson's disease, depression, anxiety, sleep, and immunological and endocrine disorders. Overall, placebo effects vary from less than 10 to over 60 percent, depending on the severity of the condition and the specific context. Generally, however, placebo effects that alter subjective "quality of life" measures are greater than the influence of placebo on the actual etiology of the biologic disease.

Nevertheless, the neural mechanisms of placebo are associated with that of the respective medical condition. For example, reduced pain ratings during placebo analgesia are accompanied by decreased activity in the classic pain-processing areas of the brain. Moreover, TeÂtreault and colleagues (2016) found that placebo pills not only produced stronger analgesia than no treatment against chronic osteoarthritis pain but that the patients who would be placebo responders could be predicted from certain measures of the brain recordings. Evidence also supports the involvement of endogenous opioid and endocannabinoid systems as well as dopaminergic activity (perhaps indicating stimulation of the reward system during pain relief) in the biological response to placebos.

Surprisingly, even when patients are told a medication they are getting is a placebo, it still can ease symptoms and pain. In one study, patients with *irritable bowel syndrome* were either given no treatment or placebo pills, honestly labeled as "sugar pills." By the end of the three-week trial, almost twice as many patients given the placebo reported sufficient symptom relief (59 percent) compared to the control (35 percent) (Kaptchuk et al., 2010). Similar results were seen in a 2014 study involving 66 migraine patients. When these patients took rizatriptan (10 milligrams) that was labeled "placebo" (a treatment that theoretically had "pure pharmacologic effects"), the outcomes did not differ from those in patients given placebos deceptively labeled "rizatriptan" (pure expectation effect). However, when rizatriptan was correctly labeled "rizatriptan," its analgesic effect increased by 50 percent (Kaptchuk and Miller, 2015). The most recent trial was conducted in patients with chronic lower back pain who had not responded to previous therapies. While normal treatment was maintained, one group, the open-label subjects, also received sugar pills twice a day. These patients were additionally told why the "dummy" pills might be effective. During the next three weeks, this group noted a dramatic pain reduction, whereas the group not given the sugar pills reported no change in their pain levels (Carvalho et al., 2016).

Evidence suggests that genetics may play a role in affecting placebo responses. Synaptic levels of dopamine are reduced by the enzyme COMT (Catechol-O-Methyltransferase, "which plays a key role in processes associated with the placebo effect such as reward, pain, memory and learning." Researchers have found different placebo effects in people with variants of the COMT gene. In one study, patients with irritable bowel syndrome were divided into three different groups. Some were put on a waiting list and didn't receive treatment (the control group), some were given fake acupuncture by a *sympathetic* therapist (the augmented placebo group), and others were given fake acupuncture by an *unsympathetic* therapist (the limited placebo group). The patients were assessed for their COMT variant. Those patients who were most likely to state that their pain was relieved by the bogus therapy had a high dopamine version of the gene (Hall et al., 2012).

Outcomes of placebo treatment are not always positive; they can also be negative, in which case the effect is termed a *nocebo*. An example of placebo expectation that also illustrates some negative aspects is a study by Espay and colleagues (2015) in which 12 Parkinson's patients were told they would each get two shots, one an expensive drug that cost $1500 a treatment and the other costing only $100. In a calculated deception, the patients were told which was which as they got their injections. Although both injections were actually saline, the "expensive" drug produced a remarkable 28 percent improvement in motor skills, or a 7-point improvement, in one motor test given following therapy. The "cheap" drug only produced a three-point improvement on the same test. As noted by Andrade (2015), one implication of this result may be that patients could have lower expectations of, and may not benefit as much from, placebo processes associated with generic drugs.

Moreover, as noted by Kaptchuk and Miller (2015), although placebos may provide relief, they rarely cure and they do not alter the pathophysiology of diseases. Nevertheless, they are not "dummy pills"; they can meaningfully enhance treatment effects. This is illustrated in a study by Benedetti and colleagues (2016), who studied 42 people undergoing brain stimulation surgery for advanced parkinsonism. Parkinsonian patients undergoing surgery were given an injection of saline, but they were told that it was the antiparkinsonian drug apomorphine. It was found that the saline injection only produced a response in those patients who had been given one to four daily doses of the apomorphine prior to surgery. Only these "preconditioned" patients responded to the saline in that their neurons (which could be studied during the operation) were more active. This neurophysiological change means that the behavioral results were not due to any bias of the patients or experimenters. A neurologist who was "blind" to the respective treatments of the groups determined that the symptoms of the experimental group decreased. In fact, the saline response was greater in those who had received more injections of apomorphine. Because it takes only a few hours for the drug to be almost completely eliminated from the body, residual amounts of drug could not account for these effects. In those who had been given four prior doses, the drug and placebo responses were the same. This result suggests that someday, a placebo paired intermittently with a subtherapeutic drug dose might produce continued therapeutic effects. Such approaches may have the potential to reduce side effects, limit problems with drug dependency and toxicity, and reduce costs.

STUDY QUESTIONS

1. Distinguish between the terms *pharmacodynamics* and *pharmacokinetics*.
2. What is a drug receptor? What are the major types and how do they differ?
3. Discuss the receptor phenomena of *upregulation* and *downregulation*.
4. What are the major components of a dose–response function and what do they represent?
5. Define the terms *full, partial,* and *inverse agonist; allosteric drug;* and *antagonist.*
6. What is the difference between a *competitive* and *noncompetitive/irreversible* antagonist?
7. Which factors influence drug safety and toxicity and how is drug safety measured?
8. What is "irrational polypharmacy" and how can it be avoided?
9. Define the placebo response and discuss the history and the major factors that influence it.

REFERENCES

Andrade, C. (2015). "Cost of Treatment as a Placebo Effect in Psychopharmacology: Importance in the Context of Generic Drugs." *Journal of Clinical Psychiatry* 67: e534–e536.

Armstrong, N., et al. (2006). "Measurement of Conformational Changes Accompanying Desensitization in an Ionotropic Glutamate Receptor." *Cell* 127: 85–97.

Beecher, H. K. (1955). "The Powerful Placebo." *Journal of the American Medical Association* 159: 1602–1606.

Benedetti, F., et al. (2016). "Teaching Neurons to Respond to Placebos." *Journal of Physiology* 594: 5647–5660. doi: 10.1113/JP271322.

Bishop, J. R., and Bishop, D. L. (2011). "How to Prevent Serotonin Syndrome from Drug-Drug Interactions." *Current Psychiatry* 10: 81–83.

Carvalho, C., et al. (2016). "Open-Label Placebo Treatment in Chronic Low Back Pain: A Randomized Controlled Trial." *Pain* 157: 2766–2772. doi: 10.1097/j.pain.0000000000000700.

Coleman, J. A., et al. (2016). "X-ray Structures and Mechanism of the Human Serotonin Transporter. *Nature* 532: 334–339. doi: 10.1038/nature17629.

Espay, A. J., et al. (2015). "Placebo Effect of Medication Cost in Parkinson Disease: A Randomized Double-Blind Study." *Neurology* 84: 794–802. doi: 10.1212/WNL.0000000000001282.

Gouaux, E., and MacKinnon, R. (2005). "Principles of Selective Ion Transport in Channels and Pumps." *Science* 310: 1461–1465.

Hall, K. T., et al. (2012). "Catechol-O-Methyltransferase val158met Polymorphism Predicts Placebo Effect in Irritable Bowel Syndrome." *PLoS One* 7: e48135.

Holmes, R. D., et al. (2016). "Mechanisms of the Placebo Effect in Pain and Psychiatric Disorders." *Pharmacogenomics Journal* 16: 491–500. doi: 10.1038/tpj.2016.15.

Iverson, L. L., et al. (2009). *Introduction to Neuropsychopharmacology.* New York: Oxford University Press.

Kaptchuk, T. J., et al. (2010). "Placebos without Deception: A Randomized Controlled Trial in Irritable Bowel Syndrome." *PLoS One* 5: e15591.

Kaptchuk, T. J., and Miller, F. G. (2015). "Placebo Effects in Medicine." *New England Journal of Medicine* 373: 8–9. doi: 10.1056/NEJMp1504023.

Lambert, D. G. (2004). "Drugs and Receptors." *Continuing Education in Anaesthesia, Critical Care & Pain* 4: 181–184.

Lasagna, L., et al. (1954). "A Study of the Placebo Response." *American Journal of Medicine* 16: 770–779.

Levine, J., et al. (1978). "The Mechanism of Placebo Analgesia." *Lancet* 2: 654–657.

Marchant, J. (2016). "Placebos: Honest Fakery." *Nature* 535: S14–S15. doi: 10.1038/535S14a.

Muller, P. Y., and Milton, M. N. (2012). "The Determination and Interpretation of the Therapeutic Index in Drug Development." *Nature Reviews Drug Discovery* 11: 751–761.

Pan, A. C., et al. (2013). "Molecular Determinants of Drug–Receptor Binding Kinetics." *Drug Discovery Today* 18: 667–673. doi: 10.1016/j.drudis.2013.02.007.

Peciña, M., and Zubieta, J.-K. (2015). "Molecular Mechanisms of Placebo Responses in Humans." *Molecular Psychiatry* 20: 416–423. doi: 10.1038/mp.2014.164.

Pin, J.-P., and Bettler, B. (2016). "Organization and Functions of mGlu and GABA Receptor Complexes." *Nature* 540: 60–68. doi: 10.1038/nature20566.

Sanders, L. (2013). "Sudden-Onset Madness." *New York Times.* February 15. http://www.nytimes .com/interactive/2013/02/17/magazine/diagnosis-sudden-onset-madness.html.

Schedlowski, M., et al. (2015). "Neuro-Bio-Behavioral Mechanisms of Placebo and Nocebo Responses: Implications for Clinical Trials and Clinical Practice." *Pharmacological Review* 67: 697–730. doi: 10.1124/pr.114.009423.

Scheindlin, S. (2009). "The Problematic Placebo." *Molecular Interventions* 9: 108–113.

Scimemi, A. (2014). "Structure, Function, and Plasticity of GABA Transporters." *Frontiers of Cellular Neuroscience* 8: 161. doi: 10.3389/.2014.00161.

TeÂtreault, P., et al. (2016). "Brain Connectivity Predicts Placebo Response across Chronic Pain Clinical Trials." *PLoS Biology* 14: e1002570. doi: 10.1371/journal.pbio.1002570.

Tummino, P. J., and Copeland, R. A. (2008). "Residence Time of Receptor-Ligand Complexes and Its Effect on Biological Function." *Current Topics in Biochemistry* 47: 5481–5492.

Wager, T. D., and Atlas, L. Y. (2015). "The Neuroscience of Placebo Effects: Connecting Context, Learning and Health." *Nature Reviews Neuroscience* 16: 403–418. doi: 10.1038/nrn3976.

Wang, K. H., et al. (2015). "Neurotransmitter and Psychostimulant Recognition by the Dopamine Transporter." *Nature* 521: 322–327. doi: 10.1038/nature14431.

Werneke, U., et al. (2016). "Conundrums in Neurology: Diagnosing Serotonin Syndrome—A Meta-Analysis of Cases." *BMC Neurology* 16: 97. doi: 10.1186/s12883-016-0616-1.

Wootten, D., et al. (2013). "Emerging Paradigms in GPCR Allostery: Implications for Drug Discovery." *Nature Reviews Drug Discovery* 12: 630–644. doi: 10.1038/nrd4052.

Yamashita, A., et al. (2005). "Crystal Structure of a Bacterial Homologue of Na$^+$/Cl$^-$Dependent Neurotransmitter Transporters." *Nature* 437: 215–223.

Xu, C., et al. (2014). "Complex GABAB Receptor Complexes: How to Generate Multiple Functionally Distinct Units from a Single Receptor." *Frontiers in Pharmacology,* 5(12): 1–8. doi: https://doi.org/10.3389/fphar.2014.00012.

Yernool, D., et al. (2004). "Structure of a Glutamate Transporter Homologue from *Pyrococcus horikoshii.*" *Nature* 431: 811–818.

Zigman, D., and Blier, P. (2012). "A Framework to Avoid Irrational Polypharmacy in Psychiatry." *Journal of Psychopharmacology* 26: 1507–1511.

PART 2

Pharmacology of Drugs of Abuse

This section is composed of seven chapters that cover the pharmacology of drugs subject to compulsive use, abuse, and dependency. The section begins with Chapter 4, an overview of the neurobiology of addiction that describes current thinking about the neuroanatomical and neurotransmitter basis of substance abuse. Chapter 5 discusses ethyl alcohol, a sedative-hypnotic quite similar in its pharmacology to the sedatives discussed later in Chapter 13. Alcohol differs, however, in that it has few medical indications and is most often used as a recreational intoxicant.

The psychostimulants are discussed in two chapters. Chapter 6 details the pharmacology of caffeine and nicotine, the most widely used recreational drugs. Neither drug has much therapeutic value, but both are used because of their psychostimulant properties. The toxicities associated with tobacco use and the treatments for nicotine dependence are included in this chapter. Chapter 7 describes the psychostimulants cocaine, amphetamine, methamphetamine, and several related agents. These drugs present significant abuse issues as well as continuing uses in medicine.

Chapter 8 presents the pharmacology of drugs characterized by their ability to produce altered states of consciousness, the so-called psychedelic drugs, including those found in nature as well as those produced synthetically.

Chapter 9 presents the pharmacology of tetrahydrocannabinol and other compounds found in the marijuana plant. Current research is uncovering medical uses of psychedelic cannabinoids (for example, THC), nonpsychedelic marijuana alkaloids (for example, cannabidiol), and cannabinoid antagonists (for example, rimonabant).

Finally, Chapter 10 addresses the opiate analgesics. Although these drugs provide significant therapeutic benefit for alleviation of pain, they also have substantial abuse liability. During the last few years, the dramatic increase in abuse of opiate medications has become a major public health problem, creating serious concerns about how to deal with an epidemic of illicit prescription opioids.

THERAPEUTIC POTENTIAL FOR DRUGS OF ABUSE

The drugs in this section have traditionally fallen into one of two categories. Some, such as alcohol, are primarily recreational, with no significant medical benefit. They are typically discussed as drugs of abuse. Other drugs in this group, such as opiates, do have significant medical uses, in addition to their abuse potential. During the last few years, however, this boundary has become blurred. For example, there has been a resurgence of interest in the medicinal properties of hallucinogens and cannabis (marijuana). Although they were once investigated as possible therapeutic agents, hallucinogens and cannabis were primarily viewed as recreational drugs, subject to abuse. More recently, however, interest in their therapeutic potential has resurfaced, as will be discussed in Chapters 8 and 9, respectively. Conversely, the recreational and illicit use of drugs that were initially recognized and approved for their medical usefulness, such as opiates and stimulants, has reached epidemic proportions. More drugs are now understood to have both medicinal and addictive properties, and this has made it much more complicated to develop guidelines for how they should be used.

One result of these changes is an explosive growth in the production of illegal varieties of drugs in all four categories. That is, in order to evade legal restrictions, suppliers have created new molecular entities or manufactured more potent versions of opiates (such as Carfentanil and U4770), stimulants (such as "bath salts"), cannabis (such as "spice" drugs) (Miliano et al., 2016), and hallucinogens (such as N-BOMe).

The term *new* or *novel psychoactive substances* (NPS) has been applied to this category of emerging drugs. Chemists covertly research the compounds linked to the effects of specific psychoactive drugs and use them to develop new, illicit compounds that mimic those effects (Baumann et al., 2014; see also Tracy et al., 2017). Schifano and colleagues (2015) write, "Overall, NPS are defined as new narcotic/psychotropic drugs which are not controlled by the United Nations' 1961 Narcotic Drugs/1971 Psychotropic Substances Conventions, but which may pose a public health threat." These substances have been reported in almost 100 countries and territories, and more than 500 NPS have been identified worldwide. In response to the crisis, the National Institute on Drug Abuse (NIDA) launched a five-year project called the National Drug Early Warning System in 2014, which aims to create a network of scientists, public health experts, and law enforcement representatives for sharing information and assisting with local drug research (Underwood, 2015).

Only about 5 percent of the adult population uses NPS, but the drugs pose a significant problem for two reasons. First, they are more likely to be used by children, adolescents, and young adults, because the drugs may (technically) be legal and easily available online. Second, their side effects may be unpredictable, severe, and more dangerous than the classic drugs of abuse. Although laws are continually passed to ban NPS, new varieties are constantly being created to evade restrictions. Because it is time-consuming for laboratories to identify the components, there is little pharmacological information about them, much of which is limited to their acute toxicity. Long-term effects and addictive liability are unknown, and most information must come from nonhuman, animal studies.

The job of figuring out what these drugs do in the brain, and how dangerous they might be, was given to a small lab at the NIDA, currently headed by neuroscientist Michael Baumann. Set up in 2012, the laboratory only analyzes drugs that have at least a thousand mentions in the National Forensic Laboratory Information System, a U.S. drug surveillance program run by the Drug Enforcement Administration (DEA). This laboratory is a crucial resource in the effort to protect our population from the current deluge of NPS.

REFERENCES

Miliano, C., et al. (2016). "Neuropharmacology of New Psychoactive Substances (NPS): Focus on the Rewarding and Reinforcing Properties of Cannabimimetics and Amphetamine-Like Stimulants." *Frontiers in Neuroscience* 10:153. doi: 10.3389/fnins.2016.00153.

Schifano, F., et al. (2015). "Novel Psychoactive Substances of Interest for Psychiatry." *World Psychiatry* 14: 15–26.

Tracy, D. K., et al. (2017). "Novel Psychoactive Substances: Types, Mechanisms of Action, and Effects." *BMJ* 356:i6848. doi: 10.1136/bmj.i6848.

Underwood, E. (2015). "A New Drug War." *Science* 347: 469–473. doi: 10.1126/science.347.6221.469.

Epidemiology and Neurobiology of Addiction

Drug abuse has been a societal problem for thousands of years, ever since grain was fermented (ethyl alcohol) and natural substances that produced euphoria (cocaine), pain relief (morphine), or altered states of consciousness for divination (psilocybin, mescaline) were found. As history suggests, as long as these drugs persist in society, they will be associated with compulsive use, dependency, and addiction. This chapter reviews the current trends in regard to drug abuse in the United States, introduces the relevant concepts and neurobiological mechanisms believed to be responsible for addiction, and summarizes current approaches to treatment of dependency and abuse. The individual drugs discussed in their respective chapters are brought together in this overview of principles that apply to all drugs of abuse. Table 4.1 describes the current schedules of categories for controlled substances included in this section.

EXTENT OF THE DRUG PROBLEM

Between related expenses (such as crime and health care) and lost productivity, the estimated cost of drug use in American society is more than half a trillion dollars annually (National Institute on Drug Abuse, 2017). But the cost is more than just monetary; in terms of social dysfunction, unemployment, academic failure, and domestic and other violence, the public health consequences are staggering.

To address the nation's drug abuse and addiction problems, in 2010 then-President Obama inaugurated the National Drug Control Strategies initiative, providing recommendations and proposals for reducing the toll of addiction in the United States. This document was based on the premise, supported by scientific evidence, that drug addiction is not a moral failing but rather a disease of the brain that can be prevented and treated. The aim of the 2010 and subsequent annual National Drug Control Strategies was to establish and promote a balance of evidence-based public health and safety initiatives focusing on key areas such as substance abuse prevention, treatment, and recovery.

TABLE 4.1 Definition of controlled substance schedules

Drugs and other substances that are considered controlled substances under the Controlled Substances Act (CSA) are divided into five schedules. An updated and complete list of the schedules is published annually in Title 21 Code of Federal Regulations (CFR) §§ 1308.11 through 1308.15. Substances are placed in their respective schedules based on whether they have a currently accepted medical use in treatment in the United States, their relative abuse potential, and likelihood of causing dependence when abused.

Schedule I

Substances in this schedule have:
- No currently accepted medical use in the United States,
- A lack of accepted safety for use under medical supervision, and
- A high potential for abuse.

Examples include: heroin, lysergic acid diethylamide (LSD), marijuana (cannabis), peyote, 3,4-methylenedioxymethamphetamine ("ecstasy"), "spice," and "bath salts."

Schedule II

Substances have a high potential for abuse, which may lead to severe psychological or physical dependence.

Examples of opiates include: methadone (Dolophine®), oxycodone (OxyContin®, Percocet®), fentanyl (Sublimaze®, Duragesic®), morphine, opium, and codeine.

Examples of stimulants include: amphetamine (Dexedrine®, Adderall®), methamphetamine (Desoxyn®), and methylphenidate (Ritalin®).

Schedule III

Substances have less potential for abuse than substances in Schedules I or II and abuse may lead to moderate or low physical dependence or high psychological dependence.

Examples include: products containing not more than 90 milligrams of codeine per dosage unit (Tylenol with Codeine®), buprenorphine (Suboxone®), ketamine, and anabolic steroids such as Depo®-Testosterone.

Schedule IV

Substances have a low potential for abuse relative to substances in Schedule III.

Examples include: alprazolam (Xanax®), clonazepam (Klonopin®), diazepam (Valium®), lorazepam (Ativan®), midazolam (Versed®), and triazolam (Halcion®).

Schedule V

Substances have a low potential for abuse relative to substances listed in Schedule IV and consist primarily of preparations containing limited quantities of certain opiates.

Examples include: cough preparations containing not more than 200 milligrams of codeine per 100 milliliters or per 100 grams (Robitussin AC®, Phenergan with Codeine®).

In 2015, the *National Drug Control Strategy* focused on seven core areas:

- Preventing drug use in our communities;
- Seeking early intervention opportunities in health care;
- Integrating treatment for substance use disorders into health care and supporting recovery;

- Breaking the cycle of drug use, crime, and incarceration;
- Disrupting domestic drug trafficking and production;
- Strengthening international partnerships; and
- Improving information systems to better address drug use and its consequences.

In addition, the current strategy specifically emphasizes a commitment to confronting the misuse of prescription opiate medications and heroin. To this end, the president's fiscal year 2016 budget included $133 million aimed at addressing the opioid epidemic, including expanding state-level prescription drug overdose prevention strategies, medication-assisted treatment programs, and access to the overdose-reversal drug naloxone (see Figure 4.1).

The Substance Abuse and Mental Health Services Administration (SAMHSA) administers a yearly survey, the National Survey on Drug Use and Health (NSDUH). Information is obtained from individuals in the United States who are 12 years or older regarding their substance use, misuse, or addiction. The questions asked are whether the individuals used the respective substances at any time in their lives, at any point in the last year, or during the last month (also termed as *current use*). The latter two periods are viewed as more accurate than lifetime use. SAMHSA reported that in 2014:

an estimated 27.0 million Americans aged 12 or older (a little more than 10 percent) were current illicit drug users, meaning that they had used an illicit drug during the month prior to the survey interview. The most commonly used illicit drug in the past month was marijuana, which was used by 22.2 million people aged 12 or older. An estimated 6.5 million people reported nonmedical use of psychotherapeutic drugs in the past month, including 4.3 million nonmedical users of prescription pain relievers.

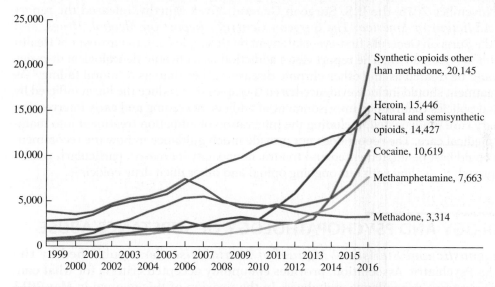

FIGURE 4.1 Drugs involved in U.S. overdose deaths. Among more than 64,000 drug overdose deaths estimated in 2016, the sharpest increase occurred among deaths related to fentanyl and fentanyl analogs (synthetic opioids) with over 20,000 overdose deaths. [Data from CDC WONDER, 2017.]

That is, the number of current nonmedical users of pain relievers was second to marijuana among specific illicit drugs. Smaller numbers of people in 2014 were current users of the other illicit drugs. More than one in five young adults aged 18 to 25 (22.0 percent) were current users of illicit drugs in 2014, [which] corresponds to about 7.7 million young adults. [Although] this value was stable between 2009 and 2014, the 2014 estimate was higher than the estimates from 2002 through 2008. (Center for Behavioral Health Statistics and Quality, 2015)

The Monitoring the Future study is the nation's largest survey of drug use, behaviors, attitudes, and values of American secondary school students, college students, and young adults. In 2006, 30 percent of undergraduates acknowledged cannabis use within the past year; in 2015, the number was modestly increased to 38 percent. Chronic cannabis use in this group, which was defined as 20 or more uses in the past month, rose from 3.5 percent in 2007 to 5.9 percent in 2014. The 5.9 percent of young people reporting chronic use in 2014 was the greatest percentage recorded since data were first collected in 1980, 34 years previously. The following year, 2015, daily use declined to 4.6 percent (Johnston et al., 2016).

As reported in the *2015 Overview of Key Findings on Adolescent Drug Use*, "the most striking finding in 2015 is that across the very broad spectrum of drugs (more than 50 classes and subclasses) none exhibited a statistically significant increase." This was also the case in 2014. The study authors further report that "cigarettes and alcohol continued to show significant declines, reaching their lowest levels in the history of the study. With regard to illicit drugs, annual prevalence declined for synthetic marijuana, heroin, MDMA (ecstasy, Molly), sedatives, and nonmedical use of any prescription drug. Annual prevalence of using *any illicit drug* remained essentially unchanged in all three grades in 2015; annual prevalence was 14.8 percent, 27.9 percent, and 38.6 percent in 8th, 10th, and 12th grades, respectively" (Johnston et al., 2016, 5).

In November 2016, the U.S. Surgeon General, Vivek Murthy, released the report *Facing Addiction in America: The Surgeon General's Report on Alcohol, Drugs, and Health*, the Surgeon General's first-ever statement on this topic (U.S. Department of Health & Human Services, 2016). The report views addiction as a chronic neurological disorder that should be treated as any other chronic disease, rather than as a "moral failing." As such, treatment should include evidence-based therapies that reduce the harm inflicted by drugs and policies that reduce imprisonment of addicts. Screening and early intervention in primary care is advocated, including the integration of addiction treatment into mainstream medical care. The report does not provide much guidance in how the recommendations could best be implemented and treatment capacity increased, particularly on the best approach to dealing with our ongoing opioid and other illicit drug epidemic.

NOSOLOGY AND PSYCHOPATHOLOGY OF SUBSTANCE ABUSE

The *Diagnostic and Statistical Manual of Mental Disorders*, published by the American Psychiatric Association, provides commonly accepted criteria for what constitutes substance dependence and abuse. In the revision of this manual in May 2013 (DSM-5; see Chapter 17), the chapter of "Substance-Related and Addictive Disorders" combined substance abuse and substance dependence into one overarching category, "Substance Use Disorder" (SUD). Substance Use Disorder is defined as mild, moderate, or severe depending on the level of severity, which is determined by the number of diagnostic criteria met by an individual. Whereas a diagnosis of substance abuse previously required only one symptom, mild substance use disorder in the DSM-5 requires two to three symptoms from a list of eleven, while four to five symptoms are required for the diagnosis of moderate, and six to seven for the diagnosis of a severe SUD.

Substance use disorders occur when the recurrent use of alcohol and/or drugs causes clinically and functionally significant impairment, such as health problems, disability, and failure to meet major responsibilities at work, school, or home. According to the DSM-5, a diagnosis of substance use disorder is based on the evidence of impaired control, social impairment, risky use, and pharmacological criteria. It was felt that looking at a continuum of severity allowed experts to diagnose people with an alcohol and/or drug problem more easily. This may also lead to earlier diagnoses, which could allow appropriate interventions to be applied more easily. The chapter also includes gambling disorder as the sole condition in a new category on behavioral addictions. In addition, a new diagnosis, "Internet Use Gaming Disorder," is included in Section 3, a category of disorders that are not yet agreed on but need further research.

Approximately, one-third of people addicted to an illicit drug or alcohol have a diagnosed *comorbid* psychiatric disorder, a situation covered by the term *dual diagnosis*. Among people with a lifetime diagnosis of schizophrenia, 47 percent have met the criteria for substance abuse or dependence; those with an anxiety disorder, 23.7 percent; those with obsessive–compulsive disorder, 32.8 percent; those with bipolar disorder, 50 percent; and those with depression, 32 percent — with distribution equal for males and females. Current evidence indicates that managing mood symptoms with pharmacotherapy can help those with a substance abuse problem, although results are not always consistent (Pettinati et al., 2013).

NEUROBIOLOGY OF ADDICTION

Recognition of the existence of a neural system responsible for the biological basis of "pleasure" originated with the discovery in the 1950s (by the scientists Olds and Milner, 1954) that rats would work (often very hard) to get electrically stimulated in certain brain sites. Gradually, the anatomical pathways and the neurochemical substances that comprised this system were determined and mapped. This circuit is believed to be the neurobiological basis for the experience of pleasure, satisfaction, or reward. Although presumably this system mediates the pleasures experienced from natural stimuli, such as food and sex, drugs that can stimulate these brain areas activate this system more intensely and directly. According to this interpretation, despite their specific pharmacological effects, all drugs of abuse act through this "reward" system, and such activation promotes repeated use. Unfortunately, in vulnerable people, repeated use can lead to addiction—a loss of control over drug use. Withdrawal of the drug will produce unpleasant emotional reactions regardless of the specific substance. Even after all traces of the specific abused drug are gone from the body (through the process of detoxification), the addicted individual experiences urges to use the drug again and is at risk of relapsing.

The development of such cravings indicates that *something in the brain has changed as a result of long-term drug use*; some process of neuroadaptation has occurred. It is these neurobiological changes that are responsible for craving and relapse, even after long periods of abstinence. Appreciation of this phenomenon, which occurs with all abused drugs, has led to increased research into the mechanisms responsible for craving and relapse; the recognition that such processes are similar to other types of learned reactions; and the realization that these mechanisms may also be relevant to other types of nondrug addictions, such as gambling and other compulsive behaviors. Efforts are currently ongoing to develop new treatments for these maladaptive learned responses. This view of the neurobiological basis of substance abuse is referred to as the *Brain Disease Model of Addiction* (BDMA). The following sections summarize the experimental evidence and conceptual arguments that led to the BDMA, and then present some of the criticisms of the theory.

Common Effects of Abused Drugs on Brain Reward Circuits

The core of the reward circuit is one of the brain pathways for dopamine, called the *mesolimbic dopamine pathway* (Figure 4.2). As shown in Figure 4.2, this pathway begins with a group of dopamine neurons in the ventral tegmental area (VTA), a structure that is located in the midbrain (see Chapter 2). The axons of these dopamine

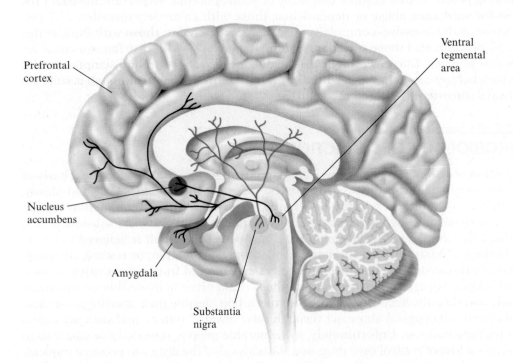

FIGURE 4.2 The reward circuit. The major structures involved in the subjective sensation of pleasure and reward. The pathway starts with dopamine-releasing neurons in the ventral tegmental area (VTA). Axons from the VTA neurons release dopamine onto the amygdala, nucleus accumbens (ventral striatum), and prefrontal cortex (Fowler, 2007).

neurons extend to several other brain structures, where they release dopamine when the VTA is activated. The most relevant structures, in this context, are the nucleus accumbens (NAc), the amygdala, the hippocampus (see Figure 4.2), and the prefrontal cortex. The nucleus accumbens is sometimes referred to as the ventral striatum. The dopamine pathway from the VTA to the NAc is critical to addiction: if these brain regions are lesioned, animals will no longer become addicted (Nestler and Malenka, 2004).

This pathway is integrated with the other structures. The amygdala is involved in mediating the emotional characteristics of drug use, the hippocampus is crucial to recording memories of such experiences, and the frontal regions of the cortex synthesize and coordinate information and are involved in planning and the inhibitory control of behavior.

In addition to dopamine neurons, there are also other neurons within the VTA that interact with the dopamine neurons. Some release the neurotransmitter GABA. The release of GABA inhibits dopamine neurons and normally suppresses dopamine release.

During the last few decades, a converging body of evidence has suggested that regardless of their specific effects, most abused drugs share a common action with respect to this mesolimbic dopamine pathway. That is, most abused drugs increase the amount of dopamine that is released from the VTA onto the NAc, amygdala, hippocampus, and frontal lobe. But they do not all increase dopamine activity in the same way. In some cases, the dopamine increase is direct; in others, dopamine is increased indirectly. Some drugs may increase dopamine by more than one mechanism and some may produce other, nondopaminergic responses as well (Pierce and Kumaresan, 2006).

For example, cocaine (and other stimulants; see Chapter 7) increases the amount of dopamine on NAc neurons by blocking dopamine reuptake into VTA neurons after the transmitter has been released. Nicotine (see Chapter 6) may stimulate dopamine neurons directly and cause them to release dopamine. Heroin and other opioids (see Chapter 10) act on receptors located on GABA neurons and inhibit GABA release. When GABA release is reduced, there is less inhibition of dopamine neurons and dopamine release increases. Opioids can also act directly on the NAc to produce a positive "reward" signal. Drugs that are CNS depressants, such as benzodiazepines (see Chapter 13) and alcohol (see Chapter 5), may also increase dopamine by inhibiting GABA release as well as by other actions (Nestler and Malenka, 2004). Benzodiazepines activate a specific subtype of $GABA_A$ receptor, a subtype that contains the α1 subunit. These specific subtypes are found on the same neurons as the receptors for opiates. In other words, both benzodiazepines and opiates increase dopamine release by inhibiting GABA neurons (and disinhibiting the VTA dopamine neurons) (Riegel and Kalivas, 2010).

How do we know that the effect of drugs on dopaminergic activity is related to their pleasurable subjective effects? Compelling and extensive evidence from studies done for over 30 years in nonhuman animals supports this relationship. In 1997, however, a particularly relevant observation was made in cocaine addicts, which showed that dopamine was also related to the sensation of pleasure in humans. In this study, methylphenidate (Ritalin; see Chapter 15) was given to cocaine addicts while they underwent a brain scan. Methylphenidate, like cocaine, blocked the dopamine transporter and increased the amount of dopamine in the synapse. The addicts rated the "high" they experienced after receiving methylphenidate while the brain scans showed the percent of transporters blocked by each dose. There was a significant correlation—the greater the subjective rating of the "high," the greater the proportion of transporters blocked, which meant the greater the increase in the amount of dopamine release (Volkow et al., 1997). Subsequent studies conducted with healthy volunteers and nondependent drug users found that administration of alcohol, tobacco, ketamine, and cannabis could also increase striatal dopamine release to some degree (see review by Nutt et al., 2015).

As noted above, the VTA–NAc pathway and the other limbic regions are also presumed to be responsible, at least in part, not only for the positive effect of drugs but also for the pleasurable effects of natural rewards, such as food, sex, and other enjoyable activities. Consequently, these same regions have also been implicated in the so-called natural addictions (that is, compulsive behaviors in regard to natural rewards), such as pathological overeating, pathological gambling, and sexual addictions (Nestler, 2005).

Research indicates that long-term, chronic exposure to any of several drugs of abuse will impair this dopamine pathway such that eventually the system becomes less responsive to normal, naturally rewarding stimuli, and they are not as enjoyable as they once were. Essentially, tolerance develops within the pathway (Nestler, 2005) and naturally rewarding stimuli do not increase dopaminergic activity as much as they used to. These changes may contribute to the unpleasant, dysphoric, emotional state that develops between drug exposures or when drugs are withdrawn. In contrast, drugs maintain their ability to increase brain levels of dopamine.

In brief, drugs, like other rewarding experiences, cause release of dopamine from VTA neurons to NAc neurons. When released, dopamine causes animals to feel good, prompting them to repeat the pleasurable action, leading to compulsive use and addiction.

But this raises another question. Many people use legal drugs, such as alcohol. Yet why do only some drug users become addicted? Is there something different about their brains? Some evidence suggests that this might be the case. In one study, normal male subjects were given methylphenidate and asked if they found the experience pleasant, unpleasant, or neutral. At the same time, they underwent a brain scan that measured their dopamine receptors. It turned out that the subjects who reported that they found methylphenidate to be pleasant had lower D_2 receptor levels than those who reported that the drug injection was unpleasant. In fact, the subjects who enjoyed the drug experience had receptor levels similar to those previously reported in cocaine abusers, even though these subjects were not abusing drugs (Volkow et al., 2004).

Does this result mean that if a person has a low density of receptors, he or she is biologically vulnerable to drug abuse? In other words, do people at risk for acquiring addictions have a weaker response to "pleasure" than people who are not as vulnerable, perhaps because of a dopamine receptor deficiency? The implication is that such individuals may have a biological deficit and may require a more powerful stimulus (a drug) to experience a normal pleasurable sensation, while for others the same drug experience may actually be too strong to be enjoyable.

This interpretation is consistent with studies in which methylphenidate (or in different experiments, amphetamine) was given to different groups of nonaddicts and either detoxified or nondetoxified addicts. In these cases, the addicts reported a less intense "high" and showed less dopamine (DA) increase in their brains, suggesting that the addict's brain is less responsive to the drug. This has been termed a "blunted" reaction to the dopaminergic challenge. Even people addicted to opiates and alcohol had reduced dopamine release after stimulant administration compared with nonaddicts (Nutt et al., 2015; Volkow et al., 2011, 2014).

From Abuse to Addiction

Regardless of the mechanism responsible, however, repeated drug use may develop into chronic drug use that can become compulsive and result in addiction. Because the frontal lobe is one of the areas of the brain that is part of the reward circuit, it is also profoundly altered by chronic drug abuse. One common change that occurs after long-term drug use is cortical "hypofrontality." This means that the normal baseline activity of several regions of the frontal cortex is reduced. Brain scans have shown that addicts not only have fewer dopamine receptors in the NAc than normal, they also have a lower metabolic rate in the frontal lobe. This has been interpreted to mean that their frontal lobe responses to normal, nondrug stimuli are "sluggish." But even though this brain area is sluggish when activated by natural rewards, the frontal lobes become more activated than normal when drug abusers are exposed to stimuli that cause craving, such as drugs or drug cues. For example, when methylphenidate was injected into addicts and nonaddicted subjects, metabolism *increased* in the frontal areas of the addicts' brains but *decreased* in the brains of nonaddicted subjects (see Volkow et al., 2004, 2016).

Did You Know?

Decreased Dopamine in Addicted Brains

These brain images indicate that there are fewer dopamine receptors (D_2) in the brain of a cocaine addict compared with a nondrug user. Dopaminergic neurons are responsible for conditioned learning and motivation, and such changes are presumed to be the basis for the decrease in sensitivity to normal rewards that occurs during the development of addictive behavior (National Institute on Drug Abuse, 2010).

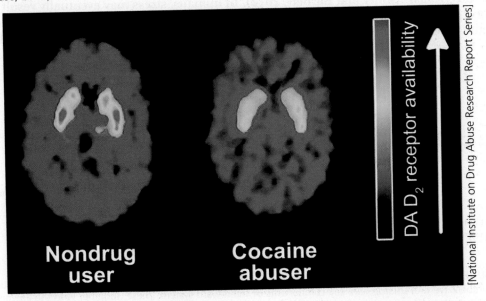

Nondrug user

Cocaine abuser

DA D_2 receptor availability

[National Institute on Drug Abuse Research Report Series]

Even after three or four months of abstinence, the prefrontal cortex may not recover. Durazzo and coworkers (2011) used magnetic resonance imaging (MRI) of the brain to examine the reward system in addicts one week after abstinence and again 12 months later. They found that the cortex of the brain was thinner in all the addicts compared with control subjects, but in addition, those with less volume and surface area were more likely to relapse after one year.

In summary, as a result of chronic drug use, natural rewards become *less* pleasurable and release less dopamine. The frontal cortex becomes inherently less active and less responsive to normal rewards, but it is *overactive* in response to drugs or the stimuli that predict drugs.

Of course, for drug use to continue, the user has to remember the positive feelings produced by the drugs and the environmental situation in which it occurred. Memory of drug use and its context is mediated by the other structures associated with the reward circuit, the amygdala and hippocampus (Figure 4.3). In fact, over time, stimuli that "predict" drugs or were associated with the environment in which drugs were used produce a greater response in the reward pathway than the rewarding stimuli themselves. It is proposed that such conditioned, or learned, responses elicit powerful *craving* sensations in the frontal cortex. The frontal lobes are said to become *sensitized* to drug-related stimuli. For example, addicted people frequently relapse after returning to an environment in which they have previously taken drugs, even after they have gone through detoxification and recently spent time in a rehabilitation program.

Furthermore, the brain structures involved in addiction are hypersensitive not only to activation by drugs of abuse and drug-associated stimuli, but also to environmental *stressors*. In fact, studies in humans and animal models indicate that stress is significantly involved in the vulnerability to develop addiction and in relapse in addicted persons (Haass-Koffler and Bartlett, 2012). In humans, stress may eventually result in a mood disorder, such as depression, especially during periods of drug withdrawal, leading to the development of a co-occurring situation (Yadid et al., 2012). An example of the

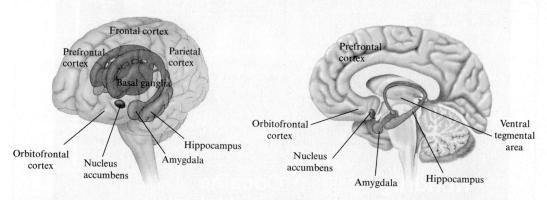

FIGURE 4.3 Major brain structures involved in addiction. The ventral tegmental area (VTA) and nucleus accumbens (ventral striatum) are key components of the reward system. These, together with the amygdala, hippocampus, and prefrontal cortex (PFC), coordinate drives, emotions, and memories.

importance of stress and learned reactions in triggering relapse is shown in Figure 4.4, a composite summary of the results of numerous animal experiments. It shows three phases of drug abuse. In the first phase, rats responded on one lever for cocaine infusions, but did not respond on a second lever that produced only a saline injection (self-administration). In the second phase, when responding no longer produced cocaine (extinction), the rats eventually stopped pressing the lever. Finally, in the third phase, separate groups of animals were exposed to (1) direct injection of cocaine, (2) an environmental stimulus previously associated with the drug, or (3) a stressful stimulus (for example, electric shock). Each of these three treatments reinstated responding on the lever that had previously been associated with cocaine injections. (Although not shown, cocaine responding also increased even more after a period of abstinence, that is, after drug injections were stopped but without the extinction responses.) This summary figure shows that even when drug abuse is extinguished, relapse can be readily elicited by three major conditions:

- Reexperience with the drug
- Conditioned drug cues
- Stress (including withdrawal-induced reactions)

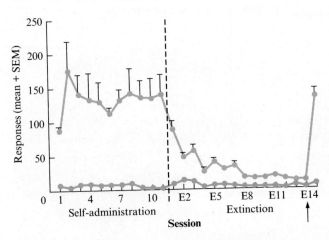

FIGURE 4.4 Variables that promote relapse. This figure illustrates the development, extinction, and relapse phases of addiction in an animal model. Some animals were trained for 12 days to self-administer cocaine in response to a lever press (blue circles). Control animals (orange circles) received no cocaine in response to a lever press. At the vertical dashed line, all animals underwent extinction training (lever presses no longer produced the drug) for 14 days. At the end of this phase (arrow at session E14), all animals were presented with (1) a cue that accompanied the previous cocaine administration in the training stage; (2) a mild stressor, such as a brief electrical stimulus; or (3) a small amount of intravenous cocaine. All three stimuli overcame extinction in animals that had received cocaine before the extinction period (blue circle at day E15). Cue, stress, or cocaine resulted in resumption of lever pressing in an attempt to obtain cocaine ("reinstatement" of drug seeking). In control animals (orange circle at days E14 and E15), presentation of a cue at day E15 did not result in drug-seeking behavior. [Data from Kalivas et al., 2006.]

Glutamatergic Substrates of Addiction

Regardless of whether they are triggered by drugs, by conditioning, or by stress, these heightened craving sensations are transmitted from the frontal cortex through downstream nerve pathways that feed back onto the reward pathway. In this case, however, the nerve fibers that connect the frontal lobe structures with the downstream reward circuit are not primarily dopaminergic. Rather, they release the transmitter *glutamate* onto the NAc and VTA (Figure 4.5). Evidence from animal experiments and from human brain scans shows that chronic exposure to any of several drugs of abuse causes complex changes in these frontal cortical regions and their glutamatergic outputs. For example, studies with rats showed that the glutamate synapse between the frontal lobes and the NAc *actually became stronger* (responded more intensely) when tested 24 hours after a single exposure to cocaine. To be specific, the increased strength was measured as an increase in the response of AMPA receptors relative to that of NMDA receptors. Most important, the increased reaction was not restricted to cocaine, but was also produced by other abused drugs including amphetamine, morphine, alcohol, nicotine, and benzodiazepines, while drugs that were not abused did not produce this increase in synaptic strength (Madsen et al., 2012).

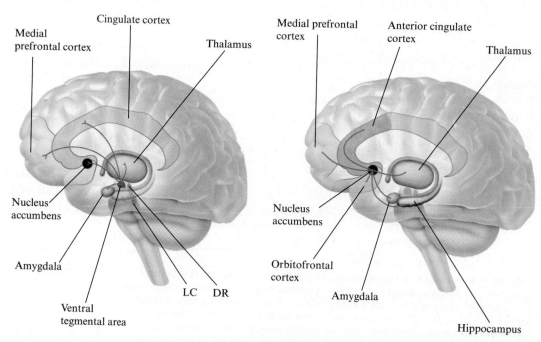

FIGURE 4.5   Schematic of the brain circuitry of addiction. The brain on the left shows the dopamine fibers that originate from the ventral tegmental area (VTA) and which release dopamine in the nucleus accumbens (NAc) (ventral striatum) and other structures in the limbic system. Other brain structures that influence these sites are also indicated: the noradrenergic nucleus of the locus coeruleus (LC) and the serotonergic dorsal raphe nucleus (DR). The right side indicates the excitatory glutamatergic structures that interact with the VTA and mediate the development of drug addiction: the medial prefrontal cortex (mPFC), the orbitofrontal cortex (OFC), the anterior cingulate cortex (ACC), the thalamus, hippocampus, and amygdala.

Other postsynaptic glutamate receptors, notably the mGluR5 subtype, are also altered in addiction. It has been shown that mice lacking this receptor were less prone to relapse after becoming addicted to cocaine (Novak et al., 2010). This was interpreted to mean that without the mGluR5 receptor, mice could not "learn" the association between drug administration and reward that occurred in normal mice (Duncan and Lawrence, 2012).

Glial cells associated with the synapse also play an important role in maintaining the normal concentration of glutamate. [There is increasing recognition that glial may be involved in the effect of a variety of addictive drugs (Cooper et al., 2012).] In particular, there are structures located on glial cells that modulate the amount of glutamate in the vicinity of the synapse. One of these is a transporter, GLT-1, which carries glutamate into the glial cell so that it can eventually be returned to the presynaptic neuron. Another structure on the glial cell is a protein, xCT. This protein pushes glutamate *out* of the glial cell in exchange for an amino acid, cystine (a variant of the amino acid cysteine), and is therefore called the *cystine–glutamate exchanger*. These two proteins, the glial–glutamate transporter-1 (GLT-1) and the cystine–glutamate exchanger (xCT), maintain a balance between glutamate inside and out of the synapse. Chronic drug exposure can decrease the levels of these two proteins. As a result, the amount of glutamate in the synapse resulting from addiction unbalances the normal regulatory processes that control glutamate release. (Shen et al., 2014, provide experimental support for this theory in an animal study of drug administration.)

In summary, the *hypersensitivity of the frontal cortex to drugs or drug cues (learning), which develops in addiction, is the basis of the phenomenon of craving. Craving is biologically mediated as increased glutamatergic reactivity within the reward circuit.* These changes are believed to be responsible for the profound impulsivity (acting on sudden urges to take a drug) and compulsivity (being driven by irresistible inner forces to take a drug) that define addiction (Kalivas, 2009).

The increased activation of these pathways also causes some biochemical changes within the VTA–NAc and other brain reward regions. One of the most dramatic examples is that chronic exposure to all drugs of abuse, including cocaine, amphetamine, opiates, alcohol, nicotine, cannabinoids, and phencyclidine, increases the amount of a protein called ΔFosB, which builds up in the NAc. In fact, chronic exposure to natural rewards, such as high ingestion of sweets, will also increase ΔFosB.

Another substance in the brain that is increased by chronic drug use is brain-derived neurotrophic factor (BDNF). In fact, blood levels of BDNF were found to be significantly increased in opiate-dependent patients, and this increase was significantly associated with craving for heroin (Heberlein et al., 2011).

The Brain Disease Model of Addiction in Summary

Regardless of the neurobiological details, the BDMA remains the most prominent theory of addiction. As currently restated by Volkow and colleagues, the overall model can be summarized as follows:

In response to natural rewards, such as food or sex, dopamine neurons eventually stop firing because chronic consumption produces satiation. Addictive drugs, however, do not produce normal satiation, they continue to elicit dopamine release with chronic use. As a result of repeated drug exposure, dopamine neurons gradually stop firing as much in response to the drug itself and instead, begin firing to the various stimuli associated with the drug context, that is, the environment, persons, and mental state associated with drug taking. These cues become conditioned to the drug. Over time, addicts do not experience the same intensity of euphoria in response to the drug as they did initially. They also lose motivation for more normal stimuli and activities that had previously been enjoyable. Furthermore, when the drug effect wears off or the drug is not available, there is an increase in stress and dysphoria as a result of withdrawal. This unpleasant state motivates the addict to further drug use. Rather than taking drugs to feel pleasure, the addict eventually takes drugs to relieve the discomfort of withdrawal. The relative significance of these two phenomena, drug-induced "high" versus withdrawal-induced dysphoria, still prompts intense discussion (Wise and Koob, 2014; Koob, 2015; Volkow and Morales, 2015; Koon and Mason, 2016; and Volkow et al., 2016).

In addition to the changes in the reward circuit and the emotional systems of the brain produced by chronic drug use, there are changes in the prefrontal cortex, which is responsible for executive control functions. That is, the dulling of the response to pleasure also impairs the capacities for self-regulation and inhibition. This development is associated with changes in glutamatergic function in the prefrontal cortex that weakens the addict's ability to resist intense urges or to maintain abstinence. Susceptibility to addiction, as with many other diseases, is only found in a minority of people who use drugs. Vulnerability is presumably due to numerous genetic, social, and environmental factors, such as family history, early drug exposure, developmental trauma, and mental illness.

Treatment approaches derived from this model, discussed below, could address any or all of these processes. For example, therapy might decrease the rewarding effect of drugs or increase the reward intensity of natural stimuli. Other approaches might be to interfere with learned associations between drugs and the environment so as to enhance motivation for nondrug-related activities, or to increase inhibitory control. In this regard, evidence has been reported that cortical stimulation reduces responding for drugs in rats that compulsively self-administered cocaine (Chen et al., 2013), and that stimulating specific dopamine receptors in the nucleus accumbens of mice reduced cocaine seeking (Bock et al., 2013).

Criticism of the Brain Disease Model of Addiction

Although the BDMA has predominated addiction research, it has not been without its critics. In particular, Nutt and colleagues have questioned the reliance on dopamine as an encompassing, neurobiological explanation (Nutt et al., 2015). They note that evidence for the dopamine hypothesis has been strongest for stimulants, which are the drugs that most directly affect dopamine levels. In contrast, dopamine release has not been as consistently reported in humans in response to alcohol, cannabis, or ketamine, nor is there a reliable association with such release and hedonic effects, particularly in regard to cannabis. Moreover, they argue, dopamine receptor blockade is not very effective in reducing the rewarding effect of stimulants or in treating human addiction, even to stimulants. They point out that neither opiate administration nor expectation of an opiate reward affected striatal dopamine levels in humans; that nicotine has a negligible effect on dopamine levels; and that even at doses that produce substantial behavioral effects, cannabis also had minimal dopaminergic effects in the brain.

With regard to the observation that cocaine users had lower striatal dopamine density than control groups, Nutt and colleagues (2015) state that this might be a result of receptor downregulation produced by the chronic drug use, rather than a preaddictive condition. Moreover, this phenomenon is not consistently and reliably seen in opiate, cannabis, or nicotine addiction, and there is apparently no data on this issue in regard to ecstasy or ketamine. Furthermore, while "blunted" dopamine release in response to a stimulant challenge has been reported in opiate- and alcohol-dependent subjects (as predicted by the model), it was not seen in cannabis-dependent subjects. Again, it is not known if any changes in dopamine function were present before the addiction, if they mediate addiction vulnerability, or if they are a *consequence* of drug dependence. Finally, they note that the theory has not led to any new treatments. They conclude by proposing that while the BDMA might be most relevant to stimulant addiction, evidence exists that other transmitter systems (such as opiate or GABAergic substrates) are involved in addiction to other drugs and that these alternatives should be further investigated.

Hall and coworkers (2015) also take issue with an overarching focus on the BDMA. They point out that most people with addiction actually recover without treatment. Even those who remain addicted can decrease their drug use in response to modest incentives, such as payment for clean urine samples. This argues against a severe compulsive disorder for the majority of users, leaving only a minority of addicts who might fit the criteria for the BDMA. When drugs are self-administered by nonhuman animals, this is usually assessed in very restricted contexts with few alternatives available, which is an artificial situation and does not parallel human drug use. Animal research also has little to say about the likelihood of recovery. Other neurobiological approaches are not more useful. For example, there is no currently reliable genetic guidance to predict addiction vulnerability. Human neuroimaging studies do not tell us if any differences in brain structure or function between addicted and nonaddicted populations is a cause or a result of drug use. In either case, these data do not prove that drug use is a compulsion. While the neurobiological model is becoming increasingly complex, the extensive research triggered by the BDMA has led to few new drugs for treatment. Even these are not any better than older drugs that preceded this model by decades. For a variety of reasons, there is little pharmaceutical interest in developing new drugs for addiction. Other approaches to treating addiction, especially brain-invasive methods (such as deep brain stimulation), are extremely expensive for a small population of addicted patients, most of whom would not be able to pay for them. Essentially, they argue that the overemphasis in neurobiological research has overshadowed more cost-effective social approaches, such as increased taxes, advertising bans, and restrictions (for example, smoking) in public spaces.

PHARMACOTHERAPY OF SUBSTANCE USE DISORDERS

As noted previously by both Nutt and Hall, in spite of its intellectual sophistication and creativity, the Brain Disease Model of Addiction has not yet produced novel treatments for this disorder. Current approaches still consist mostly of traditional, relatively specific therapies, focusing on medications that directly affect the biological actions of the primary drug of abuse (Pierce et al., 2012). Unfortunately, many people who abuse drugs do not abuse just one drug. Yet there is no universal treatment agent whose mechanism transcends a particular drug. This section includes an overview of classic approaches to drug treatment of addiction, which will be discussed further in the relevant chapters of this book, and then describes some recent efforts that fall outside of these categories.

Agonist Substitution Treatment

Prescribing a substitute drug for the abused agent is one of the most well-established pharmacological interventions for addiction. Agonists can reduce both the rewarding effect of the abused (and cross-tolerant) drugs, as well as the discomfort of withdrawal. They can also improve compliance and promote healthier behaviors. Agonists can be given by safer routes, such as oral, that reduce abuse potential, decrease the frequency of treatment sessions, and minimize the disruptions produced by the volatility of illicit drug use (Negus and Henningfield, 2015). It has long been known that the faster the subjective effect of a drug, the greater its abuse potential. (The importance of pharmacokinetic variables in addiction are reviewed by Allain et al., 2015.)

This approach has been most commonly used to treat opioid and nicotine addiction. The method originated with early studies of the opiate methadone, which was found to reduce heroin use, crime, and the spread of HIV infections, as well as helping to get addicts involved in their treatment (see Lingford-Hughes et al., 2004; Nutt and Lingford-Hughes, 2008). Methadone can substitute for heroin because it is a relatively full opioid agonist, but it has a slower onset of effect. The oral route produces less of a "rush" than does heroin; its long half-life allows once-daily dosing, which reduces both cravings for and the effect of (and the need to obtain) heroin. Nevertheless, because methadone is still a very addictive drug, which can be fatal in overdose and diverted into street use, it is usually given in supervised situations. This practice is expensive; often addicts are allowed to take doses home over the weekend, which leads to diversion and accidental overdoses, often in children.

Agonist substitution has also long been used effectively for treating nicotine addiction. A variety of formulations have been developed, including nicotine lozenges, chewing gum, and patches (see Chapter 6). Similarly, oral forms of synthetic cannabis agonists (for example, dronabinol) or their analogues (for example, nabilone) have been assessed for treatment of cannabis addiction with modest benefit (see Chapter 9). At this writing, a clinical trial is ongoing, testing a drug that inhibits the breakdown of endogenous cannabinoids. The drug, PF-04457845, blocks an enzyme that metabolizes one of these substances and may relieve cannabinoid withdrawal (Martinez and Trifilieff, 2015).

A similar approach may be seen with *disulfiram* (Antabuse), which is a traditional agent for treating alcoholism. As described in Chapter 5, disulfiram blocks an enzyme that is involved in alcohol metabolism. If alcohol is taken with disulfiram, the substance acetaldehyde is not metabolized; it builds up and produces an unpleasant reaction that presumably prevents subsequent alcohol use. But it has been shown that disulfiram can also block dopamine β-hydroxylase (DbH) in the brain, thereby increasing dopamine and depleting noradrenaline. Both changes may be beneficial in stimulant dependence (Gaval-Cruz and Weinshenker, 2009). In fact, disulfiram has shown modest benefit in treating cocaine addiction (Pani et al., 2010) and it is hypothesized that this may be due to its effects on the dopaminergic system, although clear evidence of this is needed (Preti, 2007). The effectiveness of DbH may be genetically influenced in that patients with normal levels of the enzyme responded better than those with low levels. Nepicastat, a selective DbH inhibitor, is under clinical investigation (Shorter et al., 2015). One disadvantage is that disulfiram also blocks the metabolism of cocaine as well as dopamine, which apparently increases the unpleasant anxiogenic effects of cocaine.

A "substitution" approach may also be effective for treating stimulant addiction (Herin et al., 2010). The drug *modafinil* (Provigil), currently approved for treating narcolepsy, is a mild stimulant and enhances glutamate neurotransmission. Although there is some evidence that modafinil might blunt some of the psychological and physiological effects of stimulants, clinical results have been inconsistent (see Chapter 7) and essentially negative. Similarly, administration of L-dopa was also ineffective (Shorter et al., 2015). Agonist-based treatment of cocaine dependence/use disorder with amphetamine-type stimulants has been debated by Negus and Henningfield (2015). In spite of experimental and some clinical evidence for therapeutic effectiveness, there is substantial concern about the public health consequences surrounding amphetamine treatment of cocaine abuse. The difficulty of developing a specific formulation that would be clinically reliable, politically acceptable, and commercially successful makes it very unlikely that a pharmaceutical sponsor would invest the extensive resources necessary to bring a stimulant agonist to market.

Partial Agonist Substitution Treatment

Instead of substituting one full agonist for another, an alternative approach is to use a partial agonist such as buprenorphine for opiate addiction (discussed in Chapter 10). Like methadone, such treatment reduces intravenous injecting, because the addict is exposed to sufficient drug to overcome the need for additional opiate use. Buprenorphine produces less severe withdrawal than methadone, but that may be due to its long half-life, which may "protect" an addict from heroin use for two to three days. There is still the risk of potentially fatal respiratory depression (overdose death) if buprenorphine is combined with other sedative hypnotics. This risk can be reduced if an opiate antagonist is added to buprenorphine, which has been done.

Partial agonists have also been successfully developed for nicotine addiction, for which varenicline (an $\alpha_4\beta_2$ partial nicotinic agonist) was approved (see Chapter 6). The concept is the same as with buprenorphine for opioid dependence in that the agent provides sufficient stimulation to reduce smoking, but does not support self-administration. Interestingly, there is emerging evidence that varenicline may also reduce alcohol consumption (Steensland et al., 2007). Cytisine, a plant alkaloid and a partial agonist at $\alpha_4\beta_2$ nAChRs, has been tested in various preclinical models associated with nicotine addiction and is approved for smoking cessation in Europe. Sazetidine-A, a novel nAChR desensitizing agent and partial agonist with high selectivity for $\alpha_4\beta_2$ receptors, has been shown to reduce nicotine self-administration in preclinical models. The possible usefulness of nicotinic partial agonists, antagonists, and other drugs that modulate cholinergic function for both nicotine and alcohol dependence is extensively reviewed by Rahman and colleagues (2015).

As discussed by Nutt and Lingford-Hughes (2008), dopamine partial agonists would presumably be an interesting target for stimulant addiction. Such drugs should provide enough dopamine activation to reduce the effects of withdrawal yet block the consequences of illicit stimulant use. The antipsychotic aripiprazole is such a drug and it was reportedly effective in preventing relapse in an animal model of cocaine administration (Feltenstein et al., 2007), but was not found effective in one study for stimulant abuse in addicts (Tiihonen et al., 2007).

This approach is also being investigated for treatment of cannabis addiction. That is, medications are being developed that would decrease the subjective effects of cannabis but avoid the adverse effects of an antagonist (described below) (Martinez and Trifilieff, 2015).

Antagonists as Treatments for Addiction

Another standard approach to treating addiction is to administer an antagonist of the abused drug. By directly blocking the reinforcing effect, an antagonist would eventually reduce the compulsive behavior. The opiate antagonists naloxone, naltrexone, and nalmefene have long been available for such treatment. A major difficulty with these agents, however, is compliance—because they offer no positive reinforcement, it is hard to maintain adherence. If the addict continues to take an antagonist, it will be very effective in reducing abuse. But if the patient stops the antagonist and then relapses to heroin, there is a possibility that the opiate will be even more dangerous than it was before the antagonist treatment. The tolerance that developed during prior opiate use (before the antagonist treatment) will have worn off and renewed opiate use may produce serious problems, such as respiratory depression. Nutt and Lingford-Hughes (2008) discuss the advantages of a long-acting naltrexone implant, although they acknowledge that even this formulation would not eliminate the problems produced by rapid termination of antagonist exposure.

Nevertheless, heroin addiction can be successfully treated with specific opiate blockers, such as naloxone and naltrexone. It is not self-evident that opiate antagonists would also be effective against other types of addictive drugs, such as alcohol and stimulants, but some data support that possibility. In one trial, the sustained release, implantable version of naltrexone was assessed over ten weeks in patients addicted to both heroin and amphetamine (Tiihonen, 2012). As expected, the group given naltrexone had significantly less heroin in their urine samples than the control group. But there was almost a significant difference in their amphetamine samples as well. Furthermore, in the naltrexone group, those patients who continued using the stimulant noted that its effect was reduced, suggesting that compared to placebo, the opiate antagonist blocked the "high" produced by amphetamine (Penetar, 2012).

Antagonists of other abused drugs are available, notably the benzodiazepine antagonist/partial agonist *flumazenil* (Anexate, Romazicon). There is interest in developing a long-acting formulation or protocol for treating benzodiazepine abuse (Gupta, 2015; Hood et al., 2014).

Doxazosin, a long-acting, selective α-1 adrenergic antagonist, has been examined in clinical trials for treatment of cocaine addiction. Some positive results in a pilot study have led to Phase II clinical trials (Shorter et al., 2015).

A number of potent and selective antagonists are also available for the cannabis (marijuana) CB_1 receptor. One of them, *rimonabant* (Acomplia), was approved for weight loss, but it was subsequently pulled off the market because of reports of depression and suicidality (see Chapter 9).

Additional Neurotransmitter Targets

GABAergic System

As noted above, the dopaminergic cell bodies in the ventral tegmental area are under GABAergic control, and the GABA-B receptor is involved in this interaction (Cousins et al., 2002). GABA-B agonists, such as baclofen, can reduce the reinforcing effects of several different classes of abused drugs (for example, heroin, psychostimulants, alcohol) in animal models under a variety of conditions. Studies in humans have also shown baclofen to be promising in treating cocaine addiction and alcoholism (Nutt and Lingford-Hughes, 2008), although current outcomes do not recommend its use as a first-line treatment for alcoholism (Muzyk et al., 2012). Moreover, baclofen was not effective for cannabis dependence in a human laboratory study (Haney et al., 2010).

Other GABAergic medications being tested as possible agents for preventing cocaine relapse are anticonvulsants. One such drug is *gamma-vinyl-GABA* (GVG; Vigabatrin), an anticonvulsant that blocks the enzyme that breaks down GABA. This drug had shown some benefit in small trials and was subsequently found to be effective in a randomized, placebo-controlled clinical trial (Brodie et al., 2009). Because it appears to cause visual field defects, it has not been approved for use in the United States. A novel agent, CPP-115, is more potent and specific, showed some benefit without the visual side effects, but adherence was questioned. This medication is currently under Phase II investigation for treatment of cocaine use disorders (Shorter et al., 2015).

The drug *gabapentin* (Neurontin), which increases GABA synthesis, showed some benefit in treating cannabis dependence, and a large clinical trial was recently completed (Scripps Research Institute, 2016).

Treatment Approaches Derived from the Glutamatergic Model of Addiction

The incorporation of glutamate into the BDMA as a possible mediator of learned associations between drugs and environmental stimuli is the basis for studying glutamatergic agents as antiaddiction treatments.

The proposed glial dysfunction involving the xCT exchange process and GLT-1 led to the consideration of the drug *N*-acetylcysteine for addiction. This drug is currently prescribed for pulmonary disease as well as acetaminophen overdose; it was found to *increase the brain's production of xCT*. In a similar manner, the drug ceftriaxone is an antibiotic that appears *to increase levels of GLT-1*. Laboratory experiments with these drugs indicated that they might reduce the likelihood of relapse to cocaine (Abulseoud et al., 2012; Shen et al., 2014).

Because acetylcysteine is already available for human use, several small clinical trials have been conducted in people who are nicotine addicts, marijuana users, cocaine addicts, and pathological gamblers (Dean et al., 2011). The drug is well tolerated but, even though many of the participants reported that they had less craving or desire to use their respective drug or engage in gambling, objective results from these studies were not impressive (Olive et al., 2012). Recent data from animal studies may provide an explanation. The latest experiments reveal what happens when *N*-acetylcysteine raises extracellular glutamate in the critically important nucleus accumbens region of the reward system. As predicted, at lower doses of the medication, the released glutamate stimulates presynaptic glutamate autoreceptors (mGluR2/3) on neurons. The presynaptic stimulation dampens neuronal activity in the nucleus accumbens and, in rats, reduces the tendency to respond to cocaine-associated cues. But at higher doses, more glutamate is released and an additional postsynaptic glutamate receptor, mGluR5, is also stimulated. The postsynaptic stimulation has opposite effects; it intensifies neuronal activity. The researchers proposed that a medication (or combination of medications) that both increases nonsynaptic extracellular glutamate to stimulate mGluR2/3 and inhibits mGluR5 receptors might reduce the risk of relapse more effectively than *N*-acetylcysteine alone (Kupchik et al., 2012). A large clinical trial—achieving cannabis cessation-evaluating *N*-acetylcysteine treatment (ACCENT)—was completed in July 2016 (Sherman et al., 2017).

Affecting the glial control of glutamate by ceftriaxone has also been reported to prevent relapse in laboratory animals. This drug, however, has to be given by intramuscular injection, which limits its practical benefit.

Another medication in this class is the drug *modafinil* (Provigil), used to treat narcolepsy. Although its mechanism of action is not known for certain and it seems predominantly to be a reuptake blocker of dopamine and norepinephrine, it also increases glutamate levels. In animals, it reduced responses for cocaine and amphetamine and it blocked a measure of relapse in morphine-treated animals (Mahler et al., 2012). Clinically, however, the effects of modafinil on cocaine use have been inconsistent. [One explanation of why such a drug, which increases glutamate, might be antiaddictive is that it might "normalize" glutamate function in addicts during withdrawal (Olive et al., 2012).]

Acamprosate (Campral, used clinically to maintain alcohol abstinence; see Chapter 5) has also been found in animal models to reduce glutamate overactivity or release in the nucleus accumbens and hippocampus during early ethanol withdrawal and to prevent associated toxicities (Mason and Heyser, 2010). Although electrophysiological studies of its mechanism of action have been inconsistent, it is considered to be an NMDA modulator. A large multicenter study, however, did not find that acamprosate was any more effective than placebo in treating alcohol addicts (Olive et al., 2012).

Several antiepileptic drugs also reduce glutamatergic actions and may have some benefit against addiction. Topiramate has been tested in studies of cocaine abstinence and found to be modestly effective. This drug not only facilitates GABA function, it reduces transmitter release, including glutamate, and blocks AMPA receptors. It can cause sedation and memory problems and should not be used in persons with a history of kidney stones (Johnson et al., 2007; Lingford-Hughes et al., 2004; Sofuoglu and Kosten, 2006). Several reports during the last decade found topiramate useful in reducing subjective effects, craving, and heavy consumption in alcohol addicts. There are also some positive results in regard to behavioral addictions such as gambling, overeating, and sex (Olive et al., 2012). This drug showed some benefit for cocaine abuse (Johnson et al., 2013) and cannabis abuse (Miranda et al., 2016), but the effects were modest and a majority of participants stopped taking the drug because of side effects.

Gabapentin (which increases GABA, see above) and lamotrigine are two other anticonvulsants that inhibit the release of various transmitters, including glutamate. Both drugs can relieve some somatic symptoms of alcohol withdrawal. The results of studies assessing their ability to treat addiction are inconsistent (gabapentin) and very limited (lamotrigine). Lamotrigine can also produce an uncommon but serious skin rash (Olive et al., 2012). Memantine is a noncompetitive antagonist at NMDA receptors and is used primarily to treat cognitive decline in Alzheimer's disease. Current evidence is inconsistent in regard to alcohol addiction (Olive et al., 2012).

Other approaches involving glutamate include agonists that act directly on the presynaptic glutamate autoreceptor, the mGluR2/3 subtype. As noted above, by stimulating this autoreceptor, glutamate agonists decrease glutamate release, which might prevent relapse. Interestingly, these receptors are also found on dopamine terminals, where they reduce dopamine release. This could mean that they might also reduce the probability of initiating drug use. In animals, these agents reduced the self-administration of cocaine, alcohol, and nicotine (Kalivas and Volkow, 2011). Several reviews of animal experiments have recently been published supporting the involvement of metabotropic glutamate receptors in addiction (Brown et al., 2012; Cleva and Olive, 2012; Duncan and Lawrence, 2012; Li et al., 2013). Preclinical nonhuman animal studies of drugs that affect the mGluR5 receptor are investigating this possibility (Gould et al., 2016).

In addition to the metabotropic types of glutamate receptor, studies are also examining the effects of ionotropic glutamate receptors, the AMPA and NMDA subtypes. Excessive AMPA activity may contribute to relapse. The drug tezampanel is an AMPA/kainate receptor antagonist that is being tested for relief of acute migraine, and it reduced cocaine self-administration in animal experiments. Two other drugs, talampanel (an AMPA/kainate antagonist) and perampanel (a noncompetitive AMPA antagonist, approved in 2012 for use in patients aged 12 years and older with partial-onset seizures), are being evaluated in some neurological disorders and might be usefully tested for addiction.

A group of substances called *ampakines* modulate the AMPA receptor; they maintain its sensitivity in the presence of stimulation, preventing desensitization. These compounds might counteract some of the toxic effects of drug exposure; for example, they might prevent the possible development of Parkinson's disease in people who abuse methamphetamine.

NMDA receptors might affect addiction because of a general enhancement of learning and memory (Sofuoglu et al., 2013). This would include extinction, in which an animal learns that a behavior or context is no longer associated with a drug.

For this reason, the NMDA coagonist drug D-cycloserine (DCS) has been tested in various human and nonhuman experiments in extinction procedures in an effort to help addicts "unlearn" the association between the drug and the environment of illicit use (Hammond et al., 2013). For example, in cigarette smokers, DCS facilitated extinction compared to the placebo treatment. In another study, the drug showed a slight effect in reducing cravings in cocaine addicts. So far, however, the clinical application of DCS has not been as effective as suggested by the preclinical animal models (Myers and Carlezon, 2012; Olive et al., 2012).

A specific subtype of NMDA receptor containing the NR2B subunit has been most implicated in the association between drugs and drug cues. The drug ifenprodil blocks this receptor subtype and has been reported to reduce relapse in animal models of drug abuse (Kalivas and Volkow, 2011). (For extensive discussions of glutamatergic studies related to drug abuse, see D'Souza, 2015, and Spencer et al., 2016.)

Opioid System

The μ type of MORs are also located on GABA neurons in the VTA and they play a key role in modulating ventral tegmental area dopaminergic activity. A link between alcohol use and endogenous opioid activity was suggested by animal models in which the opioid antagonist naltrexone reduced alcohol self-administration by blocking this μ-opioid receptor. Naltrexone has now been shown in several clinical trials in alcoholism to reduce the risk of a full-blown relapse (Pettinati et al., 2006). It does not work for everyone and may be most effective for people who are more severely alcohol dependent. Jayaram-Lindström and coworkers (2008) and now Tiihonen and colleagues (2012) have shown that naltrexone may also promote abstinence from amphetamines. Evidence has been reviewed showing that other drugs of abuse, such as nicotine, other stimulants, and cannabis may also interact with the endogenous opioid system. The μ-opiate receptor appears to be critically involved in the rewarding properties of several abused drugs and in the development of physical dependence to nicotine and cannabinoids (Noble et al., 2015; Trigo et al., 2010). To date, however, these neurobiological interactions have not produced new antiaddiction medications beyond those already discussed.

Cannabinoid System

Cannabinoid-opiate interactions are gaining more attention in current concepts of addiction and reward mechanisms (Robledo, 2010), including the substrates for nicotine (Maldonado and Berrendero, 2010) and alcohol (López-Moreno et al., 2010) addiction. As discussed by Parolaro and coworkers (2010), there are three primary aspects relevant to this model: (1) cannabinoids can release opioid peptides and opioids can release endogenous cannabinoids (endocannabinoids); (2) when receptors for these two systems are both located on the same cells, there is evidence for direct receptor–receptor interaction; and (3) there is an interaction between their intracellular pathways. For example, activation of either of these two systems produces a similar degree of relapse to alcohol in animal models of alcohol addiction. The cannabinoid–opioid relationship in the reward system might also differ from their interaction within other systems, such as the pain pathways.

There is also a lot of overlap between cannabis abuse and alcohol abuse. These drugs are both central nervous system depressants and produce similar behavioral reactions, such as ataxia, feelings of intoxication, motor impairments, memory problems, sleep disruption, and other neuropsychological deficits. They also show cross-tolerance with each other to some of these effects. Pava and Woodward (2012) present a comprehensive review of the interactions between alcohol (ethanol) and the endo-cannabinoid system, describing the changes in the EC receptors produced by chronic alcohol consumption.

NEW DIRECTIONS

Johnson and Lovinger (2016) comprehensively review the scientific evidence describing how presynaptic metabotropic receptors, GPCRs, exert control over neurotransmitter release. The authors focus on the receptors for the transmitters dopamine, endo-cannabinoids, and glutamate. They propose that drugs targeting these receptors may be able to influence drug-seeking behavior and might be usefully explored as addiction medications.

Vaccines are another promising therapy for relapse prevention. The approach works by stimulating the production of drug-specific antibodies (to nicotine, opiates, cocaine, or amphetamine). If the drug of abuse is still used, the antibodies bind to the drug molecules in the blood and prevent them from crossing the blood–brain barrier, thereby blocking the euphoria produced in the brain and presumably decreasing further use. Progress has been most advanced with respect to vaccines for nicotine (see Chapter 6) and cocaine addiction (see Chapter 7) and, most recently, heroin (see Chapter 10). With regard to cannabis, the THC molecule is too hard to access. Alcohol molecules themselves are too small to attach to the protein that would be necessary to deliver the immunity. But a drug that blocks the gene, which produces the alcohol-metabolizing enzyme in the liver (aldehyde dehydrogenase), is being developed. Essentially, this substance would produce a very unpleasant reaction, basically a hangover, if alcohol were taken.

Some novel approaches have come from related areas of research. For example, the overlap between drug stimuli and natural stimuli in the reward system suggests that substances that affect eating might also affect drug use. One agent is GLP-1, a glucagon-like peptide, which is released from the GI tract in response to food and is involved in the regulation of eating. An agonist drug, exenatide (Ex-4), which stimulates the GLP-1 receptor, is currently used in the treatment of diabetes. By acting on the glucagon receptor, the drug appears to reduce the rewarding effect of highly palatable food. Realizing the similarity to drug reward, researchers gave the drug to mice and found that it seemed to reduce the rewarding effect of cocaine (Graham et al., 2013).

Another novel approach, derived from other areas of behavioral treatment, is the possibility of treating addiction by administering deep brain stimulation (DBS). Luigjes and colleagues (2012) review the current evidence from animal and human studies that support this modality for refractory addiction. The primary question is: which brain area would be most effective? The authors support the NAc as the most promising site for human trials although other locations, notably the medial prefrontal cortex, have not been extensively investigated.

Neuroscientists have begun to recognize the implications of an impaired prefrontal cortex, which regulates long-term planning, decision making, and moral judgment. Researchers are now searching for ways to make these prefrontal systems more resilient. These approaches raise a question: is drug use the cause of users' prefrontal problems or do they have preexisting defects that make them susceptible to addiction? After all, a lot of people are able to use drugs in a socially controlled manner; only a certain percentage actually go on to become addicted. Perhaps part of the reason is that such people lack prefrontal-mediated control over behavior. In the protected environment of a rehabilitation center, drugs and other cues associated with drug taking are eliminated and stressful situations that suppress prefrontal activity are minimized. This environment, as much as any medication, provides the context in which prefrontal cortex function can be strengthened. Finally, religion has long been shown to have a strong inverse association with drug addiction. Some religious rituals have been found to provoke enhanced activity in prefrontal regions. It may be that the original insight behind Alcoholics Anonymous of allowing oneself to be guided by a "higher power" has a biological substrate in the frontal lobe (Schnabel, 2009).

STUDY QUESTIONS

1. What types of drug abuse problems are currently of most concern, that is, which drugs and which populations?

2. Is a propensity for abusing drugs caused by a psychopathological process in the user or is it a property of the particular drug?

3. What is the neurobiological mechanism that underlies the behavioral reinforcing properties of abused drugs?

4. How does chronic drug use eventually become addiction?

5. What types of receptor-based approaches to the pharmacotherapy of drug abuse have been developed?

6. How has our understanding of the neurobiology of addiction guided efforts to find new therapies?

REFERENCES

Abulseoud, O. A., et al. (2012). "Ceftriaxone Upregulates the Glutamate Transporter in Medial Prefrontal Cortex and Blocks Reinstatement of Methamphetamine Seeking in a Condition Place Preference Paradigm." *Brain Research* 1456: 14–21.

American Psychiatric Association. (2000). *Diagnostic and Statistical Manual of Mental Disorders,* 4th ed., text revision (DSM-IV-TR). Washington, DC: American Psychiatric Association.

American Psychiatric Association. (2013). *Diagnostic and Statistical Manual of Mental Disorders,* 5th ed. (DSM-5). Washington, DC: American Psychiatric Association.

Allain, F., et al. (2015). "How Fast and How Often: The Pharmacokinetics of Drug Use are Decisive in Addiction." *Neuroscience and Biobehavioral Reviews* 56: 166-79. doi: 10.1016/j.neubiorev.2015.06.012.

Baumann, M. H., et al. (2014). "Bath Salts, Spice, and Related Designer Drugs: The Science Behind the Headlines." *Journal of Neuroscience* 34: 15150–15158. doi: 10.1523/JNEUROSCI.3223-14.2014.

Bock, R., et al. (2013). "Strengthening the Accumbal Indirect Pathway Promotes Resilience to Compulsive Cocaine Use." *Nature Neuroscience* 16: 632–638.

Brodie, J. D., et al. (2009). "Randomized, Double-Blind, Placebo-Controlled Trial of Vigabatrin for the Treatment of Cocaine Dependence in Mexican Parolees." *American Journal of Psychiatry* 166: 1269–1277.

Brown, R. M., et al. (2012). "mGlu5 Receptor Functional Interactions and Addiction." *Frontiers in Pharmacology* 3: 1–9, article 84.

Center for Behavioral Health Statistics and Quality. (2015). "Behavioral Health Trends in the United States: Results from the 2014 National Survey on Drug Use and Health." HHS Publication No. SMA 15-4927, NSDUH Series H-50. http://www.samhsa.gov/data/.

Chen, B. T., et al. (2013). "Rescuing the Cocaine-Induced Prefrontal Cortex Hypoactivity Prevents Compulsive Cocaine Seeking." *Nature* 496: 359–362.

Cleva, R. M., and Olive, M. F. (2012). "Metabotropic Glutamate Receptors and Drug Addiction." *Wiley Interdisciplinary Reviews: Membrane Transport and Signaling* 1: 281–295.

Cooper, Z. D., et al. (2012). "Glial Modulators: A Novel Pharmacological Approach to Altering the Behavioral Effects of Abused Substances." *Expert Opinion on Investigational Drugs* 21: 169–178.

Cousins, M. S., et al. (2002). "GABA B Receptor Agonists for the Treatment of Drug Addiction: A Review of Recent Findings." *Drug and Alcohol Dependence* 65: 209–220.

Dean, O., et al. (2011). "*N*-Acetylcysteine in Psychiatry: Current Therapeutic Evidence and Potential Mechanisms of Action." *Journal of Psychiatry and Neuroscience* 36: 78–86.

D'Souza, M. (2015). "Glutamatergic Transmission in Drug Reward: Implications for Drug Addiction." *Frontiers in Neuroscience* 9: 404. doi: 10.3389/fnins.2015.00404.

Duncan, J. R., and Lawrence, A. J. (2012). "The Role of Metabotropic Glutamate Receptors in Addiction: Evidence from Preclinical Models." *Pharmacology Biochemistry and Behavior* 100: 811–824.

Durazzo, T. C., et al. (2011). "Cortical Thickness, Surface Area, and Volume of the Brain Reward System in Alcohol Dependence: Relationships to Relapse and Extended Abstinence." *Alcoholism: Clinical and Experimental Research (ACER)* 35: 1187–1200.

Feltenstein, M. W., et al. (2007). "Aripiprazole Blocks Reinstatement of Cocaine Seeking in an Animal Model of Relapse." *Biological Psychiatry* 61: 582–590.

Fowler, J. S., et al. (2007). "Imaging the Addicted Human Brain." *Addiction Science & Clinical Practice* 3: 4–16 (NIH Publication No. 07–6171).

Gaval-Cruz, M., and Weinshenker, D. (2009). "Mechanisms of Disulfiram-Induced Cocaine Abstinence: Antabuse and Cocaine Relapse." *Molecular Interventions* 9: 175–187.

Gould, R. W., et al. (2016). "Partial mGlu5 Negative Allosteric Modulators Attenuate Cocaine-Mediated Behaviors and Lack Psychotomimetic-Like Effects." *Neuropsychopharmacology* 41: 1166–1178.

Graham, D. L., et al. (2013). "GLP-1 Analog Attenuates Cocaine Reward." *Molecular Psychiatry* 18: 961–962.

Gupta, S. (2015). "Is This a Groundbreaking Cure for Opiates and 'Benzos' Addicts?" *The Independent*. April 20. http://www.independent.co.uk/life-style/health-and-families/features/is-this-a-groundbreaking-cure-for-opiates-and-benzos-addicts-10190635.html.

Haass-Koffler, C. L., and Bartlett, S. E. (2012). "Stress and Addiction: Contribution of the Corticotropin Releasing Factor (CRF) System in Neuroplasticity." *Frontiers in Molecular Neuroscience* 5: 1–13, article 91.

Hall, W., et al., (2015). "The Brain Disease Model of Addiction: Is it Supported by the Evidence and Has it Delivered on its Promises?" *Lancet Psychiatry* 2: 105–110.

Hammond, S., et al. (2013). "D-serine Facilitates the Effectiveness of Extinction to Reduce Drug-Primed Reinstatement of Cocaine-Induced Conditioned Place Preference." *Neuropharmacology* 64: 464–471.

Haney, M., et al. (2010). "Effects of Baclofen and Mirtazapine on a Laboratory Model of Marijuana Withdrawal and Relapse." *Psychopharmacology* (Berl) 211: 233–244.

Heberlein, A., et al. (2011). "Serum Levels of BDNF Are Associated with Craving in Opiate-Dependent Patients." *Journal of Psychopharmacology* 25: 1480–1484.

Herin, D. V., et al. (2010). "Agonist-Like Pharmacotherapy for Stimulant Dependence: Preclinical, Human Laboratory, and Clinical Studies." *Annals of the New York Academy of Sciences* 1187: 76–100.

Hood, S. D., et al. (2014). "Benzodiazepine Dependence and Its Treatment with Low Dose Flumazenil." *British Journal of Clinical Pharmacology* 77: 285–294.

Jayaram-Lindström, N., et al. (2008). "Naltrexone for the Treatment of Amphetamine Dependence: A Randomized, Placebo-Controlled Trial." *American Journal of Psychiatry* 165: 1442–1448.

Johnson, B. A., et al. (2007). "Topiramate for Treating Alcohol Dependence: A Randomized Controlled Trial." *JAMA* 298: 1641–1651.

Johnson, B. A., et al. (2013). "Topiramate for the Treatment of Cocaine Addiction. A Randomized Clinical Trial." *JAMA Psychiatry* 70: 1338–1346.

Johnston, L. D., et al. (2016). *Monitoring the Future National Survey Results on Drug Use, 1975–2015: Volume 2, College Students and Adults Ages 19–55.* Ann Arbor: Institute for Social Research, The University of Michigan. http://monitoringthefuture.org/pubs/monographs/mtf-vol2_2015.pdf.

Johnson, K. A., and Lovinger, D. M. (2016). "Presynaptic G Protein-Coupled Receptors: Gatekeepers of Addiction?" *Frontiers in Cellular Neuroscience* 10: 1–22, article 264. doi: 10.3389/fncel.2016.00264.

Johnston, L. D., et al. (2016). *Monitoring the Future National Survey Results on Drug Use, 1975–2015: Overview, Key Findings on Adolescent Drug Use.* Ann Arbor: Institute for Social Research, The University of Michigan. http://www.monitoringthefuture.org/pubs/monographs/mtf-overview2015.pdf.

Kalivas, P. W., et al. (2006). "Animal Models and Brain Circuits in Drug Addiction." *Molecular Interventions* 6: 339–344.

Kalivas, P. W. (2009). "The Glutamate Homeostasis Hypothesis of Addiction." *Nature Reviews Neuroscience* 10: 561–572.

Kalivas, P. W., and Volkow, N. D. (2011). "New Medications for Drug Addiction Hiding in Glutamatergic Neuroplasticity." *Molecular Psychiatry* 16: 974–986.

Koob, G. F. (2015). "The Dark Side of Emotion: The Addiction Perspective." *European Journal of Pharmacology* 753: 73–87.

Koob, G. F., and Mason, B. J. (2016). "Existing and Future Drugs for the Treatment of the Dark Side of Addiction." *Annual Review of Pharmacology and Toxicology* 56: 299–322.

Kupchik, Y. M., et al. (2012). "The Effect of *N*-Acetylcysteine in the Nucleus Accumbens on Neurotransmission and Relapse to Cocaine." *Biological Psychiatry* 71: 978–986.

Li, X., et al. (2013). "Metabotropic Glutamate 7 (mGlu 7) Receptor: A Target for Medication Development for the Treatment of Cocaine Dependence." *Neuropharmacology* 66: 12–23.

Lingford-Hughes, A. R., et al. (2004). "Evidence-Based Guidelines for the Pharmacological Management of Substance Misuse, Addiction and Comorbidity." *Journal of Psychopharmacology* 18: 293–335.

López-Moreno, J. A., et al. (2010). "Functional Interactions Between Endogenous Cannabinoid and Opioid Systems: Focus on Alcohol, Genetics and Drug-Addicted Behaviors." *Current Drug Targets* 11: 406–428.

Luigjes, J., et al. (2012). "Deep Brain Stimulation in Addiction: A Review of Potential Brain Targets." *Molecular Psychiatry* 17: 572–583.

Madsen, H. B., et al. (2012). "Neuroplasticity in Addiction: Cellular and Transcriptional Perspectives." *Frontiers in Molecular Neuroscience* 5: 1–16, article 99.

Mahler, S. V., et al. (2012). "Modafinil Attenuates Reinstatement of Cocaine Seeking: Role for Cystine-Glutamate Exchange and Metabotropic Glutamate Receptors." *Addict Biol.* 2014 January; 19(1): 1–17. doi:10.1111/j.1369-1600.2012.00506.x.

Maldonado, R., and Berrendero, F. (2010). "Endogenous Cannabinoid and Opioid Systems and Their Role in Nicotine Addiction." *Current Drug Targets* 11: 440–449.

Mameli, M., and Lüscher, C. (2011). "Synaptic Plasticity and Addiction: Learning Mechanisms Gone Awry." *Neuropharmacology* 61: 1052–1059.

Martinez, D. and Trifilieff, P. (2015) "A Review of Potential Pharmacological Treatments for Cannabis Abuse" *American Society of Addiction Medicine* (online) https://www.asam.org/resources/publications/magazine/read/article/2015/04/13/a-review-of-potential-pharmacological-treatments-for-cannabis-abuse

Mason, B. J., and Heyser, C. J. (2010). "The Neurobiology, Clinical Efficacy and Safety of Acamprosate in the Treatment of Alcohol Dependence." *Expert Opinion on Drug Safety* 9: 177–188.

Miranda, R. Jr., et al. (2017). "Topiramate and Motivational Enhancement Therapy For Cannabis Use Among Youth: A Randomized Placebo-Controlled Pilot Study." *Addiction* 22: 779–790, January, 11. doi: 10.1111/adb.12350.

Muzyk, A. J., et al. (2012). "Defining the Role of Baclofen for the Treatment of Alcohol Dependence: A Systematic Review of the Evidence." *CNS Drugs* 26: 69–78.

Myers, K. M., and Carlezon, W. A., Jr. (2012). "D-Cycloserine Effects on Extinction of Conditioned Responses to Drug-Related Cues." *Biological Psychiatry* 71: 947–955.

National Institute on Drug Abuse. (2010). *Research Reports: Cocaine Abuse and Addiction.* NIH Publication Number 10–4166. September.

National Institute on Drug Abuse. (2017). "Costs of Substance Abuse." *Trends & Statistics.* April 21. https://www.drugabuse.gov/related-topics/trends-statistics.

Negus, S. S. and Jack Henningfield, J. (2015). "Agonist Medications for the Treatment of Cocaine Use Disorder." *Neuropsychopharmacology* 40: 1815–1825. doi: 10.1038/npp.2014.322

Nestler, E. (2005). "Is There a Common Molecular Pathway for Addiction?" *Nature Neuroscience* 8: 1445–1449.

Nestler, E. J., and Malenka, R. C. (2004). "The Addicted Brain." *Scientific American* 290: 78–85.

Noble, F., et al. (2015). "The Opioid Receptors as Targets for Drug Abuse Medication." *British Journal of Pharmacology* 172: 3964–3979.

Novak, M. (2010). "Incentive Learning Underlying Cocaine-Seeking Requires mGluR5 Receptors Located on Dopamine D1 Receptor-Expressing Neurons." *Journal of Neuroscience* 30: 11973–11982.

Nutt, D., and Lingford-Hughes, A. (2008). "Addiction: The Clinical Interface." *British Journal of Pharmacology* 154: 397–405.

Nutt, D. J., et al. (2015). "The Dopamine Theory of Addiction: 40 Years of Highs and Lows." *Nature Reviews Neuroscience* 16: 305–312.

Olds, J., and Milner, P. (1954). "Positive Reinforcement Produced by Electrical Stimulation of Septal Area and Other Regions of Rat Brain." *Journal of Comparative and Physiological Psychology* 47: 419–427.

Olive, M. F., et al. (2012). "Glutamatergic Medications for the Treatment of Drug and Behavioral Addictions." *Pharmacology, Biochemistry and Behavior* 100: 801–810.

Pani, P. P., et al. (2010). "Disulfiram for the treatment of cocaine dependence." *Cochrane Database Systematic Review* CD007024. doi: 10.1002/14651858.CD007024.pub2.

Parolaro, D., et al. (2010). "Cellular Mechanisms Underlying the Interaction between Cannabinoid and Opiate System." *Current Drug Targets* 11: 393–405.

Pava, M. J., and Woodward, J. J. (2012). "A Review of the Interactions between Alcohol and the Endocannabinoid System: Implications for Alcohol Dependence and Future Directions for Research." *Alcohol* 46: 185–204.

Penetar, D. M. (2012). "Sustained-Release Opiate Blockers for Treating Heroin and Amphetamine Dependence." *American Journal of Psychiatry* 169: 5.

Pettinati, H. M., et al. (2006). "The Status of Naltrexone in the Treatment of Alcohol Dependence: Specific Effects on Heavy Drinking." *Journal of Clinical Psychopharmacology* 26: 610–625.

Pettinati, N. M., et al. (2013). "Current Status of Co-Occurring Mood and Substance Use Disorders: A New Therapeutic Target." *American Journal of Psychiatry* 170: 23–30.

Pierce, R. C., and Kumaresan, V. (2006). "The Mesolimbic Dopamine System: The Final Common Pathway for the Reinforcing Effect of Drugs of Abuse?" *Neuroscience and Biobehavioral Reviews* 30: 215–238.

Pierce, R. C., et al. (2012). "Rational Development of Addiction Pharmacotherapies: Successes, Failures, and Prospects." *Cold Spring Harbor Perspectives in Medicine* 2: a012880.

Preti, A. (2007). "New Developments in the Pharmacotherapy of Cocaine Abuse." *Addiction Biology* 12: 133–151.

Rahman, S., et al. (2015). "Nicotinic Receptor Modulation to Treat Alcohol and Drug Dependence." *Frontiers in Neuroscience* 8: 1–11, article 426.

Riegel, A. C., and Kalivas, P. W. (2010). "Lack of Inhibition Leads to Abuse." *Nature* 463: 743–744.

Robledo, P. (2010). "Cannabinoids, Opioids and NMDA: Neuropsychological Interactions Related to Addiction." *Current Drug Targets* 11: 429–439.

Schifano, F., et al. (2015). "Novel Psychoactive Substances of Interest for Psychiatry." *World Psychiatry* 14: 15–26.

Schnabel, J. (2009). "Rethinking Rehab." *Nature* 458: 25–27.

Scripps Research Institute. (2016, December). "Gabapentin Treatment of Cannabis Dependence." U.S. National Institutes of Health. https://clinicaltrials.gov/ct2/show/NCT00974376.

Shen, H-W., et al. (2014). "Synaptic Glutamate Spillover Due to Impaired Glutamate Uptake Mediates Heroin Relapse." *Journal of Neuroscience* 34: 5649. http://doi.org/10.1523/JNEUROSCI.4564-13.2014.

Sherman, B. J., et al. (2017). "Gender Differences Among Treatment-Seeking Adults with Cannabis Use Disorder: Clinical Profiles Of Women and Men Enrolled in The Achieving Cannabis Cessation—Evaluating *N*-Acetylcysteine Treatment (ACCENT) Study." *American Journal on Addiction* 26: 136–144. doi: 10.1111/ajad.12503.

Shorter, D., et al. (2015). "Emerging Drugs for the Treatment of Cocaine Use Disorder: A Review of Neurobiological Targets and Pharmacotherapy." *Expert Opinion on Emerging Drugs* 20: 15–29.

Sofuoglu, M., et al. (2013). "Cognitive Enhancement as a Treatment for Drug Addictions." *Neuropharmacology* 64: 452–463.

Sofuoglu, M., and Kosten, T. R. (2006). "Emerging Pharmacological Strategies in the Fight against Cocaine Addiction." *Expert Opinion on Emerging Drugs* 11: 91–98.

Spencer, S., et al. (2016). "The Good and Bad News about Glutamate in Drug Addiction." *Journal of Psychopharmacology*, June 28. doi: 10.1177/0269881116655248.

Steensland, P., et al. (2007). "Varenicline, an $\alpha_4\beta_2$ Nicotinic Acetylcholine Receptor Partial Agonist, Selectively Decreases Ethanol Consumption and Seeking." *Proceedings of the National Academy of Sciences USA* 104: 12518–12523.

Tiihonen, J., et al. (2007). "A Comparison of Aripiprazole, Methylphenidate, and Placebo for Amphetamine Dependence." *American Journal of Psychiatry* 164: 160–162.

Tiihonen, J., et al. (2012). "Naltrexone Implant for the Treatment of Polydrug Dependence: A Randomized Controlled Trial." *American Journal of Psychiatry* 169: 531–536.

Tracy, D. K., et al. (2017). "Novel Psychoactive Substances: Identifying and Managing Acute and Chronic Harmful Use." *BMJ* 356: i6814. doi: 10.1136/bmj.i6814.

Trigo, J. M., et al. (2010). "The Endogenous Opioid System: A Common Substrate in Drug Addiction." *Drug and Alcohol Dependence* 108: 183–194.

U.S. Department of Health & Human Services. (2016). *Facing Addiction in America: The Surgeon General's Report on Alcohol, Drugs, and Health.* https://addiction.surgeongeneral.gov/surgeon-generals-report.pdf.

Volkow, N. D., et al. (1997). "Relationship Between Subjective Effects of Cocaine and Dopamine Transporter Occupancy." *Nature* 386: 827–830.

Volkow, N. D., et al. (2004). "The Addicted Human Brain Viewed in the Light of Imaging Studies: Brain Circuits and Treatment Strategies." *Neuropharmacology* 47, Supplement 1: 3–13.

Volkow, N. D., et al. (2011). "Addiction: Beyond Dopamine Reward Circuitry." *Proceedings of the National Academy of Sciences* 108: 15037–15042.

Volkow, N. D., et al. (2014). "Stimulant-Induced Dopamine Increases Are Markedly Blunted in Active Cocaine Abusers." *Molecular Psychiatry* 19: 1037–1043.

Volkow, N. D., et al. (2016). "Neurobiologic Advances from the Brain Disease Model of Addiction." *New England Journal of Medicine* 374: 363–371.

Volkow, N. D., and Morales, M. (2015). "The Brain on Drugs: From Reward to Addiction." *CELL* 162: 712–725.

Wise, R. A., and Koob, G. F. (2014). "The Development and Maintenance of Drug Addiction." *Neuropsychopharmacology* 39: 254–262.

Yadid, G., et al. (2012). "Modulation of Mood States as a Major Factor in Relapse to Substance Use." *Frontiers in Molecular Neuroscience* 5: 1–5, article 81.

Ethyl Alcohol and the Inhalants of Abuse

ETHYL ALCOHOL

Ethyl alcohol (ethanol) is a psychoactive drug that is similar in most respects to all the other sedative-hypnotic compounds that will be discussed in Chapter 13. But there are two main differences between classical sedative-hypnotics (for example, benzodiazepines) and ethanol. First, ethanol is used primarily for recreational rather than medical purposes, and second, ethanol has unique kinetics of metabolism that separates it from most other drugs.

In spite of the recent surge in abuse of cannabis and opiates and their numerous chemical variants, alcoholism, alcohol abuse, binge drinking, and underage drinking remain significant public health issues. About 16.6 million Americans older than 18 years are estimated to have an alcohol use disorder (Editorial, *Lancet*, 2015). Globally, women, especially younger women, are now ingesting nearly as much alcohol as men. More women are also drinking "dangerously" and harming themselves as a direct result (Slade et al., 2016). Although the percentage of people in the United States who drink (about 56 percent) has not changed, the percent of heavy drinking and binge drinking is increasing. And the simultaneous use of alcohol with other drugs, such as cannabis, and energy drinks increases the risk of problems from alcohol. According to the most recent available data, the 12-month and lifetime prevalence for alcohol use disorder (AUD) in the United States were 13.9 percent and 29.1 percent, respectively (Grant et al., 2016). (See Criteria for Diagnosis of Alcohol Use Disorder in the appendix at the end of this chapter.)

Pharmacokinetics of Alcohol

Absorption

Ethyl alcohol is a very simple molecule, found in 12 to 15 percent concentrations in wines, about 5 percent in beers (as much as 7 to 10 percent in some "microbrews," and as high as 10 to 12 percent in 16- and 24-ounce cans of fortified beverages). In "hard" liquors, alcohol is present in concentrations of 40 to 50 percent, usually expressed as alcohol "proof," which is twice the percent concentration (for example, 80 proof equals 40 percent ethanol). The appendix at the end of this chapter addresses the amount of alcohol that is present in representative forms of alcohol-containing beverages.

Alcohol diffuses easily across all biological membranes. Thus, after it is consumed, alcohol is rapidly and completely absorbed from the entire gastrointestinal tract, both in the stomach and the upper intestine, although most is absorbed from the upper intestine because of its large surface area. The time from the last drink to maximal concentration in blood ranges from 15 to 60 minutes. In a person with an empty stomach, approximately 20 percent of a single dose of alcohol is absorbed directly from the stomach, usually quite rapidly. The remaining 80 percent is absorbed rapidly and completely from the upper intestine; the only limiting factor is the time it takes to empty the stomach.

In persons who have undergone gastric bypass surgery for morbid obesity, the stomach and most of the upper intestine are bypassed. In such persons, alcohol absorption occurs in the lower intestine and, in the absence of an alcohol-metabolizing enzyme normally in the stomach and upper intestine (described below), the lower intestine slowly adapts and eventually absorbs alcohol very readily. As a result, post-gastric-bypass patients have much higher peak blood alcohol concentrations (BAC) after ingesting alcohol and they require more time to become sober (Woodard et al., 2011). Such increases have not been observed in patients who have undergone gastric banding instead of a complete gastric bypass (Suzuki et al., 2012). These unexpected increases in BAC have been linked to potential increases in alcohol use disorders in gastric bypass patients (King et al., 2012), although other possibilities have been proposed, such as altered gene expression in brain regions involved in reward processing (Davis et al., 2013).

Distribution

After absorption, alcohol is evenly distributed throughout all body fluids and tissues. The blood–brain barrier is freely permeable to alcohol, so when alcohol appears in the blood and reaches a person's brain, it crosses the blood–brain barrier almost immediately. Alcohol is also freely distributed across the placenta and easily enters the brain of a developing fetus. Fetal blood alcohol levels are essentially the same as those of the drinking mother.

Metabolism and Excretion

Approximately 95 percent of the alcohol a person ingests is enzymatically metabolized by the enzyme *alcohol dehydrogenase* (ADH). The other 5 percent is excreted unchanged, mainly through the lungs.[1] Very small amounts of alcohol are excreted in the urine.

---

[1] Small amounts of alcohol are excreted from the body through the lungs; most of us are familiar with "alcohol breath." This excretion forms the basis for the breath analysis test because alcohol equilibrates rapidly across the membranes of the lung. In the Breathalyzer test, a ratio of 1:2300 exists between alcohol in inhaled air and alcohol in venous blood. The blood alcohol concentration is easily extrapolated from alcohol concentration in the expired air.

About 85 percent of the metabolism of alcohol occurs in the liver. Some alcohol metabolism is carried out by a *gastric* ADH enzyme, located in the lining of the stomach, which can decrease the blood level of alcohol by about 15 percent, obviously attenuating alcohol's systemic toxicity. Rapid gastric emptying (as by drinking on an empty stomach or by having had bariatric surgery) reduces the time that alcohol is susceptible to gastric metabolism and results in increased blood levels. Drinking on a full stomach retains alcohol in the stomach, increases its exposure to gastric ADH, and reduces the resulting peak blood level of the drug.

It is well recognized that whenever women and men consume comparable amounts of alcohol (after correction for differences in body weight), women have higher blood ethanol concentrations than men. The reasons appear to be threefold:

1. Women have about 50 percent less gastric metabolism of alcohol than men because women, whether alcoholic or nonalcoholic, have a lower level of gastric ADH enzyme. Because the gastric enzyme metabolizes about 15 percent of ingested alcohol, the blood alcohol concentration is increased by about 7 percent over that in a male drinking the same weight-adjusted amount of alcohol.

2. Men may have a greater ratio of muscle to fat than do women. Men thus have a larger vascular compartment (fat has little blood supply). Therefore, alcohol is somewhat more diluted in men, again decreasing blood alcohol levels in men compared to women.

3. Women, with higher body fat than men (fat contains little alcohol), concentrate alcohol in plasma, drink for drink, more than men, raising the apparent blood level.

The metabolism of alcohol by ADH is only the first step in a normal three-step metabolic process involved in the breakdown of alcohol (Figure 5.1):

1. Alcohol dehydrogenase functions to convert alcohol to acetaldehyde. A coenzyme called *nicotinamide adenine dinucleotide* (NAD) is required for the activity of this enzyme. The availability of NAD is the rate-limiting step in this reaction; enough is present so that the maximum amount of alcohol that can be metabolized in 24 hours is about 170 grams.

2. The enzyme acetaldehyde dehydrogenase (ALDH) converts acetaldehyde to acetic acid. The drug *disulfiram* (Antabuse) irreversibly inhibits this enzyme and is one possible treatment for alcoholism.

3. Acetic acid is broken down into carbon dioxide and water, thus releasing energy (calories).[2]

The average person metabolizes about 10 to 14 milliliters of 100 percent alcohol per hour, independent of the blood level of alcohol. This rate is fairly constant for different

---

[2] (±)-Salsolinol is a metabolite of ethanol produced by the chemical interaction of dopamine with acetaldehyde in the brain. The formation of salsolinol in the brain from the reaction of acetaldehyde and extracellular dopamine stimulates dopaminergic activity through several mechanisms. Peana and colleagues (2016) review the literature on this topic and the possibility that salsolinol may contribute to alcohol's addictive property.

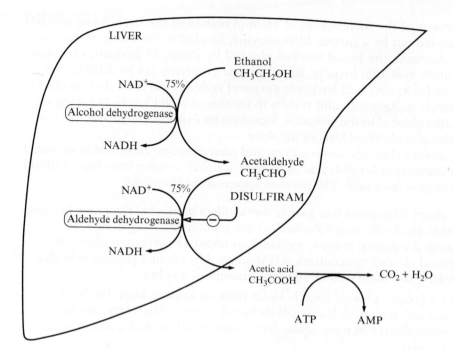

FIGURE 5.1 Metabolism of ethanol. Ethanol is oxidized by the enzyme alcohol dehydrogenase using NAD (nicotinamide adenine dinucleotide) as a cofactor to form acetaldehyde. A second oxidative step converts acetaldehyde to acetic acid, which in turn is broken down to carbon dioxide and water. The first step involving alcohol dehydrogenase (ADH) is the rate-limiting step. The drug *disulfiram* (Antabuse) blocks the second step by blocking the activity of aldehyde dehydrogenase (ALDH). ATP = adenosine phosphate; AMP = adenosine monophosphate.

people.[3] Figure 5.2 illustrates the rate of alcohol elimination for a group of 48 healthy men administered a standard dose of ethanol. Here, the blood alcohol concentration falls at a rate of about 0.011 and 0.015 grams%/hour.[4] It takes an adult 1 hour to metabolize the amount of alcohol that is contained in a 1-ounce glass of 80 proof (40 percent) whiskey, a 4-ounce glass of 12 percent wine, a 12-ounce bottle of 5 percent beer, or a 6-ounce glass of 8 to 10 percent microbrew or fortified beer. Commercially poured (for example, by bartenders) alcoholic drinks usually exceed these amounts by about 50 percent; similar variation occurs in home-poured drinks. In the United States, one "standard" drink equivalent contains roughly 14 grams of pure alcohol.

Consumption of 4 to 5 ounces of wine, 12 ounces of 5 percent beer, or 1.0 to 1.5 ounces of 80 proof whiskey per hour would keep the blood levels of alcohol in

---

[3] In biochemical terms, this is called *zero-order metabolism*. Virtually all other drugs are metabolized by first-order metabolism, which means that the amount of drug metabolized per unit time depends on the amount (or concentration) of drug in blood. Perhaps zero-order metabolism occurs because the amount of enzyme (or a cofactor required for activity of the enzyme) is limited and becomes saturated with only small amounts of alcohol in the body.

[4] Grams% is the number of grams of ethanol that would be contained in 100 milliliters of blood.

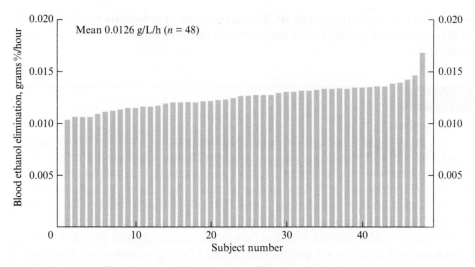

FIGURE 5.2 Individual variations in the elimination rate of ethanol as measured in 48 healthy males after they drank 0.68 gram of ethanol per kilogram of body weight. Neat whisky was ingested on an empty stomach. Values are expressed as grams of alcohol metabolized per liter of blood per hour. If expressed as grams%, 0.10 g/L/h would equate to a 0.01 grams% per hour fall in blood concentration; 0.15 g/L/hr would equal a 0.015 grams% per hour fall in blood concentration. [Data from A. W. Jones 2003.]

a person fairly constant. If a person ingests more alcohol in any given hour than is metabolized, his or her blood concentrations increase. Consequently, there is a limit to the amount of alcohol a person can consume in an hour without becoming drunk. The appendix at the end of this chapter expands on the topic of drink equivalents.

The following may serve to explain the relationship between the amounts of alcohol consumed, the resulting *blood alcohol concentration* (BAC), and the impairment of motor and intellectual functioning (here, driving ability): today, all states have set a BAC of 0.08 grams% as intoxication, and a person who drives with a BAC above this amount can be charged with driving while under the influence of alcohol. Thus, one might assume that a level of 0.07 grams% is acceptable but a level of 0.09 grams% is not. The behavioral effects of alcohol, however, are not all or none; alcohol (like all sedatives) progressively impairs a person's ability to function. Thus, the 0.08 grams% blood level is only a legally established, arbitrary value. A person whose BAC is under 0.08 grams% yet functions with impairment detrimental to operation of a motor vehicle can still suffer criminal penalties. Driving ability is minimally impaired at a BAC of 0.01 grams%, but at 0.04 to 0.08 grams%, a driver has increasingly impaired judgment and reactions and becomes less inhibited. As a result, the risk of an accident quadruples. The deterioration of a person's driving ability continues at a BAC of 0.10 to 0.14 grams%, leading to a sixfold to sevenfold increase in the risk of having an accident. At 0.15 grams% and higher, a person is 25 times more likely to become involved in a serious accident. Recognizing that over 100 countries on six continents have BAC limits set at 0.05 grams% or lower, the National Traffic Safety Board in April 2013 recommended to states that they lower the BAC content that constitutes drunken driving to the 0.05

grams% level. In fact, U.S. Department of Transportation regulations prohibit truck drivers from driving at 0.04 grams% and airline pilots from flying at 0.02 grams% after 8 hours of abstinence.

Did You Know?

Hangover-Free Alcohol

For over 10 years, psychopharmacologist Dr. David Nutt has been on a mission to develop a safe substitute for alcohol that would produce the good effects, like sociability and relaxation, but without getting people drunk. The substance is called *Alcosynth*. So far, his group has patented 90 potential compounds, with three or four possible candidates under consideration. The ultimate drug would be used like alcohol, drunk by itself or mixed into cocktails. While current prototypes can impair reflex speed and attention, they produce less unsteadiness, do not give you a hangover, won't hurt the liver, and have practically no calories! The peak effect in the brain plateaus so that you won't get a greater effect from eight drinks than from four and can't overdose. Alcosynth is currently being closely monitored for potential health risks. For example, it does not claim to remedy all of the other dangers of intoxication (such as impaired judgment and drunk driving), not only to drinkers but to those around them. But globally, alcohol misuse is the fifth leading risk factor for premature death and disability. Dr. Nutt's goal is to reduce these devastating effects of alcoholism and he hopes that his alternative will replace alcohol by 2050.

Figure 5.3 illustrates the correlation between the number of drink equivalents imbibed, gender, body weight, and the resulting blood alcohol concentration. To use the information, choose the correct chart (male or female), then find the number that is closest to your body weight in pounds. Look down the left column to find the number of drinks consumed. BAC is found by matching body weight with number of drinks ingested. Then note that BAC falls about 0.015 grams% every hour from the time that the first drink was ingested. From the total number of drinks ingested, subtract the amount of alcohol that has been metabolized from the number of hours since drinking began (remember that approximately 1 drink equivalent is metabolized in 1 hour). The final figure is the approximate BAC. By calculating this number, the degree to which driving ability is impaired can be predicted.

Factors that may alter the predictable rate of metabolism of alcohol are usually not of major clinical significance, with two exceptions. First, with long-term use, alcohol can induce drug-metabolizing enzymes in the liver, increasing the liver's rate of metabolizing alcohol (and so inducing *tolerance*) as well as its rate of metabolizing other compounds that are similar to alcohol (termed *cross-tolerance*). Second, as discussed above, ADH enzyme (termed *ADH1*) usually is responsible for alcohol metabolism. In chronic alcohol use, in very high (toxic) blood levels, and in persons with alcohol-induced liver failure, a variant of ADH1 enzyme (termed either *ADH3* or *ADH1C*) is produced as the liver becomes incapable of metabolizing alcohol by ADH (Haseba and Ohno, 2010). This enzyme variant may help persons with potentially fatal

Blood Alcohol Concentration–A Guide

One drink equals 1 ounce of 80 proof alcohol; 12-ounce bottle of beer; 2 ounces of 20% wine; 3 ounces of 12% wine.

Men

Drinks	Approximate blood alcohol percentage (grams%) Body weight (pounds)								
	100	120	140	160	180	200	220	240	
0	.00	.00	.00	.00	.00	.00	.00	.00	Only safe driving limit
1	.04	.03	.03	.02	.02	.02	.02	.02	Impairment begins
2	.08	.06	.05	.05	.04	.04	.03	.03	Driving skills significantly affected
3	.11	.09	.08	.07	.06	.06	.05	.05	
4	.15	.12	.11	.09	.08	.08	.07	.06	
5	.19	.16	.13	.12	.11	.09	.09	.08	Possible criminal penalties
6	.23	.19	.16	.14	.13	.11	.10	.09	
7	.26	.22	.19	.16	.15	.13	.12	.11	Legally intoxicated
8	.30	.25	.21	.19	.17	.15	.14	.13	
9	.34	.28	.24	.21	.19	.17	.15	.14	
10	.38	.31	.27	.23	.21	.19	.17	.16	Criminal penalties

Alcohol is "burned up" by the body at .015 grams% per hour, as follows:

Number of hours since starting first drink	1	2	3	4	5	6
Percent alcohol burned up	.015	.030	.045	.060	.075	.090

Calculate BAC
Example:
180 lb. man – 6 drinks in 4 hours
BAC = .130 grams% on chart
Subtract .060 grams% metabolized in 4 hours
BAC = .070 grams% – DRIVING IMPAIRED

Women

Drinks	Approximate blood alcohol percentage (grams%) Body weight (pounds)									
	90	100	120	140	160	180	200	220	240	
0	.00	.00	.00	.00	.00	.00	.00	.00	.00	Only safe driving limit
1	.05	.05	.04	.03	.03	.03	.02	.02	.02	Impairment begins
2	.10	.09	.08	.07	.06	.05	.05	.04	.04	Driving skills significantly affected
3	.15	.14	.11	.10	.09	.08	.07	.06	.06	
4	.20	.18	.15	.13	.11	.10	.09	.08	.08	
5	.25	.23	.19	.16	.14	.13	.11	.10	.09	Criminal penalties
6	.30	.27	.23	.19	.17	.15	.14	.12	.11	
7	.35	.32	.27	.23	.20	.18	.16	.14	.13	Legally intoxicated
8	.40	.36	.30	.26	.23	.20	.18	.17	.15	
9	.45	.41	.34	.29	.26	.23	.20	.19	.17	
10	.51	.45	.38	.32	.28	.25	.23	.21	.19	Criminal penalties

Alcohol is "burned up" by the body at .015 grams% per hour, as follows:

Number of hours since starting first drink	1	2	3	4	5	6
Percent alcohol burned up	.015	.030	.045	.060	.075	.090

Calculate BAC
Example:
140 lb woman – 6 drinks in 4 hours
BAC = .190 grams% on chart
Subtract .060 grams% metabolized in 4 hours
BAC = .130 grams% – LEGALLY INTOXICATED

FIGURE 5.3 Relation between blood alcohol concentration, body weight, and the number of drinks ingested for men and women. See text for details.

blood alcohol levels to survive toxic levels of alcohol. Protective effects of this enzyme variant appear most prominently in Asian persons (Li et al., 2012).

Finally, biological markers that detect alcohol use even when BAC levels are reported as zero have been recently developed. Because alcohol is cleared fairly rapidly from the body, these biomarkers detect minor metabolites of alcohol and are usually positive for about 80 hours following drinking. Such biomarkers are proving to be valuable tools to improve verification of abstention in alcohol-dependent persons (Albermann et al., 2012; Dahl et al., 2011). These minor metabolites include ethyl glucuronide and ethyl sulfate. The ethyl glucuronide and ethyl sulfate comprise about 0.02 and 0.010 percent of the ethanol dose, respectively, but they can be reliably detected in blood, urine, and hair samples. In addition, phosphatidylethanols (PEth) are a group of phospholipids formed only in the presence of ethanol. They have been reported to be the most sensitive substances and to show the best correlation with self-reported alcohol use (de Bejczy et al., 2015). Such testing is now being widely used in programs where abstinence from alcohol is required. False positives can be obtained when one has used alcohol-containing products such as mouthwashes (Reisfield et al., 2011a) or hand sanitizers (Reisfield et al., 2011b).

Powdered Alcohol

Palcohol is powdered alcohol, a product developed in the United States by Mark Phillips, and produced and marketed by Lipsmark, an Arizona-based company. It is generally made using microencapsulation, a process in which tiny particles or droplets are surrounded by a coating resulting in small capsules. When reconstituted with water, alcohol powder, which comes in a 4 inch by 6 inch sealable pouch, becomes an alcoholic beverage. The goal is to create five versions: rum, vodka, and three mixed drinks—Cosmopolitan, Lemon Drop, and a margarita version called "Powderita"— according to the company's Web site. Each version will be sold in single-use packets, which consumers can mix with 6 ounces of liquid, filling about a third of a standard glass tumbler, to make one drink. Each drink will have 10 percent alcohol by volume, about the equivalent of a glass of wine.

Mr. Phillips is not the first to develop a powdered form of alcohol. In 1966, Sato Foods Industries Co., Ltd. invented alcohol powderization, which has been available in Japan and Europe. Mr. Phillips's version was approved for sale in March 2015 by the Alcohol and Tobacco Tax and Trade Bureau (TTB). But the TTB declared less than two weeks later that it had issued the approval in error; Phillips maintains his company voluntarily surrendered approval because of a mistake on the product's proposed label. It is still subject to state regulation; as of April 2016, 31 states have legislated or regulated complete bans on powdered alcohol. California is next in line to ban the substance, nine other states also have bans pending, and only three states currently allow the sale of powdered alcohol (Texas, Colorado, and Arizona).

Because powdered alcohol is easily transported and combined with other alcoholic drinks, there is the concern that it will promote underage use, increase binge drinking, and illicit beverage "spiking." Furthermore, its easy concealment gives it potential for insufflation and injection. The large amounts needed, however, argue against such serious adverse outcomes.

Pharmacodynamics

Identifying the mechanism of the action of alcohol continues to be difficult. For many years, it was presumed that alcohol acted through a general depressant action on nerve membranes and synapses. Because it is both water-soluble and lipid-soluble, ethanol dissolves into all body tissues. This property led to a unitary hypothesis of action—that the drug dissolves in nerve membranes, distorting, disorganizing, or "perturbing" the membrane, similar to the action of general anesthetics (see Chapter 13). The result is a nonspecific and indirect depression of neuronal function, which would account for the nonspecific and generalized depressant behavioral effects of the drug. The hypothesis, however, does not explain the evidence that alcohol may disturb both the synaptic activity of various neurotransmitters, especially major excitatory (glutamate) and inhibitory (GABA) systems, and various intracellular transduction processes that modulate memory, cognitive performance, and motor performance.

Glutamate Receptors

Ethanol is a potent inhibitor of the NMDA subtype of glutamate receptors and glutamate receptor-mediated synaptic plasticity (Moykkynen and Korpi, 2012). Ethanol disrupts glutaminergic neurotransmission by depressing the responsiveness of NMDA receptors to released glutamate. This ethanol inhibition of glutamate receptors, however, seems to be restricted to certain brain areas such as the hippocampus, amygdala, and striatum and requires fairly high concentrations of the drug. This action may explain such effects of severe alcohol intoxication as impairments of motor performance and memory.

With chronic alcohol intake and persistent glutaminergic suppression, there is a compensatory up regulation of NMDA receptors. As a result, if alcohol is removed (such as during alcohol withdrawal), these excess excitatory receptors would elicit withdrawal signs, including seizures. Excess glutamate release during withdrawal may also be responsible for excitatory neuronal nerve damage and loss (Heinz et al., 2009).

As discussed below, the drug *acamprosate*, a structural analogue of glutamate, is an anticraving drug used to maintain abstinence in alcohol-dependent patients. By interacting with NMDA receptors, it is thought to reduce the neuronal hyperexcitability caused by chronic alcohol ingestion and withdrawal (Mann et al., 2008).

GABA Receptors

The decrease in glutamate responsiveness may be exacerbated by alcohol's enhancement of inhibitory GABA neurotransmission. Ethanol binds to a different subunit on the $GABA_A$ receptor than do other GABA agonists (Strac et al., 2012) and activates an inhibitory increase in chloride ion flows. The behavioral results of this neuronal inhibition include sedation, muscle relaxation, and impairment of cognitive and motor skills. Low doses of ethanol reduce both panic and the anxiety surrounding panic. This supports the view that drinking by those with panic disorder, stress, and anxiety is reinforced by a GABAergic agonistic effect. Thus, the use of alcohol to self-medicate one's panic or anxiety may contribute to the high rate of co-occurring alcohol use disorders with these other conditions.

Did You Know?

Rejected Male Fruit Flies Turn to Alcohol

Many animals, including mice, rats, and monkeys, are known to drink more alcohol after they have been isolated for sufficient periods of time. Mice that are victims of aggression or that are bullied also drink more. To see if stress produces similar effects in fruit flies, researchers allowed one group of males to mate with receptive females, while exposing another group to females who had previously mated and were no longer receptive to the males. Four days later, both groups of male flies were offered two diets: one was a normal liquid meal of yeast and sugar; the second contained 15 percent alcohol added to the yeast and sugar. As with some people, fruit flies will generally develop a preference for alcohol, including the diet containing the 15 percent solution. However, on average, the rejected flies drank significantly more of the alcoholic diet, drinking from that choice 70 percent of the time, while their sexually sated counterparts drank from the spiked liquid 50 percent of the time. Additional experiments were conducted to rule out other interpretations of the results. Presumably, the sexually deprived flies were using alcohol to make up for their frustration. It seems that some types of reward have not been greatly altered by evolution (Carey, 2012).

Opioid Receptors

GABA-mediated inhibition may activate opioid receptors, which, in turn, influence dopaminergic neurons. That is, ethanol may induce opioid release, which in turn triggers dopamine release in the brain reward system, especially the nucleus accumbens and orbitofrontal cortex (Mitchell et al., 2012). Administration of *naltrexone* (ReVia, Vivatrol) blocks opioid receptors and may reduce alcohol craving. Naltrexone is approved by the Food and Drug Administration (FDA) for the treatment of alcohol dependence, as discussed later in this chapter.

Serotonin Receptors

There is some literature and increasing emphasis on the role of serotonin in the actions of alcohol and as a mediator of alcohol reward, preference, dependence, and craving (Sari et al., 2011). Chronic alcohol consumption augments serotonergic activity; serotonin dysfunction has been postulated to play a role in the pathogenesis of some types of alcoholism. Today, emphasis is on the role of serotonin $5\text{-}HT_2$ and $5\text{-}HT_3$ receptors in the central effects of ethanol; these receptors are located on dopaminergic neurons in the nucleus accumbens. Serotonin reuptake-inhibiting antidepressants such as *sertraline* (Zoloft) (see Chapter 12) reduce alcohol consumption in individuals who are considered to be at a lower risk for excessive drinking. Serotonin receptors appear to be involved in impulsivity, a core behavior that contributes to the vulnerability to addiction and relapse (Kirby et al., 2011).

Cannabinoid Receptors

Within the past few years, important information has been gathered on the probable role of cannabinoid receptors (see Chapter 9) in the actions of alcohol, especially in postwithdrawal cravings and in the relapse to drinking. Chronic ingestion of ethanol stimulates the formation of the endogenous neurotransmitter for cannabinoid receptors, a substance called *anandamide*. This neurotransmitter activates the cannabinoid receptors and, with continued ethanol ingestion, eventually leads to the downregulation of these receptors. Cessation of drinking leads to a hyperactive endocannabinoid reaction, which appears to result in a craving for alcohol and a return to drinking. Blockade of cannabinoid receptors leads to loss of desire to self-administer alcohol and other drugs of abuse. As reviewed by Pava and Woodward (2012), stimulation of cannabinoid receptors contributes to the motivational and reinforcing properties of alcohol, and, conversely, chronic consumption of alcohol alters the functioning of the endogenous cannabinoid system.

Pharmacological Effects

The immediate primary neurobiological effect of alcohol is a graded, reversible neuronal depression, and impairment of mental functioning and cognition (Oscar-Berman and Marinkovic, 2007). Respiration is transiently stimulated at low doses, but as blood concentrations of alcohol increase, respiration becomes progressively depressed; at toxic doses, respiration ceases, causing death. Alcohol is also an anticonvulsant, although it is not clinically used for this purpose. On the other hand, withdrawal from chronic, high-dose, alcohol ingestion produces a prolonged period of hyperexcitability and seizures can occur; seizure activity peaks approximately 8 to 12 hours after the last drink.

In the central nervous system (CNS), the effects of alcohol are additive with those of other sedative-hypnotic compounds, resulting in more sedation and greater impairment of motor and cognitive abilities. Other sedatives (especially the benzodiazepines) and marijuana are the sedative-hypnotic drugs most frequently combined with alcohol, and they increase its deleterious effects on motor and intellectual skills (for example, driving ability), as well as alertness. In fact, a new federal study suggests alcohol has a more extreme impact on drivers than marijuana (Marsh, 2015). This report provides the most recent self-reported national estimates of driving under the influence of alcohol, marijuana, and alcohol and marijuana combined among persons aged 16 to 25 years, using data from the Substance Abuse and Mental Health Services Administration (SAMHSA) National Survey on Drug Use and Health (NSDUH) from 2002 to 2014. The participants drank alcohol to reach approximately 0.065 percent peak breath alcohol concentration, inhaled vaporized marijuana, or had a placebo. Researchers said alcohol "significantly increased lane departures/minimum and maximum lateral acceleration; these measures were not sensitive to cannabis." Researchers also concluded cannabis-influenced drivers "may attempt to drive more cautiously to compensate for impairing effects, whereas alcohol-influenced drivers often underestimate their impairment and take more risk." That said, from 2002 to 2014, the prevalence of self-reported driving under the influence of alcohol alone among persons aged 16 to 20 years and 21 to 25 years significantly *declined* by 59 and 38 percent, respectively. In addition, the reported prevalence of driving under the influence of alcohol and marijuana combined significantly declined by 39 percent in both age groups (Azofeifa et al., 2015).

Patients suffering from insomnia find alcohol to be an effective hypnotic agent, although the short duration of action of alcohol can lead to early morning awakenings, which does not alleviate the effects of insomnia.

Alcohol also affects the circulation and the heart. Alcohol dilates the blood vessels in the skin, producing a warm flush and a decrease in body temperature. Thus, it is pointless and possibly dangerous to drink alcohol to keep warm when one is exposed to cold weather. Long-term use of high doses of alcohol is associated with diseases of the heart muscle, which can result in heart failure. *Low* doses of alcohol, however, consumed daily (up to 2 drink equivalents per day for men and 0.5 to 1.0 daily drink equivalents for women) *reduce* the risk of coronary artery disease and peripheral artery disease. This protective effect on blood vessels occurs because of an alcohol-induced increase in high-density lipoprotein in blood, with a corresponding decrease in low-density lipoprotein.[5] Unfortunately, the cardioprotective effect of low doses of alcohol is lost on people who also smoke cigarettes or who are binge drinkers[6] (Ruidavets et al., 2010).

Drinking small amounts of alcohol a day may decrease the likelihood of having a stroke. Between 1.5 and 2 drink equivalents per day, totaling 20 to 30 grams of alcohol, was found to be correlated with a decrease in risk of several types of stroke (total, ischemic, and fatal). However, this apparent protective effect was reversed at higher doses. Daily amounts greater than 2 drink equivalents per day, totaling 40 to 45 grams, were associated with an increase in the likelihood of hemorrhagic stroke (Zhang et al., 2014). The mechanisms responsible for the protective effect of low doses of alcohol on stroke appear to involve increases in (protective) high-density cholesterol and an aspirinlike decrease in platelet aggregation.

In brief, there seems to be a sizable amount of evidence that moderate alcohol consumption is associated with decreased rates of cardiovascular disease, diabetes, and death. But even moderate drinking may produce cardiac damage in older persons (average age 76 years; Goncalves et al., 2015) or other impairments in persons with certain genetic makeup (Holmes et al., 2014). Also, even moderate drinking seems to be associated with increased rates, perhaps to a lesser extent, of some cancers, especially breast cancer, as well as some other diseases or conditions. Adjusted for multiple variables (including smoking) and compared with nondrinkers, relative risks for total cancer in women ranged from 1.04 (with light to moderate intake) to 1.30 (with heavy intake [≥45 grams daily]); for alcohol-related cancers, corresponding relative risks ranged from 1.13 to 1.66. These increases in relative risk, driven mainly by breast cancer, were similar for never smokers and ever smokers. Risk for total cancer in men who drank was elevated significantly only among those with daily alcohol intakes of 30 to 44.9 grams (Cao et al., 2015; Rehm, 2015).

Alcohol is high in calories but has little nutritional value; consumption of a high-alcohol diet (and little else!) slowly leads to vitamin deficiencies and nutritional diseases, which may result in physical deterioration. Alcohol abuse has been suggested as the most common cause of vitamin and trace element deficiencies in adults.

Alcohol (like all depressant drugs) is not an aphrodisiac. The behavioral disinhibition induced by low doses of alcohol may appear to cause some loss of restraint,

---

[5]The higher the concentration of high-density lipoprotein and the lower the concentration of low-density lipoprotein, the lower the incidence of development of arteriosclerosis and occlusive vascular disease.

[6]Binge drinking defined as more than 5 drink equivalents within 2 hours (by men) or more than 4 drink equivalents within 2 hours (women).

but alcohol depresses body function and interferes with sexual performance. As Shakespeare wrote in *Macbeth*: "It provokes the desire, but it takes away the performance."

Lastly, patients with chronic widespread pain (CWP) who consume moderate amounts of alcohol have lower levels of disability, according to a large new population-based study from the United Kingdom. In those with CWP, the percentage of subjects with disabling pain decreased with increasing alcohol consumption—from 47.2 percent among those who did not drink regularly to only 18.6 percent among those who drank 21 to 35 units per week. The relationship was similar for both men and women, but the lowest disability was at 11 to 20 units per week in females and 21 to 35 units per week in males (Macfarlane et al., 2015).

Psychological Effects

The short-term psychological and behavioral effects of alcohol are primarily related to a mixture of stimulant and depressant effects of low doses of the drug in the CNS. Figure 5.4 correlates the effects of alcohol with blood levels. The behavioral reaction that occurs at low doses is largely determined by the person, his or her mental expectations, and the environment in which drinking occurs. In one setting, a person may become relaxed and euphoric; in another, withdrawn or violent. Mental expectations and the physical setting become progressively less important at increasing doses because the sedative effects increase and behavioral activity decreases.

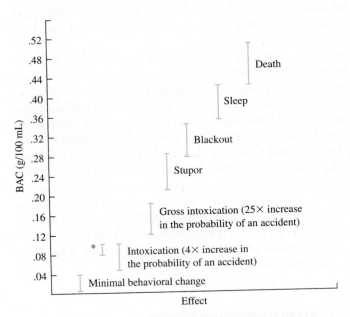

FIGURE 5.4 Correlation of the blood level of ethanol with degrees of intoxication. The legal level of intoxication (*) varies according to state law; the range of BAC values is shown. BAC = blood alcohol concentration.

Did You Know?

Which Type of Drinker Are You?

Psychology researchers have published a study that involved 374 undergraduates, drawing from literature and pop culture to propose that there are four drinking categories: the Ernest Hemingway, the Mary Poppins, the Nutty Professor, and the Mr. Hyde. The Ernest Hemingway group is the largest, consisting of about 40 percent of drinkers. The famous author was known to brag that he could consume large quantities of alcohol without becoming drunk. Therefore, the Ernest Hemingway group includes drinkers whose personalities do not seem to be altered as they consume enough alcohol to become inebriated. Individuals who are normally extroverts and who become even more sociable when they drink alcohol make up the Mary Poppins group. The Nutty Professor designation refers to the movie character portrayed by Eddie Murphy, who developed a chemically induced alter ego. Typically introverted, they become less inhibited and more effusive and social when they drink. Finally, the Mr. Hydes show a different type of transformation when they drink. Alcohol causes these individuals to become less upstanding and more hostile (Winograd et al., 2016).

As doses increase, a person may still function (although with less coordination) and attempt to drive or otherwise endanger themselves and others. Perceptual speed is markedly impaired by ethanol. At BAC values of about 0.05 to 0.09 grams%, sociability and talkativeness increase, but inhibitions, attention, judgment, and control are decreased; information processing is slowed; and there is loss of efficiency in critical performance testing. As the BAC increases, the drinker becomes progressively more incapacitated. Memory, concentration, and insight are progressively dulled and lost, even though one may remain in a state of wakefulness.

Alcohol intoxication plays a major role in a large percentage of violent crimes, including battery, rape, sexual assault, and certain kinds of deviant behaviors. Indeed, there is a dose-related increase in aggressive responsiveness in both males and females (Duke et al., 2011). Alcohol is implicated in more than half of all homicides and assaults; about 40 percent of violent offenders in jail were drinking at the time of the offense for which they were incarcerated. More than 50 percent of all motor vehicle highway accidents are alcohol related, a number that has changed little in 20 years. Many drinkers develop a type of "alcohol myopia," defined as shortsightedness in which superficially understood, immediate aspects of experience have a disproportionate influence on behavior and emotion (Giancola et al., 2011). Cognitive and attentional deficits cause a focus on the present, reduce fear and anxiety, and impair problem-solving ability. Finally, alcohol use increases concerns with power and dominance, which are linked to male violence generally and to intimate partner interactions in particular. The effect can be an inappropriate sense of mastery, control, or power.

Long-Term Effects on the Brain

It has long been known that chronic alcohol consumption is associated with severe executive function deficits, even after a protracted period of abstinence (Noel et al., 2001). Because executive functions are believed to mediate the suppression of craving and relapse, persistent executive function deficits could affect the capacity to maintain abstinence.

Persistent alcohol use harms adolescents. In the largest prospective study of its kind to date, investigators studied changes in regional brain morphology over time in heavy drinkers compared with nondrinkers. The analysis involved 134 at-risk adolescents (72 percent white; 57 percent male; mean baseline age 15 years) who were interviewed every three months and who underwent magnetic resonance imaging an average of three times (mean follow-up duration, 3.8 years). During the study, 59 participants were continuous nondrinkers and 75 initiated heavy drinking. Those who became heavy drinkers had higher baseline rates of depressive symptoms and childhood conduct disorder. Over the course of the study, heavy drinkers showed greater volume reductions than nondrinkers in frontal, lateral, and—in males only—temporal neocortical gray matter. Growth in corpus callosum and pons white matter was seen in both nondrinkers and heavy drinkers, but was less in heavy drinkers. Concurrent use of other drugs—primarily marijuana—did not significantly alter these findings (Squeglia et al., 2015). Adolescent binge ethanol exposure inhibits the development of new neurons throughout the hippocampus, which might contribute to impaired cognition (Vetreno and Crews, 2015).

Monthly binge drinking in midlife is an independent risk factor, doubling the risk of long-term cognitive impairments later in life (Jyri et al., 2010). Problematic drinking behavior in midlife produces a more rapid cognitive decline than nonproblematic drinking and was associated with severe cognitive impairment in people with low baseline cognitive scores (Kim et al., 2016). At the same time, no evidence was found to support the idea that long-term *moderate* alcohol consumption in older adults exacerbates age-related cognitive decline (Moussa et al., 2015).

Effects on Memory Formation

Alcohol's effects on memory range from mild deficits to alcohol-induced blackouts. Blackouts are of two types: *fragmentary* blackouts (where bits and pieces are remembered and much is not encoded) and *en bloc*, where nothing is remembered. Blackouts occasionally occur at BACs in excess of about 0.14 grams%, becoming more common at BACs of 0.25 to 0.30 grams% (White et al., 2004). Perry and coworkers (2006) obtained a dose-response curve for alcohol-induced blackouts (Figure 5.5). The probability of experiencing blackout at BACs below 0.2 grams% is about 20 percent. At a BAC of about 0.28 to 0.3 grams%, the probability of a blackout is 50 percent or higher. Gender, drinking experience, drinking without eating, the rate at which alcohol is ingested, and gulping of alcohol all predict blackout at lower BACs. Also, some persons may have an inherent neurobiological vulnerability to alcohol-induced memory impairments due to alcohol's effects on contextual memory processes (Wetherill et al., 2012a, 2012b). Importantly, during a blackout, one is still awake and is capable of engaging in complicated and potentially hazardous activities (for example, driving, engaging in sexual activity, etc.) without having memory of having done so, which often leads to adverse legal consequences.

The mechanism responsible for a blackout is usually ascribed to blockade of protein synthesis that is essential for the formation of long-term encoding of memory (Gold, 2008). This state is closely related to organic dementia, in which severe cognitive dysfunction occurs (Lee et al., 2009).

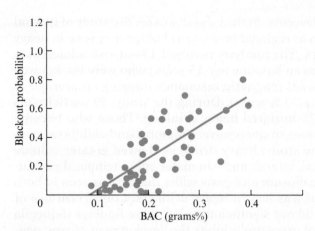

FIGURE 5.5 Probability of blackouts as a function of the blood alcohol concentration (BAC) (grams%, or grams per 100 cc whole blood). [Data from Perry et al., 2006.]

Tolerance, Dependence, and Withdrawal

The patterns and mechanisms for the development of tolerance to and psychological and physical dependence on alcohol are similar to those for other CNS depressants. The extent of tolerance depends on the amount, pattern, and extent of alcohol ingestion. People who ingest alcohol only intermittently on sprees or more regularly but in moderation develop little or no tolerance. People who regularly ingest large amounts of alcohol develop marked tolerance. The tolerance is of three types:

1. *Metabolic tolerance,* whereby the liver increases its amount of drug-metabolizing enzyme. This type accounts for at most 25 percent of the tolerance to alcohol.

2. *Tissue,* or *functional, tolerance,* whereby neurons in the brain adapt to the amount of drug present. Drinkers who develop this type of tolerance characteristically display blood alcohol levels about twice those of nontolerant drinkers at a similar level of behavioral intoxication. Note, however, that despite behavioral adaptation, impairments in cognitive function are similar at similar blood levels in both tolerant and nontolerant drinkers. In other words, at a BAC of 0.15 grams%, both tolerant and nontolerant drinkers display marked deficits in insight, judgment, cognition, and other executive functions. The tolerant person may just *appear* less intoxicated.

3. *Associative, contingent,* or *homeostatic tolerance.* A variety of environmental manipulations can counter the effects of ethanol; counterresponses are a possible mechanism of tolerance.

After physical dependence develops, withdrawal of alcohol results in a period of rebound hyperexcitability within hours that may eventually lead to convulsions, which could be life threatening. Alcohol abuse is one of the most common causes of adult-onset seizures; seizures occur in about 10 percent of adults during alcohol withdrawal. The period of seizure activity is relatively short, usually 6 hours or less, but seizures can be very severe. Blocking seizure activity during withdrawal is a major goal of detoxification and usually involves two classes of agents: the benzodiazepines and the anticonvulsants. A "kindling" model of alcohol withdrawal seizures suggests that repeated alcohol withdrawals may lead to an increase in the severity of subsequent withdrawals and a greater likelihood of withdrawal seizures with each detoxification. Indeed, the number of detoxifications is an important variable in the predisposition to withdrawal seizures. Using this concept, Malcolm and coworkers (2000) postulated that repeated detoxifications might also cause neurobehavioral alterations that affect alcohol craving. Patients who had experienced multiple detoxifications had higher scores on tests that measure obsessive thoughts about alcohol, drink urges, and drinking behaviors. Thus, recurrent detoxifications may lead to increased rates of relapse due to a "kindling" of behaviors and thoughts leading to a compulsion to return to drinking. The researchers added that the kindling effect persists despite treatment with benzodiazepines or other traditional sedative-hypnotic drugs. In fact, the medical management of alcohol detoxification may be better achieved with anticonvulsant "mood stabilizers" (see Chapter 14) than with benzodiazepines (Becker et al., 2006; Martinotti et al., 2010).

In addition to withdrawal seizures, the alcohol withdrawal syndrome can include tremulousness with hallucinations, psychomotor agitation, confusion and disorientation, sleep disorders, and a variety of associated discomforts. This syndrome is sometimes referred to as *delirium tremens* (DTs).

Toxicity

Although many adverse actions associated with alcohol have already been mentioned, abuse may cause additional problems. Acute use may produce a *reversible drug-induced dementia,* manifested as a clouded sensorium with disorientation, impaired insight and judgment, anterograde amnesia (blackouts), and diminished intellectual capabilities.

With increasing doses (or blood levels) of alcohol, a person's affect may become labile, with emotional outbursts precipitated by otherwise innocuous events. With higher doses, delusions and hallucinations may occur. In social situations, these alterations result in unpredictable states of disinhibition (drunkenness), deterioration in driving performance, and uncoordinated motor behavior. As stated earlier, only at very high doses (perhaps at BACs of 0.4 grams% and greater) is consciousness lost and a state of "anesthesia" with immobilization occurs. At this point, respiration becomes shallow and death can result.

Liver damage is a serious long-term physiological consequence of excessive alcohol consumption. Irreversible changes in both the structure and the function of the liver are common. For example, ethanol produces active oxidants during its metabolism by hepatocytes, which results in oxidative stress on liver cells. Seventy-five percent of all deaths attributed to alcoholism are caused by cirrhosis of the liver, and cirrhosis is the seventh most common cause of death in the United States.

Long-term alcohol ingestion may irreversibly cause the *destruction of nerve cells,* producing a permanent brain syndrome with dementia called *Korsakoff's syndrome.*

More subtle and persistent cognitive deficits may be present whether or not a diagnosis of Korsakoff's syndrome is made. This condition is termed *alcohol dementia* and it can involve long-term problems with memory, learning, and other cognitive skills. The *digestive system* may also be affected. *Pancreatitis* (inflammation of the pancreas) and *chronic gastritis* (inflammation of the stomach), with the development of peptic ulcers, may occur.

As noted, chronic excessive alcohol consumption is a major risk factor for *cancer* in humans. A recent statement from the American Society of Clinical Oncology (LoConte, et al., 2018) notes that 5.5 percent of all new cancer occurrences and 5.8 percent of all cancer deaths worldwide are attributed to alcohol ingestion. Heavy, long-term use holds the greatest risk. Alcohol is causally associated with oropharyngeal and larynx cancer, esophageal cancer, liver cancer, breast cancer, and colon cancer. Indeed, between 2006 and 2010, 88,000 deaths in the United States resulted from alcohol. Worldwide, about 3.3 million deaths are yearly attributable to alcohol use. Even when ethanol use alone may not be strongly carcinogenic, it appears to be a cancer promoter. For example, the risk of head and neck cancers for heavy drinkers who also smoke cigarettes is up to 15 times greater than for those who abstain from both. The risk of throat cancer is 44 times greater for heavy users of both alcohol and tobacco than for nonusers.

Teratogenic Effects

For years, we have known that alcohol is both a physical and a behavioral teratogen. *Fetal alcohol syndrome* (FAS) is a devastating developmental disorder that occurs in the offspring of mothers who have high blood levels of alcohol during critical stages of fetal development; it affects as many as 30 to 50 percent of infants born to alcoholic women. Alcohol abuse during pregnancy appears to be the most frequent known teratogenic cause of intellectual disability.

Sayal and coworkers (2009) noted that binge drinking, even in the absence of regular ingestion of alcohol, increased the risk of childhood mental health problems, primarily related to hyperactivity and inattention problems. Kot-Leibovich and Fainsod (2009) noted that alcohol interferes with the biosynthesis of retinoic acid, which is required for normal brain development. Because subtle intellectual and behavioral effects of low-level alcohol consumption may go unnoticed, no safe level of alcohol intake during pregnancy has been established and there is no threshold level of alcohol ingestion that triggers fetal alcohol syndrome (Feldman et al., 2012). Features of the full fetal alcohol syndrome include the following:

- CNS dysfunction, including microcephaly (reduced cranial circumference), mental retardation, and behavioral abnormalities (often presenting as hyperactivity and difficulty with social integration)
- Retarded body growth rate (fetal growth retardation)
- Facial abnormalities (short palpebral fissures, short nose, wide-set eyes, and small cheekbones)
- Other anatomical abnormalities (for example, congenital heart defects and malformed eyes and ears)

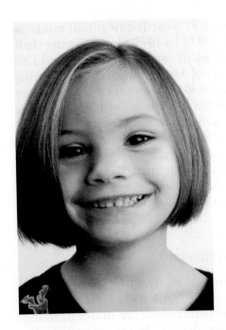

Young girl with mild symptoms of Fetal Alcohol Disorder. [Rick's Photography/Shutterstock]

In the United States, an estimated 2.6 million infants are born annually following significant in utero alcohol exposure. Many display the full features of FAS and about 1 newborn out of every 100 live births displays a lesser degree of damage, termed *fetal alcohol effects*, perhaps more correctly termed *alcohol-related neurodevelopmental disorder* (ARND). Taken together, the combined rate of FAS and ARND is estimated to be at least 9 per 1000 live births. Alcohol ingestion is thus the third leading cause of birth defects with associated intellectual disability; it is the only one that is preventable.

Although the structural abnormalities and growth retardation of FAS are well described, the behavioral and cognitive effects of prenatal alcohol exposure are less appreciated. Intelligence quotient (IQ), attention, learning, memory, language, and motor and visuospatial activities are impaired in children prenatally exposed to varying amounts of alcohol (Sayal et al., 2009). Medina (2011) discusses alcohol-induced learning and memory disorders in offspring of women who drank through the third trimester of pregnancy. This is a period during which the fetal brain goes through a period of fast growth ("brain growth spurt") and neurons are more susceptible to alcohol exposure. Here, depression of synaptogenesis and interference with brain "wiring" may lead to persistent deficits in neuronal plasticity.

In a study in Finland, Autti-Ramo (2000) followed 70 children with fetal alcohol exposure (42 with recognized cognitive and other deficits, 10 with physical growth restrictions only, and 18 classified as normal). They were assessed at age 12 for psychosocial well-being. The longer the alcohol exposure during pregnancy, the more likely the child was to have significant cognitive and social impairments. Of the 42 children with early recognition of cognitive deficits, 29 (69 percent) were in permanent foster or institutional care. Even among the children in the normal and growth-restricted groups, 10 (36 percent) were temporarily or permanently in alternative care. Behavioral problems were significant.

Baer and coworkers (2003) reported results of a 21-year longitudinal study in which they followed offspring of 500 women who, in 1974 to 1975, drank during their pregnancies (30 percent were binge drinkers). Offspring of two women displayed FAS and 31 offspring were identified as having components of ARND. When these offspring attained the age of 21, 11 percent of their mothers and 21 percent of their fathers were identified as having had a history of alcohol problems. The offspring of mothers who were binge drinkers during pregnancy exhibited three times the likelihood of at least mild alcohol dependence than did offspring of mothers who did not drink alcohol during their pregnancy (14.1 versus 4.5 percent).

The prevention of FAS and ARND obviously involves abstinence from alcohol by women who are, plan to become, or are capable of becoming pregnant. Screening questionnaires may be effective in helping to protect not only the unborn infant but also the long-term health of the mother.

Alcoholism and Its Pharmacological Treatment

The recognition of alcoholism as a multifaceted *medical and behavioral* disorder is relatively recent. In 1935, Alcoholics Anonymous was founded on a *moral model* of alcoholism; it offered a spiritual and behavioral framework for understanding, accepting, and recovering from the compulsion to use alcohol. In the late 1950s, the American Medical Association recognized the syndrome of alcoholism as an illness. In the mid-1970s, alcoholism was redefined as a *chronic, progressive, and potentially fatal disease.* In 1992, the description was expanded to acknowledge the genetic, psychosocial, and environmental contributions, and the impaired control over drinking despite negative consequences.

Several factors promote the development of alcoholism. One of the most important is drinking at an early age, especially binge drinking (Rohde et al., 2001). The National Institute on Alcohol Abuse and Alcoholism defines binge drinking as a pattern of drinking that brings a person's blood alcohol concentration (BAC) to 0.08 grams percent or above. This typically happens when men consume five or more drinks and women consume four or more drinks in about 2 hours. In contrast, moderate drinking is no more than one drink per day for women and no more than two drinks per day for men, translating to seven or fewer drinks per week for women and 14 or fewer drinks per week for men.

A second important factor in the development of alcoholism is *self-medication* of psychological distress. That is, some, if not many, alcoholics may have first used alcohol and become psychologically dependent on the drug as a self-prescribed medication to treat another, primary, disorder. Moreover, early-onset ethanol drinkers are more likely to use alcohol as a "stress reducer" than are drinkers who begin drinking at a later age (Dawson et al., 2007). Goodwin and Gabrielli (1997) stated that 30 to 50 percent of alcoholics meet criteria for major depression. People who suffer from depression have double the risk of alcohol abuse and dependence as people who don't. In bipolar disorder, the risk of an alcohol use disorder is six to seven times higher. Some antidepressants may be more dangerous than others when combined with alcohol. For example, bupropion may be preferred by patients because it has minimal sexual side effects. But when combined with alcohol, bupropion can increase the likelihood of a seizure. An older category of antidepressants, the monoamine oxidase inhibitors (MAOIs), is especially risky if combined with alcohol. Alcohol contains variable amounts of tyramine, a natural substance also found in fermented foods like aged cheese and cured meats that, when combined with MAOIs, could cause a dangerous increase in blood pressure (Petrow, 2016).

Approximately, 33 percent of alcohol drinkers have a coexisting anxiety disorder, many have antisocial personalities, some are schizophrenic (see Green et al., 2015 and commentaries), and many (36 percent) are addicted to other drugs. Kushner and coworkers (Kushner et al., 2011, 2012; Menary et al., 2011) discussed the comorbidity of current anxiety disorders and the development of alcoholism. Drinking behavior is negatively reinforced when alcohol temporarily reduces anxiety and the resulting escalation of drinking increases the risk for the development of anxiety disorders. Further, persons with anxiety disorders transition from regular drinking to alcohol dependence more rapidly than do persons without anxiety disorders.

As many as 38 percent of alcohol-dependent patients demonstrate impulse control problems. The co-occurrence of pathologic gambling (one type of impulse control disorder) was associated with a younger age of onset of alcohol dependence, a higher number of detoxifications, and a longer duration of dependence. Frye and Salloum (2006) discuss the co-occurrence of alcoholism and bipolar disorder. An overwhelmingly positive association exists between alcohol use disorder and personality disorders, especially antisocial, histrionic, and dependent disorders (Grant et al., 2004). Finally, as many as 31 percent of heavy drinkers over the age of 12 years are using illicit drugs. *Dual diagnosis* (or *comorbid illness*) must always be considered with alcohol use disorders (Tiet and Mausbach, 2007).

Pharmacotherapies for Alcohol Abuse and Dependence

According to the results of the 2015 National Survey of Drug Use and Health, 15.1 million adults (6.2 percent of those 18 years or older) had alcohol use disorder. However, only 6.7 percent of this group received treatment (NIH, 2017). Combined data from 2009 to 2012 from the National Survey on Drug Use and Health revealed why so many alcohol-dependent persons have not sought treatment. Of the survey respondents who recognized they were alcohol dependent and knew they needed treatment for their alcohol problem, almost 50 percent did not seek treatment because they were simply not ready to completely stop drinking. This is the group that might benefit most by a "harm reduction" approach (SAMHSA, 2012). Support for harm reduction comes from the evidence that alcohol-associated mortality risk increases exponentially as per diem consumption of alcohol rises above the hazardous drinking threshold. The U.S. public health official definition of hazardous drinking for men is 5 drink equivalents a day or 15 a week; for women, the threshold is 4 drink equivalents a day or 8 per week. According to estimates of Nutt and Rehm (2014), a decrease in consumption from 100 to 50 grams of daily alcohol would reduce health harms eightfold.

In other words, although eliminating alcohol ingestion is an obviously effective therapeutic goal for treating alcoholism, achieving success is extremely difficult. Over 20 years ago, Vaillant (1996) performed a remarkable 50-year follow-up of two cohorts of men who began abusing alcohol at an early age. One group consisted of university undergraduates; the second consisted of nondelinquent inner-city adolescents. By 60 years of age, 18 percent of the college alcohol abusers had died, 11 percent were abstinent, 11 percent were controlled drinkers, and 60 percent were still abusing alcohol. By 60 years of age, 28 percent of the inner-city alcohol abusers had died, 30 percent were abstinent, 12 percent were controlled drinkers, and 30 percent were still abusing alcohol.

The ideal goals of pharmacotherapy for alcohol dependence and abuse include

- Reversal of the acute pharmacologic effects of alcohol
- Treatment and prevention of withdrawal symptoms and complications, including limitation of neuronal injury during detoxification
- Maintenance of abstinence, prevention of relapse, or reduction in the number of active drinking days
- Treatment of coexisting psychiatric disorders

At this time, no agent can reverse the acute pharmacologic effects of alcohol (Akbar, et al., 2017). Acute alcohol intoxication is usually treated with supportive care and a quiet environment to protect both the intoxicated person and others at risk of injury. Some feel that caffeine can antagonize alcohol intoxication and increase alertness. Caffeine, however, does not reverse the intoxicating effects of alcohol. As a behavioral stimulant, caffeine can only increase activity, not reverse the motor, cognitive, or other dysfunctions induced by alcohol. This has practical implications in regard to the prevalent consumption of energy drinks (Chapter 6). In analyses limited to youth who ever drank alcohol, consumption of energy drinks within the past seven days was significantly associated with a higher likelihood of ever mixing energy drinks and alcohol (27 versus 7 percent) (Edmund et al., 2014). Unfortunately, combining energy drinks with alcohol increases people's desire to keep drinking more than if they drank alcohol alone (McKetin and Coen, 2014).

Pharmacotherapies for Management of Alcohol Withdrawal

The major therapeutic goal of managing acute alcohol withdrawal or detoxification is to prevent uncontrolled excitation by either reducing glutamate activity or increasing GABA activity. Classically, this has been achieved through use of either benzodiazepines (see Chapter 13) or anticonvulsant medications (see Chapter 14).

Benzodiazepines.   When alcohol ingestion is stopped, withdrawal symptoms begin within a few hours. Substituting a long-acting benzodiazepine prevents or suppresses the withdrawal symptoms and is then either maintained at a level low enough to allow the person to function or is withdrawn gradually. Their use, however, is restricted to only a few days or perhaps a month because of the potential for developing physical dependence on these drugs. Preferred drugs are the benzodiazepines with long-acting active metabolites—*chlordiazepoxide* (Librium) or *diazepam* (Valium) (Amato et al., 2011). Acute seizure activity can be controlled with the faster-onset, shorter-acting benzodiazepine, lorazepam.

Anticonvulsant Mood Stabilizers. The benzodiazepines have important limitations when used for the treatment of alcohol withdrawal: sedation, psychomotor impairments, additive interactions with alcohol, and the potential for abuse and dependence. Because seizures are common in acute alcohol withdrawal, the use of an antiepileptic drug seems intuitively appropriate. Although older anticonvulsants have significant limitations that can be deleterious in alcoholics (contributing to liver and pancreatic problems, for example), they have historically been shown to be effective. Examples include *carbamazepine* (Tegretol) and *valproic acid* (Depakote); their use, however, is limited by adverse effects on the liver. Newer anticonvulsants are much less liver toxic and include *gabapentin* (Neurontin), *pregabalin* (Lyrica), *oxcarbazepine* (Trileptal), *lamotrigine* (Lamictal), and *topiramate* (Topamax). Leggio and coworkers (2008) reviewed such use; Guglielmo and coworkers (2012) recently studied the efficacy of pregabalin for alcohol withdrawal syndrome. Rubio and coworkers (2006) and Krupitsky and coworkers (2007) reported on the efficacy of *lamotrigine* (Lamictal) to improve mood, decrease alcohol craving, and decrease alcohol consumption while reducing glutamate release and presumably exerting "brain protection" during alcohol withdrawal in patients with alcoholism.

Pharmacotherapies to Help Maintain Abstinence and Prevent Relapse

The FDA has approved three medications specifically for the treatment of alcohol dependence: disulfiram, naltrexone, and acamprosate. In addition, five drugs are commonly used off-label to help patients with alcohol use disorder: nalmefene (an opiate antagonist related to drugs like naltrexone), baclofen (a GABA_B agonist), gabapentin (an anticonvulsant), ondansetron (a serotonin type-3 antagonist), and topiramate (an anticonvulsant). Yet, even in well-controlled clinical trials, most of these drugs have only modest effects (Soyka and Müller, 2017).

Nevertheless, even modest improvement may be better than the best nonpharmacological clinical approach. Saitz and coworkers (2013) looked at how chronic care management (CCM) affected abstinence results in people with alcohol and other drug dependence. CCM involved benefits such as coordinated long-term care, motivational enhancement therapy, counseling for relapse prevention, and inclusive psychiatric, addiction, and social work support, with referrals. The alternate, control, group was given an appointment for primary care and a list of treatment resources with a phone number for scheduling counseling. The CCM and control groups did not differ in abstinence from stimulants, opioids, or heavy drinking (44 compared to 42 percent). Even secondary measures such as severity of addiction, drug difficulties, or quality of life did not show any significant differences. In people who suffered from drug and alcohol dependence, a comparison of CCM with treatment consisting of a primary care appointment but no CCM showed no improvement of abstinence after one year.

Disulfiram (Antabuse), available for over 60 years, produces an aversive reaction if the patient drinks. Disulfiram alters the metabolism of alcohol by inhibiting the liver enzyme needed to metabolize alcohol, aldehyde dehydrogenase, which causes the metabolite *acetaldehyde* to accumulate (see Figure 5.1). If the patient ingests alcohol within several days of taking this drug, the accumulation results in an acetaldehyde syndrome, characterized by flushing, throbbing headache, nausea, vomiting, chest pain, unstable blood pressure, and other miserable symptoms. However, controlled trials of disulfiram therapy to reduce alcohol consumption have been disappointing (Elbreder et al., 2010).

In one study by the U.S. Veterans Administration, 605 subjects were randomized into 3 groups. One group received a standard 250 milligram per day dose of disulfiram, one group received an inactive 1 milligram per day dose of disulfiram, and one group received riboflavin. The percentage of participants did not differ in time to first drink or in abstinence. Subjects given 250 milligrams per day, compared with the other groups, drank for fewer days after relapse. In very old subjects or those with comorbid medical conditions, medical reactions to disulfiram can be serious (Robinson et al., 2014).

A common reason that patients give for relapsing while on disulfiram is anxiety. That led Bogenschutz and coworkers (2016) to study the coadministration of the benzodiazepine *lorazepam* (Ativan) and disulfiram. Although lorazepam appeared to be a safe and effective treatment for anxiety in patients with AUD who were already taking disulfiram, adherence to disulfiram was a problem; only 26 of the original group of 41 patients were available for follow-up at 16 weeks.

Opiate Antagonists.   Opiate antagonists are believed to work by blocking the effects of the endogenous opiates that are released as a result of the rewarding effect of drinking alcohol; that is, they reduce the pleasurable effect of alcohol. Some evidence suggests that this approach works best if the antagonist is taken relatively soon (such as 1 hour) before the individual expects to drink alcohol. If taken a long time before drinking starts, the opiate blocker may not be able to interrupt the rewarding effects of alcohol.

Naltrexone is an opiate antagonist that was approved for treating alcoholism in oral formulation (as ReVia) by the FDA in 1984 and (as Vivitrol*)* in 2006, when it was approved as a once-a-month depot injectable. Naltrexone was an effective antirelapse treatment for alcoholism for brief 12-week intervals in a meta-analysis of 24 controlled randomized clinical trials ($n = 2861$). A large study—combined pharmacotherapies and behavioral interventions for alcohol dependence (COMBINE)—conducted at multiple locations ($n = 1383$) found that a dose of 100 milligrams per day, together with medical treatment, was better than a placebo over 16 weeks in increasing the percent of abstinent days from 75.1 to 80.6, and decreasing the percentage of individuals reporting heavy drinking from 73 to 66.2 percent (Robinson et al., 2014). Patients with a family history of alcohol abuse disorder, strong cravings, and a "sweet tooth" may benefit most from naltrexone (Garbutt et al., 2016). Common side effects, if they occur, appear early in therapy and include nausea, vomiting, abdominal pain, headache, and fatigue. High dosages, 100 to 300 milligrams daily, may be toxic to the liver, but when naltrexone is discontinued, recovery may occur. Ongoing use of opiates is contraindicated with naltrexone treatment because naltrexone's antagonism of opiate receptors will block opioid analgesia. A reduction in the number of daily drinks and heavy drinking days relative to placebo may occur with injected naltrexone. For patients who do not follow oral dosing instructions, injectable naltrexone has the benefit of efficacy during its prolonged steady-state drug release. Except for pain and irritation at the injection site, the side effects are comparable to oral naltrexone (Robinson et al., 2014).

The U.S. Food and Drug Administration (FDA) has not approved the naltrexone *implant*, which is surgically inserted under the skin and left in place for 2 to 6 months, but one study found this formulation to be cost effective for reduced hospitalization for at least six months after implantation (Kelty et al., 2014).

Despite evidence of effectiveness, not all studies have yielded positive results and the effect is small (Hackl-Herrwerth et al., 2010; O'Malley et al., 2015). It has been noted, however, that there are many more heavy drinkers who are not dependent as there are dependent drinkers. Heavy drinkers are less likely to choose abstinence; they will prefer moderation. And that amount of harm reduction is achievable with the current drugs (Hester, 2015).

Some research has been done with a naltrexone derivative called *nalmefene* (Revex; Selincro). Like naltrexone, nalmefene is an antagonist at the mu and delta opiate receptors, but nalmefene also is a partial agonist at the kappa opioid receptor. In a preclinical European study of nalmefene tablets taken each day of perceived alcohol craving (*as needed*), the results indicated a modest decrease of heavy drinking days (compared with placebo) over the six-month trial period (Mann et al., 2013). Dropout rates were quite high. Nalmefene was approved for an unusual "as-needed" indication (within Europe) that places control of treatment with the patient. If a patient is concerned that they may drink or has already begun to drink, one 18 milligram tablet should be taken immediately. Regulators granted this approval on the basis of results from three clinical trials in Europe, which demonstrated that this use of nalmefene by heavy drinkers, produced a more normal amount of alcohol consumption. The implication of this approval is that the strategy of harm reduction is effective (Jancin, 2015; Paille and Martini, 2014). Published studies show very limited benefit. In one case, nalmefene was more effective than placebo only after 13 months (van den Brink et al., 2014), while a systematic review found no value (Palpacuer et al., 2015). Other reports found nalmefene to be cost effective (Laramée et al., 2014) and to produce a clinically relevant decrease in mortality risk (Roerecke et al., 2015). The manufacturer has stated that the company would not seek marketing approval for nalmefene in the United States because the drug's remaining duration of patent protection makes it commercially nonviable.

Acamprosate. *Acamprosate* (Campral), approved by the FDA in 1984 for use in the treatment of alcoholism, was the first pharmacologic agent specifically designed to maintain abstinence in ethanol-dependent people after detoxification. The drug is thought to exert both a GABA-agonistic action at GABA receptors and an inhibitory action at glutaminergic NMDA receptors. It appears to act in the CNS to restore the normal activity of glutaminergic neurotransmission altered by chronic alcohol exposure (Mason and Heyser, 2010).

Spanagel and coworkers (2014), however, have provided evidence from animal models and humans that acamprosate does not interact with glutamate receptor mechanisms. They propose that acamprosate itself is biologically inactive and that its antirelapse effects are due to a calcium component of the chemical compound.

Acamprosate is poorly absorbed orally and is, therefore, given in relatively high doses (about 2 grams per day). It has a half-life of about 18 hours and is excreted unchanged by the kidneys; it is not metabolized before excretion. Diarrhea is the most common side effect of acamprosate; nervousness, fatigue, insomnia, and depression have been reported with high dosages.

In early human studies, acamprosate was thought to be about three times as effective as placebo, with drinking frequency reduced by 30 to 50 percent. Today, it is thought perhaps to be comparable to naltrexone, with efficacy increased by adding the drug to established, abstinence-based, cognitive-behavioral rehabilitation programs, or by combining the drug with naltrexone. In both situations, naltrexone and acamprosate, although less than impressive individually, can be effective when used together and/or added to intensive psychotherapies. Coadministration of acamprosate and naltrexone significantly increased the rate and extent of absorption of acamprosate, as indicated by a 33 percent increase in acamprosate blood level and a 33 percent reduction in time to peak blood level. Acamprosate did not affect the pharmacokinetics of naltrexone. Thus, when using the two drugs in combination, the dose of acamprosate, although poorly absorbed orally, can be reduced by 33 percent. Used alone in the treatment of alcohol dependence, acamprosate has had limited efficacy (Rosner et al., 2010).

In a systematic review in the *Journal of the American Medical Association* (*JAMA*), researchers examined over 120 studies of medications used for alcohol use disorders. Some 23,000 patients were enrolled, most after detoxification or a period of sobriety.

According to the study, "Both acamprosate and oral naltrexone were associated with reduction in return to drinking. When directly compared with one another, no significant differences were found between acamprosate and naltrexone for controlling alcohol consumption. Factors such as dosing frequency, potential adverse events, and availability of treatments may guide medication choice" (Jonas et al., 2014).

Baclofen.   Baclofen (Lioresal) has been available since the late 1970s for the treatment of neuromuscular spasticity. It is an agonist of the GABA$_B$ receptor. In alcohol use disorder, GABA transmission is downregulated, which is why medications under development for AUD often target the GABA transmitter. Studies during the late 1970s showed some efficacy in treating alcoholism. More recent studies produced mixed results, but that might be due to the fact that doses were too low. Very high doses, up to 270 milligrams per day, were reported to have efficacy in reducing craving and promoting abstinence from alcohol (Muzyk et al., 2012; Pastor et al., 2012; Rigal et al., 2012; Robinson et al., 2014). But this was not the case in a multicenter, double-blind, placebo-controlled trial involving 151 patients randomly assigned to high-dose baclofen (starting at a low dose and increasing to 150 mg/day), low-dose baclofen (30 mg/day), or placebo over 16 weeks. At the end of the trial, researchers found no difference in relapse rates among the three groups. In each group, about 25 percent of participants relapsed. Together, these studies indicate that baclofen may be as effective as psychosocial care, but does not seem to increase effectiveness further (Beraha et al., 2016). Baclofen is a generally safe medication with relatively mild side effects and without a risk for abuse. The adverse reactions most commonly reported are fatigue, nausea, vertigo, sleepiness, and abdominal pain (Robinson et al., 2014).

Gabapentin.   The FDA has approved gabapentin as an anticonvulsant for epilepsy and postherpetic neuralgia. Chemically similar to GABA, gabapentin may increase GABA activity in the CNS, antagonize glutamate activity, and decrease norepinephrine and dopamine release (Robinson et al., 2014). Doses of gabapentin between 400 to 1600 milligrams per day are typically safe and tolerated well. There is some evidence that gabapentin may reduce cravings and alcohol consumption, delay relapse, and improve sleep in those with AUD. It has been proposed that gabapentin may balance the GABA or glutamate dysregulation that has been reported in early alcohol abstinence which, in turn, may decrease the risk of relapse. In clinical trials, measures of abstinence and reduced heavy drinking were found at doses of 600 to 1800 milligrams per day (Furieri and Nakamura-Palacios, 2007; Mason, 2014). When up to 1200 milligrams of gabapentin were combined with 50 milligrams of naltrexone per day, results over a 6-week period were better than naltrexone plus placebo or double placebo on heavy drinking time, number of heavy drinking days, and number of drinks per day (Anton et al., 2011). Some of these effects may have been due to gabapentin's positive effects on sleep. In patients with severe liver disease or who may be likely to drink during detoxification, gabapentin is a safe alternative to benzodiazepines. Gabapentin's side effects include daytime sedation, dizziness, ataxia, fatigue, and dyspepsia (Robinson et al., 2014).

Topiramate.   FDA-approved indications for topiramate include migraine headaches and some seizure disorders. Certain glutamate receptor subtypes are blocked by the drug, while GABAergic neuronal inhibition is facilitated (Florez et al., 2011). As an anticonvulsant, topiramate is helpful in the treatment of alcohol withdrawal syndrome and, as an agent for anxiolytic, antirelapse and antianger therapy, the drug is useful in long-term alcoholism therapy. Relative to placebo, as much as 300 milligrams of topiramate a day was better at reducing the number of heavy drinking days and the number of drinks per day, and at alleviating cravings and increasing the number of abstinent days. Compared with placebo, topiramate increased "safe drinking" in a three-month trial, defined as less than 1 standard drink for women per day and less than 2 standard drinks per day for men. The drug can be given while the patient is drinking as well as through the withdrawal and maintenance phases (Johnson and Ait-Daoud, 2011). Impaired memory and concentration are the main side effects (Likhitsathian et al., 2012), but cognitive problems may be prevented by increasing doses very slowly and perhaps by keeping doses lower than 300 milligrams per day (Otto, 2014). Rapid titration or high dosage may also induce paresthesia and anorexia. Possible side effects include metabolic acidosis, kidney stones, and narrow-angle glaucoma. The teratogenic effects of cleft lip and palate preclude administration to pregnant women or in any woman of childbearing age. Because topiramate is renally excreted, doses should be reduced in patients with renal impairment.

DeSousa (2010) compares topiramate with other anticonvulsants for use in the treatment of alcoholism. Furthermore, and consistent with previous trials, Knapp and coworkers (2015) found both anticonvulsants zonisamide and topiramate reduced ethanol intake on three measures of alcohol consumption: percent days drinking per week, drinks consumed per day, and percent days heavy drinking per week. In this study, the anticonvulsant levetiracetam was also found to significantly reduce the percent days heavy drinking. Treatment with either topiramate or zonisamide was associated with increased difficulty with verbal fluency and verbal working memory; impairment of visual memory was detected in the topiramate but not the zonisamide group.

Serotonergic Agents

Pettinati and coworkers (2010) studied the combination of sertraline (an SSRI) and naltrexone in 170 depressed, alcohol-dependent patients. Patients also received weekly cognitive-behavioral therapy. In a 14-week trial, the combination was successful in producing abstinence from alcohol in a greater number of patients (53 percent) than either drug alone (about 23 to 27 percent) or placebo (23 percent). There was also a strong trend for major reductions in depressive symptomatology. Buspirone appears to be less effective, being no better than placebo (Kenna, 2010). Research continues into subtypes of alcoholics, especially age-of-onset subtypes who may be differentially sensitive to SSRIs (Kranzler et al., 2012).

Some positive results for AUD have been reported for the serotonin type-3 (5-HT3) receptor antagonist *ondansetron* (Zofran). 5-HT3 receptors may be a locus for alcohol effects in the brain, especially in its rewarding effects. In two clinical trials, ondansetron was found to be effective for *early onset alcoholism* (EOA). Early onset alcoholism is defined as alcoholism that develops by age 25 or earlier and is associated with a strong family history of AUD and notable antisocial traits. In the first trial conducted with 271 participants with EOA, researchers found a twice-daily dose of 4 micrograms per kilogram (mcg/kg) of ondansetron was better than placebo for reducing cravings and number of drinks per day, and increasing the number of abstinent days (Johnson et al., 2000). In the second trial, conducted with 321 participants with EOA at 16 mcg/kg twice daily, the intensity of symptoms of fatigue, confusion, and general emotional distress, such as depression, anxiety, and hostility, was significantly less than with placebo (Johnson et al., 2003). The common side effects of ondansetron include constipation or diarrhea, increased liver enzymes, tachycardia, headache, and fatigue. Conditions such as congenital long QT syndrome, risk of QTc prolongation, or major liver problems are contraindications (Robinson et al., 2014).

COMBINE Study

Treatment for alcohol dependence may include medications, behavioral therapies, or both. To understand how combining these treatments may impact effectiveness, a large, placebo-controlled study (1383 recently alcohol-abstinent volunteers in 11 treatment sites) was designed—the combined pharmacotherapies and behavioral interventions for alcohol dependence (COMBINE) study. In different combinations, two medications (oral naltrexone and acamprosate) and two behavioral interventions (medical management, or MM, and combined behavioral intervention, or CBI) were employed.

All treatment groups showed substantial reductions in drinking (Anton et al., 2006). Unexpectedly, acamprosate showed no evidence of efficacy. MM with naltrexone, CBI, or both fared better than placebo on drinking outcomes (percent days abstinent from alcohol and time to first heavy drinking day).

More recent studies (Gueorguieva et al., 2011, 2012; Prisciandaro et al., 2012) have added little to the previous COMBINE results.

Although current medications for alcoholism are only modestly effective, there are a few new options under investigation. One phase 2 trial examined the effectiveness of a vasopressin receptor 1B antagonist, which has anxiolytic activity and decreased alcohol intake in animal models, but the results were unimpressive (Ryan et al., 2017).

Although ketamine has approved indications for use in anesthesia and analgesia, it is also abused as a recreational drug (Chapter 7). Preliminary evidence indicated that alcoholics might be more likely to remain abstinent if treated with ketamine in addition to psychotherapy. A pilot study found that 3 doses of ketamine plus psychotherapy reduced average 12-month relapse rates to 34 from 76 percent. Scientists think ketamine's antidepressant properties may have helped. In the United Kingdom, scientists are looking for 96 individuals diagnosed with severe alcohol use disorder and who are "recently abstinent" to volunteer for research into a new therapy. For three weeks, one group (50 percent) will receive a weekly low-dose ketamine injection in addition to seven 1.5-hour psychotherapy sessions. The other group will be injected with saline over the same treatment period (Kelland, 2016). (For background information on this approach and an update see McAndrew et al., 2017.)

INHALANTS OF ABUSE

Inhalants are breathable chemical vapors that produce psychoactive (mind-altering) effects. They are among the most toxic and lethal of abused substances.[7] Inhalant abuse (also known as *huffing, sniffing,* or *bagging*) is the intentional inhalation of a volatile substance for the purposes of achieving an altered mental state (Williams et al., 2007). Although other abused substances can be inhaled (for example, nicotine, THC, cocaine, methamphetamine), the term *inhalants* is used to describe a variety of substances whose main common characteristic is that they are rarely, if ever, taken by any route other than inhalation. A variety of products common to the home and the workplace contain substances that can be inhaled. A few were developed as general anesthetics; examples include nitrous oxide and halothane. These anesthetics were never meant to be used to achieve a "recreational" intoxicating effect. Likewise, other agents were developed for home and industrial use and were never intended to be used to affect the mind. Table 5.1 lists many of the commonly encountered inhalants of abuse.

Not included in Table 5.1 are the *nitrites,* a special class of inhalants. Although other inhalants are used to alter mood, the nitrites are used primarily as sexual enhancers. Formerly, one nitrite (amyl nitrite) was used to dilate veins and reduce the workload of the heart; it relieved chest pain associated with coronary artery disease. Today, amyl nitrite is infrequently used for this purpose. Other nitrites (isobutyl nitrite

---

[7] See www.inhalants.com, sponsored by the National Inhalant Prevention Coalition.

TABLE 5.1 Chemicals commonly found in inhalants

	Inhalant	Chemical
Adhesives	Airplane glue	Toluene, ethyl acetate
	Other glues	Hexane, toluene, methyl chloride, acetone,
	Special cements	methyl ethyl ketone, methyl butyl ketone
		Trichloroethylene, tetrachloroethylene
Aerosols	Spray paint	Butane, propane (U.S.), fluorocarbons,
	Hair spray	toluene, hydrocarbons, "Texas shoe shine"
	Deodorant, air freshener	(a spray containing toluene)
	Analgesic spray	Butane, propane (U.S.), chlorofluorocarbons (CFCs)
	Asthma spray	Butane, propane (U.S.), CFCs
	Fabric spray	CFCs
	PC cleaner	CFCs
		Butane, trichloroethane
		Dimethyl ether, hydrofluorocarbons
Anesthetics	Gas	Nitrous oxide
	Liquid	Halothane, enflurane
	Local	Ethyl chloride
Cleaning agents	Dry cleaning	Tetrachloroethylene, trichloroethane
	Spot remover	Xylene, petroleum distillates,
	Degreaser	chlorohydrocarbons
		Tetrachloroethylene, trichloroethane,
		trichloroethylene
Solvents and gases	Nail-polish remover	Acetone, ethyl acetate
	Paint remover	Toluene, methyl chloride, methanol
	Paint thinner	acetone, ethyl acetate
	Correction fluid and thinner	Petroleum distillates, esters, acetone
	Fuel gas	Trichloroethylene, trichloroethane
	Lighter fluid	Butane, isopropane
	Fire extinguisher	Butane, isopropane
		Bromochlorodifluoromethane
Aerosol whipped cream canisters		Nitrous oxide
"Room odorizers"	Locker Room, Rush, poppers	Isoamyl, isobutyl, isopropyl, or butyl nitrate (now illegal), cyclohexyl

and butyl nitrite) are sold as video head cleaners, leather cleaners, and so on. These nitrites produce vasodilatation and a "flush" with reduction in blood pressure that is claimed to increase sexual satisfaction.

Inhalant abuse disproportionately affects young people. Nearly 20 percent of children in middle and high school have experimented with inhaled substances. Inhalants are frequently the first mind-altering drugs used by children, occasionally as young as three to four years of age. Inhalant abuse reaches its peak at some point during the seventh to ninth grades, with eighth graders regularly showing the highest rates of abuse. Inhalants are popular with youth because of peer influence, low cost, availability, and rapid onset of effect. When inhaled, they produce euphoria, delirium, intoxication, and alterations in mental status resembling alcohol intoxication or a "light" state of general anesthesia. Users are usually not aware of the potentially serious health consequences that can result. Especially in children, inhalant abuse is an underrecognized form of substance abuse with significant morbidity and mortality.

Why Inhalants Are Abused and Who Abuses Them

Inhalant abuse goes back at least a hundred years after ether, nitrous oxide, and chloroform were introduced into medicine as general anesthetics. Concomitant with their discovery as anesthetics was their discovery as intoxicating agents, leading to nitrous oxide and ether parties. Today, helium inhalation is common, with toxicity and even deaths resulting from displacement by helium of oxygen from the lungs.

The 2015 results of the *National Survey on Drug Use and Health: Trends in Prevalence of Inhalants* show for ages 12 or older, ages 12 to 17, ages 18 to 25, and ages 26 or older that the respective percent of lifetime use was 9.60, 9.10, 13.10, and 9.60. As indicated by these values, a few users continue their abuse of inhalants into adulthood, usually as part of a polysubstance abuse pattern. Kaar and colleagues. (2016) present research using the 2014 *Global Drug Survey* (GDS) ($n = 74,864$), the largest survey of recreational drug use in the world. The findings confirm that use of nitrous oxide gas (N_2O) is very common, in particular in the United Kingdom and United States (38.6 and 29.4 percent lifetime prevalence). Patterns of abuse resemble patterns seen in abuse of other types of substances: there are experimenters, intermittent users, and chronic

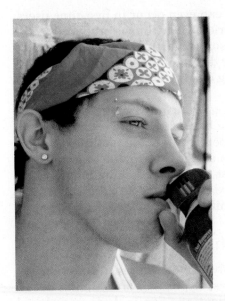

Young man using inhalant to get high.
[Available Light/Getty Images]

abusers. The majority of young inhalant abusers do not view such abuse as being risky (Perron and Howard, 2008); even so, about 20 percent of abusers will develop an inhalant substance abuse disorder (Perron et al., 2009).

Consequences of Acute Use of Inhalants

Acute consequences of inhalant use are generally divided into several types of toxicity:

- Acute hypoxic injury resulting from gaseous displacement of oxygen from one's lungs and subsequently the brain
- Acute intoxication similar to alcohol intoxication with resultant injury from motor vehicle and other accidents
- Medical emergencies such as cardiac arrhythmias leading to "sudden sniffing deaths"

Acute *hypoxia* follows from the replacement of oxygen in the lungs by gases such as nitrous oxide, found in small metal canisters used in refillable whipped cream containers ("whippets"). Reduced oxygen levels in the lungs lead to reduced oxygenation in the blood and hence in the brain. Similar effects can also follow from inhalation of helium, an inert gas often used to fill party balloons. By such displacement and the resulting hypoxia, helium can cause disorientation, blackouts, and even death. The nitrous oxide not only displaces oxygen in the lungs, but its absorption leads to an anesthetic state with disorientation, confusion, and sleep. If not administered together with oxygen (as with an anesthetic gas machine), severe hypoxia and death can result.

Acute *intoxication* is a syndrome consisting of dizziness, incoordination, slurred speech, euphoria, lethargy, slowed reflexes, slowed thinking and movement, tremor, blurred vision, stupor or coma, generalized muscle weakness, and involuntary eye movements similar to alcohol intoxication (Howard et al., 2011). This obviously impairs driving abilities.

The so-called *sudden sniffing death syndrome* can even occur in first-time users. Here, volatile hydrocarbons sensitize the heart to serious arrhythmias produced by the sudden surge of adrenalin that occurs when a person is startled or becomes excited during intoxication. This kind of episode can occur during initial experimentation or during any episode of abuse. Indeed, sudden sniffing death syndrome may account for 50 percent of fatalities from acute intoxication.

Therefore, although death is relatively rare during acute intoxication, when it does occur, it usually follows from lack of oxygen to the brain (anoxia), cardiac arrhythmias, or trauma. Gasoline fuels accounted for 46 percent of acute fatalities. Butane and propane sniffing is also associated with sudden sniffing death due to production of rapid-onset, potentially fatal cardiac arrhythmias. Currently, helium inhalation is increasingly being reported as responsible for hypoxia-associated fatalities. Alper and coworkers (2008) discuss toluene inhalation (glue sniffing) and sudden deaths.

Long-Term Consequences of Chronic Inhalant Abuse

Most inhalants produce intoxication that lasts only a few minutes. If one survives the experience, usually little damage is caused, unless hypoxia or arrhythmias occur. With *chronic abuse* of inhalants, serious complications can include peripheral and central nervous system dysfunction, including peripheral neuropathies and encephalopathy, liver and/or kidney failure, dementia, loss of cognitive, and other higher functions due to damage to the cerebellum, gait disturbances, loss of coordination, neurological disorders such as parkinsonism, and loss of muscle strength (Dingwall and Cairney, 2011; Howard et al., 2011; Lubman et al., 2008). Certainly, when abuse occurs in young persons, such CNS damage results in long-term or even permanent intellectual impairment.

Toluene is a common ingredient in a number of the substances sought out for inhalant abuse, apparently for its euphorigenic, hallucinogenic, and behaviorally rewarding effects. Indeed, toluene is taken up into and activates the central reward centers, including the mesolimbic dopaminergic reward centers and the frontal cortex. Long-term neurotoxicity includes cerebellar degeneration, encephalopathy, and dementia. Peripheral toxicities include renal (kidney) and liver dysfunction.

Inhalant misuse during pregnancy is associated with significant risks to the developing fetus, as inhalants readily cross the placental barrier; maternal hypoxia can also damage the fetus. Bowen (2011) has termed this *fetal solvent syndrome.*

Many people who abuse inhalants for prolonged periods over many days feel a strong need to continue abusing them. A mild withdrawal syndrome can follow long-term abuse, perhaps similar to withdrawal from any of many sedative-hypnotic drugs. Symptoms of long-term inhalant abuse include weight loss, muscle weakness, disorientation, incoordination, irritability, depression, and neurocognitive deficits.

Treatment of acute inhalant intoxication is primarily supportive with the administration of supplemental oxygen. Treatment of chronic inhalant abuse is much more difficult. Results of a survey of 550 drug treatment program directors indicate that most inhalant abusers have a pessimistic attitude about the treatment effectiveness and hopes for long-term recovery (Beauvais et al., 2002). The surveyed directors perceived that a great deal of neurological damage results from inhalant use and that education, preventive efforts, and treatments are inadequate. Early identification of abusers and rapid intervention are essential in preventing both short-term and long-term consequences.

Treatment programs that specialize in inhalant dependence are almost nonexistent (Konghom et al., 2010). Standard approaches are generally ineffective for inhalant abusers because of the need for long-term detoxification and adverse effects on cognitive function. Talk therapies are inappropriate for many patients with neurological dysfunction; the short attention span and poor impulse control of many patients make group therapy a poor choice as well. The best treatment is prevention.

STUDY QUESTIONS

1. Describe the metabolism of alcohol. What enzymes are involved?

2. How long does it take for an adult to metabolize the alcohol in a 1-ounce glass of 80 proof whiskey? A 4-ounce glass of wine? A 12-ounce bottle of beer? A pint of 7 percent microbrew?

3. What are the neurobiological effects of alcohol on the CNS?

4. What are the major physiological and psychological effects of alcohol?

5. Describe some of the fetal effects of alcohol. Is there a "safe" level of drinking during pregnancy?

6. Summarize some of the drugs used in treating alcoholism.

7. Summarize some of the problems associated with both acute and chronic inhalant abuse.

REFERENCES

Akbar, M., et al. (2017). "Medications for Alcohol Use Disorders: An Overview." *Pharmacology & Therapeutics*. As of March 3, 2018 doi: 10.1016/j.pharmthera.2017.11.007.

Albermann, M. C., et al. (2012). "Preliminary Investigations on Ethyl Glucuronide and Ethyl Sulfate Cutoffs for Detecting Alcohol Consumption on the Basis of an Ingestion Experiment and on Data from Withdrawal Treatment." *International Journal of Legal Medicine* 126: 757–764.

Alper, A. T., et al. (2008). "Glue (Toluene) Abuse: Increased QT Dispersion and Relation with Unexplained Syncope." *Inhalation Toxicology* 20: 37–41.

Amato, L., et al. (2011). "Efficacy and Safety of Pharmacological Interventions for the Treatment of the Alcohol Withdrawal Syndrome." *Cochrane Database of Systematic Reviews* June 15, 6: CD008537.

Anton, R. F., et al. (2006). "Combined Pharmacotherapies and Behavioral Interventions for Alcohol Dependence: The COMBINE Study: A Randomized Controlled Trial." *JAMA* 295: 2003–2017.

Anton, R. F. et al. (2011). "Gabapentin Combined with Naltrexone for the Treatment of Alcohol Dependence." *American Journal of Psychiatry* 168: 709–717. doi: 10.1176/appi.ajp.2011.10101436

Autti-Ramo, I. (2000). "Twelve-Year Follow-Up of Children Exposed to Alcohol in Utero." *Developmental Medicine and Child Neurology* 42: 406–411.

Azofeifa, A., et al. (2015). "Driving Under the Influence of Alcohol, Marijuana, and Alcohol and Marijuana Combined among Persons Aged 16–25 Years—United States, 2002–2014 Weekly." *Morbidity and Mortality Weekly Report* 64: 1325–1329. https://www.cdc.gov/mmwr/preview/mmwrhtml/mm6448a1.htm.

Baer, J. S., et al. (2003). "A 21-Year Longitudinal Analysis of the Effects of Prenatal Alcohol Exposure on Young Adult Drinking." *Archives of General Psychiatry* 60: 377–385.

Beauvais, F., et al. (2002). "A Survey of Attitudes among Drug Use Treatment Providers Toward the Treatment of Inhalant Users." *Substance Use and Abuse* 37: 1391–1410.

Becker, H. C., et al. (2006). "Pregabalin Is Effective Against Behavioral and Electrographic Seizures during Alcohol Withdrawal." *Alcohol and Alcoholism* 24: 399–406.

Beraha, E. M., et al. (2016). "Efficacy and Safety of High-Dose Baclofen for the Treatment of Alcohol Dependence: A Multicentre, Randomised, Double-Blind Controlled Trial." *European Neuropsychopharmacology* 26: 1950–1959.

Bogenschutz, M., et al. (2016). "Co-Administration of Disulfiram and Lorazepam in the Treatment of Alcohol Dependence and Co-Occurring Anxiety Disorder." *American Journal of Drug and Alcohol Abuse* 42: 490–499.

Bowen, S. E. (2011). "Two Serious and Challenging Medical Complications Associated with Volatile Substance Misuse: Sudden Sniffing Death and Fetal Solvent Syndrome." *Substance Use and Misuse* 46, Supplement 1: 68–72.

Cao, Y., et al. (2015). "Light to Moderate Intake of Alcohol, Drinking Patterns, and Risk of Cancer: Results From Two Prospective US Cohort Studies." *BMJ* 351. http://dx.doi.org/10.1136/bmj.h4238.

Carey, B. (2012). "Learning from the Spurned and Tipsy Fruit Fly." *New York Times* March 15. http://www.nytimes.com/2012/03/16/health/male-fruit-flies-spurned-by-females-turn-to-alcohol.html.

Dahl, H., et al. (2011). "Urinary Ethyl Glucuronide and Ethyl Sulfate Testing for Recent Drinking in Alcohol-Dependent Outpatients Treated with Acamprosate or Placebo." *Alcohol and Alcoholism* 46: 553–557.

Davis, J. F., et al. (2013). "Roux en Y Gastric Bypass Increases Ethanol Intake in the Rat." *Obesity Surgery* 23: 920–930. doi:10.1007/s11695-013-0884-4.

Dawson, D. A., et al. (2007). "Impact of Age at First Drink on Stress-Reactive Drinking." *Alcoholism: Clinical and Experimental Research* 31: 69–77.

de Bejczy, W. L., et al. (2015). "Phosphatidylethanol Is Superior to Carbohydrate-Deficient Transferrin and γ-Glutamyltransferase as an Alcohol Marker and Is a Reliable Estimate of Alcohol Consumption Level." *Alcoholism, Clinical and Experimental Research* 39: 2200–2208.

DeSousa, A. (2010). "The Role of Topiramate and Other Anticonvulsants in the Treatment of Alcohol Dependence: A Clinical Review." *CNS & Neurological Disorders—Drug Targets* 9: 45–49.

Dingwall, K. M., and Cairney, S. (2011). "Recovery from Central Nervous System Changes Following Volatile Substance Misuse." *Substance Use and Misuse* 46 (Supplement 1): 73–83.

Duke, A. A., et al. (2011). "Alcohol Dose and Aggression: Another Reason Why Drinking More Is a Bad Idea." *Journal of Studies on Alcohol and Drugs* 72: 34–43.

Editors. (2015). "All In for Alcohol Awareness" [editorial]. *The Lancet* 385: 1477.

Elbreder, M. F., et al. (2010). "The Use of Disulfiram for Alcohol-Dependent Patients and Duration of Outpatient Treatment." *European Archives of Psychiatry and Clinical Neuroscience* 260: 191–195.

Emond, J. A., et al. (2014). "Energy Drink Consumption and the Risk of Alcohol Use Disorder among a National Sample of Adolescents and Young Adults." *Journal of Pediatrics* 165: 1194–1200.

Feldman, H. S., et al. (2012). "Prenatal Alcohol Exposure Patterns and Alcohol-Related Birth Defects and Growth Abnormalities: A Prospective Study." *Alcoholism: Clinical & Experimental Research* 36: 670–676.

Florez, G., et al. (2011). "Topiramate for the Treatment of Alcohol Dependence: Comparison with Naltrexone." *European Addiction Research* 17: 29–36.

Frye, M. A., and Salloum, I. M. (2006). "Bipolar Disorder and Comorbid Alcoholism: Prevalence Rate and Treatment Considerations." *Bipolar Disorder* 8: 677–685.

Furieri F. A., and Nakamura-Palacios, E. M. (2007). "Gabapentin Reduces Alcohol Consumption and Craving: A Randomized, Double-Blind, Placebo-Controlled Trial." *Journal of Clinical Psychiatry* 68: 1691–1700.

Garbutt, J. C., et al. (2016). "Association of the Sweet-Liking Phenotype and Craving for Alcohol with the Response to Naltrexone Treatment in Alcohol Dependence: A Randomized Clinical Trial." *JAMA Psychiatry* 73:1056–1063. doi: 10.1001/jamapsychiatry.2016.215.

Giancola, P. R., et al. (2011). "Alcohol, Violence, and the Alcohol Myopia Model: Preliminary Findings and Implications for Prevention." *Addictive Behaviors* 36: 1019–1022.

Gold, P. E. (2008). "Protein Synthesis Inhibition and Memory: Formation vs Amnesia." *Neurobiology of Learning and Memory* 89: 201–211.

Goncalves, A., et al. (2015). "Relationship between Alcohol Consumption and Cardiac Structure and Function in the Elderly: The Atherosclerosis Risk in Communities Study." *Circulation: Cardiovascular Imaging* 8. doi: 10.1161/CIRCIMAGING.114.002846.

Goodwin, D. W., and Gabrielli, W. F. (1997). "Alcohol: Clinical Aspects." In J. H. Lowinson, P. Ruiz, R. B. Millman, and J. G. Langrod, eds. *Substance Abuse: A Comprehensive Textbook*, 3rd ed. (pp. 142–148). Baltimore: Williams & Wilkins.

Grant, B. F., et al. (2004). "Co-Occurence of 12-Month Alcohol and Drug Use Disorders and Personality Disorders in the United States." *Archives of General Psychiatry* 61: 361–368.

Grant, B. F., et al. (2016). "Epidemiology of DSM-5 Drug Use Disorder: Results From the National Epidemiologic Survey on Alcohol and Related Conditions-III." *JAMA Psychiatry* 73: 39–47. doi:10.1001/jamapsychiatry.2015.2132.

Green, A., et al. (2015). "Long-Acting Injectable vs Oral Risperidone for Schizophrenia and Co-Occurring Alcohol Use Disorder: A Randomized Trial." *Journal of Clinical Psychiatry* 10: 1359–1365.

Gueorguieva, R., et al. (2011). "Baseline Trajectories of Drinking Moderate Acamprosate and Naltrexone Effects in the COMBINE Study." *Alcoholism: Clinical and Experimental Research* 35: 523–531.

Gueorguieva, R., et al. (2012). "Baseline Trajectories of Heavy Drinking and Their Effects on Postrandomization Drinking in the COMBINE Study: Empirically Derived Predictors of Drinking Outcomes During Treatment." *Alcohol* 46: 121–131.

Guglielmo, R., et al. (2012). "Pregabalin for Alcohol Dependence: A Critical Review of the Literature." *Advances in Therapeutics* 29: 947–957.

Hackl-Herrwerth, R. S., et al. (2010). "Opioid Antagonists for Alcohol Dependence." *Cochrane Database of Systematic Reviews* 12: CD001867.

Haseba, T., and Ohno, Y. (2010). "A New View of Alcohol Metabolism and Alcoholism—Role of the High-*Km* Class III Alcohol Dehydrogenase (ADH3)." *International Journal of Environmental Research and Public Health* 7: 1076–1092.

Heinz, A., et al. (2009). "Identifying the Neural Circuitry of Alcohol Craving and Relapse Vulnerability." *Addiction Biology* 14: 108–118.

Hester, R. (2015). "Naltrexone Reduces Heavy Drinking in Problem Drinkers Across the Spectrum of Dependence." *Journal of Clinical Psychiatry* 76: e226–e227.

Holmes, M. V., et al. (2014). "Association between Alcohol and Cardiovascular Disease: Mendelian Randomisation Analysis Based on Individual Participant Data." *BMJ* 349: g4164. https://doi.org/10.1136/bmj.g4164.

Howard, M. O., et al. (2011). "Inhalant Use and Inhalant Use Disorders in the United States." *Addiction Science & Clinical Practice* 6: 18–31.

Jancin, B. (2015). "Harm-Reduction Approach to Alcoholism Gains Credibility: Abstinence Seen by Some as 'Almost Impossible' to Achieve." *Clinical Psychiatry News* 43.

Johnson, B. A., et al., (2000). "Ondansetron for Reduction of Drinking among Biologically Predisposed Alcoholic Patients: *A Randomized Controlled Trial*." JAMA 284: 963–971.

Johnson, B. A., et al. (2003). "Ondansetron Reduces Mood Disturbance among Biologically Predisposed, Alcohol-Dependent Individuals." *Alcoholism: Clinical and Experimental Research* 27: 1773–1779.

Johnson, B. A., and Ait-Daoud, N. (2011). "Topiramate in the New Generation of Drugs: Efficacy in the Treatment of Alcoholic Patients." *Current Pharmaceutical Design* 16: 2103–2112.

Jonas, D. E., et al. (2014). "Pharmacotherapy for Adults with Alcohol Use Disorders in Outpatient Settings: A Systematic Review and Meta-Analysis." *JAMA* 311: 1889–1900. doi:10.1001/jama.2014.3628.

Jyri, J., et al. (2010). "Midlife Alcohol Consumption and Later Risk of Cognitive Impairment: A Twin Follow-up Study." *Journal of Alzheimer's Disease* 22: 939–948.

Kaar, S. J., et al. (2016). "Up: The Rise of Nitrous Oxide Abuse. An International Survey of Contemporary Nitrous Oxide Use." *Journal of Psychopharmacology* 30: 395–401.

Kelland, K. (2016). "'Special K' Party Drug to be Trialed as Treatment for Alcoholics." *Reuters*. July 6. http://www.reuters.com/article/us-health-alcoholism-ketamine-idUSKCN0ZM2L8.

Kelty, E., et al. (2014). "Changes in Hospital and Out-Patient Events and Costs Following Implant Naltrexone Treatment for Problematic Alcohol Use." *Journal of Psychopharmacology* 28: 745–750.

Kenna, G. A. (2010). "Medications Acting on the Serotonergic System for the Treatment of Alcohol Dependent Patients." *Current Pharmaceutical Design* 16: 2126–2135.

Kim, S., et al. (2016). "Association between Alcohol Drinking Behaviour and Cognitive Function: Results from a Nationwide Longitudinal Study of South Korea." *BMJ Open* 6: e010494. doi: 10.1136/bmjopen-2015- 010494.

King, W. C., et al. (2012). "Prevalence of Alcohol Use Disorders Before and After Bariatric Surgery." *JAMA* 307: 2516–2525.

Kirby, L. G., et al. (2011). "Contributions of Serotonin in Addiction Vulnerability." *Neuropharmacology* 61: 421–432.

Knapp, C. M., et al. (2015). "Zonisamide, Topiramate, and Levetiracetam Efficacy and Neuropsychological Effects in Alcohol Use Disorders." *Journal of Clinical Psychopharmacology* 35: 34–42. doi: 10.1097/JCP.0000000000000246.

Konghom, S., et al. (2010). "Treatment for Inhalant Dependence and Abuse." *Cochrane Database of Systematic Reviews* December 8 (12): CD007537.

Kot-Leibovich, H., and Fainsod, A. (2009): "Ethanol Induces Embryonic Malformations by Competing for Retinaldehyde Dehydrogenase Activity During Vertebrate Gastrulation." *Disease Models and Mechanisms* 2: 295–305.

Kranzler, H. R., et al. (2012). "Comparison of Alcoholism Subtypes as Moderators of the Response to Sertraline Treatment." *Alcoholism: Clinical and Experimental Research* 36: 509–516.

Krupitsky, E. M., et al. (2007). "Antiglutamatergic Strategies for Ethanol Detoxification: Comparison with Placebo and Diazepam." *Alcoholism: Clinical and Experimental Research* 31: 604–611.

Kushner, M. G., et al. (2011). "Vulnerability to the Rapid ("Telescoped") Development of Alcohol Dependence in Individuals with Anxiety Disorder." *Journal of Studies on Alcohol and Drugs* 72: 1019–1027.

Kushner, M. G., et al. (2012). "Alcohol Dependence Is Related to Overall Internalizing Psychopathology Load Rather than to Particular Internalizing Disorders: Evidence from a National Sample." *Alcoholism: Clinical and Experimental Research* 36: 325–331.

Laramée, P., et al. (2014). "The Cost-Effectiveness and Public Health Benefit of Nalmefene Added to Psychosocial Support for the Reduction of Alcohol Consumption in Alcohol Dependent Patients with High/Very High Drinking Risk Levels: A Markov Model." *BMJ Open* 4: e005376. doi:10.1136/bmjopen-2014–005376.

Lee, H., et al. (2009). "Alcohol-Induced Blackout." *International Journal of Environmental Research and Public Health* 6: 2783–2792.

Leggio, L., et al. (2008). "New Developments for the Pharmacological Treatment of Alcohol Withdrawal Syndrome. A Focus on Non-Benzodiazepine GABA-ergic Medications." *Progress in Neuro-Psychopharmacology and Biological Psychiatry* 32: 1106–1117.

Li, D., et al. (2012). "Further Clarification of the Contribution of the ADH1C Gene to Vulnerability of Alcoholism and Selected Liver Diseases." *Human Genetics* 131: 1361–1374.

Likhitsathian, S., et al. (2012). "Cognitive Changes in Topiramate-Treated Patients with Alcoholism: A 12-Week Prospective Study in Patients Recently Detoxified." *Psychiatry and Clinical Neurosciences* 66: 235–241.

LoConte, N. K., et al. (2018). "Alcohol and Cancer: A Statement of the American Society of Clinical Oncology." *Journal of Clinical Oncology* 36: 83–93.

Lubman, D. I., et al. (2008). "Inhalant Abuse among Adolescents: Neurobiological Considerations." *British Journal of Pharmacology* 154: 316–326.

Macfarlane, G. J., et al. (2015). "Moderate Alcohol Consumption Is Associated with Lower Risk (and Severity) of Chronic Widespread Pain: Results from a UK Population-Based Study." *Arthritis Care & Research* 67: 1297–1303. doi: 10.1002/acr.22604.

Malcolm, R., et al. (2000). "Recurrent Detoxification May Elevate Alcohol Craving as Measured by the Obsessive Compulsive Drinking Scale." *Alcohol* 20: 181–185.

Mann, K., et al. (2008). "Acamprosate: Recent Findings and Future Research Directions." *Alcoholism: Clinical and Experimental Research* 32: 1105–1110.

Mann, K., et al. (2013). "Extending the Treatment Options in Alcohol Dependence: A Randomized Controlled Study of As-Needed Nalmefene." *Biological Psychiatry* 73: 706–713.

Marsh, R. (2015). "Fed study: Booze impact greater than pot on driving." *CNN.com.* June 25. http://www.cnn.com/2015/06/24/politics/marijuana-study-drivers-impact/.

Martinotti, G., et al. (2010). "Pregabalin, Tiapride and Lorazepam in Alcohol Withdrawal Syndrome: A Multi-Centre, Randomized, Single-Blind Comparison Trial." *Addiction* 105: 288–299.

Mason B. J., et al. (2014). "Gabapentin Treatment for Alcohol Dependence: A Randomized Clinical Trial." *JAMA Internal Medicine* 174: 70–77. doi: 10.1001/jamainternmed.2013.11950.

Mason, B. J., and Heyser, C. J. (2010). "The Neurobiology, Clinical Efficacy and Safety of Acamprosate in the Treatment of Alcohol Dependence." *Expert Opinion on Drug Safety* 9: 177–188.

McAndrew, A., et al. (2017). "A Proof-Of-Concept Investigation Into Ketamine as a Pharmacological Treatment for Alcohol Dependence: Study Protocol for a Randomised Controlled Trial." *Trials* 18: 159. doi: 10.1186/s13063-017-1895-6.

McKetin, R., and Coen, A. (2014). "The Effect of Energy Drinks on the Urge to Drink Alcohol in Young Adults." *Alcoholism: Clinical and Experimental Research* 38: 2279–2285. doi: 10.1111/acer.12498.

Medina, A. E. (2011). "Fetal Alcohol Spectrum Disorders and Abnormal Neuronal Plasticity." *The Neuroscientist* 17: 274–287.

Menary, K. R., et al. (2011). "The Prevalence and Clinical Implications of Self-Medication among Individuals with Anxiety Disorders." *Journal of Anxiety Disorders* 25: 335–339.

Mitchell, J. M., et al. (2012). "Alcohol Consumption Induces Endogenous Opioid Release in the Human Orbitofrontal Cortex and Nucleus Accumbens." *Science Translational Medicine* 11 January 4: 116ra6.

Moussa, M. N., et al. (2015). "Long-Term Moderate Alcohol Consumption Does Not Exacerbate Age-Related Cognitive Decline in Healthy, Community-Dwelling Older Adults." *Frontiers in Aging Neuroscience* 6: 341. doi: 10.3389/fnagi.2014.00341.

Moykkynen, T., and Korpi, E. R. (2012). "Acute Effects of Ethanol on Glutamate Receptors." *Basic Clinical Pharmacology and Toxicology* 111: 4–13.

Muzyk, A. J., et al. (2012). "Defining the Role of Baclofen for the Treatment of Alcohol Dependence: A Systematic Review of the Evidence." *CNS Drugs* 26: 69–78.

National Institute on Alcohol and Alcoholism (2017). *Alcohol Facts and Statistics.* June. https://pubs.niaaa.nih.gov/publications/alcoholfacts&stats/AlcoholFacts&Stats.pdf.

Noel, X., et al. (2001). "Supervisory Attentional System in Nonamnestic Alcoholic Men." *Archives of General Psychiatry* 58: 1152–1158.

Nutt, D. J., and Rehm, J. (2014). "Doing It by Numbers: A Simple Approach to Reducing the Harms of Alcohol." *Journal of Psychopharmacology* 28: 3–7.

O'Malley, S. S., et al. (2015). "Reduction of Alcohol Drinking in Young Adults by Naltrexone: A Double-Blind, Placebo-Controlled, Randomized Clinical Trial of Efficacy and Safety." *Journal of Clinical Psychiatry* 76: e201–e213.

Oscar-Berman, M., and Marinkovic, K. (2007). "Alcohol: Effects on Neurobehavioral Functions and the Brain." *Neuropsychology Review* 17: 239–257.

Otto, M. A. (2014). "Start Low, Go Slow with Topiramate for Alcohol Use Disorder." *Internal Medicine News.* July 5. http://www.mdedge.com/internalmedicinenews/article/89177/addiction-medicine/start-low-go-slow-topiramate-alcohol-use.

Palpacuer, C., et al. (2015). "Risks and Benefits of Nalmefene in the Treatment of Adult Alcohol Dependence: A Systematic Literature Review and Meta-Analysis of Published and Unpublished Double-Blind Randomized Controlled Trials." *PLOS Medicine* 12: e1001924. doi: 10.1371/journal.pmed.1001924.

Paille, F. and Martini, H. (2014). "Nalmefene: a new approach to the treatment of alcohol dependence." *Substance Abuse and Rehabilitation* 5: 87–94.

Pastor, A., et al. (2012). "High Dose Baclofen for Treatment-Resistant Alcohol Dependence." *Journal of Clinical Psychopharmacology* 32: 266–268.

Pava, M. J., and Woodward, J. J. (2012). "A Review of the Interactions between Alcohol and the Endocannabinoid System: Implications for Alcohol Dependence and Future Directions for Research." *Alcohol* 46: 185–204.

Peana, A. T., et al. (2016). "From Ethanol to Salsolinol: Role of Ethanol Metabolites in the Effects of Ethanol." *Journal of Experimental Neuroscience* 10: 137–146. doi:10.4137/JEN.S25099.

Perron, B. E., and Howard, M. O. (2008). "Perceived Risk of Harm and Intentions of Future Inhalant Use Among Adolescent Inhalant Users." *Drug and Alcohol Dependence* 97: 185–189.

Perron, B. E., et al. (2009). "Prevalence, Timing, and Predictors of Transitions from Inhalant Use to Inhalant Use Disorders." *Drug and Alcohol Dependence* 100: 277–284.

Perry, P. J., et al. (2006). "The Association of Alcohol-Induced Blackouts and Grayouts to Blood Alcohol Concentrations." *Journal of Forensic Science* 51: 896–899.

Petrow, S. (2016). "Drinking on Antidepressants." *New York Times*. December 20. http://nyti.ms/2i3Zdj2.

Pettinati, H. M., et al. (2010). "A Double-Blind, Placebo-Controlled Trial that Combines Sertraline and Naltrexone for Treating Co-Occurring Depression and Alcohol Dependence." *American Journal of Psychiatry* 167: 668–675.

Prisciandaro, J. J., et al. (2012). "Simultaneous Modeling of the Impact on Alcohol Consumption and Quality of Life in the COMBINE Study: A Coupled Hidden Markov Analysis." *Alcoholism: Clinical and Experimental Research* 36: 2141–2149.

Rehm, J. (2015). "Light or Moderate Drinking Is Linked to Alcohol-Related Cancers, Including Breast Cancer." *BMJ* 351: h4400. http://dx.doi.org/10.1136/bmj.h4400.

Reisfield, G. M., et al. (2011a). "Ethyl Glucuronide, Ethyl Sulfate, and Ethanol in Urine after Intensive Exposure to High Ethanol Content Mouthwash." *Journal of Analytical Toxicology* 35: 264–268.

Reisfield, G. M., et al. (2011b). "Ethyl Glucuronide, Ethyl Sulfate, and Ethanol in Urine after Sustained Exposure to an Ethanol-Based Hand Sanitizer." *Journal of Analytical Toxicology* 35: 85–91.

Rigal, L., et al. (2012). "Abstinence and 'Low-Risk' Consumption 1 Year after the Initiation of High-Dose Baclofen: A Retrospective Study among "High-Risk" Drinkers." *Alcohol and Alcoholism* 47: 439–442.

Robinson, S., et al. (2014). "Medication for Alcohol Use Disorder." *Current Psychiatry* 13: 23–32. doi: 10.1177/0269881115602487.

Roerecke, M., et al. (2015). "Clinical Relevance of Nalmefene versus Placebo in Alcohol Treatment: Reduction in Mortality Risk." *Journal of Psychopharmacology* 29: 1152–1158.

Rohde, P., et al. (2001). "Natural Course of Alcohol Use Disorders from Adolescence to Young Adulthood." *Journal of the American Academy of Child and Adolescent Psychiatry* 40: 83–90.

Rosner, S., et al. (2010). "Acamprosate for Alcohol Dependent Patients." *Cochrane Database of Systematic Reviews* 9: CD004332.

Rubio, G., et al. (2006). "Effects of Lamotrigine in Patients with Bipolar Disorder and Alcohol Dependence." *Bipolar Disorder* 8: 289–293.

Ruidavets, J.-B., et al. (2010). "Patterns of Alcohol Consumption and Ischemic Heart Disease in Culturally Divergent Countries: The Prospective Epidemiological Study of Myocardial Infarction (PRIME)." *BMJ* 341: c6077. doi: https://doi.org/10.1136/bmj.c6077.

Ryan, M. L., et al. (2017). "A Phase 2, Double-Blind, Placebo-Controlled Randomized Trial Assessing the Efficacy of ABT-436, A Novel V1b Receptor Antagonist, for Alcohol Dependence." *Neuropsychopharmacology* September 23. http://dx.doi.org/10.1038/npp.2016.214.

Saitz, R., et al. (2013). "Chronic Care Management for Dependence on Alcohol and Other Drugs: The AHEAD Randomized Trial." *JAMA* 310: 1156–1167.

Sari, Y., et al. (2011). "Role of the Serotonergic System in Alcohol Dependence: From Animal Models to Clinics." *Progress in Molecular Biology and Translational Sciences* 98: 401–443.

Sayal, K., et al. (2009). "Binge Pattern of Alcohol Consumption During Pregnancy and Childhood Mental Health Outcomes: Longitudinal Population-Based Study." *Pediatrics* 123: e289–e296.

Slade, T., et al. (2016). "Birth Cohort Trends in the Global Epidemiology of Alcohol Use and Alcohol-Related Harms in Men and Women: Systematic Review and Metaregression." *BMJ Open* 6: e011827. http://bmjopen.bmj.com/content/6/10/e011827.full.

Soyka, M., and Muller, C. A. (2017). "Pharmacotherapy of Alcoholism: An Update on Approved and Off-Label Medications." *Expert Opinions on Pharmacotherapy* 18: 1187–1199. doi: 10.1080/14656566.2017.1349098.

Spanagel, R., et al. (2014). "Acamprosate Produces Its Anti-Relapse Effects Via Calcium." *Neuropsychopharmacology* 39: 783–791. doi:10.1038/npp.2013.264.

Squeglia, L. M., et al. (2015). "Brain Development in Heavy-Drinking Adolescents." *American Journal of Psychiatry* 172: 531–542. doi: 10.1176/appi.ajp.2015.14101249.

Strac, D. S., et al. (2012). "The GABA$_A$ Receptor Alpha-2 Subunit Gene (GABARA2) Is Associated with Alcohol-Related Behavior." *BMC Pharmacology and Toxicology* 13(Supplement 1): A8.

Substance Abuse and Mental Health Services Administration. (2013). *Results from the 2012 National Survey on Drug Use and Health: Summary of National Findings.* NSDUH Series H-46, HHS Publication No. (SMA) 13-4795. Rockville, MD.

Suzuki, J., et al. (2012). "Alcohol Use Disorders after Bariatric Surgery." *Obesity Surgery* 22: 201–207.

Tiet, Q. Q., and Mausbach, B. (2007). "Treatments for Patients with Dual Diagnosis: A Review." *Alcoholism: Clinical and Experimental Research* 31: 513–536. https://www.samhsa.gov/homelessness-programs-resources/hpr-resources/alcohol-management-harm-reduction.

van den Brink, W., et al. (2014). "Long-Term Efficacy, Tolerability and Safety of Nalmefene As-Needed in Patients with Alcohol Dependence: A 1-Year, Randomised Controlled Study." *Journal of Psychopharmacology* 28: 733–744. doi: 10.1177/0269881114527362.

Vaillant, G. E. (1996). "A Long-Term Follow-Up of Male Alcohol Abuse." *Archives of General Psychiatry* 53: 243–249.

Vetreno, R. P., and Crews, F. T. (2015). "Binge Ethanol Exposure during Adolescence Leads to a Persistent Loss of Neurogenesis in the Dorsal and Ventral Hippocampus That Is Associated with Impaired Adult Cognitive Functioning." *Frontiers in Neuroscience* 9: 35. doi: 10.3389/fnins.2015.00035.

Wetherill, R. R., et al. (2012a). "Acute Alcohol Effects on Contextual Memory BOLD Response: Differences Based on Fragmentary Blackout History." *Alcoholism: Clinical and Experimental Research* 36: 1108–1115.

Wetherill, R. R., et al. (2012b). "Subjective Perceptions Associated with the Ascending and Descending Slopes of Breath Alcohol Exposure Vary with Recent Drinking History." *Alcoholism: Clinical and Experimental Research* 36: 1150–1157.

White, A. M., et al. (2004). "Experiential Aspects of Alcohol-Induced Blackouts among College Students." *American Journal of Drug and Alcohol Abuse* 30: 205–224.

Williams, J. F., et al. (2007). "Inhalant Abuse." *Pediatrics* 119: 1009–1017.

Winograd, R. P., et al. (2016). "Searching for Mr. Hyde: A Five-Factor Approach to Characterizing 'Types of Drunks.'" *Addiction Research & Theory* 24: 1–8. doi: 10.3109/16066359.2015.1029920.

Woodard, G. A. (2011). "Impaired Alcohol Metabolism after Gastric Bypass Surgery: A Case-Crossover Trial." *Journal of the American College of Surgeons* 212: 209–214.

Zhang, C., et al. (2014). "Alcohol Intake and Risk of Stroke: A Dose-Response Meta-Analysis of Prospective Studies." *International Journal of Cardiology* 174: 669–677. doi: 10.1016/j.ijcard.2014.04.225.

CHAPTER 5 **APPENDIX**

WHAT IS A DRINK? HOW MUCH ALCOHOL IS IN YOUR DRINK?

One drink equivalent, in the United States, is approximately 7 to 14 grams of alcohol, or the amount of alcohol that contains 10 cubic centimeters (1/3 ounce) of 100 percent ethanol. A 150-pound person with normal liver function metabolizes about 7 to 14 grams of alcohol per hour and reduces the blood alcohol concentration (BAC) by 0.015 grams.

This amount of alcohol is contained in about 1 to 1.5 ounces of 40 percent (80 proof) liquor, 4 ounces of 12 percent wine, or a 12-ounce bottle of 5 percent beer.

In the table below, typical alcoholic beverages are converted to their calculated drink equivalents.

If you drink	You have consumed about
One 12 oz. Budweiser (5% alcohol)	1.5 drink equivalents
One 6- pack of 12 oz. Budweiser	9 drink equivalents
Short case (12 bottles) of 12 oz. Budweiser	18 drink equivalents
One 16 oz. Budweiser	1.9 (about 2) drink equivalents
One 24 oz. Budweiser	3 drink equivalents
One 40 oz. Budweiser	5 drink equivalents
One 12 oz. Bud Light (4.2%)	1.25 drink equivalents
One 12 oz. Bud-Ice (5.5%)	1.9 (almost 2) drink equivalents
One 16 oz. Old English 800 (8%)	3.8 (almost 4) drink equivalents
One 40 oz. Old English 800	9 drink equivalents
Two 40 oz. Old English 800	18 drink equivalents (2/3 pint of whiskey)
One 16 oz. Rainier Ale (7.2%)	3.5 drink equivalents
One 40 oz. St. Ides Malt (7.3%)	8 drink equivalents
One 16 oz. microbrew (5%–7%)	2.2 to 3.4 drink equivalents
One 64 oz. pitcher of microbrew	9.5 to 13 drink equivalents
One 12 oz. Hornsby Draft Cider (6%)	2 drink equivalents
One 16 oz. barley wine (10%)	4.8 drink equivalents
One 12 oz. Zima cooler (4.6%)	1.6 drink equivalents
One 12 oz. Mike's Hard Lemonade (5%)	1.8 drink equivalents

Comments

Budweiser and the other brand names are used for illustration only. Other beers are similar, with modest differences. Their alcohol concentration may or may not be listed on the label or package. Coors, for example, is 4.9 percent alcohol, while Coors Light is 4.2 percent. Busch is 4.5 percent. Henri Weinhard Private Reserve is 4.6 percent. Red Dog is 5 percent alcohol, whereas microbrews may be as high as 7 percent alcohol.

Ice beers are made by slightly freezing the brew and removing some of the ice, increasing the alcohol content. Most are 5.9 percent alcohol, such that a 12-ounce bottle would be 5.2 drink equivalents of ethanol.

Wine coolers are classified as malt beverages and have alcohol contents from 4.6 percent to 7 percent. They are considered to be 1.5 to 2 drink equivalents per bottle.

A tavern can sell beer, ale, and malt liquor up to 14 percent alcohol, hard cider up to 10 percent alcohol, and wine up to 14 percent alcohol. Taverns and pubs often serve beer and ale in pitchers that contain from 60 to 72 ounces. If the pitcher contains regular draft beer at about 5 percent alcohol, a 64-ounce pitcher contains about 9.5 drink equivalents of ethanol.

CHAPTER 6

Caffeine and Nicotine

CAFFEINE

Caffeine is the most widely consumed psychoactive drug in the world; in the United States, it is consumed daily by up to 80 percent or more of the adult population (Childs and deWit, 2012). It belongs to a family of substances called *xanthines* that also includes theophylline and theobromine. These substances stimulate the central nervous system, act on the kidneys to produce diuresis (urine), stimulate cardiac muscle, and relax smooth muscle.

Caffeine occurs naturally in the coffee bean (which is actually a seed) (*Coffea arabica* from Arabia), the tea leaf (*Thea sinensis* from China), the kola nut (*Cola nitida* from West Africa), and the cocoa bean (*Theobroma cacao* from Mexico). Tea actually contains more caffeine than coffee by dry weight but, because it is brewed more weakly, there is less caffeine in a standard serving. (In 1688, the Dutch began the cultivation of coffee on the island of Java. It is this association with coffee production that led to the nickname "java" for a good cup of coffee!) The reason why caffeine is found in so many (at least 60) plants is not known for certain, but it is speculated that it serves as a pesticide, because caffeine is toxic to the larvae of several insects. In addition to insects, caffeine is toxic to birds, dogs, and cats.

In addition to these organic sources, caffeine is often added to soft drinks, bottled water, candies, and medications (Table 6.1). In particular, since the introduction of the energy drink Red Bull (in Austria in 1987 and the United States in 1997), many other brands of energy drinks have been marketed, containing about 80 milligrams of caffeine per serving with a range of 50 milligrams to 550 milligrams per can or bottle, although they may not list the caffeine content on the label (Ishak et al., 2012; Sepkowitz, 2013; see Torpy and Livingston, 2013, for a table of caffeine content in energy drinks and other beverages).

AeroShot Pure Energy, the first caffeine mist product available to consumers, came in a small tube—resembling an asthma inhaler—and gave a 100-milligram shot of caffeine as well as assorted B vitamins when inhaled. It was recommended to be used no more than three times per day. As a dietary supplement, AeroShot didn't require FDA approval, but the FDA issued a warning letter in March of 2012 about its dangers.

TABLE 6.1 Caffeine content in beverages, foods, and medicines

Tea (6 oz.)	
Black tea	25–110 mg
Oolong tea	12–55 mg
Green tea	8–16 mg
Coffee (8 oz.)	
Brewed	135–150 mg
Instant	60–100 mg
Decaffeinated	1–25 mg
Sodas (12 oz.)	
Coke	46 mg
Pepsi	38 mg
Jolt	59 mg
Mountain Dew	52 mg
Surge	52.5 mg
Other	
Chocolate bar (50 gm)	20 mg
Cocoa (5 oz.)	2–20 mg
Hot chocolate (220 mL)	4 mg
Vivarin (1 tablet)	200 mg
Espresso drinks	
Latte	70 mg

In comparison, the average cup of coffee contains about 135 milligrams and, among regular caffeine users, daily intake averages between 200 and 500 milligrams, correlating with two to five cups of coffee daily.[1]

The Food and Drug Administration (FDA) classifies caffeine as "generally recognized as safe," but only in beverages containing up to 0.02 percent caffeine. Yet caffeine powder, which is sold as a dietary supplement, is unregulated. The FDA's official stance is that up to 400 milligrams per day of caffeine is safe for consumers. To date, caffeine may be added to beverages and food as long as it is listed in the ingredients panel, although the amount of caffeine is not required to be stated.

Ironically, in 1911, the FDA seized 40 kegs and 20 barrels of Coca-Cola syrup because the caffeine was considered a significant health hazard. By that time, the cocaine and alcohol had already been removed. The case dragged on for years until Coca-Cola eventually reduced the amount of caffeine and the legal action was dropped (Sepkowitz, 2013).

---

[1]The caffeine content of one cup of coffee varies widely. One hundred milligrams is often used as an average. Among popular "gourmet" coffees, however, one company's coffee averages 200 milligrams per 8 fluid ounces. Thus, a 12-ounce cup of black coffee has 300 milligrams; the 16-ounce "grande" has 400 milligrams. Mixed coffee drinks have less caffeine because of added milk or flavorings. Another company's coffee averages 80 to 90 milligrams; the coffee of a third company has 100 to 125 milligrams of caffeine per 8 ounces.

Pharmacokinetics

Taken orally, caffeine is rapidly and completely absorbed. Significant blood levels are reached after oral ingestion in 15 to 20 minutes and 99 percent is taken up within 45 minutes (Persad, 2011). Caffeine is soluble in both water and oil; therefore, it is equally distributed throughout the body and the brain and, like all psychoactive drugs, freely crosses the placenta to the fetus.

Caffeine's elimination half-life varies from about 2.5 to 10 hours (Magkos and Kavouras, 2005) and is extended by alcohol and other medications, in infants, women taking oral contraceptives, pregnant women, the elderly, and patients with chronic liver disease. Conversely, in cigarette smokers, caffeine's half-life is shortened; however, when smoking is terminated, caffeine's half-life increases. The reduced metabolism of caffeine can increase plasma caffeine levels and may contribute to cigarette withdrawal symptoms in heavy coffee drinkers, particularly because caffeine can induce or intensify anxiety disorders such as panic disorder (Lambert et al., 2006).

The structure and metabolism of caffeine are shown in Figure 6.1. The two major metabolites of caffeine, paraxanthine and theophylline, behave similarly to caffeine; a third metabolite, theobromine (the main alkaloid in chocolate), does not. Because theophylline relaxes the smooth muscles of the bronchi, it is used to treat asthma. Caffeine is metabolized in the liver by the CYP-1A2 subgroup of hepatic drug-metabolizing enzymes. Certain selective serotonin reuptake inhibitor (SSRI) antidepressants, such as fluoxetine and fluvoxamine (see Chapter 12), are potent inhibitors of CYP-1A2, and people taking these antidepressants can exhibit unexpected toxicity or

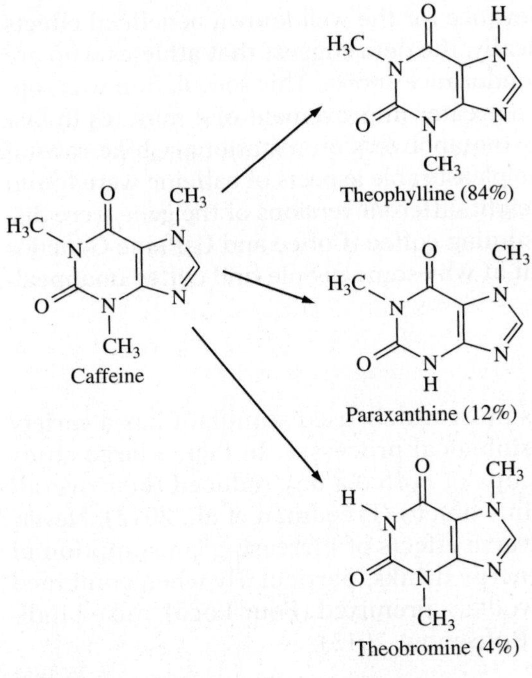

FIGURE 6.1 Metabolism of caffeine to three end products.

intolerance to caffeine as plasma levels of caffeine rise, including de novo production of "caffeinism" (defined below), with severe anxiety reactions.

Pharmacological Effects

There is a wide disparity in reactions to caffeine. Research on caffeine pharmacokinetics provides an explanation. It has been reported that the gene that controls caffeine's metabolic enzyme comes in several varieties. One version of this gene increases the rate at which caffeine is metabolized. If an individual receives a copy of this variant from both parents, that person will break down caffeine four times faster than someone who received a slow gene variant from at least one parent. The former group is termed "rapid caffeine metabolizers" and the latter group is termed "slow caffeine metabolizers." Cornelis and colleagues (2006) set out to determine the consequences of inheriting these gene variants for the risk of having a heart attack. They analyzed data from 4000 adults, half of whom had a prior heart attack. When the data from all the participants were combined, drinking 4 or more cups of coffee a day increased the risk of a heart attack by 36 percent. If the data for the slow metabolizers were removed and only the data from the fast metabolizers analyzed, then the risk was not increased. In fact, fast metabolizers had a reduced risk. Interpretation of the data suggests that the longer duration of caffeine exposure in the slow metabolizers increases the risk of heart attacks, whereas the quick elimination of caffeine by fast metabolizers reduces this adverse side effect while permitting other substances to exert beneficial actions.

Palatini and colleagues (2009) found a similar result for hypertension: slow metabolism was associated with a greater likelihood of hypertension and fast metabolism with a lesser likelihood. These results may have relevance for the well-known beneficial effects of caffeine on physical performance. Specifically, the data suggest that athletes who are fast metabolizers may have an advantage in endurance sports. This speculation was supported by a study that found caffeine led to a greater improvement of 4 minutes in fast metabolizers compared to 1 minute in slow metabolizers on a stationary bike race of 40 kilometers (Womack et al., 2012). Even the pleasurable aspects of caffeine were found to be associated with gene variants; in 2015, eight different versions of the gene were discovered that increased the likelihood of consuming coffee (Coffee and Caffeine Genetics Consortium, 2015). These outcomes may hint at why some people find coffee unappealing while others depend on it to start the day.

Beneficial Effects of Caffeine

There is mounting evidence that the world's most widely used stimulant has a variety of positive effects on both mental and physiological processes. In fact, a large study found that people who drank four to five cups of coffee a day reduced their overall risk of death by 12 (in men) to 16 percent (in women) (Freedman et al., 2012). Nevertheless, there is concern in regard to the adverse effects of increasing consumption of caffeine, especially by young people using energy drinks, particularly when combined with alcohol, such as in bars (Red Bull and vodka), premixed (Four Loco), mixed individually, or drunk separately (Howland and Rohsenow, 2013).

Cardiovascular Function.   In spite of the fact that caffeine consumption can transiently raise blood pressure when taken in coffee, the blood pressure elevations are small, and long-term risks may be mitigated by compensatory actions. In fact, drinking moderate amounts of coffee is linked to lower rates of pretty much all cardiovascular disease. Cardiovascular disease risk as a function of chronic long-term coffee ingestion was evaluated in a meta-analysis, which included 36 studies and a correspondingly large pool of over 1,270,000 subjects. It was found that three to five cups of coffee per day, which constituted a modest intake, was associated with the least cardiovascular risk. If five or more cups were drunk daily, the risk was the same as if no coffee was consumed (Ding et al., 2014). Moreover, in a small trial conducted in heart failure patients, 100 milligrams of caffeine ingested hourly for five hours did not induce arrhythmias, even during exercise (Zuchinali et al., 2016).

Coffee drinkers were also less likely to have calcium in their coronary arteries than nondrinkers, with the lowest levels occurring in people who drank three or four cups daily (Choi et al., 2015). There is also no evidence that frequent consumption of caffeine-containing foods, including coffee, tea, or chocolate, has any impact on premature atrial contractions (PACs) and premature ventricular contractions (PVCs) (Dixit et al., 2016; Wilson and Bloom, 2016).

While caffeine dilates coronary arteries, it exerts an opposite effect on cerebral blood vessels; it constricts these vessels, thus decreasing blood flow to the brain by about 30 percent and reducing pressure within the brain. This action can produce striking relief from headaches, especially migraines, and is the reason why it is an ingredient in some analgesics.

Gastrointestinal.   Regular coffee drinking has been shown to improve glucose metabolism and insulin secretion, and significantly reduce risk for type 2 diabetes (Floegel et al., 2012; Huxley et al., 2009). A statistical correlation between high consumption of black tea and low prevalence of type 2 diabetes across 50 countries has also been reported (Beresniak et al., 2012). Preliminary data also showed that overweight patients treated with unroasted coffee beans in supplement form lost an average of 17 pounds over 22 weeks. The authors speculated that the weight loss may be due in part to coffee containing chlorogenic acid, a plant compound with antioxidant properties thought to reduce glucose absorption (Vinson et al., 2012). Compared with people who drank no coffee, those who drank three cups a day, whether decaffeinated or not, were about 25 percent less likely to have abnormal liver enzyme levels (Xiao et al., 2014).

Cancer.   Evidence suggests that moderate-to-heavy coffee consumption (three to six cups a day across studies) can reduce the risk for numerous cancers, including endometrial (Je et al., 2011), prostate (Wilson et al., 2011), head and neck (Galeone et al., 2010), basal cell carcinoma (Song et al., 2012), colon (Schmit et al., 2016), and estrogen receptor-negative breast cancer (Li et al., 2011). These protective effects are believed to be at least partially due to coffee's antioxidant and antimutagenic properties (Je et al., 2011; Turati et al., 2011). Other reported benefits include protection against liver diseases (Molloy et al., 2012), decreased risk for gout (Park et al., 2016; Zhang et al., 2016), and a possible antimicrobial effect (Matheson et al., 2011).

Neurological Numerous studies, including six large prospective studies, have supported a protective effect of caffeine against Parkinson's disease in both men and women (James et al., 2011; Liu et al., 2012). It does not matter if the caffeine is in coffee or tea (but decaffeinated coffee is not effective). Caffeine intake significantly reduces the risk of Parkinson's disease much more in those with high genetic susceptibility compared to those with low genetic susceptibility (Kumar et al., 2015). Furthermore, no study has ever found that coffee increases the risk of Parkinson's disease.

Patients with the highest levels of coffee consumption, four to six cups per day, had significantly lower risks of developing multiple sclerosis (MS) (33 percent reduction compared with those who drank no coffee) over various time periods (according to an early release abstract from the 2015 American Academy of Neurology meeting). Lower odds of MS with increasing consumption of coffee were observed, regardless of whether coffee consumption occurred at disease onset or 5 or 10 years prior to disease onset (Hedström et al., 2016).

Cognition and Mental Health. Numerous epidemiological studies indicate that the risk of developing Alzheimer's disease is reduced by a lifetime of consistent consumption of coffee, and that three to five cups a day are optimum for producing the protective effect (Arab et al., 2013; Cao et al., 2012). The protective effect is thought to be due to coffee's polyphenols as well as caffeine. Both of these substances are anti-inflammatory and preserve neurons associated with memory (Vassallo et al., 2014). The development of neurofibrillary tangles and amyloid plaques, which are the main Alzheimer's markers, are also thought to be prevented by caffeine (Laurent et al., 2014). Even acute administration of 200 milligrams of caffeine was found to improve memory of pictures in humans (Borota et al., 2014), while a single dose of 60 milligrams enhanced attention and alertness in adults (Wilhelmus et al., 2016). Furthermore, Sherman and colleagues (2016) reported memory improvement in college-age adults when they drank coffee in the morning, which was their nonoptimal time of day, but not in the afternoon. This was not due to an increase in physiological arousal or a general expectancy bias. In fact, because of its cognitive-enhancing possibilities, it has been argued that caffeine should be reassessed for the treatment of ADHD (Ioannidis et al., 2014). Moreover, it has been reported that honeybees given caffeine paired with sugar water were three times more likely to remember a learned floral scent after 24 hours than bees given just the sugar water. Caffeine occurs naturally in the nectar of *Coffea* and *Citrus* plant species, and it may be that the caffeine in their nectar improves the likelihood that their pollen will be distributed (Wright et al., 2013)!

Coffee consumption might also benefit mental health (Lucas et al., 2011). Women who drank two to four cups of coffee per day had a 15 to 20 percent decreased risk for depression compared with those who drank less than one cup per week. There was no association with depression and decaffeinated coffee. This is perhaps not surprising, because caffeine is a psychostimulant and is usually taken because of its activation of mood and behavior. At low doses, caffeine increases subjective arousal and physical endurance, improves concentration, elevates mood, and enhances performance on simple motor (such as driving simulation) and cognitive tasks, especially monotonous tasks (Smith et al., 2013). Fatigue is reduced and the need for sleep is delayed (Childs and deWit, 2012). Energy drinks also improve performance on laboratory tasks of memory and cognition. While this effect might be due to the fact that these drinks also contain a lot of sugar (glucose) (Ishak et al., 2012; Wesnes et al., 2016), evidence points to caffeine, rather than taurine or glucose, for reported changes in cognitive performance following consumption of energy drinks, especially in caffeine-withdrawn habitual caffeine consumers (Giles et al., 2012). In a rare study of "real-world" conditions, it was found that long-haul truckers who reported that they used caffeinated drinks to stay awake had a 63 percent reduced likelihood of crashing compared with drivers who did not take caffeinated products (Sharwood et al., 2013).

Other Physiological Actions. Other physiological actions of caffeine include bronchial relaxation (an antiasthmatic effect), increased secretion of gastric acid (which can promote gastric reflux), and increased urine output (although this may become tolerant in habitual users).

University of Texas scientists reported that men who consumed 85 to 303 milligrams of caffeine per day (equal to the caffeine in approximately two to three cups of coffee) were up to 42 percent less likely to report the occurrence of erectile dysfunction than men who consumed less than 75 milligrams (about one cup of coffee). The results may be due to the fact that caffeine relaxes penile arteries, which causes an increase in blood flow (Lopez, et al., 2015).

Although the emphasis here has been on caffeine, similar beneficial effects have been reported for tea and cocoa. Tea may improve working memory (Schmidt et al., 2014) and may have some modest metabolic, cardiovascular, and antidiabetic benefits (Sae-tan et al., 2014). Those who drank tea were less likely to have hepatocellular carcinoma, liver steatosis, liver cirrhosis, and chronic liver disease. Laboratory tests show that chemical components of green tea inhibit cancer cell migration (Seo et al., 2016). Tea has also been associated with a lower risk of depression (Carroll, 2015).

Recent studies have reported the benefits of theobromine, which may have antitumor, anti-inflammatory, or cardiovascular potential without the undesirable side effects of caffeine. While the main mechanisms of action of theobromine, like caffeine, are inhibition of phosphodiesterases and blockade of adenosine receptors, it also has other important nonadenosinergic, antioxidant, actions (Martínez-Pinilla et al., 2015).

Adverse Effects of Caffeine

Most people adjust, or titrate, their intake of caffeine to achieve the beneficial effects while minimizing undesirable effects. Heavy consumption of coffee (12 or more cups per day or 1.5 grams of caffeine) can cause agitation, anxiety, tremors, rapid breathing, and insomnia. The lethal dose of caffeine is about 10 grams, although ingestion in a short period of time of only 3 grams might be fatal; a blood level of 80 micrograms or more is considered potentially lethal (Sepkowitz, 2013). There are documented cases of seizures and deaths associated with caffeine consumption in energy drinks (and caffeine pills), which may be exacerbated by sleep deprivation (Ishak et al., 2012; Szpak and Allen, 2012). It has been reported that within 30 minutes of consuming an energy drink, a person's systolic blood pressure may increase by an average of 6.2 percent, compared with 3.1 percent after consuming a placebo drink. The energy drink also increased diastolic blood pressure (6.8 versus 0 percent) and serum norepinephrine levels (74 versus 31 percent) (Svatikova et al., 2015).

The FDA limits caffeine content in soft drinks, but energy drinks do not always fit into that classification and, depending on the manufacturer, may be categorized as dietary supplements, because they contain "natural" substances such as ginkgo or other herbs, which are not regulated by the FDA.

According to results of Lipshultz and colleagues (2013), energy drinks such as Red Bull are involved in more than half of the calls to poison control centers in the United States involving children less than 6 years old. Some of these children suffer from seizures and heart problems. In most of these incidents, the drinks were accidentally consumed. Nevertheless, nearly a third reported serious symptoms such as tremors, nausea, vomiting or chest pain, and erratic heart rhythms. The American Medical Association recommends limited sales to people younger than 18 (Seifert et al., 2013).

People with anxiety disorders such as panic and social anxiety disorder tend to be sensitive to the anxiogenic properties of caffeine, especially if they usually avoid caffeinated products and do not develop a tolerance to caffeine's effect, but high doses can produce anxiety even in people without such disorders. The wide variability in sensitivity to the anxiogenic effect of caffeine may be due to differences in caffeine metabolism or in the amount of adenosine receptors through which caffeine exerts its effects (discussed below) (Childs and deWit, 2012).

Caffeinism is a clinical syndrome produced by the overuse or overdoses of caffeine. Central nervous system (CNS) symptoms include increases in anxiety, agitation, and insomnia, as well as mood changes. Peripheral symptoms include tachycardia, hypertension, cardiac arrhythmias, and gastrointestinal disturbances. Caffeinism is usually dose related, with doses higher than about 500 to 1000 milligrams (1 gram, or five to ten cups of coffee) causing the most unpleasant effects. After prolonged or high doses, caffeine can produce psychosis in otherwise healthy people, especially during periods of increased stress, and worsen this condition in people with schizophrenia (Childs and deWit, 2012; Crowe et al., 2011; Persad, 2011). Cessation of caffeine ingestion resolves these symptoms.

There is also some controversy in regard to the practical benefit obtained from the use of caffeine to increase alertness. While frequent consumers may feel more alert after consumption, evidence suggests that this may be due to the reversal of acute withdrawal effects (Rodgers et al., 2010).

Perhaps the most concerning adverse effect of caffeine is its effect on sleep and the consequences of the combined use of energy drinks and alcohol on alertness and risky behavior. Although caffeine reduces fatigue and improves attention, it disturbs sleep. Even when taken during the day and certainly before bedtime, caffeine may impair the duration and quality of sleep and cause repeated awakenings (Childs and deWit, 2012; Burke et al., 2015). Compared to young adults, middle-aged adults are generally more sensitive to the effects of a high dose of caffeine on sleep quantity and quality (Robillard et al., 2015). While caffeine can reduce some of the motor impairment, sedation, and intoxication produced by alcohol (Childs and deWit, 2012), which is why it is added to alcohol, it also increases sexually risky behaviors, marijuana use, fighting, prescription drug abuse, alcohol abuse, and cigarette smoking (Ishak et al., 2012). The fact that caffeine enhances alcohol tolerance and can counteract some symptoms of a hangover may also contribute to subsequent alcohol dependence (Childs and deWit, 2012).

Nevertheless, since 2010, the FDA has regarded drinks containing both caffeine and alcohol as dangerous because the caffeine masked some of the cues that people used to tell if they were intoxicated.

In 2014, almost 17 million pounds of caffeine powder was imported into the United States (Carpenter, 2015). Caffeine is commonly synthesized in pharmaceutical factories, because it is less expensive than extraction from coffee and tea plants. The majority of this large quantity of caffeine powder winds up in soft drinks, particularly in the most successful and popular brands. Regulation of caffeine differs, depending on the type of product to which it is added. Caffeine is an ingredient in dietary supplements (energy drinks), in foods and beverages, and in over-the-counter medications (NoDoz), as well as in prescription medications, particularly in drug therapy for migraine headaches.

Pure powdered caffeine—readily available from tobacco shops and the Internet for over the past decade—was packaged in the same way as protein powder and often marketed as a source of energy rather than as a stimulant. The reality is that these products are 100 percent caffeine, with a single teaspoon roughly equivalent to the amount in 25 cups of coffee. Ten grams, about a tablespoon, is a lethal dose for an adult—symptoms include rapid, erratic heartbeat, and seizures. The FDA responded to these products by posting a consumer advisory warning of the danger (Landa, 2014) and, in 2015, by sending warning letters to five producers of caffeine powder.

Did You Know?

Pure Powdered Caffeine Fatalities

Caffeine is usually thought of as a relatively safe drug with minimal risk of overdose. Unfortunately, the availability of pure powdered caffeine proves this to be an erroneous and dangerous assumption. In 2014, two young men, Logan James Stiner and James Wade Sweatt, died after ingesting too much of this stimulant. Mr. Stiner was an 18-year-old senior in high school, an athlete and prom king who was graduating in a few days. Wanting to increase his energy, he used caffeine powder that a friend had purchased through Amazon. Mr. Sweatt, 24 years old, had recently married and just graduated from the University of Alabama at Birmingham. He took the caffeine powder to avoid the sugar and sodium added to sodas and energy drinks. Each young man miscalculated the amount of the drug he took and died of an overdose. The official cause of death stated for Mr. Stiner was "cardiac arrhythmia and seizure, due to acute caffeine toxicity due to excessive caffeine ingestion." In October 2014, two U.S. senators, Sherrod Brown of Ohio and Richard Blumenthal of Connecticut, wrote to (then) FDA Commissioner Margaret Hamburg, arguing that the product should be banned by the FDA.

Mechanism of Action

Caffeine acts primarily by blocking all subtypes of adenosine receptors A_1, A_{2A}, A_3, and A_{2B}. The structure of adenosine is shown in Figure 6.2. Adenosine is a *neuromodulator* that influences the release of several neurotransmitters in the CNS. There do not

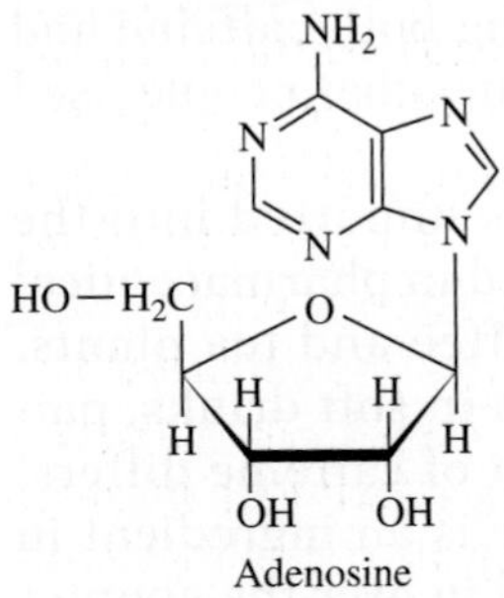

FIGURE 6.2 Structure of adenosine. Note the similarity of adenosine to caffeine (shown in Figure 6.1).

appear to be discrete adenosinergic pathways in the CNS; rather, adenosinergic neurons form a diffuse system. Adenosine levels usually increase during the day and exert a sleep-inducing effect in the brain. By blocking adenosine receptors, caffeine promotes wakefulness; it increases respiratory and heart rates, constricts blood vessels, and releases monoamines and acetylcholine.

In the striatum, type 2 adenosine receptors and type 2 dopamine receptors may combine to form a complex called a *heteromer*. When adenosine levels increase during the day, the molecules of adenosine act on this heteromer and reduce the effect of dopamine on its (associated) receptor. Caffeine blocks these adenosine receptors, which increases dopaminergic function. This may be one reason that caffeine has a beneficial effect in regard to Parkinson's disease (Bonaventura et al., 2015; Ferré et al., 2016).

Caffeine does not induce a release of dopamine in the nucleus accumbens; it leads to a release of dopamine in the prefrontal cortex, which is consistent with the drug's alerting effects and mild behavioral reinforcing properties. In addition to the direct effects of caffeine on adenosine receptors, paraxanthine, the primary metabolite of caffeine in humans, increases locomotor activity as well as extracellular levels of dopamine through a phosphodiesterase inhibitory mechanism (Ribeiro and Sebastião, 2010).

Reproductive Effects

Caffeine is consumed by at least 75 percent of pregnant women, but whether it is safe to ingest during pregnancy is an unresolved issue. As early as 1980, the FDA cautioned pregnant women to minimize their intake of caffeine. Recent reports have explored the connection between caffeine intake and rates of miscarriage (Pollack et al., 2010), fetal growth restriction (CARE Study Group, 2008), birth weight, and length of gestation (Jahanfar and Sharifah, 2009). In general, while data are limited and controversial, caffeine, at least in reasonable doses, seems to cause a modest degree of fetal growth restriction and in very large doses, may slightly increase the risk of miscarriage.

In contrast to earlier reports, a recent large epidemiological study found caffeine intake (200 to 300 milligrams per day) was consistently associated with decreased birth weight and increased odds of being small for gestational weight (Sengpiel et al., 2013). Caffeine itself does not appear to be a human teratogen, nor does it appear to affect the course of normal labor and delivery (Brent et al., 2011). One recent study, however, found that the adult offspring of mice that had been treated with caffeine while pregnant did have some neurological abnormalities, cognitive deficits, and increased susceptibility to seizures (Silva et al., 2013). Current U.S. recommendations generally advise that pregnant women limit daily intake to about 200 milligrams or less (300 milligrams per day per the World Health Organization).

Tolerance and Dependence

Chronic use of caffeine, even in regular daily doses as low as 100 milligrams, is associated with habituation and tolerance, and discontinuation may produce low-grade withdrawal symptoms. Because tolerance and dependence can occur rapidly, even after low doses, most habitual users are probably physically dependent to some degree. Individuals may become tolerant to several actions of caffeine, including diuresis, blood pressure increases, sleep disturbance, and other physiological responses, as well as subjective sensations. Tolerance is more likely with high doses of 750 to 1200 milligrams, while low doses may not produce complete tolerance (Meredith et al., 2013).

People who drink a great deal of coffee complain of headache (the most common symptom), drowsiness, fatigue, and a generally negative mood state on withdrawal. Impaired intellectual and motor performance, difficulty with concentration, and drug (caffeine) craving are also reported. Withdrawal symptoms typically begin slowly, maximize after one or two days, and cease within a few days; readministration of caffeine rapidly relieves withdrawal symptoms.

Caffeine use disorder is recognized as a diagnosable condition in the DSM-5 and three of the most significant indices from the nine criteria must be present for this diagnosis: (1) chronic craving or an inability to decrease or eliminate caffeine consumption; (2) maintained use, even after recognizing that caffeine has caused or worsened some type of mental or physical problem; and (3) elicitation of withdrawal symptoms or the prevention of withdrawal by continued consumption (Meredith et al., 2013).

NICOTINE

Epidemiology and Public Policy

Nicotine is one of the three most widely used psychoactive drugs in our society, along with caffeine and ethyl alcohol. Despite the fact that it has no current therapeutic applications in medicine, nicotine's widespread use and its well-established toxicity give it immense importance. Tobacco use continues to be the leading cause of preventable death and disease in the United States with about 45 million smokers, more than 400,000 premature deaths, and 300 billion dollars in health care expenses and lost productivity (Mohamed et al., 2015).

After stalling for several years, smoking rates started to fall after 2009 when, among many other tobacco-control interventions, the federal cigarette tax was increased, followed by the 2012 launch of the first federally funded mass media campaign aimed at reducing tobacco use (see Fiore, 2016 for a discussion). Smoking rates among adults in the United States fell to record lows in 2015, dropping to 15.1 from 16.8 percent in 2014, according to the Centers for Disease Control and Prevention in an early release of data from the National Health Interview Survey, 2015. Nevertheless, one in four adults still uses tobacco products at least occasionally, the CDC reported, and the use of tobacco products by youth, particularly snus, hookahs, and e-cigarettes, continues to increase.

The Family Smoking and Prevention and Tobacco Control Act became law in June 2009 and gave the FDA authority to regulate the manufacture, distribution, and marketing of cigarettes and several other tobacco products. However, this initial order did not include e-cigarettes, cigars, hookahs, pipe tobacco, or nicotine gels and dissolvables; these were added on August 8, 2016. Health warnings were also added to several tobacco products and free samples were banned. Products that entered the market after February 15, 2007, must be authorized by the FDA before they can be sold. Furthermore, tobacco products cannot be sold to individuals younger than 18 and require a photo ID to verify age. Vending machine sales of tobacco are only permitted in adult facilities. The law also provided support for additional tobacco control regulations by the FDA in the future.

This is just one of several significant developments regarding tobacco control. Another is Tobacco 21, a national campaign aimed at raising the tobacco and nicotine sales age in the United States to 21, produced and funded by the *Preventing Tobacco Addiction Foundation*, a public health nonprofit organization established in 1996. In September 2015, in a national initiative, the first federal Tobacco 21 legislation was introduced (Tobacco to 21 Act, S. 2100). Although in 2013 only 8 U.S. localities had adopted Tobacco 21 laws, by March 2016 at least 125 localities and the states of Hawaii and California had followed suit (Morain et al., 2016).

A no-tobacco-sale order (NTSO) is an order prohibiting the sale of tobacco products at a retail outlet, either indefinitely or for a specified time period (U.S. Food and Drug Administration, Center for Tobacco Products, 2016). The law states that this prohibition can be applied to a retailer who has violated tobacco restrictions five or more times over 36 months of compliance inspections. The FDA filed NTSO restrictions for the first time in October 2015 against several stores after numerous violations regarding the sale and distribution of tobacco products, including sales to minors.

The importance of smoking prevention in youth was reinforced by several reports concerning the long-term consequences of early onset smoking. Not surprisingly, high rates of smoking initiation during adolescence were not only associated with high lung cancer mortality decades later, but at a younger age than would normally be expected (Funatogawa et al., 2012; Whitley et al., 2012). Aside from the physiological costs, there are social costs for smoking. In March 2013, the University of Pennsylvania announced that beginning in July, it would no longer hire tobacco users to work in its health care system; this was accompanied by two articles that presented opposing views about the ethics of denying employment to people who smoke (Asch et al., 2013; Schmidt et al., 2013). In fact, unemployed smokers have a harder time finding work than job seekers who do not smoke, and researchers reported that smokers earn less than nonsmokers when they do become employed (Prochaska et al., 2016).

While nearly 70 percent of adults who smoke report wanting to quit and more than 50 percent reported making an attempt to stop in the year before they were questioned, only a little over 6 percent were successful (Malarcher et al., 2011). For those who succeed, however, the benefits of quitting can be dramatic. Life expectancy can increase on average from 10 to 4 years in those who quit between 25 and 64 years of age, respectively (Schroeder, 2013). Moreover, the cardiovascular benefits of quitting are not reduced even if those who quit subsequently gained weight (at least, if they did not have diabetes) (Clair et al., 2013).

Pharmacokinetics

Although more than 4000 compounds are released by burning cigarette tobacco, nicotine is the primary addictive substance and is responsible for tobacco dependence. The other compounds produce the adverse long-term cardiovascular, pulmonary, and carcinogenic effects of cigarettes.

Nicotine is readily absorbed from every site on or in the body, including the lungs, buccal and nasal mucosa, skin, and gastrointestinal tract. Easy and complete absorption promotes the recreational abuse of smoked or chewed tobacco as well as its therapeutic use in treating nicotine dependency in chewing gums, nasal sprays, transdermal skin patches, and smokeless inhalers.

Nicotine is suspended in cigarette smoke in the form of minute particles (tars) and is quickly absorbed into the bloodstream from the lungs when the smoke is inhaled, although absorption is much slower than once thought and arterial concentrations of nicotine rise rather slowly. It is likely that blood rapidly saturates with nicotine and blood leaving the lungs (to the left side of the heart) can carry only a modest amount of drug. Thus, the arterial concentration rises slowly, even though blood carried to the brain at the initiation of smoking is nearly saturated with nicotine, accounting for the early "rush" perceived with the first cigarette.

The average cigarette contains about 8 to 10 milligrams of nicotine, but only about 20 to 25 percent of that amount enters the bloodstream. Because a cigarette is typically smoked in 10 puffs and within 5 minutes, the average smoker will absorb 1 to 2 milligrams of nicotine, but absorption can range from 0.5 to 3 milligrams. In a typical day, the average smoker absorbs anywhere from 20 to 40 milligrams.

The lethal dose for the average adult has typically been reported as 60 milligrams, but more recently suggested to be between 500 and 1000 milligrams of ingested nicotine. A smoker can readily avoid acute toxicity because inhalation as a route of administration offers exceptional controllability of the dose. By controlling the frequency of breaths, the depth of inhalation, the time the smoke is held in the lungs, and the total number of cigarettes smoked, the smoker regulates the rate of drug intake and controls the blood level of nicotine. (People who harvest or cultivate tobacco may experience green tobacco sickness, a type of nicotine poisoning caused by dermal exposure to wet tobacco leaves).

Characteristically, smokers wake in the morning in a state of nicotine deficiency, smoke one or more cigarettes fairly rapidly to achieve a blood level of about 15 milligrams per liter, and continue smoking through the day to maintain this level. The elimination half-life of nicotine in a chronic smoker is about two hours, necessitating frequent administration of the drug to avoid withdrawal symptoms or drug craving. When nicotine is administered in the form of snuff, chewing tobacco, or gum, blood levels of nicotine are comparable to the levels achieved by smoking.

The liver metabolizes approximately 80 to 90 percent of the nicotine, primarily by the CYP-2A6 enzyme. People in whom the CYP-2A6 enzyme is absent (or inhibited by certain drugs) have higher blood levels of nicotine and lower levels of its metabolite. The constituents of tobacco smoke, however, also induce hepatic enzymes CYP1A1, 1A2, and possibly 2E1, which are involved in the metabolism of many hormones and drugs, such as caffeine, estrogen, some antidepressants, and other psychotropic agents (Fankhauser, 2013). As a result, smoking may reduce levels of these medications and smoking cessation may increase blood levels, especially in moderate or heavy smokers (10 or more cigarettes a day).

The primary metabolite of nicotine is *cotinine*, which serves as a marker of both tobacco use and exposure to environmental smoke, and is often used to measure tobacco consumption in laboratory experiments. There is some evidence that although cotinine itself is nonaddictive and has no cardiovascular effects in humans, it might have some anxiolytic and cognitive benefits (Moran, 2012).

Mechanism of Action

Nicotine exerts virtually all its CNS and peripheral effects by activating specific acetylcholine receptors (nicotinic receptors; nAChRs). These are divided into two groups: muscle receptors, found on skeletal (voluntary) muscles, and neuronal receptors, located throughout the peripheral and central nervous systems. Neuronal nicotinic receptors are composed of five subunits arranged around a central pore (which is termed a pentameric arrangement), like segments of an orange (see Chapter 3). A dozen proteins, labeled α_{2-10} and β_{2-4}, serve as subunits in nACh receptors. The most abundant and widely distributed nACh subunit proteins in the brain are the α_4 and β_2 subunits. Animal and human imaging studies have shown that nACh receptors consisting of two α_4 and three β_2 subunits are critical for the rewarding effects of nicotine (Figure 6.3). Because nicotine stimulates these receptors, it is classified as an agonist. But while stimulation occurs at low doses, nicotine at high doses can block the receptors and thus has a biphasic action. In addition, within the time it takes to finish smoking a single cigarette, these nicotinic receptors become

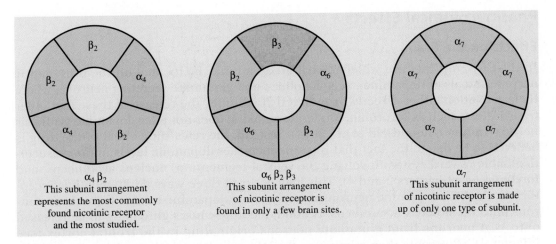

$\alpha_4 \beta_2$
This subunit arrangement represents the most commonly found nicotinic receptor and the most studied.

$\alpha_6 \beta_2 \beta_3$
This subunit arrangement of nicotinic receptor is found in only a few brain sites.

α_7
This subunit arrangement of nicotinic receptor is made up of only one type of subunit.

FIGURE 6.3 Diagram of the most common subtypes of the receptor for acetylcholine.

desensitized; that is, they temporarily do not respond to nicotine or acetylcholine. During the day, tolerance develops as nicotine builds up in the smoker's body, but this is lost overnight when the user is not smoking, which contributes to the powerful effect of the first cigarette of the day.

Menthol. Widely used as a flavoring in many products, menthol has been an additive to tobacco cigarettes since 1926. Although the concentration of menthol in cigarettes varies by brand, it is present in 90 percent of all tobacco products and used to mask the harshness of inhaled smoke, make smoking easier, and provide an oral sensation that appeals to many smokers. But smokers of menthol cigarettes are less likely to quit and have higher relapse rates than smokers of nonmenthol cigarettes. Recent studies may shed some light on the reason for this difference.

Chronic, long-term smokers of both menthol and unflavored cigarettes acquire more receptors for nicotine, particularly in neurons involved in the pathways for reward and motivation. But smokers of menthol cigarettes develop even more of these receptors (9 to 28 percent more) than smokers of unflavored cigarettes. In fact, even without nicotine, menthol increased the number of brain nicotinic receptors, especially in the ventral tegmental area, which is part of the dopamine signaling pathway that mediates addiction. Studies show that menthol directly reduces the activation of the nACh receptor by nicotine; that is, menthol decreases the ability of nicotine to activate the nACh receptor (it is an allosteric modulator of the nACh). Nicotine does not activate the receptor channel to the same extent when coapplied with menthol (Henderson et al., 2016; Kabbani, 2013; Wickham, 2015). Beginning in 2022, the European Union will ban menthol-flavored cigarettes and the U.S. Food and Drug Administration is considering taking similar measures. In June 2017, the San Francisco board of supervisors voted unanimously to ban menthol-flavored cigarettes and flavored tobacco products, effective April 2018.

Pharmacological Effects

Effects on the Brain

In the CNS, nAChRs are widely distributed and may be located on the presynaptic nerve terminals of dopamine-, acetylcholine-, and glutamate-secreting neurons, where their activation either directly or indirectly facilitates the release of these and other transmitters, such as serotonin. Moderate smoking does not alter dopamine synthesis in the striatum (Bloomfield et al., 2014). Instead, the rewarding effect of the drug is believed to be due to the fact that nicotine increases dopamine levels in the mesocorticolimbic reward system involving the ventral tegmentum, nucleus accumbens, and forebrain (see Chapters 2 and 4). This may occur in three ways. First, nicotinic receptors on the VTA dopamine neurons directly cause dopamine release from these neurons onto the nucleus accumbens. Second, nicotine causes glutamate to be released onto VTA neurons from glutamate neurons originating in the frontal cortex (see Chapter 4). Glutamate then stimulates the VTA neurons to release dopamine. Third, nicotine desensitizes nicotinic receptors that are on GABA neurons in the VTA. These receptors are normally stimulated by Ach to release GABA onto VTA dopamine neurons, and GABA normally inhibits dopamine release. When nicotine desensitizes the nAChRs, less GABA is released; the VTA is less inhibited and releases more dopamine. Moreover, it has been reported that in laboratory animals, repeated periods of exposure to and subsequent withdrawal from nicotine increased its rewarding value and also upregulated nicotinic brain receptors. It was speculated that this phenomenon might be one reason why smokers relapse frequently (Hilario et al., 2012). Morel and colleagues (2014) identified a specific alpha subunit of the nicotinic receptor that is an important regulator of nicotinic-induced dopamine activation and the genetic component that controls the expression of that subunit. This links genetics to receptor structure and to self-administration of nicotine.

Studies in humans found that the motivation to smoke (puff rate) predicted the magnitude of dopamine release in the limbic striatum and the amount of dopamine release was correlated with decreased craving and withdrawal symptoms. Results also support the preferential involvement of the limbic striatum in the motivation to smoke, anticipation of pleasure from cigarettes, and relief of withdrawal symptoms (Le Foll et al., 2014). Volume, surface area, and shape of the striatum were also related to measures of craving (Janes et al., 2015). The first demonstration of tobacco smoking-induced *cortical* dopamine release in humans was shown by Wing and colleagues (2015). Studies in the mouse found that under certain conditions, such as simultaneous intake of the two drugs, prior nicotine use promoted *cocaine* self-administration. This result suggests how nicotine in products such as e-cigarettes may be a "gateway" to other drug use (Kandel and Kandel, 2014).

Nicotine-induced release of acetylcholine may improve cognitive performance and may also be responsible for the arousal effects commonly seen with smoking. Very few studies, however, have looked at nicotine's effect on memory performance in normal *nonsmokers*. There is some evidence for the improvement of working memory in nonsmokers, but only under specific experimental conditions; one study did find that nicotine patches improved some aspects of attention in nonsmokers who had no preexisting cognitive impairments (Levin et al., 2006). Such outcomes have raised interest in the development of nicotinic drugs as "cognitive enhancers," which might be beneficial in treating Alzheimer's disease. There is stronger evidence suggesting a protective role for nicotine receptors in Parkinson's disease; as with caffeine, tobacco smoking is associated with a reduced likelihood of Parkinson's disease (Quik et al., 2012). The potential benefits of nicotine, its metabolites, and related compounds for treating Parkinson's disease are discussed by Barreto and colleagues (2015). High doses have toxic effects, but low doses may be therapeutic.

Smoking and Mental Health.   In the United States, individuals with mental disorders account for 40 to 50 percent of all cigarettes consumed (Smith et al., 2014). Unlike in those not mentally ill, smoking rates have changed little in the mentally ill (Cook et al., 2014). In fact, associations of smoking with drug and alcohol abuse, attention deficit/hyperactivity disorder, bipolar disorder, and antisocial personality disorder have each increased over the last decades (Talati et al., 2016). Moreover, tobacco smoking is an independent risk factor for developing schizophrenia and nonaffective psychoses with a dose-response association, although the risk is much lower for bipolar disorder (Kendler et al., 2015). Patients with schizophrenia, bipolar disorder, or depression also have a significantly increased risk of tobacco-related mortality (Callaghan et al., 2014) and of being diagnosed with nicotine withdrawal syndrome (Smith et al., 2014). Conversely, smokers reported more frequent symptoms compared with nonsmokers of depressed mood, poor sleep, low energy, hopelessness, lack of appetite, lack of interest, and trouble concentrating (Parikh et al., 2014). Smoking is also associated with an increased risk of panic attacks and quitting smoking helps to reduce such attacks (Bakhshaie et al., 2016).

The good news is that smoking cessation treatment can be effective in people with mental illness, even with comorbid substance abuse, and can improve the psychiatric condition (Cook et al., 2014; Taylor et al., 2014). Adding smoking cessation treatment to the treatment for illicit stimulant use did not worsen the latter and even enhanced abstinence from non-nicotine use as well as from nicotine use (Winhusen et al., 2014). However, patients with a history of substance abuse and who take antidepressants may have a lower smoking cessation rate than those without such a background (Zorick et al., 2014). Smoking cessation itself in people with no psychiatric disorders did not worsen mental health (Taylor et al., 2015).

Acute Effects on the Body

In the peripheral nervous system, nicotine causes an increase in blood pressure, heart rate, cardiac contractility, release of epinephrine (adrenaline) from the adrenal glands, and an increase in the activity of the gastrointestinal tract.

In nonatherosclerotic coronary arteries, nicotine produces vasodilation, increasing blood flow to meet the increased oxygen demand of the heart muscle. In atherosclerotic coronary arteries (which cannot dilate), however, cardiac ischemia can result when the oxygen supply fails to meet the oxygen demand created by the drug's cardiac stimulation. This occurrence can precipitate angina or myocardial infarction (heart attack).

In the early stages of smoking, nicotine causes nausea and vomiting by stimulating both the vomiting center in the brain stem and the sensory receptors in the stomach. Tolerance to this effect develops rapidly. Nicotine also reduces weight gain, probably by reducing appetite and altering taste bud sensitivity. Stomach secretions are inhibited, but bowel activity is stimulated; in people with little tobacco tolerance, the drug is a laxative.

Nicotine stimulates the hypothalamus to release antidiuretic hormone, which causes fluid retention. The activity of afferent nerve fibers coming from the muscles is reduced by nicotine, leading to a decrease in muscle tone. This action may be involved (at least partially) in the relaxation a person may experience as a result of smoking.

Tolerance and Dependence

While some of the acute effects wane, there is little tolerance to the primary rewarding effects of nicotine. On the other hand, nicotine clearly induces both physiological and psychological dependence in a majority of smokers. As early as 1988, the surgeon general of the United States (U.S. Department of Health and Human Services, 1988) concluded that tobacco use is addictive, nicotine was the substance in tobacco that causes addiction, and nicotine addiction was pharmacologically as powerful as addiction to other drugs, such as heroin and cocaine.

A well-defined withdrawal syndrome has been delineated, which is alleviated by nicotine replacement. Abstinence symptoms include a severe craving for nicotine, irritability, anxiety, anger, difficulty in concentrating, restlessness, impatience, increased appetite, weight gain, and insomnia. Symptoms usually begin within about two hours after the last use of tobacco, peak within 24 to 48 hours, and gradually decline over the next 10 days to several weeks. Mild depression (dysphoria and anhedonia) and increased appetite may persist for months. In one study, smoking cessation produced a mean increase in body weight of 4 to 5 kilograms after 12 months of abstinence, although most weight was gained in the first 3 months (Aubin et al., 2012). The difficulty in handling cigarette dependence is illustrated by the fact that cigarette smokers who seek treatment for other drug and alcohol problems often find it harder to quit cigarette smoking than to give up the other drugs. Even Sigmund Freud continued his cigar habit (20 per day) until death, in spite of an endless series of operations for mouth and jaw cancer (his jaw was eventually totally removed), persistent heart problems that were exacerbated by smoking, and numerous attempts at quitting.

Unlike other drugs that produce physical dependence, the severity of tobacco withdrawal does not seem to be related to the dose (heavy or light amount of smoking), the duration of the habit, previous attempts at quitting, sex, age, education, or alcohol and caffeine use (McKim and Hancock, 2013). On the other hand, there is some evidence that genetic factors play a role in the development of dependence, specifically the probability of smoking 20 or more cigarettes daily, earlier and faster onset of heavy smoking, and the likelihood of relapse after quitting (Belsky et al., 2013).

Toxicity

Central Nervous System

Studies of the effects of nicotine on brain anatomy report a loss of brain matter in the cerebral hemispheres in current smokers (Fritz et al., 2014; Morales et al., 2014), as well as differences between smokers and nonsmokers in the strength of some connections between various brain structures (Addicott et al., 2015; Lerman et al., 2014). Evidence suggests that enzyme activity in the brain (as opposed to the liver) could affect brain nicotine levels and influence smoking behavior (Garcia et al., 2015).

Another study also revealed the deleterious effect of smoking on the CNS in multiple sclerosis (MS); patients who continued to smoke experienced a faster onset of secondary progressive MS (SPMS) (Hillert et al., 2015).

Cardiovascular Disease

The carbon monoxide in smoke decreases the amount of oxygen delivered to the heart muscle, while nicotine increases the amount of work the heart must do (by increasing the heart rate and blood pressure). Both carbon monoxide and nicotine increase the incidence of atherosclerosis (narrowing) and thrombosis (clotting) in the coronary arteries. These three actions (among others) seem to underlie the dramatic increase in the risk of death from coronary heart disease in smokers compared to nonsmokers (Teo et al., 2006). Cigarette smokers manifest a 50 percent increase in the progression of atherosclerosis when compared with people who have never smoked.

Besides the coronary arteries, atherosclerosis occurs in other arteries as well, most notably the aorta (in the abdomen), the carotid arteries (in the neck), and the femoral and other arteries of the legs. Cigarette-induced occlusion of these vessels blocks the blood flow to important body organs and results in ischemic damage, strokes, and other disorders. However, in women who quit smoking for 20 years or more, this risk dropped to the level of those who never smoked compared to current smokers (Sandhu et al., 2012).

Pulmonary Disease

When tobacco smoke is inhaled, tar and ash are deposited on the moist membranes through which oxygen and carbon dioxide have to cross to and from the blood. Eventually, these toxins overcome the processes by which pollutants are removed and destroyed in the lung. This leaves the lung more susceptible to infections and other toxic damage. Chronic smoking results in difficulty in breathing, wheezing, chest pain, lung congestion, emphysema (a form of irreversible lung damage), and increased susceptibility to infections of the respiratory tract.

Cancer

Although nicotine itself is not carcinogenic, the relationship between smoking and cancer is now beyond question. A new study (Lortet-Tieulent et al., 2016) has found that 28.6 percent of all cancer deaths in the United States are attributable to cigarette smoking: 22.9 percent of cancer deaths in women and 33.7 in men. This is likely an underestimate because the study only included data on cigarettes and not cancers caused by secondhand smoke, pipes, hookahs, cigars, smokeless tobacco, and electronic nicotine delivery systems or deaths from many other diseases linked to smoking.

Cigarette smoke contains diverse carcinogens and cigarette smoking is the major cause of lung cancer in both men and women. Smoking is also a major cause of cancers of the mouth, voice box (larynx), and throat. Concomitant alcohol ingestion greatly increases the incidence of these problems. In addition, cigarette smoking is a primary cause of bladder cancer and pancreatic cancer, and it increases the risk of cancer of the uterine cervix twofold.

In addition to these disorders, smoking promotes many other illnesses. Among hormonal effects, smoking contributes to the development of insulin resistance and type 2 diabetes (Pan et al., 2015). It has several effects on the visual system: it increases the risk of cataract formation and Graves' ophthalmopathy, an autoimmune disease associated with too much thyroid activation, in which the eyes bulge because of swelling and inflammation (Kapoor and Jones, 2005). Smoking also causes premature aging of the skin (at least partly because of blood vessel constriction) and current smokers have a greater risk of developing cutaneous squamous cell cancer compared to nonsmokers (Leonardi-Bee et al., 2012).

Smoking even increases, by 17 percent, death from diseases that do not have established relationships with cigarette smoking (Carter et al., 2015).

The FDA has established a list of 93 harmful and potentially harmful constituents (HPHCs) that tobacco companies will eventually be required to report for every regulated tobacco product sold in the United States. All HPHCs included on the list cause or may cause serious health problems, including cancer, lung disease, and addiction to tobacco products. The complete list includes ammonia, formaldehyde, nicotine, nitrosamines, carbon monoxide, and other toxins.

Effects of Passive Smoke

Many nonsmokers are exposed to the toxic agents in the passive smoke exuded by burning and exhaled cigarettes, pipes, cigars, and like tobacco products, called *environmental tobacco smoke, secondhand smoke,* or *passive smoking.* In 1993, the Environmental Protection Agency classified secondhand smoke as a Class A carcinogen. In 2011, the first global assessment published data from 2004 across 192 countries and concluded that secondhand smoke accounted for about 1 percent, or about 603,000 deaths, worldwide (Öberg et al., 2011). Of particular concern, 165,000 children were estimated to have died from smoke-related respiratory infections, mostly in Southeast Asia and Africa. Children whose parents smoke have a higher risk of sudden infant death syndrome, ear infections, pneumonia, bronchitis, and asthma. Data from the National Health and Nutrition Examination Surveys from 2003 through 2010 of children ages 6 to 19 who had been diagnosed with asthma showed that 53 percent had cotinine in their blood. Smoke exposure increased doctor visits, disturbed sleep, and impaired physical activity (Akinbami et al., 2012). Prenatal exposure has also been found to increase subsequent psychiatric problems in offspring of smokers (Ekblad et al., 2010). There is even evidence that children who are exposed to secondhand smoke are more likely to start smoking themselves than children who are not exposed to passive smoke (Doweiko, 2012). Worldwide, 40 percent of children are regularly exposed to secondhand smoke and children account for more than a quarter of all deaths and over half of all healthy years of life lost due to exposure to secondhand smoke. Legislation to reduce the effects of secondhand smoke through public smoking bans have led to drops in both preterm births and childhood asthma hospitalizations (Been et al., 2014; Kalkhoran and Glantz, 2014).

Effects During Pregnancy

Cigarette smoking reduces oxygen delivery to the developing fetus, causing a variable degree of fetal hypoxia. This condition may underlie the reported increases in irritability and increased muscle tone in the neonate (Stroud et al., 2009) and even longer-term intellectual and physical deficiencies (Abbott and Winzer-Serhan, 2012). Furthermore, cigarette smoking produces a two- to threefold increase in being small for gestational age (SGA) or being born preterm (McCowan et al., 2009). Even women exposed to passive smoke inhalation have low-birth-weight children. In fact, when a smoking ban was introduced in northern Belgium, gradually over successive years (2006, 2007, and 2010), there was a statistical decrease in the rate of preterm births. The rate dropped the most during the last phases, when smoking was banned in restaurants and in bars selling food (Cox et al., 2013). These risks can be reversed if smoking is stopped early in pregnancy. Also, the weight of a smoker's small for gestational age offspring usually becomes normal at about 18 months of age.

Programs designed to reduce smoking behaviors and nicotine dependence during pregnancy offer special challenges because the safety of pharmacological interventions (bupropion, nicotine replacement therapies, varenicline) has not been established. Nevertheless, in a French study involving 402 pregnant women (all over 18 years old and between 12 and 20 weeks pregnant) who smoked at least five cigarettes a day, the effectiveness of 16-hour nicotine patches was evaluated. In addition to receiving behavioral support for smoking cessation, participants were randomly chosen to receive either nicotine or placebo patches throughout their pregnancy. Researchers measured birth weight and total abstinence (as confirmed by carbon monoxide levels in exhaled air from the pregnant women). Neither birth weight nor smoking cessation showed any improvement with nicotine patches compared with placebo patches. Only 11 women (5.5 percent) given the nicotine patch achieved complete abstinence, which was comparable to the 10 women (5.1 percent) who received the placebo patch (Berlin et al., 2014).

Pharmacological Approaches to Nicotine Dependence

As nicotine dependence gradually became recognized during the 1990s, a variety of pharmacological treatments were developed to "reduce the harm" of smoking, with the presumed goal of promoting cessation. These are sometimes referred to as *potentially reduced exposure products* (PREPs), developed as a means of tobacco harm reduction (THR).

According to the U.S. Public Health Service (2008) and the U.S. Preventive Services Task Force (Patnode et al., 2015), several products are considered to be first-line options for smoking cessation, also called *nicotine replacement therapy* (NRT). These include nicotine gum, lozenges, inhalers, mouth spray, nasal spray, the transdermal nicotine patch, orally dissolvable films, and low-nicotine cigarettes (Hansson et al., 2012). Dissolvable tobacco consists of fine-grained tobacco formed into pellets, strips, or toothpick-size "sticks" that dissolve in the mouth. Nontobacco, or non-NRT agents, include the antidepressant bupropion and the partial nicotine agonist varenicline (Chantix). The efficacy of other smoking cessation medications is less well established (Siu et al., 2015).[2]

---

[2]All insurers under the *Affordable Care Act* must cover screening for tobacco use and pay for at least two tobacco cessation attempts per year. That coverage would include four counseling sessions of at least 10 minutes each (including telephone, group, and individual counseling) as well as all FDA-approved tobacco cessation medications (whether prescription or over the counter) with a 90-day supply as prescribed. That coverage is to be without prior authorization or cost sharing for the patient.

Several other forms of nicotine administration have also become popular, including sublingual products, referred to as "snus,"[3] water pipes (hookahs), and electronic cigarettes.

Snus consists of moist powdered tobacco (with salt and water) sold as small mesh pouches, which are held in the mouth for about 30 minutes and then discarded. A snus user packs the tobacco into the upper lip to get the nicotine and swallows the by-product, rather than spit it out. One 2-gram portion of snus increases blood nicotine concentration to around 15 nanograms per milliliter of tobacco within 30 minutes. In contrast, a cigarette delivers about 23 nanograms per milliliter of nicotine in the first five minutes, but by 30 minutes the levels of nicotine in the body are comparable between the two. The products are promoted as a way to get a nicotine fix when you cannot smoke, like nicotine gum. Except for Sweden, the sale of snus has been banned throughout the European Union since 1992.

In the spring of 2015, the FDA denied a petition by two tobacco companies to ease up on the warnings around smokeless tobacco. For now, they will carry the same warning labels stating that they are "not a safe alternative to cigarettes" currently required for other smokeless tobacco products. As of November 2015, eight snus products have been the first to be cleared under the FDA's premarket tobacco application (PMTA) pathway, established after Congress authorized the agency to regulate tobacco products.

Using a *hookah* (also called a *shisa, narghile,* or *water pipe*) involves smoking substances through a water pipe such that the smoke passes through the water and is cooled before inhalation. Originating in northern Africa and southwest Asia, it is a tradition at least four centuries old and is now very popular among adult men in Middle Eastern countries (Brockman et al., 2012). Hookah smoking, however, is spreading worldwide; in the United States, adolescents and young adults are increasingly adopting this habit. Apparently, many hookah smokers believe it is less harmful and addictive than smoking cigarettes. Studies so far show that this is not the case, and that both short- and long-term effects of water-pipe tobacco smoking are just as harmful (Hakim et al., 2011). Secondhand exposure to hookah smoke is also an underappreciated health hazard for workers in the increasing number of venues that allow water pipes (Zhou et al., 2016). Smoking hookahs more than doubles the odds that a noncigarette smoker will begin smoking within two years, according to a recent study (Soneji et al., 2015). Using snus increases the risk of starting smoking by more than sixfold. At follow-up, among those who did not smoke cigarettes at baseline, 39 percent of hookah users had begun smoking, compared with 20 percent of those who had not used water pipes. Similarly, among baseline nonsmokers, 55 percent of smokeless tobacco users had begun smoking at follow-up, compared with 21 percent of those who did not use snus.

---

[3] To make snus, small strips of tobacco are dried, then ground into a powder, which is then treated with heat (up to 100 degrees Celsius) for 24 to 36 hours. A "wet" snuff, snus tobacco contains 50 percent water and 30 percent tobacco. It is usually sold in teabag-shaped portions that the user bundles under the upper lip. A heavy snus user may consume the product for 13 to 15 hours a day. With high levels of salt, moist oral snuff produces less saliva than dipping or chewing tobaccos such as Skoal, Copenhagen, or Red Man, and the saliva by-product is meant to be swallowed. The finished tobacco product is chilled below room temperature to keep its contents fresh. Expect to find American tobacconists installing refrigerators if they carry snus.

Vapor Products: E-cigarettes and Electronic Nicotine Devices

Perhaps the most controversial product in the PREP category is the *electronic cigarette*, or *e-cigarette*. Predecessors appeared as early as 1965 and 1986, but current versions were developed in 2003 by the Chinese pharmacist Hon Lik, a former deputy director of the Institute of Chinese Medicine in Liaoning Province (U.S. Department of Health and Human Services, 2016). The e-cigarette has no tobacco. Instead, users add drops of liquid nicotine to the battery-powered device, which delivers a propylene glycol–nicotine vapor that is inhaled. Laboratory studies suggest that e-cigarettes may be safer than tobacco products because they essentially contain fewer nonnicotinic toxic substances and they do not produce secondhand smoke. They also have the advantage of providing the behavioral stimuli that is often conditioned to smoking—the physical act of holding a cigarette and inhaling and exhaling a vapor. The presence of diethylene glycol, however, a toxic chemical found in antifreeze, raises safety concerns. Users can also modify the apparatus to produce more vapor, increase the amount of nicotine, or add other ingredients besides nicotine. The Vype eTank is a refillable e-cigarette that gives users control over the nicotine strength and flavor combinations that suit them; there are a range of Vype eLiquid flavors in a variety of nicotine strengths. There is a wide variation in the amount of nicotine, even in different samples of the same product.

Devices known as *vape-pens* are larger than typical e-cigarettes. They have bigger batteries that are capable of raising the temperature, and consequently the nicotine level, higher than the standard e-cig. These may be appealing because the blood level of nicotine is lower with e-cigs than with normal cigarettes. Unfortunately, the increased temperature also increases the level of toxins and carcinogens. Higher nicotine levels, or batteries, have also been introduced by the tobacco companies. One example is a new e-cigarette formulation that the company Njoy developed to increase lung absorption so that the nicotine level approaches 70 percent of a regular cigarette (Moyses et al., 2015).

The Voke, developed in the UK, completely does away with electronic components, batteries, and heat, relying instead on a pressurized canister containing 20 refills of pharmaceutical-grade nicotine activated by a breath-controlled microvalve. Every time the user draws on the device, they are administered a precise dose of nicotine. Basically, the Voke is an e-cigarette-shaped inhaler that does not produce any kind of visible smoke or vapor. But it does reproduce other elements of smoking, including a typical "throat catch," that is, the sensation of smoke in the back of the throat. At the beginning of 2017, this product was licensed to the company Kind Consumer, which hopes to introduce it in 2018.

Philip Morris International's newest product, the iQOS, is a hybrid between a cigarette and an e-cigarette. The Marlboro-branded iQOS uses real tobacco in the shape of small cigarettes ("heat sticks") that are inserted into the heating device and heated at high temperatures, but not actually burned. The iQOS only heats the tobacco to 350 degrees Celsius, whereas tobacco cigarettes burn at around 800 degrees, but the product delivers a mouthful of tobacco-flavored vapor without smoke or tar. Smokers who use iQOS will still have more chemical exposure than smokers who switch to one of the vapor alternatives. As of September 2017, this product was not approved in the United States.

E-cigarettes are not devoid of toxicity. In 2014, the American Association of Poison Control Centers reported that more than 3700 children were exposed to liquid nicotine, a dramatic increase from prior years. The next year, New York fined four producers of liquid nicotine made for electronic cigarettes because the packaging was too easy for children to open, which violated a 2014 law. That same year, attorneys general of 33 states in the United States argued for health warning labels to be required by the FDA on liquids containing nicotine as well as several other tobacco items. This request resulted in a new set of labeling and advertising regulations from the FDA. Between March 2013 and March 2014, the FDA received over 50 complaints of electronic cigarette injury—about the same as the number received in all of the preceding five years. Effects included difficulty breathing, headache, cough, dizziness, sore throat, nosebleeds, chest pain, and allergic reactions. At the May 2015 annual meeting of the American Thoracic Society, Dr. P. V. Dicpinigaitis reported that exposure to electronic cigarette vapors significantly reduced the sensitivity of the cough reflex in a group of healthy volunteers. In experiments on mice, scientists found that e-cigarette vapor could harm the lungs and make them more susceptible to respiratory infections, and that e-cigarette vapors appeared to increase the aggressiveness of dangerous bacteria such as methicillin-resistant *Staphylococcus aureus* (MRSA), making it more virulent (although cigarette smoke has a much greater effect) (Crotty Alexander et al., 2014). E-cigarette use is associated with higher cardiac sympathetic tone and increased oxidative stress, but it remains unclear to what extent these changes represent an increase in cardiovascular risk (Moheimani et al., 2017). Moreover, some popular e-cigarettes get so hot that they, too, can produce some of the carcinogens found in cigarettes and at similar levels.

It is generally believed that the inhaled chemicals produced from an e-cigarette are less dangerous than the nearly 300 carcinogens that are released from a regular cigarette (Shahab et al., 2017), but it is not completely clear what those chemicals are. The vaping process itself may produce a more addictive form of nicotine, called *free base*, than smoking (El-Hellani et al., 2015). The high-powered e-cigarettes, known as *tank systems*, produce formaldehyde, a known carcinogen, along with the nicotine-laced vapor. The toxin is formed when liquid nicotine and other e-cigarette ingredients are subjected to high temperatures (Jensen et al., 2015). In addition to this inherent toxicity, Krishnan-Sarin and colleagues (2017) report that many teens who use electronic cigarettes have tried "dripping," in which small amounts of e-liquid are dropped directly onto an e-cigarette's atomizer coil to vaporize the liquid at a high temperature; users then inhale the vapor immediately. The most commonly reported reasons for dripping included: it "produces thicker clouds of vapor," the "flavor tastes better," and it provides "a stronger throat hit." The authors noted that e-liquids exposed to high temperatures produce significant increases in the levels of formaldehyde, acetaldehyde, and acetone in the vapors. Dinakar and O'Connor (2016) provide a review of the health effects of electronic cigarettes.

E-Cigarettes and Smoking Cessation.   But, the most important question is, do e-cigarettes really help smokers to stop or are they merely a steppingstone to cigarettes and other tobacco products? This issue has caused much debate among the experts. The main reason for regular e-cigarette use cited in surveys has been "to kick" the tobacco habit, and some public health experts support that "harm-reduction" strategy.

Arguments in favor of e-cigarettes are that they are safer than conventional cigarettes and have the potential to promote cessation. The amount of toxic substances is lower than that in tobacco smoke, the carcinogenic content is "negligible," the risk of nicotinic poisoning is minimal if they are used as intended, and other components of the vapor are not dangerous, at least in people without respiratory difficulties. The increase in e-cigarette use is expected to be more common among people who already smoke, and e-cigarettes might help motivated smokers quit by reducing their urge to smoke.

A panel of public health experts from the United Kingdom published a report in 2015 regarding the relative effects of electronic cigarettes. They determined that e-cigarettes were 95 percent less dangerous than regular cigarettes. In addition, they did not believe that there was sufficient evidence to argue that e-cigarette use led to subsequent use of other tobacco products (Green et al., 2016). In January 2016, UK drug regulators gave the go-ahead for a British American Tobacco (BAT) e-cigarette, the e-Voke, to be sold as a therapy for quitting smoking.

Those against e-cigarettes argue that all forms of nicotine are addictive and substantially more harmful than not smoking at all. Moreover, opponents argue that e-cigarettes or similar alternatives might be used by smokers to increase their consumption of nicotine, rather than discontinue conventional cigarettes. Regulatory authorities could make e-cigarettes safer by requiring child-proof packaging, prohibiting the addition or production of potentially dangerous contaminants in products with nicotine, and by capping the voltage and temperature specifications of these devices, which would reduce formaldehyde exposure. It is generally acknowledged that while e-cigarettes are less harmful than conventional cigarettes, they are still more risky than total abstention from tobacco and could be made safer (Lindblom, 2015).

The hope that cigarette smokers would switch to e-cigarettes and benefit from lower rates of heart disease, lung disease, and cancer assumes that the only persons who use e-cigarettes would be current tobacco users looking for a safer cigarette. But there is concern that e-cigarettes serve as the entryway for young nontobacco users to become addicted to nicotine. This concern is supported by data showing that a third of e-cigarette users were nonsmokers and 1.4 percent were never smokers (Avdalovic and Murin, 2015). According to one Web-based survey, electronic cigarettes did not help smokers quit or even smoke less. Of course, these respondents were not trying to quit. On the other hand, one small placebo-controlled trial suggested that although e-cigarettes were at least as good as nicotine patches in helping smokers quit, cessation rates were low either way at 6 to 7 percent (Grana et al., 2014). In fact, the results of a subsequent study suggested that e-cigarettes are linked with *less* smoking cessation: individuals who used e-cigarettes had 28 percent lower odds of quitting cigarettes compared with those who did not use e-cigarettes. It did not even matter if smokers had an interest in quitting or not; there was no difference in e-cigarette use between the two groups (Kalkhoran and Glantz, 2016).

In the 2015 National Youth Tobacco Survey, e-cigarettes were the most commonly used tobacco product among teens for the second year in a row. According to the Surgeon General's Report, e-cigarette use among high school students increased "an astounding 900 percent" from 2011 to 2015. In 2015, nearly 38 percent of high schoolers reported having tried an e-cigarette at least once. Researchers found that 67 percent of respondents considered e-cigarettes to be "healthier" than regular cigarettes (Wills et al., 2015). The most common reasons teens gave for initially trying e-cigarettes were curiosity, a cool factor, and because of their friends. But six months later, none of those reasons were significant predictors of continued e-cigarette use. Only 5.9 percent of students said they tried e-cigarettes in an effort to quit smoking, but smoking cessation was the only reason that was significantly associated with continued e-cigarette use. The authors also noted that after 6 months, 80 percent of teens who said they were using e-cigarettes to quit smoking were still smoking traditional cigarettes (Bold et al., 2016). Adolescents who vaped frequently, defined as weekly smoking or more than two cigarettes per day, were more likely to be more frequent and heavier smokers six months later. Vaping was not associated with smoking reductions (Leventhal et al., 2016). A 2016 analysis of teenagers in Hawaii showed e-cigarette use to be positively associated with both tobacco initiation and increased smoking frequency. E-cigarettes had no benefit in reducing tobacco use in teens who smoked (Wills et al., 2017).

Moreover, a survey of Connecticut high school students in the spring of 2014 found about 18 percent of e-cigarette users and cannabis users used e-cigarettes to vaporize cannabis (Morean et al., 2015).

Nicotine Replacement Therapies

As noted above, while most smokers say they want to quit, only a small percent are successful. Current tobacco dependence treatments have a 12-month abstinence success rate of 22 percent at best, but the relapse rate within 1 year is high and over 90 percent of over-the-counter nicotine replacement therapy (NRT) users relapse within 6 months (Mohamed et al., 2015). Whether cessation occurs by a gradual reduction in the number of cigarettes smoked or by quitting abruptly with no prior decrease, the quit rates are the same (Lindson-Hawley et al., 2012). People who used reduced-nicotine cigarettes (≤ 2.4 milligrams per gram of tobacco) did decrease the number of cigarettes they smoked per day compared with people who smoked their regular brand (or 15.8 milligrams per gram of tobacco) over a six-week trial, but the difference was not impressive (Donny et al., 2015). Nevertheless, the benefit might be cost effective (Fiore and Baker, 2015).

To alleviate the symptoms of nicotine withdrawal while the smoker quits the smoking habit, NRT products offer nicotine exposure in the absence of tobacco. In the United States, the patch, lozenge, and gum can be sold over the counter, while the nasal spray and oral inhaler are only available with a prescription. Some countries sell a nicotine mouth spray and sublingual tablet, but these are not available in the United States. It is important to avoid smoking while using NRTs; psychological counseling in conjunction can be useful. Smokers, however, who were sent nicotine patches in the mail were more than twice as likely as smokers who did not receive the posted patches to report that they were no longer smoking six months later, even though they received no behavioral support. This suggests that NRT alone is an effective strategy to help smokers stop smoking (Cunningham et al., 2016). Burghardt and Ellingrod (2012) describe clinical applications for the therapeutic use of NRTs.

The second category of medications used for smoking cessation consists of drugs not considered to be NRTs, although they may act on the nicotinic receptor. Currently, these include antidepressants, primarily bupropion (Zyban), and *partial nicotine receptor agonists*, such as varenicline, dianicline, and cytosine (trade name Tabex).

In their review, Hughes and coworkers (2007) concluded that the antidepressants *bupropion* (Wellbutrin, Zyban) and *nortriptyline* (Pamelor) double a person's chances of giving up smoking and have an acceptable rate of side effects. SSRI antidepressants such as *fluoxetine* (Prozac) are not effective. Of the two, bupropion is the most studied and most widely used. Bupropion delays smoking relapse and also results in less weight gain. Interestingly, bupropion and nortriptyline appear to work equally well in both depressed and nondepressed smokers; this suggests that these drugs help smokers quit in some way other than through their action as antidepressants. Bupropion inhibits $\alpha_4\beta_2$ and α_7 nAChRs, inhibits nicotine-induced dopamine release, and reduces nicotine self-administration—pharmacological properties that may contribute to the smoking cessation effect (Slemmer et al., 2000).

Partial Nicotinic Agonists

In late 2006, a new approach to treating nicotine dependence was introduced. *Varenicline* (Chantix) (Jorenby et al., 2006) and two other drugs, cytisine (West et al., 2011) and dianicline (Tonstad et al., 2011), are pharmacologically classified as *partial nicotine receptor agonists*. By partially stimulating the receptor, they reduce withdrawal symptoms, but block access of nicotine to the receptor. Continued smoking is less satisfying and may help the person to quit and maintain abstinence. Because nicotine indirectly induces the release of dopamine (which produces its stimulant and reinforcing action), these drugs also enable a low-level release of dopamine (Zierler-Brown and Kyle, 2007). Figure 6.4 compares the effect on nicotinic receptors and dopamine release of smoking, smoking abstinence, and varenicline administration.

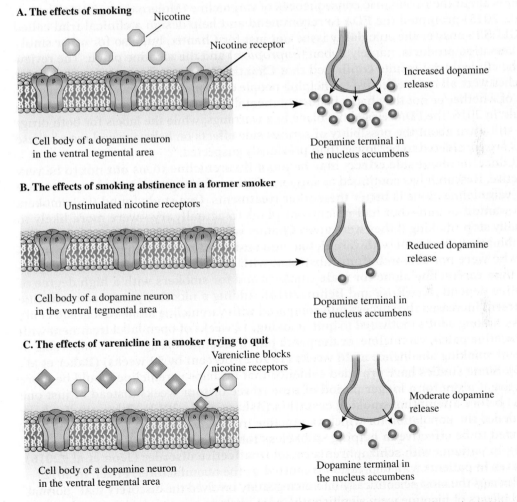

A. The effects of smoking

Nicotine

Nicotine receptor

Increased dopamine release

Cell body of a dopamine neuron in the ventral tegmental area

Dopamine terminal in the nucleus accumbens

B. The effects of smoking abstinence in a former smoker

Unstimulated nicotine receptors

Reduced dopamine release

Cell body of a dopamine neuron in the ventral tegmental area

Dopamine terminal in the nucleus accumbens

C. The effects of varenicline in a smoker trying to quit

Varenicline blocks nicotine receptors

Moderate dopamine release

Cell body of a dopamine neuron in the ventral tegmental area

Dopamine terminal in the nucleus accumbens

FIGURE 6.4   The effect on nicotine receptors and dopamine release of **A.** nicotine from cigarettes, **B.** nicotine withdrawal, and **C.** varenicline administration.

Although initial reports were positive, subsequent outcomes were less impressive. Dianicline was not very effective in promoting abstinence and is no longer under development. Cytisine is an unusual compound extracted from the seeds of *Cytisus laborinum* (Golden Rain acacia) (West et al., 2011). It was first marketed in Bulgaria in 1964 and has been available in former Eastern Bloc countries for over 40 years under the brand name Tabex; it is not available in the United States. Cytisine results have been very modest in achieving the cessation of nicotine addiction (Walker et al., 2014).

A long debate over Chantix and its safety began soon after its 2006 approval. Patients and their doctors started reporting suicidal thoughts, aggression, depression, and agitation. After reviewing the evidence, the FDA gave the drug a black box warning in 2009, which it updated in 2011. In 2015, the FDA added the warning that until patients knew how Chantix affected their ability to tolerate alcohol, they should decrease the amount of alcohol they drink, and that patients who had a seizure while taking Chantix should stop the medicine and seek medical attention immediately. That year, conflicting publications about the psychiatric consequences of varenicline (Molero et al., 2015; Thomas et al., 2015) prompted the FDA to recommend and help design a clinical trial called EAGLES to answer the suicidality issue not just for Chantix, but also for other smoking cessation products, namely Zyban (*bupropion*) and the nicotine patch. The review of the clinical trial results confirmed that Chantix, Zyban, and nicotine replacement patches were all more effective for helping people quit smoking than a placebo, regardless of whether or not they had a history of mental illness (Anthenelli et al., 2016). As a result, in 2016, the FDA revised the black box warnings; while the labels for both drugs will still warn about the possibility of serious side effects on behavior and mood, these risks are considered to be "lower than previously suspected."

Concerns about side effects may be moot if varenicline turns out not to be very effective. Research has continued to support efficacy, although it is not always the case that varenicline alone is better than other treatments. One study found that smokers who wanted to quit—but had no current plans to actually try—were more likely to actually stop smoking if they were given Chantix versus a placebo (Ebbert et al., 2015). Combination treatment with varenicline and sustained-release bupropion for smokers who were not able to become abstinent with the nicotine patch was more effective than varenicline alone for male smokers and for smokers with a high degree of nicotine dependence (Rose and Behm, 2014). Adding a nicotine patch to varenicline treatment increased the success rate compared with varenicline alone (Coenraad et al., 2014). Among adults motivated to quit smoking, 12 weeks of open-label treatment with the nicotine patch, varenicline, or the patch plus a nicotine lozenge was comparable in rates of smoking abstinence at 26 weeks (19 to 21 percent by 52 weeks) (Baker et al., 2016). Some studies have provided evidence that perhaps varenicline would be more effective if given for a longer period of time (three or four weeks instead of just one week) before attempting smoking cessation (Ashare et al., 2012). Other studies have broadened the population for which varenicline treatment might be useful: it has been reported to be effective in helping smokeless tobacco users quit (Fagerström et al., 2010), in patients with schizophrenia or schizoaffective disorder (Jeon et al., 2016), and even in patients with depression (reported by the manufacturer, Pfizer, in 2012).

Perhaps the most scientifically interesting study involved the discovery that "normal" metabolizers of nicotine were significantly more likely to remain abstinent with varenicline compared to the nicotine patch for up to six months. In contrast, varenicline was equal to the nicotine patch at helping "slow" metabolizers quit, but there were more overall side effects reported with the drug. Medications like varenicline may be more effective in smokers who are normal metabolizers. This could be due to the fact that dopamine levels are increased by varenicline, which may reduce the cravings elicited by the rapid drop in nicotine experienced by normal metabolizers. In one such group of normal metabolizers, 22 percent of those on the patch were abstinent when the treatment was completed, versus almost 40 percent of those taking varenacline (Lerman et al., 2015).

Vaccine Therapy

A nicotine vaccine (similar to a cocaine vaccine; see Chapter 7) is one novel approach. Nicotine itself is a nonimmunogenic molecule and must be conjugated (attached) to a carrier protein to induce antibodies. The idea is that, once bound to antibodies, nicotine cannot cross the blood–brain barrier. This reduces its rewarding effect, which should promote abstinence. But a vaccine does not reduce the drug craving; it only blocks the drug's access to the brain.

Currently, two products, NicVAX and NIC002 (formerly NicQbeta) have been sufficiently tested. Results have been disappointing; none of the included studies detected a statistically significant difference in long-term cessation between participants receiving vaccine and those receiving placebo (Hartman-Boyce et al., 2012). Selecta Biosciences has taken over the project from the original company, Nabi. Selecta is using a slightly different technology involving synthetic vaccine particles (SVP), but has not yet started clinical trials.

Alternative Therapies to Smoking Cessation

Unfortunately, the long-term prognosis for smoking abstinence remains poor. Alpert and colleagues (2013) found that NRT products were no better in preventing relapse, even when used in conjunction with counseling (or combined with the opiate antagonist naltrexone (David et al., 2014)), than no treatment. These authors argue that public health policies, based on mass-media campaigns and no-smoking laws, are more effective in the long-term. Even in combination, drugs and counseling to help patients stop smoking, while doubling the odds of success relative to no intervention, still rarely exceeds a 20 percent success rate (Ong, 2012).

Other agents that have been developed and found ineffective or no better than NRTs for smoking cessation include cytisine derivatives, nicotinic full agonists, and nicotinic antagonists. Sazetidine A is a new class of nAChR ligand. It does not activate the receptor, block nicotine-induced activities, or upregulate the receptor. Rather, it desensitizes the nAChR for prolonged periods without activation. It is called a "silent desensitizer." As yet, there is no published information on smoking cessation effectiveness. One problem is that it is hard to develop agents that are sufficiently *selective* for the respective nAChR subtype, primarily because there are overlapping binding sites across subtypes. This has prompted the search for positive allosteric modulators (PAMS), which do not bind to the ACh binding site or activate nAChRs in the absence of ACh. In the presence of ACh, PAMs increase the response to the transmitter. Such drugs are not reinforcing on their own, "but replace the subjective reinforcement effect of nicotine" without abuse liability of their own (Mohamed et al., 2015, 5).

Possibly opening up a different approach, researchers have discovered an enzyme, NicA2, found in bacteria known as *Pseudomonas putida*, which lives in soils from tobacco fields. The bacteria depend on nicotine as their only source of the carbon and nitrogen they need to live. In testing the enzyme as a possible aid to smoking cessation, researchers added nicotine to a blood sample at a level corresponding to smoking one cigarette, then added the NicA2 enzyme. The half-life of the nicotine was reduced from 2 to 3 hours to 9 to 15 minutes. Higher doses, along with some chemical alterations, might even work faster, perhaps keeping nicotine in the blood from ever reaching the brain. The fact that the enzyme remained stable for up to three weeks at body temperature supports its development as a viable drug candidate (Xue et al., 2015).

One of the most unusual observations in regard to nicotine addiction was a report several years ago that some patients who were smokers and who had experienced a stroke in a part of the brain called the *insular cortex* had lost their desire to smoke. These patients were able to quit easily one day after surgery and did not have an urge to resume smoking. The involvement of this site in nicotine addiction has since been supported by experiments in rats, which have shown the phenomenon to be specific to the insular region (Pushparaj et al., 2013). Although unexpected, this accidental discovery may lead to new approaches to treating this difficult addiction.

A summary table of clinical guidelines for cessation of tobacco smoking, compiled by the Preventive Services Task Force, can be found at Siu et al. (2015).

STUDY QUESTIONS

1. Describe the mechanism of action of caffeine. How does this mechanism explain the clinical effects of the drug?

2. What are the positive and negative effects of caffeine?

3. Discuss the political, health, and economic issues related to tobacco. Should the FDA regulate nicotine as a drug? Should tobacco be banned?

4. What are the psychoactive effects of nicotine? How do they contribute to cigarette dependence?

5. Discuss the clinical uses and limitations of nicotine replacement devices. How might their efficacy be boosted?

6. Compare and contrast the pharmacotherapeutic options for smoking cessation.

REFERENCES

Abbott, L. C., and Winzer-Serhan, U. H. (2012). "Smoking During Pregnancy: Lessons Learned from Epidemiological Studies and Experimental Studies Using Animal Models." *Critical Reviews in Toxicology* 42: 279–303.

Addicott, M. A., et al. (2015). "Increased Functional Connectivity in an Insula-Based Network is Associated with Improved Smoking Cessation Outcomes." *Neuropsychopharmacology* 40: 2648–2656.

Akinbami, L. J., et al. (2012). "Impact of Tobacco Smoke Exposure on Children Ages 6–19 Years with Asthma in the US, 2003–2010." *Pediatric Academic Societies.* Abstract 4340.2.

Alpert, H., et al. (2013). "A Prospective Cohort Study Challenging the Effectiveness of Population-Based Medical Intervention for Smoking Cessation." *Tobacco Control* 22: 32–37.

Anthenelli, R. M., et al. (2016). "Neuropsychiatric Safety and Efficacy of Varenicline, Bupropion, and Nicotine Patch in Smokers with and Without Psychiatric Disorders (EAGLES): A Double-Blind, Randomised, Placebo-Controlled Clinical Trial." *The Lancet* 387: 2507–2520.

Arab, L., et al. (2013). "Epidemiologic Evidence of a Relationship Between Tea, Coffee, or Caffeine Consumption and Cognitive Decline." *Advances in Nutrition* 4: 115–122.

Asch, D. A., et al. (2013). "Conflicts and Compromises in Not Hiring Smokers." *New England Journal of Medicine* 368: 1369–1371.

Ashare, R. L., et al. (2012). "Effects of 21 Days of Varenicline Versus Placebo on Smoking Behaviors and Urges Among Non-Treatment Seeking Smokers." *Journal of Psychopharmacology* 26: 1383–1390.

Aubin, H. J., et al. (2012). "Weight Gain in Smokers After Quitting Cigarettes: Meta-Analysis." *BMJ* 345: e4439.

Avdalovic, M. V., and Murin, S. (2015). "Point: Does the Risk of Electronic Cigarettes Exceed Potential Benefits? Yes." *Chest* 148: 580–582. doi: 10.1378/chest.15-0538.

Baker, T. B., et al. (2016). "Effects of Nicotine Patch vs Varenicline vs Combination Nicotine Replacement Therapy on Smoking Cessation at 26 Weeks: A Randomized Clinical Trial." *JAMA* 315: 371–379.

Bakhshaie, J., et al. (2016). "Cigarette Smoking and the Onset and Persistence of Panic Attacks During Mid-Adulthood in the United States: 1994–2005." *Journal of Clinical Psychiatry* 77: e21–e24.

Barreto, G. E., et al. (2015). "Beneficial Effects of Nicotine, Cotinine and its Metabolites as Potential Agents for Parkinson's Disease." *Frontiers in Aging Neuroscience* 6: Article 340.

Been, J. V., et al. (2014). "Effect of Smoke-Free Legislation on Perinatal and Child Health: A Systematic Review and Meta-Analysis." *Lancet* 383: 1549. http://dx.doi.org/10.1016/S0140–6736(14)60082–9.

Belsky, A., et al. (2013). "Polygenetic Risk and the Developmental Progression to Heavy, Persistent Smoking and Nicotine Dependence: Evidence from a 4-Decade Longitudinal Study." *JAMA Psychiatry* 70: 534–542.

Beresniak, A., et al. (2012). "Relationships Between Black Tea Consumption and Key Health Indicators in the World: An Ecological Study." *BMJ Open* 2: e000648.

Berlin, I., et al. (2014). "Nicotine Patches in Pregnant Smokers: Randomised, Placebo Controlled, Multicentre Trial of Efficacy." *BMJ* 348. doi: 10.1136/bmj.g1622.

Bloomfield, M. A. P., et al. (2014). "Dopamine Function in Cigarette Smokers: An [18F]-DOPA PET Study." *Neuropsychopharmacology* 39: 2397–2404.

Bold, K. W., et al. (2016). "Reasons for Trying E-cigarettes and Risk of Continued Use." *Pediatrics* 138: e20160895.

Bonaventura, J., et al. (2015). "Allosteric Interactions Between Agonists and Antagonists Within the Adenosine A2A Receptor-Dopamine D2 Receptor Heterotetramer." *Proceedings of the National Academy of Science USA* 112: E3609–E3618.

Borota, D., et al. (2014). "Post-Study Caffeine Administration Enhances Memory Consolidation in Humans." *Nature Neuroscience* 17: 201–203. doi: 10.1038/nn.3623.

Brent, R. L., et al. (2011). "Evaluation of the Reproductive and Developmental Risks of Caffeine." *Birth Defects Research (Part B)* 92: 152–187.

Brockman, L. N., et al. (2012). "Hookah's New Popularity Among US College Students: A Pilot Study of the Characteristics of Hookah Smokers and Their Facebook Displays." *BMJ Open* 2: e001709.

Burghardt, K., and Ellingrod, V. L. (2012). "Smoking Cessation: What to Tell Patients About Over-the-Counter Treatments." *Current Psychiatry* 11: 43–47.

Burke, T. M., et al. (2015). "Effects of Caffeine on the Human Circadian Clock in Vivo and in Vitro." *Science Translational Medicine* 7: 305ra146. http://www.ncbi.nlm.nih.gov/pubmed/26378246.

Callaghan, R. C., et al. (2014). "Patterns of Tobacco-Related Mortality among Individuals Diagnosed with Schizophrenia, Bipolar Disorder, or Depression." *Journal of Psychiatric Research* 48: 102–110. doi: http://dx.doi.org/10.1016/j.jpsychires.2013.09.014.

Cao, C., et al. (2012). "High Blood Caffeine Levels in MCI Linked to Lack of Progression to Dementia." *Journal of Alzheimer's Disease* 30: 559–572.

CARE Study Group. (2008). "Maternal Caffeine Intake During Pregnancy and Risk of Fetal Growth Restriction: A Large Prospective Observational Study." *BMJ* 337: a2332.

Carter, B. D., et al. (2015). "Smoking and Mortality—Beyond Established Causes." *New England Journal of Medicine* 372: 631–640. doi: 10.1056/NEJMsa1407211.

Carpenter, M. (2015). "Caffeine Powder Poses Deadly Risks." *New York Times*. May 18. https://well.blogs.nytimes.com/2015/05/18/caffeine-powder-poses-deadly-risks-2/.

Carroll, A. E. (2015). "Health Benefits of Tea? Here's What the Evidence Says." *New York Times*. October 5. https://www.nytimes.com/2015/10/06/upshot/what-the-evidence-tells-us-about-tea.html.

Childs, E., and deWit, H. (2012). "Potential Mental Risks." In Yi-Fang Chu, ed., *Coffee: Emerging Health Effects and Disease Prevention*, pp. 293–306. Hoboken, NJ: John Wiley & Sons.

Choi, Y., et al. (2015). "Coffee Consumption and Coronary Artery Calcium in Young and Middle-Aged Asymptomatic Adults." *Heart* 101: 686–691. doi: 10.1136/heartjnl-2014–306663.

Clair, C., et al. (2013). "Association of Smoking Cessation and Weight Change with Cardiovascular Disease Among Adults with and without Diabetes." *Journal of the American Medical Association* 309: 1014–1021.

Coenraad, F. N., et al. (2014). "Efficacy of Varenicline Combined with Nicotine Replacement Therapy vs Varenicline Alone for Smoking Cessation: A Randomized Clinical Trial." *JAMA* 312: 155–161. doi: 10.1001/jama.2014.7195.

Coffee and Caffeine Genetics Consortium (2015). *Molecular Psychiatry* 20: 647–656. doi: 10.1038/mp.2014.107.

Cook, B. L., et al. (2014). "Trends in Smoking Among Adults with Mental Illness and Association Between Mental Health Treatment and Smoking Cessation." *JAMA* 311: 172–182. doi: 10.1001/jama.2013.284985.

Cornelis, M. C., et al. (2006). "Coffee, CYP1A2 Genotype, and Risk of Myocardial Infarction." *JAMA* 295: 1135–1141. doi: 10.1001/jama.295.10.1135.

Cox, B., et al. (2013). "Impact of a Stepwise Introduction of Smoke-Free Legislation on the Rate of Preterm Births: Analysis of Routinely Collected Birth Data." *BMJ* 346: f441.

Crotty Alexander, L., et al. (2014). "Electronic Cigarette Vapor Exposure Decreases Staphylococcus Aureus Susceptibility to Macrophage and Neutrophil Killing." *American Thoracic Society Conference*. Abstract A6624.

Crowe, S. F., et al. (2011). "The Effect of Caffeine and Stress on Auditory Hallucinations in a Non-Clinical Sample." *Personality and Individual Differences* 50: 626.

Cunningham, J. A., et al. (2016). "Effect of Mailing Nicotine Patches on Tobacco Cessation Among Adult Smokers: A Randomized Clinical Trial." *JAMA Internal Medicine* 176: 184–190. doi: 10.1001/jamainternmed.2015.7792.

David, S. P., et al. (2014). "Systematic Review and Meta-Analysis of Opioid Antagonists for Smoking Cessation." *BMJ* 4: e004393.

Dicpinigaitis, P. V. (2017). "Effect of Tobacco and Electronic Cigarette Use on Cough Reflex Sensitivity." *Pulmonary Pharmacology & Therapeutics* 47: 45–48. doi: 10.1016/j.pupt.2017.01.013.

Dinakar, C., and O'Connor, G. T. (2016). "The Health Effects of Electronic Cigarettes." *New England Journal of Medicine* 375: 1372–1381. October 6, 2016 doi: 10.1056/NEJMra1502466.

Ding, M., et al. (2014). "Long-Term Coffee Consumption and Risk of Cardiovascular Disease: A Systematic Review and A Dose-Response Meta-Analysis of Prospective Cohort Studies." *Circulation* 129: 643–659.

Dixit, S., et al. (2016). "Consumption of Caffeinated Products and Cardiac Ectopy." *Journal of the American Heart Association* 5: e002503. doi: 10.1161/JAHA.115.002503.

Donny, E. C., et al. (2015). "Randomized Trial of Reduced-Nicotine Standards for Cigarettes." *New England Journal of Medicine* 374: 394–397. doi: 10.1056/NEJMc1513886.

Doweiko, H. E. (2012). *Concepts of Chemical Dependency,* 8th ed. Belmont, CA: Brooks/Cole.

Ebbert, J. O., et al. (2015). "Effect of Varenicline on Smoking Cessation Through Smoking Reduction: A Randomized Clinical Trial." *JAMA* 313: 687–694. doi: 10.1001/jama.2015.280.

Ekblad, M., et al. (2010). "The Effect of Prenatal Smoking Exposure on Adolescents' Use of Psychiatric Drugs." *Pediatric Academic Societies*. Abstract 4401.56.

El-Hellani, A., et al. (2015). "Free-Base and Protonated Nicotine in Electronic Cigarette Liquids and Aerosols." *Chemical Research in Toxicology* 28: 1532–1537. doi: 10.1021/acs.chemrestox.5b00107.

Fagerström, K., et al. (2010). "Stopping Smokeless Tobacco with Varenicline: Randomized Double-Blind Placebo Controlled Trial." *BMJ* 341: c6549.

Fankhauser, M. P. (2013). "Drug Interactions with Tobacco Smoke: Implications for Patient Care." *Current Psychiatry* 12: 12–16.

Ferré, S., et al. (2016). "Allosteric Mechanisms within the Adenosine A2A-Dopamine D2 Receptor Heterotetramer." *Neuropharmacology* 104: 154–160. doi: 10.1016/j.neuropharm.2015.05.028. PMID 26051403.

Ferré, S. (2016). "Mechanisms of the Psychostimulant Effects of Caffeine: Implications for Substance Use Disorders." *Psychopharmacology (Berl.)* 233: 1963–1979. doi: 10.1007/s00213-016-4212-2.

Fiore, M., and Baker, T. (2015). "Reduced-Nicotine Cigarettes—A Promising Regulatory Pathway." *New England Journal of Medicine* 373: 1289–1291.

Floegel, A., et al. (2012). "Coffee Consumption and Risk of Chronic Disease in the European Prospective Investigation into Cancer and Nutrition (EPIC) Germany Study." *American Journal of Clinical Nutrition* 95: 901–908.

Freedman, N. D., et al. (2012). "Association of Coffee Drinking with Total and Cause-Specific Mortality." *New England Journal of Medicine* 366: 1891–1904.

Fritz, H.-C., et al. (2014). "Current Smoking and Reduced Gray Matter Volume—a Voxel-Based Morphometry Study." *Neuropsychopharmacology* 39: 2594–2600.

Funatogawa, I., et al. (2012). "Impacts of Early Smoking Initiation: Long-term Trends of Lung Cancer Mortality and Smoking Initiation from Repeated Cross-Sectional Surveys in Great Britain." *BMJ Open* 2: e001676.

Galeone, C., et al. (2010). "Coffee and Tea Intake and Risk of Head and Neck Cancer: Pooled Analysis in the International Head and Neck Cancer Epidemiology Consortium." *Cancer Epidemiology, Biomarkers & Prevention* 19: 1723–1736.

Garcia, K. L. P., et al. (2015). "Effect of Brain CYP2B Inhibition on Brain Nicotine Levels and Nicotine Self-Administration." *Neuropsychopharmacology* 40: 1910–1918. doi: 10.1038/npp.2015.40.

Giles, G. E., et al. (2012). "Differential Cognitive Effects of Energy Drink Ingredients: Caffeine, Taurine, and Glucose." *Pharmacology, Biochemistry and Behavior* 102: 569–577.

Goldman, M. D., and Stuve, O. (2015). "Smoking beyond Multiple Sclerosis Diagnosis: A Risk Factor Still Worth Modifying." *JAMA Neurology* 72: 1105–1106. doi: 10.1001/jamaneurol.2015.1805.

Grana, R. A., et al. (2014). "A Longitudinal Analysis of Electronic Cigarette Use and Smoking Cessation." *JAMA Internal Medicine* 174: 812–813. doi: 10.1001/jamainternmed.2014.187.

Green, S. H., et al. (2016). "Evidence, Policy and E-Cigarettes—Will England Reframe the Debate?" *New England Journal of Medicine* 374: 1301–1303. doi: 10.1056/NEJMp1601154.

Hakim, F., et al. (2011). "The Acute Effects of Water-Pipe Smoking on the Cardiorespiratory System." *Chest* 139: 775–781.

Hansson, A., et al. (2012). "Effects of Nicotine Mouth Spray on Urges to Smoke, a Randomized Clinical Trial." *BMJ* 2: e001618.

Hartman-Boyce, J., et al. (2012). "Nicotine Vaccines for Smoking Cessation." *Cochrane Database Systems Review* 8: CD007072.

Hedström, A. K., et al. (2016). "High Consumption of Coffee Is Associated with Decreased Multiple Sclerosis Risk; Results from Two Independent Studies." *Journal of Neurology, Neurosurgery & Psychiatry* 87: 1–7. doi: 10.1136/jnnp-2015-312176.

Henderson, B. J., et al. (2016). "Menthol Alone Upregulates Midbrain nAChRs, Alters nAChR Subtype Stoichiometry, Alters Dopamine Neuron Firing Frequency, and Prevents Nicotine Reward." *Journal of Neuroscience* 6: 2957–2974. doi: 10.1523/JNEUROSCI.4194-15.2016.

Hilario, M. R. F., et al. (2012). "Reward Sensitization: Effects of Repeated Nicotine Exposure and Withdrawal in Mice." *Neuropsychopharmacology* 37: 2661–2670.

Hillert, J., et al. (2015). "Effect of Smoking Cessation on Multiple Sclerosis Prognosis." *JAMA Neurology* 72: 1117–1123. doi: 10.1001/jamaneurol.2015.1788.015.

Hopkins, M., et al. (2012). "Comprehensive Smoke-Free Laws—50 Largest U. S. Cities, 2000 and 2012." *Morbidity and Mortality Weekly Report* 61: 914–917.

Howland, J., and Rohsenow, D. H. (2013). "Risks of Energy Drinks Mixed with Alcohol." *JAMA* 309: 245–246.

Hughes, J. R., et al. (2007). "Antidepressants for Smoking Cessation." *Cochrane Database of Systematic Reviews* 1: CD000031.

Huxley, R., et al. (2009). "Coffee, Decaffeinated Coffee, and Tea Consumption in Relation to Incident Type 2 Diabetes Mellitus: A Systematic Review with Meta-Analysis." *Archives of Internal Medicine* 169: 2053–2063.

Ioannidis, K., et al. (2014). "Ostracising Caffeine from the Pharmacological Arsenal for Attention-Deficit Hyperactivity Disorder – Was This a Correct Decision? A Literature Review." *Journal of Psychopharmacology* 28: 830–836. doi: 10.1177/0269881114541014.

Ishak, W. W., et al. (2012). "Energy Drinks: Psychological Effects and Impact on Well-Being and Quality of Life—A Literature Review." *Innovations in Clinical Neuroscience* 9: 25–34.

Jahanfar, S., and Sharifah, H. (2009). "Effects of Restricted Caffeine Intake by Mother on Fetal, Neonatal and Pregnancy Outcome." *Cochrane Database of Systematic Reviews* 15: CD006965.

James, J. E., et al. (2011). "The Putative Neuroprotective Effects of Caffeine." *Journal of Caffeine Research* 1: 91–96.

Janes, A. C., et al. (2015). "Striatal Morphology is Associated with Tobacco Cigarette Craving." *Neuropsychopharmacology* 40: 406–411. doi: 10.1038/npp.2014.185.

Jensen, R. P., et al. (2015). "Hidden Formaldehyde in E-Cigarette Aerosol." *New England Journal of Medicine* 372: 392–393. doi: 10.1056/NEJMc1413069.

Jeon, D., et al. (2016). "Adjunctive Varenicline Treatment for Smoking Reduction in Patients with Schizophrenia: A Randomized Double-Blind Placebo-Controlled Trial." *Schizophrenia Research* 176: 206–211. doi: 10.1016/j.schres.2016.08.016.

Je, Y., et al. (2011). "A Prospective Cohort Study of Coffee Consumption and Risk of Endometrial Cancer over a 26-Year Follow-Up." *Cancer Epidemiology Biomarkers and Prevention* 20: 1–9.

Jorenby, D. E., et al. (2006). "Efficacy of Varenicline, an $\alpha_4\beta_2$ Nicotinic Acetylcholine Receptor Partial Agonist, vs Placebo or Sustained-Release Bupropion for Smoking Cessation: A Randomized Controlled Trial." *JAMA* 296: 56–63.

Kabbani, N. (2013). "Not so Cool? Menthol's Discovered Actions on the Nicotinic Receptor and Its Implications for Nicotine Addiction." *Frontiers in Pharmacology* 4: 95. doi: 10.3389/fphar.2013.00095.

Kalkhoran, S., and Glantz, S. A. (2014). "Smoke-Free Policies: Cleaning the Air with Money to Spare." *Lancet* 383: 1526. doi: http://dx.doi.org/10.1016/S0140–6736(14)60224–5.

Kalkhoran S., and Glantz, S. A. (2016). "E-cigarettes and Smoking Cessation in Real-World and Clinical Settings: A Meta-Analysis." *Lancet Respiratory Medicine* 4: 116–128. doi: http://dx.doi.org/10.1016/S0140-6736(14)60224-5.

Kandel, E. R., and Kandel, D. B. (2014). "A Molecular Basis for Nicotine as a Gateway Drug." *New England Journal of Medicine* 371: 932–43. doi: 10.1056/NEJMsa1405092.

Kapoor, D., and Jones, T. H. (2005). "Smoking and Hormones in Health and Endocrine Disorders." *European Journal of Endocrinology* 152: 491–499.

Kendler, K. S. et al. (2015). "Smoking and Schizophrenia in Population Cohorts of Swedish Women and Men: A Prospective Co-relative Control Study." *American Journal of Psychiatry* 172: 1092–1100. doi: http://dx.doi.org/10.1176/appi.ajp.2015.15010126.

Krishnan-Sarin, S., et al. (2017). "E-Cigarettes and "Dripping" Among High-School Youth." *Pediatrics* 139: e20163224.

Kumar, P. K., et al. (2015). "Differential Effect of Caffeine Intake in Subjects with Genetic Susceptibility to Parkinson's Disease." *Scientific Reports* 5: 15492. doi: 10.1038/srep15492.

Lambert, R. A., et al. (2006). "A Pragmatic, Unblinded, Randomized, Controlled Trial Comparing an Occupational Therapy-Led Lifestyle Approach and Routine GP Care for Panic Disorder Treatment in Primary Care." *Journal of Affective Disorders* 99: 63–71.

Landa, M. M. (2014). "Tragic Deaths Highlight the Dangers of Powdered Pure Caffeine." *FDA Voice* [blog]. December 16. http://blogs.fda.gov/fdavoice/index.php/2014/12/tragic-deaths-highlight-the-dangers-of-powdered-pure-caffeine/#sthash.u4NRQft7.dpuf.

Laurent, C., et al. (2014). "Beneficial Effects of Caffeine in a Transgenic Model of Alzheimer's Disease-like Tau Pathology." *Neurobiology of Aging* 35: 2079–2090. doi: http://dx.doi.org/10.1016/j.neurobiolaging.2014.03.027.

Le Foll, M., et al. (2014). "Elevation of Dopamine Induced by Cigarette Smoking: Novel Insights from a [^{11}C]-(+)-PHNO PET Study in Humans." *Neuropsychopharmacology* 39: 415–424. doi: 10.1038/npp.2013.209.

Leonardi-Bee, J., et al. (2012). "Smoking and the Risk of Nonmelanoma Skin Cancer: Systematic Review and Meta-Analysis." *Archives of Dermatology* 148: 939–946.

Lerman, C., et al. (2015). "Use of the Nicotine Metabolite Ratio as a Genetically Informed Biomarker of Response to Nicotine Patch or Varenicline for Smoking Cessation: A Randomised, Double-Blind Placebo-Controlled Trial." *Lancet Respiratory Medicine* 3: 131–138. doi: 10.1016/S2213–2600(14)70294–2.

Lerman, C., et al. (2013). "Large-Scale Brain Network Coupling Predicts Acute Nicotine Abstinence Effects on Craving and Cognitive Function." *JAMA Psychiatry* 71: 523–530. doi: 10.1001/jamapsychiatry.2013.4091.

Leventhal, A. M., et al. (2016). "Association of e-Cigarette Vaping and Progression to Heavier Patterns of Cigarette Smoking." *JAMA* 316: 1918–1920. doi: 10.1001/jama.2016.14649.

Li, J., et al. (2011). "Coffee Consumption Modifies Risk of Estrogen-Receptor Negative Breast Cancer." *Breast Cancer Research* 13: R49.

Lindblom, E. N. (2015). "Effectively Regulating E-Cigarettes and Their Advertising—and the First Amendment." *Food and Drug Law Journal* 70: 57–94.

Lindson-Hawley, N., et al. (2012). "Reduction versus Abrupt Cessation in Smokers Who Want to Quit." *Cochrane Database System Review* 11: CD008033.

Liu, R., et al. (2012). "Caffeine Intake, Smoking and Risk of Parkinson Disease in Men and Women." *American Journal of Epidemiology* 175: 1200–1207.

Lortet-Tieulent, J., et al. (2016). "State-Level Cancer Mortality Attributable to Cigarette Smoking in the United States." *JAMA Internal Medicine* 176: 1792–1798. doi: 10.1001/jamainternmed.2016.6530.

Lucas, M., et al. (2011). "Coffee, Caffeine, and Risk of Depression Among Women." *Archives of Internal Medicine* 171: 1571–1578.

Magkos, F., and Kavouras, S. A. (2005). "Caffeine Use in Sports, Pharmacokinetics in Man, and Cellular Mechanisms of Action." *Critical Reviews in Food Science and Nutrition* 45: 535–562.

Malarcher, A., et al. (2011). "Quitting Smoking Among Adults—United States 2001–2010." *Morbidity and Mortality Weekly Report* 60: 1513–1519.

Martínez-Pinilla, E., et al. (2015). "The Relevance of Theobromine for the Beneficial Effects of Cocoa Consumption." *Frontiers in Pharmacology* 6: 1–5. doi: 10.3389/fphar.2015.00030.

Matheson, E. M., et al. (2011)."Tea and Coffee Consumption and MRSA Nasal Carriage." *Annals of Family Medicine* 9: 299–304.

McCowan, L. M. E., et al. (2009). "Spontaneous Preterm Birth and Small for Gestational Age Infants in Women Who Stop Smoking Early in Pregnancy: Prospective Cohort Study." *BMJ* 338: b1081.

McKim, W. A., and Hancock, S. (2013). *Drugs and Behavior,* 7th ed. Upper Saddle River, NJ: Pearson Prentice Hall.

Meredith, S. E., et al. (2013). "Caffeine Use Disorder: A Comprehensive Review and Research Agenda." *Journal of Caffeine Research* 3: 114–130. doi: 10.1089/jcr.2013.0016.

Mohamed, T. S., et al. (2015). "Orthosteric and Allosteric Ligands of Nicotinic Acetylcholine Receptors for Smoking Cessation." *Frontiers in Molecular Neuroscience* 8: 71. doi: 10.3389/fnmol.2015.00071.

Moheimani, R. S., et al. (2017). "Increased Cardiac Sympathetic Activity and Oxidative Stress in Habitual Electronic Cigarette Users Implications for Cardiovascular Risk." *JAMA Cardiology* doi: 10.1001/jamacardio.2016.5303.

Molero, Y., et al. (2015). "Varenicline and Risk of Psychiatric Conditions, Suicidal Behaviour, Criminal Offending, and Transport Accidents and Offences: Population Based Cohort Study." *BMJ* 350: h2388. doi: https://doi.org/10.1136/bmj.h2388.

Molloy, J. W., et al. (2012). "Association of Coffee and Caffeine Consumption with Fatty Liver Disease, Nonalcoholic Steatohepatitis, and Degree of Hepatic Fibrosis." *Hepatology* 55: 429–436.

Moran, V. E. (2012). "Cotinine: Beyond That Expected, More Than a Biomarker of Tobacco Consumption." *Frontiers in Pharmacology* 3: 173.

Morain, S. R., et al. (2016). "Have Tobacco 21 Laws Come of Age?" *New England Journal of Medicine* 374: 1601–1604. doi: 10.1056/NEJMp1603294.

Morales, A. M., et al. (2014). "Cigarette Exposure, Dependence, and Craving Are Related to Insula Thickness in Young Adult Smokers." *Neuropsychopharmacology* 39: 1816–1822. doi: 10.1038/npp.2014.48.

Morean, M. E., et al. (2015). "High School Students' Use of Electronic Cigarettes to Vaporize Cannabis." *Pediatrics* 136: 611–616. doi: 10.1542/peds.2015-1727.

Morel, C., et al. (2014). "Nicotine Consumption Is Regulated by a Human Polymorphism in Dopamine Neurons." *Molecular Psychiatry* 19: 930–936. doi: 10.1038/mp.2013.158.

Moyses, C., et al. (2015). "Evaluation of a Novel Nicotine Inhaler Device: Part 1. Arterial and Venous Pharmacokinetics." *Nicotine & Tobacco Research* 17: 18–25.

Öberg, M., et al. (2011). "Worldwide Burden of Disease from Exposure to Second-Hand Smoke: A Retrospective Analysis of Data from 192 Countries." *Lancet* 377: 139–146.

Ong, M. (2012). "Smoking Cessation and Alcoholism." *American College of Physicians*. The ACP Internal Medicine 2012 Conference Session: 852–276.

Pan, A., et al. (2015). "Relation of Active, Passive, and Quitting Smoking with Incident Type 2 Diabetes: A Systematic Review and Meta-Analysis." *Lancet Diabetes & Endocrinology* 3: 958–967. doi: 10.1016/S2213–8587(15)00316–2.

Parikh, R., et al. (2014). "Impact of Smoking on Mental Health Symptoms in Adults with Depressive Disorders." *American Academy of Addiction Psychiatry*. Abstract 48.

Park, K., et al. (2016). "Effects of Coffee Consumption on Serum Uric Acid." *Seminars in Arthritis and Rheumatism* 45: 580–586. doi: 10.1016/j.semarthrit.2016.01.003.

Patnode, C. D., et al. (2015). "Behavioral Counseling and Pharmacotherapy Interventions for Tobacco Cessation in Adults, Including Pregnant Women: A Review of Reviews for the U.S. Preventive Services Task Force." *Annals of Internal Medicine* 163: 608–621. doi: 10.7326/M15–0171.

Persad, L. A. B. (2011). "Energy Drinks and the Neurophysiological Impact of Caffeine." *Frontiers in Neuroscience* 5: 1–8.

Pollack, A. Z., et al. (2010). "Caffeine Consumption and Miscarriage: A Prospective Cohort Study." *Fertility and Sterility* 93: 304–306.

Prochaska, J. J., et al. (2016). "Likelihood of Unemployed Smokers vs Nonsmokers Attaining Reemployment in a One-Year Observational Study." *JAMA Internal Medicine* 176: 662–670. doi: 10.1001/jamainternmed.2016.0772.

Pushparaj, A., et al. (2013). "Electrical Stimulation of the Insular Region Attenuates Nicotine-Taking and Nicotine-Seeking Behaviors." *Neuropsychopharmacology* 38: 690–698.

Quik, M., et al. (2012). "Nicotine as a Potential Neuroprotective Agent for Parkinson's Disease." *Movement Disorders* 27: 947–957.

Ribeiro, J. A., and Sebastião, A. M. (2010). "Caffeine and Adenosine." *Journal of Alzheimer's Disease* 20: Suppl. 1: S3–S15.

Robillard, R., et al. (2015). "Sleep is More Sensitive to High Doses of Caffeine in the Middle Years of Life." *Journal of Psychopharmacology* 29: 688–697.

Rodgers, P. J., et al. (2010). "Association of the Anxiogenic and Alerting Effects of Caffeine with ADORA2A and ADORA1 Polymorphisms and Habitual Level of Caffeine Consumption." *Neuropsychopharmacology* 35: 1973–1983.

Rose, J. E., and Behm, F. M. (2014). "Combination Treatment With Varenicline and Bupropion in an Adaptive Smoking Cessation Paradigm." *American Journal of Psychiatry* 171: 1199–205. doi: 10.1176/appi.ajp.2014.13050595.

Sae-tan, S., et al. (2014). "Voluntary Exercise and Green Tea Enhance the Expression of Genes Related to Energy Utilization and Attenuate Metabolic Syndrome in High Fat-Fed Mice." *Molecular Nutrition & Food Research* 58: 1156–1159.

Sandhu, R., et al. (2012). "Smoking, Smoking Cessation and Risk of Sudden Cardiac Death in Women." *Circulation: Arrhythmia and Electrophysiology* 5: 1091–1097. doi: 10.1002/mnfr.201300621.

Schmidt, H., et al. (2013). "The Ethics of Not Hiring Smokers." *New England Journal of Medicine* 368: 1369–1371.

Schmidt, A., et al. (2014). "Green Tea Extract Enhances Parieto-Frontal Connectivity During Working Memory Processing." *Psychopharmacology* 231: 3879–3888.

Schmit, S. L., et al. (2016). "Coffee Consumption and the Risk of Colorectal Cancer." *Cancer Epidemiology, Biomarkers & Prevention* 25: 634–639. doi: 10.1158/1055-9965.

Schroeder, S. A. (2013). "New Evidence That Cigarette Smoking Remains the Most Important Health Hazard." *New England Journal of Medicine* 368: 389–390.

Seifert, S. M., et al. (2013). "An Analysis of Energy-Drink Toxicity in the National Poison Data System." *Clinical Toxicology* 51: 566–574. doi: 10.3109/15563650.2013.820310.

Sengpiel, V., et al. (2013). "Maternal Caffeine Intake During Pregnancy Is Associated with Birth Weight but Not with Gestational Length: Results from a Large Prospective Observational Study." *BMC Medicine* 11: 42.

Seo, E.-J., et al. (2016). "Both Phenolic and Non-Phenolic Green Tea Fractions Inhibit Migration of Cancer Cells." *Frontiers in Pharmacology* 7: 398. doi: 10.3389/fphar.2016.00398.

Sepkowitz, K. A. (2013). "Energy Drinks and Caffeine-Related Adverse Events." *JAMA* 309: 243–244.

Sharwood, L. N., et al. (2013). "Use of Caffeinated Substances and Risk of Crashes in Long Distance Drivers of Commercial Vehicles: Case-Control Study." *BMJ* 346: f1140.

Shahab, L., et al. (2017). "Nicotine, Carcinogen, and Toxin Exposure in Long-Term E-Cigarette and Nicotine Replacement Therapy Users: A Cross-sectional Study." *Annals of Internal Medicine* 166: 390-400. doi: 10.7326/M16-1107.

Sherman, S. M., et al. (2016). "Caffeine Enhances Memory Performance in Young Adults during Their Non-optimal Time of Day." *Frontiers in Psychology* 7: 1764. doi: 10.3389/fpsyg.2016.01764.

Silva, C. G., et al. (2013). "Adenosine Receptor Antagonists Including Caffeine Alter Fetal Brain Development in Mice." *Science Translational Medicine* 5: 197ra104.

Siu, A. L., et al., for the U.S. Preventive Services Task Force* (2015). "Behavioral Counseling and Pharmacotherapy Interventions for Tobacco Cessation in Adults, Including Pregnant Women: A Review of Reviews for the U.S. Preventive Services Task Force." *Annals of Internal Medicine* 163: 622–634.

Slemmer, J. E., et al. (2000). "Bupropion Is a Nicotinic Antagonist." *The Journal of Pharmacology and Experimental Therapeutics* 295: 321–327.

Smith, A. P., et al. (2013). "Acute Effects of Caffeine on Attention: A Comparison of Non-Consumers and Withdrawn Consumers." *Journal of Psychopharmacology* 27: 77–83.

Smith, P. H., et al. (2014). "Cigarette Smoking and Mental Illness: A Study of Nicotine Withdrawal." *American Journal of Public Health* 104: e127–e133. doi: 10.2105/AJPH.2013.301502.

Soneji, S., et al. (2015). "Associations Between Initial Water Pipe Tobacco Smoking and Snus Use and Subsequent Cigarette Smoking Results From a Longitudinal Study of US Adolescents and Young Adults." *JAMA Pediatrics* 169: 129–136.

Song, F., et al. (2012). "Increased Caffeine Intake Is Associated with Reduced Risk of Basal Cell Carcinoma of the Skin." *Cancer Research* 72: 3282–3289.

Stroud, L. R., et al. (2009). "Maternal Smoking during Pregnancy and Neonatal Behavior: A Large-Scale Community Study." *Pediatrics* 123: e842–e848.

Svatikova, A., et al. (2015). "A Randomized Trial of Cardiovascular Responses to Energy Drink Consumption in Healthy Adults." *JAMA* 314: 2079–2082.

Szpak, A., and Allen, D. (2012). "A Case of Acute Suicidality Following Excessive Caffeine Intake." *Journal of Psychopharmacology* 26: 1502–1510.

Talati, A., et al. (2016). "Changing Relationships Between Smoking and Psychiatric Disorders Across Twentieth Century Birth Cohorts: Clinical and Research Implications." *Molecular Psychiatry* 21: 464–471. doi: 10.1038/mp.2015.224.

Taylor, G., et al. (2014). "Change in Mental Health After Smoking Cessation: Systematic Review and Meta-Analysis." *BMJ* 348: g1151.

Taylor, G., et al. (2015). "Does Smoking Reduction Worsen Mental Health? A Comparison of Two Observational Approaches." *BMJ* 5: e007812.

Teo, K. K., et al. (2006). "Tobacco Use and Risk of Myocardial Infarction in 52 Countries in the INTERHEART Study: A Case-Controlled Study." *Lancet* 368: 642–658.

Thomas, K. H., et al. (2015). "Risk of Neuropsychiatric Adverse Events Associated with Varenicline: Systematic Review and Meta-Analysis." *BMJ* 350: h1109.

Tonstad, S., et al. (2011). "Dianicline, a Novel $\alpha_4\beta_2$ Nicotinic Acetylcholine Receptor Partial Agonist, for Smoking Cessation: A Randomized Placebo-Controlled Clinical Trial." *Nicotine Tobacco Research* 13: 1–6.

Torpy, J. M., and Livingston, P. H. (2013). "Energy Drinks." *JAMA* 309: 297.

Turati, F., et al. (2011). "Coffee and Cancers of the Upper Digestive and Respiratory Tracts: Meta-Analyses of Observational Studies." *Annals of Oncology* 22: 536–544.

U.S. Department of Health and Human Services. (1986). "The Health Consequences of Involuntary Smoking: A Report of the Surgeon General." Centers for Disease Control and Prevention, Office of Smoking and Health. U.S. Government Printing Office. www.cdc.gov/tobacco.

U.S. Department of Health and Human Services. (1988). "The Health Consequences of Smoking—Nicotine Addiction: A Report of the Surgeon General." Centers for Disease Control and Prevention, Office of Smoking and Health. U.S. Government Printing Office. www.cdc.gov/tobacco.

U.S. Department of Health and Human Services. (2006). "The Health Consequences of Involuntary Exposure to Tobacco Smoke: A Report of the Surgeon General." Centers for Disease Control and Prevention, Office of Smoking and Health. U.S. Government Printing Office. www.cdc.gov/tobacco.

U.S. Department of Health and Human Services. (2012). "Preventing Tobacco Use Among Youth and Young Adults: A Report of the Surgeon General." Centers for Disease Control and Prevention, Office of Smoking and Health. U.S. Government Printing Office. www.cdc.gov/tobacco.

U.S. Department of Health and Human Services. (2016). "*E-Cigarette Use Among Youth and Young Adults*, Chapter 1. Introduction, Conclusions, and Historical Background Relative to E-Cigarettes." Centers for Disease Control and Prevention, Office of Smoking and Health. U.S. Government Printing Office. https://www.cdc.gov/tobacco/data_statistics/sgr/e-cigarettes/pdfs/2016_SGR_Chap_1_508.pdf.

U.S. Food and Drug Administration, Center for Tobacco Products. (2016). *Civil Money Penalties and No-Tobacco-Sale Orders for Tobacco Retailers Responses to Frequently Asked Questions (Revised)*. https://www.fda.gov/downloads/tobaccoproducts/labeling/rulesregulationsguidance/ucm447310.pdf.

Vassallo, N., et al. (2014). "Good Things in Life: Can Coffee Consumption Reduce the Risk of Developing Alzheimer's Disease?" Institute for Scientific Information on Coffee, from 24th annual Alzheimer Europe Conference on 23rd October 2014. http://coffeeandhealth.org/2014/11/moderate-coffee-consumption-may-lower-risk-alzheimers-disease-20-per-cent/.

Vinson, J. A., et al. (2012). "Randomized Double-Blind Placebo-Controlled Crossover Study to Evaluate the Efficacy and Safety of a Green Coffee Bean Extract in Overweight Subjects." Program and Abstracts of the 243rd American Chemical Society National Meeting and Exposition; March 25–29, 2012; San Diego, California. Abstract 92.

Walker, N., et al. (2014). "Cytosine vs Nicotine for Smoking Cessation." *New England Journal of Medicine* 371: 2353–2362.

Wesnes, K. A., et al. (2016). "Effects of the Red Bull Energy Drink on Cognitive Function and Mood in Healthy Young Volunteers." *Journal of Psychopharmacology* 31: 211–221.

West, R., et al. (2011). "Placebo-Controlled Trial of Cytisine for Smoking Cessation." *New England Journal of Medicine* 365: 1193–1200.

Whitley, E., et al. (2012). "Association of Cigarette Smoking from Adolescence to Middle-Age with Later Total and Cardiovascular Disease Mortality: The Harvard Alumni Health Study." *Journal of the American College of Cardiology* 60: 1839–1840.

Whitten, L. (2009). "Studies Link Family of Genes to Nicotine Addiction." National Institute on Drug Abuse. December 1. https://www.drugabuse.gov/news-events/nida-notes/2009/12/studies-link-family-genes-to-nicotine-addiction.

Wickham, R. J. (2015). "How Menthol Alters Tobacco-Smoking Behavior: A Biological Perspective." *Yale Journal of Biology and Medicine* 88: 279–287.

Wilhelmus, M. M. M., et al. (2016). "Effects of a Single, Oral 60 Mg Caffeine Dose on Attention in Healthy Adult Subjects." *Journal of Psychopharmacology* 31: 222–232.

Wills, T. A., et al. (2015). "Risk Factors for Exclusive E-Cigarette Use and Dual E-Cigarette Use and Tobacco Use in Adolescents." *Pediatrics* 135: e43-e51. doi: 10.1542/peds.2014–0760.

Wills, T. A., et al. (2017). "Longitudinal Study of E-Cigarette Use and Onset of Cigarette Smoking among High School Students in Hawaii." *Tobacco Control* 26: 34–39. doi: 10.1136/tobaccocontrol-2015–052705.

Wilson, P. W. F., and Bloom, H. L. (2016). "Caffeine Consumption and Cardiovascular Risks: Little Cause for Concern." *Journal of the American Heart Association* 5: e003089. doi: 10.1161/JAHA.115.003089.

Wilson, K. M., et al. (2011). "Coffee Consumption and Prostate Cancer Risk and Progression in the Health Professionals Follow-up Study." *Journal of the National Cancer Institute* 103: 876–884.

Winhusen, T. M., et al. (2014). "A Randomized Trial of Concurrent Smoking Cessation and Substance Use Disorder Treatment in Stimulant Dependent Smokers." *Journal of Clinical Psychiatry* 75: 336–343.

Wing, V. C., et al. (2015). "Measuring Cigarette Smoking-Induced Cortical Dopamine Release: A [^{11}C]FLB-457 PET Study." *Neuropsychopharmacology* 40: 1417–1427. doi: 10.1038/npp.2014.327.

Womack, C. J., et al. (2012). "The Influence of a CYP1A2 Polymorphism on the Ergogenic Effects of Caffeine." *Journal of International Society of Sports Nutrition* 9: 7. doi: 10.1186/1550–2783–9–7.

Wright, G. A., et al. (2013). "Caffeine in Floral Nectar Enhances a Pollinator's Memory of Reward." *Science* 339: 1202–1204.

Xiao, Q., et al. (2014). "Inverse Associations of Total and Decaffeinated Coffee with Liver Enzyme Levels in National Health and Nutrition Examination Survey 1999–2010." *Hepatology* 60: 2090–2097.

Xue, S., et al. (2015). "A New Strategy for Smoking Cessation: Characterization of a Bacterial Enzyme for the Degradation of Nicotine." *Journal of the American Chemical Society* 137: 10136–10139.

Zhang, Y., et al. (2016). "Is Coffee Consumption Associated with a Lower Risk of Hyperuricaemia or Gout? A Systematic Review and Meta-Analysis." *BMJ* 6: e009809. doi: 10.1136/bmjopen-2015–009809.

Zhou, S., et al. (2016). "Secondhand Hookah Smoke: An Occupational Hazard for Hookah Bar Employees." *Tobacco Control* 0: 1-6. doi: 10.1136/tobaccocontrol-2015–052505.

Zierler-Brown, S. L., and Kyle, J. A. (2007). "Oral Varenicline for Smoking Cessation." *Annals of Pharmacotherapy* 41: 95–99.

Zorick, T., et al. (2014). "A Naturalistic Study of the Association Between Antidepressant Treatment and Outcome of Smoking Cessation Treatment." *Journal of Clinical Psychiatry* 75: e1433–e1438.

Zuchinali, P. et al. (2016). "Short-Term Caffeine Use Isn't Associated with Arrhythmias in Heart Failure Patients." *JAMA Internal Medicine* 176: 1752–1759.

CHAPTER 7

Cocaine, the Amphetamines, and Other Psychostimulants

The psychostimulants are drugs that exert their primary behavioral effects by augmenting the action of the monoamine (biogenic amine) neurotransmitters, the most important of which is dopamine. Sometimes these drugs are referred to as *sympathomimetics* because they activate the transmitters that stimulate the sympathetic nervous system and mimic sympathetic arousal.

In addition to cocaine and amphetamines (including methamphetamine), the psychostimulants include the naturally occurring plant products, such as ephedrine and cathinone, as well as the synthetic drugs methylphenidate and modafinil (and its active isomer, armodafinil). Although these latter substances have approved medical uses, this chapter primarily concerns their recreational use as drugs of abuse. Most recently, recreational use of the group of synthetic stimulants, colloquially known as "bath salts," has become a serious public health concern and this development has received the greatest attention among the drugs in this category.

COCAINE

History

Cocaine is derived from the leaves of the *Erythroxylon coca* plant, grown in the high altitude of the Peruvian and Bolivian Andes of South America. In fact, methodology has been developed that can identify which of the 19 known coca-growing regions in Bolivia, Colombia, and Peru is the origin of a sample of cocaine (Mallete et al., 2016). It has been suggested that this substance may have arisen naturally because it is toxic to insects that eat the leaves of the plant and therefore protects it from damage. Nevertheless, at least 5000 years ago, humans discovered the psychoactive properties of the plant, and its ability to reduce fatigue, thirst, and hunger was appreciated for many centuries by the indigenous Indian population. In fact, the practice of chewing the leaves or brewing a tea from the leaves persists even today. When chewed, the leaves are usually mixed with lime (often from sea shells), which interacts with saliva to release the cocaine and reduce its bitter taste, resulting in a daily dose of about 200 milligrams. When the Incas conquered the region in about the tenth century C.E., they adopted it as a sacred substance, restricted to the priests and nobility for special ceremonies. When the Spanish conquered the Incas in the sixteenth century, they initially banned coca use, but then realized how useful it was as a form of money and as a way of increasing the productivity of the native workers.

The Spanish sent samples of the plant to Europe, where eventually Carl Linnaeus classified it in its own family (*Erythroxylaceae*) and the most important species was named *Erythroxylon coca* by Jean-Baptiste Lamarck. Europeans, however, were unaware of the psychoactive properties of the plant, perhaps because its potency deteriorated during the long trip from South America to Europe. It was not until 1857 (or 1859) that the compound was isolated and named cocaine by the chemist Albert Nieman, who noted its anesthetic effect on his tongue.

Cocaine soon became very popular as an additive to drinks and elixirs, most famously when added to wine by Angelo Mariani in 1863. This product, Vin Mariani, was extremely successful and was endorsed by a long list of celebrities, including presidents, kings, and even the Pope. In the United States, a Georgia pharmacist, John Pemberton, developed a similar product called "French Wine of Cola, Ideal Tonic." But when the city of Atlanta prohibited the sale of alcohol, he changed the formulation, removing alcohol, adding soda water, and combining the coca (about 60 milligrams in 8 ounces) with syrup of the kola nut, containing 2 percent caffeine. This drink, named Coca-Cola, was promoted as a health drink and is one reason why soda fountains in the United States were located in drug stores, that is, with other medicinal products.

At the same time, the introduction of the syringe and hypodermic needle prompted many attempts to use cocaine to produce local anesthesia for surgery. Perhaps the first medical report of cocaine's local anesthetic action was made in 1880[1] and cocaine became widely used for topical anesthesia, spinal anesthesia, and nerve blocks from about 1884 until about 1918, when *procaine* (Novocaine) was developed as the first synthetic local anesthetic. Procaine is devoid of psychological and dependence-producing effects.

In 1884, Sigmund Freud advocated the use of cocaine to treat depression and to alleviate chronic fatigue. He described cocaine as a marvelous drug with the ability even to cure opioid (morphine and heroin) addiction. While using cocaine to relieve his own depression, Freud described the drug as inducing exhilaration and lasting euphoria that was no different from the normal euphoria of the healthy person. Unfortunately, he did not immediately perceive its side effects—tolerance, dependence, a state of psychosis, and withdrawal depression. But eventually, in his later writings, Freud called cocaine the "third scourge" of humanity, after alcohol and heroin.

Around the end of the nineteenth century in the United States, there were no restrictions on the sale or consumption of cocaine, and it became popular with writers and other artists. Robert Louis Stevenson is said to have conceived of Dr. Jekyll and Mr. Hyde with cocaine in mind, and some of the behavioral effects of the drug were

[1]At that time, no other anesthetics (general or local) had been discovered. Surgery was limited to brief procedures conducted without anesthetic or with the patient under alcohol intoxication.

exhibited by Sir Arthur Conan Doyle's character Sherlock Holmes, under the supervision of his companion, Dr. Watson. In the late 1800s, however, concern about cocaine's toxicities increased, with several hundred reports of cocaine intoxication and several reported deaths. About 1910, President Taft proclaimed cocaine to be "Public Enemy Number One," and in 1914, the Harrison Narcotic Act banned the incorporation of cocaine into patent medicines and beverages. With the enforcement of the Narcotic Act, cocaine use decreased during the 1930s, largely replaced by the newly available amphetamines, which were cheaper and produced longer-lasting yet similar effects. Cocaine all but disappeared until the late 1960s, when tight federal restrictions on the distribution of amphetamines raised the cost, once again making cocaine attractive.

In the 1980s, a new epidemic of cocaine use began with the widespread availability of crack cocaine, intended for use by inhalation (smoking) rather than injection. This stimulant epidemic continues today, although the relatively inexpensive and widely available methamphetamine is currently more commonly encountered. With the increased availability of lower-cost methamphetamine, the number of cocaine users has stabilized (for more historical information, see Doweiko, 2012; Levinthal, 2012; McKim and Hancock, 2013).

Forms of Cocaine

The leaf of *E. coca* contains about 1 percent cocaine. When the leaves are soaked and mashed, cocaine is extracted in the form of coca paste (60 to 80 percent cocaine). *Basuco* is a residual paste that is a by-product of cocaine production. It produces a very brief (2-minute) "high" when smoked. This induces binge, which results in rapid addiction. Coca paste is usually treated with hydrochloric acid to form the less potent, water-soluble salt *cocaine hydrochloride* before it is exported. The powdered hydrochloride salt can be absorbed through the nasal mucosa ("snorted," that is, by nasal insufflation) and, because this salt form is water soluble, it can be injected intravenously. In the hydrochloride form, however, cocaine decomposes when it is heated and is destroyed at the temperature of smoke, making it unsuitable for use by inhalation. In contrast, cocaine base, also known as *freebase*, is insoluble in water, but is soluble in alcohol, acetone, or ether. Heating the freebase converts cocaine to a stable vapor that can be inhaled, allowing the drug to reach the brain within less than 10 seconds, a very potent, addictive characteristic. Unfortunately, this process can be dangerous and there is considerable risk of fire or an explosion. It was appreciated that it might be very profitable to offer a safer smokeable form of cocaine. This product, called *crack cocaine*, or simply *crack*, is essentially cocaine base that is prepared for smoking before it is sold to the user. In illicit factories, cocaine hydrochloride is mixed with baking soda and water and heated until cocaine crystals precipitate. The name *crack* is derived from the sound of the crystals popping when smoked. (Interestingly, this is a variant of the method used by the Incas. By mixing the coca leaves with lime, they made saliva more basic, which enhanced absorption.)

Cocaine hydrochloride ("crystal" or "snow"), when snorted as a line of drug, provides a dose of about 25 milligrams; a user might sniff about 50 to 100 milligrams of drug at a time. The smoking of crack cocaine yields average doses in the range of 250 milligrams to 1 gram (Table 7.1).

TABLE 7.1 Pharmacokinetics of cocaine administration

Administration route	Mode	Initial onset of action (sec.)	Duration of "high" (min.)	Average acute dose (mg)	Peak plasma levels (ng/mL)	Purity (%)	Bioavailability (% absorbed)
Oral	Coca leaf chewing	300–600	45–90	20–50	150	0.5–1	25
Oral	Cocaine HCl	600–1800		100–200	150–200	20–80	20–30
Intranasal	Snorting cocaine HCl	120–180	30–45	5–30	150	20–80	20–30
Intravenous	Cocaine HCl	30–45	10–20	25–50	300–400	10–100	100
				>200	1000–1500		
Smoking	Coca paste	8–10	5–10	60–250	300–800	40–85	6–32
	Free base	8–10	5–10	250–1000	800–900	90–100	6–32
	Crack	8–10	5–10	250–1000	?	50–95	6–32

SOURCE: M. S. Gold, "Cocaine (and Crack): Clinical Aspects," in J. H. Lowinson, P. Ruiz, R. B. Millman, and J. G. Langrod, eds., *Substance Abuse: A Comprehensive Textbook*, 3rd ed. (Baltimore: Williams & Wilkins, 1997), p. 185.

Pharmacokinetics

Absorption
Cocaine is absorbed from all sites of application, including mucous membranes, the stomach, and the lungs. Table 7.1 presents some pharmacokinetic data for common methods of administration. Cocaine hydrochloride crosses the mucosal membranes poorly because the drug is a potent vasoconstrictor (one of its defining pharmacological actions), constricting blood vessels and limiting its own absorption. In addition, anywhere from 70 to 80 percent of the amount absorbed may be biotransformed by the liver before it reaches the brain. As a consequence, only about 20 to 30 percent of the snorted drug is absorbed through the nasal mucosa into blood. When cocaine base is vaporized and smoked, absorption is rapid and quite complete; effects begin within seconds and peak at 5 minutes. Intravenous injection of cocaine hydrochloride bypasses all the barriers to absorption, placing the total dose of drug immediately into the bloodstream. The 30- to 60-second delay in the onset of action simply reflects the time it takes the drug to travel from the site of injection through the pulmonary circulation and into the brain.

Distribution
Cocaine penetrates the brain rapidly; initial brain concentrations far exceed the concentrations in plasma. After it penetrates the brain, cocaine is rapidly redistributed to other tissues. Cocaine freely crosses the placental barrier, achieving levels in the fetus equal to those in the mother.

Metabolism and Excretion
Cocaine has a biological half-life in plasma of only about 50 minutes; enzymes located both in plasma and in the liver rapidly and almost completely metabolize it. Butyrylcholinesterase is the major enzyme for metabolizing cocaine in humans. Although cocaine is rapidly removed from plasma, it is more slowly removed from the brain, in which it can be detected for eight or more hours after initial use. Urine can test positive for cocaine for up to 12 hours. The major metabolite of cocaine is the inactive compound *benzoylecgonine* (BE) (see Figure 7.1), which can be detected in the urine for about 48 hours and much longer (up to two weeks) in chronic users, and forms the primary basis of drug testing for cocaine use. The persistence of BE in urine implies that high-dose, long-term users might accumulate drug in their body tissues. Cocaine and BE can also be detected in hair for several months; hair closest to the scalp takes three to four months to become negative (Garcia-Bournissen et al., 2009).

There is an important metabolic interaction between cocaine and ethanol. In people who use cocaine and concurrently drink alcohol, the liver enzymes that metabolize the two drugs produce a unique ethyl ester of benzoylecgonine. This metabolite (called *cocaethylene*) (see Figure 7.1) is pharmacologically as active as cocaine in blocking the presynaptic dopamine reuptake transporter (see below), potentiating the euphoric effect of cocaine, increasing the risk of dual dependency, and increasing the severity of withdrawal with chronic use (Bunney et al., 2001). Cocaethylene is actually more toxic than cocaine, as it is a potent calcium channel blocker in the heart and exacerbates cocaine's toxicity (Farooq et al., 2009). The half-life of cocaethylene is about 150 minutes, outlasting cocaine in the body.

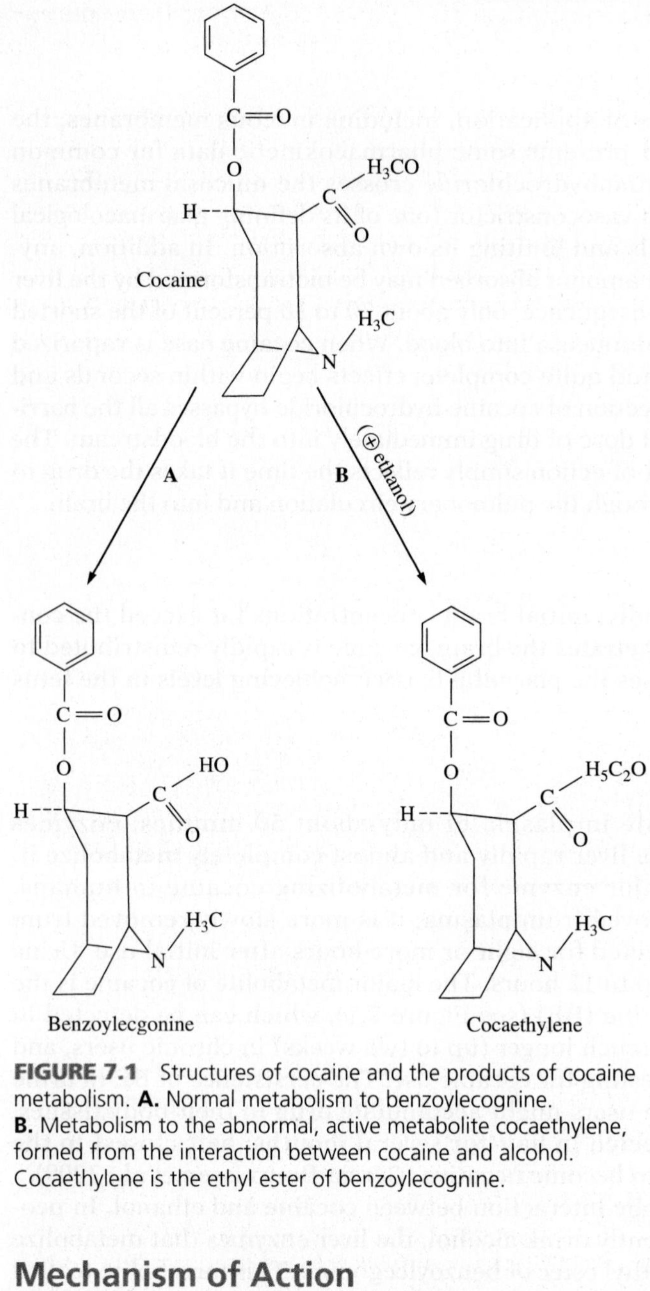

FIGURE 7.1 Structures of cocaine and the products of cocaine metabolism. **A.** Normal metabolism to benzoylecognine.
B. Metabolism to the abnormal, active metabolite cocaethylene, formed from the interaction between cocaine and alcohol.
Cocaethylene is the ethyl ester of benzoylecognine.

Mechanism of Action

Pharmacologically, cocaine has three prominent actions that account for virtually all its physiological and psychological effects. Cocaine is the only drug that possesses these three characteristics: it is a potent *local anesthetic*; it is a *vasoconstrictor*, strongly constricting blood vessels and raising blood pressure; and it is a powerful *psychostimulant.* Its vasoconstrictive and cardiac effects contribute to severe cardiovascular and cerebrovascular toxicities (Phillips et al., 2009), while the stimulant action is responsible for its addictive potency.

Cocaine blocks the reuptake of all the monoamine neurotransmitters, although most of its effects appear to be due to the blockade of dopamine reuptake (see Figure 7.2). Blockade of the dopamine transporter markedly increases the levels of dopamine within the synaptic cleft. Increased dopamine levels in the nucleus accumbens (NAc) and other components of the dopaminergic reward system seem to be responsible for the euphoric effects of the drug (see Chapter 4). Brain imaging studies suggest that at least 47 percent of the transporters must be blocked for cocaine to produce the "high" and that the doses of cocaine commonly abused block about 60 to 77 percent of dopamine transporters.

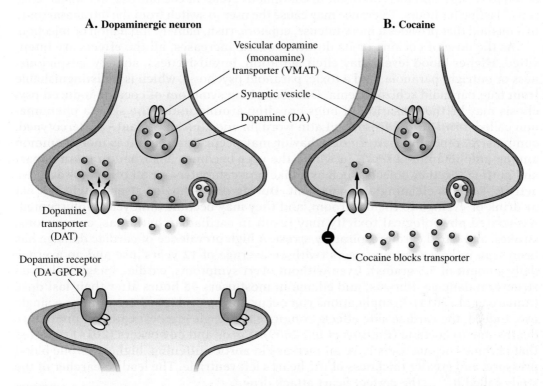

FIGURE 7.2 Dopamine nerve terminal and transporter proteins involved in the active uptake of dopamine (DA). **A.** Two transporters are shown. The first is a vesicular dopamine transporter (VMAT), located in the cytoplasm of the presynaptic neuron, bound to dopamine-containing storage vesicles. This transporter carries dopamine from the cytoplasm into storage. The second type of dopamine transporter (the DAT) is found on the synaptic membrane of the presynaptic neuron and functions to transport dopamine from the synaptic cleft into the presynaptic nerve terminal, recycling the transmitter and ending the process of synaptic transmission. **B.** The dopamine transporter is blocked by cocaine, prolonging the action of DA in the synaptic cleft.

Pharmacological Effects in Human Beings

Because the psychostimulants activate the sympathetic nervous system, they produce the characteristic physiological effects of an increased heart rate, blood pressure, vasodilation, and bronchodilation. (In fact, as discussed below, this last action was a primary reason for the development of amphetamine.) Body temperature rises, pupils dilate, blood glucose increases, and blood flow to the muscles increases. Subjective effects of low doses of cocaine (25 to 75 milligrams) include increased energy and alertness, with a decrease in fatigue, increased libido, and a general feeling of euphoria or elevation of mood. Appetite is reduced, activity is increased, and sleep is prevented. If snorted, there may first be a numbing sensation (termed the "freeze"); if injected or inhaled, the euphoric effect is so rapid, it is called the "rush." The typical duration of the positive feelings may be 10 to 20 minutes, followed by a mild depression, called the "letdown," or "comedown" (McKim and Hancock, 2013). Tolerance to the euphoric effects of cocaine develops rapidly, and this can result in continuous cycles of cocaine use, known as "coke runs," lasting for hours. Tolerance may cause the user to switch from the intranasal route to a method that provides a more intense, euphoric rush, namely, inhalation or injection.

As the dose of cocaine or its duration of use increases, all the effects are intensified. Higher blood levels may elicit agitation, impulsiveness, anxiety, suspiciousness or outright paranoia, and a toxic, paranoid psychosis, which is indistinguishable from true paranoid schizophrenia. One disturbing symptom of cocaine-induced psychosis may be the sensation of bugs crawling around under the skin, a phenomenon called *formication*, from the Latin word *formica*, meaning "ant." A stereotyped, compulsive, repetitive pattern of behavior may occur (although it is more common among amphetamine users), in which the user becomes absorbed in taking apart and putting together objects, such as a bike or a computer—or an otherwise aversive activity, such as cleaning an apartment. During this behavior, users might not eat or drink or even go to the bathroom, and they may become annoyed if interrupted. Associated physiological toxicity may result in cardiac arrhythmias, convulsions, strokes, and lethal cardiorespiratory arrest. A high prevalence of cardiac damage has been seen in heavy cocaine users (with an average of 12 years' use and an average daily amount of 5.5 grams). Even without overt symptoms, cardiac imaging showed structural damage, fibrosis, and edema in most users 48 hours after their last dose (Aquaro et al., 2011). Complications can occur during prolonged use or after a single use. Indeed, the cardiac side effects comprise the single greatest cause of premature deaths due to cocaine (Phillips et al., 2009). Kozor and coworkers (2014) reported that chronic cocaine users have an increase in aortic stiffening, higher systolic blood pressure, and greater thickness of the heart's left ventricle. The lead researcher of the study called it ". . . the perfect heart attack drug."

When the acute effects wear off, depression, dysphoria, anxiety, somnolence, and drug craving follow the CNS activation. Although using cocaine may heighten sexual interest and high doses (injected or smoked) are sometimes described as orgasmic, cocaine is not an aphrodisiac. Sexual dysfunction is common in heavy users because they lose interest in interpersonal and sexual interactions.

Dependence on cocaine can produce changes in the brain. Ersche and colleagues (2011) scanned the brains of 120 people, half of whom were cocaine dependent. Not only was there widespread loss of gray matter (neurons), the decrease was related to the duration of the cocaine abuse. That is, the longer they had been abusing the drug, the greater the loss of gray matter, and the volume of the reduction was associated with greater compulsion to take cocaine. Although cocaine-dependent persons performed normally on a computer-based spatial learning task, they had abnormal neural responses in cortical areas that mediated reward (Tau et al., 2014). Studies have also shown a deficiency in D_2 receptors in the brains of cocaine-dependent persons and one report found higher D_3 levels than controls, suggesting that this might be a biomarker relevant to addiction (Payer et al., 2014). Nevertheless, if cocaine-dependent users continue taking the drug, cognitive function deteriorates. Within one year of increasing cocaine use (almost a threefold increase), users showed a decrease in memory function. Those who stopped taking cocaine, however, appeared to recover completely, although drug use at an early age hampers recovery (Vonmoos et al., 2014). Studies in animals have consistently shown that repeated exposure to psychostimulant drugs, such as cocaine, activates the immune response and leads to inflammatory changes in the brain. But an examination in chronic cocaine-abusing humans did not show evidence of microglial activation (suggesting no immune reaction or inflammatory change) in the brain (Narendran et al., 2014).

Finally, in cocaine-positive emergency room patients, 24 percent of chief complaints were related to violent trauma and an autopsy study found that the most common cause of death among cocaine-positive patients (37 percent) was violent injury (Walton et al., 2009).

An acutely toxic dose of cocaine has been estimated to be about 2 milligrams per kilogram of body weight. Thus, 150 milligrams of cocaine is a toxic one-time dose for a 150-pound (70-kilogram) person.

Comorbidity

Cocaine-dependent people are typically young (12 to 39 years of age), male, and dependent on at least three drugs. They tend to have coexisting psychopathology (30 percent have anxiety disorders, 67 percent suffer from clinical depression, and 25 percent exhibit paranoia). Other comorbidities include bipolar disorder, antisocial personality disorder, posttraumatic stress disorder, and attention deficit/hyperactivity disorder (ADHD) (Kaye et al., 2013). Intravenous drug users often take cocaine and heroin together in a mixture known as a *speedball*. The heroin reduces the jitteriness and hypervigilance caused by the cocaine, while the cocaine reduces the sleepiness caused by the heroin.

Cocaine and Pregnancy

If a pregnant mother uses cocaine, her fetus will absorb a higher concentration of the drug than she does. The drug crosses the placenta very quickly. There, cocaine and its metabolites are stored in the uterine wall and the placental membrane and, by diffusion, provide continuous drug delivery to the amniotic fluid (De Giovanni and Marchetti, 2012). It is well established that when pregnant women use cocaine, their children will be smaller in size, weight, and head circumference (Gouin et al., 2011).

According to Malek (2012), cocaine use during the early months of pregnancy can also cause "spontaneous abortion, probably due to an increase in maternal plasma norepinephrine, which increases uterine contractility, constricts placental vessels, and decreases blood flow to the fetus." Spontaneous abortions are more likely to occur if the drug is ingested in binges rather than in typical fashion. Malek also notes that congenital anomalies, such as brain malformation and cardiovascular abnormalities, are common with maternal cocaine use and " have been reported to occur in 7 to 40 percent of infants exposed to cocaine in utero." Withdrawal symptoms may occur in about one-third of babies born to cocaine-using mothers. These include seizures, lethargy, hyperactive reflexes, vomiting, diarrhea, high-pitched crying, and restlessness. Such babies have a harder time feeding and are more likely to be sick in their first year of life. Prenatal cocaine exposure may impair attentiveness and emotional expressivity in offspring, producing a condition that resembles attention deficit/hyperactivity disorder (Thompson et al., 2009). Although one study found that intrauterine cocaine was not a strong predictor of adolescent delinquent behaviors (Gerteis et al., 2011), another group of researchers reported that adolescents between the ages of 14 and 17 exposed to cocaine in utero had lower gray matter volume in brain regions involved in emotion, reward, memory, and executive function compared with nonexposed adolescents. Amazingly, each 1 milliliter decrease in gray matter volume increased the probability of initiating substance use by 69 to 83 percent (Rando et al., 2013).

In addition to suffering the deleterious direct effect of the drug, the infant born of a cocaine-using mother is more likely to be abused and neglected. Prenatal care is often poor and tobacco and alcohol use is prevalent. Because of the decreased appetite produced by cocaine, both the mother and the fetus are at risk of malnutrition (Keegan et al., 2010). Many negative effects of cocaine on offspring are due to psychiatric problems of the mothers, which may be mediated by depression. Cocaine-using mothers are less attentive and interactive with their infants during the first six months. As the number of environmental risk factors (depression, domestic abuse, psychiatric symptoms, and absence of a significant other) increases, a substance-abusing mother may be overwhelmed and have little time for effective parenting. High levels of cocaine use are strongly associated with failure to maintain custody of children due to neglect and/or abuse (Nephew and Febo, 2012).

AMPHETAMINES

Like cocaine, the amphetamines (Figure 7.3) produce a variety of sympathomimetic effects on both the CNS and the autonomic nervous system.[2] The amphetamine molecule has two isomers. The more potent one is *dextroamphetamine*, or

---

[2]The *autonomic nervous system* (ANS) is frequently called the visceral nervous system because it regulates and maintains the homeostasis of the body's internal organs. It controls the function of the heart, the flow of blood, and the functioning of the digestive tract, and it regulates other internal functions that are essential for maintaining the balance necessary for life. The ANS comprises two subdivisions—the *sympathetic* and the *parasympathetic*. The function of the parasympathetic nervous system can be viewed as maintaining our "vegetative" functions, while the sympathetic nervous system handles the body's reaction to stress, fear, and other responses that demand an immediate alerting response. Neurotransmitters in the sympathetic division of the ANS include epinephrine (adrenaline), norepinephrine, and dopamine.

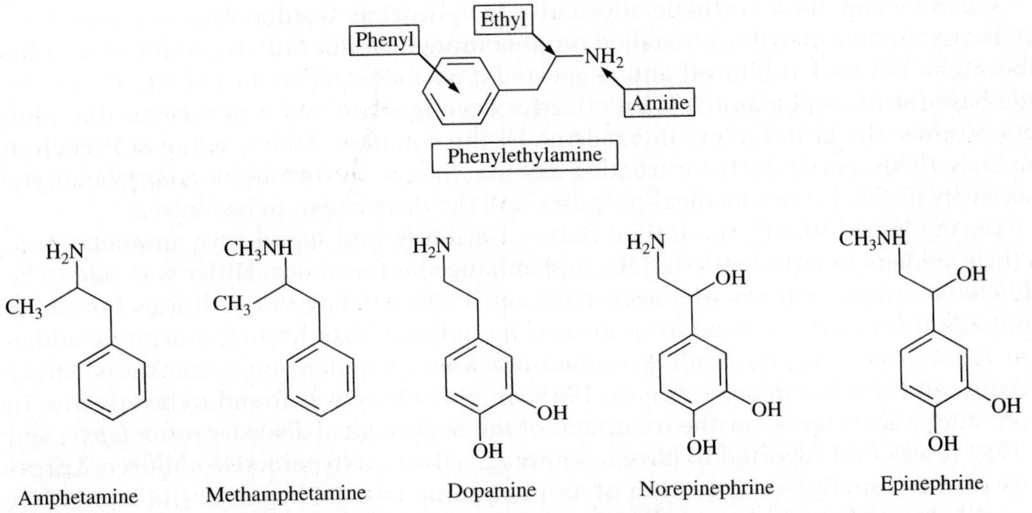

FIGURE 7.3 The basic sympathomimetic amine nucleus (phenylethylamine), the neurotransmitters dopamine, norepinephrine, and epinephrine, and the structures of amphetamine and methamphetamine.

d-amphetamine (Dexedrine, DextroStat); the less potent is the levo- or l-amphetamine isomer. The two isomers are combined in the medication Adderall, approved for treatment of ADHD (see Chapter 15). A modified version of d-amphetamine is formed by substituting CH_3 (called a *methyl group*) for the H at one end, producing methamphetamine (see Figure 7.3). This change allows the drug to cross the blood–brain barrier much faster.

History

The Romanan chemist Lazar Edeleanu first developed the drug amphetamine—which he called *phenylisopropylamine*—in 1887. Its structure was similar to the natural substance ephedrine, which had been separated from the herb *ma-huang* source around the same time by Nagayoshi Nagai. But the actions of amphetamine were not studied until 1910, when the pharmacologists Barger and Dale wrote about its effects. Because there was no therapeutic use for amphetamine at that time, it was not developed further. In 1918, over 30 years after Edeleanu's work, the chemist Akira Ogata developed the related agent, methamphetamine, from the same plant source *ma-huang*.

In 1924, ephedrine's structure was determined and it was found to have an effect similar to our transmitter epinephrine. Epinephrine was already being used to treat asthma, but it was short-lived and had to be injected. Ephedrine was better because it could be taken orally and was longer-lasting. Being a natural plant product, however, there were concerns that supplies would run out, and intense efforts were made to find an alternative.

When looking for a synthetic alternative to ephedrine, Gordon Alles, a seminal figure in psychopharmacology, recalled amphetamine. He not only reproduced it in his laboratory, but took it himself and suggested it as a cheaper replacement. As the volatile base form, amphetamine is an effective decongestant and was sold for that indication under the brand name Benzedrine by the company Smith, Kline & French in the early 1930s, particularly for treating asthma. In ampule formulation, amphetamine was easily usable for nonmedical purposes and the drug began to be abused.

During World War II, the United States, Germany, and Japan gave amphetamines to their soldiers to fight battle fatigue and enhance performance. Hitler was said to be addicted to amphetamines. Between 1935 and 1946, a list of 39 conditions for which amphetamines could be used in treatment included schizophrenia, morphine addiction, tobacco smoking, head injury, radiation sickness, hypotension, seasickness, severe hiccups, and caffeine dependence. In 1935, amphetamine was found to be effective in promoting wakefulness, for the treatment of the neurological disorder *narcolepsy*, and in 1937 it was first reported to have a "calming" effect on hyperactive children. Large-scale abuse (usually oral ingestion of amphetamine tablets) began in the late 1940s, primarily by students and truck drivers to maintain wakefulness, temporarily increase alertness, and delay sleep. In the 1960s, amphetamines were also used as diet pills and as antidepressants. Their anorexic and antidepressant actions, however, become tolerant within weeks, and they are no longer approved for those uses. Today, legitimate use is largely restricted to the clinical treatment of ADHD and occasionally in the treatment of narcolepsy.

In the late 1960s, the abuse pattern changed with the advent of injectable forms of the drug. During the next decades there was an epidemic of abuse (especially in Japan) that saw the appearance of the "speed freak"—users who took IV doses continuously for days.

After decades of reported abuse, the Food and Drug Administration (FDA) restricted amphetamine to prescription use in 1965, but nonmedical use remained widespread. Amphetamine became a Schedule II drug under the Controlled Substances Act in 1971. Eventually the epidemic receded for several reasons. First, users saw the dangers of compulsive use and this understanding was expressed in the phrase "speed kills." Second, at the same time, the government exerted pressure on drug companies to decrease their legal production of the drug; medical use was inhibited and unethical physicians were prosecuted. Third, more effective and legal medical alternatives to depression were discovered. And fourth, cocaine reappeared. During the 1970s and 1980s, more people could afford cocaine. In 1974, 5 million people said they had tried it; by 1985, 25 million people had done so. Although cocaine use began leveling off in the mid-1980s, it rose again after "crack" appeared—the smokeable version of cocaine. And then, in the mid-1990s, amphetamine abuse resurfaced, becoming even more of a scourge when the smokeable form of methamphetamine, "ice," was developed.

Currently, there is much concern about the abuse of prescription stimulants by college students and young adults. It is especially difficult to get reliable data about how many nonstudent adult workers misuse stimulants, although substance abuse treatment facilities report seeing an increase in adults in the age range from 25 to 45 years (Schwarz, 2015). A survey released in November 2014 (*Under Pressure: College*

Students and the Abuse of Rx Stimulants: Partnership for Drug-Free Kids) found that 20 percent of college students and 17 percent of young adults (ages 18 to 25) reported the abuse of stimulants at least once in their lifetime. The most common reason for taking the drugs was to improve their performance in school or on the job while pursuing an active social life. A substantial proportion of young people are using these drugs in an effort to balance their academic or professional work and time with friends and family. (For a discussion of this issue, see Gerlach et al., 2014.)

In January 2015, the drug *lisdexamfetamine* (Vyvanse), which is already approved for ADHD, became the first drug approved for binge-eating disorder. Lisdexamfetamine is a combination of the stimulant dextroamphetamine and the amino acid L-lysine. In this form, the drug is inactive. When swallowed, the amino acid is metabolically separated from dextroamphetamine in the gut, which activates the stimulant. Doses of 50 or 70 milligrams per day reduced the number of binge-eating days per week, with body weight reductions between 5.2 percent and 6.25 percent. Most common adverse effects were dry mouth, decreased appetite, insomnia, and headache (Citrome, 2015). Although the FDA had previously forbidden the promotion of this drug for obesity (which is common in cases of binge-eating disorder), the administration said Vyvanse was granted priority approval because there was no other drug treatment available for the disorder. And it did not ask an advisory committee to review the issue because Vyvanse is already sold as an ADHD drug and its safety profile is well known.

Pharmacokinetics of Amphetamine Compared with Cocaine

Most of the pharmacokinetic differences between cocaine and amphetamine are minor. Both are very lipid soluble and well absorbed from all sites in the body. Amphetamine has a longer duration of effect than cocaine. The half-life of cocaine is short, 30 to 90 minutes, which promotes repeated use. Enzymes in the plasma and liver rapidly and almost completely metabolize cocaine. Amphetamine's half-life is in hours. Moreover, individuals differ in their pharmacokinetic response to oral amphetamine. About 20 to 25 percent are early peak responders (within 60 minutes), who have an earlier rise in plasma levels and more sustained heart rate elevation than late peak responders (more than 60 minutes; 50 to 55 percent) (Smith et al., 2016). Such differences in the temporal pattern of response might influence abuse potential.

Mechanism of Action

Similar to cocaine, amphetamine modifies the action of dopamine and norepinephrine in the brain (see Figure 7.4). But amphetamine does this in several ways. At low doses, (1) it binds to the presynaptic membrane of dopaminergic neurons and induces the release of dopamine from the nerve terminal; (2) it binds to the dopamine reuptake transporter, causing it to not only block reuptake, but also to act in reverse and transport free dopamine out of the nerve terminal; (3) at high doses, it interacts with dopamine containing synaptic storage vesicles, releasing free dopamine, perhaps

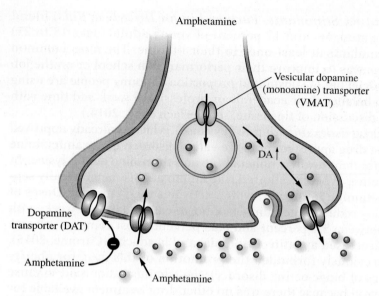

FIGURE 7.4 Mechanism of action of amphetamine on dopamine nerve terminals. Amphetamine blocks the dopamine (DA) transporter (DAT), preventing the reuptake of dopamine. Amphetamine is also taken up into the terminal by the DAT, where it interferes with the dopamine transporter of the synaptic vesicles (VMAT). This depletes the vesicles and increases DA levels in the cytoplasm of the terminal. As a result, the direction of the DAT reverses, which means more dopamine is released into the synaptic cleft. Not shown is an additional effect of amphetamine, a weak block of the enzyme MAO. Amphetamine also has comparable effects on the norepinephrine transporter (NET).

into the nerve terminal, although exocytotic release has been questioned (Siciliano et al., 2014); and (4) also at high doses, amphetamine binds to monoamine oxidase (MAO) in dopaminergic neurons and prevents the degradation of dopamine, leaving free dopamine in the nerve terminal. It has further been shown that as few as five days of amphetamine self-administration reduced the ability of D_2 autoreceptors to inhibit dopamine release in the nucleus accumbens (Calipari et al., 2014). This would also be expected to increase extracellular dopamine. High-dose amphetamine has a similar effect on noradrenergic neurons; it can induce the release of norepinephrine into the synaptic cleft and inhibit the norepinephrine reuptake transporter.

Pharmacological Effects

Both cocaine and amphetamine have the net effect of increasing the amount of dopamine available (although through different mechanisms); therefore, cocaine abusers have difficulty distinguishing between the subjective effects of 8 to 10 milligrams of cocaine and 10 milligrams of dextroamphetamine when the doses are administered intravenously.

Pharmacological responses to amphetamines vary with the specific drug, the dose, and the route of administration. In general, with amphetamine itself, effects may be categorized as those produced by low to moderate doses (5 to 50 milligrams), usually administered orally, and those observed at high doses (more than approximately 100 milligrams), often administered intravenously. These dose ranges are not the same for all amphetamines. For example, dextroamphetamine is three to four times more potent than amphetamine; low-to-moderate doses range from 2.5 to 20 milligrams, while high doses are 50 milligrams or more. Amphetamine metabolites are excreted in the urine and are detectable for up to 48 hours. Methamphetamine is even more potent, although methamphetamine-dependent people who have developed a tolerance to the drug take massive doses.

At low doses, all amphetamines increase blood pressure and heart rate, relax bronchial muscle, and produce a variety of other actions that follow from the body's alerting response. In the CNS, amphetamine is a potent stimulant, producing alertness; euphoria; excitement; wakefulness; a reduced sense of fatigue; loss of appetite; increased mood, motor and speech activity; and a feeling of power. Interestingly, some subjective effects of amphetamine, such as "arousal" and "euphoria," are related to personality traits, such as "impulsivity" (Kirkpatrick et al., 2013). In fact, it has been reported that pathological gamblers had different blood pressure and cortisol responses to amphetamine than healthy controls (Zack et al., 2015), suggesting noradrenergic disturbances that may be more affected by the drug. During short-duration, high-intensity activity, such as an athletic competition, performance may be enhanced despite impairment of dexterity and fine motor skills.

At moderate doses (20 to 50 milligrams), additional effects of amphetamines include stimulation of respiration, slight tremors, restlessness, and a greater increase in motor activity, insomnia, and agitation. As doses increase, this reaction is accompanied by the worsening or de novo production of anxiety disorders, possibly progressing from restlessness and nonspecific anxiety to obsessive behaviors, panic disorders, paranoia, and eventually a paranoid psychosis. Recreational use of amphetamine is also associated with neuronal dopamine system dysfunction—such as less dopamine binding, blunted release, and blunted subjective response to an amphetamine challenge relative to nonusers (Schrantee et al., 2015).

Chronic high doses produce additional effects. Stereotypical behaviors include continual, purposeless, repetitive acts; sudden outbursts of aggression and violence; paranoid delusions; and severe anorexia. Weight loss, skin sores, infections from neglected health care, and a variety of other consequences occur both because of the drug itself and because of poor eating habits, lack of sleep, or the use of unsterile equipment for intravenous injections. Most high-dose users show a progressive deterioration in their social, personal, and occupational affairs.

The toxic dose of amphetamine varies widely. Severe reactions can occur even from low doses (20 to 30 milligrams). On the other hand, people who have developed tolerance have survived doses of 400 to 500 milligrams. Even larger doses are tolerated by chronic users. The slogan "speed kills" refers not only to a direct fatal effect of single doses of amphetamine, but also to the deteriorating mental and physical condition of the addicted user.

Methamphetamine

It has been estimated that 35 percent of methamphetamine in the United States comes from clandestine laboratories (Talbert et al., 2012). It is easily synthesized from readily obtainable chemicals, including pseudoephedrine. Methamphetamine was originally an approved drug, effective in the treatment of ADHD. Today, however, it is rarely used legitimately and has clearly demonstrated neurotoxicity.

Like cocaine hydrochloride, methamphetamine (the hydrochloride salt) is broken down at temperatures required for smoking. But when converted to its crystalline form, methamphetamine can be effectively vaporized and inhaled in smoke. It also known as ice, speed, crystal, crank, and go, with considerable overlap in nomenclature with other amphetamines except for ice, which refers to the smokeable form. Thus, ice is to methamphetamine as crack is to cocaine: the crystalline, smokeable form of the parent compound. Unlike cocaine, however, methamphetamine has an extremely long half-life (about 12 hours), resulting in an intense, persistent drug action.

Pharmacokinetics

Smoking ice results in its near-immediate absorption into plasma, with additional absorption continuing over the next 4 hours. The blood level then progressively declines. The biological half-life of methamphetamine is more than 11 hours. After distribution to the brain, about 60 percent of the methamphetamine is slowly metabolized in the liver and the end products are excreted through the kidneys, along with unmetabolized methamphetamine (about 40 percent is excreted unchanged) and small amounts of its pharmacologically active metabolite, amphetamine.

Neurotoxicity

Methamphetamine produces acute delusional and psychotic behavior. Psychotic symptoms in one study were just over five times more likely to occur during episodes of methamphetamine use. The risk was dose dependent and doubled if the addict also used marijuana or alcohol (McKetin et al., 2013). More than 75 percent of methamphetamine-induced-psychosis inpatients exhibited some form of violence. The most common psychotic symptoms were persecutory delusions and auditory hallucinations. Recovery can take more than a month and, in addition to antipsychotics, electroconvulsive therapy was administered for patients with psychoses lasting more than a month (Zarrabi et al., 2016). Hsieh and colleagues (2014) suggest that methamphetamine-induced psychosis may be caused by damage to cortical interneurons. The process involves an overflow of dopamine in the striatum, leading to excessive cortical glutamate release, ultimately damaging interneurons. Interneuronal damage would impair thalamocortical signals, which would manifest as psychotic symptoms.

Methamphetamine users are also at risk for various types of cardiac toxicity, such as strokes, heart attack, and tears of the aorta (aortic dissection) (Huang et al., 2016; Westover and Nakonezny, 2010). Furthermore, methamphetamine abuse reduces immunity and increases the risk of acquiring numerous infectious diseases, such as AIDS, hepatitis, MRSA, STDs, and fungal diseases (Salamanca et al., 2015).

Neurotoxicity includes damage to serotonin and dopamine nerve terminals, neuronal death, and replacement with astroglial and microglial cells in the brain (Cadet and Krasnova, 2009; Sekine et al., 2008). Dopaminergic defects have been associated with slower motor function and memory deficits, perhaps with predisposition to future development of neurodegenerative disorders such as Parkinson's disease (Callaghan et al., 2012). In fact, Ares-Santos and colleagues (2014) showed that methamphetamine killed neurons in the striatum of mice within 30 days after administration. There was a partial recovery of dopamine terminals starting three days after treatment, and motor activity and coordination also showed some recovery in parallel with the dopaminergic terminals. Nevertheless, there was long-lasting loss and degeneration of dopaminergic cell bodies in the substantia nigra and dopaminergic terminal destruction in the striatum.

Thompson and coworkers (2004) first identified the structural defects in the human brain associated with chronic methamphetamine abuse. The authors noted an 11 percent reduction in gray matter (neurons), a 7 percent increase in white matter volume (due to inflammation), and a 20 percent increase in ventricular (fluid chamber) volumes. These data indicate neuronal loss with scar replacement (white matter) and a compensatory increase in ventricle size. In brief, the limbic region, involved in drug craving, reward, mood, and emotion, lost 11 percent of its tissue. "The cells are dead and gone," Dr. Thompson stated. Addicts were depressed, anxious, and unable to concentrate. The 8 percent tissue loss in the hippocampus, the brain's center for making new memories, was comparable to the brain deficits in early Alzheimer's. Methamphetamine addicts also performed significantly worse on memory tests than healthy people of the same age. Nevertheless, whether or not abuse causes cognitive decline in humans is not certain and the evidence is mixed. Overall, most of the data argue for intellectual decline for some duration in some users (Dean et al., 2013).

The molecular basis of this neurotoxic effect includes "oxidative stress (metabolic activation), activation of genetically based transcription factors, DNA damage, excitotoxicity, blood–brain barrier (BBB) breakdown, glial cell activation, and neuronal degeneration" (Cadet and Krasnova, 2009, 101). Acute and chronic methamphetamine "induces robust, widespread, but structure-specific leakage of the blood–brain barrier, acute glial cell activation, and increased water content (edema), which are related to drug-induced brain hyperthermia (elevated temperature)" (Kiyatkin and Sharma, 2009, 65). The "leaky" blood–brain barrier ultimately increases the migration of reactive oxygen molecules, such as white blood cells, into the brain, initiating the neuronal damage. The increased brain temperature produced by methamphetamine potentiates these toxic effects (Kiyatkin et al., 2007; Kiyatkin and Sharma, 2012; Turowski and Kenny, 2015). This same action (and potential for brain injury) is also caused by methamphetamine derivatives, including MDMA ("ecstasy") and 5-MeO-DiPT ("Foxy") (Gouzoulis-Mayfrank and Daumann, 2009; Nakagawa and Kaneko, 2008).

The review by Northrop and Yamamoto (2015) describes the blood–brain barrier disruptions produced by methamphetamine as a starting point for developing treatments, which may improve the long-lasting neural and cognitive damage. It has even been suggested that because methamphetamine can break down the blood–brain barrier, it might be used to help transport other drugs into the CNS, especially considering that it is already an FDA-approved medication under the trade name Desoxyn, for treating ADHD and obesity. The FDA, however, warns that prescribers must carefully weigh the inherent risks of Desoxyn against the limited therapeutic benefits. (For a thorough review of the history, epidemiology, pathophysiology, and clinical presentation and treatment of methamphetamine abuse and toxicity, see Richards et al., 2016.)

Effects in Pregnancy

As with cocaine, there is no clear-cut pattern of congenital abnormalities, although infants born to methamphetamine-abusing mothers exhibit growth retardation and lower birth weights (Smith et al., 2006), and an increased rate of intracerebral hemorrhage. Sowell and colleagues (2010) reported that brain structures known to be sites of neurotoxicity in adult methamphetamine abusers are more vulnerable to prenatal methamphetamine exposure than to alcohol exposure, and more severe cortical damage is associated with more severe cognitive deficits in offspring. Although there is some empirical evidence for amphetamine-induced neurotoxicity and neurodevelopmental deficits, the data are scarce and it is difficult to separate from the other factors of poverty, neglect, and other drug use (Behnke and Smith, 2013; Oei et al., 2012).

Good and colleagues (2010) reported on the demographic variables associated with pregnancy in methamphetamine-using mothers. While 17 percent of nonmethamphetamine users gave birth to preterm babies, that number jumped to 50 percent in drug users. More of the users gave birth via C-sections and suffered uncontrolled high blood pressure and placental abruption. The majority of pregnant methamphetamine users (about 66 percent) also had fewer prenatal care visits, and more of their babies died soon after birth (4 percent) or responded poorly on newborn health measures (6 percent) than the offspring of nonusers (1 percent). Almost 25 percent of the drug-using mothers had been abused during their pregnancy; and 40 percent of the babies born of methamphetamine using mothers were removed from their birth mother and placed in foster care, another care facility, or adopted.

The first study of behavioral effects of children born to methamphetamine-using mothers was published by LaGasse and colleagues in 2012. They found that at age 3, scores for anxiety, depression, and moodiness were slightly higher in children of methamphetamine users, with differences persisting at age 5. The older children who had been exposed to methamphetamine also had more aggression and attention problems similar to ADHD (attention deficit/hyperactivity disorder). Another recent study found some subtle deficits in children aged 5.5 years pre-exposed to methamphetamine in utero, which also suggested a risk for ADHD (Kiblawi et al., 2013).

Tolerance and Dependence

Tolerance to the euphoria rapidly develops and can necessitate higher and higher doses, which starts a vicious cycle of drug use and withdrawal. Comer and coworkers (2001) studied the effects of 5 and 10 milligrams of methamphetamine twice daily on nonusers in a controlled setting. Positive feelings toward the drug were experienced only on day 1; on subsequent days, the subjects felt a loss of positive effects and increases in negative feelings (dizziness, nausea, depression, and so on). (For a review, see Panenka et al., 2013.)

Amphetamines are prone to compulsive abuse and physical dependence is readily induced. Once drug use is stopped, a person experiences a withdrawal syndrome. Withdrawal symptoms include increased appetite, weight gain, decreased energy, and increased need for sleep. Paranoid symptoms may persist, but generally do not develop as a result of withdrawal. On the other hand, patients suddenly discontinuing amphetamine use may develop severe depression and become suicidal. Early in abstinence, chronic methamphetamine users have low brain levels of stored dopamine. In some abstinent users, dopamine levels recover, raising the question of whether users who cannot maintain abstinence have a more persistent dopamine depletion (Boileau et al., 2016).

Management of amphetamine withdrawal does not require detoxification, but it does require appropriate and cautious clinical observation of the patient, recognition of depression, and treatment with an appropriate antidepressant drug if clinically necessary. Antipsychotic drugs (see Chapter 11) may be necessary to treat paranoid or psychotic reactions or behaviors (Shoptaw et al., 2009).

NONAMPHETAMINE BEHAVIORAL STIMULANTS

Nonamphetamine stimulants include ephedrine (found in nature in the Chinese herb ma-huang), pseudoephedrine, the herbal substance *khat*, the related cathinones ("bath salts"), DMAA, methylphenidate, pemoline, *modafinil* (Provigil), and *armodafinil* (Nuvigil).

Ephedrine today has little use in medicine other than intravenous use in anesthesiology to temporarily elevate blood pressure and heart rate when such action is needed. Ephedrine also transiently reduces appetite. Most use of ephedrine has been in herbal medicine, incorporated into herbal and dietary supplements for energy increase and weight loss. Unfortunately, the drug can be toxic or even fatal when combined with other stimulant drugs such as caffeine and was banned in dietary supplements by the FDA in 2004. Pseudoephedrine is used in cough and cold medicines to relieve nasal congestion. But as a compound used in the illicit manufacture of methamphetamine, it has been placed under prescription-only restriction.

Catha edulis is a flowering shrub in East Africa. The leaves and fresh shoots are commonly known as *khat*. Khat can be chewed (like loose tobacco) or brewed as a tea at a daily dose of up to several hundred grams. Khat has stimulant properties and is said to cause excitement, loss of appetite, and euphoria, similar to the effects of amphetamine or cocaine. The active components of khat are cathinone (see Figure 7.5) and cathine (closely related in structure). Khat must be used fresh because cathinone, the pharmacologically more active substance, deteriorates within about 48 hours after harvest. The cathine appears to be a mild psychostimulant, comparable to caffeine in potency. Khat is being increasingly encountered as a substance of abuse in the United States and elsewhere.

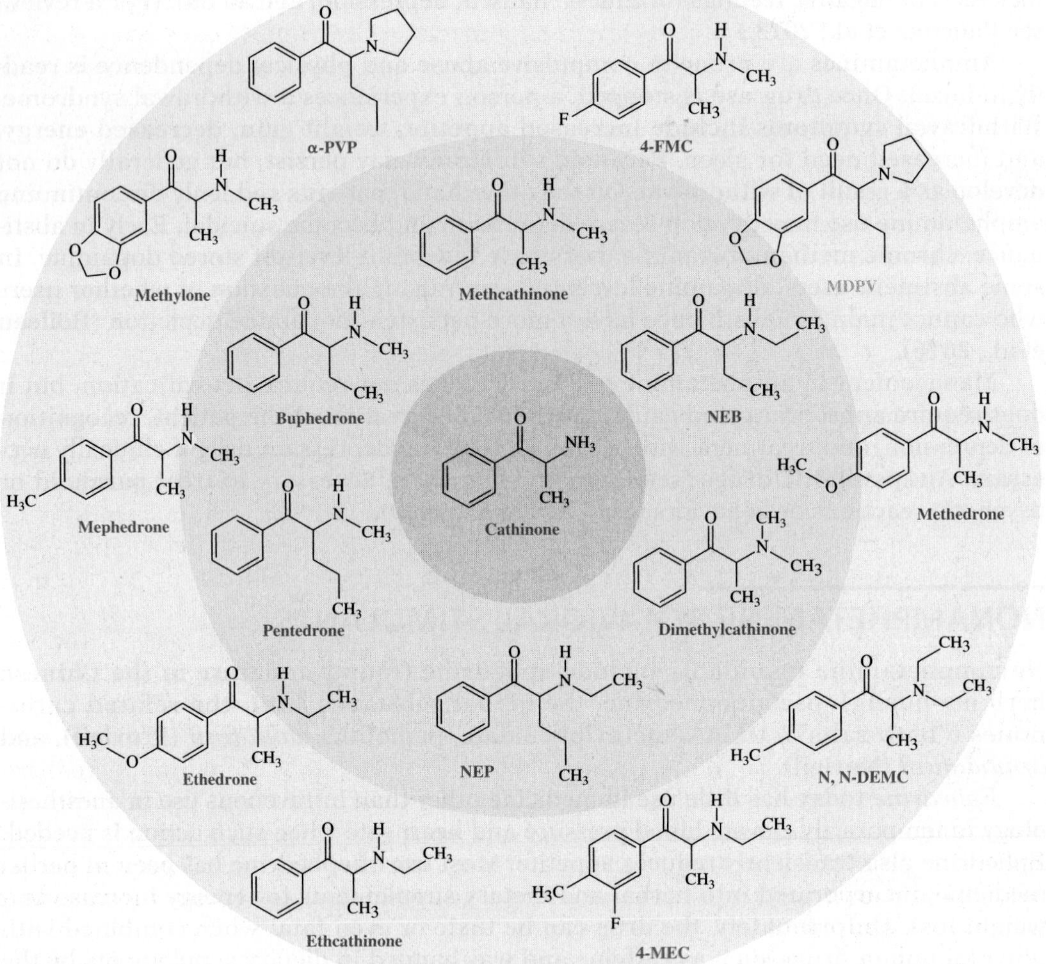

FIGURE 7.5 Chemical structures of a small sample of some synthetic cathinones.

Synthetic Cathinones (Bath Salts)

By far, the most concerning development in stimulant abuse in the past few years has been the increased use of derivatives of cathinone ((S)-2-amino-1-phenyl-1-propanone), the naturally occurring beta-ketone amphetamine analogue found in the leaves of the *Catha edulis* (khat) plant. Synthesis of cathinone derivatives (sometimes referred to as *bk-amphetamines*) has been reported since the late 1920s; for example, methcathinone was synthesized in 1928 and mephedrone in 1929

(Prosser and Nelson, 2012; Rosenbaum et al. 2012). By 1933, the League of Nations was already raising concerns about detrimental effects. But it was not until the 1990s that outbreaks occurred globally, eventually reaching the United States around 2009.

In early 2011, emergency rooms began to see an increase in admissions from ingestion of bath salts–synthetic cathinone that paralleled the sharp rise in reported overdoses (Aarde et al., 2015). In September of that year, the Drug Enforcement Administration (DEA) gave notice that it intended to temporarily "schedule" the three drugs that were the main synthetic cathinones. Mephedrone, methylone, and MDPV (methylenedioxypyrovalerone) were officially classified as Schedule I drugs on April 12, 2013. Legal regulation of bath salts is difficult because each compound has to be individually banned (Beaman and Hayes, 2013). Although some bath salt materials only contain a single compound, others contain two or more combinations of pure cathinone. In addition, they may be contaminated with other substances such as caffeine, lidocaine, and piperazines (Baumann, 2014).

Several routes of exposure are effective, including nasal insufflation, oral ingestion, rectal insertion, and intravenous and intramuscular injection. According to user input, mephedrone and methylone doses are 100 to 200 milligrams orally; effects begin about 30 to 45 minutes after ingestion and last about 2 to 5 hours. MDPV appears more potent, with effects elicited 15 to 30 minutes after a typical oral dose of 10 to 15 milligrams and lasting 2 to 7 hours. These drugs produce amphetamine-like or cocainelike subjective effects due to catecholaminergic activation in the central and peripheral nervous systems and MDMA-like ("ecstasylike") effects from serotonergic activation (Baumann, 2014). Papaseit and colleagues (2016) have conducted the first human clinical trial (ClinicalTrials.gov, NCT02232789) comparing mephedrone and MDMA (mephedrone dose of 200 milligrams; MDMA dose 100 milligrams). Mephedrone produced a significant increase in blood pressure, heart rate, and pupillary diameter. It elicited stimulantlike effects of euphoria and well-being, and induced mild changes in perceptions with similar ratings to those observed after MDMA administration. But mephedrone blood levels peaked earlier and its duration of effect was briefer than MDMA, which might account for its more compulsive abuse liability.

Among the dangerous toxic reactions produced by high doses or long-term use of synthetic cathinones are hyperthermia and hallucinations, which may be associated with aggressive behaviors. Typical clinical effects include agitation and anxiety, paranoia, impaired concentration and memory, headache, rapid heart rate, hypertension, vertigo, abdominal pain, rhabdomyolysis (muscle damage), and convulsions, which can be lethal (for a review, see Karila et al., 2015).

In rat brain synaptosomes, mephedrone and methylone release dopamine, norepinephrine, and serotonin, similar to MDMA. MDPV, however, antagonizes the uptake of dopamine and noradrenaline, and minimally affects serotonin. Importantly, MDPV is 50 times more potent than cocaine as a blocker of DAT and 10 times more potent as a blocker of NET (Baumann et al., 2014). Compared with mephedrone or methylone, MDPV has been found to be anywhere from 3 to 10 times more potent in potentiating motor activity. Most of the fatal bath salt overdoses in the United States reported MDPV in either urine or blood. MDPV-specific urine and blood tests conducted on patients admitted to the emergency room showed a tenfold increase in overall dopamine levels compared with those who took cocaine (Islam et al., 2015).

Rats readily self-administer MDPV across a range of doses (0.05 to 0.5 milligram per kilogram infusion) and will increase their intake at certain concentrations, which is similar to what is seen with methamphetamine and other drugs of compulsive use in humans (such as cocaine and heroin). While rats will also self-administer methylone, they usually do not escalate their dosage over time. This observation implies that the addictive effects of the methylone may be mediated by its release of serotonin. Such data have led to the speculation that the actions of stimulant drugs in humans might be predicted by considering the inhibition ratio of the dopamine transporter to the serotonin transporter as well as the potency at which dopamine and serotonin are secreted by neurons, where "a relative activation of the serotonin system would be linked to a reduction in abuse potential" (Miliano et al., 2016).

Repeated use of high doses of synthetic cathinones will result in tolerance, dependence, and craving. Sudden termination of chronic methcathinone, mephedrone, and MDPV may elicit symptoms of withdrawal (Miliano et al., 2016). No specific antidote is available. Bath salt–induced agitation often is treated with IV benzodiazepines. Mephedrone produces a delirious state in conjunction with psychotic symptoms. Antipsychotic therapy has been suggested for addressing ongoing agitation. Symptomatic treatment of tachycardia involves beta blockers, such as labetalol (Islam et al., 2015).

After mephedrone became illegal, it was replaced by several "second-generation" chemical formulations. These included 4-methyl-N-ethylcathinone (4-MEC), which releases serotonin and blocks dopamine reuptake, and 49-methyl-α-pyrrolidino-propiophenone (4-MePPP), which can block both dopamine and serotonin reuptake, although it is more potent at the dopamine transporter. This distinction is derived from rat studies that showed that the drug 4-MEC greatly increased serotonin while it only slightly raised dopamine levels and did not alter motor activity. In contrast, 4-MePPP produced selective increases in dopamine and robust motor stimulation (Saha et al., 2015). Concentrations of methylone, mephedrone, and MBPV are reportedly higher in placental blood and fetal brains of mice than they are in either maternal brains or plasma (Strange et al., 2017). Therefore, fetal risk from these compounds is a cause for concern. As yet, there are no reported studies of possible teratogenesis from use of these compounds.

Flakka (α-pyrrolidinovalerophenone)

Although reports of MDPV dropped precipitously after it was banned in 2011, at about the same time, DEA surveillance reports of a drug with the street name "flakka" (α-pyrrolidinovalerophenone, α-PVP) increased from about 20 to more than 3000. In 2013, Dr. Michael Baumann, the head of NIDA's drug analysis laboratory, found that it acted almost exactly like the banned drug—a finding that supported the DEA's decision to outlaw α-PVP in 2014 (Underwood, 2015).

The name "flakka" (from the Spanish word *flaca*) is a Hispanic colloquial expression that means either a slender woman or a beautiful, elegant woman "who charms all she meets." Originally synthesized in the 1960s, flakka is a synthetic stimulant structurally related to other bath salts, such as 3,4-methylenedioxypyrovalerone (MDPV), and may be described as a "second-generation bath salt." It comes in the form of crystals of different colors that dissolve in the mouth, which gives it another nickname, "gravel," because of its similar appearance to white–pink aquarium gravel. Because it is cheap and may elicit some strange behaviors, flakka is sometimes called "$5 insanity." It can be taken by mouth, injected, snorted, or vaporized, and in this state, it may substitute for nicotine in e-cigarettes. Overdoses are more likely as a result of vaporization, because this approach increases the rate at which the drug enters the bloodstream. Flakka is more potent than cocaine or amphetamine in blocking dopamine and norepinephrine transporters. Heart rate and blood pressure might be dangerously elevated by the rapid increase in norepinephrine, while sudden increases in dopamine may elicit euphoria, along with delusions, hallucinations, and agitation. Other behavioral effects of flakka are comparable to those of stimulants, such as alertness and energy, and may progress to include delirium accompanied by paranoia and possibly delusions of great power and strength (Olson, 2015).

Intoxication due to flakka is treated with supportive care to reverse the effects and prevent further problems. Therapy includes intravenous benzodiazepines to sedate the patient and mitigate seizures until the effects of the drug wear off. Intravenous fluids are also administered, especially if rhabdomyolysis is evident. It is difficult to identify flakka intoxication with a laboratory assay because standard urine drug testing does not detect the substance. Flakka and its metabolites, however, may be recognized by special testing of blood or urine through the use of gas and liquid chromatographic mass spectrometric methods (Melton, 2015).

One agent that shares some structural components of ephedrine and amphetamine is *DMAA* (1,3-dimethylamylamine or methylhexaneamine). This drug was initially patented in 1944 and marketed as Forthane for decongestion. Forthane was withdrawn in the 1970s, but DMAA returned in 2004 after the FDA banned the sale of the stimulant ephedra in dietary supplements (because of thousands of adverse event reports). Supplement manufacturers used DMAA as a substitute for ephedra and claimed it was a natural component of the geranium plant (Gregory, 2013).

In April 2012, the FDA sent letters to ten companies that manufactured and distributed 16 dietary supplements containing DMAA, stating that it is not a "dietary ingredient." The FDA said it had received 42 adverse event reports on products containing DMAA. It raises blood pressure and may cause a heart attack because it constricts blood vessels. The U.S. Army has pulled DMAA supplements from all of its on-base stores after the deaths of two soldiers were linked to its use. Several lawsuits regarding DMAA have also been filed and it has now been added to the group of banned substances by the World Anti-Doping Agency.

Some manufacturers have removed DMAA from their products, but others have insisted that the substance is a natural component of the geranium plant and is safe when used as directed. This is questionable, however, since the only study cited was a Chinese report from 1996 in a journal that is no longer in existence. Moreover, the authors simply speculated that it was a component, without any analyses to confirm their findings.

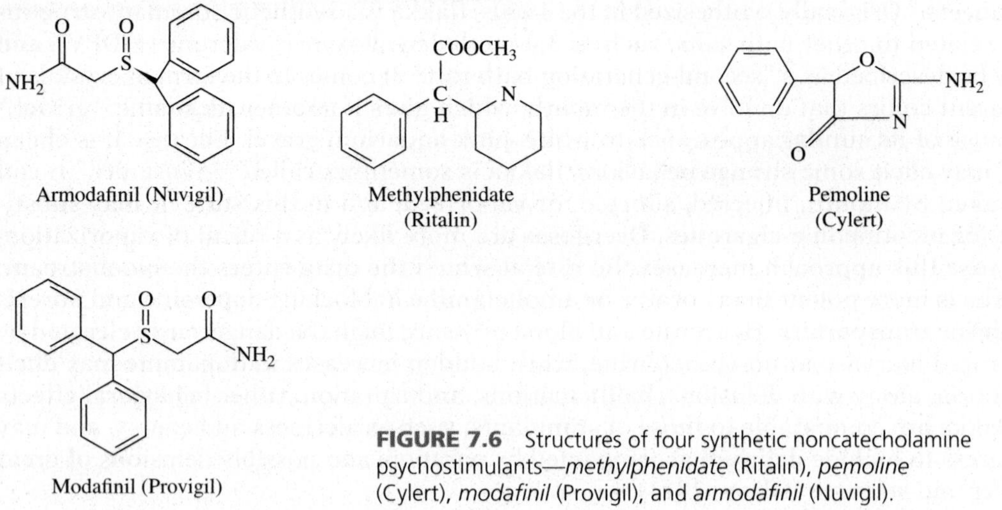

Armodafinil (Nuvigil)

Methylphenidate
(Ritalin)

Pemoline
(Cylert)

Modafinil (Provigil)

FIGURE 7.6 Structures of four synthetic noncatecholamine psychostimulants—*methylphenidate* (Ritalin), *pemoline* (Cylert), *modafinil* (Provigil), and *armodafinil* (Nuvigil).

Armstrong and colleagues (as cited in Zhang et al., 2012) have found no detectable DMAA in eight different geranium oils and other studies have not been able to confirm its presence. DMAA is not accepted as an herbal substance by the American Botanical Council, and both DMAA and methylhexaneamine, are not permitted to be identified on labels as "geranium" by the American Herbal Products Association.

Methylphenidate (Ritalin) (Figure 7.6) is a nonamphetamine behavioral stimulant in which the regular-release formulation has a half-life of 2 to 4 hours. Its primary medical use is in the treatment of ADHD (see Chapter 15). Methylphenidate increases the synaptic concentration of dopamine by blocking the presynaptic dopamine transporter (a cocainelike action) and also perhaps by slightly increasing the release of dopamine (an amphetaminelike or ephedrinelike action). When methylphenidate is injected intravenously, experienced cocaine users report a cocainelike or amphetaminelike rush, an action not usually experienced with oral dosage. At clinically relevant doses, methylphenidate blocks more than 50 percent of the dopamine transporters 60 minutes after oral administration. A slow uptake of methylphenidate into the brain after oral administration accounts for its low level of positive reinforcement effects.

Pemoline (Cylert) is a CNS stimulant structurally dissimilar to either methylphenidate or amphetamine (see Figure 7.6). Its use for the treatment of ADHD is limited by reports of rare instances of hepatitis, necessitating close monitoring of liver function. Indeed, the risks of pemoline outweigh its usefulness and it has been removed from the market.

Modafinil (Provigil) (see Figure 7.6) is a nonamphetamine psychostimulant whose primary characteristic is "wakefulness promotion." Its mechanism of action is not well established; it does block dopamine transporters in the human brain in a manner similar to that exerted by cocaine (Volkow et al., 2009), but perhaps less potently (Loland et al., 2012). Modafinil shares common neurobiological mechanisms with psychostimulants. Recent studies have shown that modafinil can also be reinforcing to humans and that the reinforcing effects of modafinil may be related to the dopaminergic system, as in most drugs with abuse potential. It has been shown that modafinil increased dopamine levels in the nucleus accumbens shell and core of mice at levels similar to those induced by typical psychostimulants, and that this enhancement was due to blockade of DAT (Wuo-Silva et al., 2016). A potentially serious skin rash limits its use.

The FDA has approved modafinil for the treatment of three disorders: narcolepsy, shift-work sleep disorder, and obstructive sleep apnea with residual excessive sleepiness despite the use of a continuous positive airway pressure device. Modafinil has also been used in the treatment of ADHD, although the FDA has not approved it for this use. One recent study did not find it effective for ADHD in adults (Arnold et al., 2014). Although it also had no significant cognitive effects in methamphetamine addicts except in a test of sustained attention (Dean et al., 2011), it has been used for enhancing cognition even in the absence of a therapeutic diagnosis.[3]

Laboratory investigations of putative cognitive enhancement from modafinil in healthy volunteers have shown consistent but relatively modest benefit. The drug, however, increased "motivation" in that participants described feeling more pleasure in performing the experimental tasks (Müller et al., 2013). This effect may have produced the cognitive improvement. Battleday and Brem (2015) provided the first review of modafinil's actions in non-sleep-deprived people since 2008. They argue that the cognitive effects of this drug may depend on the type of assessment used. Benefits are not consistent or very impressive when "basic" tests are used, but more "complex assessments" show enhancement of attention, executive function, and learning. They did not observe any substantial evidence for side effects or mood changes. However, according to Nicholson and coworkers (2015), this is not consistent with other reports of headache, dizziness, tachycardia, nervousness and insomnia, and GI complaints. Post-marketing surveys report Stephens-Johnson syndrome, a potentially fatal skin eruption. Nicholson and coworkers (2015) also discuss serious adverse events associated with modafinil and note that almost half occur when used for nonindicated reasons. Andrade (2016) provides the results of an extensive literature in humans, concluding that there is no serious risk of seizure with either modafinil or armodafinil (below), even in patients with ADHD, head injury, brain tumors, or seizure disorders. But he notes that either modafinil or armodafinil may affect the levels of some anticonvulsant drugs by pharmacokinetic interactions and that this possibility needs to be considered in individual situations.

Armodafinil (Nuvigil; Figure 7.6) is the active (R)-isomer of the racemic drug modafinil. As with citalopram/escitalopram, methylphenidate/dexmethylphenidate, and amphetamine/dextroamphetamine, when an older racemic medicine goes generic and becomes less expensive, a manufacturer can market the active "half" of the drug under a new patent (making it more expensive). That seems to be the situation with armodafinil, making it twice as "potent" as the racemic counterpart (therefore, one uses half of the milligram dosage). Nuvigil is protected by a U.S. patent that expires in 2023. Armodafinil has the same FDA indications as modafinil (Krystal et al., 2010)

---

[3] Drugs considered to be cognitive enhancers are referred to as *neuroenhancers* or *nootropics*.

and at least one formulation has been generic since 2012, while others were released in 2016. Armodafinil is also approved for the treatment of sleepiness due to jet lag, a lower dose of 50 to 150 milligrams being recommended.

Pharmacological Treatment of Stimulant Dependency

At the outset, it should be stated that there are no pharmacotherapies for stimulant addiction that have been proven or approved by the FDA (Haile et al., 2012a; Ling et al., 2014; Shorter and Kosten, 2011). Pharmacological strategies include blocking euphoria, reducing withdrawal and negative mood symptoms (such as depression), and ameliorating craving by enhancing the prefrontal glutaminergic cortical projections that seem to be impaired in drug dependency (discussed in more detail in Chapter 4) (Elkashef and Montoya, 2012; Elkashef and Vocci, 2011; Karila et al., 2011; Olive et al., 2012).

Dopaminergic/Adrenergic Treatment Approaches

The subjective effects and euphoria of cocaine are believed to be due to the blockade of the dopamine transporter and consequent buildup and release of dopamine in the reward pathways. But even a single cocaine dose may cause an upregulation of the transporter that can last as long as a month. This means that even after acute use, there is a decrease in dopamine molecules in the synapse, which may lead to drug craving and seeking (Zheng and Zhan, 2012a). There is also experimental evidence that low dopamine receptor function is correlated with a greater likelihood of relapse in methamphetamine abusers (Wang et al., 2012). Therefore, drugs that are either direct or indirect dopaminergic agonists might replace the drug-induced dopaminergic stimulation and reduce both craving and relapse. An extraordinary number of such drugs has been assessed, but results are not impressive. One review of clinical trials examined three direct dopamine agonists (amantadine, bromocriptine, and L-dopa/carbidopa) and concluded that none of them were effective for the treatment of cocaine abuse or dependence (Amato et al., 2011). Another study found little benefit for the dopamine agonist ropinirole or the antipsychotic partial dopamine agonist aripiprazole (Meini et al., 2011). Aripiprazole was also ineffective for the treatment of methamphetamine dependence (Coffin et al., 2013). The antidepressant drug *bupropion* (Wellbutrin, Zyban, and other brand names) acts primarily to block the uptake of dopamine, although it also has some effect on norepinephrine. *Bupropion* is approved by the FDA for treatment of nicotine addiction. It has not shown substantial effectiveness, however, against either cocaine (Shoptaw et al., 2008) or methamphetamine addiction (Elkashef et al., 2008; Heinzerling et al., 2013). The serotonergic antidepressants are also not very effective in this regard (Shorter and Kosten, 2011). Similarly, the sustained release formulation of *methylphenidate* (Ritalin), which is a well-established stimulant treatment for ADHD, has been investigated in cocaine abusers with and without comorbid ADHD. Although it appears effective in regard to reducing ADHD symptoms, methylphenidate does not seem to be very useful against cocaine addiction (Grabowski et al., 1997; Haile et al., 2012a). In parallel with the success of "agonist replacement" treatment for nicotine and opioid addiction, amphetamine and methamphetamine have also been tested for treatment of cocaine abuse. Sustained-release amphetamine and methamphetamine agents are being studied as possible "replacement" options, but understandably only in certain patients who would not be considered at risk for abuse and diversion (Grabowski et al., 2001; Herin et al., 2010; Mariani and Levin, 2012; Rush and Stoops, 2012). Heroin-dependent persons also addicted to cocaine used less cocaine when given sustained-release dexamfetamine. The effect, however, was modest (44.9 days versus 60.6 days) (Nuijten et al., 2016).

The "wakefulness-promoting" drug *modafinil* (Provigil) has also generated interest, especially because it was shown not to be reinforcing on its own in cocaine abusers (Vosburg et al., 2010). Unfortunately, it was not effective in reducing either methamphetamine abuse (Anderson et al., 2012) or cocaine abuse (Dackis et al., 2012; Nuijten et al., 2015). Modafinil might be helpful in improving the sleep quality of people undergoing stimulant withdrawal (Shorter and Kosten, 2011). The fact that psychostimulants have noradrenergic effects as well as dopaminergic actions has prompted studies of adrenergic antagonists for cocaine abuse. The α-1 receptor antagonist doxazosin has a long half-life of 22 hours and has been found to decrease positive subjective effects of cocaine in cocaine-dependent persons who have not sought treatment (Newton et al., 2012), which suggests that it may have some therapeutic benefit. Finally, the drug *buspirone* (BuSpar), a nonbenzodiazepine anxiolytic that acts on both serotonin and dopamine, was shown to selectively reduce responding for cocaine (but not food) in rhesus monkeys (Mello et al., 2013), but was not effective in a clinical trial in cocaine-dependent persons (Winhusen et al., 2014).

GABAergic/Glutamatergic Treatment Approaches

In addition to the dopaminergic class of possible antiaddiction medicines, the GABA system has received substantial interest. This is derived from the fact that GABA has an inhibitory effect on dopamine release in the brain reward pathways (see Chapter 4). Unfortunately, because GABA is so widespread within the central nervous system, it has been difficult to develop effective antiaddiction drugs without unacceptable side effects.

Gamma-vinyl-GABA vigabatrin (Sabril), an antiepileptic drug available in Europe, is an irreversible inhibitor of the metabolic enzyme *GABA transaminase*; it increases GABA activity and reduces drug-induced increases in extracellular nucleus accumbens dopamine. Vigabatrin shows anticraving effects against abused drugs, including cocaine (Brodie et al., 2009). Its use is limited by a drug-induced loss of some portion of the visual field (peripheral vision), although one study demonstrated that short-term use of vigabatrin is less damaging to visual fields than originally thought (Fechtner et al., 2006). Baclofen is a GABA_B receptor agonist, that had shown some signs of efficacy in clinical trials with cocaine abusers. Subsequent results, however, have been modest, although it may have a place in helping to prevent relapse in severe cocaine addiction (Shorter and Kosten, 2011). Several anticonvulsants that act to increase GABA levels or to decrease glutamate (or both) have also been evaluated for cocaine addiction. Agents include valproate, tiagabine, topiramate (Baldacara et al., 2016; Elkashef et al., 2012; Johnson et al., 2013), and lamotrigine (Brown et al., 2012), as well as vigabatrin (Somoza et al., 2013). Although in some cases the drugs may affect subjective reports of drug craving, none of these studies have found significant decreases in cocaine use. In regard to glutamate, the broad effects of this excitatory transmitter make it even more difficult to isolate a drug that would exert a specific antiaddictive action. But the substance N-acetylcysteine has received some attention because it appears to modulate the presynaptic control of cortical glutamate release (on the reward pathway) that is regulated by the metabotropic glutamate autoreceptor, mGluR2/3 (see Chapter 4). By improving the function of this autoreceptor, N-acetylcysteine may help to reduce glutamate release and thereby decrease drug craving (Amen et al., 2011). Other glutamatergic agents relevant to this approach are also being assessed (Xia et al., 2013).

Miscellaneous Agents

Disulfiram (Antabuse) is used to treat alcoholism because it blocks the enzyme aldehyde dehydrogenase, which metabolizes alcohol (see Chapter 5). This inhibition causes the metabolite acetaldehyde to build up, which is very unpleasant and produces several noxious symptoms. It has been discovered that disulfiram also blocks the enzyme dopamine-beta-hydroxylase (DBH; DβH), which converts dopamine (DA) to norepinephrine (NE), thereby decreasing the levels of norepinephrine relative to dopamine. In addition, this drug also inhibits enzymes that metabolize cocaine and has other biochemical actions that have produced conflicting outcomes in both laboratory and clinical experiments that complicate predictions about its antiaddictive actions (Gaval-Cruz and Weinshenker, 2009; Pani et al., 2010). Apparent conflicts in the data might be resolved by a recent clinical study that revealed a bimodal effect of this drug in cocaine users. These investigators found that the effect of disulfiram on cocaine use depended on the dose relative to body weight. Specifically, participants given 4 milligrams per kilogram of body weight self-administered the smallest amount of cocaine and those given 2 milligrams per kilogram self-administered the most (Haile et al., 2012b). Currently, a more selective inhibitor of DβH called nepicastat is being studied as a possible treatment for cocaine addiction.

Inhibition of the enzyme aldehyde dehydrogenase by another drug, ALDH2i, has also been found to reduce cocaine use and relapse in laboratory animals. Here, the mechanism seems to be due to a series of biochemical reactions initiated by antagonism of the enzyme that leads to production of the substance tetrahydropapaveroline. This substance in turn blocks the enzyme tyrosine hydroxylase, which is the first step in dopamine synthesis. As a result, less dopamine is produced. It is hypothesized that the decrease in dopamine production and release is responsible for suppressing cocaine-seeking behavior in laboratory studies (Yao et al., 2010).

Another agent of current interest is *tetrahydropalmatine* (THP), an alkaloid found in several different plant species, including the *Corydalis* family and the plant *Stephania rotunda*. These plants have traditional uses in Chinese herbal medicine as treatment for anxious insomnia and chronic pain. The pharmaceutical industry has synthetically produced the more potent enantiomer levo-tetrahydropalmatine (*l*-THP), which has been marketed worldwide under different brand names as an alternative to anxiolytic and sedative drugs of the benzodiazepine group and analgesics such as opiates. It is also sold as a dietary supplement. *l*-THP has several neurobiological actions: it antagonizes DA_1 and DA_2 receptors and perhaps DA_3 receptors also. It may also block the alpha-1 type of adrenergic receptor and it may modulate $GABA_A$ receptors. In laboratory experiments, it reduces cocaine self-administration and relapse (Shorter and Kosten, 2011; Wang and Mantsch, 2012).

Several drug combinations have also been assessed in efforts to find effective treatments for stimulant abuse. One example is the medication Prometa, which is a combination of three drugs: the benzodiazepine antagonist flumazenil, for recovery from sedation; the drug *gabapentin* (Neurontin), believed to reduce glutamate and relieve cravings; and the antihistamine agent hydroxyzine, believed to help manage withdrawal symptoms. In a randomized, double-blind, placebo-controlled 108-day study trial, 120 methamphetamine-dependent patients were administered this cocktail. Although drug use declined in the Prometa and placebo groups, there was no difference between them in any measure (Ling et al., 2012).

Another combination that has blocked cocaine use in laboratory animals is that of the opiate antagonist naltrexone and the partial opiate agonist buprenorphine. The concept behind this approach is that chronic cocaine use produces a negative emotional state of stress and a dysphoric mood that is actually mediated by the endogenous opiate dynorphin (see Chapter 10). It remains to be seen if this indirect method of reducing stimulant-induced stress will be useful (Wee et al., 2012a). Some positive outcomes, however, were seen in a clinical trial that evaluated the effect of a naltrexone–bupropion combination to treat methamphetamine use disorder. Out of 49 participants with methamphetamine addiction, 11 were considered responders with a majority of negative urine screens during the last four weeks (out of an eight-week trial) (Mooney et al., 2016). Sushchyk and colleagues (2016) have reported that naltrexone and *l*-THP reduced cocaine relapse in laboratory animals.

Because methamphetamine activates the hypothalamic-pituitary-adrenal (HPA) axis, which causes an increase in the release of stress hormones, it may promote a stress-related increase in anxiety and depression and subsequent relapse. Drugs that reduce HPA dysfunction might be useful in the treatment of methamphetamine addiction (Zuloaga et al., 2015). Along those lines, Kablinger and colleagues (2012) conducted a preliminary study in 45 cocaine-dependent patients of two drugs, *metyrapone*, a drug that blocks the synthesis of the stress hormone cortisol, and the drug *oxazepam*, a benzodiazepine. The combination was well tolerated and was found to reduce craving and cocaine use. An earlier study had shown that metyrapone did not alter the pleasurable effect of methamphetamine in humans and produced some serious adverse reactions (Harris et al., 2003), but perhaps the addition of the benzodiazepine mitigated those effects.

The more general approach of trying to heal the neural damage produced by stimulant abuse is also the rationale for an ongoing clinical investigation of the drug *ibudilast* for methamphetamine abuse, summarized below. When individuals first become abstinent from methamphetamine, an inflammatory process occurs in brain cells, especially glial cells. By dampening inflammation in glial cells, it was proposed that ibudilast may preserve glial and other nerve cells during early abstinence. Ibudilast has been used safely in humans for 18 years in Japan and South Korea as a treatment for asthma and pulmonary and cardiovascular diseases; therefore, it is safe to use as a potential treatment for methamphetamine dependence.

The 11 methamphetamine addicts in this trial, all paid volunteers, were housed in a hospital unit and not allowed to leave for three weeks. They were intravenously injected with methamphetamine while being treated with ibudilast. After the initial results found that the combination was safe, the second phase of the study, a 12-week trial of 140 treatment-seeking human methamphetamine addicts, was started. Half the volunteers took ibudilast twice a day and the other half took a placebo. They visited the trial unit three times a week for drug-craving monitoring, urine drug screens, and medication adherence monitoring. In March 2016, results were published from the first phase of the clinical trial. The authors reported that ibudilast significantly reduced the subjective effects of methamphetamine in persons with methamphetamine dependence (Worley et al., 2016). A second phase of the study will determine if the drug can maintain abstinence during at least the final 2 weeks of a 12-week trial. (For a review of ibudilast, see Rolan et al., 2013.)

Interestingly, in nonhuman laboratory animals, modafinil also showed some protection from the toxic effect of methamphetamine on dopamine neurons (Raineri et al., 2012). On the other hand, another compound, citicoline, known as *cytidine diphosphate-choline* (CDP-choline) or cytidine 5-diphosphocholine, had no effect on cocaine use or craving (Brown et al., 2015; Licata et al., 2011). This agent is a substance found in the biochemical pathways involving choline (used for making acetylcholine). It was hypothesized to be helpful because it has some benefit for treating neuronal damage from stroke or brain injury. Finally, there is evidence that the hormone *oxytocin* modulates behavioral effects of psychostimulants in rodents and might be a possible candidate for addiction treatment (Carson et al., 2013).

Pharmacokinetic Approaches to Psychostimulant Abuse—Metabolizing Enzymes

One novel approach to addressing cocaine abuse that has recently undergone rapid development is to intercept the drug molecule before it reaches the brain. These pharmacokinetic (PK) methods do not involve direct effects on either transporters or receptors. Rather, this approach counteracts cocaine either by binding to it as an antibody that prevents it from crossing the blood–brain barrier or as a cocaine-metabolizing enzyme, that breaks down the drug to inactive metabolites in the plasma so that only a small amount of the drug reaches the CNS (Gorelick, 2012). With regard to the antibody method, antibodies can be obtained "actively" through a vaccine or "passively" with antibodies produced in another host and then administered to the addict-patient. The disadvantage is that "passive" vaccines have a shorter half-life.

With regard to enzymes, the cocaine-metabolizing enzyme can be administered as an exogenous drug therapy or it can be provided as a gene therapy, which means the persons receiving the modified gene can then make the modified enzyme for themselves. In the exogenous enzyme approach, two types have been developed: one is a mutation of the butyrylcholinesterase enzyme found in humans, while the other comes from bacteria associated with the soil in which coca plants are grown. The breakdown of cocaine occurs more rapidly with these substances and they reduce the adverse actions of the drug in nonhuman animal models. Because the human-derived mutants of butyrylcholinesterase would presumably not elicit an immune response if given to humans, it might be the better candidate. The past decade has seen rapid progress with alteration of butyrylcholinesterase-producing enzymes that destroy cocaine so efficiently that even though the enzyme is restricted to the blood, they prevent or interrupt drug actions in the CNS. During the same time, gene-transfer technology has also been improved such that enzymes can be delivered by endogenous gene transduction at high levels for periods of a year or longer after a single treatment (Brimijoin and Gao, 2012; Narasimhan et al., 2012; Schindler and Goldberg, 2012; Zheng and Zhan, 2012b; Zlebnik et al., 2014).

Cocaine-metabolizing enzymes have one advantage over vaccines and antibodies. At sufficiently high concentrations of cocaine, the antibodies may be saturated, leaving enough of the drug left over to produce the desired effect. In contrast, even if the cocaine-metabolizing enzyme is saturated, it maintains its effectiveness. That is, because it degrades the drug, each enzyme molecule can metabolize many cocaine molecules. One molecule of a currently available enzyme can metabolize 5700 cocaine molecules a minute (Zheng and Zhan, 2012a).

The short half-life of cocaine might seem to make this approach impractical. But because the half-life of cocaine is proportional to the dose, the half-life increases and becomes much longer under cocaine overdose conditions and there is enough time for an enzyme injection to be effective. Furthermore, because the drug is distributed equally in plasma, brain, and heart tissue, metabolism of cocaine molecules in the blood will rapidly cause the molecules in the brain and heart to return to the plasma to maintain equilibrium. Clinical trials of cocaine-metabolizing enzymes for cocaine addiction treatment have shown that it is safe and that it reduces many of the positive subjective effects of the drug (Zheng and Zhan, 2012a). Furthermore, the combination of enzyme *and* antibody administration gave an even better blockade of cocaine-induced behavioral stimulation in rodents (Carroll et al., 2012). Research is continuing to develop drugs that remain active in the body for longer periods of time and are more efficient (Smethells et al., 2016; Zheng et al., 2015).

Pharmacokinetic Approaches to Psychostimulant Abuse—Vaccines

The cocaine vaccine (termed *TA-CD*) is a cocaine derivative (succinyl norcocaine) coupled to recombinant cholera toxin B. It is designed to generate drug-specific antibodies that bind to cocaine and prevent it from traveling to the brain from the blood, thereby neutralizing its psychoactive effect. The molecules are then broken down by cholinesterases in the blood to inactive metabolites and excreted. The concept is intriguing and promising but, as with all vaccines, the problems are (1) getting the concentration of antibodies high enough to block any amount of drug that might be used; and (2) compliance—getting the patients to return for the necessary number of injections to produce the required amount of antibody. Patients need to receive five vaccinations over the course of two to three months, during which time they are vulnerable to relapse. Incentives such as counseling and an escalating payment for successive vaccinations can improve adherence (Stitzer et al., 2010; Whitten, 2010).

The amount of antibody produced predicts clinical effectiveness. Antibody levels of 43 micrograms per milliliter (μg/mL) or higher resulted in more cocaine-free urine samples than those with levels less than 43 μg/mL. Unfortunately, only 31 percent of the vaccinated cocaine users attained antibody levels greater than 43 μg/mL (Shen et al., 2012) and even those had only two months of adequate cocaine blockade. The most common adverse effect was local injection site irritation. Even if the vaccine is successful, a cocaine-dependent person who has these antibodies in the blood may move to another drug or use large amounts of cocaine. Nevertheless, the methodology is improving and a recent version produced a high amount of antibody, which lasted for about four months in laboratory rats (Wee et al., 2012b). This may be one of the first antiaddiction vaccines approved by the FDA for human use. Improvements in vaccine development are ongoing (Lockner et al., 2015).

Vaccines for use in methamphetamine addiction are also in development, with several laboratories working on specific parameters. One problem is that the methamphetamine molecule is simple, which makes it unnoticeable to the immune system. Furthermore, both methamphetamine and its metabolite amphetamine also have a long half-life, which makes it difficult for vaccine development. Passive administration of antibodies has already been found to reduce methamphetamine self-administration in rats and to decrease stimulant-induced motor activity. Behavioral assays that are better at measuring the effectiveness of the vaccine are also needed. At present, vaccines capable of producing enough antibody to bind a sufficient amount of drug for a sufficient amount of time are not yet available. One new agent, however, named MH6 is most likely just the beginning of a successful effort to find more effective treatment options for psychostimulant abuse (Miller et al., 2013). Kosten and colleagues (2013) provide a review of current developments in vaccines for cocaine and methamphetamine.

STUDY QUESTIONS

1. Compare and contrast the pharmacological history of cocaine and amphetamine.

2. Compare and contrast the pharmacological effects of cocaine and amphetamine.

3. How do cocaine and amphetamine differ in their mechanism of action?

4. What are the effects of psychostimulants on the fetus?

5. Describe the behavioral consequences of chronic high doses of psychostimulants.

6. What are the neurotoxic effects of methamphetamine on the brain?

7. What are the most common psychostimulants besides cocaine and amphetamine, and how do they differ among themselves?

8. What types of pharmacological approaches have been tried to treat stimulant addiction? How successful are they?

REFERENCES

Aarde, S., et al. (2015). "In Vivo Potency and Efficacy of the Novel Cathinone A-Pyrrolidinopentio-phenone and 3,4-Methylenedioxypyrovalerone: Self-Administration and Locomotor Stimulation in Male Rats." *Psychopharmacology (Berl)* 232: 3045–3055. doi: 10.1007/s00213-015-3944-8.

Amato, L., et al. (2011). "Dopamine Agonists for the Treatment of Cocaine Dependence." *Cochrane Database Systemic Reviews:* CD003352. PMID: 22161376.

Amen, S. L., et al. (2011). "Repeated N-Acetyl Cysteine Reduces Cocaine Seeking in Rodents and Craving in Cocaine-Dependent Humans." *Neuropsychopharmacology* 36: 871–878.

Anderson, A. L., et al. (2012). "Modafinil for the Treatment of Methamphetamine Dependence." *Drug and Alcohol Dependence* 120: 135–141.

Andrade, C. (2016). "A Method for Deciding About the Possible Safety of Modafinil and Armodafinil in Patients with Seizure Disorder." *Journal of Clinical Psychiatry* 77: e25–e28. doi: 10.4088/JCP.15f10580.

Aquaro, G. D., et al. (2011). "Silent Myocardial Damage in Cocaine Addicts." *Heart* 97: 2056–2062.

Ares-Santos, S., et al. (2014). "Methamphetamine Causes Degeneration of Dopamine Cell Bodies and Terminals of the Nigrostriatal Pathway Evidenced by Silver Staining." *Neuropsychopharmacology* 39: 1066–1080. doi: 10.1038/npp.2013.307.

Arnold, V. K., et al. (2014). "A 9-Week, Randomized, Double-Blind, Placebo-Controlled, Parallel-Group, Dose-Finding Study to Evaluate the Efficacy and Safety of Modafinil as Treatment for Adults with ADHD." *Journal of Attention Disorders* 18: 133–144. doi: 10.1177/1087054712441969.

Baldacara, L., et al. (2016). "Efficacy of Topiramate in the Treatment of Crack Cocaine Dependence: A Double-Blind, Randomized, Placebo-Controlled Trial." *Journal of Clinical Psychiatry* 77: 398–406.

Battleday, R. M., and Brem, A.-K. (2015). "Modafinil for Cognitive Neuroenhancement in Healthy Non-Sleep-Deprived Subjects: A Systematic Review." *European Neuropsychopharmacology* 25: 1865–1881. doi: 10.1016/j.euroneuro.2015.07.028.

Baumann, M. H., et al. (2014). "Bath Salts, Spice, and Related Designer Drugs: The Science behind the Headlines." *The Journal of Neuroscience* 34: 15150–15158. doi: 10.1523/JNEUROSCI.3223-14.2014.

Beaman, J., and Hayes, E. (2013). "Synthetic Cathinones: Signs, Symptoms, and Treatment." *Psychiatric Times* 30.

Behnke, M., and Smith, C. (2013). "Prenatal Substance Abuse: Short- and Long-Term Effects on the Exposed Fetus." *Pediatrics* 131: e1009–1024. doi: 10.1542/peds.2012-3931.

Boileau, I., et al. (2016). "Rapid Recovery of Vesicular Dopamine Levels in Methamphetamine Users in Early Abstinence." *Neuropsychopharmacology* 41: 1179–1187. doi:10.1038/npp.2015.267.

Brimijoin, S., and Gao, Y. (2012). "Cocaine Hydrolase Gene Therapy for Cocaine Abuse." *Future Medicinal Chemistry* 4: 151–162.

Brodie, J. D., et al. (2009). "Randomized, Double-Blind, Placebo-Controlled Trial of Vigabatrin for the Treatment of Cocaine Dependence in Mexican Parolees." *American Journal of Psychiatry* 166: 1269–1277.

Brown, E. S., et al. (2012). "A Randomized, Double-Blind, Placebo-Controlled Trial of Lamotrigine Therapy in Bipolar Disorder, Depressed or Mixed Phase and Cocaine Dependence." *Neuropsychopharmacology* 37: 2347–2354.

Brown, E. S., et al. (2015). "A Randomized, Double-Blind, Placebo-Controlled Trial of Citicoline for Cocaine Dependence in Bipolar I Disorder." *American Journal of Psychiatry* 172: 1014–1021.

Bunney, E. B., et al. (2001). "Electrophysiological Effects of Cocaethylene, Cocaine, and Ethanol on Dopaminergic Neurons of the Ventral Tegmental Area." *Journal of Pharmacology and Experimental Therapeutics* 297: 696–703.

Cadet, J. L., and Krasnova, I. N. (2009). "Molecular Basis of Methamphetamine-Induced Neuro-degeneration." *International Review of Neurobiology* 88: 101–119.

Calipari, E. S., et al. (2014). "Amphetamine Self-Administration Attenuates Dopamine D2 Autore-ceptor Function." *Neuropsychopharmacology* 39: 1833–1842. doi: 10.1038/npp.2014.30.

Callaghan, R. C., et al. (2012). "Increased Risk of Parkinson's Disease in Individuals Hospitalized with Conditions Related to the Use of Methamphetamine or Other Amphetamine-Type Drugs." *Drug and Alcohol Dependence* 120: 35–40.

Carroll, M. E, et al. (2012). "Combined Cocaine Hydrolase Gene Transfer and Anti-Cocaine Vac-cine Synergistically Block Cocaine-Induced Locomotion." *PLoS One* 7:e43536.

Carson, D. S., et al. (2013). "A Brief History of Oxytocin and Its Role in Modulating Psychostimu-lant Effects." *Journal of Psychopharmacology* 27: 231–247.

Citrome, L. (2015). "Lisdexamfetamine for Binge Eating Disorder in Adults: A Systematic Review of the Efficacy and Safety Profile for This Newly Approved Indication—What Is the Number Needed to Treat, Number Needed to Harm and Likelihood to be Helped or Harmed?" *International Journal of Clinical Practice* 69: 410–421. doi: 10.1111/ijcp.12639.

Coffin, P. O., et al. (2013). "Aripiprazole for the Treatment of Methamphetamine Dependence: A Randomized, Double-Blind, Placebo-Controlled Trial." *Addiction* 108: 751–761.

Comer, S. D., et al. (2001). "Effects of Repeated Oral Methamphetamine Administration in Humans." *Psychopharmacology* 155: 397–404.

Dackis, C. A., et al. (2012). "A Double-Blind, Placebo-Controlled Trial of Modafinil for Cocaine Dependence." *Journal of Substance Abuse Treatment* 43: 303–312.

Dean, A. C., et al. (2011). "Acute Modafinil Effects on Attention and Inhibitory Control in Methamphetamine-Dependent Humans." *Journal of Studies on Alcohol and Drugs* 72: 943–953.

Dean, A. C., et al. (2013). "An Evaluation of the Evidence That Methamphetamine Abuse Causes Cognitive Decline in Humans." *Neuropsychopharmacology* 38: 259–274.

De Giovanni, N., and Marchetti, D. (2012). "Cocaine and Its Metabolites in the Placenta: A Sys-tematic Review of the Literature." *Reproductive Toxicology* 33: 1–14.

Doweiko, H. E. (2012). *Concepts of Chemical Dependency,* 8th ed. Belmont, CA: Brooks/Cole.

Elkashef, A., and Montoya, I. (2012). "Pharmacotherapy of Addiction." *Drug Abuse and Addic-tion in Medical Illness* Part 1: 107–119.

Elkashef, A., and Vocci, F. (2011). "Pharmacotherapy of Cocaine Addiction." *Addiction Medicine* Part 8: 1017–1128.

Elkashef, A. M., et al. (2008). "Bupropion for the Treatment of Methamphetamine Dependence." *Neuropsychopharmacology* 33: 1162–1170.

Elkashef, A. M., et al. (2012). "Topiramate for the Treatment of Methamphetamine Addiction: A Multi-Center Placebo-Controlled Trial." *Addiction* 107: 1297–1306.

Ersche, K. D., et al. (2011). "Abnormal Structure of Frontostriatal Brain Systems Is Associated with Aspects of Impulsivity and Compulsivity in Cocaine Dependence." *Brain* 134: 2013–2024.

Farooq, M. U., et al. (2009). "Neurotoxic and Cardiotoxic Effects of Cocaine and Ethanol." *Journal of Medical Toxicology* 5: 134–138.

Fechtner, R. D., et al. (2006). "Short-Term Treatment of Cocaine and/or Methamphetamine Abuse with Vigabatrin: Ocular Safety Pilot Results." *Archives of Ophthalmology* 124: 1257–1262.

Garcia-Bournissen, F., et al. (2009). "Pharmacokinetics of Disappearance of Cocaine from Hair After Discontinuation of Drug Use." *Forensic Science International* 189: 24–27.

Gaval-Cruz, M., and Weinshenker, D. (2009). "Mechanisms of Disulfiram-Induced Cocaine Abstinence: Antabuse and Cocaine Relapse." *Molecular Interventions* 9: 175–187.

Gerlach, K. K., et al. (2014). "Epidemiology of Stimulant Misuse and Abuse: Implications for Future Epidemiologic and Neuropharmacologic Research." *Neuropharmacology* 87: 91–96. doi: 10.1016/j.neuropharm.2014.04.020.

Gerteis, J., et al. (2011). "Are There Effects of Intrauterine Cocaine Exposure on Delinquency During Early Adolescence? A Preliminary Report." *Journal of Developmental and Behavioral Pediatrics* 32: 393–401.

Gold, M. S. (1997). "Cocaine (and Crack): Clinical Aspects." In J. H. Lowinson, P. Ruiz, R. B. Millman, and J. G. Langrod, eds., *Substance Abuse: A Comprehensive Textbook,* 3rd ed. Baltimore: Williams & Wilkins.

Good, M. M., et al. (2010). "Methamphetamine Use During Pregnancy." *Obstetrics & Gynecology* 116: 330–334.

Gorelick, D. A. (2012). "Pharmacokinetic Strategies for Treatment of Drug Overdose and Addiction." *Future Medicinal Chemistry* 4: 227–243.

Gouin, K., et al. (2011). "Effects of Cocaine Use during Pregnancy on Low Birthweight and Preterm Birth: Systematic Review and Meta-analyses." *American Journal of Obstetrics & Gynecology* 204: 340.e1–340.e12.

Gouzoulis-Mayfrank, E., and Daumann, J. (2009). "Neurotoxicity of Drugs of Abuse—The Case of Methylenedioxyamphetamines (MDMA, Ecstasy) and Amphetamines." *Dialogues in Clinical Neuroscience* 11: 305–317.

Grabowski, J., et al. (1997). "Replacement Medication for Cocaine Dependence: Methylphenidate." *Journal of Clinical Psychopharmacology* 17: 485–488.

Grabowski, J., et al. (2001). "Dextroamphetamine for Cocaine-Dependence Treatment: A Double-Blind Randomized Clinical Trial." *Journal of Clinical Psychopharmacology* 21: 522–526.

Gregory, P. J. (2013). "Availability of DMAA Supplements Despite U. S. Food and Drug Administration Action." *JAMA Internal Medicine* 173: 164–165.

Haile, C. N., et al. (2012a). "Pharmacotherapeutics Directed at Deficiencies Associated with Cocaine Dependence: Focus on Dopamine, Norepinephrine and Glutamate." *Pharmacology and Therapeutics* 134: 260–277.

Haile, C. N., et al. (2012b). "The Impact of Disulfiram Treatment on the Reinforcing Effects of Cocaine: A Randomized Clinical Trial." *PLoS One* 7: e47702.

Harris, D. S., et al. (2003). "Altering Cortisol Level Does Not Change the Pleasurable Effects of Methamphetamine in Humans." *Neuropsychopharmacology* 28: 1677–1684.

Heinzerling, K. G., et al. (2013). "Pilot Randomized Trial of Bupropion for Adolescent Methamphetamine Abuse/Dependence." *Journal of Adolescent Health* 52: 502–505.

Herin, D. V., et al. (2010). "Agonist-Like Pharmacotherapy for Stimulant Dependence: Preclinical, Human Laboratory, and Clinical Studies." *Annals of the New York Academy of Sciences* 1187: 76–100.

Hsieh, J. H., et al. (2014). "The Neurobiology of Methamphetamine Induced Psychosis." *Frontiers in Human Neuroscience* 8: 537. doi: 10.3389/fnhum.2014.00537.

Huang, M.-C., et al. (2016). "Risk of Cardiovascular Diseases and Stroke Events in Methamphetamine Users: A 10-Year Follow-Up Study." *Journal of Clinical Psychiatry* 77: 1396–1403. doi: 10.4088/JCP.15m09872.

Islam, F. A., et al. (2015). "What to Do When Adolescents with ADHD Self-Medicate with Bath Salts." *Current Psychiatry* 14: e3–e4.

Johnson, B. A., et al. (2013). "Topiramate's Effects on Cocaine-Induced Subjective Mood, Craving and Preference for Money over Drug Taking." *Addiction Biology* 18: 405–416.

Kablinger, A., et al. (2012). "Effects of the Combination of Metyrapone and Oxazepam on Cocaine Craving and Cocaine Taking: A Double-Blind, Randomized, Placebo-Controlled Pilot Study." *Journal of Psychopharmacology* 26: 973–998.

Karila, L., et al. (2011). "Pharmacological Treatments for Cocaine Dependence: Is There Something New?" *Current Pharmaceutical Design* 17: 1359–1368.

Karila, L., et al. (2015). "Synthetic Cathinones: A New Public Health Problem." *Current Neuropharmacology* 13: 12–20.

Kaye, S., et al. (2013). "Attention Deficit Hyperactivity Disorder (ADHD) Among Illicit Psychostimulant Users: A Hidden Disorder?" *Addiction* 108: 923–931.

Keegan, J., et al. (2010). "Addiction in Pregnancy." *Journal of Addictive Diseases* 29: 175–191.

Kiblawi, Z. N., et al. (2013). "The Effect of Prenatal Methamphetamine Exposure on Attention as Assessed by Continuous Performance Tests: Results from the Infant Development, Environment, and Lifestyle Study." *Journal of Developmental Behavioral Pediatrics* 34: 31–37.

Kirkpatrick, M. G., et al. (2013). "Personality and the Acute Subjective Effects of *d*-Amphetamine in Humans." *Journal of Psychopharmacology* 27: 256–264.

Kiyatkin, E. A., et al. (2007). "Brain Edema and Breakdown of the Blood-Brain Barrier During Methamphetamine Intoxication: Critical Role of Brain Hyperthermia." *European Journal of Neuroscience* 26: 1242–1253.

Kiyatkin, E. A., and Sharma, H. S. (2009). "Acute Methamphetamine Intoxication: Brain Hyperthermia, Blood-Brain Barrier, Brain Edema, and Morphological Cell Abnormalities." *International Review of Neurobiology* 88: 65–100.

Kiyatkin, E. A., and Sharma, H. S. (2012). "Environmental Conditions Modulate Neurotoxic Effects of Psychomotor Stimulant Drugs of Abuse." *New Perspectives of Central Nervous System Injury and Neuroprotection* 102: 147–171.

Kosten, T., et al. (2013). "Vaccines against Stimulants: Cocaine and Methamphetamine." *British Journal of Clinical Pharmacology* 77: 368–374. doi: 10.1111/bcp.12115.

Kozor, R., et al. (2014). "Regular Cocaine Use Is Associated with Increased Blood Pressure, Aortic Stiffness, and Ventricular Mass in Young Otherwise Healthy Individuals." *PLos One* 9: e89710. doi: 10.1371/journal.pone.0089710.

Krystal, A. D., et al. (2010). "A Double-Blind, Placebo-Controlled Study of Armodafinil for Excessive Sleepiness in Patients with Treated Obstructive Sleep Apnea and Comorbid Depression." *Journal of Clinical Psychiatry* 71: 32–40.

LaGasse, L. L., et al. (2012). "Prenatal Methamphetamine Exposure and Childhood Behavior Problems at 3 and 5 Years of Age." *Pediatrics* 129: 681–688.

Levinthal, C. F. (2012). *Drugs, Behavior and Modern Society,* 7th ed. New York: Allyn & Bacon.

Licata, S. C., et al. (2011). "Effects of Daily Treatment with Citicoline: A Double-Blind, Placebo-Controlled Study in Cocaine-Dependence Volunteers." *Journal of Addiction Medicine* 5: 57–64.

Ling, W., et al. (2012). "Double-Blind Placebo-Controlled Evaluation of the Prometa Protocol for Methamphetamine Dependence." *Addiction* 107: 361–369.

Ling, W., et al. (2014). "Treating Methamphetamine Abuse Disorder." *Current Psychiatry* 13: 36–44.

Lockner, J. W., et al. (2015). "Flagellin as Carrier and Adjuvant in Cocaine Vaccine Development." *Molecular Pharmaceutics* 12: 653–662. doi: 10.1021/mp500520r.

Loland, C. J., et al. (2012). "R-Modafinil (Armodafinil): A Unique Dopamine Uptake Inhibitor and Potential Medication for Psychostimulant Abuse." *Biological Psychiatry* 72: 405–413.

Malek, A. (2012). "Effects of Prenatal Cocaine Exposure on Human Pregnancy and Postpartum." *Pharmaceutica Analytica Acta* 3: 1–8. doi: 10.4172/2153-2435.1000191.

Mallete, J. R., et al. (2016). "Geographically Sourcing Cocaine's Origin—Delineation of the Nineteen Major Coca Growing Regions in South America." *Scientific Reports* 6: 23520. doi: 10.1038/srep23520.

Mariani, J. J., and Levin, F. R. (2012). "Psychostimulant Treatment of Cocaine Dependence." *Psychiatric Clinics of North America* 35: 425–439.

McKetin, R., et al. (2013). "Dose-Related Psychotic Symptoms in Chronic Methamphetamine Users: Evidence from a Prospective Longitudinal Study." *JAMA Psychiatry* 70: 319–324.

McKim, W. A., and Hancock, S. (2013). *Drugs and Behavior,* 7th ed. Upper Saddle River, NJ: Pearson Prentice Hall.

Meini, M., et al. (2011). "Aripiprazole and Ropinirole Treatment for Cocaine Dependence: Evidence from a Pilot Study." *Current Pharmaceutical Design* 17: 1376–1383.

Mello, N. K., et al. (2013). "Effects of Chronic Buspirone Treatment on Cocaine Self-Administration." *Neuropsychopharmacology* 38: 455–467.

Melton, S. T. (2015). "$5 Insanity: A New Drug of Abuse." *MedScape.* November 23. http://www.medscape.com/viewarticle/854616.

Miliano, C., et al. (2016). "Neuropharmacology of New Psychoactive Substances (NPS): Focus on the Rewarding and Reinforcing Properties of Cannabimimetics and Amphetamine-Like Stimulants." *Frontiers in Neuroscience* 10: 153. doi: 10.3389/fnins.2016.00153.

Miller, M. L., et al. (2013). "A Methamphetamine Vaccine Attenuates Methamphetamine-Induced Disruptions in Thermoregulation and Activity in Rats." *Biological Psychiatry* 73: 721–728.

Mooney, L. J., et al. (2016). "Utilizing a Two-stage Design to Investigate the Safety and Potential Efficacy of Monthly Naltrexone Plus Once-daily Bupropion as a Treatment for Methamphetamine Use Disorder." *Journal of Addiction Medicine* 10: 236–243. doi: 10.1097/ADM.0000000000000218.

Müller, U., et al. (2013). "Effects of Modafinil on Non-Verbal Cognition, Task Enjoyment and Creative Thinking in Healthy Volunteers." *Neuropharmacology* 64: 490–495.

Nakagawa, T., and Kaneko, S. (2008). "Neuropsychotoxicity of Abused Drugs: Molecular and Neural Mechanisms of Neuropsychotoxicity Induced by Methamphetamine, 3,4-Methylenedioxymethamphetamine (Ecstasy) and 5-Methoxy-N,N-Diisopropyltryptamine (Foxy)." *Journal of Pharmaceutical Sciences* 106: 2–8.

Narasimhan, D., et al. (2012). "Bacterial Cocaine Esterase: A Protein-Based Therapy for Cocaine Overdose and Addiction." *Future Medicinal Chemistry* 4: 137–150.

Narendran, B. J., et al. (2014). "Cocaine Abuse in Humans Is Not Associated with Increased Microglial Activation: An 18-kDa Translocator Protein Positron Emission Tomography Imaging Study with [^{11}C]PBR28." *Journal of Neuroscience* 34: 9945–9950. doi: 10.1523/JNEUROSCI.0928-14.2014.

Nephew, B. C., and Febo, M. (2012). "Effects of Cocaine on Maternal Behavior and Neurochemistry." *Current Neuropharmacology* 10: 53–63.

Newton, T. F., et al. (2012). "Noradrenergic α_1 Receptor Antagonist Treatment Attenuates Positive Subjective Effects of Cocaine in Humans: A Randomized Trial." *PLoS One* 7: e30854.

Nicholson, P. J., et al. (2015). "Correspondence Arising: Modafinil for Cognitive Neuroenhancement in Healthy Non-Sleep-Deprived-Subjects." *European Neuropsychopharmacology* 26: 390. doi: 10.1016/j.euroneuro.2015.12.024.

Northrop, N. A., and Yamamoto, B. R. (2015). "Methamphetamine Effects on Blood–Brain Barrier Structure and Function." *Frontiers in Neuroscience* 9: 69. doi: 10.3389/fnins.2015.00069.

Nuijten, M., et al. (2015). "Modafinil in the Treatment of Crack-Cocaine Dependence in the Netherlands: Results of an Open-Label Randomised Controlled Feasibility Trial." *Psychopharmacology* 29: 678–687. doi: 10.1177/0269881115582151.

Nuijten, M., et al. (2016). "Sustained-Release Dexamfetamine in the Treatment of Chronic Cocaine-Dependent Patients on Heroin-Assisted Treatment: A Randomised, Double-Blind, Placebo-Controlled Trial." *Lancet* 387: 2226–2234. doi: 10.1016/S0140-6736(16)00205-1.

Oei, J. L., et al. (2012). "Amphetamines, the Pregnant Woman and Her Children: A Review." *Journal of Perinatology* 32: 737–747.

Olive, M. F., et al. (2012). "Glutamatergic Medications for the Treatment of Drug and Behavioral Addictions." *Pharmacology Biochemistry and Behavior* 100: 801–810.

Olson, S. (2015). "New Designer Drug Flakka Works Like Bath Salts, Causes 'Excited Delirium.'" *Medical Daily*. April 6. http://www.medicaldaily.com/new-designer-drug-flakka-works-bath-salts-causes-excited-delirium-328224.

Panenka, W. J., et al. (2013). "Methamphetamine Use: A Comprehensive Review of Molecular, Preclinical and Clinical Findings." *Drug and Alcohol Dependence* 129: 167–179.

Pani, P. P., et al. (2010). "Disulfiram for the Treatment of Cocaine Dependence." *Cochrane Database of Systematic Reviews:* CD007024.

Papaseit, E., et al. (2016). "Human Pharmacology of Mephedrone in Comparison with MDMA." *Neuropsychopharmacology* 41: 2704–2713. doi:10.1038/npp.2016.75.

Payer, D. E., et al. (2014). "Heightened D_3 Dopamine Receptor Levels in Cocaine Dependence and Contributions to the Addiction Behavioral Phenotype: A Positron Emission Tomography Study with [^{11}C]-(+)-PHNO." *Neuropsychopharmacology* 39: 321–328. doi: 10.1038/npp.2013.192.

Phillips, K., et al. (2009). "Cocaine Cardiotoxicity: A Review of the Pathophysiology, Pathology, and Treatment Options." *American Journal of Cardiovascular Drugs* 9: 177–196.

Prosser, J. M., and Nelson, L. S. (2012). "The Toxicology of Bath Salts: A Review of Synthetic Cathinones." *Journal of Medical Toxicology* 8: 33–42.

Raineri, M., et al. (2012). "Modafinil Abrogates Methamphetamine-Induced Neuroinflammation and Apoptotic Effects in the Mouse Striatum." *PLoS One* 7: e46599.

Rando, K., et al. (2013). "Prenatal Cocaine Exposure and Gray Matter Volume in Adolescent Boys and Girls." *Biological Psychiatry* 74: 482–489.

Richards, J. R. (2016). "Methamphetamine Toxicity." *Medscape.* http://emedicine.medscape.com/article/820918-overview.

Rolan, P., et al. (2013). "Ibudilast: A Review of Its Pharmacology, Efficacy and Safety in Respiratory and Neurological Disease." *Expert Opinion on Pharmacotherapy* 10: 2897–2904. doi: 10.1517/14656560903426189.

Rosenbaum, C. D., et al. (2012). "Here Today, Gone Tomorrow . . . and Back Again? A Review of Herbal Marijuana Alternatives (K2, Spice), Synthetic Cathinones (Bath Salts), Kratom, *Salvia Divinorum*, Methoxetamine, and Piperazines." *Journal of Medical Toxicology* 8: 15–32.

Rush, C. R., and Stoops, W. W. (2012). "Agonist Replacement Therapy for Cocaine Dependence: A Translational Review." *Future Medicinal Chemistry* 4: 245–265.

Saha, K., et al. (2015). "'Second-Generation' Mephedrone Analogs, 4-MEC and 4-MePPP, Differentially Affect Monoamine Transporter Function." *Neuropsychopharmacology* 40: 1321–1331. doi:10.1038/npp.2014.325.

Salamanca, S. A., et al. (2015). "Impact of Methamphetamine on Infection and Immunity." *Frontiers of Neuroscience* 8: 445. doi: 10.3389/fnins.2014.00445.

Schindler, C. W., and Goldberg, S. R. (2012). "Accelerating Cocaine Metabolism as an Approach to the Treatment of Cocaine Abuse and Toxicity." *Future Medicinal Chemistry* 4: 163–175.

Schrantee, A., et al. (2015). "Dopaminergic System Dysfunction in Recreational Dexamphetamine Users." *Neuropsychopharmacology* 40: 1172–1180. doi: 10.1038/npp.2014.301.

Schwarz, A. (2015). "Workers Seeking Productivity in a Pill Are Abusing A.D.H.D. Drugs." *New York Times*. April 18. https://www.nytimes.com/2015/04/19/us/workers-seeking-productivity-in-a-pill-are-abusing-adhd-drugs.html.

Sekine, Y., et al. (2008). "Methamphetamine Causes Microglial Activation in the Brains of Human Abusers." *Journal of Neuroscience* 28: 5756–5761.

Shen, X. Y., et al. (2012). "Vaccines Against Drug Abuse." *Nature* 91: 60–70.

Shoptaw, S. J., et al. (2008). "Bupropion Hydrochloride Versus Placebo, in Combination with Cognitive Behavioral Therapy, for the Treatment of Cocaine Abuse/Dependence." *Journal of Addictive Disorders* 27: 13–23.

Shoptaw, S. J., et al. (2009). "Treatment for Amphetamine Psychosis." *Cochrane Database of Systematic Reviews* CD003026.

Shorter, D., and Kosten, T. R. (2011). "Novel Pharmacotherapeutic Treatments for Cocaine Addiction." *BMC Medicine* 9: 119–128.

Siciliano, C. A., et al. (2014). "Biphasic Mechanisms of Amphetamine Action at the Dopamine Terminal." *The Journal of Neuroscience* 34: 5575–5582. doi: 10.1523/JNEUROSCI.4050–13.2014.

Smethells, J. R., et al. (2016). "Long-Term Blockade of Cocaine Self-Administration and Locomotor Activation in Rats by an Adenoviral Vector–Delivered Cocaine Hydrolase." *Journal of Pharmacology and Experimental Therapeutics* 357: 375–381. doi: 10.1124/jpet.116.232504

Smith, L. M., et al. (2006). "The Infant Development, Environment, and Lifestyle Study: Effects of Prenatal Methamphetamine Exposure, Polydrug Exposure, and Poverty on Intrauterine Growth." *Pediatrics* 118: 1149–1156.

Smith, C. T., et al. (2016). "Individual Differences in Timing of Peak Positive Subjective Responses to D-amphetamine: Relationship to Pharmacokinetics and Physiology." *Journal of Psychopharmacology* 30: 330–343. doi: 10.1177/0269881116631650.

Somoza, E. C., et al. (2013). "A Multisite, Double-Blind, Placebo-Controlled Clinical Trial to Evaluate the Safety and Efficacy of Vigabatrin for Treating Cocaine Dependence." *JAMA Psychiatry* 10: 1–8.

Sowell, E. R., et al. (2010). "Differentiating Prenatal Exposure to Methamphetamine and Alcohol versus Alcohol and Not Methamphetamine Using Tensor-Based Brain Morphometry and Discriminant Analysis." *Journal of Neuroscience* 30: 3876–3885.

Stitzer, M. L., et al. (2010). "Drug Users' Adherence to a 6-Month Vaccination Protocol: Effects of Motivational Incentives." *Drug and Alcohol Dependence* 107: 76–79.

Strange, L. G., et al. (2017). "The Pharmacokinetic Profile of Synthetic Cathinones in a Pregnancy Model." *Neurotoxicology and Teratology* 63: 9–13. doi: 10.1016/j.ntt.2017.08.001.

Sushchyk, S., et al. (2016). "Combination of Levo-Tetrahydropalmatine and Low Dose Naltrexone: A Promising Treatment for the Prevention of Cocaine Relapse." *Journal of Pharmacology and Experimental Therapeutics* 357: 248–257. doi: 10.1124/jpet.115.229542.

Talbert, J., et al. (2012). "Pseudoephedrine Sales and Seizures of Clandestine Methamphetamine Laboratories in Kentucky." *JAMA* 308: 1524–1526.

Tau, G. Z., et al. (2014). "Neural Correlates of Reward-Based Spatial Learning in Persons with Cocaine Dependence." *Neuropsychopharmacology* 39: 545–555. doi: 10.1038/npp.2013.189.

Thompson, B. L., et al. (2009). "Prenatal Exposure to Drugs: Effects on Brain Development and Implications for Policy and Education." *Nature Reviews Neuroscience* 10: 303–312.

Thompson, P. M., et al. (2004). "Structural Abnormalities in the Brains of Human Subjects Who Use Methamphetamine." *Journal of Neuroscience* 24: 6028–6036.

Turowski, P., and Kenny, B. A. (2015). "The Blood–Brain Barrier and Methamphetamine: Open Sesame?" *Frontiers in Neuroscience* 9: 156. doi: 10.3389/fnins.2015.00156.

Underwood, E. (2015). "A New Drug War." *Science* 347: 469–473.

Volkow, N. D., et al. (2009). "Effects of Modafinil on Dopamine and Dopamine Transporters in the Male Human Brain: Clinical Implications." *JAMA* 301: 1148–1154.

Vonmoos, L. M., et al. (2014). "Cognitive Impairment in Cocaine Users Is Drug-Induced but Partially Reversible: Evidence from a Longitudinal Study." *Neuropsychopharmacology* 39: 2200–2210. doi: 10.1038/npp.2014.71.

Vosburg, S. K., et al. (2010). "Modafinil Does Not Serve as a Reinforcer in Cocaine Abusers." *Drug and Alcohol Dependence* 106: 233–236.

Walton, M. A., et al. (2009). "Predictors of Violence Following Emergency Department Visit for Cocaine-Related Chest Pain." *Drug and Alcohol Dependence* 99: 79–88.

Wang, G. J., et al. (2012). "Decreased Dopamine Activity Predicts Relapse in Methamphetamine Abusers." *Molecular Psychiatry* 17: 918–925.

Wang, J. B., and Mantsch, J. R. (2012). "*l*-Tetrahydropalamatine: A Potential New Medication for the Treatment of Cocaine Addiction." *Future Medicinal Chemistry* 4: 177–186.

Wee, S., et al. (2012a). "A Combination of Buprenorphine and Naltrexone Blocks Compulsive Cocaine Intake in Rodents Without Producing Dependence." *Science Translational Medicine* 4: 146ra110.

Wee, S., et al. (2012b). "Novel Cocaine Vaccine Linked to a Disrupted Adenovirus Gene Transfer Vector Blocks Cocaine Psychostimulant and Reinforcing Effects." *Neuropsychopharmacology* 37: 1083–1091.

Westover, A. N., and Nakonezny, P. A. (2010). "Aortic Dissection in Young Adults Who Abuse Amphetamines." *American Heart Journal* 160: 315–321.

Whitten, L. (2010). "Cocaine Vaccine Helps Some Reduce Drug Abuse." *National Institute on Drug Abuse*. December 1. https://www.drugabuse.gov/news-events/nida-notes/2010/12/cocaine-vaccine-helps-some-reduce-drug-abuse.

Winhusen, T. M., et al. (2014). "Multisite, Randomized, Double-Blind, Placebo-Controlled Pilot Clinical Trial to Evaluate the Efficacy of Buspirone as a Relapse-Prevention Treatment for Cocaine Dependence." *Journal of Clinical Psychiatry* 75: 757–764. doi: 10.4088/JCP.13m08862.

Worley, M. J., et al. (2016). "Ibudilast Attenuates Subjective Effects of Methamphetamine in a Placebo-Controlled Inpatient Study." *Drug and Alcohol Dependence* 162: 245–250. doi: http://dx.doi.org/10.1016/j.drugalcdep.2016.02.036.

Wuo-Silva, R., et al. (2016). "Modafinil Induces Rapid-Onset Behavioral Sensitization and Cross-Sensitization with Cocaine in Mice: Implications for the Addictive Potential of Modafinil." *Frontiers in Pharmacology* 7: 420. doi: 10.3389/fphar.2016.00420.

Xia, L., et al. (2013). "Metabotropic Glutamate 7 (mGlu7) Receptor: A Target for Medication Development for the Treatment of Cocaine Dependence." *Neuropharmacology* 66: 12–23.

Yao, L., et al. (2010). "Inhibition of Aldehyde Dehydrogenase-2 Suppresses Cocaine Seeking by Generating THP, a Cocaine Use–Dependent Inhibitor of Dopamine Synthesis." *Nature Medicine* 16: 1024–1028.

Zack, M., et al. (2015). "Differential Cardiovascular and Hypothalamic Pituitary Response to Amphetamine in Male Pathological Gamblers versus Healthy Controls." *Journal of Psychopharmacology* 29: 971–982. doi: 10.1177/0269881115592338.

Zarrabi, H., et al. (2016). "Clinical Features, Course and Treatment of Methamphetamine-Induced Psychosis in Psychiatric Inpatients." *BMC Psychiatry* 16: 44. doi: 10.1186/s12888-016-0745-5.

Zhang, Y., et al. (2012). "1,3-Dimethylamylamine (DMAA) in Supplements and Geranium Products: Natural or Synthetic?" *Drug Testing and Analysis* 4: 986–990.

Zheng, F., and Zhan, C. G. (2012a). "Are Pharmacokinetic Approaches Feasible for Treatment of Cocaine Addiction and Overdose?" *Future Medicinal Chemistry* 4: 125–128.

Zheng, F., and Zhan, C. G. (2012b). "Modeling of Pharmacokinetics of Cocaine in Human Reveals the Feasibility for Development of Enzyme Therapies for Drugs of Abuse." *PLoS Computational Biology* 8: e1002610. doi: 10.1371/journal.pcbi.1002610.

Zheng, F., et al. (2015). "R6236—Long-Acting Cocaine Hydrolase as Enzyme Therapy for Cocaine Addiction." Presented at the 2015 American Association of Pharmaceutical Scientists Annual Meeting and Exposition, Orlando, FL.

Zlebnik, N. E., et al. (2014). "Long-Term Reduction of Cocaine Self-Administration in Rats Treated with Adenoviral Vector-Delivered Cocaine Hydrolase: Evidence for Enzymatic Activity." *Neuropsychopharmacology* 39: 1538–1546. doi: 10.1038/npp.2014.3.

Zuloaga, D. G., et al. (2015). "Methamphetamine and the Hypothalamic-Pituitary-Adrenal Axis." *Frontiers in Neuroscience* 9: 178. doi: 10.3389/fnins.2015.00178.

CHAPTER 8

Psychedelic Drugs

This chapter introduces a class of drugs that act on various neurotransmitter pathways in the central nervous system (CNS) to produce hallucinatory perceptual experiences, which may be accompanied by marked changes in cognition and mood. In contrast to other drugs of abuse, many of these drugs are taken specifically to alter subjective states of consciousness rather than for a direct reinforcing effect. A current term applied to a person who uses these drugs is *psychonaut*, to indicate the exploratory nature of the experience. In fact, it is not uncommon for these substances to produce a dysphoric, rather than euphoric, subjective experience. Moreover, unlike their response to classically rewarding drugs, nonhuman animals are less likely to self-administer these drugs and may sometimes even work to avoid them. Primarily for this reason, there has been less research on these drugs than on drugs considered to have more therapeutic potential. This situation, however, is beginning to change, as this chapter describes.

Because of the unusual subjective, psychological, and physiological effects they produce, the best term for classifying these drugs has been debated for a long time. The term *hallucinogen* is used because these agents can, in high enough doses, induce hallucinations, defined as *perceptions in the absence of the appropriate sensations*. However, that is somewhat misleading because illusory phenomena and perceptual distortions are more common than are true hallucinations. The term *psychotomimetic* has also been used because of the alleged ability of these drugs to mimic psychoses or induce psychotic states. However, previous assumptions that psychedelic drugs might induce a psychotic reaction are incorrect. According to analyses of data obtained from the U.S. National Survey on Drug Use and Health (NSDUH) covering the years 2008 to 2012, people who used any of the three psychedelics drugs—LSD, psilocybin, and mescaline—were not at risk of developing symptoms of mental health problems (Hendricks et al., 2015; Johansen and Krebs, 2015). In fact, Hendricks and colleagues found that people who had used LSD and psilocybin had *lower* lifetime rates of suicidal thoughts and attempts.

In this chapter, the term *psychedelic* (mind-manifesting) is used because it allows for more flexibility in grouping together a disparate array of effects into a recognizable syndrome. Many psychedelic agents occur in nature; others are synthetically produced.

TABLE 8.1 Classification of psychedelic drugs

Anticholinergic	Scopolamine
Catecholaminelike	Mescaline
	Myristicin, elemicin
	DOM, MDA, DMA, MDMA (Ecstasy), TMA, MDE
Serotoninlike	Lysergic acid diethylamide (LSD)
	Dimethyltryptamine (DMT), AMT, 5-MeO-DIPT
	Psilocybin, psilocin, bufotenine
	Ololiuqui
	Harmine
Glutaminergic NMDA receptor antagonists	Phencyclidine (Sernyl)
	Ketamine (Ketalar)
	Dextromethorphan
Opioid kappa receptor agonist	Salvinorin A

Regardless of their origin, most psychedelic drugs act on one of the known neurotransmitter systems. Similarities in structure and in neurochemical and psychological effects lead to the major categories of psychedelic drugs (Table 8.1): *anticholinergic, monoaminergic* (*catecholaminelike* and *serotoninlike*), *glutaminergic NMDA receptor antagonists* (the two psychedelic anesthetics as well as dextromethorphan), and the *opioid kappa receptor agonist* salvinorin A. Finally, there are some additional substances, derivatives that are related to these compounds, which are described in their respective sections.

SCOPOLAMINE: THE PROTOTYPE ANTICHOLINERGIC (ACh) PSYCHEDELIC

This class of drugs might more appropriately be called *antimuscarinic* because they are competitive antagonists of the muscarinic type of ACh receptor (see Chapter 3). The three most common anticholinergics are *scopolamine, atropine*, and *l-hyoscyamine*. Scopolamine (Figure 8.1) is the classic example of an anticholinergic drug with psychedelic properties. Medically, scopolamine is found in some travel-sickness products, including motion-sickness–prevention patches.[1] More commonly, exposure occurs because of the anticholinergic side effects produced by many psychotropic medications such as antidepressants (see Chapter 12) and antipsychotics (see Chapter 11).

---

[1] Certain medicines also have anticholinergic properties and can cause similar effects. Examples include antihistamines, such as diphenhydramine, Benadryl, and certain medicines used in the treatment of parkinsonism (for example, Cogentin).

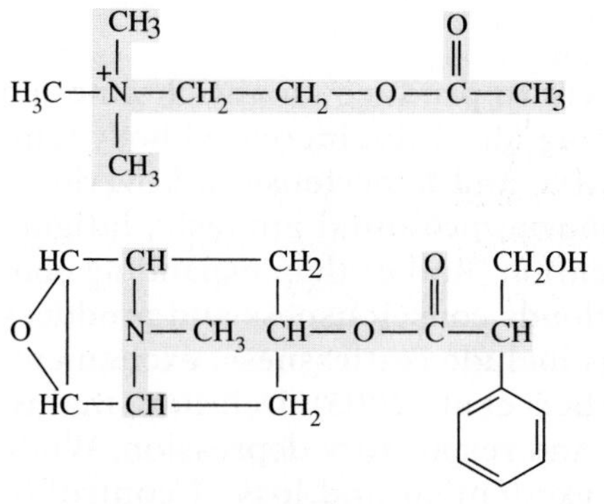

FIGURE 8.1 Structural formulas of acetylcholine (a chemical transmitter) and the anticholinergic psychedelic scopolamine, which acts by blocking acetylcholine receptors. The shaded portion of each molecule illustrates structural similarities, which presumably contribute to receptor fit.

Historical Background

The history of scopolamine is long and colorful (Holzman, 1998). The drug is distributed widely in nature; it is found in especially high concentrations in the plants *Atropa belladonna* (belladonna, or deadly nightshade), *Datura stramonium* (Jamestown weed, jimsonweed, stinkweed, thorn apple, or devil's apple), *Mandragora officinarum* (mandrake), and *Datura inoxia* (moonflower). Both professional and amateur poisoners of the "since antiquity" frequently used deadly nightshade as a source of poison. In fact, the plant's name, *Atropa belladonna*, is derived from Atropos, one of the three Fates, who supposedly cut the thread of life. *Belladonna* means "beautiful woman," which refers to the drug's ability to dilate the pupils when it is applied topically to the eyes (eyes with widely dilated pupils were presumably a mark of beauty). Accidental ingestion of berries from *Datura* has even been associated with the incapacitation of whole armies, for example, the defeat of Marc Antony's army in 36 BCE. Ingestion of tea made from this plant was said to have contributed to the defeat of British soldiers by settlers in the rebellion known as Bacon's Revolution near Jamestown, Virginia, in 1676 (hence the name Jamestown weed, or jimson weed).

Scopolamine-containing plants have been used and misused for centuries. For example, the delirium caused by scopolamine may have persuaded certain people that they could fly—associated with the Halloween images of flying witches. Marijuana and opium preparations from the Far East were once fortified with material from *D. stramonium*. Today, cigarettes made from the leaves of *D. stramonium* and *A. belladonna* are smoked occasionally to induce intoxication. Throughout the world, leaves of plants that contain atropine or scopolamine are still used to prepare intoxicating beverages.

Pharmacological Effects

Scopolamine acts on the peripheral nervous system to produce an anticholinergic syndrome consisting of dry mouth, reduced sweating, dry skin, increased body temperature, dilated pupils, blurred vision, tachycardia, and hypertension. Low doses reaching the CNS produce drowsiness, mild euphoria, profound amnesia, fatigue, mental confusion, dreamless sleep, and loss of attention. Rather than expanding consciousness, awareness, and insight, scopolamine clouds consciousness and produces amnesia. As doses increase, psychiatric symptoms include restlessness, excitement, hallucinations, euphoria, and disorientation (DeFrates et al., 2005). Delirium, that is, mental confusion, may progress to stupor, coma, and respiratory depression. While scopolamine intoxication can convey a sense of excitement and loss of control to the user, the clouding of consciousness and the reduction in memory of the episode render scopolamine rather unattractive as a psychedelic drug. Although historically used as poisons, the margin of safety for these drugs is large and death is usually a result of accidents (wandering into traffic or falling), or of inadvertent ingestion (for example, of the berries by children). There is a classic phrase describing the effects of scopolamine, which states that it makes you "hot as a hare, blind as a bat, dry as a bone, red as a beet, and mad as a hen." Typically, sensorium and psychosis usually clear within 36 to 48 hours. If necessary, the antidote to anticholinergic poisoning is the drug physostigmine, which blocks the enzyme acetylcholinesterase (AChE). AChE metabolizes ACh in the synaptic cleft. By blocking this metabolism, physostigmine may increase the concentration of ACh sufficiently to overcome the lethal effects of scopolamine.

Tolerance to anticholinergics is generally modest and psychological dependence uncommon. Physical dependence can develop, particularly in conjunction with long-term use of medications that have anticholinergic actions or side effects. Withdrawal symptoms include vomiting, excessive sweating and salivation, and general malaise.

MONOAMINERGIC PSYCHEDELICS

As the name indicates, these drugs share a neurochemical similarity with the biogenic amine neurotransmitters, such as serotonin (5-HT), dopamine, and norepinephrine. Examples of the serotonergic category are LSD, psilocybin, and DMT, whereas the catecholamine type includes mescaline and MDMA (ecstasy). Within their respective effective dose ranges, the subjective effects of these drugs are quite similar, although they vary greatly in potency and in duration of action. Essentially, the actions range from amphetaminelike (more stimulatory and less hallucinogenic) to LSD like (more hallucinatory and less stimulatory). Tolerance usually develops rapidly to the effects of most of these drugs within three or four successive daily exposures and they are often cross-tolerant with each other—although not with the drugs in the other psychedelic classes. In addition to sharing many psychological effects, these drugs also produce similar physiological actions, notably sympathomimetic effects such as increases in blood pressure and heart rate, pupil dilation, increased body temperature, tremors, nausea, and other reactions as noted.

CATECHOLAMINERGIC PSYCHEDELICS

A large group of psychedelic drugs are structurally similar to both catecholamine neurotransmitters and the amphetamine stimulants (Figure 8.2). They differ structurally from the normal neurotransmitters by the addition of one or more methoxy (–OCH_3)

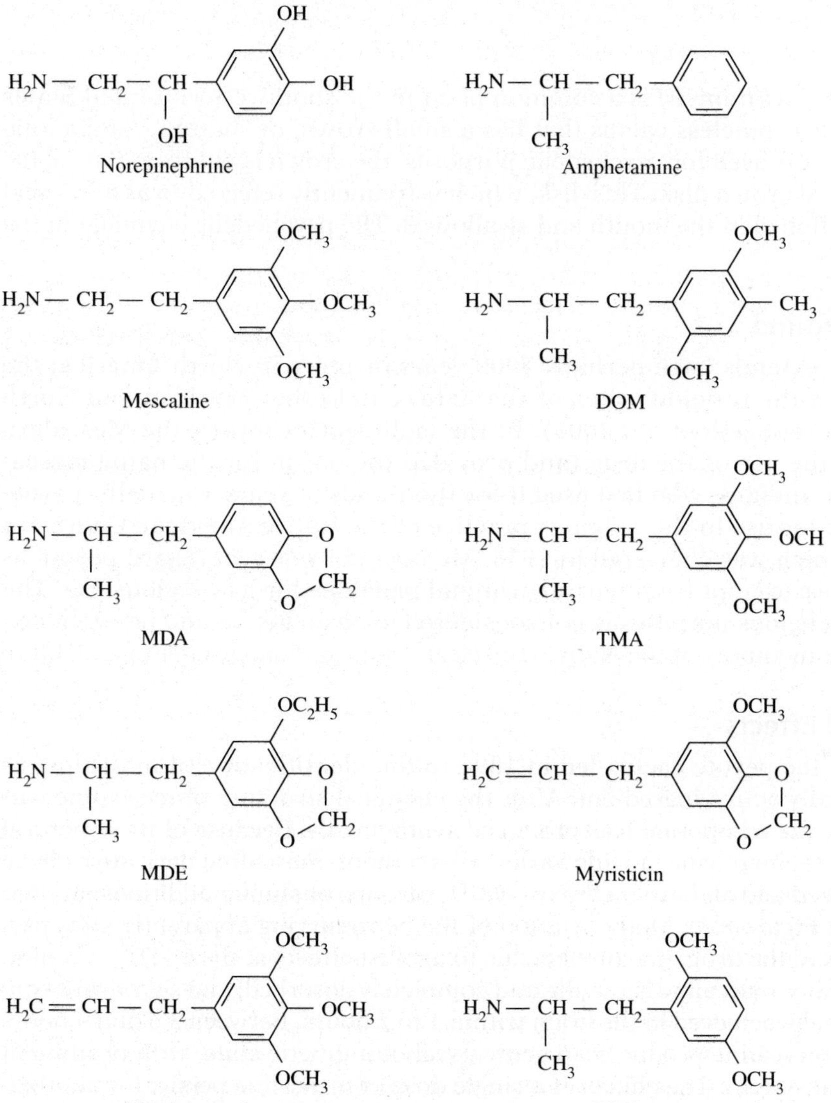

FIGURE 8.2   Structural formulas of norepinephrine (a chemical transmitter), amphetamine, and eight catecholaminelike psychedelic drugs. These eight drugs are structurally related to norepinephrine and are thought to exert their psychedelic actions by altering the transmission of nerve impulses at norepinephrine and serotonin synapses in the brain.

groups to the phenyl ring structure, which confer psychedelic properties in addition to their amphetaminelike psychostimulant properties. Methoxylated amphetamine derivatives include mescaline, DOM (also called STP), MDA, MDE, MDMA (ecstasy), MMDA, DMA, and certain drugs that are obtained from nutmeg (myristicin and elemicin). As a group, these drugs that exhibit a blend of stimulant and hallucinogenic actions have classically been referred to as *entactogens*.

Mescaline

Peyote (*Lophophora williamsii*) is a common plant in the southwestern United States and in Mexico. It is a spineless cactus that has a small crown, or "button," and a long root. When the plant is used for psychedelic purposes, the crown is cut from the cactus and dried into a hard brown disk. This disk, which is frequently referred to as a "mescal button," is later softened in the mouth and swallowed. The psychedelic chemical in the button is mescaline.

Historical Background

The use of peyote extends back perhaps 5000 years or more in North America; the cactus was used in the religious rites of the Aztecs and other Mexican and North American Indians (el-Seedi et al., 2005). In the eighteenth century, the Mescalero Apaches adopted the use of the drug (and provided the origin for the name mescaline) from Mexican Indians, who had used it for thousands of years. Currently, peyote is legally available for use in the religious practice of the Native American Church of North America, which was chartered in 1918. Members of this sect regard peyote as sacramental and are exempt from federal criminal penalties for its religious use. The use of peyote for religious purposes is not considered to be an abuse, and peyote is seldom abused by the members of the Native American Church (Fickenscher et al., 2006).

Pharmacological Effects

Early research on the peyote cactus led in 1896 to the identification of mescaline as its pharmacologically active ingredient. After the chemical structure of mescaline was elucidated in 1918, the compound was produced synthetically. Because of its structural resemblance to norepinephrine, a wide variety of synthetic mescaline derivatives have now been synthesized and all have methoxy ($-OCH_3$) groups or similar additions on their benzene rings (see Figure 8.2). Methoxylation of the benzene ring apparently adds psychedelic properties to the drug, presumably due to agonist effects at the $5-HT_{2A}$ receptor.

When taken orally, mescaline is rapidly and completely absorbed, and significant concentrations are usually achieved in the brain within 1 to 2 hours. Between 3.5 and 4 hours after drug intake, mescaline produces an acute psychotomimetic state, with prominent effects on the visual system. The effects of a single dose of mescaline persist for approximately 10 hours. The drug does not appear to be metabolized before it is excreted.

The usual oral dose (5 milligrams per kilogram body weight) in the average normal subject causes anxiety, sympathomimetic effects, hyperreflexia of the limbs, tremors, and visual hallucinations that consist of brightly colored lights, geometric designs, animals, and occasionally people; color and space perception is often concomitantly impaired, but otherwise the sensorium is normal and insight is retained.

Synthetic Amphetamine Derivatives

Methylenedioxymethamphetamine (MDMA), 2C-B, DOM, MDA, DMA, MDE, TMA, AMT, and 5-MeO-DIPT are structurally related to mescaline and methamphetamine (see Figure 8.2) and, as might be expected, produce similar effects. They have moderate behavioral stimulant effects at low doses, but as with LSD, psychedelic effects dominate as doses increase. These derivatives are considerably more potent and more toxic than mescaline.

MDMA: The Prototype Catecholamine Psychedelic

The German pharmaceutical company E. Merck developed methylenedioxymethamphetamine in about 1914 as an appetite suppressant, but this indication was not pursued. In the 1950s, during the Cold War, the United States military tested it on animals as a possible "brainwashing" drug. By the 1970s, there was interest in it as a therapeutic aid for patients undergoing psychological treatment and by the 1980s, college students started experimenting with the drug. Today it is known by its street name, "ecstasy," and is associated with the social phenomenon of the "rave," a large dance party, often with hundreds of participants, accompanied by loud electronic music, videos, light shows, and the like.

MDMA resembles MDA in structure, but may be less hallucinogenic. It is a releaser and/or reuptake inhibitor of the monoamines (5-HT, dopamine, and norepinephrine) as well as acetylcholine (Grilly and Salamone, 2012). As with other psychedelic compounds, the psychological experience is not always predictable. Nevertheless, this drug is most commonly associated with reports of "empathy," "insight," "enhanced communication," and "transcendent religious experiences." Most frequent adverse reactions are physiological, such as an increase in blood pressure and heart rate, muscle tension and jaw clenching, fatigue, insomnia, sweating, blurred vision, loss of motor coordination, and anxiety. When used during periods of intense activity, however, such as the all-night dancing that occurs during a rave, symptoms of a potentially fatal syndrome called *malignant hyperthermia* may occur. In addition to hyperthermia, the symptoms include tachycardia, disorientation, dilated pupils, convulsions, rigidity, breakdown of skeletal muscle, kidney failure, cardiac arrhythmias, and death (Hall and Henry, 2006). MDMA-precipitated malignant hyperthermia may be blocked by a drug called *dantrolene* (Duffy and Ferguson, 2007) and should an MDMA-intoxicated hyperthermic patient be taken to an emergency room in time, dantrolene can be lifesaving. (For a review of the thermal effects of MDMA in humans, see Parrott, 2012.)

Perhaps because tolerance develops rapidly to MDMA, the drug is not conducive to frequent use. In addition to tolerance, other self-reported long-term effects include the inability to concentrate, depression of mood, and (paradoxically) "feeling more open toward people" (Grilly and Salamone, 2012, 332).

More disturbing are the issues raised by chronic MDMA use. Although categorized as a catecholaminelike psychedelic, it has been established that MDMA is a potent and selective serotonin neurotoxin in both animals and humans (Gouzoulis-Mayfrank and Daumann, 2009; Urban et al., 2012). Even low doses may be neurotoxic, resulting in small but significant effects on brain microvasculature, white matter maturation, and possible axonal damage (deWin et al., 2008). In regard to specific neural structures, there is some evidence that chronic ecstasy use may produce damage to the hippocampus (den Hollander et al., 2012). Brain scans of 10 male ecstasy users, with a mean age of 25.4 years, were compared with scans of 7 non-drug–using, matched control persons, with a mean age 21.3 of years. The ecstasy users had taken an average of 281 tablets during the last 6.5 years, but were drug-free for a mean of 2 months when tested. The hippocampal volume of the ecstasy users was on average 10.5 percent smaller than that of the control group. Even though this might be considered a modest (albeit statistically significant) difference, the fact that all participants were still young adults and presumably had many more years of life is disturbing.

Although the behavioral consequences of such damage are not clear, numerous studies in humans have reported that a variety of memory functions are impaired during MDMA intoxication (Grilly and Salamone, 2012; Kuypers et al., 2011; Kuypers and Ramaekers, 2005, 2007), including everyday, real-world memory function (Hadjiefthyvoulou et al., 2011).

While it may not be surprising that acute MDMA intoxication would impair memory acutely, there is some conflict in regard to the important question of whether or not more long-lasting memory impairment is caused by chronic MDMA use. Many studies of this issue have been criticized because they did not determine if the groups of drug users and nonusers had the same initial performance on the memory tasks before drug use began. Wagner and colleagues (2013) addressed this by testing a cohort of new MDMA users between 2006 and 2009, then following up with a second assessment after 12 months. Of the initial group of 149 individuals, 109 were available 1 year later. Among these, the only illicit drug used by 43 participants was cannabis, while 23 participants used 10 or more pills of MDMA. When tested with various assessments of learning and memory, these two groups differed only on a task involving recall of visual stimuli. However, even this modest degree of cognitive impairment was not seen by Halpern and colleagues (2011), who compared illicit ecstasy users with nonusers on a battery of 15 neuropsychological tests. This study was designed to minimize the defects of other investigations by excluding persons with "significant" lifetime exposure to other illicit drugs or alcohol; requiring that all participants be members of the rave subculture; and testing breath, urine, and hair samples of all participants at the time of evaluation to exclude possible surreptitious substance use. By implementing these measures, they found little evidence of impaired cognitive function.

The issue of whether MDMA produces cognitive deficits is especially relevant because there is interest in its possible therapeutic use, as described later in this chapter. Related to that development, a series of experiments have examined the effect of MDMA on noncognitive, emotional, or social processes, often with the intent of determining possible therapeutic benefit. One study compared the different emotional states elicited by MDMA and methylphenidate in human participants. MDMA elicited what is termed *empathogenic reactions*, such as a feeling of closeness to others, openness, and trust; methylphenidate did not affect emotional reactions or empathy. MDMA increased blood levels of oxytocin and prolactin (hormones believed to be related to empathic states), but methylphenidate did not. Neither drug influenced moral judgment (Schmid et al., 2014). Another study reported that participants who ingested MDMA increased their "trustworthiness" rating of pictures of faces and increased their cooperative behavior on experimental games relative to their ratings without the drug. Ratings of "euphoria, energy, and jaw clenching," made after taking the drug, contrasted with the scores of less empathy, compassion, and trust in the absence of the drug (Stewart et al., 2014).

Baggott and colleagues (2015) investigated the effect of MDMA on speech content in 35 healthy volunteers, who received 1.5 milligrams per kilogram of oral MDMA or placebo on two successive sessions, followed by a 5-minute standardized talking task. The conversations involved a close personal relationship and were analyzed for specific categories, such as affect, social interaction, and cognition. Consistent with other reports, the drug increased the use of social words and words relating to both positive and negative emotions supporting the view that MDMA increases the "willingness to disclose." In a follow-up study, MDMA decreased anxiety about expressing emotional memories; that is, the drug had a "prosocial" action and facilitated emotional disclosure (Baggott et al., 2016). Using a laboratory test in which participants determine whether they or another person will receive money, Kirkpatrick and colleagues (2015) reported that MDMA increased generosity, supporting a "prosocial" action of the drug. According to Kamboj and colleagues (2015), MDMA elicited effects that were described as "increases in self-compassion and reductions in self-criticism."

MDMA-Related Substances

Occasionally, new MDMA-related drugs emerge. For example, *2,5-dimethoxy-4-propylthiophenethylamine* (Schifano et al., 2005) is known as "blue mystic," "2C-T-7," "T7," "tripstay," and "Tweety-Bird mescaline"; *4-bromo-2,5-dimethoxyphenethylamine* is known as "2C-B," "nexus," "2s," "toonies," "bromo," "spectrum," and "Venus." These drugs produce hallucinogenic actions with the side effects of nausea, anxiety, panic attacks, and paranoid ideation. A related agent is *4-methylmethcathinone*, or mephedrone ("M-smack"), which has been reported to be substituting for MDMA in Europe (Brunt et al., 2011) and is described in Chapter 7. This drug seems to be a cheaper and less-regulated alternative to cocaine and ecstasy, and its use is currently increasing as abuse of other drugs such as heroin, cannabis, and amphetamine decreases. Mephedrone was banned in the United Kingdom in April 2010 and almost immediately, an alternative agent, 5,6-methylenedioxy-2-aminoindane, or MDAI, took its place. (After the ban, a survey of over 300 clubbers found that users were more likely to add mephedrone to other agents, rather than replace established drugs [Moore et al., 2013]).

MDAI

First synthesized in the 1990s by Dr. David Nichols at Purdue University in the United States, MDAI was discovered accidentally during investigations of MDMA, of which it is an analogue. It is a reuptake inhibitor of serotonin, dopamine, and norepinephrine and also appears to release serotonin as well, although without producing the neurotoxicity associated with MDMA. In low doses, the drugs MDA, MDMA, and MDAI are hallucinogenic, but at higher doses they exert amphetaminelike pharmacological effects. Proponents speak of enhancing the recreational state, particularly in regard to entheogenic (spiritual) experiences, a phenomenon common to this class of drugs. In other words, users describe effects similar to those of MDMA—euphoria, empathy, and intensification of sensory experiences. However, MDAI has also been linked to reports of renal failure, acute respiratory distress, and hepatic failure. Because the first reports of its recreational use are so recent, not appearing until 2011, there is not yet much information about its prevalence and pattern of use (Gallagher et al., 2012).

The Piperazines

Another category of drugs used as an ecstasy replacement is the *piperazines*. Piperazine was originally developed as an antihelminthic (a deworming drug), but the amphetaminelike actions were eventually recognized. The best known are 1-benzylpiperazine (BZP), 1-(3-trifluoromethylphenyl) piperazine (TFMPP), and meta-chlorophenylpiperazine (mCPP) (Bossong et al., 2010). The first two drugs, BZP and TFMPP, are often taken together as a combination "party pill." Both facilitate catecholamine release from sympathetic neurons, especially from dopamine neurons. This stimulates postsynaptic alpha and beta adrenergic receptors in the central and peripheral nervous systems. BZP also blocks the reuptake of 5-HT (Schep et al., 2011). This drug was initially proposed as an antidepressant in the early 1970s, but it lacked efficacy. TFMPP affects serotonin more directly and releases it from neurons (Rosenbaum et al., 2012). There is minimal information about the pharmacokinetics of these drugs. BZP doses are typically 75 to 150 milligrams and the effects last about 6 to 8 hours. Because onset of effect may take up to 2 hours, with peak plasma concentrations reached 60 to 90 minutes after oral administration, users sometimes take multiple doses before experiencing intoxication, which can be dangerous. Both drugs presumably cross the blood–brain barrier. Elimination is essentially complete in 44 hours for BZP (which is excreted unchanged) and 24 hours for TFMPP (which undergoes many metabolic changes). When taken recreationally, low doses cause stimulant effects, while hallucinogenic actions predominate at higher doses (Rosenbaum et al., 2012). The most frequently noted symptoms include palpitations, QT prolongation, agitation, anxiety, confusion, dizziness, headache, tremor, mydriasis, insomnia, urine retention, and vomiting. Even at low doses, seizures may be elicited in some individuals and have been reported up to 8 hours after administration, for which benzodiazepine treatment alone may be sufficient. While there is not conclusive evidence of fatalities, toxicity may cause numerous organs to fail and supportive care is essential (Schep et al., 2011).

mCPP

Meta-chlorophenylpiperazine (mCPP) is a major metabolite of the psychotropic drug trazodone and may be responsible for some of its side effects, such as headaches and migraines induced many hours after initial consumption; in fact, it has been used for testing potential antimigraine medications. As a recreational substance, mCPP is actually generally considered to be an unpleasant experience and is not desired by drug users. It lacks any reinforcing effects, produces depressive and anxiogenic effects in rodents and humans, and can induce panic attacks in susceptible individuals. It also worsens obsessive-compulsive symptoms in people with the disorder. It is an agonist at practically all serotonergic receptors and may also block reuptake of and release serotonin. Its potent anorectic effects have prompted the development of selective 5-HT_{2C} receptor agonists for the treatment of obesity.

2C-B

4-Bromo-2,5-dimethoxyphenethylamine (2C-B) is a psychoactive analog of mescaline that is appearing more frequently at raves and club venues. Reported oral doses of about 20 milligrams produce perceptual effects similar to those of serotonergic agents and positive effects similar to MDMA (Caudevilla-Gálligo et al., 2012).

DOM

DOM (dimethoxymethamphetamine) has effects that are similar to those of mescaline; doses of 1 to 6 milligrams produce euphoria, which is followed by a 6- to 8-hour period of hallucinations. DOM is 100 times more potent than mescaline, but much less potent than LSD. The use of DOM is associated with a high incidence of overdose (because it is potent and street doses are poorly controlled). Acute toxic reactions are common; they consist of tremors that may eventually lead to convulsive movements, prostration, and even death. Because toxic reactions are common, the use of DOM is not widespread.

Designer Psychedelics

MDA (methylenedioxyamphetamine), *DMA* (dimethoxymethylamphetamine), *MDE* (methylenedioxyethylamphetamine), *TMA* (trimethoxyamphetamine), and other structural variations of amphetamine are encountered as "designer psychedelics." MDA is also a metabolite of MDMA, and much of MDMA's effect may be due to the presence of MDA. In general, the pharmacological effects of these drugs resemble those of mescaline and LSD; they reflect a mix of catecholamine and serotonin interactions. Side effects and toxicities (including fatalities) are similar to those of MDMA. MDA is sometimes represented as MDMA; when this occurs, MDA is more lethal in lower doses and its effects are longer lasting than those of MDMA. Confirmation of the well-established visual effects of MDA was recently obtained from the first human study to be conducted with this drug in over 30 years (Baggott et al., 2010). Consistent with typical anecdotal descriptions, MDA increased self-reports of "mystical" types of hallucinogenic effects, including visual alterations.

AMT and 5-MeO-DIPT.   In April 2003, the Drug Enforcement Administration (DEA) designated alpha-methyltryptamine (AMT) and 5-methoxy-diisopropyltryptamine (5-MeO-DIPT, or "Foxy") as Schedule I substances under the Controlled Substances Act. Administered orally, both drugs cause hallucinations, mood elevation, nervousness, insomnia, and pupillary dilation. AMT is of slow onset (3 to 4 hours) after oral administration and prolonged duration (12 to 24 hours). It is also a potent reuptake inhibitor of norepinephrine, dopamine, and serotonin (Nagai et al., 2007).

Foxy is of more rapid onset (20 to 30 minutes) and shorter duration (3 to 6 hours). It has been reported to induce an acute confusional state for several hours (Itokawa et al., 2007) and to substitute for MDMA.

Myristicin and Elemicin

Nutmeg and mace are common household spices sometimes abused for their hallucinogenic properties. Myristicin and elemicin, the pharmacologically active ingredients in nutmeg and mace, are responsible for the psychedelic action. Ingestion of large amounts (1 to 2 teaspoons—5 to 15 grams—usually brewed in tea) may, after a delay of 2 to 5 hours, induce feelings of unreality, confusion, disorientation, impending doom, depersonalization, euphoria, visual hallucinations, and acute psychotic reactions. Considering the close structural resemblance of myristicin and elemicin to mescaline (see Figure 8.2), these psychedelic actions are not unexpected. Ingestion of large quantities of nutmeg, however, produces many unpleasant side effects, including vomiting, nausea, and tremors, although deaths are infrequent.

SEROTONERGIC PSYCHEDELICS

The predominant serotoninlike psychedelic drugs are *lysergic acid diethylamide* (LSD), *psilocybin* and *psilocin*, *dimethyltryptamine* (DMT), and *bufotenine* (Figure 8.3). Because of their structural resemblance to one another and to serotonin, it has been presumed that these agents exert their effects through interactions at serotonin 5-HT$_2$ receptors (Geyer and Vollenweider, 2008). Nevertheless, their specific mechanism of action has been difficult to determine. It is generally accepted that the subjective effects are mediated by postsynaptic 5-HT$_2$ receptors. This is consistent with the observation that the affinity for these receptors is highly correlated with their hallucinogenic potency in humans and with the fact that many, but not all, 5-HT$_2$ antagonists block this effect. Current evidence suggests that 5-HT$_{1A}$, 5-HT$_{2A}$, and 5-HT$_{2C}$ receptor subtypes may all be involved in the hallucinogenic effects, that some of these receptors may be located presynaptically and some postsynaptically, and that depending on the receptor, some of the drugs may act as agonists, partial agonists, or antagonists (Grilly and Salamone, 2012). There is also evidence from nonhuman studies that these drugs exert their hallucinogenic effects in the brain by acting on the locus coeruleus and the cerebral cortex.

Lysergic Acid Diethylamide (LSD): The Prototype Serotonergic Psychedelic

During the mid-1960s and early 1970s, LSD became one of the most remarkable and controversial drugs known. In doses that are so small that they might even be considered infinitesimal, LSD induces remarkable psychological changes, enhancing self-awareness and altering internal reality, while causing relatively few alterations in the general physiology of the body.

Historical Background

LSD was first synthesized in 1938 by Albert Hofmann (who died in 2008 at the age of 102), a Swiss chemist. His work was part of an organized research program to investigate possible therapeutic uses of compounds obtained from ergot, a natural product derived from a fungus (*Claviceps purpurea*). Early pharmacological studies of LSD in animals failed to reveal anything unusual; the psychedelic action was neither sought nor expected. Thus, LSD remained unnoticed until 1943, when Hofmann (1994) had an unusual experience:

> In the afternoon of 16 April, 1943, . . . I was seized by a peculiar sensation of vertigo and restlessness. Objects, as well as the shape of my associates in the laboratory, appeared to undergo optical changes. I was unable to concentrate on my work. In a dream-like state I left for home, where an irresistible urge to lie down overcame me. I drew the

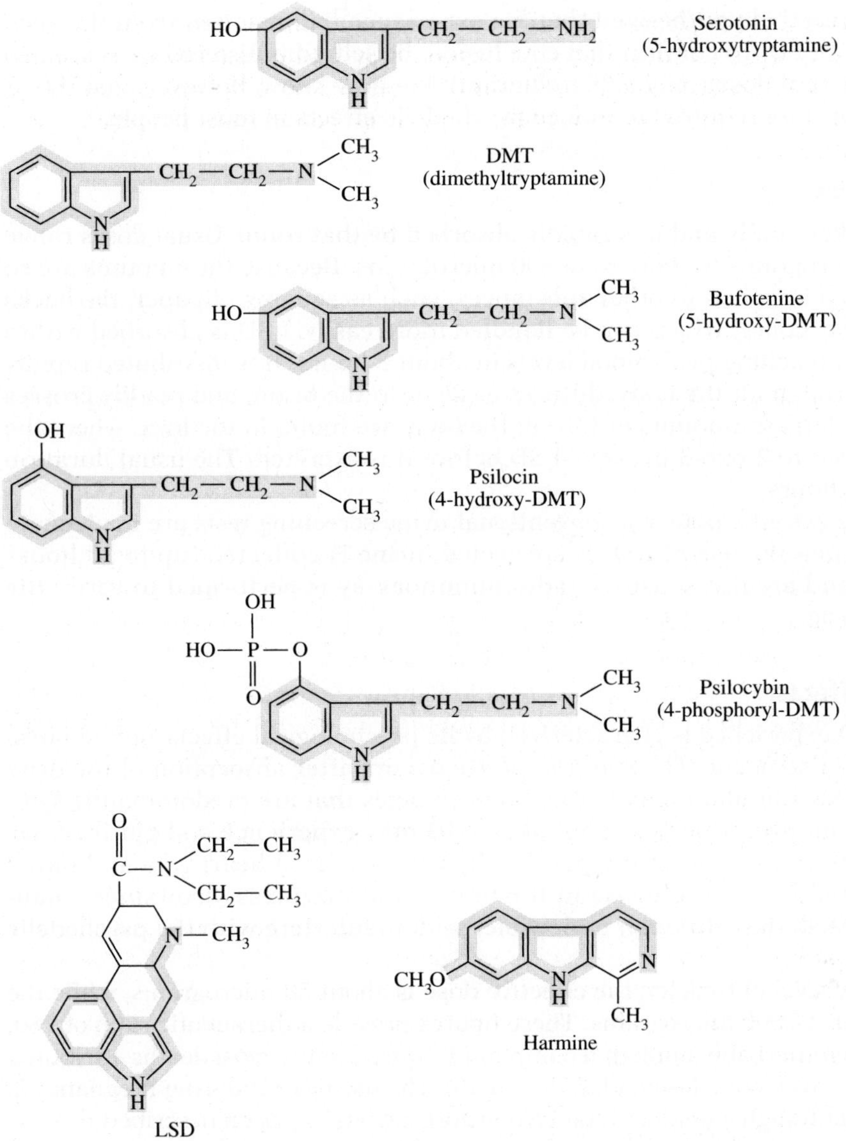

FIGURE 8.3 Structural formulas of serotonin (a chemical transmitter) and six serotoninlike psychedelic drugs. These six drugs are structurally related to serotonin (as indicated by the shading) and are thought to exert their psychedelic actions through alterations of serotonin synapses in the brain. Although LSD is structurally much more complex than serotonin, the basic similarity of the two molecules is apparent.

curtains and immediately fell into a peculiar state similar to drunkenness, characterized by an exaggerated imagination. With my eyes closed, fantastic pictures of extraordinary plasticity and intensive color seemed to surge toward me. After two hours, this state gradually wore off. (80)

Hofmann correctly hypothesized that his experience had resulted from the accidental ingestion of LSD. To confirm that conclusion, he self-administered what seemed to be a minuscule oral dose (only 0.25 milligram). We now know, however, that this is about 10 times the dose required to induce psychedelic effects in most people.

Pharmacokinetics

LSD is usually taken orally and it is rapidly absorbed by that route. Usual doses range from about 25 micrograms to more than 300 micrograms. Because the amounts are so small, LSD is often attached to other substances, such as squares of paper, the backs of stamps, or sugar cubes, which can be handled more easily. LSD is absorbed within about 60 minutes, reaching peak blood levels in about 3 hours. It is distributed rapidly and efficiently throughout the body, diffuses easily into the brain, and readily crosses the placenta. The largest amounts of LSD in the body are found in the liver, where the drug is metabolized to 2-oxo-3-hydroxy-LSD before it is excreted. The usual duration of action is 6 to 8 hours.

Because of its extreme potency, conventional urine screening tests are inadequate to detect LSD. When the use of LSD is suspected, urine is collected (up to 30 hours after ingestion) and an ultrasensitive radioimmunoassay is performed to verify the presence of the drug.

Physiological Effects

Although the LSD experience is characterized by its psychological effects, subtle physiological changes also occur. The *somatic phase* occurs after absorption of the drug and consists of CNS stimulation and autonomic changes that are predominantly sympathomimetic in nature. A person who takes LSD may experience a slight increase in body temperature; dilation of the pupils; slightly increased heart rate and blood pressure; increased levels of glucose in the blood; and dizziness, drowsiness, nausea, and other effects that although noticeable, seldom interfere with the psychedelic experience.

LSD has a low level of toxicity; the effective dose is about 50 micrograms, while the lethal dose is about 14,000 micrograms. These figures provide a therapeutic ratio of 280, making the drug a remarkably nonlethal compound; consequently most deaths attributed to LSD result from accidents, homicides, or suicide. The use of LSD during pregnancy is certainly unwise, although a distinct fetal LSD syndrome has not been described.

Psychological Effects

The psychological effects of LSD are intense. Doses of 25 to 50 micrograms produce alterations in perception, thinking, emotion, arousal, and self-image. The *sensory* (or *perceptual*) *phase* is characterized by sensory distortions and pseudohallucinations, which are the effects desired by the drug user. Time is slowed or distorted. Sensory input is intensified, with enhanced visualization of previously seen or imagined objects and decreased vigilance and logical thought. Visual alterations are the most characteristic phenomena; they typically include colored lights, distorted perceptions, and vivid and fascinating images and shapes. Colors can be heard and sounds may be seen.

The *psychic phase* signals a maximum drug effect, with changes in mood, disruption of thought processes, altered perception of time, depersonalization, true hallucinations, and psychotic episodes. The loss of boundaries and the fear of fragmentation create a need for a structuring or supporting environment and experienced companions. During the "trip," distressing thoughts and memories can emerge. Mood may be labile, shifting from depression to gaiety, from elation to fear. Tension and anxiety may mount and reach panic proportions. Such an experience is considered a "bad trip."

Carhart-Harris and colleagues (2016) from Dr. Nutt's laboratory have investigated the neurobiological effects of the drug. As might be expected, LSD, given to 20 healthy volunteers, increased activity in the visual areas of the brain, which was associated with the perceived hallucinations. But under the influence of the drug, many other brain areas were also activated, even though the participants closed their eyes. In effect, the drug appeared to enhance the visual experience of their imagination by increasing the connectivity between the visual cortex and other brain regions. The effect was described as producing a more "integrated and unified" brain (Figure 8.4.) Listening to music while taking LSD also intensified the neural responses as well as the visual imagery (Kaelen et al., 2016).

On the basis of their neuroimaging studies, Dr. Nutt and colleagues have proposed a general model of psychedelic action. Their theory considers the mental state produced by psychedelics to be an example of a "primitive" consciousness. Primitive states of consciousness are considered to be less structured and less organized than normal waking states. The experience is similar to primitive states that are not drug induced, such as REM (rapid eye movement or dream) sleep or some psychotic conditions, and they argue that studying psychedelic-induced experiences might offer some insight into these non-drug–induced primitive states (Carhart-Harris et al., 2014; Nour et al., 2016).

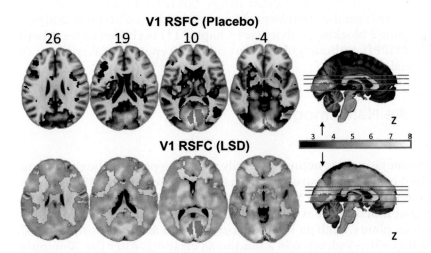

FIGURE 8.4 The areas that contributed to vision were more active under LSD, as seen by the increased color in the brain images, which was linked to hallucinations. [Dr. Robin Carhart-Harris, Imperial College London.]

Tolerance and Dependence

Tolerance of both the psychological and physiological alterations induced by LSD readily and rapidly develops, and cross-tolerance occurs between LSD and other psychedelics. Tolerance is lost within several days after the user stops taking the drug.

Physical dependence on LSD does not develop, even when the drug is used repeatedly for a prolonged period of time. In fact, most heavy users of the drug say that they ceased using LSD because they tired of it, had no further need for it, or had had enough. Even when the drug is discontinued because of concern about bad trips or about physical or mental harm, few withdrawal signs are exhibited. Laboratory animals do not self-administer LSD.

Adverse Reactions and Toxicity

Unpleasant experiences with LSD may involve an uncontrollable drift into confusion or dissociative, psychotic, or acute panic reactions, perhaps triggered by a reliving of earlier traumatic experiences. LSD and related substances have a unique action: after the acute effect of these drugs dissipates, some of the symptoms that occurred during the intoxicated state may return (Lerner et al., 2002). These symptoms are mainly visual and defined by either of two terms, flashback, or hallucinogen persisting perception disorder (HPPD), which are used fairly synonymously. As explained by Lerner, a "flashback is usually a short-term, nondistressing, spontaneous, recurrent, reversible, and benign condition accompanied by a pleasant affect … HPPD is a generally long-term, distressing, spontaneous, recurrent, pervasive, either slowly reversible or irreversible nonbenign condition accompanied by an unpleasant dysphoric affect" (Lerner et al., 2002; see also Johnson et al., 2008). Although these phenomena can occur without warning, they are most likely to appear just before sleep or when a person enters a dark environment.

Treatment of flashbacks and HPPD has been symptomatic. Case reports note the success of benzodiazepines as well as other drugs, but there is no consensus on appropriate therapy and no specific treatment. Most commonly, an atypical antipsychotic drug with serotonin-2 blocking activity (see Chapter 11) is chosen to treat both acute LSD toxicity and HPPD, although older literature has reported exacerbation of LSD-like panic and visual symptoms.

Other Serotoninlike Hallucinogens

DMT

DMT (dimethyltryptamine) is a short-acting, naturally occurring psychedelic compound that can be synthesized easily and is structurally related to serotonin. DMT produces LSD-like effects in the user, and like LSD, it is a partial agonist at $5\text{-}HT_2$ receptors. Widely used throughout much of the world, DMT is an active component of various types of South American plants, such as *Virola calophylla* and *Mimosa hostilis*. Used by itself, DMT is snorted or smoked, often in a marijuana cigarette. After the 30-minute period of effect, the user returns to normal feelings and perceptions—thus the nicknames "lunch-hour drug," "businessman's lunch," and "businessman's LSD."

Interestingly, although DMT is commonly thought to exert its psychedelic effect through action of 5-HT_{2A} receptors, Su and coworkers (2009) demonstrated binding to sigma-1 receptors as a possible mode of action.[2]

In 1994, Strassman and coworkers conducted controlled investigations of DMT in "highly motivated," experienced hallucinogen users. When it was administered intravenously (0.04 to 0.4 milligram per kilogram of body weight), onset of action occurred within 2 minutes and was negligible at 30 minutes. DMT elevated blood pressure, heart rate, and temperature; dilated pupils; and increased body endorphin and hormone levels. The psychedelic threshold dose was 0.2 milligram per kilogram of body weight. Hallucinogenic effects included a rapidly moving, brightly colored visual display of images. Auditory effects were less common. "Loss of control" associated with a brief but overwhelming "rush" led to a dissociated state in which euphoria alternated or coexisted with anxiety.

DMT is one of two main ingredients in *ayahuasca* (also called *hoasca*), a psycho-active beverage that has been drunk as a tea for centuries in religious, spiritual, and medicinal contexts by Amazon Indians in the rainforests of South America. The other main ingredient is harmine, a substance that is a potent monoamine oxidase, or MAO, inhibitor. Effects have an onset of about 30 to 60 minutes, peak at 1 to 2 hours, and persist for about 3 to 4 hours. In most cases, effects are well tolerated, but disorientation, paranoia, and anxiety may occur. In religious ceremonial use, such reactions are unusual (Gable, 2007).

Bufotenine

Bufotenine (5-hydroxy DMT or dimethylserotonin), like LSD and DMT, is a potent serotonin agonist hallucinogen with an affinity for several types of serotonin receptors, especially the 5-HT_{2A} receptor. The name *bufotenine* comes from the name for a toad of the genus *Bufo*, whose skin and glandular secretions supposedly produce hallucino-genic effects when ingested.

After subcutaneous injection into rats, the half-life of bufotenine is about 2 hours, with MAO responsible for metabolism. Bufotenine is not found in the bodies of normal people. However, it can be produced in an alternative and unusual pathway for the metabolic breakdown of serotonin. Indeed, some have attempted to correlate the presence of bufotenine in urine with various psychiatric disorders, although this theory is not generally accepted.

Psilocybin

Psilocybin (4-phosphoryl-DMT) and psilocin (4-hydroxy-DMT) are two psychedelic agents that are found in many species of mushrooms that belong to the genera *Psilo-cybe, Panaeolus, Copelandia,* and *Conocybe*. As Figure 8.3 shows, the only difference between psilocybin and psilocin is that psilocybin contains a molecule of phosphoric acid. After the mushroom has been ingested, phosphoric acid is enzymatically removed from psilocybin, thus producing psilocin, the active psychedelic agent.

---

[2] Formerly thought to be a type of opioid receptor, the sigma-1 receptor is actually an endoplasmic reticulum protein implicated in neuroprotection, neuronal plasticity, anxiety, and depression (Hashimoto, 2009; Maurice and Su, 2009; Paschos et al., 2009).

Psilocybin exerts an agonist effect at serotonin 5-HT$_{2A}$ and 5-HT$_{1A}$ receptors, similar to the effects of other serotonin psychedelics, at about 0.25 milligram per kilogram of body weight when ingested. Psilocybin-containing mushrooms grow throughout much of the world, including the northwestern United States. Psilocin and psilocybin are approximately 1/200th as potent as LSD; their effects peak in about 2 hours and last about 6 to 10 hours. Unlike DMT, psilocin and psilocybin are absorbed effectively when taken orally; the mushrooms are eaten raw to induce psychedelic effects.

There is great variation in the concentration of psilocybin and psilocin among the different species of mushrooms, as well as significant differences among mushrooms of the same species. For example, the usual oral dose of *Psilocybe semilanceata* (liberty caps) may consist of 10 to 40 mushrooms, while the dose for *Psilocybe cyanescens* may be only 2 to 5 mushrooms. Also, some extremely toxic species of mushrooms are not psychoactive, but they bear a superficial resemblance to the mushrooms that contain psilocybin and psilocin. Because the effects of psilocybin so closely resemble those produced by LSD, the "psilocybin" sold illicitly may *be* LSD, and ordinary mushrooms laced with LSD may be sold as "magic mushrooms."

Although the psychedelic effects of *Psilocybe mexicana* are part of Indian folklore, *Psilocybe* intoxication was not described until 1955, when Gordon Wasson, a New York banker, traveled through Mexico. He mingled with native tribes and was allowed to participate in a *Psilocybe* ceremony, during which he consumed the magic mushroom and described his own hallucinatory experience.

Ololiuqui

Ololiuqui is a naturally occurring substance in morning glory seeds that is used by Central and South American Indians as an intoxicant and hallucinogen. The drug is used ritually for spiritual communication, as are the extracts of most plants that contain psychedelic drugs. The use of ololiuqui seeds in Central and South America was first described by the sixteenth-century Spanish explorer Francisco Hernandez de Cordoba, who is said to have reported, "When the priests wanted to commune with their Gods, [they ate ololiuqui seeds and a thousand visions and] satanic hallucinations appeared to them" (Brecher, 1972).

The seeds were analyzed in Europe by Albert Hofmann, the discoverer of LSD, who identified several components, one of which was lysergic acid amide (not LSD). The lysergic acid amide that Hofmann identified is approximately one-tenth as active as LSD as a psychoactive agent. However, considering the extreme potency of LSD, lysergic acid amide is still quite potent.

Side effects of ololiuqui include nausea, vomiting, headache, increased blood pressure, dilated pupils, and sleepiness. These side effects are usually quite intense and serve to limit the recreational use of ololiuqui. Ingestion of 100 or more seeds produces sleepiness, distorted perception, hallucinations, and confusion. Flashbacks have been reported, but they are infrequent.

Harmine

Harmine is a psychedelic agent that is obtained from the seeds of *Peganum harmala*, a plant native to the Middle East, and from *Banisteriopsis caapi* of the South American tropics. Intoxication by harmine is usually accompanied by nausea.

Therapeutic Applications of the Monoaminergic Hallucinogens

The first North American study of LSD in humans was conducted in 1949 and during the 1950s, large quantities of LSD were distributed to scientists for research purposes. A significant impetus for research was the notion that the effects of LSD might constitute a model for psychosis, which would provide some insight into the biochemical and physiological processes of schizophrenia and its treatment (Passie et al., 2008; see Liester, 2014, and Das et al., 2016 for historical descriptions of therapeutic applications of LSD). But that was not the case. Drug-induced hallucinations are mostly visual and usually involve distortions of the environment that are generally considered pleasant or neutral. The person taking LSD is very suggestible and concerned about relationships to other people. In contrast, schizophrenic hallucinations are usually auditory, often unpleasant and threatening, and are derived from the user's internal mental state, not from the external environmental context. Schizophrenic patients are not very suggestible and are not greatly affected by interpersonal interactions. People with schizophrenia who have taken LSD acknowledge that it is different from a psychotic experience (Grilly and Salamone, 2012).

Alternatively, as early as the 1950s, a few psychiatrists began to study the drug as a possible treatment for alcoholism and other mental disorders. One of these, Humphrey Osmund, coined the term *psychedelic*, meaning "mind manifesting." Between the 1950s and 1960, Osmund and various colleagues treated about 2000 alcoholic patients, concluded that a single large dose of LSD could be an effective treatment for alcoholism, and noted that between 40 and 45 percent of their patients given the drug had not experienced a relapse after a year. Similar outcomes were reported by another psychiatrist, Ronald Sandison, who treated psychiatric patients with LSD (although years later, in 2002, 43 of those patients received an out-of-court-settlement from the British National Service).

Two types of therapeutic methods were developed during this time. In one approach, called *psychedelic therapy*, a large dose of LSD was administered in conjunction with psychotherapy; in the other method, called *psycholytic therapy*, several smaller doses, gradually increasing in amount, were administered together with psychoanalysis. Between 1950 and 1965, some 40,000 patients were prescribed one of these forms of LSD therapy as part of treatments for a variety of psychological and psychiatric disorders, including autism. Although the studies may not have been as rigorous as a clinical trial, the results seemed promising. In 1960, a physician named Sydney Cohen reported on the results of 44 physicians who had administered 25,000 doses of LSD or mescaline to 5000 people under widely varying conditions. He found no serious adverse outcomes or addictive signs that he attributed to the drug.

Nevertheless, this therapeutic approach died out. Several reasons have been proposed for this lack of follow-up. First, the psychiatric profession did not develop reliable protocols and measures for the consistent therapeutic use of these agents. Second, the dramatic increase in recreational use of the psychedelic drugs in the 1960s, epitomized by the phrase coined by Dr. Timothy Leary, "turn on, tune in, and drop out," led to the perception that such drugs were a public health problem. When new safety rules for drugs were approved by Congress in 1962, LSD was listed as an experimental agent by the FDA, which meant that research involving its actions became restricted. Within the year, the drug was sold on the street, often in sugar cubes soaked with the liquid formulation. As a drug of abuse, it was associated with antiwar protests, and subsequently prohibited by the federal government in 1968, which made it a felony for anyone to possess it (Costandi, 2014).

The third reason for the lack of therapeutic study of psychedelics was the top-secret experiments (code named MKUltra) conducted by the Central Intelligence Agency (CIA) and other governmental and military entities. From about 1953 and throughout the 1970s, high doses of potent psychedelic drugs were given to unwitting servicemen as part of research programs prompted by concerns about Cold War enemies. Some of these soldiers eventually sued the United States government with varied success for mental or emotional problems they suffered as a result of these involuntary drug exposures. One of the most dramatic cases resulting from those unethical experiments was the case of Frank Olsson, an Army scientist who died after falling out of a New York hotel window in 1953, nine days after he was given LSD without his knowledge. His family was told he committed suicide, but in 1975 a commission appointed by then-President Ford disclosed for the first time that Olsson had been an unwitting drug subject. In 1996, the Manhattan District Attorney's Office opened a homicide investigation, but was unable to bring charges.

As a result of these social and cultural developments, LSD and similar psychedelic drugs were placed in the Schedule I category of abused substances not generally considered useful in a therapeutic context.

The situation began to change in the 1990s when the Food and Drug Administration (FDA) approved the first human clinical studies of psychedelic drugs in a quarter of a century. After more than two decades, Dr. Rick Strassman studied DMT in 1992. Unlike the more widely known psychedelics, DMT had much less of a stigma, allowing Strassman to get his studies approved far more easily. In the same year, the FDA also passed the Prescription Drug User Fee Act, which encouraged research on new drugs.

In addition, since 1986, a nonprofit research organization, the Multidisciplinary Association for Psychedelic Studies (MAPS), has tried to get permission to study the therapeutic potential of psychedelic drugs such as ecstasy and cannabis. In 2004, Michael Mithoefer, a psychiatrist in Charleston, South Carolina, was the first to win FDA approval for clinical studies using MDMA to treat posttraumatic stress disorder (PTSD). In 2011, the results of the first completed clinical trial were published, assessing MDMA as a therapeutic addition to psychotherapy (Mithoefer et al., 2011, 2013). Twenty patients with chronic PTSD received psychotherapy over 20 to 30 sessions; 12 patients also received the drug and 8 received placebo in 2 of these sessions (lasting 8 hours) scheduled a few weeks apart. Two months later, 10 out of 12 patients who had received the drug responded to treatment, while only 2 out of the 8 placebo patients showed improvement. These 12 patients, plus 7 of the initial placebo patients who subsequently chose to take the drug, participated in a long-term follow-up session. After a mean of 45.4 months since the MDMA session, 16 of those 19 maintained their clinical benefit. While a subsequent effort to replicate this result with 12 different patients suffering from treatment-resistant PTSD did not produce any significant benefit from the drug, some positive effects have been supported (Oehen et al., 2013). Amoroso and Workman (2016) found that MDMA-assisted psychotherapy for PTSD was significantly more effective and resulted in fewer dropouts than the alternate option of exposure therapy. In 2017, MAPS will test MDMA as a treatment for PTSD. If it is successful, the FDA may move to legalize MDMA-assisted therapy. Presumably this decision will take into account the evidence cited earlier regarding brain damage from chronic MDMA exposure.

Similarly, there has been a resurgence of studies with psilocybin as an adjunct to psychotherapy for obsessive-compulsive disorder (Moreno, 2006) and depression and end-of-life anxiety in cancer (Grob et al., 2011). (This drug may have been chosen because although chemically similar to LSD, it does not have the same negative historical associations). As little as one dose of psilocybin—sufficient to induce changes in perception and mysticallike experiences—significantly decreased anxiety and depression for up to six months in patients with life-threatening cancer (Griffiths, 2015). Patients who received a high dose of psilocybin showed significantly less anxiety and depression at follow-up five weeks later compared with patients who received a low dose of the drug, and maintained the benefit for six months. One group of 12 patients had been clinically depressed for a significant amount of time—17.8 years on average—and had not responded to standard medications, such as selective serotonin reuptake inhibitors (SSRIs). A week after receiving an oral dose of psilocybin, all patients experienced a marked improvement in their symptoms. After three months, five patients were in complete remission (Carhart-Harris et al., 2016). Patients with anxiety associated with life-threatening diseases gained significant relief from LSD-associated psychotherapy that lasted for at least 12 months (Gasser et al., 2015). Further support for the benefit of psilocybin in treating depression and anxiety in patients with life-threatening cancer was provided by two clinical trials: Griffiths and colleagues (2016) and Ross and colleagues (2016). In each case, a single dose of the drug (approximately 0.3 to 0.43 milligrams per kilograms across the two studies) relieved significant symptoms of depression and anxiety for up to six months or more in 60 to 80 percent of the patients. A review of psychedelics in the treatment of unipolar mood disorder, even in the absence of a life-threatening disease, found an overall average of 79.2 percent of patients exhibited clinically relevant improvement (Rucker et al., 2016). These reviews and a series of corresponding commentaries were published in a single issue of the *Journal of Psychopharmacology*, which exclusively discussed the resurgence of interest in the neuropsychiatric possibilities of psychedelic agents.

Psilocybin has also shown promise in treating addiction to drugs such as tobacco (Johnson et al., 2014) or alcohol (Bogenschutz and Pommy, 2012; Bogenschutz et al., 2015). One review of clinical trials for alcoholism concluded that even one dose of LSD given in conjunction with other treatment was useful in reducing alcohol misuse (Krebs and Johansen, 2012).

Even ayahuasca has been re-evaluated for a variety of therapeutic applications, including psychiatric disorders. In a recent study, researchers gave one mild dose of ayahuasca to six volunteers who had been diagnosed with mild to severe depression that was unresponsive to at least one conventional antidepressant drug. None had drunk ayahuasca before. According to the investigators, the drink began to reduce depression in patients within hours and the effect was still present after three weeks. Because there were no placebo controls, it cannot be assumed that improvements were due solely to the pharmacological properties of the drug independent of the ritualistic spiritual and sociological context (Frood, 2015). Further trials are planned although understandably, it is not easy to conduct placebo-controlled studies with hallucinogenic compounds. Frecska and colleagues (2016) provide an extensive review of the biochemical and pharmacological characteristics of this plant combination, including possible benefits for numerous neurodegenerative, metabolic, and psychiatric disorders. A systematic review of human studies was conducted by dos Santos and colleagues

(2016), who evaluated the current evidence for neuropsychiatric effects of ayahuasca. According to their assessment, the drug was well tolerated and improved mood, altered visual perception, increased introspection, and had positive long-term effects on cognition and on spirituality.

Some studies conducted in healthy persons have replicated historical descriptions of "mystical experiences" (McLean et al., 2011) and other emotionally positive effects of vivid imagery (Carhart-Harris et al., 2012a; Studerus et al., 2012). In one study, researchers injected volunteers with psilocybin and then observed their brains via functional magnetic resonance imaging (fMRI) (Carhart-Harris et al., 2012b). They were surprised to see that instead of an increase in brain activity (which they expected), they saw decreases in brain activity, which were negatively correlated with the intensity of the psychedelic experience. Psilocybin produced responses that looked like the brain of someone in deep meditation. The areas with decreased activity were the same as those that are overactive in depression. A study published in October 2014 compared brain scans of subjects given psilocybin with scans of their brains without the drug. The drug appeared to change connectivity of cortical brain sites; areas were linked that were not typically connected. These kinds of rearrangements might be therapeutically beneficial, for example, in helping people to reprocess anxiety or depression.

People with depressed moods have a tendency to dwell on the past, a characteristic referred to as "mental time travel." It is thought that the brain circuit which mediates this phenomenon, the default-mode network (DMN), may be stronger in people with depression. To determine whether LSD could reduce the extent of "mental time travel," researchers gave nondepressed volunteers either LSD or a placebo, took fMRI brain scans, and interviewed the participants. They reported that subjects given LSD made fewer references to the past and had weaker DMN connections than those given placebo (Speth et al., 2016).

Several books have now been published in this area (Brown, 2013; Roberts, 2013; Sessa, 2012); and Bogenschutz and Johnson (2016) provide an update on the therapeutic applications of psychedelic drugs for addiction.

Did You Know?

Documenting the Complex Relationship Between Humans and Psychoactives
Founded in 1995, Erowid is a nonprofit educational and harm-reduction resource with 60,000 pages of online information about psychoactive plants and chemicals including over 350 drugs (https://www.erowid.org/). Erowid's mission is to "provide and facilitate access to objective, accurate, and non-judgmental information" about psychoactive substances (Erowid, n.d.). Begun by a couple, a man called "Earth Erowid" and a woman called "Fire Erowid," now in their forties, it has grown from only a few "hits" a day to at least 17 million unique inquiries in 2014 (Witt, 2015). The core of the site is called "Plants and Drugs," which has sections ("vaults") that provide information on individual drugs, including both positive and negative effects, history, and legal status. The contents are a combination of experiential reports submitted by individuals who have used the substances as well as information from the scientific literature. Each submission undergoes examination and review by trained volunteers, ranging from college students to computer scientists, before being posted. Descriptions of each substance include benefits and risks as well as warnings about dangerous activities during intoxication.

GLUTAMINERGIC NMDA RECEPTOR ANTAGONISTS

Phencyclidine and Ketamine

Phencyclidine (PCP, angel dust) and ketamine ("Special K"), shown in Figure 8.5, are structurally unrelated to other psychedelic drugs. They were first developed as safer surgical anesthetics because they produce less respiratory depression. This was successful in that unlike other anesthetics, the lethal dose of PCP is 10 times the anesthetic dose and, at appropriate doses, it also reduces pain reactions while maintaining blood pressure and heart rate. Unfortunately, however, it was later found that these two drugs also produced a unique psychedelic or dissociative state.

Phencyclidine was developed in 1956 and was briefly used as an anesthetic in humans before being abandoned because of a high incidence of psychiatric reactions (described below), but is still used as a veterinary anesthetic. *Ketamine* (Ketalar), which resembles phencyclidine structurally, was developed as a replacement shortly after the prominent psychedelic properties of phencyclidine were identified. Introduced in 1960, ketamine induces a phencyclidinelike anesthetic state in low doses, with similar but less severe psychiatric side effects. Ketamine is still used in special situations, such as in pediatric and veterinary anesthesia, and in the field (where there is limited equipment to counter respiratory depression). It is also occasionally used in patients who cannot tolerate the cardiovascular depressant effects of other anesthetics.

Currently, ketamine has shown some evidence that it might represent a new class of antidepressant. Injections of ketamine appear to produce rapid antidepressant effects in treatment-resistant patients. Unfortunately, so far, even patients who responded repeatedly relapsed within weeks. Nevertheless, research into this possible therapeutic action is ongoing, as discussed in Chapter 12.

In addition to possible antidepressant use, the altered perception, disorganized thought, cognitive dysfunction, suspiciousness, confusion, and lack of cooperation elicited by these drugs resembles both the positive and negative symptoms of a schizophrenic state. In fact, both PCP and ketamine can induce symptoms that are almost indistinguishable from those associated with schizophrenia (Mouri et al., 2007) and they exacerbate psychosis in schizophrenia patients, although infrequent users do not develop schizophrenia. Nevertheless, this phenomenon has led to a glutamatergic model of schizophrenia (see Chapter 11) and experimental evaluation of glutamatergic agents as antipsychotic medications.

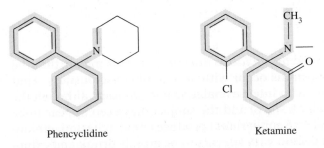

Phencyclidine   Ketamine

FIGURE 8.5 Structural formulas of the psychedelic anesthetic drugs phencyclidine and ketamine.

Abuse of phencyclidine and ketamine began in the mid-1960s (Wolff and Winstock, 2006), but was not common until the 1990s, when ketamine showed up as an adulterant to ecstasy tablets. Phencyclidine may be sold as "crystal," "angel dust," "hog," "PCP," "THC," "cannabinol," or "mescaline." When sold as crystal or angel dust (street names for methamphetamine), concentrations vary between 50 and 90 percent; when purchased under other names or in concoctions, the amount of PCP falls to between 10 and 30 percent; the typical street dose is about 5 milligrams. Phencyclidine can be eaten, snorted, or injected (usually intramuscularly, rarely intravenously), but it is most often smoked, or sprinkled on tobacco, parsley, or marijuana. Ketamine is typically not taken orally because it is metabolized to norketamine, which is less psychedelic and more sedative. Currently, these are increasing in popularity as club drugs.

Pharmacokinetics

When smoked, peak effects occur in about 15 minutes, when about 40 percent of the dose appears in the user's bloodstream. Oral absorption of PCP is slow; maximum blood levels are reached in about 2 hours. The elimination half-life is about 18 hours but ranges from about 11 to 51 hours. A positive urine assay is assumed to indicate that PCP was used within the previous week. Because false-positive test results are common, a positive assay requires secondary confirmation.

Mechanism of Action

Phencyclidine and ketamine both exert their psychotomimetic, analgesic, and amnestic actions primarily as a result of binding as noncompetitive antagonists of the *N*-methyl-*D*-aspartate (NMDA)/glutamate receptors. In addition, these drugs may block acetylcholine receptors and dopamine reuptake, induce dopamine release, and act as a partial agonist at dopamine 2 receptors (Morgan and Curran, 2011). These actions support the current view that NMDA receptor dysfunction is involved in the pathophysiology of schizophrenia (see Chapter 11).

Phencyclidine and ketamine inhibit NMDA receptors by two mechanisms: (1) blockade of the open channel by occupying a site within the channel in the receptor protein (as discussed earlier for phencyclidine); and (2) reduction in the frequency of NMDA channel opening by binding to a second attachment site on the outside of the receptor protein. As noted, PCP and ketamine are powerful analgesic drugs. The mechanism seems to be twofold: these two drugs (1) block NMDA-glutamate receptors in the spinal cord; and (2) activate descending analgesic pathways, pathways that appear to involve norepinephrine and dopamine.

Psychological Effects

Phencyclidine and ketamine are termed *dissociative anesthetics*. This means that the analgesia, amnesia, and sensory distortions occur without loss of consciousness. That is, they produce an unresponsive state with intense analgesia and amnesia, although the subject's eyes remain open (with a blank stare) and the subject may even appear to be awake. Phencyclidine in low doses (1 to 5 milligrams) produces mild agitation, euphoria, disinhibition, or excitement in a person who appears to be grossly drunk and exhibits a blank stare. The subject may be rigid and unable to speak. In many cases, however, the subject is communicative but does not respond to pain. At low doses, ketamine

produces similar effects; distortions of time and space, hallucinations, and mild dissociative effects. Users reportedly describe its effects as "melting into the surroundings,"
"visual hallucinations," "out-of-body experiences," and "giggliness" (Stewart, 2011).
At large doses, ketamine induces a more severe dissociation referred to as the "k-hole,"
in which the detachment experienced by users is so intense that their perceptions
appear completely divorced from their previous reality (Morgan and Curran, 2011).
Subjects may become withdrawn, negativistic, and unable to maintain a cognitive set;
they manifest concrete, impoverished, idiosyncratic, and bizarre responses to questions.

High doses induce a state of coma or stupor. However, abusers tend to titrate their
dose to maximize the intoxicant effect while attempting to avoid unconsciousness.
Blood pressure usually becomes elevated, but respiration does not become depressed.
The patient may recover within 2 to 4 hours, although a state of confusion and cognitive poverty may last for 8 to 72 hours. The disruption of sensory input by PCP causes
unpredictable, exaggerated, distorted, or violent reactions to environmental stimuli,
which may be augmented by PCP-induced analgesia and amnesia. Massive oral overdoses involving up to 1 gram of street-purchased PCP result in prolonged periods of
stupor or coma, followed by a prolonged recovery phase marked by confusion and
delusions lasting as long as 2 weeks. In some people, this state of confusion may be
followed by a psychosis that lasts from several weeks to a few months.

Side Effects and Toxicity

With regard to lethality, these drugs have a wide margin of safety. Ketamine, for example, has exhibited no adverse outcomes, even in medical settings with marked overdoses.
Even coughing and swallowing reflexes are maintained. The highest mortality risk comes
from accidental death due to dissociation and analgesia, but there is little scientific data
available, even on emergency room (ER) presentations of ketamine toxicity. Ng and colleagues (2010), however, reported on 233 ER cases (with an average age of 22 years, two-
thirds of whom were male) with impaired consciousness in 45 percent; abdominal pain
in 21 percent; lower urinary tract symptoms in 12 percent; and dizziness in 12 percent.

On the other hand, ketamine-induced ulcerative colitis of the bladder is a recently
identified and potentially severe condition of chronic use. Symptoms include frequency
and urgency of urination, incontinence, and sometimes painful passing of blood in the
urine. Although it is difficult to get accurate information, there is some evidence that 50
percent of users have sought medical attention for ketamine-induced cystitis. One-third of
the cases resolved after cessation of drug use, one-third stabilized, and one-third
continued to worsen (Muetzelfeldt et al., 2008). Another emerging condition of high-
dose ketamine use is water on the kidney (hydronephrosis). According to Muetzelfeldt
and colleagues (2008), one-third of chronic users also reported "k-cramps," intense
abdominal pain associated with bile duct abnormality (Muetzelfeldt et al., 2008).

Cognitive impairment occurs in humans even with a single dose, but recreational
use is not associated with long-term cognitive impairment, as 1-year abstinent former
ketamine users did not show deficits (Morgan and Curran, 2011).

Treatment of Intoxication

Therapy for PCP and ketamine intoxication is aimed at reducing the systemic level of
the drug, keeping the patient calm and sedated, and preventing severe adverse medical effects. Sensory inputs should be minimized by placing the intoxicated person in a

quiet environment, with physical restraint if necessary to prevent self-injury. Agitation can be reduced with either a benzodiazepine or an atypical antipsychotic. Hyperthermia, hypertension, convulsions, renal failure, and other medical consequences should be treated as necessary. PCP and ketamine-induced psychotic states may be long-lasting, especially in people with a history of schizophrenia.

Tolerance to PCP and ketamine does develop, but gradually; escalation of abused doses may be due to behavioral adaptations that compensate for the disruptive effects of the drug rather than a direct physiological action. The incidence of dependence is not known. A specific withdrawal syndrome has not been described and cravings seem to be the most common symptom.

Methoxetamine

This ketamine analogue first appeared in 2010 and there is not much medical literature as yet. Presumably it acts like ketamine, as a noncompetitive antagonist of the NMDA receptor with dopamine reuptake properties. Recent research (Hondebrink et al., 2017) shows a variety of neuronal actions, including potent uptake inhibition of all three monoaminergic transmitters (dopamine, norepinephrine, and serotonin) as well as other effects, some of which differ from that of ketamine. In an animal model of depression (Botanas et al., 2017), methoxetamine showed antidepressant effects within 30 minutes of administration, which lasted for at least 24 hours. This action was blocked by either an AMPA antagonist or a serotonergic antagonist. Methoxetamine also produced changes in glutamatergic and serotonergic gene expression in the hippocampus. These actions are consistent with a possible antidepressant action of methoxetamine. It is taken orally, inserted rectally, insufflated (snorted), or injected intramuscularly. Doses depend on the route of administration: 20 to 100 milligrams orally and 10 to 50 milligrams by intramuscular injection. After insufflation, the effect may be delayed, prompting users to take more because they believe the first dose was inadequate. Users have stated that the effects begin about 5 to 10 minutes after injection and last from 1 to 2 hours, compared with 5 to 7 hours after insufflation. Effects include euphoria and the perceptual hallucinations typical of ketamine, as well as an opiatelike effect. It seems to have weaker analgesic and anesthetic properties than ketamine, but a longer duration of action (Corazza et al., 2012). Undesirable reactions are primarily gastrointestinal (nausea, vomiting, diarrhea), paranoia and anxiety, tachycardia, and nystagmus. Respiratory depression, reduction of phantom limb pain, and antidepressant effects have also been reported. As with ketamine and PCP, treatment consists of supportive care, benzodiazepines, fluids, and antiemetics as needed (Rosenbaum et al., 2012; Troy, 2013).

Dextromethorphan (DXM)

DXM is a common ingredient in more than 140 varieties of over-the-counter cough suppressants such as various Coricidin products, Robitussin DM, Vicks 44, Tylenol DM, and many others. Recreational ingestion is referred to as "roboing," "dexing," "robo-tripping," or "robo-copping." In a recent study in human volunteers, high doses between 5.7 and 11.4 milligrams per kilogram produced hallucinations that participants identified as being comparable to classic hallucinogens, such as psilocybin (Reissig et al., 2012). However, DXM acts through NMDA receptor blockade, an action similar to that of PCP and ketamine. In fact, DXM and its metabolite dextrorphan (DXO) can substitute for PCP and exert PCP-like effects (and the active metabolite DXO may be responsible for many of the high-dose effects of DXM; Miller, 2005). These findings imply that both serotonergic and glutamatergic neurotransmitter systems may be involved in the perceptual, cognitive, and mood-altering effects of many hallucinogenlike compounds, including dissociative anesthetics such as ketamine and PCP (Reissig et al., 2012).

DXM increased blood pressure and heart rate and produced psychological/behavioral activation (such as increased ratings of arousing/stimulating, shaky/jittery, nervous/anxious, restless, and talkative) as well as other somatic effects (lightheadedness/dizziness, numbness/tingling, queasiness/feeling sick to the stomach, and headache). DXM also increased ratings of distance from reality, visual effects with eyes open and closed, restless/fidgety, joy/euphoria/peace, nausea/vomiting, and psychological discomfort. At the maximum dose only, DXM increased the ratings of unresponsiveness to questions, anxiety or fearfulness, and confusion/disorientation. Nevertheless, participants also endorsed positive effects in regard to "mysticism" (Reissig et al., 2012). Acute psychotic reactions have occasionally been reported (Martinak et al., 2017).

SALVINORIN A

Salvia divinorum ("magic mint," "diviner's sage," "Sally-D"), a member of the mint family of perennial herbs, is a psychoactive plant that has been used for curing and divination in traditional spiritual practices by the Mazatec peoples of Oaxaca, Mexico, for many centuries (Vortherms and Roth, 2006). Among the various species of *Salvia*, only this plant is known to contain the active hallucinogen salvinorin A. Generally, the leaves of the plant are chewed or brewed in a tea, but the dried leaves can also be smoked in the manner of marijuana or cocaine freebase. When smoked in doses of 200 to 500 micrograms, *Salvia* has been used as a short-acting (approximately 30 minutes), legal hallucinogen for several years. Ingestion typically does not produce hallucinogenic effects, either because of first-pass metabolism or enzyme breakdown.

In recent years, users of *S. divinorum* have posted YouTube videos of themselves under the influence, with the mainstream news media occasionally also broadcasting these clips. This agent received much media attention after the singer–actress Miley Cyrus was photographed smoking it. Jared Loughner, the perpetrator of the 2011 Tucson, Arizona, mass shooting (which included Congresswoman Gabby Gifford), was said to be a long-term user (Rosenbaum et al., 2012).

A compilation of descriptions from the Erowid Center (Erowid.org) includes: "Laughter, visions, peace/understanding, experiencing multiple realities/travel to other places or time/contacting other entities/spirits, entering 'realm of the dead,' feeling of being underground, flying, floating, twisting, loss of individuality/connected to a larger 'whole.'" Adverse effects include intense anxiety, dysphoria and confusion, and a hangover with headache and drowsiness for several hours. There are no characteristic physical signs except for some tachycardia and hypertension. But because the drug is often taken with other substances, specific reactions are difficult to determine. Addiction and dependence liability are unknown and there is no recognized antidote for intoxication.

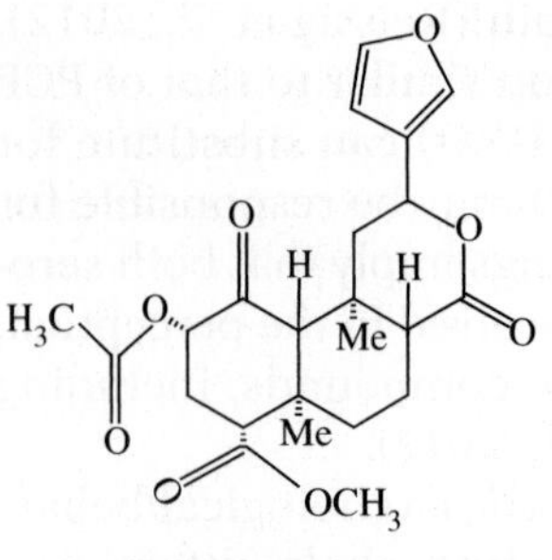

FIGURE 8.6   Structure of salvinorin A, the active drug in *Salvia divinorum*.

Laboratory studies in healthy adult human subjects confirm that smoking salvia rapidly elicits intense and unique sensory effects in which the users lose normal awareness of themselves and their surroundings, and may experience delusional phenomena (Addy et al., 2015; Johnson et al., 2016).

Mechanism of Action

The molecular structure (Figure 8.6), mechanism of action, and perhaps clinical effects of salvinorin A are distinct from other naturally occurring or synthetic hallucinogens (Butelman et al., 2010). Unlike classical hallucinogens, salvinorin A has no action at the serotonin 5-HT$_{2A}$ receptor but is classified as a *kappa opioid agonist*, the first naturally occurring compound known to exhibit such an action (Roth et al., 2002). Laboratory studies in nonhuman animals confirm that salvinorin A's effects differ from 5-HT$_2$ agonists, LSD, psilocybin, THC, NMDA antagonists, and delta or mu opiate agonists, but are similar to the effects of other kappa agonists and are blocked by kappa antagonists (Addy, 2012). This is unusual because the drug is not *structurally* like other kappa agonists and because its effects are also similar to those of 5-HT$_{2A}$ agonists (Cunningham et al., 2011; Johnson et al., 2011). The high density of κ-opioid receptors in the claustrum suggests that by studying the subjective experience of salvinorin A in humans, the role of the claustrum in consciousness might be better understood (Stiefel et al., 2014).

Potential Therapeutic Uses of Salvinorum Derivatives

Hanes (2001) reported on one patient with severe depression unrelieved by traditional antidepressant medications who chewed two or three leaves at a time three times per week and claimed total remission of depressive symptoms. As a kappa agonist, however, the drug has the potential to induce (rather than relieve) depressive reactions. Braida and coworkers (2009) expand on potential antidepressant and anxiolytic effects of salvinorin A. Historically, *Salvia* preparations have been used to treat gastrointestinal disorders, including diarrhea. Fichna and coworkers (2009) expand on this topic and demonstrate that salvinorin A inhibits colonic contractions and motility through actions on gastric kappa receptors and cannabinoid-2 receptors. The authors postulate use in the treatment of lower intestinal disorders associated with increased intestinal transit and diarrhea. Salvinorin A has therapeutic potential as a treatment for pain, mood and personality disorders, substance abuse, and gastrointestinal disturbances, which suggests that nonalkaloids may be potential options for new therapeutic drug development (Cunningham et al., 2011).

STUDY QUESTIONS

1. What is a psychedelic drug?

2. List the major classes of psychedelic drugs presented in this chapter and the respective mechanisms of action that differentiate them.

3. How do the psychedelic drugs differ in their psychological/subjective effects?

4. What therapeutic benefits, if any, have been proposed for the psychedelic hallucinogens?

5. What acute adverse psychological reactions are produced by the various psychedelic drugs?

6. Are there any long-term physical, neurological, or psychological consequences of the psychedelics?

7. How does salvinorin A differ from other drugs in this category in its mechanism of action and its psychological effects?

REFERENCES

Addy, P. H. (2012). "Acute and Post-Acute Behavioral and Psychological Effects of Salvinorum A in Humans." *Psychopharmacology* 220: 195–204.

Addy, P. H., et al. (2015). "The Subjective Experience of Acute, Experimentally-Induced Salvia Divinorum Inebriation." *Journal of Psychopharmacology* 29: 426–435.

Amoroso, T., and Workman, M. (2016). "Treating Posttraumatic Stress Disorder with MDMA-Assisted Psychotherapy: A Preliminary Meta-Analysis and Comparison to Prolonged Exposure Therapy." *Journal of Psychopharmacology* 30: 595–600.

Baggott, M. J., et al. (2010). "Investigating the Mechanisms of Hallucinogen-Induced Visions Using 3,4-Methylenedioxyamphetamine (MDA): A Randomized Controlled Trial in Humans." *PLoS One* 5: e14074.

Baggott, M. J., et al. (2015). "Intimate Insight: MDMA Changes How People Talk About Significant Others." *Journal of Psychopharmacology* 29: 669–677.

Baggott, M. J., et al. (2016). "Effects of 3,4-Methylenedioxymethamphetamine on Socioemotional Feelings, Authenticity, and Autobiographical Disclosure in Healthy Volunteers in a Controlled Setting." *Journal of Psychopharmacology* 30: 378–387.

Bogenschutz, M. P., and Pommy, J. M. (2012). "Therapeutic Mechanisms of Classic Hallucinogens in the Treatment of Addictions: From Indirect Evidence to Testable Hypotheses." *Drug Testing and Analysis* 4: 543–555.

Bogenschutz, M. P., et al. (2015). "Psilocybin-Assisted Treatment for Alcohol Dependence: A Proof-Of-Concept Study." *Journal of Psychopharmacology* 29: 289–299.

Bogenschutz, M. P., and Johnson, M. W. (2016). "Classic Hallucinogens in the Treatment of Addictions." *Progress in Neuro-Psychopharmacology and Biological Psychiatry* 64: 250–258.

Bossong, M. G., et al. (2010). "mCPP: An Undesired Addition to the Ecstasy Market." *Journal of Psychopharmacology* 24: 1395–1401.

Botanas, C. J., et al. (2017). "Methoxetamine Produces Rapid and Sustained Antidepressant Effects Probably via Glutamatergic and Serotonergic Mechanisms." *Neuropharmacology* 126: 121–127. doi: 10.1016/j.neuropharm.2017.08.038.

Braida, D., et al. (2009). "Potential Anxiolytic- and Antidepressant-Like Effects of Salvinorin A, the Main Active Ingredient of *Salvia divinorum*, in Rodents." *British Journal of Pharmacology* 157: 844–853.

Brecher, E. M., and the Editors of Consumer Reports Magazine. (1972). *Licit and Illicit Drugs: The Consumers Union Report on Narcotics, Stimulants, Depressants, Inhalants, Hallucinogens, and Marijuana - Including Caffeine, Nicotine, and Alcohol.* New York: Little, Brown. http://www.druglibrary.org/schaffer/library/studies/cu/cumenu.htm.

Brown, D. J. (2013). *Psychedelic Drug Research: A Comprehensive Review.* N.p.: Reality Sandwich Singles. http://realitysandwich.com/163342/psychedelic_drug_research/.

Brunt, T. M., et al. (2011). "Instability of the Ecstasy Market and a New Kid on the Block: Mephedrone." *Journal of Psychopharmacology* 25: 1543–1547.

Butelman, E. R., et al. (2010). "The Discriminative Effects of the Kappa-Opioid Hallucinogen Salvinorin A in Nonhuman Primates: Dissociation from Classic Hallucinogen Effects." *Psychopharmacology* 210: 253–262.

Carhart-Harris, R. L., et al. (2012a). "Implications for Psychedelic-Assisted Psychotherapy: Functional Magnetic Resonance Imaging with Psilocybin." *British Journal of Psychiatry* 200: 238–244.

Carhart-Harris, R. L., et al. (2012b). "Neural Correlates of the Psychedelic State as Determined by FMRI Studies with Psilocybin." *Proceedings of the National Academy of Sciences USA.* 109: 2138–2143.

Carhart-Harris, R. L., et al. (2014). "The Entropic Brain: A Theory of Conscious States Informed by Neuroimaging Research with Psychedelic Drugs." *Frontiers in Human Neuroscience* 8: 20. doi: 10.3389/fnhum.2014.00020.

Carhart-Harris, R. L., et al. (2016). "Neural Correlates of the LSD Experience Revealed by Multimodal Neuroimaging." *Proceedings of the National Academy of Sciences* 113: 4853–4858.

Caudevilla-Gálligo, F., et al. (2012). "4-Bromo-2,5-Dimethoxyphenethylamine (2C-B): Presence in the Recreational Drug Market in Spain, Pattern of Use and Subjective Effects." *Journal of Psychopharmacology* 26: 1026–1035.

Corazza, O., et al. (2012). "Phenomenon of New Drugs on the Internet: The Case of Ketamine Derivative Methoxetamine." *Human Psychopharmacology Clinical and Experimental* 27: 145–149.

Costandi, M. (2014). "A Brief History of Psychedelic Psychiatry." *The Psychologist* 27: 714–716. https://issuu.com/thepsychologist/docs/psy09_14web/84?e=1106616/9079836.

Cunningham, C. W., et al. (2011). "Neuropharmacology of the Naturally Occurring κ-Opioid Hallucinogen Salvinorin A." *Pharmacological Reviews* 63: 316–347.

Das, S., et al. (2016). "Lysergic Acid Diethylamide: A Drug of 'Use'?" *Therapeutic Advances in Psychopharmacology* 6: 214–228.

DeFrates, L. J., et al. (2005). "Antimuscarinic Intoxication Resulting from the Ingestion of Moonflower Seeds." *Annals of Pharmacotherapy* 39: 173–176.

den Hollander, B., et al. (2012). "Preliminary Evidence of Hippocampal Damage in Chronic Users of Ecstasy." *Journal of Neurology Neurosurgery and Psychiatry* 83: 83–85.

deWin, M. M. L., et al. (2008). "Sustained Effects of Ecstasy on the Human Brain: A Prospective Neuroimaging Study in Novel Users." *Brain* 131: 2936–2945.

dos Santos, R. G., et al. (2016). "The Current State of Research on Ayahuasca: A Systematic Review of Human Studies Assessing Psychiatric Symptoms, Neuropsychological Functioning, and Neuroimaging." *Journal of Psychopharmacology* 30:1230–1247. doi: 10.1177/0269881116652578.

Duffy, M. R., and Ferguson, C. (2007). "Role of Dantrolene in Treatment of Heat Stroke Associated with Ecstasy Ingestion." *British Journal of Anaesthesia* 98: 148–149.

el-Seedi, H. R., et al. (2005). "Prehistoric Peyote Use: Alkaloid Analysis and Radiocarbon Dating of Archaeological Specimens of *Lophophora* from Texas." *Journal of Ethnopharmacology* 101: 238–242.

Erowid. (n.d.). "About Erowid" https://www.erowid.org/general/about/about.shtml.

Fichna, J., et al. (2009). "Salvinorin A Inhibits Colonic Transit and Neurogenic Ion Transport in Mice by Activating Kappa-Opioid and Cannabinoid Receptors." *Neurogastroenterology and Motility* 21: 1326e–1328e.

Fickenscher, A., et al. (2006). "Illicit Peyote Use among American Indian Adolescents in Substance Abuse Treatment: A Preliminary Investigation." *Substance Use and Misuse* 41: 1139–1154.

Frecska, E., et al. (2016). "The Therapeutic Potentials of Ayahuasca: Possible Effects Against Various Diseases of Civilization." *Frontiers in Pharmacology* 7: 35. doi: 10.3389/fphar.2016.00035.

Frood, A. (2015). "Ayahuasca Psychedelic Tested for Depression. Pilot Study with Shamanic Brew Hints at Therapeutic Potential." *Nature.* April 6. doi: 10.1038/nature.2015.17252.

Gable, R. S. (2007). "Risk Assessment of Ritual Use of Oral Dimethyltryptamine (DMT) and Harmala Alkaloids." *Addiction* 102: 24–34.

Gallagher, C. T., et al. (2012). "5,6-Methylenedioxy-2-aminoindane: From Laboratory Curiosity to 'Legal High.'" *Human Psychopharmacology Clinical and Experimental* 27: 106–112.

Gasser, P., et al. (2015). "LSD-Assisted Psychotherapy for Anxiety Associated with a Life-Threatening Disease: A Qualitative Study of Acute and Sustained Subjective Effects." *Journal of Psychopharmacology* 29: 57–68.

Geyer, M. A., and Vollenweider, F. X. (2008). "Serotonin Research: Contributions to Understanding Psychosis." *Trends in Pharmacological Sciences* 29: 445–453.

Gouzoulis-Mayfrank, E., and Daumann, J. (2009). "Neurotoxicity of Drugs of Abuse—The Case of Methylenedioxyamphetamines (MDMA, Ecstasy), and Amphetamines." *Dialogues in Clinical Neuroscience* 11: 305–317.

Griffiths, R. (2015). "A Single Dose of Psilocybin Produces Substantial and Enduring Decreases in Anxiety and Depression in Patients with a Life-Threatening Cancer Diagnosis: A Randomized Double-Blind Trial." Poster presented at: American College of Neuropsychopharmacology Annual Meeting, Hollywood, Florida.

Griffiths, R. R., et al. (2016). "Psilocybin Produces Substantial and Sustained Decreases in Depression and Anxiety in Patients with Life-Threatening Cancer: A Randomized Double-Blind Trial." *Journal of Psychopharmacology* 30:1181-1197. doi: 10.1177/0269881116675513.

Grilly, D. M., and Salamone, J. D. (2012). *Drugs, Brain and Behavior.* New York: Pearson.

Grob, C. S., et al. (2011). "Pilot Study of Psilocybin Treatment for Anxiety in Patients with Advanced-Stage Cancer." *Archives of General Psychiatry* 68: 71–78.

Hadjiefthyvoulou, F., et al. (2011). "Everyday and Prospective Memory Deficits in Ecstasy/ Polydrug Users." *Journal of Psychopharmacology* 25: 453–464.

Hall, A. P., and Henry, J. A. (2006). "Acute Toxic Effects of 'Ecstasy' (MDMA) and Related Compounds: Overview of Pathophysiology and Clinical Management." *British Journal of Anaesthesia* 96: 678–685.

Halpern, J. H., et al. (2011). "Residual Neurocognitive Features of Long-Term Ecstasy Users with Minimal Exposure to Other Drugs." *Addiction* 106: 777–786.

Hanes, K. R. (2001). "Antidepressant Effects of the Herb *Salvia divinorum:* A Case Report." *Journal of Clinical Psychopharmacology* 21: 634–635.

Hashimoto, K. (2009). "Can the Sigma-1 Receptor Agonist Fluvoxamine Prevent Schizophrenia?" *CNS & Neurological Disorders—Drug Targets* 8: 470–474.

Hendricks, P. S., et al. (2015). "Classic Psychedelic Use Is Associated with Reduced Psychological Distress and Suicidality in the United States Adult Population." *Journal of Psychopharmacology* 29: 1041–1043. doi: 10.1177/0269881115598338.

Hofmann, A. (1994). "Notes and Documents Concerning the Discovery of LSD." *Agents and Actions* 43: 79–81.

Holzman, R. S. (1998). "The Legacy of Atropos, the Fate Who Cut the Thread of Life." *Anesthesiology* 89: 241–249.

Hondebrink, L., et al. (2017). "Neuropharmacological Characterization of The New Psychoactive Substance Methoxetamine." *Neuropharmacology* 123: 1–9. doi: 10.1016/j.neuropharm.2017.04.035.

Imperial College London. (2016). "Brain on LSD Revealed: First Scans Show How the Drug Affects the Brain." *ScienceDaily*. April 11. https://www.sciencedaily.com/releases/2016/04/160411153006.htm.

Itokawa, M., et al. (2007). "Acute Confusional State after Designer Tryptamine Abuse." *Psychiatry and Clinical Neurosciences* 61: 196–199.

Johansen, P. Ø., and Krebs, T. S. (2015). "Psychedelics Not Linked to Mental Health Problems or Suicidal Behavior: A Population Study." *Journal of Psychopharmacology* 29: 270–279.

Johnson, M., et al. (2008). "Human Hallucinogen Research: Guidelines for Safety." *Journal of Psychopharmacology* 22: 603–620.

Johnson, M. W., et al. (2011). "Human Psychopharmacology and Dose-Effects of Salvinorin A, a Kappa Opioid Agonist Hallucinogen Present in the Plant *Salvia Divinorum*." *Drug and Alcohol Dependence* 115: 150–155.

Johnson, M. W., et al. (2014). "Pilot Study of the 5-HTR Agonist Psilocybin in the Treatment of Tobacco Addiction." *Journal of Psychopharmacology* 28: 983–992.

Johnson, M. W., et al. (2016). "Time Course of Pharmacokinetic and Hormonal Effects of Inhaled High-Dose Salvinorin A in Humans." *Journal of Psychopharmacology* 30: 323–329.

Kaelen, M., et al. (2016). "P.3.039 Effects of LSD and Music on Brain Activity." *European Neuropsychopharmacology* 26: Supplement 1: S80–S81. doi: 10.1016/S0924-977X (16)70088-5.

Kamboj, S. K., et al. (2015). "Recreational 3,4-Methylenedioxy-N-methylamphetamine (MDMA) or 'Ecstasy' and Self-Focused Compassion: Preliminary Steps in the Development of a Therapeutic Psychopharmacology of Contemplative Practices." *Journal of Psychopharmacology* 29: 961–970.

Kirkpatrick, M., et al. (2015). "Prosocial Effects of MDMA: A Measure of Generosity." *Journal of Psychopharmacology* 29: 661–668.

Krebs, T. S., and Johansen, P. O. (2012). "Lysergic Acid Diethylamide (LSD) for Alcoholism: Meta-Analysis of Randomized Controlled Trials." *Journal of Psychopharmacology* 26: 994–1002.

Kuypers, K. P. C., and Ramaekers, J. G. (2005). "Transient Memory Impairment after Acute Dose of 75 mg 3,4-Methylenedioxymethamphetamine." *Journal of Psychopharmacology* 19: 633–639.

Kuypers, K. P. C., and Ramaekers, J. G. (2007). "Acute Dose of MDMA (75 mg) Impairs Spatial Memory for Location but Leaves Contextual Processing of Visuospatial Information Unaffected." *Psychopharmacology* 189: 557–563.

Kuypers, K. P. C., et al. (2011). "MDMA Intoxication and Verbal Memory Performance: A Placebo-Controlled Pharmaco-MRI Study." *Journal of Psychopharmacology* 25: 1053–1061.

Lerner A. G., et al. (2002). "Flashback and Hallucinogen Persisting Perception Disorder: Clinical Aspects and Pharmacological Treatment Approach." *The Israel Journal of Psychiatry and Related Sciences* 39: 92–99.

Liester, M. B. (2014). "A Review of Lysergic Acid Diethylamide (LSD) in the Treatment of Addictions: Historical Perspectives and Future Prospects." *Current Drug Abuse Review* 7: 146–156.

Martinak, B., et al. (2017). "Dextromethorphan in Cough Syrup: The Poor Man's Psychosis." *Psychopharmacology Bulletin* 47: 59–63.

Maurice, T., and Su, T. P. (2009). "The Pharmacology of Sigma-1 Receptors." *Pharmacology and Therapeutics* 124: 195–206.

McLean, K., et al. (2011). "Mystical Experiences Occasioned by the Hallucinogen Psilocybin Lead to Increases in the Personality Domain of Openness." *Journal of Psychopharmacology* 25: 1453–1461.

Miller, S. C. (2005). "Dextromethorphan Psychosis, Dependence and Physical Withdrawal." *Addiction Biology* 10: 325–327.

Mithoefer, M. C., et al. (2011). "The Safety and Efficacy of ±3,4-Methylenedioxymethamphet-amine-Assisted Psychotherapy in Subjects with Chronic, Treatment-Resistant Posttraumatic Stress Disorder: The First Randomized Controlled Pilot Study." *Journal of Psychopharmacology* 25: 439–452.

Mithoefer, M. C., et al. (2013). "Durability of Improvement in Post-Traumatic Stress Disorder Symptoms and Absence of Harmful Effects or Drug Dependency After 3,4-Methylenedioxymeth-amphetamine-Assisted Psychotherapy: A Prospective Long-Term Follow-Up Study." *Journal of Psychopharmacology* 27: 28–39.

Moore, K., et al. (2013). "Do Novel Psychoactive Substances Displace Established Club Drugs, Supplement Them or Act as Drugs of Initiation: The Relationship Between Mephedrone, Ecstasy and Cocaine." *European Addiction Research* 19: 276–282.

Moreno, F. A., et al. (2006). "Safety, Tolerability, and Efficacy of Psilocybin in 9 Patients with Obsessive-Compulsive Disorder." *Journal of Clinical Psychiatry* 67: 1735–1740.

Morgan, C. J. A., and Curran, H. V. (2011). "Ketamine Use: A Review." *Addiction* 107: 27–38.

Mouri, A., et al. (2007). "Phencyclidine Animal Models of Schizophrenia: Approaches from Abnor-mality of Glutamatergic Neurotransmission and Neurodevelopment." *Neurochemistry Interna-tional* 51: 173–184.

Muetzelfeldt L., et al. (2008). "Journey through the K-hole: Phenomenological Aspects of Ket-amine Use." *Drug and Alcohol Dependence* 95: 219–329. doi: 10.1016/j.drugalcdep.2008.01.024.

Nagai, F., et al. (2007). "The Effects of Non-Medically Used Psychoactive Drugs on Monoamine Neurotransmission in Rat Brain." *European Journal of Pharmacology* 559: 132–137.

Ng, S. H., et al. (2010). "Emergency Department Presentation of Ketamine Abusers in Hong Kong: A Review of 233 Cases." *Hong Kong Medical Journal* 16: 6–11.

Nour, M. N., et al. (2016). "Ego-Dissolution and Psychedelics: Validation of the Ego-Dissolution Inventory (EDI)." *Frontiers in Human Neuroscience* 10: 269.

Oehen, P., et al. (2013). "A Randomized, Controlled Pilot Study of MDMA (±3,4-Methylenedioxy-methamphetamine)-Assisted Psychotherapy for Treatment of Resistant, Chronic Post-Traumatic Stress Disorder (PTSD)." *Journal of Psychopharmacology* 27: 40–52.

Parrott, A. C. (2012). "MDMA and Temperature: A Review of the Thermal Effects of 'Ecstasy' in Humans." *Drug and Alcohol Dependence* 121: 1–9.

Paschos, K. A., et al. (2009). "Neuropeptide and Sigma Receptors as Novel Therapeutic Targets for the Pharmacotherapy of Depression." *CNS Drugs* 23: 755–772.

Passie, T., et al. (2008). "The Pharmacology of Lysergic Acid Diethylamide: A Review." *CNS Neuroscience & Therapeutics* 14: 295–314.

Reissig, C. J., et al. (2012). "High Doses of Dextromethorphan, an NMDA Antagonist, Produce Effects Similar to Classic Hallucinogens." *Psychopharmacology* 223: 1–15.

Roberts, T. B. (2013). *The Psychedelic Future of the Mind: How Entheogens Are Enhancing Cognition, Boosting Intelligence, and Raising Values.* South Paris, ME: Park Street Press.

Rosenbaum, C. D., et al. (2012). "Here Today, Gone Tomorrow . . . and Back Again? A Review of Herbal Marijuana Alternatives (K2, Spice), Synthetic Cathinones (Bath Salts), Kratom, *Salvia Divinorum*, Methoxetamine, and Piperazines." *Journal of Medical Toxicology* 8: 15–32.

Ross, S., et al. (2016). "Rapid and Sustained Symptom Reduction Following Psilocybin Treatment for Anxiety and Depression in Patients with Life-Threatening Cancer: A Randomized Controlled Trial." *Journal of Psychopharmacology* 30: 1165–1180. doi: 10.1177/0269881116675512.

Roth, B. L., et al. (2002). "Salvinorin A: A Potent Naturally Occurring Nonnitrogenous Opioid Selective Agonist." *Proceedings of the National Academy of Sciences* 99: 11934–11939.

Rucker, J. J. H., et al. (2016). "Psychedelics in the Treatment of Unipolar Mood Disorders: A Systematic Review." *Journal of Psychopharmacology* 30: 1220–1229. doi: 10.1177/0269881116679368.

Schep, L. J., et al. (2011). "The Clinical Toxicology of the Designer "Party Pills" Benzylpiperazine and Trifluoromethylphenylpiperazine." *Clinical Toxicology* 49: 131–141.

Schifano, F., et al. (2005). "New Trends in the Cyber and Street Market of Recreational Drugs? The Case of 2C-T-7 ("Blue Mystic")." *Journal of Psychopharmacology* 19: 675–679.

Schmid, Y., et al. (2014). "Differential Effects of MDMA and Methylphenidate on Social Cognition." *Journal of Psychopharmacology* 28: 847–856.

Sessa, B. (2012). *The Psychedelic Renaissance: Reassessing the Role of Psychedelic Drugs in 21st Century Psychiatry and Society.* London: Muswell Hill Press.

Speth, J., et al. (2016). "Decreased Mental Time Travel to the Past Correlates with Default-Mode Network Disintegration Under Lysergic Acid Diethylamide." *Journal of Psychopharmacology* 30: 344–353.

Stewart C. E. (2011). "Ketamine as a Street Drug." *Emergency Medical Services* 30: 30, 32, 34 passim.

Stewart, L. H., et al. (2014). "Effects of Ecstasy on Cooperative Behaviour and Perception of Trustworthiness: A Naturalistic Study." *Journal of Psychopharmacology* 28: 1001–1008.

Stiefel, K. M., et al. (2014). "The Claustrum's Proposed Role in Consciousness is Supported by the Effect and Target Localization of Salvia Divinorum." *Frontiers in Integrative Neuroscience* 8: 20.

Strassman, R. J., et al. (1994). "Dose-Response Study of N,N-Dimethyltryptamine in Humans. II: Subjective Effects and Preliminary Results of a New Rating Scale." *Archives of General Psychiatry* 51: 98–108.

Studerus, E., et al. (2012). "Prediction of Psilocybin Response in Healthy Volunteers." *PLoS One* 7: e30800.

Su, T. P., et al. (2009). "When the Endogenous Hallucinogenic Trace Amine N, N-Dimethyltryptamine Meets the Sigma-1 Receptor." *Science Signaling* 2: pe12.

Troy, J. D. (2013). "New 'Legal' Highs: Kratom and Methoxetamine." *Current Psychiatry* 12: E1–E2.

Urban, N. B. L., et al. (2012). "Sustained Recreational Use of Ecstasy Is Associated with Altered Pre- and Postsynaptic Markers of Serotonin Transmission in Neocortical Areas: A PET Study with [^{11}C]DASB and [^{11}C]MDL 100907." *Neuropsychopharmacology* 37: 1465–1473.

Vortherms, T. A., and Roth, B. L. (2006). "Salvinorin A: From Natural Product to Human Therapeutics." *Molecular Interventions* 6: 257–265.

Wagner, D., et al. (2013). "A Prospective Study of Learning, Memory, and Executive Function in New MDMA Users." *Addiction* 108: 136–145.

Witt, E. (2015). "The Trip Planners." *The New Yorker.* November 23. http://www.newyorker.com/magazine/2015/11/23/the-trip-planners.

Wolff, K., and Winstock, A. R. (2006). "Ketamine: From Medicine to Misuse." *CNS Drugs* 20: 199–218.

CHAPTER 9

Cannabis
A New Look at an Ancient Plant

Although the hemp plant, *cannabis*, commonly called *marijuana*, has an ancient history of medical, utilitarian, and recreational use, we have only recently begun to understand how it acts in the brain to produce its effects. Cannabis—or, more specifically, its main psychoactive ingredient, *tetrahydrocannabinol* (THC)—is unique because it has stimulatory, sedating, analgesic, and hallucinatory effects, yet is not chemically related to the classical psychostimulants, sedative/hypnotics, analgesics, or hallucinogens. Moreover, during the past few years, social, legal, and economic changes have created several additional challenges in efforts to study this drug. First, advances in cultivation have produced much more varied and potent strains of the plant than in the past. This has made the older literature less relevant to the effects of current use. Second, changes in social attitudes and legal status at the state level have exposed a greater number of people, especially young people, to cannabis than ever before. At the same time, at the national level, cannabis is still placed in the most restrictive legal category, making scientific study more difficult. Third, synthetic cannabinoid use has become much more common and dangerous because of dozens of new formulations, collectively known as spice (or herbal incense)

Spice is dried, shredded plant material treated with a synthetic cannabinoid analog (an *analog* is one of a group of chemical compounds that are similar in structure and pharmacology). These novel compounds are designed to avoid legal penalties and the speed with which they appear on the street makes it very difficult to characterize their toxic effects. For example, by February 2015, more than 250 new substances appeared in the place of the first synthetic cannabinoids to be banned by the Drug Enforcement Administration in 2011 (Fattore, 2016). Finally, the increased acceptance of cannabis for medical applications has rejuvenated pharmacological research into its therapeutic possibilities (Kendall and Yudowski, 2016). In particular, one of the many ingredients in cannabis, *cannabidiol* (CBD), has continued to show medicinal promise. CBD is devoid of psychoactive properties, but appears to have potential for wide medical use, possibly including treatments for anxiety, epilepsy, schizophrenia, pain, and perhaps other disorders (Whiting et al., 2015). All these developments will be discussed in this chapter.

EPIDEMIOLOGY

Information about drug use comes from a variety of sources and at different points in time. Although large-scale surveys provide the best available evidence, they are understood to be only best-guess estimates. According to data from 596,500 adults, who participated in the annual U.S. National Survey on Drug Use and Health from 2002 to 2014, the number of adults who said they used marijuana in the previous year increased from 10.4 percent of respondents to 13.3 percent. Meanwhile, the proportion of adults who perceived great risk of harm from smoking marijuana once or twice a week dropped from 50.4 percent to 33.3 percent. Overall, it was estimated that the number of U.S. adults who use marijuana grew from 21.9 million in 2002 to 31.9 million in 2014. In 2002, 823,000 adults used marijuana for the first time in the past year; in 2014, that number grew to 1.4 million. The number of daily or near-daily users was 8.4 million in 2014, compared with 3.9 million in 2002 (Compton et al., 2016). Evidently, the increased use of cannabis is accompanied by a perceived decrease in risk.

In adolescents, from 1996 to 2016, past-month marijuana use was mostly steady among 8th, 10th, and 12th graders. In 2016, that value for 12th grade was 22.5 percent; for 10th grade, 14.0 percent; and for 8th grade, 5.4 percent. Although 68.9 percent of high school seniors do not view regular marijuana smoking as harmful, 68.5 percent say they disapprove of regular marijuana smoking. In contrast, annual prevalence of synthetic marijuana, such as "spice" and "K2," in 2015, was down for the three grades, reflecting a considerable drop in use; in college students, past-year use of synthetic marijuana fell 80 percent between 2011 and 2015 (Johnston et al., 2016; National Institute on Drug Abuse, 2016).

HISTORY

Cannabis may be the oldest cultivated plant not used for food; the earliest known evidence of cannabis use consists of fibers found in China that date to about 4000 BCE. The ancient cultures of China, India, and Tibet treated numerous ailments with the plant, including gastrointestinal illness, seizures, malaria, pain of childbirth, and snakebite. Various religious groups, such as Buddhists and Hindus, incorporated cannabis into their religious ceremonies, and recreational use was also widespread. Gradually, cannabis use spread to Asia and the Middle East. The plant had many applications and its primary behavioral effects were well known; it was used for fiber (to make rope and cloth), oil, and medicine, as well as for intoxication. For example, the ancient Greek physician Galen cautioned that its use might lead to "senseless talk." During the Middle Ages, it came to the Muslim world and Africa, where its use did not fall under the Muslim prohibition of alcohol. Over centuries, cannabis was said to have many, sometimes contradictory, properties. It could make you crave sweets, get "high," improve sex and creativity, and also decrease the sex drive, produce insanity, and cause an "amotivational" syndrome. The word *assassin* is thought to derive from the word *hashishiyya*, believed to describe common criminals who also used hashish.

Spaniards brought cannabis to America in 1545, where it was cultivated to manufacture rope for naval use—crucial for overseas empires dependent on sailing ships.

For this reason, and since cannabis did not grow well in England, Sir Walter Raleigh was ordered to cultivate hemp in Virginia in 1611 alongside another important cash crop: tobacco. From that time onward, hemp became a staple crop of the American colonists for making rope, clothes, and paper. Even George Washington grew hemp on his plantation. Before the cotton gin was introduced at the end of the eighteenth century, hemp was grown on more acreage than cotton.

After Napoleon's army brought cannabis back from Egypt in the early nineteenth century, its use for both medical and recreational purposes began to spread in the West. In the United States, drug companies marketed cannabis tinctures for medicinal use until the Pure Food and Drug Act of 1906 and the Harrison Narcotic Act of 1914 began to impose constraints. Not specifically outlawed, recreational cannabis use increased in the United States when the Eighteenth Amendment of 1920 prohibited alcohol consumption, facilitated in part by migrant workers coming from Mexico to the United States. In 1930, Harry Anslinger, the first commissioner of the Federal Narcotics Bureau, tried to eradicate cannabis. In the wake of the repeal of the Eighteenth Amendment and the end of Prohibition in 1933, he devised dramatic media attacks that led to the Marijuana Tax Act of 1937. This law did not directly outlaw cannabis, but imposed a tax on it, and it effectively ended legal medicinal use of cannabis until 1969, when the Supreme Court declared the law illegal because imposing a tax on someone who wants to possess an illegal substance is a form of self-incrimination. In 1970, the Comprehensive Drug Abuse Prevention and Control Act (also called the "Controlled Substances Act") reduced the federal penalty for possession from a felony to a misdemeanor.

In November 1996, California passed Proposition 215, the Compassionate Use Act, into law, which allowed patients with a valid physician's prescription to possess and cultivate marijuana in the state for medical use in the treatment of severe conditions, including cancer, acquired immunodeficiency syndrome (AIDS), chronic pain, and spasticity. As of December 2016, 28 states and the District of Columbia have laws legalizing marijuana for medicinal purposes. Currently, seven of these states and the District of Columbia have also adopted laws legalizing marijuana for recreational use; three of these states—California, Massachusetts, and Nevada—passed measures in November 2016 (for details and updates, see Governing.com, 2016; ProCon.org, 2017, Kilmer, 2017).

Recently, the governors of Rhode Island and Washington and a New Mexico resident, Bryan A. Krumm, petitioned the Drug Enforcement Administration (DEA) to remove marijuana from Schedule I classification. The agency had previously rejected a similar request in 2011, touching off a legal battle to force reclassification in which the DEA ultimately prevailed. In August 2016, the DEA again denied the petition to reclassify cannabis, ruling "there is no substantial evidence that marijuana should be removed from Schedule I" of the Controlled Substances Act. The DEA said in a letter that the drug has a high potential for abuse, has no currently accepted medical use in treatment in the United States, and lacks accepted safety for use under medical supervision.

The DEA, however, also announced a relaxation of its policy on growing cannabis for federally approved research. According to the *Washington Post* (Bernstein, 2016), scientists in academic institutions argue that the regulations imposed on research of Schedule I drugs make it harder to assess whether they may be useful. The new policy, designed to foster research, expands the number of manufacturers that can register with the DEA, although the exact number is not known. Nevertheless, it is thought that the National Institute on Drug Abuse (NIDA) and the University of Mississippi will lose their exclusive control of cannabis cultivation, increasing the amount and diversity of the compounds for investigation. At that point, the DEA, rather than NIDA, would be responsible for allowing the plant to be grown. In September 2017, Senator Orrin Hatch (R-UT) proposed a bill, The Marijuana Effective Drug Study Act of 2017, which would "streamline" the procedure for registering and increase the quota of marijuana allowed for medical and scientific research.

The current inconsistent legal status of cannabis has produced some problems in the cultural response to this drug. Even in those states in which it is medically allowed, the accuracy of the dose and label of these products is poor. Vandrey and colleagues (2015) found that of 75 products purchased (47 different brands), only 17 percent accurately labeled the amount of THC content they contained; 23 percent contained more THC than labeled; and 60 percent contained less THC than labeled. Two commercially available e-cigarette liquid formulations reported to contain 3.3 mg/mL of the cannabis component, cannabidiol, as the active ingredient, instead were found to contain 6.5 and 7.6 milligrams per microliter (mg/mL) of cannabidiol, along with a variety of flavoring agents (Peace et al., 2016). Similar results were reported by Bonn-Miller and coworkers (2017), who found that the labeled content of CBD and THC was incorrect in about 20 percent of products bought online. For example, the amount of CBD was only accurate in 31 percent of the samples, while 43 percent of the test samples contained more CBD and 26 percent contained less than indicated in the label.

At the same time, the ongoing epidemic of opiate use (see Chapter 10) has put pressure on the medical establishment to limit prescriptions for those analgesics. With increasing constraints on opiates and a more liberal approach to cannabis, it is not surprising that the latter drug may be viewed as a substitute and that patients may seek guidance on this issue from practitioners (Choo et al., 2016). In fact, it is already the case that marijuana is being used in place of FDA-approved drugs in states that have legalized marijuana's medical use, according to a Health Affairs study. Prescription-drug use in conditions thought to benefit from marijuana use (for example, anxiety, pain, and sleep disorders) has dropped in states that legalized medical marijuana, compared to states without legalization (Bradford and Bradford, 2016). The use of drugs not associated with a marijuana benefit, such as antibiotics and anticoagulants, did not differ between the groups of states. It was estimated that Medicare spending, both by the program and by its beneficiaries, fell by some $165 million in 2013 as the result of marijuana substitution. It has been noted that clinicians have been put in an untenable position of being asked to prescribe a drug that is a controlled substance with undocumented benefits and known harms (D'Souza and Ranganathan, 2015). As argued by Richter and Levy (2014), it may be time to devise governmental regulatory policy in preparation for eventual legalization. Towards that goal, Thomas and Pollard (2016) discuss aspects of a regulatory system that need to be put in place to ensure standardization for the researcher and to reduce the hazards of contamination and inaccurate dosage. Kilmer (2017) provides a thoughtful analysis of the public health and legal consequences that need to be considered as a result of cannabis legalization.

WHAT IS CANNABIS?

The plant genus for cannabis includes three accepted species: *Cannabis sativa*, *Cannabis indica*, and *Cannabis ruderalis*. Cannabis sativa grows throughout the world and flourishes in most temperate and tropical regions. There are at least 400 different compounds in the plant, of which more than 60 are psychoactive. In 1964, Gaoni and Mechoulam first identified the primary active ingredient, delta-9-tetrahydrocannabinol (THC) (Figure 9.1A), which renewed interest in the field and led to the discovery of the endogenous endocannabinoids (Figure 9.1B).

The components of the cannabis plant include marijuana, hashish, charas, bhang, ganja, and sinsemilla. Hashish and charas, which consist of the dried resinous exudates of the female flowers, are the most potent preparations; ganja and sinsemilla refer to the dried material found in the tops of the female plants, where the THC content is less. Bhang and marijuana are preparations taken from the dried remainder of the plant, and their THC content is the lowest. However, with advances in cultivation techniques, the concentration of THC in marijuana has increased from about 3 percent in the 1980s to about 12 percent in 2014 (ElSohly et al., 2016). Among the other cannabis constituents with biologic activity, one, cannabidiol, has attracted recent attention in the medical community. Unlike THC, CBD does not produce a psychedelic effect. In general, as shown in Figure 9.2, as strains of cannabis increase in THC concentration, amounts of CBD decrease. The reverse is also true: as levels of CBD increase, THC amounts tend to decrease. Therefore, certain strains are more potent as psychedelics, while other strains have little psychedelic action and perhaps more therapeutic potential.

Forms of THC and CBD in Cannabis

THC and CBD do not naturally occur in cannabis. Instead, they occur as acidic forms called *tetrahydrocannabinolic acid* (THCa) and *cannabidiolic acid* (CBDa). When burned in a cigarette or heated in cooking or extraction, THCa and CBDa are converted to their active forms, THC and CBD, in a reaction called *decarboxylation*. Perhaps this is why merely chewing the marijuana leaves does not result in a psychedelic effect, in contrast to chewing raw coca leaves. Of note, drying

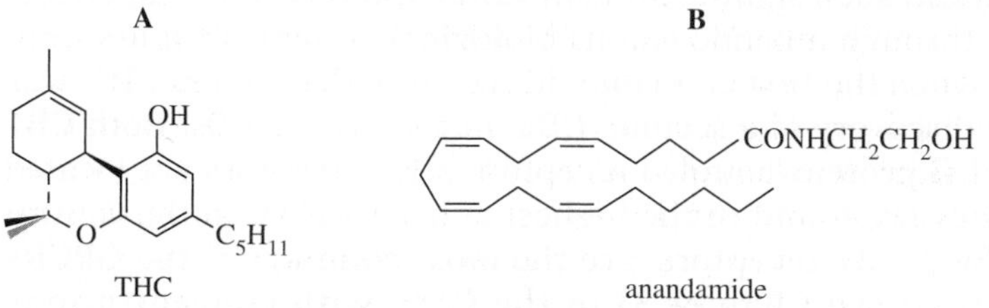

FIGURE 9.1 Structures of delta-9-tetrahydrocannabinol (THC) and anandamide, the endogenous ligand (neurotransmitter) of the cannabinoid receptor.

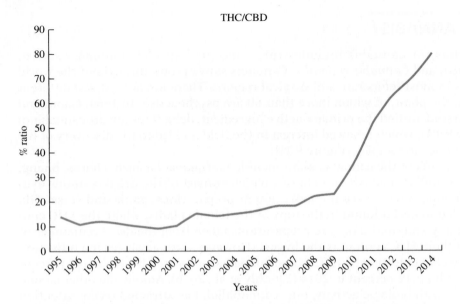

FIGURE 9.2   The THC-to-CBD ratio over time. During the period 1995 to 2014, as strains of cannabis increased in THC concentration, the amounts of CBD decreased. [Data from ElSohly et al., 2016.]

marijuana leaves slowly converts THCa to THC—heat expedites the conversion. Interestingly, this same process of decarboxylation that converts THCa to THC converts THC into an inactive metabolite, carboxy-THC, which is slowly excreted in the urine, forming the basis for urine detection of marijuana use. (As a side note, CBDa appears, like THC and CDB, to have anti-inflammatory and antiproliferative properties.)

MECHANISM OF ACTION: CANNABINOID RECEPTORS

The fact that cannabis produced such significant behavioral and physiological effects implies that the drug acted through an endogenous biological system. That assumption was confirmed in 1988 when the first cannabinoid receptor, designated CB1, was discovered, followed by the discovery of a second, CB2, in the early 1990s. Both CB1 and CB2 are in the family of G protein–coupled receptors. CB1 receptors are located throughout the body, but they are found in the highest concentration in the central nervous system (CNS). In fact, CB1 receptors; are the most common of the GPCRs (G protein–coupled receptors; see Chapter 3) in the CNS, with concentrations similar to GABA and glutamate (Seely et al., 2011). They are most abundant in the hippocampus, l ganglia, cerebellum, and frontal cortex, which is consistent with their well-known effects on memory, motor coordination, perceptual processing, and

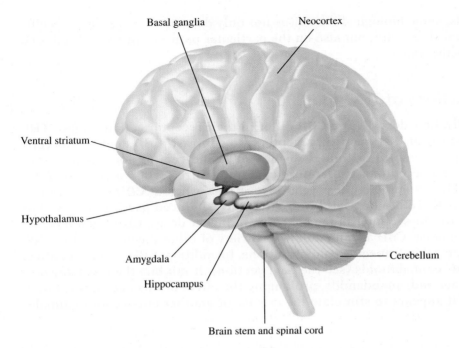

FIGURE 9.3   Cannabis produces its psychoactive effects by binding to receptors in several brain sites. These receptors are most concentrated in brain structures that regulate higher-order functions, such as judgment (neocortex), learning and memory (the hippocampus), anxiety (amygdala), drug "high" (ventral striatum), movement (basal ganglia and cerebellum), ingestion (hypothalamus), pain, and the vomiting reflex (brain stem and spinal cord).

attention, which are the respective functions of these brain structures (Figure 9.3). Because there are relatively few cannabis receptors in the brain stem, THC and other agonists have very low toxicity, except at extremely high concentrations. CB2 receptors are mostly (but not completely) found outside the CNS, primarily in tissues of the immune system, such as the tonsils and thymus. In inflammatory conditions, however, CB2 receptors can be found on the microglia cells that are activated to protect the brain.

Dopaminergic neurons are responsible for many of the positive subjective effects of THC. But the relationship between cannabinoid and dopamine systems is so complicated that it has produced conflicting evidence from research in humans and animals. Dopaminergic activity is increased by short-term THC use, while chronic use reduces such effects, although the details of long-term use are not yet clear (Bloomfield et al., 2016).

One reason it has been difficult to specify the precise effects of cannabis may be due to a phenomenon known as "functional selectivity" or "biased agonism." It has been shown that for most G protein–coupled receptors, individual agonists can have different effects on several signaling pathways through the same receptor by selectively activating different intracellular effectors (Diez-Alarcia, et al., 2016, Hebert-Chatelain et al., 2016).

In other words, some biological responses not only depend on targeting a specific G protein–coupled receptor, but also on the particular pathway, inside the cell, that this receptor activates.

Receptor Actions of THC and CBD

Mechanistically, how do THC and CBD differ in their receptor actions? First, THC is a *partial agonist* at CB1 and CB2 receptors. In contrast, CBD does not directly stimulate either receptor, although it may have indirect actions as a *partial antagonist* at CB1 receptors. It therefore can antagonize certain actions of THC. For example, THC can precipitate psychotic reactions, whereas CBD may block this action and may therefore be useful in treating THC-induced psychosis as well as schizophrenia (discussed later in the chapter). In higher doses, CBD functions as a serotonin-1A agonist. CBD also modulates a variety of other receptors in the CNS, such as a receptor that transmits pain sensations. In addition, CBD appears to affect the endogenous cannabinoids (see the next section): it inhibits the breakdown of one endocannabinoid, anandamide, prolonging the effect of this neurotransmitter. Furthermore, it appears to stimulate the release of another endogenous cannabinoid, 2-AG.

ENDOCANNABINOIDS

The discovery of the receptors through which THC produces its effects had significant implications. According to Dr. Raphael Mechoulam (2010):

> So now we are sure of two receptors that are present, and THC acts on them and stimulates them. . . . Now receptors are not present in the body because there is a plant outside there. They are present in the body in order to be activated by something the body produces when and where needed. So we went ahead looking for the compounds in the brain and periphery that would activate these receptors. And in 1992 and 1995, we reported the most important ones. One of them we called anandamide. Ananda comes from the Sanskrit name supreme joy, we were happy after working so hard identifying the compound. Which has, it turns out, to have a different chemical structure from the compound in the plant. It was rather strange, I would say, because the two compounds do exactly the same.

In Dr. Mechoulam's laboratory, Devane and coworkers (1992) isolated the first endogenous cannabinoid (eCB), anandamide, also known as *N*-arachidonoyl-ethanolamine (AEA) (see Figure 9.1B). Its pharmacology is similar to THC, although its chemical structure is different. Anandamide binds to the central (CB1) and, to a lesser extent, peripheral (CB2) cannabinoid receptors. It is found in nearly all tissues in a wide range of animals. AEA is a partial agonist at CB1 receptors and a partial agonist, or antagonist, at CB2 receptors (Seely et al., 2011).

Soon after the discovery of AEA, a second endogenous cannabinoid (eCB) was found, 2-arachidonoyl glycerol (2-AG). 2-AG binds as a full agonist to both CB1 and

CB2 receptors. It is found in even higher concentration in the brain than AEA. Since then, five more substances have been reported to function as endogenous, biologically active cannabinoid substances. Their names and chemical structures are shown in Figure 9.4.

As endogenous neurotransmitters, the eCBs are produced, released, removed, and inactivated by processes similar to those of other neurotransmitters. There are important differences, however. First, unlike typical neurotransmitters, AEA and 2-AG are not produced ahead of time and stored in the vesicles of neuronal terminals. Rather, they are synthesized on demand. What this means is that only after a postsynaptic endocannabinoid neuron is stimulated (for example, by transmitter released from a presynaptic neuron) does it begin to produce AEA or 2-AG. The transmitter opens calcium channels in the postsynaptic eCB neuron. Calcium entry activates specific enzymes, which then produce either AEA or 2-AG. Once these compounds are synthesized, they immediately diffuse out of the neuron into the synaptic space because they are very lipid soluble.

The second way this system differs from a classical transmitter function is that once the eCBs are produced and diffuse out of the postsynaptic neuron, they move back to the presynaptic neuronal terminal, where they bind to CB receptors. That is, eCBs move in a *retrograde* direction and attach to receptors on the presynaptic neuron. By binding to presynaptic CB receptors, they ultimately inhibit further release of transmitter from the presynaptic terminal. In summary, eCBs are released from depolarized postsynaptic neurons and then travel back to presynaptic neurons, where they activate CB receptors to further reduce transmitter release, such as GABA or glutamate. This represents an important way of modulating neuronal excitability and maintaining equilibrium (Battista et al., 2012: see also, Battista et al., 2015).

After the eCBs produce their effects, it is believed that they are taken back up into neurons by an endocannabinoid membrane transporter (EMT). Back in the neuron, specific enzymes metabolize them. For AEA, the major enzyme is fatty acid amide hydrolase (FAAH), which is found in the postsynaptic neuron. For 2-AG, the enzyme is monoacylglycerol lipase (MGL), which is found in the presynaptic neuron.

Drugs that inhibit uptake of eCBs as well as FAAH inhibitors have been developed that can increase brain levels of anandamide in rodents and produce analgesia and benzodiazepinelike effects in vivo, making FAAH a possible target for pain and anxiety treatment.

So, what is the function of eCBs? It has been proposed that the endocannabinoid system is involved in the normal incentives elicited, for example, by good food or other pleasurable behavior. Abnormal forms of reward, either to natural substances or drugs, are associated with dysregulated eCB signaling (Covey, 2016). According to Parsons and Hurd (2015), "[i]mpaired eCB signaling contributes to dysregulated synaptic plasticity, increased stress responsivity, negative emotional states, and cravings that propel addiction. Understanding the contributions of eCB disruptions to behavioral and physiological traits provides insight into the eCB influence on addiction vulnerability" (579). (For a review of cannabis receptors, endocannabinoids, and their postulated role in neurologic disorders such as multiple sclerosis, Huntington's disease, traumatic brain injury, and Alzheimer's disease, see Kendall and Yudowski, 2016.)

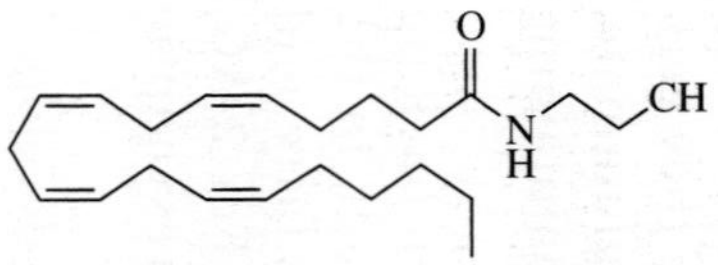

N-Arachidonoylethanolamine
(Anandamide, AEA)

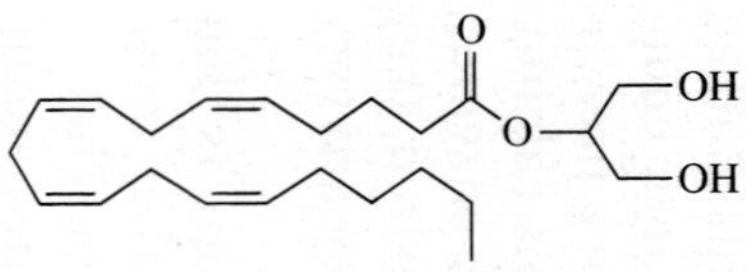

2-Arachidonoylglycerol
(2-AG)

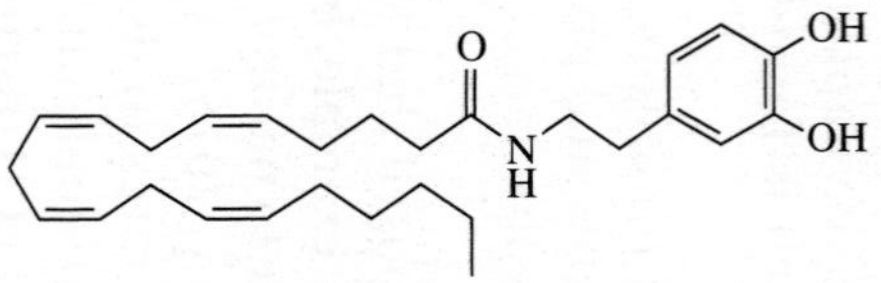

N-Arachidonoyldopamine
(NADA)

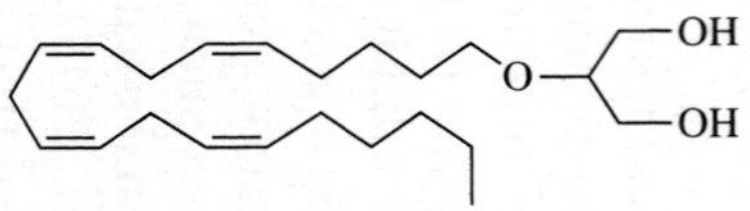

2-Arachidonoylglycerylether
(Noladin ether)

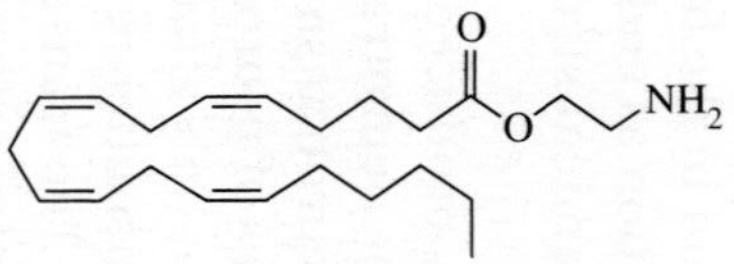

O-Arachidonoylethanolamine
(Vinodhamine)

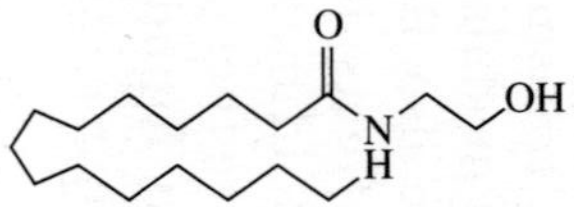

N-Palmitoylethanolamine
(PEA)

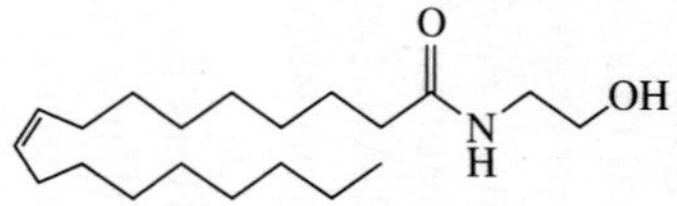

N-Oleoylethanolamine
(OEA)

FIGURE 9.4 Chemical structures of the biologically active endogenous cannabinoid compounds.

PHARMACOKINETICS

THC

THC is usually administered in the form of a hand-rolled marijuana cigarette (called a "joint") or a pipe. In general, about one-fourth to one-half of the THC is actually available in the smoke. In practice, the amount absorbed into the bloodstream depends on the amount of THC, how deeply the smoker inhales, and how long the smoke is kept in the lungs. Estimates range from 5 to 60 percent of the available THC being absorbed into the body. Whatever the amount, absorption of THC from smoking is rapid and complete. Once absorbed, THC is distributed to the various organs of the body, especially those that have significant concentrations of fatty material, such as the brain. The behavioral effects occur almost immediately after smoking begins and correspond with the rapid attainment of peak concentrations in plasma. Because of its fast and thorough metabolism, only minor amounts of THC are ultimately eliminated. The initial metabolite, 11-hydroxy-THC, is comparably psychoactive and is quickly broken down into the inactive compound, 11-nor-9-carboxy-THC (THC-COOH).

Other methods of administration include "dabbing" and "vaping." Dabbing involves preparing highly concentrated THC by passing butane through a tube packed with dried cannabis ("blasting"). Once the butane evaporates, the remaining product, butane hash oil (BHO), can reach THC concentrations up to 80 percent. BHO is then vaporized by heating it (such as with a blow torch) and inhaled ("dabbed") through a water pipe apparatus ("oil rig"). Fires, explosions, and severe burns have been attributed to this process. In addition, little is known about the long-term risks of inhaling concentrated BHO or the by-products (solder, rust, benzene) produced from heating the titanium rod ("nail") that holds the BHO during vaporization.

Another practice similar to dabbing involves putting hash oil or marijuana in a vape device or e-cigarette (see Chapter 6). Some vape devices use regular marijuana, heated to a temperature sufficient to release the active ingredients—mostly THC and CBD—as an aerosol, while preventing actual combustion. Others use concentrates such as hash oil, which can contain toxic ingredients such as lighter fluid and pesticides. For people who have not smoked before, the high concentrations of THC from vaping hash oil requires caution (Giroud et al., 2015). This is especially important when vaping BHO, which tends to be much stronger than regular marijuana. Typical BHO is at least 60 percent THC, whereas most marijuana is around 12 percent (although some strains may be as high as 28 percent).

Because much of the THC taken into the body is stored in body fat, from which it is slowly released, very low, clinically insignificant amounts of THC in blood may be maintained for a considerable time after drug use ceases; this release can last from several days to about 2 weeks and even longer in chronic smokers and obese smokers (Huestis, 2005). Such a delay tends to prolong and intensify the activity of subsequently smoked marijuana, forming a type of "reverse tolerance" to the drug, where the persistent low levels are increased by subsequently smoked THC cigarettes.

Urine testing for THC focuses on identification of its inactive metabolite, carboxy-THC. Carboxy-THC is only slowly excreted, and its half-life in urine varies. In infrequent smokers (less than twice per week), urine samples will generally be positive for 1 to 3 days. In regular smokers (those who smoke several times per week), urine specimens can test positive for 7 to 21 days. In chronic smokers, daily use for prolonged periods of time can yield positive results for 30 days or longer. Thus, a positive urine test does not necessarily mean that a person was under the influence of marijuana at the time the urine specimen was collected; there is little or no correlation between the presence of carboxy-THC in urine and the presence of a pharmacologically significant amount of THC in the blood. This can become quite important in certain legal situations, such as charges of driving while under the influence of marijuana. Exposure to secondhand smoke will usually not result in a positive result for cannabinoid metabolites in urine.

According to data from the National Institute on Drug Abuse (2017), the average marijuana extract contains over 50 percent THC, with some samples exceeding 80 percent. It is difficult to know how much the typical consumer uses, that is, if they modify their consumption depending on the potency of the material. Because the potency in prior research might have been lower, results from past studies and current studies may differ (Cressey, 2015). A recent study by DiForti and colleagues (2015) found an association between high-potency (but not low-potency) cannabis and a greater, indeed triple, risk of psychosis.

In regard to potency and research, scientists have argued that the NIDA-supplied cannabis is not comparable to that used for medicinal or recreational purposes. The only legal source of this cannabis for scientific study is the University of Mississippi, which is the only institution that has exclusive permission from the federal government to grow the plant for experimentation. Until recently, the allowed amount for research was only 21 kilograms, but it has been increased to 650 kilograms (Carroll, 2015).

Marijuana can also be taken orally, which delays onset. Acidic degradation, enzyme action, and "first-pass metabolism" may reduce the potency by two-thirds (Grilly and Salamone, 2012). However, once absorbed, the effects will last longer, and there are no associated smoking effects on the lung or any odor. With an estimated 45 percent of Colorado's marijuana sales coming in the edible form, the consequences of eating compared with smoking marijuana have become more problematic. Eating food products with THC results in a more intense and longer-lasting "high." It also takes more time for the drug to get through the liver, which means it takes longer to get "high." As a result, people often ingest more of it while they sit around waiting to feel "stoned." (In contrast, when you reach a certain level of "high" from smoking, you may forget to keep smoking.) Moreover, according to Vandrey and colleagues (2015), even where cannabis is legal, product labeling may be questionable. They report that in one study, only 17 percent of the consumable THC products in San Francisco, Los Angeles, and Seattle was correctly labeled. Greater than 50 percent had less, and some substantially more, THC than indicated. The consequence can be serious. After retail sales of recreational marijuana in Colorado began in 2014, emergency room visits increased significantly among nonresidents from 2013 to 2014 (from 85 to 168 per 10,000 emergency room visits), but not among residents (106 to 112 per 10,000 emergency room visits) (Kim et al., 2016; Kim and Monte, 2016).

Did You Know?

Maureen Dowd's Experience with Edible Marijuana

The *New York Times* editorial columnist Maureen Dowd (2014) describes her experience with edible marijuana in the form of a caramel and chocolate-flavored candy bar—and how easy it is to consume too much of a THC-infused food product and suffer the consequences:

> I nibbled off the end and then, when nothing happened, nibbled some more. . . . For an hour, I felt nothing. . . . But then I felt a scary shudder go through my body and brain. I barely made it from the desk to the bed, where I lay curled up in a hallucinatory state for the next eight hours. I was thirsty but couldn't move to get water. Or even turn off the lights. I was panting and paranoid, sure that when the room-service waiter knocked and I didn't answer, he'd call the police and have me arrested for being unable to handle my candy. . . . I strained to remember where I was or even what I was wearing, touching my green corduroy jeans and staring at the exposed-brick wall. As my paranoia deepened, I became convinced that I had died and no one was telling me. . . . It took all night before it began to wear off, distressingly slowly. The next day, a medical consultant at an edibles plant where I was conducting an interview mentioned that candy bars like that are supposed to be cut into 16 pieces for novices; but that recommendation hadn't been on the label.

Cannabidiol

Cannabidiol (CBD) is the most abundant nonpsychoactive ingredient in marijuana. It attracted interest when a strain of marijuana that was high in CBD, relative to THC, appeared to help reduce convulsions in a 3-year-old girl, Charlotte Figi, who suffered from intractable epileptic seizures (Dravet syndrome). When her mother started treating Charlotte with a laboratory-tested oil (given under the tongue in a measured amount) derived from a specific, unusual strain of cannabis, called "Charlotte's Web," the improvement was remarkable. The result prompted renewed pressure for scientific investigation of medicinal marijuana properties.

The pharmacokinetic effects of CBD are not well identified. However, Wertlake and Henson (2016) reported a technique for the identification of CBD in urine. Urinary CBD was detected for a 24-hour period (Figure 9.5). (Forensic testing currently does not identify CBD in urine, which is not necessary because CBD is not psychoactive.) It is known that following oral intake, CBD undergoes first-pass metabolism, leading to a number of metabolites, most notably 7-hydroxy-CBD (Zhornitsky and Potvin, 2012). The half-life following intravenous administration appears to be between 8 and 33 hours; 27 to 35 hours following smoking; and 2 to 5 days following oral administration. CBD is a potent inhibitor of multiple cytochrome enzymes and this may result in elevated blood concentrations of other drugs (Geffrey et al., 2015).

With regard to how CBD works within the cell, it was initially suggested that CBD blocked the metabolizing enzyme FAAH and thereby increased the levels of anandamide, an endogenous cannabinoid. It has been reported, however, that CBD does not directly block FAAH. Rather, it has been found that intracellular fatty acid

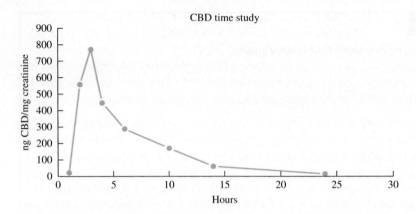

FIGURE 9.5 Twenty-four-hour time study, single individual, following a single dose of CBD oil capsules. Notes: Peak urinary level achieved approximately 3 hours postdose. Urine continued to test positive at 24 hours postdose CBD. Quantitative result corrected for creatinine concentration. [Data from Wertlake and Henson, 2016.]

binding proteins (FABPs) carry both THC and CBD from the cell membrane to the interior of the cell. FABPs also transport anandamide to its enzyme, FAAH, to be metabolized. By interacting with FABPs, THC and CBD are thought to interfere with the transport of anandamide to FAAH. In other words, THC or CBD can bind to FABPs and block anandamide from attaching to FABPs. This will reduce the amount of anandamide that gets transported to FAAH, resulting in less metabolism. Competition for FABPs may in part or wholly explain the increased circulating levels of endocannabinoids reported after consumption of cannabinoids (Elmes et al., 2015). (If both THC and CBD act this way, it is not clear why CBD has greater therapeutic effects.)

As noted, CBD reduces the psychoactive effect of THC, improving its tolerability and reducing the likelihood of adverse psychiatric side effects. In addition, the relative lack of side effects and absence of psychoactive effects allow evaluation of potential therapeutic benefits without the toxicities associated with THC. The following section describes the major pharmacological effects of THC and CBD, as well as current research developments in the medical application of these cannabinoids.

PHARMACOLOGICAL EFFECTS OF CANNABIS

Our understanding of cannabis pharmacology has become more complicated as a result of (1) the realization of the opposing actions of CBD and THC; (2) the variability of the CBD-to-THC ratio among diverse cannabis plant products; and (3) the increased potency of these and perhaps other components of the cannabis plant. An additional concern will be the issue of drug interactions between cannabis and standard medications (see Medscape review by Melton, 2017). Current discussions of physiological and psychoactive actions of cannabis will most likely need to be revised as more information is acquired about the relative contribution of these variables. The following sections summarize the major effects of cannabis and, where evidence is available, information on the specific actions of CBD, most of which comes from therapeutic applications.

Acute and Chronic Physiological Effects

Effects on the Cardiovascular System

Perhaps the most well-known cardiovascular effects of smoking marijuana are blood-shot eyes (due to dilation of the corneal blood vessels) and pupillary dilation. Smoking marijuana also elicits an initial dose-dependent increase in heart rate. Blood pressure might increase, decrease, or remain the same, depending on whether the user is standing, sitting, or lying down. Marijuana may increase the likelihood of stroke in those with other predisposing factors (Hackam, 2015). The first study (Wolff et al., 2015) to compare stroke characteristics and prognosis in younger patients (less than 45 years old) who do and do not smoke marijuana found that strokes produced by intracranial arterial stenosis were more likely to occur in those who did use the drug. This would be predicted from the cerebral vasoconstriction that is known to be elicited by cannabis. We know little about the consequences in older persons who might have compromised cardiovascular functions.

Effects on Respiration

Marijuana smoking involves repetitive, deep inhalation of unfiltered material, which is usually smoked as completely as possible in order not to waste any of the drug. So, it is no surprise that a single marijuana cigarette may be more harmful than a single tobacco cigarette in altering lung tissues and causing bronchial irritation and inflammation (Lutchmansingh et al., 2014). After controlling for tobacco use, however, there is no definitive evidence that marijuana smokers have an increase in lung cancer. This conclusion may still be premature because, in general, users smoke fewer marijuana cigarettes than nicotine, and the cohort of users may only now be reaching the age when such cancers appear. Turcotte and colleagues (2016) discuss current information on the effect of cannabis, cannabinoids, and endocannabinoids on lung function.

Effects on Sleep

Several types of sleep disturbances have been linked to chronic cannabis use, such as trouble falling asleep, maintaining sleep, feeling groggy during the next day, and the like, particularly if use began before the age of 15. If use began after the age of 18, the only difficulty was in nonrestorative sleep (Grandner, 2014). Even in adults, however, chronic daily marijuana use is significantly associated with sleep difficulties (Conroy et al., 2016).

Effects on the Immune System

Given that CB2 receptors are found primarily in the immune system, it should not be surprising that long-term marijuana use is associated with a degree of immuno-suppression, which might potentially render the smoker susceptible to infections or disease (Hegde et al., 2010). Currently, cannabinoid-induced immunosuppression does not seem to be involved in any diseases, although anti-inflammatory actions might be an important target in combating human disease (Chiurchiu et al., 2015).

Effects on Appetite, Nausea or Vomiting, and Gastrointestinal Disorders

One of the classic effects attributed to marijuana use is appetite stimulation, especially for sweet and fattening foods. This ancient association has been confirmed by modern research. THC and other CB1 receptor agonists stimulate appetite in test animals, even when the animals are sated (Seely et al., 2011). In wasting disorders, such as AIDS or cancer, cannabis may increase appetite and weight gain, but not more than the amount produced by other medications. It is possible that cannabis may actually regulate body weight, having no effect when weight is normal or excessive, but increasing it in those who are underweight. Alternately, the effect of the drug on body weight may be associated with long-term versus short-term use, the presence of other drugs, or the competition between cannabis and food for brain sites that mediate reward (Sansone and Sansone, 2014).

Appetite stimulation has been used to clinical advantage. In 1981, *nabilone* (Cesamet), a synthetic derivative of THC and the first licensed cannabis medical product, was approved to treat nausea and vomiting associated with cancer chemotherapy. In 1985, *dronabinol* (Marinol), which is synthetic THC, was approved as an antiemetic for similar situations and, in 1992, approval was extended to stimulate appetite in wasting conditions, such as AIDS. In August 2017, Syndros was approved as the first dronabinol solution for oral use, making it easy to swallow and allowing the dosage to be titrated to clinical effect. Whether other components of cannabis have antiemetic properties has not yet been determined and may be worth investigation (Rock and Parker, 2016). A cannabinoid *antagonist*, *rimonabant* (Acomplia), was developed as a diet drug, but its safety was unacceptable and it was removed from the market (Lee et al., 2009). (These drugs are discussed later in this chapter.)

Recent anecdotal evidence suggests that *cannabinoids* may affect gastric emptying and colonic motility, and strong evidence exists of an intestinal anti-inflammatory effect (Esposito et al., 2013; Izzo et al., 2015; Naftali et al., 2014). Therefore, CBD seems to have the potential to target treatment of gastrointestinal tract disorders such as irritable bowel syndrome and inflammatory bowel disease in addition to its possible role in inhibiting colon cancers (Romano et al., 2014).

Acute and Chronic Psychoactive Effects

Subjective Effects

The psychological and psychiatric effects of THC vary with dose, route of administration, experience of the user, vulnerability to psychoactive effects, and the setting in which administration occurs. Users report an increased sense of well-being, mild euphoria, relaxation, and relief from anxiety. In an interesting side note, moderate use of marijuana by married couples was associated with less intimate partner violence (Smith et al., 2014). Sometimes anxiety is increased, which may be at least partly due to the perceived increase in heart rate. In general, the senses may be enhanced and the perception of time is usually altered. Often, events seem especially funny, and laughter is easily elicited. Mundane ideas can seem profound and the loosening of associations and thought intrusions can produce an inflated sense of creativity. Illusions and hallucinations occur infrequently, possibly more at high doses.

Psychomotor Effects

Cannabis can produce impairments in coordination, perception, reaction time, and divided attention that persist for several hours beyond one's perception of the "high." This alone has obvious implications for the operation of a motor vehicle as well as impairments in performance in the workplace or at school. Driving under the influence of marijuana doubles or triples the risk of a crash. People driving under the influence of marijuana tend to compensate by driving slower, but, when the task intensity of driving increases, the driver becomes more impaired. Specifically, cannabis use increases lane weaving and impairs critical-tracking tasks, reaction time, and divided attention (MacDonald and Pappas, 2016). This increased risk is greatly potentiated by concomitant use of alcohol, even though guidelines for concomitant use have not been legislated. Doucette and coworkers (2017) offer a proposal to use an oral fluid assay to determine the degree of cannabinoid-induced driving impairment.

Rewarding Effects

It is not really known why marijuana is so rewarding. In humans, there is a range of THC doses that is pleasurable; below that there is no effect, above that, the reaction is unpleasant (Grilly and Salamone, 2012). Nonhuman primates will self-administer THC, AEA, and 2-AG (Justinova et al., 2011), substances that activate the mesolimbic dopaminergic reward system (Cooper and Haney, 2009). Barkus and colleagues (2011), however, found that intravenous injection of THC did not increase dopamine release in the brain of male volunteers, even though it was sufficient to elicit psychotic symptoms in the participants.

Filbey and Dewitt (2012) demonstrated that in abstinent marijuana users, marijuana cues activated reward neurocircuitry and the magnitude of activation was associated with the severity of problems related to marijuana use. In contrast, the intravenous administration of a synthetic CB1 agonist, Org-26828, to healthy male volunteers produced drowsiness at low doses, but caused unpleasant effects of anxiety, paranoia, and hallucinations at higher doses (Zuurman et al., 2010).

Huestis and colleagues (2001) demonstrated in humans that a specific antagonist for cannabinoid receptors produced a dose-dependent blockade of marijuana-induced intoxication and tachycardia. This suggested that cannabinoid antagonists might be used to reverse cannabinoid intoxication in people who experience unpleasant reactions (for example, panic and psychosis) or to treat cannabis addiction, similar to the use of naloxone for opioid overdose or addiction (see Chapter 10). Although cannabis, even when it is the only drug ingested, produces numerous drug-related emergency room visits each year, it is not a lethal substance. Estimates are that a fatal dose would have to be 20,000 to 40,000 times the typically ingested dose (Levinthal, 2012).

Moreover, even chronic use does not inevitably produce physical ill health. Laboratory measures of physical health (periodontal health, lung function, systemic inflammation, and metabolic health), as well as self-reported physical health status, showed that moderate cannabis use, even after 20 years, is not associated with physical health problems in early midlife, except for periodontal disease (Meier et al., 2016).

Cognitive Effects

Perhaps the best-known psychoactive effect of marijuana is that it produces memory impairment. THC impairs all stages of memory, including encoding, consolidation, and retrieval. The ability to focus attention and filter out irrelevant information is disrupted. Marijuana users' speech and presumably their underlying thought patterns become fragmented. Because of the distracting intrusions of other ideas, users forget what they or others have recently said. This difficulty in concentration impairs performance on many cognitive tasks. Furthermore, marijuana may also reduce the motivation to perform well. Even nabilone has been shown to cause impairments in attention and memory in computerized laboratory tasks in healthy male volunteers (Wesnes et al., 2010).

The memory-disrupting effects appear to be mediated by CB1 receptors in the hippocampus (Wise et al., 2009), perhaps by actions on mitochondrial CB1 receptors in that structure (Hebert-Chatelain et al., 2016). One large study of nearly a thousand marijuana users, as well as healthy controls for comparison, found that the drug was associated with abnormally low blood flow in virtually every area of the brain, but especially in the hippocampus, which might increase the risk of ultimately developing Alzheimer's disease (Amen et al., 2017). Long-term, heavy cannabis use in MS patients (with a mean duration of 27 years) may affect cognition beyond what might occur as a result of the disease itself (Honarmand et al., 2011; Pavisian et al., 2014). One intriguing finding is that the memory impairment produced by smoking marijuana may be inversely correlated with the amount of CBD in the product (Morgan et al., 2010).

Although cognitive deficits can persist for at least one month following discontinuation of heavy use, it is generally believed that only minimal effects are likely to persist. One study, however, has found that heavy cannabis users have smaller hippocampi and amygdalae than control subjects, and that this was associated with having a certain form of the CB1 gene (Schacht et al., 2012). Given the importance of these two structures for cognition, such long-term changes are troubling, especially considering that the mean age of the men and women in the study was between 27 and 28. These data are consistent with the findings of Meier and colleagues (2012), that people with comparable IQs at age 7, who were persistently diagnosed with cannabis abuse when they were teenagers, had statistically significant decreases in IQ by the age of 38. If heavy cannabis use began in adulthood, there was no change in IQ.

Effects on the Reproductive System and Pregnancy

In Western culture, marijuana is often reported to enhance sexual responsivity, whereas other cultures consider the drug to be a sexual depressant. This difference may be an example of the strong influence of expectation on cannabis's effects. But it is also possible that there is a dose-related mechanism in that low doses may enhance libido while higher doses depress it. Chronic use of marijuana by males can reduce levels of the hormone testosterone and reduce sperm count and viability (duPlessis et al., 2015). Reductions in male fertility and sexual potency, however, have not been reported. On the other hand, there is some evidence that smoking marijuana is associated with a mild increase in testicular cancer (Gurney et al., 2015). This is the most common malignancy diagnosed in young men between the ages of 15 and 45. In females, the levels of follicle-stimulating hormone and luteinizing hormone are reduced by the use of marijuana. Menstrual cycles can be affected and anovulatory cycles have been reported. All these actions reverse when drug use is discontinued.

Marijuana is the most widely used illicit drug during pregnancy and its use is increasing. Aside from recreational use, pregnant women are increasingly using marijuana to treat nausea, particularly during the first trimester of pregnancy, which is the riskiest period for deleterious effects of drug exposure to the fetus. Endogenous cannabinoids are present by day 16 of gestation, at the beginning of central nervous system development, when neural circuitry is forming. Moreover, the concentration of THC is increasing, not only in marijuana but also in other formulations, such as hash oil. Pregnant women, and those considering becoming pregnant, should be advised to avoid using marijuana or other cannabinoids either recreationally or to treat their nausea (Volkow et al., 2016).

THC freely crosses the placenta and is found in breast milk. Therefore, the developing brain is susceptible to cannabis during gestation and it would be expected to have some neurodevelopmental consequences. But the data are sparse and conflicting. While some reviewers conclude that cannabis increases the likelihood of preterm birth and small size for gestational age (Fantasia, 2017), others report only a small, nonclinically important drop in birth weight, with no difference even in preterm births or neurodevelopmental outcome for at least the first three years (Zhang et al., 2017). Although cannabis use does not appear to increase the incidence of birth defects (Mark and Terplan, 2017), one report concluded that newborns of women who smoked marijuana when pregnant may display mild, transient withdrawal signs, such as hyperactivity, reduced cognitive functioning, and changes in dopaminergic functioning (Metz and Stickrath, 2015).

The problems with information about the effects of cannabis and synthetic cannabinoids during pregnancy are that (1) the data are obtained from self-reports and (2) that it is often complicated by concurrent use of other drugs, including tobacco and alcohol (Orsolini et al., 2017). It has been reported that the majority of women reduce their consumption of or terminate cannabis use while they are pregnant (Mark and Terplan, 2017). In this regard, a survey of current cannabis use among pregnant women found that 35 percent of women were using cannabis when their pregnancy was confirmed and of those, 34 percent continued to use the drug, even though 70 percent believed that cannabis during pregnancy could be harmful. If a pregnant woman believed that cannabis was not harmful during pregnancy, she was more likely to use the drug (Mark et al., 2017). Lamy and colleagues (2017) tested the stool (meconium) of newborns to determine what the fetus ingested during the third trimester of gestation. They then compared the results with the self-reports of the mothers. The levels of cannabis metabolites were low and were not well correlated with maternal reports of cannabis use, whereas the levels of the tobacco metabolite cotinine were highly correlated with maternal smoking reports. Recently, Kim and coworkers (2017) "developed and validated a specific and sensitive method for the simultaneous determination of THC, its metabolites, . . . and CBD in umbilical cord samples," which should provide a more accurate method for determining fetal exposure. There is a need to obtain more information on its gestational and postnatal effects (Grant et al., 2017).

Therapeutic Applications of Cannabinoids

According to a recent survey, in spite of minimal clinical evidence for such indications (see next section), a substantial number of people decrease their use of medications for pain, anxiety, migraines, and insomnia after starting medical cannabis use (Piper et al., 2017).

Nonpsychiatric Disorders

Effects on Pain and Spasticity

In both humans and animals, THC and cannabinoids have been reported to be analgesic, especially against pain resulting from persistent inflammation or neuropathic pain, an action distinct from that of opioids such as morphine (Boychuk et al., 2015). Patients using medical marijuana to control chronic pain reported a 64 percent reduction in their use of more traditional, opioid prescription pain medication (Boehnke et al., 2016), although clinical data are still scarce (Nielsen et al., 2017; Nugent et al., 2017). Efforts to develop a cannabis-derived analgesic agent for clinical use, however, are yet to be successful and there is a great deal of conflicting experimental results. One systematic review of randomized trials concluded that smoking marijuana was not efficacious for managing chronic noncancer pain (Deshpande et al., 2015). In contrast, compelling evidence exists that CBD can reduce sensations of painful burning, pins and needles, numbness, neuropathic pain, and other painful conditions (Jensen et al., 2015). Fine and Rosenfeld (2013) review the analgesic effects of cannabinoids, focusing on CBD.

Smoking marijuana may, however, specifically reduce spasticity-related pain in people diagnosed with multiple sclerosis (MS). An oral medication, *nabiximols* (Sativex), is approved in Canada, New Zealand, and eight European countries for the relief of muscle spasms and poor sleep quality associated with MS as well as pain associated with end-stage cancer. Sativex contains THC and CBD in a 1:1 mixture, delivered in an oromucosal (mouth) spray. Patti and coworkers (2016) reviewed the efficacy of Sativex: 60 percent of patients reported efficacy, 26 percent discontinued the drug for lack of effectiveness, and 18 percent for side effects. The data suggest that any analgesic effect of cannabis may be due to the muscle relaxation as a result of its antispastic action rather than a direct analgesic action.

The American Academy of Neurology (AAN) supported nabiximols for MS pain and spasticity (Koppel et al., 2014) and recommended nabiximols and dronabinol for spasticity and central pain, and nabiximols for urinary disorders of MS as well (Hill, 2015). In contrast, Whiting and colleagues (2015) concluded that there was only moderate-quality evidence to support the use of cannabinoids for the treatment of chronic pain and spasticity (see also Otero-Romero et al., 2016), and that there was only low-quality evidence suggesting that cannabinoids were associated with improvements in nausea and vomiting due to chemotherapy, weight gain in HIV infection, sleep disorders, and Tourette syndrome.

Epilepsy

In the popular press, there are numerous uncontrolled clinical cases reporting medical marijuana as a treatment for epilepsy. Many of these are anecdotal accounts of children with refractory epilepsies, such as Dravet syndrome, Lennox-Gastaut syndrome (LGS), and Doose syndrome. Interest in the "Charlotte's Web" form of marijuana surged after its reported benefit in Charlotte Figi. The "Charlotte's Web" strain of medical marijuana has very little THC, with greater than a minimum 30:1 CBD-to-THC ratio (Kaur et al., 2016; Kolikonda et al., 2016; Saad and Joshi, 2015).

In 2016, several positive clinical studies were reported in conference abstracts. That same year, GW Pharmaceuticals announced positive results of the first randomized, double-blind, placebo-controlled Phase 3 clinical trial of its investigational medicine Epidiolex (CBD) for the treatment of LGS. In this trial, Epidiolex, when added as an adjunct to the patient's current treatment, significantly reduced the monthly frequency of drop seizures assessed over the entire 14-week treatment period compared with placebo ($p = 0.0135$). Epidiolex has "Orphan Drug Designation" from the FDA for the treatment of LGS and Dravet syndrome. Devinsky and coworkers (2017) have recently reported positive results for cannabidiol in Dravet syndrome.

Neuroprotection

Cannabinoids and their derivatives have been postulated to possess neuroprotective effects following brain injury (Fernandez-Ruiz et al., 2012; Nguyen et al., 2014). This action is based on the ability of THC to inhibit glutaminergic transmission and reduce reactive oxygen intermediates, which may mediate neuronal damage after head injury. One synthetic cannabinoid derivative, however, dexanabinol, was not efficacious in the treatment of traumatic brain injury in humans (Maas et al., 2006).

Cancers

The use of marijuana to treat the nausea and vomiting, anorexia, and pain associated with cancer chemotherapy led to studies of possible antitumor effects of cannabis. McAllister and colleagues (2015) and Huang and colleagues (2015) reviewed the antitumor properties of CBD and discussed its potential beneficial effects on many types of cancer, including glioblastoma, breast, lung, prostate, and colon cancer. This may be an important advance beyond the symptomatic treatment of cancer-associated nausea, vomiting, and pain. Soderstrom and coworkers (2017) provide an extensive review of cannabinoids and cancer, emphasizing actions that are not mediated by CB receptors.

Glaucoma

In 2014, the American Academy of Ophthalmology (AAO) reiterated that it does not recommend the use of medical marijuana or other cannabis products to treat glaucoma, particularly when standard therapies are available and effective. The AAO used findings from an analysis by the National Eye Institute and the Institute of Medicine as the basis for its position. Reductions in intraocular pressure following medical marijuana use were short-lived.

Psychiatric Disorders

Alzheimer's Disease

In patients already diagnosed with Alzheimer's disease, up to 4.5 milligrams daily of oral THC daily showed no benefit in reducing neuropsychiatric symptoms in dementia, such as aggression and agitation, but it was well tolerated (Van den Elsen et al., 2015). In contrast, early work in animals has shown that CBD can reverse cognitive deficits (Booz, 2011). CBD may blunt beta-amyloid-induced neuroinflammation and may be a promising agent for reducing the neuronal loss seen in Alzheimer's disease (Esposito et al., 2007; Martin-Moreno et al., 2011). Results of preliminary experiments by researchers at the Salk Institute have indicated that THC and other constituents of cannabis may facilitate the elimination of amyloid beta from brain cells. Although these data came from neurons developed in the laboratory, the implications may promote new treatments for Alzheimer's disease (Currais et al., 2016).

Anxiety Disorders

One of the indications allowed for medicinal marijuana in some states is posttraumatic stress disorder (PTSD). Although there are some scattered reports that the drug may decrease symptoms of PTSD, definitive conclusions are premature because there is insufficient clinical trial data (O'Neil et al., 2017; Yarnell, 2015). Wilkinson and colleagues (2016) conclude that we do not have satisfactory information on the safety and efficacy of marijuana for the psychiatric conditions of Tourette's syndrome, PTSD, or Alzheimer's disease. Anxiety is positively associated with cannabis use or cannabis use disorder (CUD) in cohorts drawn from some 112,000 noninstitutionalized members of the general population of 10 countries (Kedzior and Laeber, 2014). Wilkinson and coworkers (2015) found that chronic marijuana use in war veterans actually worsened PTSD and was associated with more outbursts of violent behavior and alcohol use. Nevertheless, there is some evidence that cannabis has some therapeutic effect for social anxiety (Blanco et al., 2016), possibly by reducing negative emotional states in those with this disorder (Buckner and Schmidt, 2009).

The DEA recently approved the first U.S. clinical trial to develop the marijuana plant into a prescription medicine to treat PTSD symptoms. The randomized controlled trial—sponsored by the Multidisciplinary Association for Psychedelic Studies (MAPS), a nonprofit organization dedicated to alternative medicine—will document the effects of smoked marijuana on 76 war veterans who have chronic, treatment-resistant PTSD. With DEA approval, the study has been given the green light from every relevant federal agency, including the Food and Drug Administration, the National Institute on Drug Abuse, and the Public Health Service. According to MAPS, the study started in 2016, and as of April 2017, had 12 subjects.

In contrast to marijuana, and perhaps because of its antagonistic action, early evidence strongly supports CBD as a treatment for a variety of anxiety disorders, including generalized anxiety disorder (Sarris et al., 2013), panic disorder (Soares and Campos, 2017), and social anxiety disorders (Bergamaschi et al., 2011; see also Blessing et al., 2015). But few studies have investigated chronic CBD dosing or compared CBD with drugs known to also be effective, such as benzodiazepines. One interesting aspect of this issue is the recent report of a genetic variant that influences the synthesis of the endogenous cannabinoid, anandamide (Dincheva et al., 2015). That is, some people (as well as mice) have a mutation of the gene that is responsible for making the enzyme FAAH, which deactivates anandamide. In other words, anyone with this mutation has less of the FAAH enzyme and, consequently, more anandamide. This suggests that such individuals may be generally less anxious or less likely to find cannabis as rewarding than people who naturally have more of the FAAH enzyme and less anandamide.

Schizrenia

There is compelling epidemiological evidence that cannabis is a risk factor for the onset of psychosis (Hamilton, 2017; Wilkinson et al., 2015). It has long been known that schizophrenia patients have a greater history of cannabis abuse (25 percent) than people in the general population (4 percent). As early as 1958, a published study described psychoticlike behavior in healthy volunteers after a single ingestion of cannabis, and it has been reported that up to 15 percent of cannabis users experience acute psychotic symptoms. In 1987, a comprehensive review of over 45,000 Swedish military conscripts found that those who consumed high amounts of cannabis (used more than 50 times) by the age of 18 years were 6 times more likely to have schizophrenia, even after controlling for contributing variables. In 2002, this result was replicated, showing that the risk of schizophrenia had increased to 6.7 times. This has prompted numerous efforts to determine whether psychotic symptoms predate the drug or vice versa. One extensive survey, conducted proactively on a birth cohort of persons in New Zealand, collected information about psychotic symptoms at age 11 and drug use by age 15. The results showed that early cannabis use did increase the risk of psychosis. However, whether this was due to the fact that drug exposure occurred during a time when the brain was still developing was a result of longer exposure to the drug in early users is not clear, and both factors may contribute (Lynch et al., 2012).

These and many other longitudinal studies indicate some relationship between chronic, perhaps high-dose, cannabis use and psychotic disorder (Malone et al., 2010). According to Bechtold and coworkers (2016), the effects of previous weekly cannabis use are retained in adolescents for as long as one year after they have stopped using the drug. This is not simply due to drug abuse in general; for example, alcohol use does not show this association (Large et al., 2011). Cannabis use by young people increased the risk of a psychotic experience even in those who had no prior psychotic event (Kuepper et al., 2011). In subjects who have a clinically high risk for psychosis, earlier lifetime use is associated with earlier symptomatology (Tosato et al., 2013). Even without a family history of psychosis, cannabis use is associated with the onset of schizophrenia spectrum disorder occurring three years earlier compared with drug abstinence (Helle et al., 2016), and with a more severe course and progno-sis than schizophrenia cases in general (Manrique-Garcia et al., 2014). Furthermore, continued use of cannabis after onset of psychosis was associated with more relapses compared with both discontinued use and never having used cannabis at all (Schoeler et al., 2016a, 2016b; see Andrade, 2016, for a review). One study found that cannabis users at baseline had lower body mass index, smaller waist circumference, lower dia-stolic blood pressure, and more severe psychotic symptoms than nonusers; all these parameters decreased in patients who discontinued their cannabis use after the first assessment (Bruins et al., 2016), which suggests some metabolic interactions of canna-bis with either schizophrenia or, perhaps, antipsychotics.

Possible causes for the relationship between early onset cannabis use and psycho-sis are controversial. One factor is the increased potency of cannabis (DiForti et al., 2015). During the last 20 to 30 years, the percent of THC in all parts of the marijuana plant has increased, with some reports of up to 18 percent or more, compared to past levels of 3 percent. It is not known whether or not cannabis users modify their behav-ior if the potency increases, for example, by smoking less, or changing the way they inhale. There is some data showing that users with more experience may alter their intake, depending on how strong they think the material is, but they are not capable of making accurate adjustments when potency varies or on overcoming the negative emo-tional effects of the drug (Freeman, et al., 2014; van der Pol, et al., 2014).

Some studies suggest that the risk of developing schizophrenia is an impetus for the onset of cannabis use (Gage et al., 2016). Other findings suggest that a small part of the association between schizophrenia and cannabis is due to a shared genetic etiol-ogy (Power et al., 2014), although a common genetic risk could not explain the entire association with symptoms of psychosis (Nesvåg et al., 2017).

Another factor involved in cannabis-induced psychosis may be the concentra-tion of CBD. Leweke and colleagues (2012) report that this component of cannabis reduces psychotic symptoms in patients with acute schizophrenia. Similarly, another study found that healthy people had fewer psychotic reactions to intravenous THC if they were pretreated with CBD (Evins et al., 2012). Englund and colleagues (2013) also found that in normal volunteers, CBD inhibited psychotic and paranoid symptoms and even improved the memory impairment produced by THC. Indeed, CBD appears to have therapeutic potential in the treatment of schizophrenia as well as in the acute treatment of THC-induced psychosis (Fakhoury, 2016; Manseau and Goff, 2015). Clinical trials of CBD in schizophrenia are currently under way. Unpublished results were reported of a six week trial of CBD (GW42003, 1000 milligrams per day). Used as adjunct therapy in 88 patients diagnosed with schizophrenia or a related condition, CBD outperformed placebo in reducing symptoms without any problematic side effects (Leweke et al., 2016; Rohleder et al., 2016; Schubart et al., 2014).

In 2017 the National Academies of Sciences, Engineering, and Medicine authored *The Health Effects of Cannabis and Cannabinoids: The Current State of Evidence and Recommendations for Research*, a comprehensive review of scientific evidence related to the health effects and potential therapeutic benefits of cannabis. This report pro-vides a research agenda—outlining gaps in current knowledge and opportunities for providing additional insight into these issues—that summarizes and prioritizes pressing research needs.

For the majority of users, cannabis use does not promote psychiatric problems. Frequent use, however, may increase the likelihood of depression and suicidality (Agrawal et al., 2017). At the same time, among people with mental illness, reporting at least weekly use, the rate of cannabis use was especially high for those with bipolar disorder, personality disorder, and, perhaps not surprisingly, other substance use disorders, such as alcohol (Blanco et al., 2016; Lev-Ran et al., 2013; Weinberger et al., 2016). In bipolar patients, recent studies have noted that cannabis use preceded the onset of mania (Gibbs et al., 2015; Tyler et al., 2015). Current cannabis users were less likely to have periods of recovery and remission and more likely to have recurrence, relapse, and attempted suicide; previous users' patterns closely resembled the patterns of those who never used cannabis (Zorrilla et al., 2015).

SYNTHETIC CANNABINOID AGONISTS OF ABUSE

In 1964, after THC was determined to be the active ingredient of *Cannabis sativa*, efforts were made to develop synthetic cannabinoids (SC) for possible therapeutic applications. By 1985, this had been accomplished and *dronabinol* (Marinol) was approved in the United States as an antiemetic drug. Several other agents that are chemically similar to THC have also been produced, notably *nabilone* (Cesamet) and HU-210 (synthesized at the Hebrew University in the 1960s). Nabilone is almost as potent as THC and is the only THC analog that has ever been approved as an antiemetic in the United States. HU-210 has not been approved, mainly because it is 100 to 800 times as potent as THC (Seely et al., 2011).

Additional SC compounds that differ chemically from THC were also synthesized. Chemists at the drug company Pfizer developed a group of drugs known as *cyclohexylphenols* (CP). These include substances designated as CP-50,556-1 and CP-47,497, and a related form, (C8)-CP-47,497, all of which are 30 times more potent than THC. Perhaps the newest cyclohexylphenol is NE-CHMIMO (Angerer et al., 2016), which has been found along with 5F-ADB (also known as 5F-MDMB-PINACA, another synthetic cannabinoid) in a so-called herbal mixture branded as "Jamaican Gold Extreme."

A third group of related drugs is categorized as aminoalkylindoles (AAI). This includes a drug called *pravadoline* and similar compounds, such as WIN-55212–2, developed by Sterling Drug Company. These drugs have a high affinity for both types of cannabis receptors, produce effects similar to those of THC in laboratory animals, and are blocked by cannabinoid antagonists. Nearly 20 years ago, John W. Huffman, a research chemist at Clemson University, created three of these AAIs, designated JWH-018 (1-pentyl-3-(1-naphthoyl)-indole), JWH-073, and JWH-015. These drugs have different binding affinities to the two CB receptors, but generally have similar pharmacological effects as THC, with JWH-018 having the greater relative potency (Seely et al., 2011).

Last, a fourth group of compounds that act at CB receptors, called *benzoylindoles*, include the substances AM-694 and RCS-4 (Fattore and Fratta, 2011). (For a more detailed list of chemical subdivisions, see Rosenbaum et al., 2012.)

Current Abuse

In the early 2000s, several SC compounds became available and were sold widely by "head shops" and convenience stores as well as through Internet vendors. By 2007, these compounds gained the attention of U.S. authorities. Generically called "spice" as well as other names,[1] these products are usually sold as dried leaves, resin, or powder, and without age restriction (Papanti et al., 2013; Rosenbaum et al., 2012). (See Seely et al., 2011, for a list of the herbs that are used in these products.)

The process by which spice is manufactured was compellingly described by the *New York Times* reporter Alan Schwarz (2015). After production in China, SC drugs are transported to U.S. wholesalers in the form of powder, packed in containers, and stamped as fertilizer or industrial solvents. At these sites, the powder is dissolved in alcohol or acetone, sprayed on plant material that can be smoked, and then packaged in metallic bags, which often contain the warning "Not for human consumption." Sometimes the plant material is prepared in containers that held animal feed, in cement mixers, or in other unprotected locations, which could be contaminated with hazardous substances, mold, and the like.

The chemicals are also now available as liquid cartridges used in electronic cigarettes (Castellanos and Gralnik, 2016). Typically, about 3 grams of vegetable matter are mixed in a synthetic cannabinoid package, which can be smoked or drunk as an infusion. The vegetable matter (the "herbals") in these preparations is not psychoactive; it is the synthetic drugs (the "spice") that produce the psychoactive effects.

Several factors make treatment of SC abuse difficult. There is no antidote yet, which means that no matter how intense or unexpected the reactions, the only available remedies are intravenous electrolytes and other basic medical support. Because the symptoms of intoxication can also be elicited by other types of abused stimulants or hallucinogenic drugs, it is not easy to diagnose the syndrome produced by SC agents, especially in someone who has not used them before. The problem in identifying SC intoxication is made even more difficult because there are no quick laboratory assays to confirm the presence of the drug. There is no standard urine screen for SC agents and exposure can only be verified by complicated analyses in specialized laboratories (Trecki et al., 2015). Furthermore, even the metabolic products of these substances may be psychoactive and elicit some of the symptoms (Seely et al., 2012). The difficulty of determining the active ingredients in spice products is also due to the addition of natural substances, such as tocopherol (Vitamin E) and some agents, such as nicotine, that might be stated as an ingredient, but are not actually present. In an effort to avoid federal and state prohibitions, additives are frequently changed. Furthermore, it takes time for various laboratories to calibrate and verify their in-house techniques, even after the initial agent and its metabolites are identified (Papanti et al., 2013; Trecki et al., 2015).

In summary, these drugs have gained worldwide popularity because they produce psychoactive effects; may still be legal, are easily available, and cheap; and are still

---

[1] Other variants of spice with high CBD and low THC are also available: (1) "Harlequin," which contains CBD/THC ratios of about 5:2; (2) "Sour Tsunami," which contains CBD and THC in a roughly equal amount (10 to 11 percent each); (3) "Pennywise," which is similar to Sour Tsunami; (4) "Harle-Tsu," which contains CBD and THC, is about a 20:1 ratio; (5) "ACTC," which is similar to Harle-Tsu, with up to 19 percent CBD, and (6) "Cannatonic," which contains 6 to 17 percent CBD at a THC concentration of about 6 percent.

difficult to detect, even though their negative psychoactive effects are now generally well known (Lauritsen and Rosenberg, 2016). Several European countries have banned these compounds. In the United States, synthetic cannabinoids have been classified as Schedule I compounds and are now banned in all states.

Pharmacological, Physiological, and Psychoactive Effects and Toxicity

In general, the basic pharmacology and pharmacokinetics of synthetic cannabinoids is unknown. Likewise, effects in pregnancy have not been reported. Presley and coworkers (2016) review what little is known about their metabolism in the body. Miliano and coworkers (2016) review the rewarding effects of these cannabinoid agonists as dopaminergic signaling agents in the nucleus accumbens. Cooper (2016) reviews the adverse effects of both acute intoxication as well as long-term abuse and subsequent withdrawal problems.

According to Papanti and colleagues (2013), "[t]he available evidence suggests that SCs can trigger the onset of acute psychosis in vulnerable individuals and the exacerbation of psychotic episodes in those with a previous psychiatric history" (379). Significantly, more symptoms ($p = 0.03$) were reported by respondents seeking treatment for SCs than for cannabis (Winstock and Barratt, 2013). Clinical symptoms include excited delirium, acute kidney injury (AKI), seizures, psychosis, hallucinations, cardiotoxic effects, coma, and death. Deaths from SC use have ranged from 13 to 56 years of age (Trecki et al., 2015; see their summary table of major episodes and outbreaks of SCs).

Shalit and colleagues (2016) compared SC users to cannabis users. Figure 9.6 provides some information about the increase in adverse reactions to these compounds. SC users were generally younger males who had greater severity of psychotic symptoms at admission, were more likely to be admitted by criminal court order, and required longer hospitalization periods in comparison to cannabis users. Cited motives for SC use included curiosity or experimentation (91 percent), a desire to feel good or get high (89 percent), to relax (71 percent), and to get high without risking a positive drug test (71 percent) (Bonar et al., 2014).

As noted, there is no pharmacologically specific antidote for these substances, especially because the actual contents are usually unknown. Spice blends do not contain CBD and the use of CBD as an antidote to spice intoxication has not yet been reported. In addition to supportive care, benzodiazepines may be helpful for anxiety and agitation caused by spice intoxication.

Tolerance and a cannabinoid withdrawal syndrome have been reported. Withdrawal symptoms are typical of cannabis withdrawal, namely, internal unrest, sweating, drug craving, nightmares, tremor, palpitations, nausea, and vomiting. Psychotic symptoms may be elicited in normal individuals, and recovered psychotic patients may relapse. Gastrointestinal reactions are common, and several cases of AKI from these agents were reported across the United States (Murphy et al., 2013). Five of the patients needed hemodialysis. There was no single brand associated with all the cases, but a new, previously unreported fluorinated agent was discovered, methanone (XLR-11), which was a potent CB agonist. Coma and suicide have been reported. In the United States, for example, two adolescents died after taking a spice product, one from a coronary ischemic event and the other from suicide due to extreme anxiety (Fattore and Fratta, 2011).

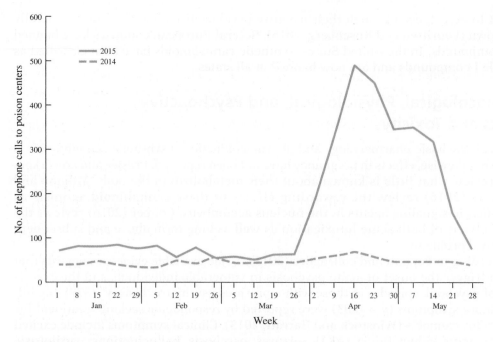

FIGURE 9.6 A line graph comparing the number of weekly telephone calls to poison centers in the United States reporting adverse health effects related to synthetic cannabinoid use from January to May 2014 and the same period in 2015. [Data from Law et al., 2015.]

Did You Know?

Mass Intoxication from Synthetic Cannabinoids

In July 2016, 33 people in a New York City neighborhood consumed a synthetic cannabinoid drug that produced intoxicated behavior likened to a "zombie" outbreak. The substance they took was the "incense" compound AK-4724 Karat Gold, that is, AMB-FUBINACA or MMB-FUBINACA, which stands for methyl 2-(1-(4-fluorobenzyl)-1H-indazole-3-carboxamido)-3-methylbutanoate). In the serum or whole blood of eight individuals, the metabolite concentrations ranged from 77 to as high as 636 nanograms per milliliter (Adams et al., 2017).

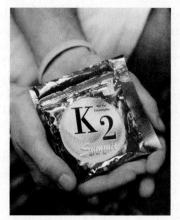

A three gram package of K_2, a synthetic cannabinoid. [Associated Press]

CANNABIS TOLERANCE, WITHDRAWAL, ADDICTION, AND DEPENDENCE

Experienced users of marijuana often report that they become more sensitive to its psychoactive effects (sensitized) rather than less (tolerant) with continued use. That is, they become "high" more quickly. However, tolerance to cannabis routinely develops in laboratory studies. This difference between experimental and "real-world" exposure is believed to be due to several factors. First, novice users have to learn how to get enough of the smoke into the lungs to provide a sufficient THC dose. Second, new users have to learn to be aware of the subjective effects of the drug. Third, because the drug accumulates in fat tissue, regular smokers have some residual amount of THC in their bodies, which increases the total amount with each cigarette, producing a quicker "high." Nevertheless, tolerance does occur to cannabis. Some degree of tolerance results from learning how to adapt to the drug's disruptive effects. Rodent studies had shown that CB1 receptors were downregulated after chronic cannabis exposure, which would also mediate tolerance. Hirvonen and colleagues (2012) have shown reversible and regionally specific downregulation of CB1 receptors in cortical brain regions of human subjects who chronically smoke cannabis. Downregulation correlated with years of smoking and receptor density returned to normal after about four weeks of monitored abstinence.

Withdrawal symptoms include irritability, anxiety, marijuana craving, disrupted sleep and strange dreams, anger and aggression, depressed mood, restlessness, decreased appetite, and weight loss. Less common symptoms include chills, headache, physical tension, sweating, stomach pain, and general physical discomfort (Vandrey and Haney, 2009). Symptoms begin within 48 hours after drug use stops and last at least 2 days, usually about 7 to 10 days, and perhaps longer; electroencephalography (EEG) changes associated with withdrawal persist for at least 28 days. Although withdrawal from cannabis has been compared to recovering from the flu or similar to nicotine withdrawal, the intensity, as with other drugs of abuse, depends on the severity of the dependence. The greater the dependence, the more severe the withdrawal syndrome, and the more likely that relapse will occur (Allsop et al., 2012). As would be expected, reinstituting marijuana use relieves withdrawal discomfort.

Originally thought to be a relatively benign and infrequent occurrence, cannabis dependence occurs in about one of every ten persons who start smoking the drug and is a common reason for admission to a drug treatment program (Benyamina et al., 2008; Cooper and Haney, 2009; Elkashef et al., 2008). When cannabis users were asked to rate the effects of their own use as positive, neutral, or negative, they gave overwhelmingly negative ratings of the effects that cannabis had on their social life (70 percent), their physical health (81 percent), their cognition (91 percent), their memory (91 percent), and their career (79 percent) (Elkashef et al., 2008). It has been estimated that 13 million individuals globally have an addiction to cannabis, with relapse rates comparable to those of other substance use disorders (Lorenzetti et al., 2016). The

DSM-5 now includes a designation of *Cannabis Use Disorder* (CUD), which can be diagnosed as mild, moderate, or severe.[2]

MacDonald and Pappas (2016) present a very compelling case for concern regarding cannabis addiction. They note that increasing decriminalization, legalization, and medicalization of cannabis in many states will most likely increase use. More frequent use by current users, more new users, and the substantial increase in potency may lead to a greater frequency of cannabis-related harms. Although the percentage of first-time cannabis users who develop dependence (9 percent) is relatively low compared to other commonly abused drugs—such as first-time stimulant (11 percent), alcohol (15 percent), cocaine (17 percent), heroin (23 percent), and nicotine (32 percent)—the absolute number of people who will become addicted is still large. Furthermore, the long half-life of THC (25 to 57 hours) means that even compulsive use may not be as obvious as with other drugs. In other words, the addicted marijuana user may only use pot at breakfast, lunch, and in the evening, whereas a person addicted to nicotine may need to smoke a cigarette every hour or two. Finally, because marijuana withdrawal is often relatively mild, with little direct organ toxicity and no known overdose, there is less deterrence for chronic use. These considerations may mask the significant harms of cannabis.

MacDonald and Pappas discuss three general areas of concern. First, they predict an increase in the number of people driving under the influence of cannabis and of cannabis plus alcohol. Second, they summarize the evidence of profound underachievement associated with cannabis addiction in education, employment, income, interpersonal relationships, and reduced overall life satisfaction, especially with

---

[2]The DSM-5 defines Cannabis Use Disorder as:

- A problematic pattern of cannabis use leading to clinically significant impairment or distress, as manifested by at least 2 of the following, occurring within a 12-month period:
  - Cannabis is often taken in larger amounts or over a longer period than was intended.
  - There is a persistent desire or unsuccessful efforts to cut down or control cannabis use.
  - A great deal of time is spent in activities necessary to obtain cannabis, use cannabis, or recover from its effects.
  - Craving, or a strong desire or urge to use cannabis.
  - Recurrent cannabis use resulting in a failure to fulfill major role obligations at work, school, or home.
  - Continued cannabis use despite having persistent or recurrent social or interpersonal problems caused or exacerbated by the effects of cannabis.
  - Important social, occupational, or recreational activities are given up or reduced because of cannabis use.
  - Recurrent cannabis use in situations in which it is physically hazardous.
  - Cannabis use is continued despite knowledge of having a persistent or recurrent physical or psychological problem that is likely to have been caused or exacerbated by cannabis.
  - Tolerance, as defined by either a (1) need for markedly increased cannabis to achieve intoxication or desired effect or (2) markedly diminished effect with continued use of the same amount of the substance.
  - Withdrawal, as manifested by either (1) the characteristic withdrawal syndrome for cannabis or (2) cannabis is taken to relieve or avoid withdrawal symptoms.

adolescent-onset use (see also Cerdá et al., 2016). Third, they describe the cannabis–psychosis link, as well as the negative effect of cannabis on other mental disorders. Finally, the authors cite evidence that cannabis produces neuropsychological impairments found with other abused substances, including blunted dopamine function (see also Sherman and McRae-Clark, 2016).

TREATMENT ISSUES

There are as yet no evidence-based pharmacotherapies available for the management of cannabis dependence (Allsop et al., 2015; Balter et al., 2014; Gorelick, 2016; Marshall et al., 2014; Martinez and Trifilieff, 2015; Sherman and McRae-Clark, 2016). The most effective approaches so far have been psychotherapy treatments, specifically motivational enhancement therapy, cognitive behavioral therapy, and contingency management. Nevertheless, abstinence rates remain modest and decline after treatment. More recently, pharmacotherapy trials have been conducted as adjuncts to psychosocial treatment (Sherman and McRae-Clark, 2016). Unfortunately, many of the drugs have proven ineffective, including antidepressants, antipsychotics, baclofen (a GABA-B agonist), and the cannabis antagonist rimonabant (Martinez and Trifilieff, 2015).

One study of addicted marijuana users (Miranda et al., 2017) found that taking the epilepsy drug *topiramate* (Topamax) in addition to psychological counseling was more effective than counseling alone. The side effects (depression, anxiety, incoordination, weight loss, and unusual sensations), however, were so unpleasant that 21 out of 50 participants dropped out of the trial.

Dronabinol, the oral form of synthetic THC that is approved by the FDA to treat chemotherapy-induced nausea and AIDS wasting syndrome, may reduce cannabis withdrawal symptoms. This would be comparable to the substitution approach used in other drug abuse treatments, such as with nicotine and opiates. In laboratory settings, 50 to 120 milligrams per day reduced anxiety, misery, chills, sleep disturbance, and loss of appetite. But it did not reduce self-administration, even when combined with behavioral therapies or when combined with lofexidine (an alpha-2 agonist used to treat sympathetic hyperactivity during withdrawal) (Levin et al., 2016). In contrast, nabilone, a synthetic analogue of THC, which the FDA also approved to treat chemotherapy-induced nausea, seemed to be more promising. This was suggested to be due to the fact that nabilone has better bioavailability (greater than 60 percent) than dronabinol (less than 20 percent) because it is not metabolized as quickly and because it has a longer duration of action (greater than 6 hours, compared with 4 hours) (Allsop et al., 2015; Martinez and Trifilieff, 2015).

The enzymes fatty acid amide hydrolase (FAAH) and monoacylglycerol lipase (MGAL), which metabolize the respective endogenous cannabinoids, AEA and 2-AG, can be pharmacologically inhibited. Inhibition of these enzymes increases the levels of the endogenous cannabinoids and stimulates the CB1 receptor. Laboratory experiments in mice chronically exposed to THC show that inhibiting these enzymes reduces withdrawal. Human research to investigate the safety and efficacy of a FAAH inhibitor (PF-04457845) is now being conducted at the Yale School of Medicine (the clinical trial identification number is NCT01618656) and is scheduled to be completed in December 2018 (Martinez and Trifilieff, 2015).

Naltrexone (an opioid antagonist; see Chapter 10) can be modestly effective in specific circumstances, but its effects can be overcome with higher doses of cannabis (Haney et al., 2015; Vandrey and Haney, 2009). According to Martinez and Trifilieff (2015), research is now being conducted to develop a cannabinoid agent that would only partially block the CB1 receptor such that it would decrease the subjective effects of cannabis, but avoid the negative side effects produced by the antagonist rimonabant.

Results of studies in animal models have shown that THC, acting on the CB1 receptor, influences both GABA and glutamate transmission. This has prompted assessment of drugs that produce their effects through these systems. *Gabapentin* is an antiepileptic and analgesic for neuropathic pain. While its mechanism of action is unclear (it binds poorly to GABA receptors, even though its structure is similar to GABA), it was found to increase GABA biosynthesis. Gabapentin had some positive effects in a clinical trial (1200 milligrams per day) although the dropout rate was high. A larger clinical trial, conducted at the Scripps Research Institute, completed data collection in May 2016.

N-acetylcysteine (NAC) is an over-the-counter supplement that is thought to restore the normal glutamate activity that is disrupted by chronic drug use. A recent clinical trial investigating NAC administration (1200 milligrams twice daily), in combination with the behavioral treatment of contingency management, showed that subjects receiving NAC were more likely to reduce their cannabis consumption compared to contingency management alone. A multisite trial of NAC for the treatment of cannabis dependence was completed in July 2016. So far, gabapentin and NAC appear to hold some promise, although the outcome of these treatments has not yet been fully evaluated (Gorelick, 2016; Sherman and McRae-Clark, 2016).

The potential role for CBD in a variety of chemical addictions has been recognized. Prud'homme and coworkers (2015) reviewed the antiaddictive potential of cannabidiol in opioid, cocaine, and methamphetamine dependence as well as in tobacco and cannabis dependence. Morgan and coworkers (2013) in a small study also noted a 40 percent reduction in the number of cigarettes smoked. As a CB1 antagonist, the rationale for CBD antagonism of THC effects is obvious.

STUDY QUESTIONS

1. Summarize the history of cannabis.
2. What are the endocannabinoids? How do cannabis and the endocannabinoid system work?
3. What are the major acute and chronic physiological effects of cannabis on the body?
4. What are the cognitive effects of cannabis?
5. What are the psychological/psychiatric effects of cannabis?
6. Discuss evidence regarding current and possible future medical uses of THC and CBD. Should therapeutic uses be pursued?

7. Should cannabis be legalized for either medical or recreational use? If so, how should it be regulated or restricted?

8. What are synthetic cannabinoids? Where did they come from and what are their effects?

9. What pharmacological approaches are being taken to treat cannabis abuse?

REFERENCES

Adams, A. J., et al. (2017). 'Zombie' Outbreak Caused by the Synthetic Cannabinoid AMB-FUBINACA in New York." *New England Journal of Medicine* 376: 235–242.

Agrawal, A., et al. (2017). "Major Depressive Disorder, Suicidal Thoughts and Behaviours, and Cannabis Involvement in Discordant Twins: A Retrospective Cohort Study." *Lancet Psychiatry*: 706.

Allsop, D. J., et al. (2012). "Quantifying the Clinical Significance of Cannabis Withdrawal." *PLoS One* 7: e44864.

Allsop, D. J., et al. (2015). "Cannabinoid Replacement Therapy (CRT): Nabiximols (Sativex) as a Novel Treatment for Cannabis Withdrawal." *Clinical Pharmacology and Therapeutics* 97: 571–574.

Amen, D. G., et al. (2017). "Discriminative Properties of Hippocampal Hypoperfusion in Marijuana Users Compared to Healthy Controls: Implications for Marijuana Administration in Alzheimer's Dementia." *Journal of Alzheimer's Disease* 56: 261–273. doi: 10.3233/JAD-160833.

Andrade, C. (2016). "Cannabis and Neuropsychiatry, 2: The Longitudinal Risk of Psychosis as an Adverse Outcome." *Journal of Clinical Psychiatry* 77: e739–e742.

Angerer, V., et al. (2016). "Separation and Structural Characterization of the New Synthetic Cannabinoid JWH-018 Cyclohexyl Methyl Derivative 'NE-CHMIMO' Using Flash Chromatography, GC-MS, IR and NMR Spectroscopy." *Forensic Science International* 266: e93–e98.

Balter, R. E., et al. (2014). "Novel Pharmacologic Approaches to Treating Cannabis Use Disorder." *Current Addiction Reports* 1: 137–143. doi: 10.1007/s40429-014-0011-1.

Barkus, E., et al. (2011). "Does Intravenous Delta-9-Tetrahydrocannabinol Increase Dopamine Release? A SPET Study." *Journal of Psychopharmacology* 25: 1462–1468.

Battista, N., et al. (2012). "The Endocannabinoid System: An Overview." *Frontiers in Behavioral Neuroscience* 6: 1–7.

Battista, N., et al. (2015). "Endocannabinoids and Reproductive Events in Health and Disease." *Handbook of Experimental Pharmacology* 231: 341–365.

Bechtold, J., et al. (2016). "Concurrent and Sustained Cumulative Effects of Adolescent Marijuana Use On Subclinical Psychotic Symptoms." *American Journal of Psychiatry* 173: 781–789. doi: 10.1176/appi.ajp.2016.15070878.

Benyamina, A., et al. (2008). "Pharmacotherapy and Psychotherapy in Cannabis Withdrawal and Dependence." *Expert Reviews in Neurotherapy* 8: 479–491.

Bergamaschi, M. M., et al. (2011). "Cannabidiol Reduces the Anxiety Induced by Simulated Public Speaking in Treatment-Naïve Social Phobia Patients." *Neuropsychopharmacology* 36: 1219–1226.

Bernstein, L. (2016). "U.S. Affirms its Prohibition on Medical Marijuana." *August* 11, The Washington Post.

Blanco, C., et al. (2016). "Cannabis Use and Risk of Psychiatric Disorders: Prospective Evidence from a US National Longitudinal Study." *JAMA Psychiatry* 73: 388–395. doi: 10.1001/jamapsychiatry.2015.3229.

Blessing, E. M., et al. (2015). "Cannabidiol as a Potential Treatment for Anxiety Disorders." *Neurotherapeutics* 12: 825–836.

Bloomfield, M. A., et al. (2016). "The Effects of Δ9-Tetrahydrocannabinol on the Dopamine System." *Nature* 539: 369–377. doi: 10.1038/nature20153.

Boehnke, K. F., et al. (2016). "Medical Cannabis Use Is Associated with Decreased Opiate Medication Use in a Retrospective Cross-Sectional Survey of Patients with Chronic Pain." *Journal of Pain.* 17: 739–744. doi: 10.1016/j.jpain.2016.03.002.

Bonar, E. E., et al. (2014). "Synthetic Cannabinoid Use Among Patients in Residential Substance Use Disorder Treatment: Prevalence, Motives, and Correlates." *Drug and Alcohol Dependence* 143: 268–271. doi: 10.1016/j.drugalcdep.2014.07.009

Bonn-Miller, M. O., et al. (2017). "Labeling Accuracy of Cannabidiol Extracts Sold Online." *JAMA* 318: 1708–1709. doi: 10.1001/jama.2017.11909.

Booz, G. W. (2011). "Cannabidiol as an Emergent Therapeutic Strategy for Lessening the Impact of Inflammation on Oxidative Stress." *Free Radical Biology & Medicine* 51: 1054–1061. doi: 10.1016/j.freeradbiomed.2011.01.007.

Boychuk, D. G., et al. (2015). "The Effectiveness of Cannabinoids in the Management of Chronic Nonmalignant Neuropathic Pain: A Systematic Review." *Journal of Oral & Facial Pain and Headache* 29: 7–14.

Bradford, A. C., and Bradford, W. D. (2016). "Medical Marijuana Laws Reduce Prescription Medication Use in Medicare Part D." *Health Affairs* 35: 1230–1236. doi: 10.1377/hlthaff.2015.1661.

Bruins, J., et al. (2016). "Cannabis Use in People with Severe Mental Illness: The Association with Physical and Mental Health—A Cohort Study. A Pharmacotherapy Monitoring and Outcome Survey Study." *Journal of Psychopharmacology* 30: 354–362. doi: 10.1177/0269881116631652.

Buckner J., and Schmidt, N. (2009). "Social Anxiety Disorder and Marijuana Use Problems: The Mediating Role of Marijuana Effect Expectancies." *Depression and Anxiety* 26: 864–870. doi: 10.1002/da.20567.

Carol, Aaron A. (2015). "How Medical Is Marijuana?" *New York Times.*

Carroll, A. E. (2015). The Upshot. "How 'Medical' Is Marijuana?" THE NEW HEALTH CARE JULY 20, The New York Times.

Castellanos, D., and Gralnik, L. (2016). "Synthetic Cannabinoids 2015: An Update for Pediatricians in Clinical Practice." *World Journal of Clinical Pediatrics* 5: 16–24. doi: 10.5409/wjcp.v5.i1.16.

Cerdá, M., et al. (2016). "Persistent Cannabis Dependence and Alcohol Dependence Represent Risks for Midlife Economic and Social Problems: A Longitudinal Cohort Study." *Clinical Psychological Science* 4: 1028–1046. doi: 10.1177/2167702616630958.

Chiurchiu, V., et al. (2015). "Cannabinoid Signaling and Neuroinflammatory Diseases: A Melting Pot for the Regulation of Brain Immune Responses." *Journal of Neuroimmune Pharmacology* 10: 268–280.

Choo, E. K., et al. (2016). "Opioids Out, Cannabis In: Negotiating the Unknowns in Patient Care for Chronic Pain." *JAMA* 316: 1763–1764. doi: 10.1001/jama.2016.13677.

Compton, W. M., et al. (2016). "Marijuana Use and Use Disorders in Adults in the USA, 2002–14: Analysis of Annual Cross-Sectional Surveys." *Lancet Psychiatry* 3: 954–964. doi: http://dx.doi.org/10.1016/S2215-0366(16)30208-5.

Conroy, D. A., et al. (2016). "Marijuana Use Patterns and Sleep among Community-Based Young Adults." *Journal of Addictive Diseases* 35: 135. doi: 10.1080/10550887.2015.1132986.

Cooper, Z. D. (2016). "Adverse Effects of Synthetic Cannabinoids: Management of Acute Toxicity and Withdrawal." *Current Psychiatry Reports* 18: 52.

Cooper, Z. D., and Haney, M. (2009). "Actions of Delta-9-Tetrahydrocannabinol in Cannabis: Relation to Use, Abuse, Dependence." *International Review of Psychiatry* 21: 104–112.

Covey, D. P., et al. (2016). "Endocannabinoid Regulation of Cocaine Reinforcement: An Upper or Downer?" *Neuropsychopharmacology* 41: 2189–2191.

Cressey, D. (2015). "The Cannabis Experiment." *Nature* 524: 280–283. doi:10.1038/524280a

Currais, A., et al. (2016). "Amyloid Proteotoxicity Initiates an Inflammatory Response Blocked by Cannabinoids." *Aging and Mechanisms of Disease* 2: 16012. doi: 10.1038/npjamd.2016.12.

D'Souza, D. C., and Ranganathan, M. (2015). "Medical Marijuana: Is the Cart before the Horse?" *JAMA* 313: 2431. doi: http://dx.doi.org/10.1001/jama.2015.6407.

Deshpande, A., et al. (2015). "Efficacy and Adverse Effects of Medical Marijuana in Chronic Non-Cancer Pain: Systematic Review of Randomized Controlled Trials." *Canadian Family Physician* 61: e372–e381.

Devane, W. A., et al. (1992). "Isolation and Structure of a Brain Constituent That Binds to the Cannabinoid Receptor." *Science* 258: 1946–1949.

Devinsky, O., et al., for the Cannabidiol in Dravet Syndrome Study Group. (2017). "Trial of Cannabidiol for Drug-Resistant Seizures in the Dravet Syndrome." *New England Journal of Medicine* 376: 2011–2020.

Diez-Alarcia, R., et al. (2016). "Biased Agonism of Three Different Cannabinoid Receptor Agonists in Mouse Brain Cortex." *Frontiers in Pharmacology* 7: 415. doi: 10.3389/fphar.2016.00415.

DiForti, M., et al. (2015). "Proportion of Patients in South London with First-Episode Psychosis Attributable to Use of High Potency Cannabis: A Case-Control Study." *Lancet* 2: 233–238. doi: http://dx.doi.org/10.1016/S2215-0366(14)00117-5.

Dincheva, I., et al. (2015). "FAAH Genetic Variation Enhances Fronto-Amygdala Function in Mouse and Human." *Nature Communications* 6: 6395. doi: 10.1038/ncomms7395.

Doucette, M. L., et al. (2017). "Oral Fluid Testing for Marijuana Intoxication: Enhancing Objectivity for Roadside DUI Testing." *Injury Prevention* Published Online First: 01 June 2017. doi: 10.1136/injuryprev-2016-042264

Dowd, M. (2014). "Don't Harsh Our Mellow, Dude." *New York Times*. June 3. https://www.nytimes.com/2014/06/04/opinion/dowd-which-harsh-our-mellow-dude.html?_r=0.

DuPlessis, S. S., et al. (2015). "Marijuana, Phytocannabinoids, the Endocrine System, and Male Fertility." *Journal of Assisted Reproduction and Genetics* 32: 1575–1588.

Elkashef, A., et al. (2008). "Marijuana Neurobiology and Treatment." *Substance Abuse* 29: 17–29.

Elmes, M. W., et al. (2015). "Fatty Acid Binding Proteins (FABPs) Are Intracellular Carriers for Δ9-Tetrahydrocannabinol (THC) and Cannabidiol (CBD)." *Journal of Biological Chemistry* 290: 8711–8721. doi: 10.1074/jbc.M114.618447.

ElSohly, M. A., et al. (2016). "Changes in Cannabis Potency Over the Last 2 Decades (1995–2014): Analysis of Current Data in the United States." *Biological Psychiatry* 79: 613–619.

Englund, A., et al. (2013). "Cannabidiol Inhibits THC-Elicited Paranoid Symptoms and Hippocampal-Dependent Memory Impairment." *Journal of Psychopharmacology* 27: 19–27.

Esposito, G., et al. (2007). "Cannabidiol *in vivo* Blunts β-Amyloid Induced Neuroinflammation by Suppressing IL-1β and iNOS Expression." *British Journal of Pharmacology* 151: 1272–1279.

Esposito, G., et al. (2013). "Cannabidiol in Inflammatory Bowel Diseases." *Phytotherapeutic Research* 27: 633–636.

Evins, A. E., et al. (2012). "The Effect of Marijuana Use on the Risk for Schizophrenia." *Journal of Clinical Psychiatry* 73: 1463–1468.

Fakhoury, M. (2016). "Could Cannabidiol Be Used as an Alternative to Antipsychotics?" *Journal of Psychiatric Research* 80: 14–21.

Fantasia, H. C. (2017). "Pharmacologic Implications of Marijuana Use During Pregnancy." *Nursing for Women's Health* 21: 217–223.

Fattore, L., and Fratta, W. (2011). "Beyond THC: The New Generation of Cannabinoid Designer Drugs." *Frontiers in Behavioral Neuroscience* 5: 1–12.

Fattore, L. (2016). "Synthetic Cannabinoids-Further Evidence Supporting the Relationship Between Cannabinoids and Psychosis." *Biological Psychiatry* 79: doi: 10.1016/j.biopsych.2016.02.001

Fernandez-Ruiz, J., et al. (2012). "Cannabidiol for Neurodegenerative Disorders: Important New Clinical Applications for This Phytocannabinoid?" *British Journal of Clinical Pharmacology* 75: 323–333.

Filbey, F. M., and DeWitt, S. J. (2012). "Cannabis Cue-Elicited Craving and the Reward Neurocircuitry." *Progress in Neuro-Psychopharmacology & Biological Psychiatry* 38: 30–35. doi: 10.1016/j.pnpbp.2011.11.001.

Fine, P. G., and Rosenfeld, M. J. (2013). "The Endocannabinoid System, Cannabinoids, and Pain." *Rambam Maimonides Medical Journal* 4: e0022. doi: 10.5041/RMMJ.10129.

Freeman, D., et al. (2014). "How Cannabis Causes Paranoia: Using the Intravenous Administration of Δ^9-Tetrahydrocannabinol (THC) to Identify Key Cognitive Mechanisms Leading to Paranoia." *Schizophrenia Bulletin* 41: 391–399.

Gage, S. H., et al. (2016). "Assessing Causality in Associations between Cannabis Use and Schizophrenia Risk: A Two-Sample Mendelian Randomization Study." *Psychological Medicine* 47: 971–980. doi: 10.1017/S0033291716003172.

Geffrey, A. L., et al. (2015). "Drug–Drug Interaction between Clobazam and Cannabidiol in Children with Refractory Epilepsy." *Epilepsia* 56: 1246–1251.

Gibbs, M. et al. (2015). "Cannabis Use and Mania Symptoms: A Systematic Review and Meta-Analysis." *Journal of Affective Disorders* 171: 39–47.

Giroud, C., et al. (2015). "E-Cigarettes: A Review of New Trends in Cannabis Use." *International Journal of Environmental Research and Public Health* 12: 9988–10008.

Gorelick, D. A. (2016). "Pharmacological Treatment of Cannabis-Related Disorders: A Narrative Review." *Current Pharmaceutical Design* 22: 6409–6419. doi: 10.2174/1381612822666160822150822.

Governing.com. (2016). "State Marijuana Laws in 2016 Map." January 30. http://www.governing.com/gov-data/state-marijuana-laws-map-medical-recreational.html.

Grandner, M. (2014). "Marijuana Use May Lead to Impaired Sleep Quality and Other News from the 28th Annual Meeting of the Associated Professional Sleep Societies." *Neurology Reviews* 22(7): 5.

Grant, K. S., et al. (2017). "Cannabis Use During Pregnancy: Pharmacokinetics and Effects on Child Development." *Pharmacology and Therapeutics* pii: S0163-7258(17)30224-3. doi: 10.1016/j.pharmthera.2017.08.014. 182: 133–151.

Grilly, D. M., and Salamone, J. D. (2012). *Drugs, Brain and Behavior*, 6th ed. Upper Saddle River, NJ: Pearson.

Gurney, J., et al. (2015). "Cannabis Exposure and Risk of Testicular Cancer: A Systematic Review and Meta-Analysis." *BMC Cancer* 15: 897. doi: 10.1186/s12885-015-1905-6.

Hackam, D. C. (2015). "Cannabis and Stroke: Systematic Appraisal of Case Reports." *Stroke* 46: 852–856.

Hamilton, I. (2017). "Cannabis, Psychosis and Schizophrenia: Unravelling a Complex Interaction." *Addiction* 112: 1653–1657.

Haney, M., et al. (2015). "Naltrexone Maintenance Decreases Cannabis Self-Administration and Subjective Effects in Daily Cannabis Smokers." *Neuropsychopharmacology* 40: 2489–2498.

Hebert-Chatelain, E., et al. (2016). "A Cannabinoid Link between Mitochondria and Memory." *Nature* 539: 555–559. doi: 10.1038/nature20127.

Hegde, V. L., et al. (2010). "Cannabinoid Receptor Activation Leads to Massive Mobilization of Myeloid-Derived Suppressor Cells with Potent Immunosuppressive Properties." *European Journal of Immunology* 40: 3358–3371.

Helle, S., et al. (2016). "Cannabis Use Is Associated with 3 Years Earlier Onset of Schizophrenia Spectrum Disorder in a Naturalistic, Multi-Site Sample (N = 1119)." *Schizophrenia Research* 170: 217–221. doi: 10.1016/j.schres.2015.11.027.

Hill, K. P. (2015). "Medical Marijuana for Treatment of Chronic Pain and Other Medical and Psychiatric Problems. A Clinical Review." *JAMA* 313: 2474–2483. doi: 10.1001/jama.2015.6199.

Hirvonen, J., et al. (2012). "Reversible and Regionally Selective Downregulation of Brain Cannabinoid CB1 Receptors in Chronic Daily Cannabis Smokers." *Molecular Psychiatry* 17: 642–649.

Honarmand, K., et al. (2011). "Effects of Cannabis on Cognitive Function in Patients with Multiple Sclerosis." *Neurology* 76: 1153–1160.

Huang, Y. H., et al. (2015). "An Epidemiologic Review of Marijuana and Cancer: An Update." *Cancer Epidemiology, Biomarkers and Prevention* 24: 15–31.

Huestis, M. A. (2005). "Pharmacokinetics and Metabolism of the Plant Cannabinoids, Delta9-Tetrahydrocannabinol, Cannabidiol, and Cannabinol." *Handbook of Experimental Pharmacology* 168: 657–690.

Huestis, M. A., et al. (2001). "Blockade of Effects of Smoked Marijuana by the CB1 Selective Cannabinoid Receptor Antagonist SR141716." *Archives of General Psychiatry* 58: 322–328.

Izzo, A. A., et al. (2015). "Endocannabinoids and the Digestive Tract and Bladder in Health and Disease." *Handbook of Experimental Pharmacology* 231: 423–447.

Jensen, B., et al. (2015). "Medical Marijuana and Chronic Pain: A Review of Basic Science and Clinical Evidence." *Current Pain and Headache Reports* 19: 50.

Johnston, L. D., et al. (2016). *Monitoring the Future National Survey Results on Drug Use, 1975– 2015: Volume 2, College Students and Adults Ages 19–55*. Ann Arbor: Institute for Social Research, The University of Michigan. http://monitoringthefuture.org/pubs/monographs/mtf-vol2_2015.pdf.

Justinova, Z., et al. (2011). "The Endogenous Cannabinoid 2-Arachidonoylglycerol Is Intravenously Self-Administered by Squirrel Monkeys." *Journal of Neuroscience* 31: 7043–7048.

Kaur, R., et al. (2016). "Endocannabinoid System: A Multi-Facet Therapeutic Target." *Current Clinical Pharmacology* 11: 110–117.

Kedzior, K. K., and Laeber, L. T. (2014). "A Positive Association between Anxiety Disorders and Cannabis Use or Cannabis Use Disorders in the General Population—A Meta-Analysis of 31 Studies." *BMC Psychiatry* 14: 136. doi: 10.1186/1471-244X-14-136.

Kendall, D. A., and Yudowski, G. A. (2016). "Cannabinoid Receptors in the Central Nervous System: Their Signaling and Roles in Disease." *Frontiers in Cellular Neuroscience* 10: 294. doi: 10.3389/fncel.2016.00294.

Kilmer, B. (2017). "Recreational Cannabis—Minimizing the Health Risks from Legalization." *New England Journal of Medicine* 376: 705–707.

Kim, H. S., and Monte, A. A. (2016) "Colorado Cannabis Legalization and Its Effect on Emergency Care." *Annals of Emergency Medicine* 68: 71–75. doi: 10.1016/j.annemergmed.2016.01.004.

Kim, H. S., et al. (2016). "Marijuana Tourism and Emergency Department Visits in Colorado." *New England Journal of Medicine* 374: 797–798. doi: 10.1056/NEJMc1515009.

Kim, J., et al. (2017). "Detection of in Utero Cannabis Exposure by Umbilical Cord Analysis." *Drug Testing and Analysis*. doi: 10.1002/dta.2307. [Epub ahead of print]

Kolikonda, M. K., et al. (2016). "Medical Marijuana for Epilepsy?" *Innovations in Clinical Neuroscience* 13: 23–26.

Koppel, B. S., et al. (2014). "Systematic Review: Efficacy and Safety of Medical Marijuana in Selected Neurologic Disorders." *Neurology* 82: 1556–1563.

Kuepper, R., et al. (2011). "Continued Cannabis Use and Risk of Incidence and Persistence of Psychotic Symptoms: 10-Year Follow-Up Cohort Study." *BMJ* 342: d738.

Lamy, S., et al. (2017). "Assessment of Tobacco, Alcohol and Cannabinoid Metabolites in 645 Meconium Samples of Newborns Compared to Maternal Self-Reports." *Journal of Psychiatric Research* 90: 86–93.

Large, M., et al. (2011). "Cannabis Use and Earlier Onset of Psychosis." *Archives of General Psychiatry* 68: 555–561.

Lauritsen, K. J., and Rosenberg, H. (2016). "Comparison of Outcome Expectancies for Synthetic Cannabinoids and Botanical Marijuana." *American Journal of Drug and Alcohol Abuse* 42: 377–84. doi: 10.3109/00952990.2015.1135158.

Law, R., et al. (2015). "Notes from the Field: Increase in Reported Adverse Health Effects Related to Synthetic Cannabinoid Use—United States, January–May 2015." *Morbidity and Mortality Weekly Report* 64: 618–619. https://www.cdc.gov/mmwr/preview/mmwrhtml/mm6422a5.htm.

Lee, H. K., et al. (2009). "The Current Status and Future Prospects of Studies of Cannabinoid Receptor 1 Antagonists as Anti-Obesity Agents." *Current Topics in Medicinal Chemistry* 9: 482–503.

Levin, F. R., et al. (2016). "Dronabinol and Lofexidine for Cannabis Use Disorder: A Randomized, Double-Blind, Placebo-Controlled Trial." *Drug and Alcohol Dependence* 159: 53–60. doi: 10.1016/j.drugalcdep.2015.11.025

Levinthal, C. F. (2012). *Drugs, Behavior and Modern Society,* 7th ed. Boston: Allyn & Bacon.

Lev-Ran, S., et al. (2013). "Cannabis Use and Cannabis Use Disorders among Individuals with Mental Illness." *Comprehensive Psychiatry* 54: 589–598.

Leweke, F. M., et al. (2012). "Cannabidiol Enhances Anandamide Signaling and Alleviates Psychotic Symptoms of Schizophrenia." *Translational Psychiatry* 2: e94.

Leweke, F. M., et al. (2016). "Therapeutic Potential of Cannabinoids in Psychosis." *Biological Psychiatry* 79: 604–612.

Lorenzetti, V., et al. (2016). "The Neurobiology of Cannabis Use Disorders: A Call for Evidence." *Frontiers in Behavioral Neuroscience* 10: 86. doi: 10.3389/fnbeh.2016.00086.

Lutchmansingh, D., et al. (2014). "Legalizing Cannabis: A Physician's Primer on the Pulmonary Effects of Marijuana." *Current Respiratory Care Reports* 3: 200–205.

Lynch, M. J., et al. (2012). "The Cannabis-Psychosis Link." *Psychiatric Times* 29: 1–5.

Maas, A., et al. (2006). "Efficacy and Safety of Dexanabinol in Severe Traumatic Brain Injury: Results of a Phase III Randomised, Placebo-Controlled, Clinical Trial." *Lancet Neurology* 1: 38–45.

MacDonald, K., and Pappas, K. (2016). "Why Not Pot? A Review of the Brain-based Risks of Cannabis." *Innovations in Clinical Neuroscience* 13: 13–22.

Malone, D. T., et al. (2010). "Adolescent Cannabis Use and Psychosis: Epidemiology and Neurodevelopmental Models." *British Journal of Pharmacology* 160: 511–522.

Manrique-Garcia, E., et al. (2014). "Prognosis of Schizophrenia in Persons with and without a History of Cannabis Use." *Psychological Medicine* 44: 2513–2521. doi: 10.1017/S0033291714000191.

Manseau, M. W., and Goff, D. C. (2015). "Cannabinoids and Schizophrenia: Risks and Therapeutic Potential." *Neurotherapeutics* 12: 816–824.

Mark, K., and Terplan, M. (2017). "Cannabis and Pregnancy: Maternal Child Health Implications During a Period of Drug Policy Liberalization." *Preventive Medicine* pii: S0091-7435(17)30175-5.

Mark, K., et al. (2017). "Pregnant Women's Current and Intended Cannabis Use in Relation to Their Views Toward Legalization and Knowledge of Potential Harm." *Journal of Addiction Medicine* 11: 211–216.

Marshall, K., et al. (2014). "Pharmacotherapies for Cannabis Dependence." *Cochrane Database of Systemic Reviews* 12. Art. No. CD008940. doi: 10.1002/14651858.CD008940.pub2.

Martin-Moreno, A. M., et al. (2011). "Cannabidiol and Other Cannabinoids Reduce Microglial Activation in Vitro and in Vivo: Relevance to Alzheimer's Disease." *Molecular Pharmacology* 79: 964–973.

Martinez, D., and Trifilieff, P. (2015). "A Review of Potential Pharmacological Treatments for Cannabis Abuse." *American Society of Addiction Medicine Magazine*. April 13. http://www.asam.org/magazine/read/article/2015/04/13/a-review-of-potential-pharmacological-treatments-for-cannabis-abuse.

McAllister, S. D., et al. (2015). "The Antitumor Activity of Plant-Derived Non-Psychoactive Cannabinoids." *Journal of Neuroimmune Pharmacology* 10: 255–267.

Mechoulam, R. (2010). Qtd. in "Dr. Raphael Mechoulam." *Medical Marijuana 411*. May 7. https://medicalmarijuana411.com/dr-raphael-mechoulam_part-one/.

Meier, M. H. (2016). "Associations between Cannabis Use and Physical Health Problems in Early Midlife: A Longitudinal Comparison of Persistent Cannabis vs Tobacco Users." *JAMA Psychiatry* 73: 731–740. doi: 10.1001/jamapsychiatry.2016.0637.

Meier, M., et al. (2012). "Persistent Cannabis Users Show Neuropsychological Decline from Childhood to Midlife." *Proceedings of the National Academy of Sciences* 109: E2657–E2664.

Melton, S. (2017). "Stirring the Pot: Potential Drug Interactions with Marijuana." *Medscape*. Jun 08.

Metz, T. D., and Stickrath, E. H. (2015). "Marijuana Use in Pregnancy and Lactation: A Review of the Evidence." *American Journal of Obstetrics and Gynecology* 213: 761–778.

Miliano, C., et al. (2016). "Neuropharmacology of New Psychoactive Substances (NPS): Focus on the Rewarding and Reinforcing Properties of Cannabinimimetics and Amphetamine-Like Stimulants." *Frontiers in Neuroscience* 10: 153.

Miranda, R., Jr., et al. (2017). "Topiramate and Motivational Enhancement Therapy for Cannabis Use Among Youth: A Randomized Placebo-Controlled Pilot Study." *Addiction Biology* 22: 779–790. doi: 10.1111/adb.12350.

Morgan, C. J., et al. (2010). "Impact of Cannabidiol on the Acute Memory and Psychotomimetic Effects of Smoked Cannabis: Naturalistic Study." *British Journal of Psychiatry* 197: 285–290.

Morgan, C. J., et al. (2013). "Cannabidiol Reduces Cigarette Consumption in Tobacco Smokers: Preliminary Findings." *Addiction Behaviors* 38: 2433–2436.

Murphy, T. D., et al. (2013). "Acute Kidney Injury Associated with Synthetic Cannabinoid Use—Multiple States, 2012." *Morbidity and Mortality Weekly Report* 62: 93–98.

Naftali, T., et al. (2014). "Cannabis for Inflammatory Bowel Disease." *Digestive Diseases* 32: 468–474.

National Academies of Sciences, Engineering, and Medicine. (2017). *The Health Effects of Cannabis and Cannabinoids: The Current State of Evidence and Recommendations for Research*. Washington, DC: The National Academies Press. doi: 10.17226/24625.

National Institute on Drug Abuse. (2016). "Drug and Alcohol Use in College-Age Adults in 2015." https://www.drugabuse.gov/related-topics/trends-statistics/infographics/drug-alcohol-use-in-college-age-adults-in-2015.

National Institute on Drug Abuse. (2017). "Is Marijuana Addictive?" https://www.drugabuse.gov/publications/research-reports/marijuana/marijuana-addictive.

Nesvåg, R., et al. (2017). "Genetic and Environmental Contributions to the Association between Cannabis Use and Psychotic-Like Experiences in Young Adult Twins." *Schizophrenia Bulletin* 43: 644–653. doi: 10.1093/schbul/sbw101.

Nguyen, B. M., et al. (2014). "Effect of Marijuana Use on Outcomes in Traumatic Brain Injury." *American Surgery* 10: 979–983.

Nielsen, S., et al. (2017). "Opioid-Sparing Effect of Cannabinoids: A Systematic Review and Meta-Analysis." *Neuropsychopharmacology* 42: 1752–1765.

Nugent, S. M., et al. (2017). "The Effects of Cannabis Among Adults with Chronic Pain and an Overview of General Harms: A Systematic Review." *Annals of Internal Medicine* 167: 319–331.

O'Neil, M. E., et al. (2017). "Benefits and Harms of Plant-Based Cannabis for Posttraumatic Stress Disorder: A Systematic Review." *Annals of Internal Medicine* 167: 332–340.

Orsolini, L., et al. (2017). "Is There a Teratogenicity Risk Associated with Cannabis and Synthetic Cannabimimetics' ('Spice') Intake?" *CNS & Neurological Disorders-Drug Targets* 16: 585–591.

Otero-Romero, S., et al. (2016). "Pharmacological Management of Spasticity in Multiple Sclerosis: Systematic Review and Consensus Paper." *Multiple Sclerosis* 22: 1386–1396. doi: 10.1177/13524585166 43600.

Papanti, D., et al. (2013). "'Spiceophrenia': A Systematic Overview of 'Spice'-related Psychopathological Issues and a Case Report." *Human Psychopharmacology* 28: 379–389.

Parsons, L. H., and Hurd, Y. L. (2015). "Endocannabinoid Signalling in Reward and Addiction." *Nature Reviews Neuroscience* 16: 579–594. doi: 10.1038/nrn4004.

Patti, F., et al. (2016). "Efficacy and Safety of Cannabinoid Oromucosal Spray for Multiple Sclerosis Spasticity." *Journal of Neurology, Neurosurgery & Psychiatry* 87: 944–951. doi: 10.1136/jnnp-2015-312591.

Pavisian, B., et al. (2014). "Effects of Cannabis on Cognition in Patients with MS: A Psychometric and MRI Study." *Neurology* 82: 1879–1887. doi: 10.1212/WNL.0000000000000446.

Peace, M. R., et al. (2016). "Evaluation of Two Commercially Available Cannabidiol Formulations for Use in Electronic Cigarettes." *Frontiers in Pharmacology* 7: 279. doi: 10.3389/fphar.2016.00279.

Piper, B. J., et al. (2017). "Substitution of Medical Cannabis for Pharmaceutical Agents for Pain, Anxiety, and Sleep." *Journal of Psychopharmacology* 31: 569–575.

Power, R. A., et al. (2014). "Genetic Predisposition to Schizophrenia Associated with Increased Use of Cannabis." *Molecular Psychiatry* 19: 1201–1204. doi: 10.1038/mp.2014.51.

Presley, B. C., et al. (2016). "Metabolism and Toxicological Analysis of Synthetic Cannabinoids in Biological Fluids and Tissues." *Forensic Science Reviews* 28: 103–169.

ProCon.org. (2017). "28 Legal Medical Marijuana States and DC." March 2. http://medicalmarijuana.procon.org/view.resource.php?resourceID=000881.

Prud'homme, M., et al. (2015). "Cannabidiol as an Intervention for Addictive Behaviors: A Systematic Review of the Evidence." *Substance Abuse Research and Treatment* 9: 33–39. doi: 10.4137/SART.S25081.

Richter, K. P., and Levy, S. (2014). "Big Marijuana—Lessons from Big Tobacco." *New England Journal of Medicine* 371: 399–401. doi: 10.1056/NEJMp1406074.

Rock, E. M., and Parker, L. A. (2016). "Cannabinoids as Potential Treatment for Chemotherapy-Induced Nausea and Vomiting." *Frontiers in Pharmacology* 7: 221. doi: 10.3389/fphar.2016.00221.

Rohleder, C., et al. (2016). "Cannabidiol as a Potential New Type of an Antipsychotic: A Critical Review of the Evidence." *Frontiers in Pharmacology* 7: 422. doi: 10.3389/fphar.2016.00422.

Romano, B., et al. (2014). "Inhibition of Colon Carcinogenesis by a Standardized Cannabis Sativa Extract with a High Content of Cannabidiol." *Phytomedicine* 21: 631–639.

Rosenbaum, C. D., et al. (2012). "Here Today, Gone Tomorrow . . . and Back Again? A Review of Herbal Marijuana Alternatives (K2, Spice), Synthetic Cathinones (Bath Salts), Kratom, Salvia Divinorum, Methoxetamine, and Piperazines." *Journal of Medical Toxicology* 8: 15–32.

Saad, D., and Joshi, C. (2015). "Pure Cannabidiol in the Treatment of Malignant Migrating Partial Seizures in Infancy: A Case Report." *Pediatric Neurology* 52: 544–547.

Sansone, R. A., and Sansone, L. A. (2014). "Marijuana and Body Weight." *Innovations in Clinical Neuroscience* 11: 50–54.

Sarris, J., et al. (2013). "Plant-Based Medicines for Anxiety Disorders, Part 2: A Review of Clinical Studies with Supporting Preclinical Evidence." *CNS Drugs* 27: 301–319.

Schacht, J. P., et al. (2012). "Associations between Cannabinoid Receptor-1 (CNR1) Variation and Hippocampus and Amygdala Volumes in Heavy Cannabis Users." *Neuropsychopharmacology* 37: 2368–2376.

Schoeler, T., et al. (2016a). "Association between Continued Cannabis Use and Risk of Relapse in First-Episode Psychosis: A Quasi-Experimental Investigation Within an Observational Study." *JAMA Psychiatry* 73: 1173–1179. doi: 10.1001/jamapsychiatry.2016.2427.

Schoeler, T., et al. (2016b). "Continued versus Discontinued Cannabis Use in Patients with Psychosis: A Systematic Review and Meta-Analysis." *Lancet Psychiatry* 3: 215–225. doi: 10.1016/S2215-0366(15)00363-6.

Schubart, C. D., et al. (2014). "Cannabidiol as a Potential Treatment for Psychosis." *European Neuropsychopharmacology* 24: 51–64.

Schwartz, A. (2015). "Arrest Underscores China's Role in the Making and Spread of a Lethal Drug." May 15.

Schwarz, A. (2015). "Arrest Underscores China's Role in the Making and Spread of a Lethal Drug." MAY 28, The New York Times.

Seely, K. A., et al. (2011). "Marijuana-Based Drugs: Innovative Therapeutics Designer Drugs of Abuse?" *Molecular Interventions* 11: 36–50.

Seely, K. A., et al. (2012). "Spice Drugs Are More Than Harmless Herbal Blends: A Review of the Pharmacology and Toxicology of Synthetic Cannabinoids." *Progress in Neuropsychopharmacology and Biological Psychiatry* 39: 234–243. doi: 10.1016/j.pnpbp.2012.04.017

Shalit, N., et al. (2016). "Characteristics of Synthetic Cannabinoid and Cannabis Users Admitted to a Psychiatric Hospital: A Comparative Study." *Journal of Clinical Psychiatry* 77: e989–e995. doi: 10.4088/JCP.15m09938.

Sherman, B. J., and McRae-Clark, A. L. (2016). "Treatment of Cannabis Use Disorder: Current Science and Future Outlook." *Pharmacotherapy* 36: 511–535. doi: 10.1002/phar.1747.

Smith, P. H., et al. (2014). "Couples' Marijuana Use Is Inversely Related to Their Intimate Partner Violence over the First 9 Years of Marriage." *Psychology of Addictive Behaviors* 28: 734–742. doi: 10.1037/a0037302.

Soares, V. P., and Campos, A. C. (2017). "Evidence for the Anti-Panic Actions of Cannabidiol." *Current Neuropharmacology* 15: 291–299.

Soderstrom, K., et al. (2017). "Cannabinoids Modulate Neuronal Activity and Cancer by CB1 and CB2 Receptor-Independent Mechanisms." *Frontiers in Pharmacology* 8: 720.

Thomas, B. F., and Pollard, G. T. (2016). "Preparation and Distribution of Cannabis and Cannabis-Derived Dosage Formulations for Investigational and Therapeutic Use in the United States." *Frontiers in Pharmacology* 7: 285. doi: 10.3389/fphar.2016.00285.

Tosato, S., et al. (2013). "The Impact of Cannabis Use on Age of Onset and Clinical Characteristics in First-Episode Psychotic Patients. Data from the Psychosis Incident Cohort Outcome Study (PICOS)." *Journal of Psychiatric Research* 47: 438–444.

Trecki, J., et al. (2015). "Synthetic Cannabinoid–Related Illnesses and Deaths." *New England Journal of Medicine* 373: 103–107.

Turcotte, C., et al. (2016). "Impact of Cannabis, Cannabinoids, and Endocannabinoids in the Lungs." *Frontiers in Pharmacology* 7: 317. doi: 10.3389/fphar.2016.00317.

Tyler, E., et al. (2015). "The Relationship between Bipolar Disorder and Cannabis Use in Daily Life: An Experience Sampling Study." *PLoS ONE* 10: e0123953. doi: 10.1371/journal.pone.0118916.

Van den Elsen, G., et al. (2015). "Tetrahydrocannabinol for Neuropsychiatric Symptoms in Dementia: A Randomized Controlled Trial." *Neurology* 84: 2338–2346.

van der Pol, P., et al. (2014). "Cross-Sectional and Prospective Relation of Cannabis Potency, Dosing and Smoking Behaviour with Cannabis Dependence: An Ecological Study." Addiction 109: 1101–1109. doi: 10.1111/add.12508.

Vandrey, R., and Haney, M. (2009). "Pharmacotherapy for Cannabis Dependence: How Close Are We?" *CNS Drugs* 23: 543–553.

Vandrey, R., et al. (2015). "Cannabinoid Dose and Label Accuracy in Edible Medical Cannabis Products." *JAMA* 313: 2491. doi: http://dx.doi.org/10.1001/jama.2015.6613.

Volkow, N. D., et al. (2016). "The Risks of Marijuana Use During Pregnancy." *JAMA* 317: 129–130. doi: 10.1001/jama.2016.18612.

Weinberger, A. H., et al. (2016). "Is Cannabis Use Associated with an Increased Risk of Onset and Persistence of Alcohol Use Disorders? A Three-Year Prospective Study among Adults in the United States." *Drug and Alcohol Dependence* 161: 363–637. doi: 10.1016/j.drugalcdep.2016.01.014.

Wertlake, P. T., and Henson, M. D. (2016). "A Urinary Test Procedure for Identification of Cannabidiol in Patients Undergoing Medical Therapy with Marijuana." *Journal of Pain Research* 9: 81–85.

Wesnes, K. A., et al. (2010). "Nabilone Produces Marked Impairments to Cognitive Function and Changes in Subjective State in Healthy Volunteers." *Journal of Psychopharmacology* 24: 1659–1669.

Whiting, P. F., et al. (2015). "Cannabinoids for Medical Use: A Systematic Review and Meta-Analysis." *JAMA* 313: 2456–2473.

Wilkinson, S. T., et al. (2015). "Impact of Cannabis Use on the Development of Psychotic Disorders." *Current Addiction Reports* 1: 115–128.

Wilkinson, S. T., et al. (2016). "A Systematic Review of the Evidence for Medical Marijuana in Psychiatric Indications." *Journal of Clinical Psychiatry* 77: 1050–1064.

Winstock, A. R., and Barratt, M. J. (2013). "Synthetic Cannabis: A Comparison of Patterns of Use and Effect Profile with Natural Cannabis in a Large Global Sample." *Drug and Alcohol Dependence* 131: 106–111.

Wise, L. E., et al. (2009). "Hippocampal CB1 Receptors Mediate the Memory Impairing Effects of Delta-9-Tetrahydrocannabinol." *Neuropsychopharmacology* 34: 2072–2080.

Wolff, V., et al. (2015). "Characteristics and Prognosis of Ischemic Stroke in Young Cannabis Users Compared with Non-Cannabis Users." *Journal of the American College of Cardiology* 66: 2052–2053. doi: 10.1016/j.jacc.2015.08.867.

Yarnell, S. (2015). "The Use of Medicinal Marijuana for Posttraumatic Stress Disorder: A Review of the Current Literature." *Primary Care Companion for CNS Disorders* 17(3). doi: 10.4088/PCC.15r01786.

Zhang, A., et al. (2017). "What Effects—If Any—Does Marijuana Use During Pregnancy Have on the Fetus or Child?" *The Journal of Family Practice* 66: 462–464.

Zhornitsky, S., and Potvin, S. (2012). "Cannabidiol in Humans: The Quest for Therapeutic Targets." *Pharmaceuticals* (Basel) 21: 529–552.

Zorrilla, I., et al. (2015). "Cannabis and Bipolar Disorder: Does Quitting Cannabis Use during Manic/Mixed Episode Improve Clinical/Functional Outcomes?" *Acta Psychiatrica Scandinavica* 131: 100–110. doi: 10.1111/acps.12366.

Zuurman, L., et al. (2010). "Pharmacodynamic and Pharmacokinetic Effects of the Intravenous CB1 Receptor Agonist Org 26828 in Healthy Male Volunteers." *Journal of Psychopharmacology* 24: 1689–1696.

CHAPTER 10

Opioid Analgesics

Pain is one of the most common of human experiences and one of the most common reasons people seek medical care. Nevertheless, as a sensory phenomenon, pain is very difficult to measure because it is such a subjective and personal experience. The International Association for the Study of Pain (IASP) defines pain as a "highly unpleasant sensory and emotional experience associated with actual or potential tissue damage" (Stone and Molliver, 2009, 237).

Acute, short-acting pain is biologically useful because it provides a warning system against real or potential damage to the body, and it resolves once the injury heals.

Chronic pain, generally defined as pain lasting more than 3 months and not caused by cancer, is typically not useful, causes suffering, restricts activities of daily living, and increases the costs of health care and disability. Common noncancerous or non-terminal chronic pain conditions include migraine, back pain, arthritis, neuropathic pain (defined as pain produced by damage to the nervous system, such as that which occurs in diabetes), AIDS, postherpetic neuralgia, multiple sclerosis, and fibromyalgia, among other disorders. Chronic nonmalignant pain is perhaps the single most common complaint brought by patients to physician offices. Chronic pain complaints are commonly treated with nonopioid analgesics, either alone or with nonprescription modalities, such as exercise, weight loss, physical therapy, psychological interventions, and so forth. Pain due to cancer and other terminal conditions, however, should be aggressively treated. A patient suffering the chronic pain of terminal illness should not be denied opioids, despite the inevitable development of tolerance and dependence as well as a potential for hastening the end of life.

OPIOID MISUSE AND ABUSE

In any given year, about 100 million people in the United States suffer from pain, with about 12 million reporting chronic pain (Califf et al., 2016). Over the past decade, physicians and patients alike have presumed that "no pain" should be the goal of therapy of chronic nonmalignant pain (Lee, 2016). Recently, it has been recognized that this "zero pain" goal has led to thousands of overdose deaths and millions of addicted persons (Ray et al., 2016). The prescribing of opioid pain relievers has quadrupled since 1999, which is in parallel with the surge in opioid fatalities. The number of annual prescriptions written for chronic pain in the United States roughly equals the number of persons in our population. The number of drug overdose deaths in the United States has more than doubled since 1999—from 6.1 to 16 per 100,000 population. In the 6-year period between 2009 and 2015, admissions to intensive care units (ICU) for opioid overdoses increased by 46 percent, and opioid deaths saw an 86 percent increase (Stevens et al., 2016). Specifically, dramatic increases in opioid deaths have occurred from heroin and synthetic opioids such as fentanyl (both discussed later in this chapter), according to new data from the Centers for Disease Control and Prevention (CDC) (Figure 10.1). In 2015, the most recent data year available, people aged 45 to 54 had the highest rate of overdose death (30 per 100,000), but the greatest percentage increase occurred in those aged 55 to 64, with an annual increase of 11 percent, partly because persons often underestimate their risk for overdoses and death (Wilder et al., 2016). Brady and colleagues (2016) review the extent of the opioid epidemic, including the evaluation, treatment, and prevention of prescription opioid abuse and dependence.

In response to this epidemic, the U.S. Food and Drug Administration (FDA) in 2016 released sweeping changes to opioid prescribing policies (Califf et al., 2016), and Congress passed the *Comprehensive Addiction and Recovery Act of 2016*, with provisions addressing the total range of care from primary prevention to recovery support. The act includes important changes to increase access to addiction treatment and medications that reverse overdoses. It also includes provisions dealing with criminal justice and law enforcement. In March 2016, the CDC released its *Guideline for Prescribing Opioids for Chronic Pain*, which provides policies for a safer, more effective treatment regimen (Frieden and Houry, 2016). In spite of these efforts, the CDC reported that 64,000 people died from overdose deaths in 2016, the majority from opiate drugs.

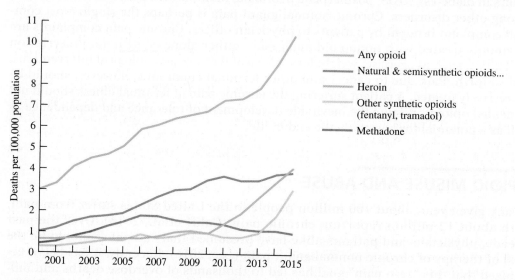

FIGURE 10.1 Overdose deaths involving opioids, by type of opioid, United States, 2000–2015. [Data from Centers for Disease Control and Prevention, 2016.]

Consequently, on October 26, 2017, the president directed the acting Secretary of Health and Human Services, Eric Hargan, to declare the opiate epidemic to be a public health emergency, as defined under the Public Health Services Act. This designation means that federal agencies can provide more grant money to address the epidemic. The order lasts 90 days and can be renewed indefinitely as long as it is considered necessary. The administration will need to work with Congress to find money for the Public Health Emergency fund.

OPIOID TERMINOLOGY

An *opioid* is any exogenous drug (natural, semisynthetic, or synthetic) that binds to an opiate receptor, produces analgesia, and is blocked by an opiate antagonist. An opioid drug may sometimes be referred to as a *narcotic*, a word derived from the Greek word *narke*, meaning "numbness," "sleep," or "stupor." Originally referring to any drug that induced sleep, the term later also became associated with opioids such as morphine and heroin. Narcotic is an inaccurate term, however, because it is sometimes used in a legal context to refer to a wide variety of abused substances that includes nonopioids such as cocaine and marijuana. The term is not useful in a pharmacological context and its use in referring to opioids is discouraged.

Opioid drugs can be categorized in different ways. Four naturally occurring alkaloids (plant-derived amines) can be isolated from the poppy plant: *morphine, codeine, papaverine,* and *thebaine* (Pathan and Williams, 2012). Chemical modification of these opiate alkaloids produced many *semisynthetic* opiates; totally *synthetic* (manmade) opiates then followed.

In regard to their action at opiate receptors, opioids can also be classified as *agonists, partial agonists, mixed agonists-antagonists,* or *antagonists*:

- *Full agonists.* All clinically used opioids produce their effects at least partly by attaching to and activating the receptors upon which our own endogenous opioids bind. Morphine is the prototype opioid full agonist, but there are many others, as shown in Table 10.1.

  Partial agonists. A partial agonist is a drug that binds to opioid receptors, but has a lower intrinsic activity (lower efficacy) than a full agonist. Therefore, a partial agonist exerts an analgesic effect, but the effect has a ceiling at less than the maximal effect produced by morphine. (Here, a *ceiling effect* is defined as a phenomenon in which a drug action reaches a maximum, such that increasing the drug dosage does not increase its effectiveness.)

- *Buprenorphine* is the prototype partial opioid agonist. When administered to a person who is not opioid dependent, it produces analgesia. When administered to an opioid-dependent person, however, buprenorphine may compete with a full agonist, preventing its full effect, and withdrawal may be precipitated. Buprenorphine has become very important in opioid dependence treatment programs, which is discussed later in this chapter.

- *Mixed agonist-antagonists.* A mixed agonist-antagonist drug produces an agonistic effect at one opioid receptor and an antagonistic effect at another. Like a partial

TABLE 10.1 Classification of Commonly Used Opiate Analgesic Agonist and Antagonist Medications

Opioid (Trade Name)	Origin	Chemical Class	Opioid Receptor Mechanism(s)	Nonopioid Mechanisms
Morphine	Natural	Morphinan	Full Agonist μ	
Codeine	Natural	Morphinan	Full Agonist μ	
Levorphanol (Levo Dromoran)	Synthetic	Morphinan	Full Agonist μ, κ	NE Reuptake block; NMDA receptor antagonist
Oxycodone (Oxycontin)	Semisynthetic	Morphinan	Full Agonist μ	
Hydrocodone (Vicodin)	Semisynthetic	Morphinan	Full Agonist μ	
Hydromorphone (Dilaudid)	Semisynthetic	Morphinan	Full Agonist μ	
Oxymorphone (Opana)	Semisynthetic	Morphinan	Full Agonist μ	
Fentanyl (Abstral, Actiq, et al.)	Synthetic	Phenylpiperidine	Full Agonist μ	
Meperidine (Demerol)	Semisynthetic	Phenylpiperidine	Full Agonist μ	
Methadone (Dolophine)	Synthetic	Diphenylheptane	Full Agonist μ	NE Reuptake block; NMDA receptor antagonist
Buprenorphine (Subutex)	Semisynthetic	Morphinan	Partial Agonist μ	
Tapentadol (Nucynta)	Synthetic		Agonist μ	NE Reuptake block
Tramadol (Ultram)	Semisynthetic		Agonist μ	NE Reuptake block; 5-HT Release
Butorphanol (Stadol)	Synthetic	Morphinan	Mixed Ag κ/Antag μ	
Pentazocine (Talwin)	Synthetic	Benzomorphan	Mixed Ag κ/Antag μ	
Naloxone (Narcan)	Semisynthetic		Antagonist μ	
Naltrexone (ReVia; Vivitrol)	Semisynthetic		Antagonist μ	
Nalmefene (Revex)	Semisynthetic		Partial Ag κ/Antag μ	

agonist, a mixed agonist-antagonist usually displays a ceiling effect for analgesia; in other words, it has decreased efficacy compared to a full agonist, such as morphine, and usually is not as effective in treating severe pain. Also, when a mixed agonist-antagonist is administered to an opioid-dependent person, the antagonistic effect precipitates an acute withdrawal syndrome. *Pentazocine* (Talwin) is the prototype mixed agonist-antagonist. Today, mixed agonist-antagonist opioids are infrequently used clinically.

- *Antagonists.* Antagonists have *affinity* for an opioid receptor, but, after attaching, they elicit no change in cellular functioning (for example, they lack intrinsic activity). Antagonists compete with the agonist for the receptor, precipitating withdrawal in an opioid-dependent person and reversing any analgesia caused by the agonist. An example of this is the clinical use of the opioid antagonist *naltrexone* in treatment programs for heroin addicts, where heroin taken after naltrexone elicits no analgesic or euphoric effects. Naloxone is another example of an antagonist. Recently, the FDA approved a nasal spray containing naloxone as an easy-to-use product to treat opioid overdose (Krieter et al., 2016; Strang et al., 2016).

Finally, opiates can be classified according to the type of receptor through which they exert their effects. Some of the most commonly used opiate drugs discussed in this chapter are shown in Table 10.1.

HISTORY

Opium, from which morphine is extracted, is an ancient drug, and there is evidence that the opium poppy, *Papaver somniferum*, was cultivated 10,000 years ago, although definite use as an analgesic is dated to about 3500 to 3000 years ago. Obtained from the sap of the seedpod of the poppy (Figure 10.2), opium has been used for thousands of years to produce euphoria, analgesia, sleep, and relief from diarrhea and cough.[1] The English word *opium* is derived from the Greek word *opion*, which means

---

[1] For thousands of years, the only way to obtain morphine has been by harvesting the milky exudate of the opium poppy. But soon not only drug companies, but drug traffickers as well, can synthesize it because of the development of genetically modified yeast (McNeil, 2015). In the last 8 years, the various steps in the process have been achieved. In 2015, the last biochemical procedure was made public, detailing an efficient method by which the morphine precursor, (S)-reticuline, could be grown in brewer's yeast, *Saccharomyces cerevisiae*. Actually, the researchers were not trying to make morphine, but rather, they were trying to determine if they could make antibiotics or anticancer drugs from the 2500 other alkaloids for which reticuline is a precursor. The question is, who will find this discovery more useful, the pharmaceutical companies or drug cartels? Since the 1960s, India, Turkey and Australia, where licensed farmers can legally grow poppies, have provided an ample and inexpensive amount of opium for drug companies. These growers depend on the sales for their livelihood. Moreover, the drug companies are already able to synthesize many other opiates more powerful than morphine. In contrast, drug cartels would benefit immensely if they could brew their product near their customers and not risk the cost of illegal production and distribution. Scientists have suggested several possible steps that can be taken to prevent misuse of the technology so as to mitigate this concern.

"poppy juice" (Doweiko, 2012, 137). In ancient times, opium was used primarily for its constipating effect and later for its sleep-inducing properties (noted by writers such as Homer, Hippocrates, Dioscorides, Virgil, and Ovid). Although it was used recreationally, not much is known about this aspect before the eighteenth century (Doweiko, 2012). During the Middle Ages, opium was used for practically every known disease and its beneficial effects earned it the name "stone of immortality." Opium, too, was often combined with alcohol, a mixture that the sixteenth-century Swiss physician Paracelsus called *laudanum,* meaning "something to be praised."

Morphine, isolated from opium by the chemist Friedrich Sertürner in 1806, is considered the model opioid analgesic against which all others are compared. Its chemical formula was determined in 1847 and, after the invention of the hypodermic needle in 1853, its use in medicine increased, especially in the battlefield and military hospitals, where it was used liberally—and that often resulted in morphine addiction. (During and after the American Civil War, morphine addiction was referred to as "the soldier's disease.")

During the second half of the nineteenth century, both clinical and recreational use of morphine and opium saw further expansion. Being unregulated, morphine could easily be added to patent medicines and elixirs as an unidentified ingredient, which resulted in addiction among the civilian population. Opium smoking,

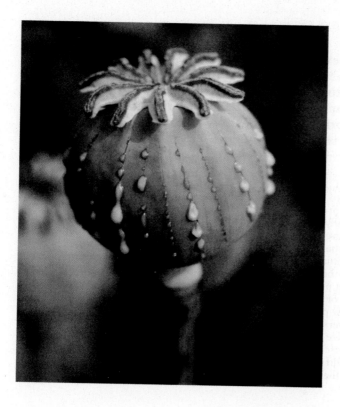

FIGURE 10.2 Photograph of the opium poppy, showing the sap (resin) released from the scored immature seedpod. The dried powder of the resin is opium. [Dr. Jeremy Burgess/Science Source.]

however, a practice introduced by Chinese immigrant workers in the United States, was more obviously recreational than therapeutic.[2] By the year 1900, more than 4 percent of the entire U.S. population was addicted to opium or another opiate (Doweiko, 2012). In one survey of 35 Boston drugstores in 1888, 78 percent of the prescriptions that had been refilled three or more times contained opium (Levinthal, 2012).

By the turn of the century, physicians became increasingly aware of the opioid addiction, especially in regard to the overprescription of opioid drugs and the widespread use of opioids in patent medicine. That concern—and the increasingly epidemiclike abuse of opioids in the United States—led to the passage of the Pure Food and Drug Act of 1906, which required that manufacturers list the ingredients of their products on the labels. This allowed people to see that their medicines contained questionable compounds and the unregulated use of opioids began to decline.

The Harrison Narcotic Act of 1914 provided legislation that had more impact on the use of morphine and opium. The new law stated that only licensed physicians and dentists could prescribe opioids (and cocaine). The law also required medical professionals to register with the Internal Revenue Service (IRS) to write such prescriptions. Gradually, this law was interpreted by court decisions to mean that opioids could only be prescribed and taken for a medically approved purpose and not for *nonmedical* reasons; that is, it ultimately became illegal for opiate addicts to get the drug just to maintain a drug habit.

Since the early twentieth century, periodic cycles of opioid abuse have been followed by efforts to reduce the recreational use of opioids—but without much success. An important part of such efforts has been an ongoing search for drugs that would alleviate pain without the potential for addiction. This search has produced an expanding formulary of natural, semisynthetic, and synthetic opiate analgesics as described in this chapter. So far, however, the goal to separate the analgesic and euphoric–addictive properties of opiates has not been reached. Nevertheless, the ongoing epidemic abuse of prescription opiates, with the epicenter in the United States, is prompting further development of opioid formulations that are pharmacologically designed to prevent recreational misuse (Coplan et al., 2016).

Moreover, there is additional concern about the concomitant use of multiple medications that depress the central nervous system (CNS). On August 31, 2016, the FDA issued a warning about the combined use of opioid and benzodiazepine medications, as well as other drugs that inhibit the CNS. The agency added their strongest alert, the

[2] The habit of smoking opium was acquired by the Chinese as a result of trade with the West, especially Britain, early in the nineteenth century. The British needed to balance their large purchases of tea from China. They did this by trading opium, grown in India, for tea. The Chinese government saw what the opium trade did to its people and had it outlawed throughout the Chinese Empire. The British, however, did not want to lose this valuable source of income and forced China to accept the opium trade. This led to the First Opium War of 1839–1842 and the Second Opium War of 1856–1860. Britain and its allies won the wars because of British naval superiority. Not only did the trade resume, China ceded the island of Hong Kong to Britain as a treaty port. (Hong Kong was ultimately returned to the People's Republic of China in 1999.)

"Boxed Warnings," to the labeling of prescription opioid pain and prescription opioid cough medicines as well as benzodiazepines in an effort to reduce the use of these combinations. Subsequently, on September 20, 2017, after additional review, the FDA published a modification of the warning. This revision stated that "the opioid addiction medications buprenorphine and methadone should not be withheld from patients taking benzodiazepines or other drugs that depress the central nervous system" (U.S. Food and Drug Administration, 2017). While the FDA acknowledged that these drug combinations can result in serious adverse reactions, it also recognized that untreated opiate addiction is also a significant risk. Information to this effect will be added to the buprenorphine and methadone drug labels in addition to specific recommendations for reducing the combined use of these drugs.

PAIN SIGNALING

Normal pain transmission is triggered when a noxious (harmful or unpleasant) stimulus activates neurons that innervate a structure in the body, such as the skin, a joint, or an internal organ. These neurons are called *primary afferent nociceptive sensory neurons* (or just *primary afferents*); their cell bodies are located in ganglia, called *dorsal root ganglia* (DRG) (Figure 10.3), which are parallel to the spinal cord. Primary afferents send information about noxious stimulation from the body to the spinal cord, specifically to the *dorsal horn*.

The terminals of the primary afferent neurons synapse onto neurons in the dorsal horn of the spinal cord. Those spinal neurons then send the message up to the thalamus, which in turn projects to (makes contact with) the cortex in the forebrain. Here is where the subjective experience of pain occurs. As the dorsal horn neurons ascend to the cortex (Figure 10.3), their axonal fibers also send out branches that synapse with other neurons in the hindbrain—called the *rostral ventral medulla* (RVM)—and neurons in the midbrain—called the *periaqueductal gray* (PAG). In addition, neurons in the cortex and other structures in the brain, such as the limbic structures, send descending fibers (axons) back down to the same midbrain, hindbrain, and spinal centers that transmitted the pain message. In this way, various brain structures can either inhibit or facilitate the experience of pain.

All of these sites may provide a target for analgesic medications. For example, drugs may provide pain relief by reducing the firing of the primary afferent neurons at the periphery; that is, at the site of the injury. This might be accomplished by antagonizing the neurochemical substances that are triggered by pain (the inflammatory reactions), which stimulate the primary afferents. This is essentially how nonsteroidal anti-inflammatory drugs (NSAIDs) such as aspirin work. Alternatively, drugs such as the anticonvulsants gabapentin and pregabalin act to reduce the excitation of the primary afferent axons and thereby decrease the signal that is transmitted to the spinal cord. Other drugs may reduce the transmission of the pain signal from within the spinal cord to the brain. Another approach is to activate the descending pathways from the brain to the spinal cord that inhibit ascending pain signals. Some of these descending pathways release the neurotransmitters serotonin and norepinephrine. The reason why some antidepressants can reduce pain (see Chapter 12) is because they increase the

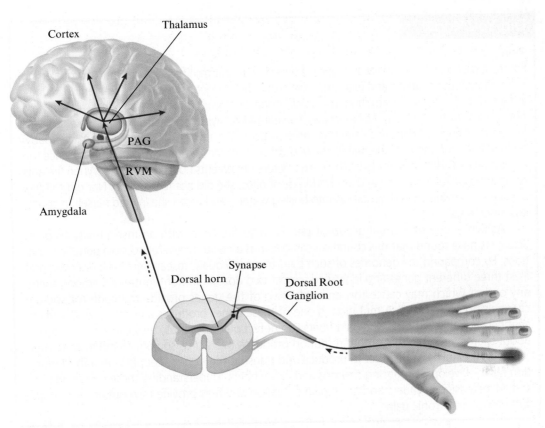

FIGURE 10.3 Overview of pain transmission. Pain signals arise from the periphery (outside of the central nervous system)., when noxious (painful) stimuli activate sensory endings of nociceptive, primary afferent, neurons. These neurons have their cell bodies (not shown) in the dorsal root ganglia (DRG) of the spinal cord. The pain signal is transmitted along the axons of the DRG neurons, which synapse on neurons in the dorsal horn of the spinal cord. Spinal cord neurons relay the pain signal to several structures as it ascends to the brain, including the hindbrain (the rostral ventral medulla, RVM), the midbrain (periaqueductal gray, PAG) and the thalamus. The thalamus projects to the higher brain areas in the cortex, where pain perception is ultimately experienced. Inhibitory and excitatory pathways (not shown) descend from the brain back to the spinal cord, modulating the same sites that were activated by the ascending pathways. Opiate drugs affect the pain signal through opiate receptors located at each of these levels in the periphery, the spinal cord, and other sites, such as the amygdala (part of the limbic system), involved in the emotional reaction to pain, as well as other supraspinal sites. Other drugs, such as antidepressants, anticonvulsants, and ion channel blocking agents, can reduce pain by acting on different mechanisms involved in signal transmission.

amount of these transmitters in the descending pathways. Finally, by acting on higher brain structures, analgesic drugs also alter the emotional reaction to pain and reduce the suffering it causes, independently of influencing the sensory phenomenon itself. This is what opioids do.

> ### Did You Know?
>
> **Pain**
>
> For most people, pain is usually an unpleasant sensation. But pain has a crucial function of alerting us to dangerous situations and without, it we would be at risk of serious, life-threatening injuries. In fact, that is exactly the situation in a small group of individuals who, for various reasons, are not capable of feeling pain. For example, 16-year-old Ashlyn Blocker has been unable to sense any kind of physical pain since the day she was born (Costandi, 2015). When her milk (baby) teeth started coming out, she nearly chewed off part of her tongue. Growing up, she once ran around on a broken ankle for two whole days before her parents noticed the injury. When fire ants swarmed over Ashlyn's body and left hundreds of bites, she did not feel a thing. Nor did she feel any pain when she dipped her hands into boiling water—and when she injured herself in countless other ways.
>
> Ashlyn is one of a small group of people who are born with an insensitivity to pain. Scientists have found that this condition can occur as a result of several possible genetic mutations. By comparing the genomes of such pain-free individuals, researchers have discovered at least three different genes and identified almost two dozen different mutations among them, any one of which may cause this anomaly. Two of the genes provide the code for sodium channels on nerve fibers. A mutation in one of these genes produces a nonfunctional sodium channel such that although the pain fibers can detect painful stimuli, they cannot send signals about them to the brain. Another mutation produces overactive sodium channels that interfere with the ability of the fiber to produce and transmit the signals. People with a third mutation fail to develop painsensing neurons and nerve fibers. Understanding these rare conditions should increase our understanding of pain sensation and may provide new options for people suffering from chronic pain.

Unfortunately, in spite of an expanding knowledge of the underlying pathology and a growing range of therapeutic options, current treatment of chronic pain remains inadequate. One review found that across all treatments, only about half of the patients responded to therapy and the reduction in pain was only about 30 percent (Turk et al., 2011). Efforts are currently directed toward nonopioid medications as well as non-pharmacological modalities that act in conjunction to alleviate the suffering in chronic pain patients (Volkow and McLellan, 2016).

OPIOID RECEPTORS

There is general agreement on the existence of at least three types of opioid receptors, all of them G-protein coupled receptors (GPCRs) (see Chapter 3). They are mu (after morphine), kappa (after the first agent known to act at this receptor, ketocyclazocine), and delta (after vas deferens, the tissue in which it was first isolated) (Pathan and Williams, 2012). In 2000, the nomenclature was changed and the respective receptor types are now also identified as MOP, KOP, and DOP. The genes encoding these three families of opioid receptors, as well as the receptors themselves, have been cloned and sequenced.

Each receptor type—mu, kappa, and delta—arises from its own gene and is expressed through a specific messenger RNA (mRNA). Each receptor is a chain of approximately 400 amino acids, and the amino acid sequences are about 60 percent identical to one another and 40 percent different. Some authorities support the existence of subtypes for the receptors, but this is not universally accepted.

The three classical opioid receptors are distributed widely throughout the central nervous system and, to a lesser extent, in the periphery (including the vas deferens, knee joint, gastrointestinal tract, and other sites). The existence of receptors on which the natural substance opium could exert such significant effects implied that there must be some inherent, endogenous substance or substances within our body that normally acted on these receptors. Presumably the receptors did not evolve just to respond to an extract of the poppy plant! Soon after the opioid receptors were discovered, these endogenous substances were also determined. Each comes from a precursor compound shown in Table 10.2. As indicated in this table, the prohormone proenkephalin is cleaved to form *met-enkephalin* and *leu-enkephalin*, which have the greatest affinity for the DOP receptor. *Dynorphin A* and *B* are agonists at the KOP receptor and are derived from the prohormone prodynorphin.[3] The parent compound of the endogenous agonist for the MOP receptor, β-*endorphin*, is pro-opiomelanocortin (POMC). There are two other MOP agonists, endomorphin 1 and 2, but their precursor has not yet been identified.

As seen in Table 10.2, a fourth type of opiate receptor has also been identified, for which an endogenous ligand and a precursor substance has been determined. However, because this receptor, the nociceptin (NOP) receptor, does not respond to the classical opiate antagonist, naloxone, its categorization has been questioned. It is considered to be a nonopioid "branch" of the opioid receptor family (Pathan and Williams, 2012).

What is the consequence of the binding of an opioid agonist to a mu (MOP) receptor? Figure 10.4 summarizes this process. As is generally the case with GPCRs,

TABLE 10.2 Classification of Opioid Receptors, Their Precursors, and Endogenous Ligands

Receptor	Precursor	Peptide
The mu receptor (MOP)	Proopiomelanocortin (POMC) Unknown	β-endorphin Endomorphin-1 Endomorphin-2
The kappa receptor (KOP)	Prodynorphin	Dynorphin-A Dynorphin-B
The delta receptor (DOP)	Proenkephalin	[Met]-enkephalin [Leu]-enkephalin
The nociceptin receptor (NOP)	Prepronociceptin	Nociceptin/orphanin FQ

SOURCE: Pathan and Williams (2012)

---

[3]The hallucinogenic agent *salvinorin A*, from the psychedelic mint plant *Salvia divinorum*, is a potent agonist of the kappa opioid receptor (discussed in Chapter 8).

the G-protein consisting of the α, β, and γ subunits breaks off from the rest of the receptor—that is, dissociates—and separates into two parts, the α component and the βγ components. These components interact with other parts of the neuron: they *activate* potassium channels, *inhibit* calcium channels, and *reduce* the amount of the substance cyclicAMP inside the neuron (by inhibiting the enzyme adenylyl cyclase), as indicated in Figure 10.4. These actions hyperpolarize the neuron; that is, the neuron is inhibited. Activating potassium channels will allow more of the positively charged potassium ions to leave the neuron; blocking calcium channels will prevent more of the positively charged calcium ions from entering the neuron. Both of these

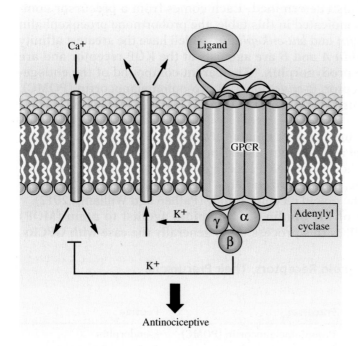

FIGURE 10.4 Schematic of the opiate receptor. The opiate receptor is a G-protein coupled receptor (GPCR). When a molecule of an opiate (ligand), such as morphine, attaches to its binding site on the receptor, it activates the G-protein, causing it to dissociate into its α component and the dual βγ component. The α component inhibits the activity of the enzyme, adenylyl cyclase. The βγ component does two things. First, it opens a channel in the membrane through which potassium ions (K$^+$) flow out. The movement of positively charged potassium ions *out of the neuron* makes the inside more negative, which means the neuron is inhibited and is less likely to fire. Second, the βγ component *inhibits* channels through which positively charged calcium ions flow *into the neuron*. This reduces neurotransmitter release. All of these processes contribute to reduce the transmission of pain.

actions will make the inside of the neuron more negative, relative to the outside. This means the neuron is less likely to fire when stimulated or, if active, it will release less transmitter.

Exogenous and endogenous opiates exert their effects throughout the body, including the periphery (outside of the central nervous system), on neurons in the dorsal horn of the spinal cord, and within various brain sites. In the spinal cord, opioid receptors are located on the presynaptic terminals of the nociceptive primary afferents. When activated by an opioid agonist, the result will be to block the release of pain-producing substances such as glutamate, substance P, and calcitonin gene-related peptide (CGRP). By blocking the release of pain-producing substances, opiates reduce ascending pain signals to higher brain centers.

In the brain, opioid analgesia is believed to be mediated by the activation of mu receptors in the midbrain and hindbrain. High densities of opiate receptors are found in midbrain periaqueductal gray (PAG) neurons, and in hindbrain nuclei located in the rostral ventral medulla (RVM). Opiate agonists indirectly activate the descending inhibitory input from these sites onto the pain processing neurons of the spinal cord. As noted, these pathways release serotonin, norepinephrine, and enkephalin, which further suppress the transmission of pain signals (Figure 10.3).

MAJOR PHARMACOLOGICAL EFFECTS OF OPIATES

Analgesia

Opiates produce analgesia and indifference to pain, reducing the intensity of pain and thus reducing the associated distress by altering the central processing of pain. Analgesia occurs without loss of consciousness and without affecting other sensory modalities. The pain may actually persist as a sensation, but patients feel more comfortable and are able to tolerate it. In other words, the perception of the pain is significantly altered.

Euphoria

Opiates produce a euphoric state, which includes a strong feeling of contentment, well-being, and lack of concern. Regular users of morphine describe the effects of intravenous injection in ecstatic and often sexual terms, but the euphoric effect becomes progressively less intense after repeated use. As with other drugs of abuse, opiates produce their rewarding effects by increasing dopamine release in the limbic reward pathway. It is postulated that opiates act indirectly in the ventral tegmental area by inhibiting GABA neurons via mu opioid receptors. The GABA neurons exert an inhibitory effect on dopamine neurons. Thus, opiates are believed to be rewarding at least partly because they disinhibit dopaminergic neurons and increase dopamine input in the nucleus accumbens and other areas (see Chapter 4).

Depression of Respiration

Opiates cause a profound depression of respiration by decreasing the brain stem respiratory center's sensitivity to higher levels of carbon dioxide in the blood. Respiratory rate is reduced even at therapeutic doses. At higher doses, the rate slows even further, respiratory volume decreases, breathing patterns become shallow and irregular and, at sufficiently high levels, breathing ceases and death follows (Figure 10.5).

Respiratory depression is the single most important acute side effect of morphine and is the cause of death from acute opioid overdosage. A respiratory rate of eight breaths per minute or less in a patient who is not actually sleeping strongly suggests acute opioid intoxication, particularly if miosis (pinpoint pupils) and/or stupor are also present. Treatment, in adults, consists of 0.4 to 2.0 milligrams of the antagonist naloxone, which can be increased up to a maximum of 10 milligrams. If respiratory depression persists after 10 milligrams of naloxone, it is unlikely that it is due to opioid overdose. Because naloxone is short-acting, reversal of opioid analgesic toxicity might require continuous infusion (Boyer, 2012). As discussed later in this chapter, this is an important consideration in regard to the current opioid epidemic. Until recently, naloxone had to be injected, which was a drawback. However, as mentioned, a nebulized (nasal spray) formulation was approved and marketed in 2016. Of course, naloxone, as an opioid antagonist, precipitates withdrawal symptoms.

Tolerance of respiratory depression appears to develop at a slower rate than analgesic tolerance. Because of this delay, patients with a long history of opioid use are, paradoxically, at increased risk for respiratory depression. Methadone may confer greater risk of overdose toxicity than other opiates because respiratory depression may occur *later* than the analgesic effect. A patient may believe that an analgesic dose is too low and then take more of the drug before it has time to take effect. Moreover, patients

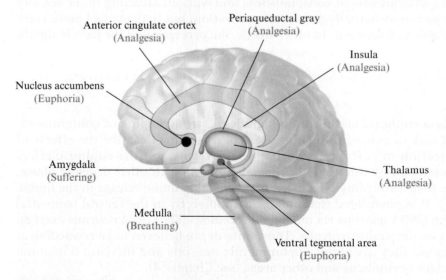

FIGURE 10.5 Brain structures where morphine acts to produce analgesia, respiratory depression, or euphoria.

tolerant to high doses of other opiates may not be tolerant to methadone (Stachnik, 2011). This may be relevant to recent efforts to understand the current dramatic increase in opiate overdose deaths. Reviews have found that overdose deaths are more likely to occur when patients are "rotated" from one opioid to another, when higher dosages are prescribed, or when drug addicts either begin or terminate opiate use. That is, loss of tolerance (after abstinence), overconfidence about dosage, or ignorance of the ingested formulation often kill relapsing opioid addicts (Courtwright, 2015).

Suppression of Cough

Opiates suppress the cough center in the hindbrain and have historically been used as cough suppressants. This is termed an antitussive action. Codeine is particularly popular for this purpose. Today, however, less-addicting drugs are used as cough suppressants and opioids have become inappropriate choices for treating persistent cough.

Sedation and Anxiolysis

Opiates reduce anxiety and produce sedation and drowsiness, but the level of sedation is not so deep as that produced by other CNS depressants. Although people who take morphine will doze, they can usually be awakened readily. During this state, cognitive slowing is prominent, accompanied by a lack of concentration, apathy, complacency, lethargy, and a sense of tranquility. This effect becomes tolerant with repeated use. Nevertheless, this action may be therapeutically useful, as it has been reported that morphine has helped to reduce the development of posttraumatic stress disorder (PTSD) in soldiers who were injured in combat during the Iraq war (Holbrook et al., 2010). That said, concern has been raised about the relatively high use of opiates in returning members of the military (Toblin et al., 2014).

Nausea and Vomiting

Opioids stimulate receptors in an area of the medulla called the *chemoreceptor trigger zone.* Stimulation of this area produces nausea and vomiting, which are characteristic and unpleasant side effects of morphine and other opioids, but they are not life-threatening. Like drowsiness, this effect becomes tolerant with chronic use.

Gastrointestinal Symptoms

As a result of their direct actions on the intestine, opiates relieve diarrhea, the most important action of opioids outside the central nervous system (CNS). These drugs cause intestinal tone to increase, motility to decrease, feces to dehydrate, and intestinal spasm (and cramping). The combination of decreased propulsion, increased intestinal tone, decreased rate of movement of food, and dehydration hardens the stool and further retards the advance of fecal material. Nothing more effective than opioids has yet been discovered for treating severe diarrhea. Two opioids have been developed that only very minimally cross the blood–brain barrier into the CNS. One is *diphenoxylate* (the primary active ingredient in Lomotil) and the other is *loperamide* (Imodium). These two drugs are exceedingly effective opioid antidiarrheals. The reason that loperamide (and other substances) cannot get into the systemic circulation or the brain is that P-glycoprotein (P-gp) blocks entry. However, opioid abusers have discovered that when taken in amounts of 10 times or more the therapeutic dose, loperamide can overcome the protective effects of P-gp and reach the brain. Use of huge-dose loperamide to relieve opioid withdrawal systems or to get high is increasing. Unfortunately, loperamide can cause cardiotoxic effects, and several deaths have been reported, possibly from this cause. In June 2016, the FDA issued a "Drug Safety Communication," warning about high-dose loperamide (Lasoff et al., 2016; Vakkalanka et al., 2016).

Opioid-induced constipation is a common and undesirable adverse consequence of chronic use, estimated to occur in 40 to 90 percent of patients (Peppin, 2012). Moreover, there appears to be little tolerance to this side effect. Treatment generally consists of administering an anticonstipatory agent together with the opiate. Although there are numerous options, in the context of this chapter, the opioid antagonists are most relevant. Naloxone, while not officially approved for this indication, is still commonly used. However, because it crosses the blood–brain barrier, naloxone can also reverse the analgesic effect of opiates and precipitate withdrawal symptoms. Therefore, newer agents have been developed that have a methyl group added to the opioid antagonist naltrexone. This prevents the antagonist from entering the brain and limits the effects to the periphery. *Methylnatrexone* (Relistor) was the first such drug and is intended to restore bowel function in adults with advanced illnesses who are receiving opioids on a continuous basis and suffer from their constipating effects (Siemens and Becker, 2016). Another injectable opiate antagonist, *alvimopan* (Entereg) is intended to restore normal bowel function in hospitalized patients who have undergone bowel surgery. *Naloxegol* (Movantik) is a third peripherally acting opioid antagonist approved by the FDA and indicated for the treatment of opioid-induced constipation in adult patients with chronic noncancer pain.

A nonopioid laxative agent, *lubiprostone* (Amitiza), already approved in 2013 for chronic idiopathic constipation in adults and in adult women with irritable bowel syndrome, was also approved for opioid-induced constipation in chronic pain patients. Although not an opioid antagonist, lubiprostone increases fluid in the gastrointestinal (GI) tract and helps one pass stool (Holder and Rhee, 2016).

Pupillary Constriction

Opiates cause pupillary constriction (miosis). Indeed, pupillary constriction in the presence of analgesia is characteristic of opioid ingestion. As noted later in this chapter, one opiate drug that does not elicit this effect is meperidine.

Endocrine Effects

Opiates exert subtle but important effects on the functioning of the endocrine system. Effects include reduced libido in men and menstrual irregularities and infertility in women. These actions occur secondary to drug-induced reductions in sex hormone-releasing agents from the hypothalamus. As a result, testosterone levels in males fall, as do the levels of luteinizing and follicle-stimulating hormones in females. If a person is taking an opioid for chronic pain, both the reduction in sex hormones and the chronic pain may result in loss of sexual desire and impaired performance, alterations in gender role, fatigue, mood alterations, loss of muscle mass and strength, abnormal menses, infertility, and osteoporosis and fractures. However, it is not always clear whether the opioid-induced hypogonadism or the chronic pain is responsible (Brennan, 2013). In addition to changes in sex hormones, patients maintained on opiates for many years may have a variety of hormonal abnormalities (Tennant, 2012).

Other Effects

Opiates can release histamine from its storage sites in mast cells in the blood, which may elicit localized itching or more severe allergic reactions, including bronchoconstriction. Opioids also affect white blood cell function, producing complex alterations in the immune system. It is advisable, perhaps, to avoid the use of morphine in patients with compromised immune function.

GENETIC OPIOID METABOLIC DEFECTS

With the current dramatic increase in opioid prescription abuse and concern about the accidental overdose of these medications, the phenomenon of genetic anomalies in opiate metabolism is receiving increasing attention (Kapur et al., 2014; Tennant, 2010, 2011, 2016; Trescott and Faynboym, 2014; Tverdohleb et al., 2016). The primary pathways for opioid metabolism involve the cytochrome P450 (CYP) 2D6 and 3A4 isoenzymes. These two isoenzymes account for over 90 percent of opiate metabolism; CYP-3A4 alone accounts for 40 to 60 percent. Although the evidence is somewhat indirect, estimates are that 20 to 30 percent of pain patients have a genetic opioid metabolic defect (GOMD) in one of these enzymes.

In some cases, the enzyme is too active. Such patients are termed "rapid" or "ultrarapid" metabolizers in whom the opioid is rapidly metabolized and pain returns much quicker than usual. These patients require a higher than normal dosage of opiate, which may cause them to be mislabeled as addicts and undertreated. Singa (2016) recently described a case history of such a patient. In other cases, the metabolic enzyme is either inactive or absent, which results in slower than normal rates of drug metabolism, causing the opioid to accumulate in the blood and increasing its toxicity from drug-induced respiratory depression.

According to Tennant (2010), it is possible that many of the numerous overdose deaths that have occurred since opioid pain prescriptions became popular in the last decade were due to this phenomenon. Tennant also discusses simple ways to diagnose and treat these conditions. One very helpful approach is to use opiates that bypass the CYP450 system and are metabolized by glucuronidation. These include oxymorphone, hydromorphone, and tapentadol (Tennant, 2016).

Even without a genetic metabolic defect, interactions between opioids and other psychotropic drugs are prevalent and can be dangerous as well as fatal. Many of the metabolic enzymes involved in opiate metabolism are either inhibited or induced by other medications, especially antidepressants and benzodiazepines, and these effects have important implications for pain prescriptions. Pierce and Brahm (2011) provide a useful discussion of these relationships and some of the most relevant specific interactions.

TOLERANCE AND DEPENDENCE

The development of tolerance and dependence with repeated use is a characteristic feature of all opioid drugs. This reflects a progressive failure of the receptors to initiate a signal after long-term opioid binding, a phenomenon termed *receptor desensitization.* The process is thought to involve the uncoupling of the receptors from the G-protein, after which the receptors are taken inside the neuron until they are eventually returned to the membrane and resensitized to opioid binding. It is believed that this cycle limits the degree of tolerance of the mu opioid receptors to their own endogenous opioid ligands. Endogenous opiates are released intermittently and they are metabolized very quickly after being released. As a result, binding of endogenous opiates is short lived. In contrast, when opioid analgesics are administered for long periods of time, they facilitate tolerance because they are constantly attached to the receptors and interfere with receptor recycling and resensitization (Boyer, 2012).

In other words, when morphine or other opioids are used only intermittently, little if any tolerance develops and the opioids retain their initial efficacy. When administration is repeated, tolerance becomes so marked that massive doses have to be administered to either maintain a degree of euphoria or prevent withdrawal discomfort. The degree of tolerance is illustrated by the fact that the dose of morphine can be increased from clinical doses (50 to 60 milligrams per day) to 500 milligrams per day over as short a period as 10 days.

Tolerance to one opioid leads to cross-tolerance for all other natural and synthetic opioids, even if they are chemically dissimilar. Cross-tolerance, however, does not develop between the opioids and the sedative hypnotics. In other words, a person who has developed a tolerance for morphine will also have a tolerance for other opiate agonists (Table 10.1) but not for alcohol or benzodiazepines.

Physical dependence is an altered physiological state induced by a drug, whereby withdrawal of a drug elicits biological reactions typical for that class of drugs. Generally, symptoms of withdrawal are the opposite of pharmacological effects. (For opiate withdrawal, see Table 10.3.) The magnitude of these acute withdrawal symptoms depends on the dose of opioid that had been used, the frequency of previous drug administration, and the duration of drug dependence. Acute opioid withdrawal is not considered life-threatening.

To help alleviate the symptoms of acute withdrawal, several approaches have been tried. These approaches include clonidine-assisted detoxification, buprenorphine-assisted detoxification, and rapid anesthesia-aided detoxification. Clonidine is a drug that acts on the sympathetic nervous system to reduce some of the physical manifestations of withdrawal. Buprenorphine will be discussed later in this chapter.

TABLE 10.3 Prominent acute opioid reactions and rebound withdrawal symptoms

Opioid Action	Symptom of withdrawal
Analgesia	Pain, irritability, hyperalgesia
Respiratory depression (decreased breathing)	Rapid breathing
Euphoria	Dysphoria, depression
Relaxation, tranquilization, and sleep	Agitation, anxiety, insomnia
Constipation	Diarrhea
Pupillary constriction	Pupillary dilation
Peripheral vasodilation; flushed and warm skin	Chilliness and goosebumps
Decreased sex drive	Spontaneous ejaculation
Drying of secretions	Lacrimation, runny nose

SOURCE: Feldman et al. (1997)

In *rapid anesthesia-aided detoxification* (RAAD), a pure opioid antagonist, such as naloxone or naltrexone, and the sympathetic blocker clonidine are administered intravenously to the opioid-dependent person while he or she is asleep under general anesthesia. The procedure continues for about 72 hours, during which time the withdrawal signs are blunted. The objective is to enable the patient to tolerate high doses of an opioid antagonist and thus undergo complete detoxification while unconscious. After awakening, the patient is maintained on naltrexone and undergoes supportive psychotherapy and group therapies for relapse prevention and to address the underlying causes of addiction. The RAAD technique is controversial, in part because it is expensive, involves the risks of anesthesia, and focuses only on short-term dependence rather than on long-term cravings and social adjustments. Thus, this technique for treating opioid addiction is infrequently used now.

Regardless of the method, there is a protracted opiate *abstinence syndrome* following acute withdrawal that can persist as long as 6 months. Symptoms include depression, abnormal responses to stressful situations, drug hunger, anxiety and other psychological disturbances, as well as other psychiatric disorders. Risk of relapse and overdosing is high, even following release from prison or from a detoxification program (Volkow and McLellan, 2016).

FULL OPIOID AGONISTS

Morphine: The Prototype Full Opioid Agonist

Among the analgesics found in the opium poppy, morphine is the most potent and represents about 10 percent of the crude exudate (in other words, the juice or sap that is harvested from the mature poppy flower). Codeine is much less potent and constitutes only 0.5 percent of the crude exudate. Despite decades of research, no other drug has been found that exceeds morphine's effectiveness as an analgesic, and no other drug is clinically superior for treating severe pain.

Morphine can be administered by injection, inhalation, or taken orally or rectally. Rylomine, an intranasal delivery system, remains under development. This product is intended to have a rapid onset of action in situations where oral use is not desired.

Orally, morphine is available in immediate-release formulation and as a long-acting, time-release product (MS-Contin). In January 2017, the FDA approved Arymo ER, the first product developed using an abuse-deterrent technology—a physical and chemical barrier approach—creating tablets that are difficult to crush, cut, grind, or break for the purpose of misuse and abuse.

In general, absorption of morphine from the gastrointestinal tract is slow and incomplete compared to absorption following injection or inhalation. Only about 20 percent of orally administered morphine reaches the CNS. Absorption through the rectum is adequate, and several opioids (morphine, hydromorphone, and oxymorphone) are available in suppository form.[4]

The risk of an overdose increases in a dose–response manner. It will nearly double at 50 to 99 morphine milligram equivalents (MME) per day and increase by a factor of up to 9 at 100 MME or more per day compared with doses of less than 20 MME per day (Frieden and Houry, 2016).

The presence of opioid receptors in the spinal cord means administration of morphine directly onto the spinal cord, an intrathecal route through small surgically implanted catheters, is effective. This route places the drug right at its site of action and may avoid its effects both on higher CNS centers (maintaining wakefulness and avoiding respiratory depression) and in the periphery (avoiding drug-induced constipation). A variation of this approach is the epidural route, in which the drug is introduced above the dura mater of the spinal cord, and diffuses across the dural membrane to bind with spinal opiate receptors. In medicine, the epidural and intrathecal techniques are used to control the pain of obstetric labor and delivery, to treat postoperative pain, and (for long-term use) to relieve terminal cancer and other forms of intractable pain. In these situations, an implantable programmed pump for intraspinal infusion is available.

Morphine crosses the blood–brain barrier fairly slowly, as it is more water-soluble than lipid soluble. Other opioids cross the blood–brain barrier much more rapidly.

Opioids reach all body tissues, including the fetus. Infants born to addicted mothers are physically dependent on opioids and exhibit withdrawal symptoms. The habitual use of morphine or other opioids during pregnancy does not seem to increase the risk of congenital anomalies; thus, these drugs are not considered to be teratogenic. However, there are increased risks of birth-related problems and fetal growth retardation.

The liver metabolizes morphine and as much as 40 to 60 percent of the drug may not reach the systemic circulation because of first-pass metabolism. One of morphine's metabolites (morphine-6-glucuronide) is actually 10 to 20 times more potent as an analgesic than morphine itself, and much of morphine's analgesic action is mediated

---

[4]This kind of preparation might be indicated for patients suffering from muscle-wasting diseases who cannot tolerate other routes of administration.

by this active metabolite. The half-lives of morphine and morphine-6-glucuronide are both 3 to 5 hours. Patients with impaired kidney function tend to accumulate the metabolite and thus may be more sensitive to morphine administration.

Urine screening tests can be used to detect codeine (discussed in the next section) and morphine as well as their metabolites. Because heroin (discussed later in the chapter) is metabolized to monoacetylmorphine and then to morphine, heroin use is suspected when monoacetylmorphine, morphine, and codeine are present in either blood or urine. Frequently, urinalysis cannot accurately determine which specific drug (heroin, codeine, or morphine) has been used. However, a specific metabolite of heroin, 6-monoacetylmorphine, is also at times detected and would definitely confirm illicit drug (such as heroin) use. Even poppy seeds contain small amounts of morphine. Depending on the drug that was taken, morphine and codeine metabolites may be detected in a patient's urine for two to four days.

Codeine

Codeine is a prodrug, which must be metabolized by the enzyme CYP 2D6 in the body to morphine, the pharmacologically active drug. Hence, the efficacy and safety of codeine is governed by CYP 2D6 activity (Crews et al., 2012). Codeine used to be widely prescribed as a low-potency opioid, but in recent years has fallen out of favor because of more reliable and stronger opioids such as hydrocodone and oxycodone. Codeine was usually combined with aspirin or acetaminophen for the relief of mild to moderate pain. These combination products were frequently sought drugs of abuse. Because it has been used for so long, codeine never underwent the safety studies required for new drugs. The plasma half-life and duration of action is about 3 to 4 hours, but codeine's pharmacokinetics are unpredictable. Moreover, almost 1 in 10 Americans have a genetic variation that causes very rapid metabolism of codeine. As a result, abnormally high levels of morphine may accumulate, leading to drowsiness and respiratory depression. Furthermore, morphine may also be passed to infants through breast milk. In 2013, the FDA warned that products containing codeine should not be used for pain relief in children after tonsillectomy or adenoidectomy because of the risk for adverse effects or death. This was based on medical reports of three deaths and one life-threatening case of respiratory depression in children with sleep apnea given codeine after one of the aforementioned surgeries. All the children were ultrarapid metabolizers.

In addition to its inherent pharmacokinetic disadvantages, four of the six selective serotonin reuptake inhibitor (SSRI) antidepressants (fluoxetine, fluvoxamine, sertraline, and paroxetine; see Chapter 12) can block the pain relief of codeine because they block the conversion of codeine to morphine. For patients taking one of these drugs, an analgesic drug other than codeine may be necessary.

Heroin

Heroin (diacetylmorphine) is three times more potent than morphine and is produced from morphine by a slight modification of its chemical structure. The increased lipid solubility of heroin leads to faster penetration of the blood–brain barrier, producing an intense rush when the drug is either smoked or injected intravenously. Heroin is metabolized to monoacetylmorphine and morphine; morphine is eventually metabolized and excreted.

Although initially developed as an analgesic in the late nineteenth century in Germany—as a more *heroisch* (heroic or valiant) intervention to pain than aspirin—heroin is rarely used medicinally or clinically except, as in the case of the United Kingdom, under restricted clinical guidelines. In the United States, heroin is illegal and anyone who manufactures, sells, distributes, and uses heroin does so illicitly.

When heroin is smoked together with crack cocaine, euphoria is intensified, the anxiety and paranoia associated with cocaine are tempered, and the depression that follows, after the effects of cocaine wear off, seems to be reduced. Unfortunately, this combination creates a multidrug addiction that is extremely difficult to treat.

According to the National Center for Health Statistics (2017), between 2010 and 2015, the increased potency of heroin and the drop in the price of the drug resulted in the dramatic fourfold rise in the annual number of lethal heroin overdoses in the United States from 3036 to 12,989. This increase occurred in all age groups, but the largest percentage was seen in those aged 55 to 64.

Studies have shown a positive relationship between high rates of prescription opioid analgesic use and heroin abuse. The concurrent use of prescription opiates and heroin is increasing, and more people are alternating between these two drugs, depending on which one is available (Cicero et al., 2015). This progression of heroin use from prescription opioid abuse appears to be a new phenomenon. In the 1960s, more than 80 percent of opioid abusers noted that they started with heroin; this was nearly reversed by the 2000s, when 75 percent started using prescription opioids before initiating heroin use (Compton et al., 2016). Most of the few studies that have been done, show that heroin use increased before policies were in place that made opioid prescriptions more difficult to obtain. The fact that heroin increased in purity and accessibility, and became cheaper, has been considered important reasons for the increased use, especially in a subgroup of people with opiate dependence who frequently misuse prescribed opiates.

Compton and colleagues (2016) describe several approaches being developed to stem prescription opioid abuse. These initiatives involve educational efforts, monitoring programs for prescription drugs, increased enforcement to deal with illegal prescribers, and development of new abuse-deterrent drug formulations, which are discussed later in this chapter.

Hydrocodone

Hydrocodone is one of the most commonly prescribed and abused opioid medications. Like codeine, hydrocodone (dihydrocodeinone) is a relatively weak analgesic. CYP 2D6 converts much of the hydrocodone to the more active compound *hydromorphone* (Dilaudid). Short-acting hydrocodone is commonly found in combination with acetaminophen in formulations such as Vicodin, Norco, and Lortab. In October 2014, these compounds, because of their high abuse risk, were rescheduled from Schedule III to Schedule II, which is a more restricted category. In addition to some other restrictions, this means that doctors cannot call in a prescription to a pharmacy Instead, they must write a prescription that the patient must, in most cases, present in person to a pharmacist in order to receive these drugs. In the first year following the rescheduling, there were 26.3 million fewer prescriptions (a 22 percent decline) and 1.1 billion fewer tablets sold (a 16 percent decline). The decrease was mostly due to the fact that patients were not able to get refills over the phone. Further analysis also revealed there was no increase in prescriptions for the synthetic opioid tramadol (see below) after hydrocodone rescheduling (Jones et al., 2016), indicating that the new restrictions were effective in reducing overall opiate use.

Long-acting hydrocodone formulations are sold under the trade names Hysingla and Zohydro. The FDA approved Zohydro (developed by Zogenix) for the treatment of moderate to severe pain, in October 2013. A year later, in November 2014, the FDA also approved Hysingla (made by Purdue Pharma), the second single-entity hydrocodone product for the treatment of moderate to severe pain. The term "single entity" means that each drug contains only hydrocodone, without any other medication, such as acetaminophen. The use of products containing acetaminophen in high doses over long periods of time has the potential for causing liver injury. Hysingla ER was originally approved with abuse deterrent technology. But the initial approval of Zohydro ER was extremely controversial because the original formulation did not contain abuse deterrent technology. In order to prescribe Zohydro ER, clinicians were required to complete a risk assessment and pain management treatment agreement. In January 2015, Zohydro ER was reformulated to contain BeadTek technology, which causes the drug to form a viscous gel when crushed or dissolved in liquids, which makes the hydrocodone difficult to inject. The new formulation of Zohydro ER, which was approved in February 2015, maintains the same pharmacokinetic and efficacy profiles as the older formulations, but includes the abuse deterrent technology.

One agent under development, KP201, is currently under FDA review as an alternative form of hydrocodone. In February 2016, the FDA granted the manufacturer of KP201 combined with acetaminophen (also known as APAP for the active ingredient acetyl-para-aminophenol) priority review status. Clinical studies have not yet been published. Guenther and coworkers (2016) reported KP201 to have similarity in abuse potential to hydrocodone (for example, Norco). In June 2016, this drug, with the trade name Apadaz, received a positive evaluation as an extended release formulation of hydrocodone and acetaminophen, but not with abuse deterrent properties and, as of March 2, 2017, had not been approved by the FDA.

In January 2017, another extended release hydrocodone compound was approved by the FDA. This product, with the trade name Vantrela, was made by the Teva pharmaceutical company. It claims to have abuse deterrent potential whether administered by oral, intranasal, or intravenous routes.

Oxycodone

Oxycodone (Percodan, OxyContin; Xtampza-ER, Remoxy) is another semisynthetic opioid similar in action to morphine. The short-acting, generic preparation is widely prescribed for the treatment of acute pain. The enzyme CYP3A4 metabolizes oxycodone to the opioid agonist noroxycodone, which is not very potent, and the enzyme CYP2D6 metabolizes oxycodone to oxymorphone, which is more potent. In most patients, analgesia is primarily due to oxycodone, but data suggests that analgesic effects in individuals with CYP2D6 abnormalities might be different.

The long-acting formulations of oxycodone (OxyContin, Xartemis-XR, Xtampza-ER, Remoxy) contain oxycodone in doses to 80 milligrams (normal acute doses are about 5 to 10 milligrams). Since 1999, OxyContin has been widely abused and responsible for numerous overdose fatalities. Abusers crushed the pill, destroying the time-release mechanisms, and either snorted the powder, smoked the drug, or diluted it in water and injected it. The abuse of OxyContin led to the development of a new formulation approved in April 2010, intended to prevent it from being cut, broken, chewed, crushed, frozen, heated, or dissolved to release more medication. Evidence from human pharmacokinetic studies shows that the drug is not rapidly released if it is dissolved in ethanol or other common drinks or solvents. Two other products, Remoxy and Xtampza-ER, are now available.

The new formulations of oxycodone did successfully reduce abuse liability. A year after the new formula was marketed, it was reported to sell for 28 percent less than the original OxyContin on the black market and abuse fell significantly. However, the use of other opioids, such as fentanyl, heroin, and *oxymorphone* (Opana; see the next section) increased. While 24 percent of drug users said they found a way around the tamper-proof mechanism, most (66 percent) said they just switched to another opioid (Cicero et al., 2012).

Hydromorphone and Oxymorphone

Hydromorphone (Dilaudid, Palladone) and *oxymorphone* (Numorphan, Opana-ER) are both structurally related to morphine and are 6 to 10 times more potent. They produce somewhat less sedation but equal respiratory depression. Palladone (not to be confused with *paliperidone*; see Chapter 11) and Exalgo are trade names for two long-acting formulations of hydromorphone that are taken once daily for treatment of chronic pain in patients who have developed a tolerance to opioids and thus can tolerate the high doses of 10 to 32 milligrams per day (the dose of short-acting hydromorphone is about 1 to 2 milligrams). The half-life of both Palladone and Exalgo is about 18 hours, providing analgesia for up to 24 hours (Weinstein, 2009). Palladone is formulated as an immediately dissolving capsule containing controlled-release pellets. Exalgo contains hydromorphone in the OROS osmotic delivery system similar to that used for Concerta (see Chapter 15).

The long-acting formulation of oxymorphone has been controversial. The FDA first approved Opana-ER in 2006. In 2010, following the reformulation of OxyContin, abuse of Opana skyrocketed, since Opana could be crushed and snorted, allowing a full 12-hour dose delivered in minutes. In response, in 2012, the manufacturer developed a crush-resistant formulation similar to that of OxyContin. One adverse effect of injection was the occurrence of thrombotic thrombocytopenic purpura (TTP). TTP is characterized by the occurrence of blood clots in small vessels throughout the body, which can damage organs. Even worse, while the new formulation appeared to deter abuse by snorting the powdered drug, abusers found they could cook the pills and adminis-ter it by injection. This has led to wide abuse and multiple deaths. Indeed, the current street cost of a single Opana pill can be up to $200 depending on the tablet strength. Martin and coworkers (2016) reviewed the technology behind controlled-release formulations for long-acting opioid pain products. Hopefully, as new guidelines for opioid prescribing are implemented, overprescription for these products will decrease (Alford, 2016; Califf et al., 2016).

Propoxyphene

Propoxyphene (Darvon) is an analgesic compound that is structurally similar to meth-adone; it is less potent than codeine but more potent than aspirin. Darvon was mar-keted in 1957 when there were few alternatives for treating pain, except aspirin and strong opioids. In 2010, the FDA determined that the drug should be removed from commercial sale because of concerns about potentially fatal heart rhythm abnormali-ties, drug overdose suicide, and overdoses.

Meperidine

Meperidine (Demerol) is a synthetic opioid whose structure differs from that of mor-phine. Because of this structural difference, meperidine was originally thought to be free of many of the undesirable properties of the opioids. However, meperidine is addictive and it can be substituted for morphine or heroin in addicts. It is one-tenth as potent as morphine, produces a similar type of euphoria, and is equally likely to cause dependence. Meperidine's side effects differ from morphine's and include more excitatory effects, such as tremors, delirium, hyperreflexia, and convulsions. These excitatory actions are produced by a metabolite of meperidine (normeperi-dine). Unlike other opiates, meperidine does not cause pinpoint pupils, but it may dilate the pupils because of an anticholinergic action. Meperidine and normeperidine can accumulate in people who have kidney dysfunction or who use only meperi-dine for their opioid addiction. Following discontinuation, withdrawal symptoms develop more rapidly than with morphine because of meperidine's shorter duration of action.

Fentanyl and Its Derivatives

Fentanyl (Sublimaze) and three related compounds, *sufentanil* (Sufenta), *alfentanil* (Alfenta), and *remifentanyl* (Ultiva) are short-acting, intravenously administered opi-oid agonists that are structurally related to meperidine. They are meant to be used during and after surgery to relieve surgical pain. Carfentanil, an even more potent compound, is used to immobilize large animals, such as elephants, in veterinary prac-tice. Fentanyl and its derivatives are multiple times more potent than morphine and frequently combined with heroin to increase its potency, usually resulting in fatalities in unsuspecting heroin users.

In addition to its intravenous formulation, fentanyl is also available in numerous other forms: a transdermal skin patch (Durapatch; Ionsys); a dissolvable buccal tablet (Fentora), which is placed between the upper cheek and gum; a fentanyl buccal soluble film (Onsolis); a sublingual tablet (Abstral); a sublingual spray (Subsys); an oral lozenge on a stick (Actiq), which is often referred to as a "lollipop"; and a nasal spray (Lazanda). The transdermal route of drug delivery offers prolonged, rather steady levels of drug in blood; the buccal tablet, the lollipop, and the nasal spray are short-acting products intended for the treatment of breakthrough cancer pain in opioid-dependent patients who are intolerant of injections (Paech et al., 2012). A sublingual, 30 microgram tablet formulation of sufentanil has been developed to treat moderate to severe acute pain. Its administration is restricted to medically supervised situations, to prevent diversion. Although sufentanil is usually given by IV infusion, it is short acting, whereas the new sublingual formulation lasts longer and does not produce a spike in blood levels. On October 12, 2017, the FDA informed the company (AcelRX Pharmaceutical) that it could not approve the drug until certain modifications were made (Minkowitz and Candiotti, 2015).

As an analgesic, fentanyl and its derivatives are 80 to 500 times as potent as morphine and profoundly depress respiration. Death from these agents is invariably caused by respiratory failure. Because they are so lipid soluble, these drugs may accumulate in fat stores, which means they need an extended period of time to leave the body; that is, to move from the fat cells to the blood and then to the liver. Remifentanil differs from fentanyl in this regard. Although it is also very lipid soluble, remifentanil is metabolized quickly outside of the liver, in the blood and tissues. For this reason, the drug is used for rapid, short-acting analgesia, which can be given for long periods but is cleared quickly (Pathan and Williams, 2012).

Fentanyl has been used illicitly under various nicknames (for example, "china white"). Numerous derivatives, such as *alpha fentanyl,* have been manufactured illegally; they emerge periodically and have been responsible for many fatalities (Lozier et al., 2015). In March 2015, a surge in overdose deaths around the country from heroin laced with fentanyl prompted the Drug Enforcement Agency (DEA) to issue a nationwide alert. Similarly, in September 2016, the DEA also issued a public warning and notified law enforcement agencies about the dangers of carfentanil, a synthetic opioid that is 10,000 times more potent than morphine and 100 times more potent than fentanyl.

Tapentadol

Tapentadol (Nucynta) was released in 2009 as a Schedule II analgesic, similar to tramadol (discussed below) because it has two types of action. First, it activates the mu opioid receptor and second, it inhibits the reuptake of norepinephrine. Tapentadol is a full mu agonist, but its binding affinity is 18 times less than morphine. Furthermore, it is only two to three times less potent than morphine, presumably because of the noradrenergic reuptake block. It differs from tramadol in that it only slightly inhibits serotonin reuptake. Because it is weakly serotonergic, it is unlikely to result in serotonin syndrome if administered with SSRI-type antidepressants. Tapentadol is not a prodrug and has no known active metabolites. As a result, it does not have to be metabolized to elicit its therapeutic effects. Consequently, there is less risk of drug–drug and cytochrome P450 interactions. This characteristic is advantageous for patients who are poor metabolizers of CYP3A4 and CYP2D6, and therefore have an unsatisfactory reaction to standard opiates. For control of moderate to severe pain, 75 milligrams of tapentadol is equivalent to 10 milligrams of oxycodone (Raffa et al., 2012; Xiao et al., 2017).

To date, the abuse potential of tapentadol appears to be modest, with abuse being reported significantly less than that of other opioids (Butler et al., 2015; Dart et al., 2016).

An extended-release formulation of tapentadol was approved in 2011 for treatment of severe chronic pain (such as severe low back pain and knee pain) and, in 2014, it became the first opioid approved for patients with diabetic peripheral neuropathy (Vadivelu et al., 2015).

Methadone

Methadone (Dolophine) is a synthetic mu agonist opioid very similar to morphine. Methadone was first shown to block the effects of heroin withdrawal in 1948. In 1965, it was introduced as a substitute treatment for opioid dependency. The outstanding properties of methadone are its effective analgesic activity, efficacy by the oral route, extended duration of action in suppressing withdrawal symptoms in physically dependent people, and tendency to show persistent effects with repeated administration.

Today, methadone has two primary legitimate uses: (1) as an orally administered substitute for heroin in methadone maintenance treatment programs; and (2) as a long-acting analgesic for the treatment of chronic pain syndromes (Krueger, 2012). This effect is thought to be partly due to an antagonistic activity at the NMDA glutamatergic receptor (see Table 10.1). Federal prescription regulations clearly separate these two uses. Physicians who do not practice in federally licensed methadone treatment programs may not prescribe the drug for the maintenance of opioid dependency; the drug may be prescribed only through licensed methadone maintenance treatment program centers. However, office-based physicians may prescribe methadone for the treatment of either acute or chronic pain. Unfortunately, such prescriptions may have contributed to the recent opioid epidemic. In 2009, only 2 percent of opioid prescriptions were for methadone, but this drug was implicated in about 30 percent of opioid overdose deaths. Although the death rate from methadone overdoses peaked for most demographic groups from 2005 to 2007 and declined thereafter, this was not the case for those aged 55 to 64 years, whose methadone overdose death rates maintained an increase through 2014 (Jones et al., 2016).

The main objectives of methadone maintenance treatment programs are rehabilitation of the dependent person and reduction of diseases associated with needle use, illicit drug use, and crime. Randomized controlled trials have shown that these aims are generally accomplished. Moreover, long-term use is relatively safe, for example, it does not impair cognitive function. Comparison between methadone patients, opiate users, and normal control persons in laboratory tests showed that cognitive function in methadone maintenance patients improved compared to those dependent on illicit opiates (Wang et al., 2014).

Although there are a number of predictors of the success of a program, the most important is the magnitude of the daily methadone dose. Programs that prescribe average daily doses exceeding 100 milligrams have higher retention rates and lower illicit drug use rates than those in which the average dose is less. Methadone is one of the most well-studied, safe, and effective available medications. Methadone overdose deaths are usually caused by high doses, an increase in dose that occurs too rapidly, or an interaction of methadone with another drug. One report provided risk-reduction suggestions to alleviate these situations (Baxter et al., 2013).

Even where liberal doses are used (sometimes up to 160 milligrams per day or higher), about one-third of the clients regularly experience withdrawal (known as "nonholders") and two-thirds (known as "holders") do not experience withdrawal on a once-daily dosing schedule. The generally accepted half-life of methadone is 24 hours.

Multiple CYP hepatic enzymes are required to metabolize methadone. Therefore, methadone is the opioid most susceptible to serious drug interactions resulting from drug-induced enzyme inhibition. For example, some sedatives and antidepressants inhibit methadone's metabolism, resulting in large elevations in blood concentrations, often resulting in unexpected fatalities (Tennant, 2010).

As well as some methadone maintenance programs may work, they reach only 170,000 of the estimated 810,000 opioid-dependent people in the United States. In recent years, diversion of methadone (from methadone clinic programs and from physicians' prescriptions for analgesic effects) has become a major problem. When the large doses prescribed for an opioid-dependent person (40 to 100 milligrams) are taken by a nonopioid-dependent person, severe respiratory depression and death frequently result.

Levo-Alpha Acetylmethadol

Levo-alpha acetylmethadol (LAAM) is related to methadone. It is an oral opioid analgesic that was approved in mid-1993 for the clinical management of opioid dependence in heroin addicts. LAAM has a slow onset and a long duration of action (about 72 hours). Its primary advantage over methadone is its long duration of action; in maintenance therapy it is administered by mouth three times a week.

In general, LAAM and methadone are of equal efficacy as measured by opioid-free urine samples in heroin-dependent persons. Higher doses of methadone (60 to 100 milligrams) and 75 to 115 milligram doses of LAAM both substantially reduced the use of heroin. Kiselica (2013) reviewed the comparable efficacies of methadone and LAAM in the treatment of opioid addiction. LAAM is currently not available due to possible serious cardiac complications.

PARTIAL AGONISTS

Tramadol

Tramadol is the active ingredient in such brand name opioids as Ultram, Ultracet, ConZip, Ryzolt, and Rybix ODT. Like codeine, tramadol is a prodrug and is converted (metabolized) by both CYP3A4 and CYP2D6 to *O*-desmethyltramadol, which is the active form of the drug. Patients with deficiencies in CYP2D6 production (that is, poor metabolizers) will tend to get reduced analgesic effects from tramadol. Those who produce increased quantities of CYP2D6 (rapid metabolizers) may experience increased pharmacologic and unexpected adverse effects. Drug interactions with CYP2D6 inhibitors may also reduce the analgesic efficacy of tramadol.

It had been generally assumed that tramadol was less liable to abuse than opioid painkillers. With an increase in tramadol prescriptions, however, came an increase in reported problems with abuse and addiction. After several years, the DEA officially moved tramadol from Schedule V to Schedule IV in 2014, which was comparable to the benzodiazepines. The original designation was based on studies in which the drug was injected and on its benign abuse record in Europe. But it was subsequently realized that taken orally in high doses, tramadol was as prone to abuse as OxyContin, which is one of the most addictive drugs in the United States. Furthermore, withdrawal of tramadol, especially rapid discontinuation, sometimes elicited symptoms unusual for opiate withdrawal, such as hallucinations, paranoia, extreme anxiety, panic attacks, confusion, and unusual sensory experiences, such as numbness and tingling in one or more extremities (Seney et al., 2003). Because it was thought to be safer than other opiates, tramadol was often prescribed to older patients. This cohort, however, accounted for the largest number of emergency room visits associated with this drug, possibly because older adults are often prescribed multiple medicines that can interact with tramadol to produce seizures and the serotonin syndrome (Chapter 12). Nevertheless, the extended-release formulation of tramadol was recently found to be effective in suppressing opiate withdrawal in a small clinical trial (Dunn et al., 2017).

A metabolite of tramadol, *O*-desmethyltramadol (*O*-DSMT), has been synthesized and is presently a legal alternative to illegal opioid drugs, packaged as a powder, or combined with other agents. One example, discussed later in the chapter, is marketed as the blend "Krypton," which consists of powdered kratom leaf (*Mitragyna speciosa*) laced with O-DSMT. It has been linked to several accidental overdose deaths (Kronstrand et al., 2011).

Buprenorphine

Buprenorphine was developed in about 1980. As a single agent, it had analgesic effects with blunted abuse liability. Indeed, buprenorphine can be used to treat both acute pain (Kumar et al., 2016) and chronic pain (Gimbel et al., 2016). In addition, buprenorphine has become invaluable in helping to reduce opioid cravings in individuals who are addicted to opiates. In its chemical structure, buprenorphine is related to several other opioid agents, including oxycodone, hydromorphone, and oxymorphone.

But buprenorphine works in a different way. It is both, a partial agonist at mu opioid receptors and an antagonist at kappa receptors. The analgesic action is mediated by stimulation of mu opioid receptors, while the kappa receptors are simultaneously blocked. While therapeutic doses provide sufficient analgesia, there is a ceiling that limits respiratory depression and the partial agonistic action plateaus with an increase in dose.

Although methadone has long been the mainstay of opiate dependence treatment, it is subject to diversion, and the federal government requires patients to receive the drug daily in federally licensed clinics. This makes it difficult for patients with full-time jobs and those who live at a distance to participate. The situation changed dramatically with the approval of *buprenorphine* and then a *buprenorphine-naloxone* (Suboxone) combination product for use in the treatment of opioid addiction. Buprenorphine as a single agent is now available in multiple preparations, each under a different trade name:

1. Buprenex was marketed in the United States in 1985 for the treatment of moderate to severe pain as an injectable buprenorphine formulation.
2. Subutex, a sublingual tablet, was approved in 2002 as a treatment for opioid addiction, especially during the initial therapeutic period. Additionally, it has an off-label application in chronic pain patients who cannot tolerate long-acting, full opioid agents or for whom such agents are inappropriate. Because of abuse problems, the manufacturer discontinued sale in 2011, but not for reasons of safety or effectiveness. Therefore, it is still available in generic form.
3. Bunavail, Suboxone, and Zubsolv: These three trade-named products are transmucosal films to be placed under the tongue from where the medication is absorbed. Each product, with Suboxone being the most popular, is formulated in conjunction with the opioid antagonist naloxone. These are treatments for dependence on any opioid, both at the beginning of opioid withdrawal and for maintenance therapy.
4. Butrans is a transdermal patch, which is approved for pain treatment that is not sufficiently alleviated by other drugs, and therefore warrants around-the-clock, long-term opioid administration. Available doses range from 5 to 20 micrograms per hour; however, for opioid-naive patients, only the 5 micrograms per hour dose is recommended. This formulation is also indicated for maintaining opioid abstinence. Butrans patches should remain on for a week before they are removed.
5. Belbuca, similar to Butrans, is indicated for around-the-clock treatment of pain that is not sufficiently relieved with alternative drugs. It is a newer formulation, available as a buccal film in doses of 75 to 900 micrograms, each lasting about 12 hours. This formulation was developed to adhere to the buccal mucosa and dissolve completely within 30 minutes. The time to peak concentration is 2.5 to 3 hours and the elimination half-life is 27.6 hours.
6. The first buprenorphine implant for maintenance treatment of opioid dependence was approved by the FDA in 2016. This formulation, Probuphine, releases a constant, low-level amount of the drug for 6 months in patients who have been stabilized on low to moderate doses of another buprenorphine agent. This alleviates the

need to take daily medication, and may increase patient compliance. This product consists of four 1-inch rods which are implanted under the skin on the inside of the upper arm, providing treatment for 6 months. No data is yet available on misuse, diversion, or reimplantation after the initial 6 months.

The most common side effects of buprenorphine are flulike symptoms, including headache, sweating, sleeping difficulties, nausea, vomiting, and mood swings. Rosenthal and coworkers (2016), in a carefully controlled trial, compared sublingual buprenorphine (90 persons) with the implanted buprenorphine pellets (Probuphine, 87 persons). About 90 percent of each group achieved a good response over a 6-month period. Modestly more (85 versus 72 percent) maintained opioid abstinence with the implant. New formulations continue to be developed. RBP-6000, developed by Indivior, is a buprenorphine formulation that is injected once a month for the treatment of adults with opiate addiction. It was effective in producing greater rates of abstinence than placebo and was generally well tolerated. The most common side effects included fatigue, constipation, headache, nausea and vomiting, and itching and pain at the injection site. The FDA approved this formulation, as Sublocade on November 30, 2017 (see Nasser et al., 2016).

A weekly, subcutaneous buprenorphine depot formulation, CAM2038, is also in development (Walsh et al., 2017). It was recently tested in adults with moderate to severe opioid use disorder, and doses of 24 and 32 milligrams were well tolerated and effective in blocking the positive subjective effects of the opiate agonist, hydromorphone, and in suppressing withdrawal symptoms. The depot formulation has the benefit of stabilizing the patient undergoing withdrawal and minimizing the likelihood of diversion. Schuckit (2016) reviewed the treatment of opioid use disorders with buprenorphine.

In addition to its indication for analgesia and addiction treatment at low doses, buprenorphine has also been reported to have an antisuicidal benefit in patients who do not have substance abuse problems (Yovell et al., 2015). It was also more effective than opioids alone in improving symptoms of PTSD in veterans with chronic pain who also have an opioid-use disorder (Seal et al., 2016).

Use of Buprenorphine for the Treatment of Opioid Dependence

In July 2016, the Substance Abuse and Mental Health Services Administration (SAMHSA) announced regulations that increased access to buprenorphine and the combination *buprenorphine* and *naloxone* (Suboxone) medications in office-based settings. The new rules permitted practitioners to dispense or prescribe Schedule III, IV, or V controlled substances already approved by the FDA without requiring a separate registration to dispense narcotic maintenance and detoxification drugs. Qualified practitioners who filed an initial notification of intent (NOI) were also allowed to treat a maximum of 30 patients at a time. After 1 year, practitioners may file a second NOI indicating an intent to treat up to 100 patients at a time, while the final rule (July 2016) expanded this access to medication-assisted treatment (MAT) for up to 275 patients. The final rule also incorporates efforts to provide all aspects of evidence-based MAT and to reduce the likelihood that the drugs are misused or diverted. These rules mean, unlike methadone, a physician in his or her office can prescribe Suboxone for the treatment of opioid dependence. Also, patients can take the drug home instead of appearing at a clinic every day. The buprenorphine-naloxone combination (in a 4:1 ratio) is less liable to abuse, not only because buprenorphine is a partial agonist, but also because the naloxone causes withdrawal if Suboxone is crushed and injected. When used correctly, however, the naloxone is not well absorbed through the GI tract or mucosa and has a minimal effect. Currently, only physicians may prescribe the drug. The proposed 2017 federal budget also includes a proposal for a buprenorphine demonstration program that would allow advanced practice providers (for example, nurse practitioners) to prescribe buprenorphine. SAMHSA will also review formulations newly approved by the FDA, developed to treat opioid use disorder.

Results are already available. For example, Tanum and colleagues (2017) compared monthly intramuscular injections of extended-release naltrexone with the oral buprenorphine-naloxone formulation in opioid-dependent patients. During the 12-week trial, the treatments were comparable in maintaining abstinence. Similarly, Lee and colleagues (2017) compared monthly intramuscular injections of extended-release naltrexone with daily, self-administered, sublingual buprenorphine-naloxone over 24 weeks in opioid-dependent patients. They found that more patients were unable to be "initiated" into the naltrexone treatment than into the buprenorphine-naloxone treatment. For those who could successfully tolerate naltrexone, however, the results for abstinence were comparable to the results of the buprenorphine plus naloxone treatment. SAMHSA strongly supports creative ways to increase access to medication-assisted treatment.

Since the introduction of buprenorphine for opioid dependence, it has become clear that this drug is not a panacea. Buprenorphine itself can be abused by intravenous injection. It was thought that adding naloxone to the tablet would precipitate withdrawal if it was crushed and injected. However, it turns out that the effect of naloxone is short lived, and the overall effect is more like taking buprenorphine alone. Both buprenorphine and buprenorphine-naloxone may be diverted and misused (for example, intravenously injected or intranasally administered). Likewise, when illicitly injected, both can cause infectious complications as well as result in death from overdose. Moreover, even though buprenorphine alone has a ceiling effect, the risk of death with buprenorphine overdose is increased if either benzodiazepines or sedative-hypnotics are taken at the same time. In fact, the use of sustained-release naltrexone pellets have been used for treatment of buprenorphine dependence (Jhugroo et al., 2014). Sansone and Sansone (2015) review issues concerning buprenorphine for opiate addiction, and Sontag (2013) describes the history of this treatment and the real-world consequences of attempts to overcome opiate addiction with buprenorphine.

Buprenorphine and Pregnancy

Opioid abuse during pregnancy increases negative outcomes for both mother and infant, not only because of the biological actions of the drug, but also because of the accompanying medical, mental health, and related social problems associated with illicit drug use (Wilder and Winhusen, 2015). Methadone had been a mainstay of maintenance therapy of opioid treatment for nearly 50 years and has been shown to be safe and effective in pregnant females compared with the use of heroin or prescription opioids. Recently, buprenorphine has become the first-line treatment for many opioid-dependent pregnant women (Brogly et al., 2015). Comparisons between methadone and buprenorphine indicate moderately strong evidence for lower risk of preterm birth, increased birth rate and larger head circumference with buprenorphine, and no greater harm (Zedler et al., 2016). Both drugs were nearly equivalent regarding the extent of neonatal abstinence syndrome following delivery. While some minor birth abnormalities can be seen, maltreatment, physical abuse, and medical neglect appear to be the greatest problems associated with postnatal care of the newborns (Kivisto et al., 2015).

MIXED AGONIST-ANTAGONIST OPIOIDS

Four approved drugs are classified as mixed agonist-antagonist opioids: *pentazocine*, *butorphanol*, *nalbuphine*, and *dezocine*. *Dezocine* (Dalgan) was discontinued in the United States as of 2011. Each of these drugs binds with varying affinity to the mu and kappa receptors. The drugs are weak mu antagonists; most of their limited analgesic effectiveness results from their stimulation of kappa receptors (see Table 10.1). Low doses cause moderate analgesia; higher doses produce little additional analgesia. In opioid-dependent people, these drugs precipitate withdrawal. A high incidence of adverse psychotomimetic side effects (dysphoria, anxiety reactions, hallucinations, and so on) is associated with these agents, limiting their therapeutic use.

Pentazocine (Talwin) and *butorphanol* (Stadol) are prototypical mixed agonist-antagonists. Neither has much potential for producing respiratory depression or physical dependence. In 1993, butorphanol, previously available for use by injection, became available as a nasal spray (Stadol NS), the first analgesic so formulated. After it is sprayed into the nostrils, peak plasma levels (and maximal effect) are achieved in 1 hour, with duration of 4 to 5 hours. Use of the nasal spray can result in euphoria and abuse of butorphanol spray can occur, but has not been a major problem. The brand name *Stadol* was discontinued by the manufacturer, so that only the generic formulations are available.

Pentazocine was first approved for use in the United States in 1967 and is still available, but not often used. Pentazocine abuse developed, particularly when the drug was combined with tripelennamine, an antihistamine. This combination of drugs, called "Ts and blues," caused serious medical complications, including seizures, psychotic episodes, skin ulcerations, abscesses, and muscle wasting. (The latter three effects are caused by the repeated injections rather than by the drugs themselves.) Following recognition of this abuse, pentazocine was combined with naloxone to prevent injection misuse and the reported incidence of misuse declined precipitously.

Nalbuphine (Nubain) is primarily a kappa agonist of limited analgesic effectiveness. Because it is also a mu antagonist, it is not likely to produce either respiratory depression or patterns of abuse. It is only available in an injectable formulation. It is currently mainly used as a treatment for morphine-induced pruritus (itching), which is a common side effect of mu agonist opioids. Abuse of nalbuphine is unusual.

PURE OPIOID ANTAGONISTS

Three opioid antagonists are clinically available: *naloxone, naltrexone,* and *nalmefene.* Each is a structural derivative of oxymorphone, a pure opioid agonist. All three have an affinity for opioid receptors (especially mu); however, after binding, they exert no agonistic effects of their own. Therefore, they antagonize the effects of opioid agonists.

Naloxone (Narcan) is the prototype pure opioid antagonist: it has no effect when injected into people who do not use opioids, but it rapidly precipitates withdrawal when injected into opioid-dependent people. Naloxone is neither analgesic nor subject to abuse. Because naloxone is neither absorbed from the GI tract nor the oral mucosa, it must be given by injection. Naloxone injection was first approved in 1971 for reversing opiate intoxication or overdose, and generic versions have been available since 1985 in two doses: 0.4 milligram per milliliter and 1 milligram per milliliter. Naloxone's duration of action is very brief, in the range of 15 to 30 minutes. Thus, for continued opioid antagonism, it must be reinjected at short intervals to avoid return of the depressant effects caused by the longer-acting agonist opioid. Naloxone is used to reverse the respiratory depression that follows acute opioid intoxication (overdoses) and to reverse opioid-induced respiratory depression in newborns of opioid-dependent mothers.

Enteen and coworkers (2010) studied opioid overdose deaths in San Francisco from 2003 through 2009 as well as results of the DOPE (Drug Overdose and Prevention and Education) project. Over 1900 persons were trained and prescribed take-home naloxone and 11 percent reported using naloxone to treat an overdose. Of 399 overdose events, 89 percent of overdoses were successfully treated with naloxone injection to prevent deaths.

In 2013, some federal agencies suggested that access to naloxone should be increased, in particular, for those prescribed opiate drugs. This was prompted by the observation that, although twice as many people died from prescription opioid overdose, more than 80 percent of naloxone was used for treating heroin overdose. In that year, a toolkit for overdose prevention was packaged by SAMHSA for use by clinicians treating patients at risk of overdose. A year later, the first autoinjector formulation, Evzio, received fast-track FDA approval. This was a fixed-dose single injection product developed so that people without medical expertise could reverse an opiate overdose. The first nasal spray formulation (a 4 milligram dose) was fast-tracked in 2015, followed by a second 2 milligram dose (also marketed as Narcan) in January 2017. Before then, naloxone injections of 1 milligram per milliliter had commonly been used off label with an atomizer for nasal delivery. Each of these products—two injection doses, Narcan nasal spray and the Evzio auto-injector—essentially has one supplier. Although the FDA has approved three manufacturers for injections of the 0.4 milligrams per milliliter dose, most are sold by Hospira, which has raised the price by 129 percent since 2012; the Evzio package cost $690 in 2014 but was $4500 in 2016 (Gupta et al., 2016; Wermeling, 2015). For a life-saving drug, the expense of this medication has been extremely controversial.

Naltrexone (ReVia) became clinically available in 1985 as the first orally absorbed, pure opioid antagonist approved for the treatment of heroin dependence. An extended release injectable formulation taken once a month is marketed under the trade name Vivitrol. The actions of naltrexone resemble those of naloxone, but naltrexone is well absorbed orally and has a long duration of action, necessitating only a single oral daily dose of about 40 to 100 milligrams. In people who take naltrexone daily, injection of an opioid agonist such as heroin is ineffective. Naltrexone can cause nausea (which can be quite severe in some people) and dose-dependent liver toxicity (Substance Abuse and Mental Health Services Administration, 2016). One problem with naltrexone is that the drug must be taken in order to be effective. Trite as that sounds, the opioid-dependent person must choose between taking naltrexone or returning to heroin use. Therefore, only highly motivated addicts take the drug. A recent trial of extended release naltrexone was disappointing in keeping criminal addicts from relapsing (Lee et al., 2016).

Today, naltrexone is used primarily to treat alcoholism. Naltrexone reportedly decreases heavy drinking, the number of days that alcohol is consumed, and the total amount of alcohol consumed, although the overall benefit has been described as "modest." The mechanism is believed to be due to antagonism of endorphin, elicited by drinking alcohol, rather than from an as-yet unidentified action outside the opioid system.

Naltrexone has also been reported to have benefits in some other medical conditions, for example, a preventive role in reducing self-injurious behaviors. Effects, however, are weak.

Nalmefene (Selincro) is a pure opioid antagonist. Developed in the early 1970s, it is used mainly to treat alcohol dependence and has been investigated for the treatment of other addictions such as pathological gambling. Compared to naltrexone, the advantages of nalmefene include longer half-life, greater oral bioavailability, and no reported dose-dependent liver toxicity. If given to people who are dependent on opiates or postoperatively for reversal of surgically administered opioids, nalmefene can precipitate acute withdrawal symptoms.

Agonist-Antagonist Combinations

One option for addressing opiate addiction is to make opiate pain medications resistant to tampering. The development of abuse-deterrent formulations is an ongoing effort, supported by the federal government, and there are numerous approaches under evaluation. One solution is to combine an agonist with an antagonist. In late 2009, the FDA approved the first of these types of medications, a combination of *morphine* and *naltrexone* (Embeda-ER). Embeda extended-release capsules are for oral use and contain pellets of morphine sulfate that surround a core of naltrexone. The naltrexone does not interfere with the analgesic action of morphine, but morphine's abuse potential is considerably reduced. Different dosing regimens are commercially available, all with a morphine-to-naltrexone ratio of 100:4. Embeda was the first FDA-approved long-acting opioid designed to reduce recreational abuse when tampered with by crushing or chewing.

As discussed earlier in this chapter, an abuse-deterrent version of OxyContin was introduced in 2010, which, when combined with water, produced a gellike substance that was hard to inject. Misuse by injecting, snorting, and smoking fell by two-thirds within 2 years. Another combination product using extended release oxycodone and naloxone was marketed in 2014 under the trade name Targiniq-ER. With this formulation, the oxycodone provides analgesic action, but the naloxone remains in the intestine (not being absorbed when taken orally) and blocks the constipating effect of the oxycodone. When crushed, and subsequently injected, the oxycodone remains active but some naloxone is absorbed, which antagonizes the opiate. This product is meant to deter, but not prevent, abuse.

A combination of oxycodone and low-dose naltrexone was developed by the same company that made Embeda. The new drug, Troxyca, was approved in August 2016. The capsules contain pellets in which a core of naltrexone is surrounded by extended-release oxycodone hydrochloride. When used as directed, the oxycodone is released as intended while the naltrexone remains sequestered. If the pellets are crushed in an effort to abuse the opiate, naltrexone is released and blocks the effect of the oxyco-done. If the dose of naltrexone in the product is sufficient and if the drug is abused by injection, the antagonist would precipitate withdrawal symptoms. Taylor and cowork-ers (2014) reviewed several oxycodone-naloxone products.

Another approach to preventing oral misuse is to develop a prodrug, which would be inactive until swallowed. In the gut, digestion would release the opiate, but this would not happen if the drug was injected. A hydromorphone prodrug (see the next section) is under development (Dolgin 2015).

NOVEL OPIOID-BASED COMPOUNDS UNDER DEVELOPMENT

In 2012, Moorman-Li and coworkers reviewed abuse-deterrent and novel opioids for the treatment of chronic pain. Four years later, Gudin and Nalamachu (2016) reviewed the development of opiate prodrugs (see below) as abuse deterrents. Here, we describe novel options for pain relief, claimed to have lower side effects and less abuse potential of currently available opioids.

- HS665 is a pure kappa agonist (Guerrieri et al., 2015; Spetea et al., 2012). Clinical trials with HS665 have not yet been reported. Being devoid of mu receptor agonism, abuse liability should be low, although analgesic activity may also be low. As a kappa agonist, this drug appears to resemble nalbuphine, an older, mixed agonist-antagonist with prominent kappa agonist activity. A recent review updates the current status of kappa agonist analgesics and describes experimental agents that have greater selectivity and potency (Erli et al., 2017).

- CR845 (difelikefalin) and nalfurafine are two other kappa receptor agonists that appear to possess both analgesic and antipuritic (anti-itch) activity (Cowan et al., 2015; Inui, 2012). CR845 poorly crosses the blood–brain barrier and thus its anal-gesic and antipuritic actions are restricted to the periphery, bypassing many of the abuse and side effect issues of centrally acting agents. Clinical trials have not been published and, as of January 2017, CR845 was still undergoing Phase II clinical testing.

    The lack of scientific publications for this drug has been the topic of an exten-sive critical review of its developmental history. According to Hesselink (2017), "[a]lthough the clinical development phase started in 2008, primary scientific data on CR845 in peer reviewed journals to date are absent. The only sources for information and valuation of the company available are some abstracts and posters, written by company employees, and many press releases of CARA Therapeutics."

Since 2009, *nalfurafine* (Remitch) has been used intravenously in several countries to treat uremic itching (see Inui, 2015, for this indication). In October 2017, information regarding a clinical trial of nalfurafine for this condition was updated on the site clinicaltrials.gov. Some data, however, suggest that this drug might have additional therapeutic benefit. Both oxycodone and nalfurafine elicited an analgesic effect in animal studies, and the combination of the two drugs was additive. Yet nalfurafine also decreased the reinforcing and respiratory depressant effect of oxycodone, suggesting that it might have some important selective actions (Townsend et al., 2017).

- NKTR-181 is a mu opioid agonist analgesic with a very slow rate of entry into the CNS. Its analgesic effect is purportedly similar to that of oxycodone, with a 90 percent slower delivery rate into the brain. Because of this, its abuse and euphoric effects are thought to be low. In addition, respiratory depression should be low compared to other mu agonists. The drug is in early clinical trials. The FDA has now granted fast-track status for NKTR-181. As of September 2017, however, only one clinical trial had been completed, successfully reducing lower back pain in humans. It may possibly be on the market by 2019.

- PF329 (ER hydromorphone) is a prodrug that is converted in the body to hydromorphone. When PF329 reaches the small intestine, an amino acid that was bonded to the hydromorphone is cleaved off by the digestive enzyme trypsin, which then activates controlled release of the drug. The molecular bonds cannot be severed by crushing or dissolving. This makes the half-life of the drug slower than that of hydromorphone. Positive results were reported by Fisher and coworkers (2012). A newer agent, PF614, is an extended-release oxycodone prodrug, for which a Phase I clinical trial was initiated in November 2016. Evidence of its deterrence potential was reported by Kirkpatrick and colleagues (2017).

- UMB-425 is a mixed mu agonist–delta antagonist that theoretically results in potent analgesic effects without tolerance liabilities (Healy et al., 2013). Results in mice were encouraging; studies in humans have not been reported. As of May 2017, studies of toxicity and pharmacokinetics had not yet been conducted.

FUTURE PHARMACOTHERAPY OF OPIOID DEPENDENCE

In 1994, Goldstein reviewed more than 20 years of administering methadone maintenance therapy to heroin addicts in New Mexico. More than half the patients were traced and analyzed. Of these 5001 patients, more than one-third had died from violence, overdose, or alcoholism. About one-quarter were still enmeshed in the criminal justice system. Another one-quarter had gone on and off methadone maintenance. Data indicated that opioid dependence is a lifelong condition for a considerable fraction of the addict population.

Similarly, in 2001, Hser and coworkers reported a remarkable 33-year follow-up of 581 male heroin addicts who were first identified in the early 1960s. At follow-up in 1996–1997, 284 were dead and 242 were interviewed; the mean age at interview was 57 years. Of the 242, 20 percent tested positive for heroin (an additional 9.5 percent refused to provide a urine sample and 14 percent were incarcerated, so urinalysis was unavailable); 22 percent were daily alcohol drinkers; 67 percent smoked; many reported illicit drug use (heroin, cocaine, marijuana, and amphetamines). The group also reported high rates of physical health, mental health, and criminal justice problems. Although long-term heroin abstinence was associated with less criminality, morbidity, and psychological distress, and with higher employment, only a minority of people who were dependent on opioids attained this goal.

Other ways of dealing with opiate addiction continue to be explored. One approach now employed is to try to mitigate the likelihood of overdose death by distributing naloxone to heroin users. Nasal naloxone is representative of such an attempt.

Another approach, which has also been applied to nicotine and cocaine addiction, is the development of a heroin vaccine. While positive results can be demonstrated in rats, human research is fraught with difficulties.

Other research has, in fact, suggested that the immune system might hold the key to preventing opiate addiction (Hutchinson et al., 2012). Investigators have reported that opiate drugs, in addition to binding classic opiate receptors, also attach to a type of receptor associated with the immune system, called *TLR4* (which stands for Toll-Like Receptor 4), which activates a biochemical pathway called *MyD88*. When the TLR4 receptor was blocked by the "unnatural" isomer of naloxone—(+)-naloxone (dextro-naloxone)—in laboratory animals, the rewarding effects of opiate drugs were reduced. The animals no longer made the effort to get opiate injections and they no longer preferred the location where they used to get the opiate. These results suggest a new direction for development of addiction treatments.

Opiate overdose deaths are caused by the respiratory depression produced when the drugs activate opiate receptors in the brain stem. Development of an opiate that would provide potent analgesia without this lethal reaction has been a long-term pharmaceutical goal. In November 2017, the drug company Trevena submitted an intravenous opioid called *oliceridine* (Olinvo) for FDA approval, which may produce such a selective effect. Oliceridine is one of a number of novel opiate compounds called "biased agonists."

This new phenomenon occurs when typical opiate agonists bind to the mu receptor and activate G-proteins to produce their effects. But such stimulation also activates another intracellular protein, β-arrestin2, which reduces G-protein action so that it does not remain activated indefinitely. β-arrestin2 also mediates opioid-induced respiratory depression and constipation, albeit the mechanism is not yet clear. Nevertheless, opioid drugs that bind to receptors in such a way that they activate the G-protein, but do not stimulate β-arrestin2 as much, might provide pain relief without the unwanted side effects. Thus, oliceridine represents the first of a new class of opiate that has a "bias" toward such selective activation. Although it remains to be seen if such drugs induce less tolerance, or are less likely to produce addiction and dependence, they represent a significant advance in opioid pain therapy (Waldman, 2017).

ILLICIT OPIOIDS OF ABUSE

In addition to the abuse of prescription opiates, the current abuse problems with opioid drugs include several substances that are not prescribed medications.

Desomorphine

Desomorphine (dihydrodesoxymorphine) is an opiate-derived compound, developed in the United States in 1932. It can be synthesized from codeine with other ingredients such as gasoline, paint thinner, hydrochloric acid, iodine, and red phosphorus (from the striking pads of matchboxes), in a manner similar to the production of methamphetamine from pseudoephedrine. This designer drug began to appear in Russia several years ago after first showing up in Siberia in 2002, perhaps because codeine is commonly sold over the counter in Russia. Unfortunately, this homemade mixture has many contaminants, is very toxic, and, when injected, can produce severe tissue damage (for example, phlebitis and gangrene) that can sometimes require limb amputation. The addict's skin becomes greenish and scaly at the injection site because the blood vessels burst and the tissue dies; this has led to the street name of "krokodil" or "crocodile" in English.

Kratom

Kratom (also known as "thang," "kakuam," "thom," "ketum," and "biak") comes from the leaves of the medicinal plant *Mitragyna speciosa*, which is native to Southeast Asia and used for thousands of years by chewing, smoking, brewing in a tea, and oral ingestion. In low doses, kratom has a stimulant action, but high doses produce sedation and opiate effects. Despite the isolation of over 40 other alkaloids, most research has been conducted on the predominant alkaloid mitragynine, which was first isolated in 1921 (Adkins et al., 2011; Troy, 2013).

Mitragynine is believed to be an agonist at the mu opiate receptor and an antagonist at the delta opiate receptor. Váradi and colleagues (2016) were able to show in mice that mitragynine pseudoindoxyl, a semisynthetic opioid obtained from the mitragynine found in kratom, was a more effective pain reliever than morphine and produced less tolerance, addiction, and dependence usually associated with opioids. Furthermore, kratom did not suppress their breathing and did not seem to produce constipation.

In humans, kratom appears to have analgesic effects and has been used to treat opioid addiction (Boyer et al., 2007). According to the American Kratom Association, an organization founded in 2014 to represent kratom users, it may help people with addiction, depression, anxiety, and PTSD. Swogger and colleagues (2015) have published a qualitative review of descriptions provided by kratom users. Nevertheless, addiction to kratom itself has also been reported.

The sale of kratom cannot be restricted by the FDA. This is because the substance is designated as a botanic dietary supplement and, in order to be banned, it would have to be proved dangerous, or producers would have to claim it was medically useful. The importation of kratom into the United States, however, was

372 CHAPTER 10 OPIOID ANALGESICS

banned in 2014; the federal government seized 25,000 pounds of kratom that year from a storage site in Los Angeles. In the summer of 2016, the CDC a report calling the plant "an emerging public-health threat," noting a surge in kratom-related calls to poison control centers (660 calls over a 5-year period) with such symptoms as tachycardia, agitation, drowsiness, nausea, and hypertension. The DEA reported that 15 kratom-related deaths had occurred between 2014 and 2016 (although 14 of those included an additional substance). In August 2016, the DEA announced its plan to temporarily ban the substance. By October, however, following weeks of complaints, the DEA withdrew that plan and instead invited the public to submit their testimonies about using the product. By the December 1 deadline, more than 22,000 people had responded, mostly telling stories about how they relied on the plant for easing their anxiety, PTSD, chronic pain, or struggles with opioid withdrawal, and how restricting access to it would destroy their lives. In November 2017, the FDA released a public health advisory related to potential concerns regarding risks associated with the use of kratom or any of its active ingredients (mitragynine and 7-hydroxymitragynine). For now, kratom remains legal in the United States with the exception of a few states.

In addition to exerting its own opiate effect, as discussed earlier in the chapter, kratom is often combined with another mu agonist, O-desmethyltramadol, the active metabolite of tramadol (a combination referred to as "krypton").

Synthetic Fentanyl Derivatives

Although numerous fentanyl analogs have been synthesized, we still do not know a great deal about their effects, in spite of the fact that their structure activity relationships have been characterized (Vardanyan and Hruby, 2014). Drug dealers have added semilegal versions of fentanyl to increase the potency of heroin on the street since the 1970s. During that period, an analog known as alpha-methylfentanyl was identified in heroin that was found in users who had overdosed. Although alpha-methylfentanyl was placed into the Schedule I category in the United States in 1981, it was detected in contaminated amounts of heroin until the 1990s, accompanied by another, even more potent analog, 3-methyl-fentanyl (TMF). TMF had been made illegal in 1986, but continued to show up intermittently for a number of years. At least 10 more unique analogs of fentanyl have now been identified by toxicologists. The DEA banned a rare type of fentanyl, acetylfentanyl, in 2015, two years after it was first detected in Maine. In early 2016, the DEA placed two other analogs into emergency scheduling, butyryl-fentanyl and beta-hydroxythiofentanyl. At the same time, the DEA emergency scheduled a weak synthetic opioid, AH-7921, after noting increased interest in online chat rooms. However, a legal substitute, furanyl-fentanyl, was already gaining attention; since the beginning of 2016, this drug has been identified in 10 overdose deaths in Pennsylvania and it has recently been responsible for an emergency room incident involving two North Dakota high school students. Later, in September 2016, a nationwide warning to the public and law enforcement, was issued by the DEA in regard to carfentanyl (4-carbomethoxyfentanyl), a synthetic opioid that is 10,000 times more potent than morphine, which was first synthesized in 1974. Due to its potency—hence carfentanyl's street name, "elephant tranquilizer"—a significant number of overdose deaths across the United States have been connected with this drug.

U-47700

U-47700 (3,4-dichloro-N-[2-(dimethylamino)cyclohexyl]-N-methylbenzamide) is a synthetic opioid that was patented by the Upjohn Company in 1978 as an analgesic, although studies in humans had not been published. U-47700, which is known on the street as "pink," "pinky," and "U4," has 7.5 times greater binding affinity for mu opioid receptors than morphine. Effects are said to be very similar to those of morphine and heroin. Information linking U-47700 to at least 46 overdose deaths in 2015 and 2016 has been acknowledged by the DEA. Citing "an imminent hazard to the public safety," the DEA classified U-47700, which was freely available on the Internet, as a Schedule I substance in November 2016.

W-18

In February 2016, while raiding a suspected drug dealer, police in Florida confiscated 2.5 pounds of a potent,, albeit legal, synthetic fentanyllike opioid called *W-18*. This substance is approximately 10,000 times more potent than morphine and 1000 times more potent than fentanyl. Although it was developed in Alberta, Canada, as an alternative painkiller, it was not manufactured and sold until a Chinese chemist discovered the formula. Nonmedical use—there is no medical use—of W-18 by individuals without opiate tolerance is extremely dangerous and has resulted in numerous deaths. It is potentially fatal at high dosages and even opiate tolerant users are at high risk for overdoses. Because we do not know if the opioid antagonist naloxone also blocks W-18, it may be difficult to counteract the drug's effect after it has been taken.

STUDY QUESTIONS

1. How are pain impulses transmitted and modulated within the central nervous system?

2. Describe the opioid receptors. What are the endogenous ligands for those receptors? What happens when an opiate agonist activates its receptor?

3. Define an opioid agonist, antagonist, mixed agonist-antagonist, and partial agonist. Give an example of each and how they are therapeutically useful.

4. In addition to analgesia, what are the major physiological effects of opioid drugs?

5. How have opiate analgesics been reformulated to reduce undesirable side effects?

6. How have opiate analgesics been reformulated to reduce their abuse potential?

7. Discuss the various options for the pharmacological management of opioid dependence and relapse.

8. What are some of the new opiate approaches to pain relief?

9. What are krocodil, kratom, and krypton? What other opiates are now being abused?

REFERENCES

Adkins, J. E., et al. (2011). "Mitragyna Speciosa, a Psychoactive Tree from Southeast Asia with Opioid Activity." *Current Topics in Medicinal Chemistry* 11: 1165–1175.

Alford, D. P. (2016). "Opioid Prescribing for Chronic Pain: Achieving the Right Balance through Education." *New England Journal of Medicine* 374: 301–303.

Baxter, L. E., Sr., et al. (2013). "Safe Methadone Induction and Stabilization. Report of an Expert Panel." *Journal of Addiction Medicine* 7: 377–386. doi: 10.1097/01.ADM.0000435321.39251.d7.

Boyer, E. W., et al. (2007). "Self-Treatment of Opioid Withdrawal with a Dietary Supplement, Kratom." *American Journal on Addictions* 16: 352–356.

Boyer, E. W. (2012). "Management of Opioid Analgesic Overdose." *New England Journal of Medicine* 367: 146–155.

Brady, K. T., et al. (2016). "Prescription Opioid Misuse, Abuse, and Treatment in the United States: An Update." *American Journal of Psychiatry* 173: 18–26. doi: 10.1176/appi.ajp.2015.15020262.

Brennan, M. J. (2013). "The Effect of Opioid Therapy on Endocrine Function." *American Journal of Medicine* 126 (Suppl. 1): S12–S18.

Brogly, S. B., et al. (2015). "Confounding of the Comparative Safety of Prenatal Opioid Agonist Therapy." *Journal of Addiction Research and Therapy* 6: 252–256.

Butler, S. F., et al. (2015). "Tapentadol Abuse Potential: A Postmarketing Evaluation using a Sample of Individuals Evaluated for Substance Abuse Treatment." *Pain Medicine* 16: 119–130.

Califf, R. M., et al. (2016). "The Proactive Response to Prescription Opioid Abuse." *New England Journal of Medicine* 374: 1480–1485.

Centers for Disease Control and Prevention. (2017). "Opioid Overdose: Opioid Data Analysis." February 9. https://www.cdc.gov/drugoverdose/data/analysis.html.

Cicero, T. J., et al. (2012). "Effect of Abuse-Deterrent Formulation of OxyContin." *New England Journal of Medicine* 367: 187–189.

Cicero, T., et al. (2015). "Shifting Patterns of Prescription Opioid and Heroin Abuse in the United States." *New England Journal of Medicine* 373: 1789–1790. doi: 10.1056/NEJMc1505541.

Compton, W. M., et al. (2016). "Relationship between Nonmedical Prescription-Opioid Use and Heroin Use." *New England Journal of Medicine* 374: 154–163. doi: 10.1056/NEJMra1508490.

Coplan, P. M., et al. (2016). "The Effect of an Abuse-Deterrent Opioid Formulation (OxyContin) on Opioid Abuse-Related Outcomes in the Postmarketing Setting." *Clinical Pharmacology and Therapeutics* 100: 275–286.

Costandi, M. (2015). "Uncomfortably Numb: The People Who Feel No Pain." *Guardian*. May 25. https://www.theguardian.com/science/neurophilosophy/2015/may/25/the-people-who-feel-no-pain.

Cowan, A., et al. (2015). "Targeting Itch with Ligands Selective for k-Opioid Receptors." *Handbook of Experimental Pharmacology* 226: 291–314.

Crews, K. K., et al. (2014). "Clinical Pharmacogenetics Implementation Consortium Guidelines for Cytochrome P450 2D6 Genotype and Codeine Therapy: 2014 Update." *Clinical Pharmacology & Therapeutics* 95: 376–381.

Dart, R. C., et al. (2015). "Trends in Opioid Analgesic Abuse and Mortality in the United States." *New England Journal of Medicine* 372: 241–248.

Dart, R. C., et al. (2016). "Diversion and Illicit Sale of Extended Release Tapentadol in the United States." *Pain Medicine* 17: 1490–1496. doi: 10.1093/pm/pnv032.

Dolgin, E. (2015). "Technology: Barriers to Misuse." *Nature* 522: S60–S61 doi: 10.1038/522S60a.

Doweiko, H. E. (2012). *Concepts of Chemical Dependency*, 8th edition. Belmont, CA: Brooks/Cole.

Enteen, L., et al. (2010). "Overdose Prevention and Naloxone Prescription for Opioid Users in San Francisco." *Journal of Urban Health: Bulletin of the New York Academy of Medicine* 87: 931–941.

Feldman, R. S., et al. (1997). *Principles of Neuropsychopharmacology* Sunderland, MA: Sinauer.

Frieden, T. R., and Houry, D. (2016). "Reducing the Risks of Relief—The CDC Opioid-Prescribing Guideline." *New England Journal of Medicine* 374:1501–1504. doi: 10.1056/NEJMp1515917.

Gimbel, J., et al. (2016). "Efficacy and Tolerability of Buccal Buprenorphine in Opioid-Experienced Patients with Moderate to Severe Chronic Low Back Pain: Results of a Phase 3, Enriched Enrollment, Randomized Withdrawal Study." *Pain* 157: 2517–2526. doi: 10.1097/j.pain.0000000000000670.

Goldstein, A. (1994). *Addiction: From Biology to Drug Policy.* New York: Freeman.

Guenther, S. (2016). "Oral Abuse Potential of Benzhydrocodone: A Novel Prodrug of Hydrocodone." Presented at the 2016 Annual Meeting of the American Academy of Pain Medicine.

Guerrieri, E., et al. (2015). "Synthesis and Pharmacological Evaluation of [(3)H]HS665, a Novel, Highly Selective Radioligand for the Kappa Opioid Receptor." *ACS Chemical Neuroscience* 18: 456–463.

Gupta, R., et al. (2016). "The Rising Price of Naloxone—Risks to Efforts to Stem Overdose Deaths." *New England Journal of Medicine* 375: 2213–2215.

Healy, J. R., et al. (2013). "Synthesis, Modeling, and Pharmacological Evaluation of UMB 425, a Mixed Mu Agonist/Kappa Antagonist Opioid Analgesic with Reduced Tolerance Liabilities." *ACS Chemical Neuroscience* 4: 1256–1266.

Holbrook, T. L., et al. (2010). "Morphine Use after Combat Injury in Iraq and Post-Traumatic Stress Disorder." *New England Journal of Medicine* 362: 110–117.

Holder, R. M., and Rhee, D. (2016). "Novel Oral Therapies for Opioid-Induced Bowel Dysfunction in Patients with Chronic Noncancer Pain." *Pharmacotherapy* 36: 287–299.

Hser, Y-I., et al. (2001). "A 33-Year Follow-Up of Narcotic Addicts." *Archives of General Psychiatry* 58: 503–508.

Hutchinson, M. R., et al. (2012). "Opioid Activation of Toll-Like Receptor 4 Contributes to Drug Reinforcement." *Journal of Neuroscience* 32: 11187–11200.

Inui, S. (2012). "Nalfurafine Hydrochloride for the Treatment of Pruritus." *Expert Opinions in Pharmacotherapy* 13: 1507–1513.

Jhugroo, A., et al. (2014). "Naltrexone Implant Treatment for Buprenorphine Dependence: Mauritian Case Series." *Journal of Psychopharmacology* 28: 800–803.

Jones, C. M., et al. (2016). "Trends in Methadone Distribution for Pain Treatment, Methadone Diversion, and Overdose Deaths—United States, 2002–2014." *Morbidity and Mortality Weekly Report* 65: 667–671.

Kapur, B. M., et al. (2014). "Pharmacogenetics of Chronic Pain Management." *Clinical Biochemistry* 47: 1169–1187.

Kiselica, A. (2013). "Methadone Maintenance vs LAAM Maintenance: Efficacy for Treating Opiate Addiction." *TCNJ Journal of Student Scholarship* 15: 1–8.

Krieter, P., et al. (2016). "Pharmacogenetic Properties and Human Use Characteristics of an FDA Approved Intranasal Naloxone Product for the Treatment of Opioid Overdose." *Journal of Clinical Pharmacology* 56:1243–1253. doi: 10.1002/jcph.759.

Kivisto, K., et al. (2015). "Prenatally Buprenorphine-Exposed Children: Health to 3 Years of Age." *European Journal of Pediatrics* 174: 1525–1533.

Kronstrand, R., et al. (2011). "Unintentional Fatal Intoxications with Mitragynine and O-Desmethyltramadol from the Herbal Blend Krypton." *Journal of Analytical Toxicology* 35: 242–247.

Krupitsky, E., et al. (2011). "Injectable Extended-Release Naltrexone for Opioid Dependence: A Double-Blind, Placebo-Controlled, Multicentre Randomized Trial." *Lancet* 377: 1506–1513.

Kumar, S., et al. (2016). "Transdermal Buprenorphine Patches for Postoperative Pain Control in Abdominal Surgery." *Journal of Clinical Diagnostic Research* 10: UC05–UC08. doi: 10.7860/JCDR/2016/18152.7982.

Lasoff, D. R., et al. (2016). "Loperamide Trends in Abuse and Misuse Over 13 Years: 2002–2015." *Pharmacotherapy* 37: 249–253.

Lee, J. D., et al. (2016). "Opioid Relapse in Criminal Justice Offenders." *New England Journal of Medicine* 374: 1232–1242. doi: 10.1056/NEJMoa1505409.

Lee, T. H. (2016). "Zero Pain is Not the Goal." *JAMA* 315: 1575–1577.

Levinthal, C. F. (2012). *Drugs, Behavior and Modern Society,* 7th ed. New York: Allyn & Bacon.

Lozier, M. J., et al. (2015). "Acetyl Fentanyl: A Novel Fentanyl Analog, Causes 14 Overdose Deaths in Rhode Island, March-May 2013." *Journal of Medical Toxicology* 11: 208–217.

Martin, C., et al. (2016). "Controlled-Release of Opioids for Improved Pain Management." *Materials Today* 19: 491–502.

McNeil, D. G. (2015). "A Way to Brew Morphine Raises Concerns over Regulation." *New York Times*. May 18. https://www.nytimes.com/2015/05/19/health/a-way-to-brew-morphine-raises-concerns-over-regulation.html?_r=0.

Minkowitz, H. S., and Candiotti, K. (2015). "The Role of Sublingual Sufentanyl Nanotabs for Pain Relief." *Expert Opinions in Drug Development* 12: 845–851.

Moorman-Li, R., et al. (2012). "A Review of Abuse-Deterrent Opioids for Chronic Nonmalignant Pain." *Pharmacology & Therapeutics* 37: 412–418.

National Center for Health Statistics. (2017). "Drug Overdose Deaths in the United States, 1999–2015." *NCHS Data Brief* No. 273. https://www.cdc.gov/nchs/products/databriefs/db273.htm.

Paech, M. J., et al. (2012). "New Formulations of Fentanyl for Acute Pain Management." *Drugs Today* 48: 119–132.

Pathan, H., and Williams, J. (2012). "Basic Opioid Pharmacology: An Update." *British Journal of Pain* 6: 11–16.

Peppin, J. F. (2012). "Opioid-Induced Constipation." *Practical Pain Management* 12: 59–66.

Pierce, A. M., and Brahm, N. C. (2011). "Opiates and Psychotropics: Pharmacokinetics for Practitioners." *Current Psychiatry* 10: 83–86.

Raffa, R. B., et al. (2012). "Mechanistic and Functional Differentiation of Tapentadol and Tramadol." *Expert Opinion in Pharmacotherapy* 13: 1437–1449.

Ray, W. A., et al. (2016). "Prescription of Long-Acting Opioids and Mortality in Patients with Chronic Noncancer Pain." *JAMA* 315: 2415–2423.

Rosenthal, R. N., et al. (2016). "Effect of Buprenorphine Implants on Illicit Opioid Use Among Abstinent Adults with Opioid Dependence Treated with Sublingual Buprenorphine: A Randomized Clinical Trial." *JAMA* 316: 282–290.

Sansone, R. A., and Sansone, L. A. (2015). "Buprenorphine Treatment for Narcotic Addiction: Not Without Risks." *Innovations in Clinical Neuroscience* 12: 32–36.

Schuckit, M. A. (2016). "Treatment of Opioid-Use Disorders." *New England Journal of Medicine* 375: 357–368.

Senay, E. C., et al. (2003). "Physical Dependence on Ultram (Tramadol Hydrochloride): Both Opioid-Like and Atypical Withdrawal Symptoms Occur." *Drug and Alcohol Dependence* 69: 233–241.

Siemens, W., and Becker, G. (2016). "Methylnaltrexone for Opioid-Induced Constipation: Review and Meta-Analysis for Objective plus Subjective Efficacy and Safety Outcomes." *Therapeutic and Clinical Risk Management* 12: 401–412.

Singa, R. M. (2016). "Genetic Testing: Adjunct in the Medical Management of Chronic Pain." *Practical Pain Management* 16: 28–31.

Soergel, D. G., et al. (2014). "Biased Agonism of the μ-Opioid Receptor by TRV130 Increases Analgesia and Reduces On-Target Adverse Effects versus Morphine: A Randomized Double-Blind, Placebo-Controlled, Crossover Study in Healthy Volunteers." *Pain* 155: 1829–1835.

Sontag, D. (2013). "Addiction Treatment with a Dark Side." *New York Times*. November 16. http://www.nytimes.com/2013/11/17/health/in-demand-in-clinics-and-on-the-street-bupe-can-be-savior-or-menace.html.

Spetea, M., et al. (2012). "Discovery and Biological Evaluation of a Diphenethylamine Derivative (HS665), a Highly Potent and Selective κ Opioid Receptor Agonist." *BMC Pharmacology and Toxicology* 13 (Suppl 1): A43.

Stachnik, J. M. (2011). "Medications for Chronic Pain—Opioid Analgesics." *Practical Pain Management* 11: 110–119.

Stevens, J. P., et al. (2016). "The Critical Care Crisis of Opioid Overdoses in the U.S." American Thoracic Society Abstract 8080. http://www.atsjournals.org/doi/abs/10.1164/ajrccm-conference.2016.193.1_MeetingAbstracts.A6146.

Stone, L. S., and Molliver, D. C. (2009). "In Search of Analgesia." *Molecular Interventions* 9: 234–251.

Strang, J., et al. (2016). "Naloxone without the Needle: Systematic Review of Candidate Routes for Non-Injectable Naloxone for Opioid Overdose Reversal." *Drug and Alcohol Dependence* 163: 16–23.

Substance Abuse and Mental Health Services Administration (2016). "Medication Assisted Treatment for Opioid Use Disorders. Final Rule." *Federal Register* 81: 44711–44739, 48821–48822.

Swogger, M. T., et al. (2015). "Experiences of Kratom Users: A Qualitative Analysis." *Journal of Psychoactive Drugs* 47: 360–367. doi: 10.1080/02791072.2015.1096434.

Taylor, R., et al. (2014). "Opioid Formulations with Sequestered Naltrexone: A Perspective Review." *Therapeutic Advances in Drug Safety* 5: 129–137.

Tennant, F. (2010). "Making Practical Sense of Cytochrome P450." *Practical Pain Management* 10: 12–18.

Tennant, F. (2011). "Genetic Screening for Defects in Opioid Metabolism: Historical Characteristics and Blood Levels." *Practical Pain Management* 11: 26–30.

Tennant, F. (2012). "Endocrine Abnormalities after 20 Years of Opioid Therapy." Presented at the 2012 American Association of Pain Medicine Annual Meeting, Poster 248.

Tennant, F. (2016). "Genetic Testing in High-Dose Opioid Patients." *Practical Pain Management* 16: 10–18.

Trescot, A. M., and Faynboym, S. (2014). "A Review of the Role of Genetic Testing in Pain Medicine." *Pain Physician* 17: 425–445.

Troy, J. D. (2013). "New 'Legal' Highs: Kratom and Methoxetamine." *Current Psychiatry* 12: e1–e2.

Turk, D., et al. (2011). "Treatment of Chronic Non-Cancer Pain." *Lancet* 377: 2226–2235.

Tverdohleb, T., et al. (2016). "The Role of Cytochrone P450 Pharmacogenomics in Chronic Non-Cancer Pain Patients." *Expert Opinions on Drug Metabolism and Toxicology* 15: 1–9.

Vadivelu, N., et al. (2015). "Tapentadol Extended Release in the Management of Peripheral Diabetic Neuropathic Pain." *Therapeutics and Clinical Risk Management* 11: 95–105.

Vakkalanka, J. P., et al. (2017). "Epidemiologic Trends in Loperamide Abuse and Misuse." *Annals of Emergency Medicine* 69: 73–78.

Váradi, A., et al. (2016). "Mitragynine/Corynantheidine Pseudoindoxyls as Opioid Analgesics with Mu Agonism and Delta Antagonism, Which Do Not Recruit β-Arrestin-2." *Journal of Medicinal Chemistry* 59: 8381–8397. doi: 10.1021/acs.jmedchem.6b00748.

Vardanyan, R. S., and Hruby, V. J. (2014). "Fentanyl-Related Compounds and Derivatives: Current Status and Future Prospects for Pharmaceutical Applications." *Future Medicinal Chemistry* 6: 385–412.

Viscusi, E. R., et al. (2016). "A Randomized, Phase 2 Study Investigating TRV130, A Biased Ligand of the μ-Opioid Receptor, for the intravenous Treatment of Acute Pain." *Pain* 157: 264–272. doi: 10.1097/j.pain.0000000000000363.

Volkow, N. D. and McLellan, A. T. (2016). "Opioid Abuse in Chronic Pain: Misconceptions and Mitigation Strategies." *New England Journal of Medicine.* 374: 1253–1263.

U.S. Food and Drug Administration. (2017). *FDA Drug Safety Communication: FDA Urges Caution about Withholding Opioid Addiction Medications from Patients Taking Benzodiazepines or CNS Depressants: Careful Medication Management Can Reduce Risks.* September 20. https://www.fda.gov/Drugs/DrugSafety/ucm575307.htm.

Wadman, M., et al. (2017). "Biased' Opioids Could Yield Safer Pain Relief." *Science* 358: 847–848. DOI: 10.1126/science.358.6365.847.

Wang, G. Y., et al. (2014). "Neuropsychological Performance of Methadone-Maintained Opiate Users." *Journal of Psychopharmacology* 28: 789–799.

Weinstein, S. M. (2009). "A New Extended Release Formulation (OROS) of Hydromorphone in the Management of Pain." *Therapeutics and Clinical Risk Management* 5: 75–80.

Wermeling, D. P. (2015). "Review of Naloxone Safety for Opioid Overdose: Practical Considerations for New Technology and Expanded Public Access." *Therapeutic Advances in Drug Safety* 6: 20–31.

Wilder, C. M., and Winhusen, T. (2015). "Pharmacological Management of Opioid Use Disorder in Pregnant Women." *CNS Drugs* 29: 625–636.

Wilder, C. M., et al. (2016). "Risk Factors for Opioid Overdose and Awareness of Overdose Risk among Veterans Prescribed Chronic Opioids for Addiction or Pain." *Journal of Addiction Diseases* 35: 42–51.

Xiao, J. P., et al. (2017). "Efficacy and Safety of Tapentadol Immediate Release Assessment in Treatment of Moderate to Severe Pain: A Systematic Review and Meta-Analysis." *Pain Medicine* 18: 14–24. doi: https://doi.org/10.1093/pm/pnw154.

Yovell, Y., et al. (2015). "Ultra-Low-Dose Buprenorphine as a Time-Limited Treatment for Severe Suicidal Ideation: A Randomized Controlled Trial." *American Journal of Psychiatry* 173: 491–498. doi: 10.1176/appi.ajp.2015.15040535.

Zedler, B. K., et al. (2016). "Buprenorphine Compared with Methadone to Treat Pregnant Women with Opioid Use Disorder: A Systematic Review and Meta-Analysis of Safety in the Mother, Fetus and Child." *Addiction* 111: 2115–2128. doi: 10.1111/add.13462.

PART 3

Psychotherapeutic Drugs

The chapters in this part introduce the drugs that are used to treat psychological disorders. These medications include the traditional and "atypical" antipsychotics (Chapter 11), the antidepressants (Chapter 12), the medications used classically to treat anxiety and insomnia (Chapter 13), and the "mood stabilizers" for treating bipolar disorder (Chapter 14).

Since the 1950s, important advances have been made in the pharmacological treatment of psychological disorders, allowing affected people to lead much more "normal" lives than ever before in human history. Progress began with the first wave, or first generation, of antipsychotic drugs (for the treatment of schizophrenia), the first two categories of antidepressant drugs, anxiolytics, and mood stabilizers. The first modern precursor of all these psychiatric medications was discovered prior to the 1970s. The next wave of development occurred in the late 1980s with the advent of the second-generation drugs for the treatment of schizophrenia and depression. Nevertheless, since those early periods of rapid development of successful drugs to treat schizophrenia, depression, anxiety, and bipolar disorder, further progress has stalled. There have been no real advances in the treatment of schizophrenia, depression, anxiety, and bipolar disorder since the advent of the second-generation agents. The goals of these next four chapters are to impart a sense of the historical development of therapeutics for each of these disorders, to describe the pharmacology of drugs currently being used to treat these disorders, to convey the disappointment in the lack of current progress in these areas, but to also show that research is still ongoing to find new and better treatment options. The drugs are organized in these chapters under descriptive headings (antidepressants, mood stabilizers, antipsychotics, and so forth), but their application is much broader than indicated by these headings. For example, besides being used to relieve major depression, antidepressants are used as antianxiety drugs and analgesics. Many of the mood stabilizers, besides being used to treat bipolar disorder, are used to treat chronic pain syndromes, psychological disorders associated with agitation and aggression, and even substance abuse. Antipsychotic drugs, besides being used to treat schizophrenia, are being used to treat bipolar disorder, explosive and aggressive disorders, autism, and other pervasive developmental disorders. Newer antipsychotic agents are being used to treat depression and dysthymia. Nevertheless, the artificial distinctions are maintained to present the pharmacology of the drugs in a logical manner.

CHAPTER 11

Antipsychotic Drugs

The drugs discussed in this chapter can be used to treat a variety of psychiatric disorders, particularly those disorders that present with psychotic symptoms. But, as you will see later in this chapter, many of the newer drugs can be used to treat other psychiatric disorders, even if no psychotic symptoms are present.

SCHIZOPHRENIA

The class of drugs we call *antipsychotics* were first found to be effective for the treatment of individuals who have schizophrenia. The criteria for the diagnosis of schizophrenia in the *Diagnostic and Statistical Manual of Mental Disorders*, 5th ed. (DSM-5), include the presence of positive symptoms (such as hallucinations and delusions); negative symptoms (such as diminished emotional expression and lack of motivation); disorganized behavior; and disturbed speech that may reflect disorganized thinking. Cognitive deficits may also be an associated feature of schizophrenia (American Psychiatric Association, 2013). Specified combinations of these symptoms must be present for at least 6 months and cause significant impairment in a person's level of functioning in one or more major life area (such as work, interpersonal relations, self-care, etc.). The onset of schizophrenia occurs primarily in late adolescence to early adulthood (Lieberman et al., 2001). According to the Centers for Disease Control and Prevention (CDC), the worldwide prevalence of schizophrenia is 0.5 to 1.0 percent; and according to the National Institute of Mental Health (NIMH), the 12-month prevalence rate for the U.S. population is 1.1 percent.

The cause—or causes—of schizophrenia are currently unknown. At present, schizophrenia is considered a polygenetic disorder, meaning it has many different causes. Genetics plays a large role. When one parent has the disorder, the probability of any child having the disorder is 7 percent; when both parents have the disorder, the probability that any child will have the disorder increases to 27 percent. In fraternal twins, if one twin has the disorder, the risk the other twin will also have the disorder is 6 to 14 percent. In identical twins, the risk rises to 33 to 60 percent that if one twin has the disorder, the other twin will also have the disorder (Gottesman et al., 2010; Hilker et al., 2017; Mulle, 2012). Large-scale genetic studies have identified 108 genetic markers that are associated with an increased risk for developing schizophrenia (Schizophrenia Working Group of the Psychiatric Genomics Consortium, 2014). Schizophrenia shares some common risk variants with other disorders such as major depressive disorder (MDD) and attention deficit/hyperactivity disorder (ADHD) (see Owen et al., 2016, and references therein). However, even though genetic technology has advanced the study of mental illness, at present, genetic testing cannot be used to diagnosis a disorder, select treatment medications, or predict response to treatment (Geschwind and Flint, 2015; Zhang and Malhotra, 2013). Ethical issues have also been raised about the use of these tests to predict that an individual will develop disorders such as schizophrenia and base treatment upon the findings (DeLisi, 2014). For example, there could be potential harm to the individual if antipsychotic medications are used as pre-emptive treatment based on the results of the test, without knowing if the individual would actually develop the disorder; or exposing the individual to the stigma of attaching a diagnostic label based on a genetic test that could affect their ability to get a job or health insurance.

Much of the recent research has suggested the influence of an array of risk factors beyond genetics for developing schizophrenia. These risk factors occur during the prenatal, perinatal, and postnatal periods and include maternal stress, maternal infections, nutritional deficiencies, and pregnancy and birth complications. Socioeconomic factors such as childhood poverty, other childhood adversities, immigration status, a late winter or early spring birth, and having an older father have also been linked to an increased risk for developing schizophrenia (Owen et al., 2016). Lastly, adolescents who are frequent users of marijuana may be at risk for developing psychotic symptoms in later years even after they discontinue using marijuana (Bechtold et al., 2016).

In general, individuals with schizophrenia have a life span that is 20 to 25 years less than individuals who do not have schizophrenia (Owen et al., 2016; van Os and Kapur, 2009). This mortality risk is related more to life-style and comorbidity risk factors than to the genetic aspects of the disorder. These risk factors include higher rates of smoking, higher rates of substance use disorders, poor diets, lack of exercise, lack of access to primary healthcare, poor attention to treatment for chronic medical conditions such as diabetes, and increased cardiometabolic and cardiovascular diseases. Some of these risk factors, like diabetes and cardiometabolic diseases, may be related to or exacerbated by the side effects of the treatment medications for schizophrenia. An interesting study from Finland suggests that use of antipsychotic medications regularly, and in particular, the long-acting depot formulations, can actually reduce mortality rates of individuals with schizophrenia by up to 40 to 50 percent compared to individuals with schizophrenia who do not take their medications regularly (Taipale et al., 2017).

Neurochemistry and Genetics

The most frequently studied neurotransmitters in schizophrenia have been dopamine and glutamate (GLU). The focus on these neurotransmitters has stemmed from the following observations: that (1) stimulant drugs like amphetamine may produce some symptoms similar to schizophrenia in normal individuals and exacerbate underlying positive symptoms in individuals who have schizophrenia; that (2) drugs such as phencyclidine (PCP) and ketamine can also exacerbate positive symptoms in individuals who have schizophrenia; and that (3) stimulants release dopamine and phencyclidine and ketamine antagonize NMDA (glutamate) receptors. So, based on these observations and the synaptic relationship among these neurotransmitter systems, there continues to be interest in understanding if any of these neurotransmitters or combinations of neurotransmitters can be involved in the pathophysiology of schizophrenia. However, although there have been numerous hypotheses or theories about neurochemical disturbances that would explain the development of schizophrenia, none of the neurochemical models completely explain the phenotypic presentation of behaviors associated with schizophrenia.

Dopamine Involvement

The dopamine system is involved in the pathophysiology of schizophrenia in some way. All drugs that have efficacy as antipsychotics block dopamine receptors. Furthermore, of all the different types of dopamine receptors (D_1, D_2, D_3, D_4, and D_5), all effective antipsychotic drugs block the D_2 receptor. Not only do all antipsychotic drugs have an affinity for the D_2 receptor, this affinity is the single best predictor of the effective clinical dose of an antipsychotic (Figure 11.1). Although there have been no consistent findings of absolute changes in dopamine levels in the brains of individuals with schizophrenia, there

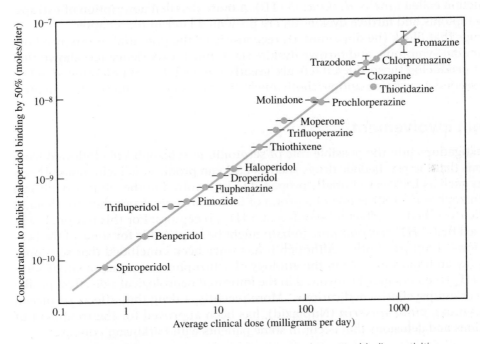

FIGURE 11.1 Correlation between the clinical potency and receptor-binding activities of neuroleptic drugs. Clinical potency is expressed as the daily dose used in treating schizophrenia and binding activity is expressed as the concentration needed to produce 50 percent inhibition of haloperidol binding. Haloperidol binds to dopamine D_2 receptors; other antipsychotic drugs compete for the same receptors. Thus, measuring the competitive inhibition of haloperidol binding correlates with potency of an antipsychotic drug.

have been intriguing data that suggest that it is the episodic release of dopamine from presynaptic terminals in certain parts of the brain that cause the pathological symptoms we see (Laruelle et al., 2003). Laruelle and Abi-Dargham (1999) infused individuals who were diagnosed with schizophrenia with amphetamine. Using SPECT (single photon emission computed tomography), they found that the amphetamine caused an increased release of dopamine in one area of the brain, the striatum, and also caused a worsening of symptoms. This effect was only observed at the beginning of the person's illness, when he or she had acute symptoms, or at times when there was an exacerbation of symptoms to the point that the person was considered acutely ill. No such changes were found when the individual was stable and not expressing symptoms. The authors interpreted these results to suggest that the expression of schizophrenic symptoms in individuals with the disorder is related in part to an underlying dysregulation in dopamine transmission that may be state related, that is, acutely ill versus stable.

Dopamine, released by neurons in the basal ganglia of the brain, is crucial for maintaining normal coordination of movement. In fact, the loss of these neurons in the basal ganglia is responsible for the neurological disorder Parkinson's disease. Similarly, by blocking dopamine receptors, antipsychotic drugs produce neurological side effects similar to Parkinson's disease, known as *extrapyramidal symptoms* (EPS), because the drugs affect the dopamine neurons in the extrapyramidal motor system. Long-term antipsychotic administration may also elicit another syndrome of abnormal motor function called *tardive dyskinesia* (TD). A more detailed description of extrapyramidal symptoms and tardive dyskinesia are presented later in this chapter.

All drugs that block the dopamine D_2 receptor have the potential to produce both extrapyramidal symptoms and tardive dyskinesia. Clinical experience has shown that the risk of producing these side effects are greatly reduced, but not eliminated, when using the second-generation antipsychotic medications discussed later in this chapter.

Serotonin Involvement

Early investigations into the possible role of serotonin in schizophrenia followed from observations that the psychedelic drugs such as LSD can produce hallucinations. Therefore, drugs such as LSD were initially proposed to be involved in the clinical syndrome seen in schizophrenia. LSD is one of a group of hallucinogenic drugs that are thought to exert their psychedelic effect as agonists at $5\text{-}HT_{2A}$ receptors. For this reason, it was hypothesized that *5-HT$_2$ receptor antagonism* might be responsible for some of the beneficial actions of antipsychotics. Although it has since been concluded that serotonin does not play an important role in the etiology of schizophrenia, antagonism of serotonin at $5\text{-}HT_2$ receptors may be involved in the improved neurological side effect profile of the newer antipsychotic medications.[1] More recently, a drug that affects serotonin $5\text{-}HT_{2A}$ receptors, *pimavanserin* (Nuplazid), has been approved for the treatment of hallucinations and delusions that occur in some patients with Parkinson's disease.

---

[1]For a detailed discussion of the relationship of the various serotonin receptors to the symptoms observed in schizophrenia, see Meltzer (2012). This review also discusses the differences between the first-generation antipsychotics and the newer second-generation antipsychotics based on the differences in their mechanism of action at the various dopamine and serotonin receptors.

Glutamate Involvement

As discussed above, the two psychedelic drugs *phencyclidine* (PCP) and *ketamine* produce some schizophrenialike symptoms, such as hallucinations, out-of-body experiences, negative symptomatology, and cognitive deficits. The mechanism responsible for these effects is a potent blockade of NMDA-type glutamate receptors. Based on this effect, it has been hypothesized that NMDA receptor hypofunction results in downstream effects on striatal dopamine, glutamate, and GABA that may underlie the deterioration seen in patients with schizophrenia.[2]

Genetic Involvement

As discussed, there has been substantial advancement in the technology for studying genetics. In particular, genome-wide association studies (GWAS) have been employed to examine the human genome in an effort to detect the genetic locus of the major psychiatric disorders such as schizophrenia and link a disease risk with a specific area of the genome. This is a highly technical and complex process which searches the genome for evidence of variations that are called *single-nucleotide polymorphisms* (SNPs) or *copy number variants* (CNVs). GWAS technology is used to identify which SNPs or CNVs occur more frequently in individuals who have a particular disorder compared to those individuals without the disorder. Using this information, researchers attempt to pinpoint genes or sections of genes that may increase the risk for having the disorder. Using GWAS, researchers report that genes that code for the dopamine receptor, such as the DRD2 gene, are involved in the pathophysiology of schizophrenia, as are genes associated with the glutamate neurotransmitter system. These findings are important because they continue to support the role of the neurotransmitter dopamine in schizophrenia and drugs that block the dopamine receptor, particularly the D_2 receptor, as effective antipsychotic drugs. In addition, recent clinical trials have focused on testing drugs that affect the glutamate system. Although these trials have not yielded positive results, glutamate remains an area for continued examination for its involvement in the treatment for schizophrenia.

Another study has pointed to the *major histocompatibility complex* (MHC), a region of the genome containing genes associated with the body's immune system, as also playing a role in the pathophysiology of schizophrenia (Schizophrenia Working Group of the Psychiatric Genomics Consortium, 2014). More recently, researchers have shown that within the major histocompatibility complex, the risk of schizophrenia is most closely linked to the C4 gene, such that the higher the expression of the C4A subtype, the greater the risk of developing schizophrenia (Dhindsa and Goldstein, 2016; Sekar et al., 2016). The relationship of the C4A gene to the developmental process of synaptic pruning make this finding especially intriguing. Humans are born with redundancies in synaptic connections and as the brain develops, it goes through a process of eliminating unneeded or unused synapses. The C4 gene is thought to be involved in this pruning process. Sekar and colleagues (2016) found that an upregulation of the expression of the C4 gene results in a greater degree of synaptic pruning. Since there is

---

[2]For a review of glutamate involvement in the pathophysiology of schizophrenia, see Kantrowitz and Javitt (2010), Kantrowitz and Javitt (2012), Poels et al. (2014), and Schwartz et al. (2012).

evidence of loss of cortical grey matter or cortical thinning in individuals with schizophrenia (Cannon et al., 2015), this finding of an abnormally energetic pruning process may help explain the neuroanatomical findings. This loss of neuronal connections due to excessive pruning may also relate to the expression of both negative symptoms and cognitive deficits in schizophrenia.

None of these genetic or neurochemical models completely explain the phenotypic presentation of behaviors associated with schizophrenia. Schizophrenia is understood to be multiple related disorders involving multiple genetic markers. Furthermore, serotonin antagonists alone are not effective in the treatment of schizophrenia, nor are GABA or glutamate antagonists effective antipsychotics. The only consistent finding thus far is that any drug shown to be effective in the treatment of schizophrenia has to block dopamine receptors, primarily the D_2 receptor (Howes et al., 2015; Paparelli et al., 2011).

HISTORICAL BACKGROUND AND CLASSIFICATION OF ANTIPSYCHOTIC DRUGS

The first drug to be used as a treatment for schizophrenia was developed from a class of compounds known as *phenothiazines*. The first phenothiazine was derived from antihistamines. Antihistamines were being used at the time to reduce the agitation of patients experiencing postsurgical shock due to their sedative effect and the understanding that histamine release was involved in the shock reaction. The antihistamines first used were not completely effective, so the search went on for a better antihistamine. In 1951, Paul Charpentier, working for a French pharmaceutical company, synthesized a new phenothiazine, *chlorpromazine*. Once released to the market in 1952, the French anesthesiologist and surgeon Henri Laborit used *chlorpromazine* in his "lytic cocktail," an anesthetic mix of drugs administered prior to surgery to deepen anesthesia and reduce body temperature with the goal of preventing postsurgical shock. Laborit found that adding chlorpromazine to his anesthetic cocktail had several beneficial effects: reducing the amount of anesthetic drugs a patient needed; producing sedation without clouding of consciousness; and producing a state of indifference, analgesia, and hypothermia, which reduces oxygen demand, inflammation, and intracranial pressure.

Later the same year, based on Laborit's report of the effect of chlorpromazine on his surgical patients, the French research psychiatrists Jean Delay and Pierre Deniker began to use it to treat their agitated patients at Sainte-Anne's Hospital in Paris. Delay and Deniker are credited with introducing the use of chlorpromazine to psychiatry. Although it did not provide a permanent cure, chlorpromazine was found to be remarkably effective in alleviating the clinical manifestations of psychosis in psychiatric patients (Lopez-Munoz et al., 2005). Chlorpromazine was marketed in France under the trade name *Largactil* in 1952 and later in the United States under the trade name *Thorazine* in 1954.[3]

---

[3] For a review of the history of the discovery of chlorpromazine, see Ban (2007) and Lopez-Munoz and colleagues (2005).

In the continuing search for more effective drugs with fewer side effects, alternatives to the phenothiazines were developed for the treatment of psychosis. Pharmaceutical companies came to market with their own products that were variations on the chemical structure of chlorpromazine. In addition to the phenothiazines, butyrophenones, thioxanthenes, dihydroindolones, dibenzepines, and diphenylbutylpiperidines were developed. The drugs in these chemical classes constitute what is now known as the *first-generation antipsychotics* (FGAs) or *typical* or *conventional antipsychotics*. They all block the dopamine D_2 receptor as well as other neurotransmitter receptors. As discussed, blockade of the dopamine D_2 receptor is necessary for the antipsychotic effect of these drugs. But this blockade also produces some of the observed neurological side effects these drugs cause, such as extrapyramidal symptoms and tardive dyskinesia; and their activity at other neurotransmitter receptors produce additional side effects.

Due to the range of side effects related to these FGAs, drug companies continued to search for drugs that would not only be effective as antipsychotic agents, but would have fewer neurological side effects. Clozapine was discovered in 1959 to have antipsychotic efficacy and was remarkable in that it did not seem to produce any of the neurological side effects seen with the FGAs. Research with this compound started in Europe in 1959. The first human trials of the drug in Europe began in 1962. Research was also begun in the United States by the drug company Sandoz in 1974. But, interestingly, the fact that it did not produce neurological side effects dampened enthusiasm for clozapine. This was due to the mistaken notion at the time that in order for a drug to be an effective antipsychotic, it had to produce neurological side effects. In addition, during clinical trials using clozapine in Finland during 1975, 18 subjects developed a blood disorder known as *agranulocytosis* and nine of them died. Agranulocytosis occurs when the body does not produce enough white blood cells to fight off infections. This side effect was attributed to clozapine and, as a result, restrictions were placed on its use in Europe beginning in 1975 and the development and testing process in the United States was halted in 1976 for some time. The restrictions imposed in Europe included the requirement for regular laboratory blood work to measure white blood cells. Between 1976 and 1982, the use of clozapine in Europe actually expanded and by measuring white blood cell levels during treatment, the onset of agranulocytosis was detected early enough to stop the medication and avoid mortality. Furthermore, during this time, researchers and clinicians were reporting remarkable outcomes in those patients who were able to continue treatment with clozapine without developing agranulocytosis. Based on these continued reports of positive outcomes coming out of Europe, Sandoz again resumed its efforts to get Food and Drug Administration (FDA) approval to test clozapine in the United States. In 1984, the FDA approved the studies on clozapine, but required more stringent monitoring for agranulocytosis. Under these conditions, the clinical trials demonstrated clozapine's effectiveness as an antipsychotic and the absence of neurological side effects. In 1990, clozapine was approved for the U.S. market and became the first of the so-called *second-generation antipsychotics* (SGAs). SGAs, also referred to as *atypical antipsychotics*, when compared to the FGAs or typical antipsychotics, do not produce or have a much lower risk of producing neurological side effects. Following clozapine's approval, pharmaceutical companies began marketing other drugs that had properties similar to clozapine but without the risk of agranulocytosis.

The distinguishing characteristic of the SGAs' mechanism of action is that although they still block the dopamine D_2 receptor, they also block one of the serotonin receptors, the 5-HT_2 receptor. Also, their potency at these serotonin receptors is greater than their potency at the dopamine receptor. This greater affinity for the serotonin receptor over the dopamine receptor allows a separation between antipsychotic efficacy and induction of extrapyramidal symptoms or other movement disorders (with the exception of risperidone at higher doses) (Horacek et al., 2006; Kapur and Remington, 2001; Kapur and Seeman, 2001). Thus, these drugs have shown that, unlike previously thought, it is possible to separate therapeutic benefit from the neurological side effects (Advokat, 2005).[4] The SGAs will be discussed in detail later in this chapter.

FIRST-GENERATION ANTIPSYCHOTICS

The *first-generation* (or *typical*) *antipsychotics* (FGAs) are drugs that were most frequently used to treat schizophrenia (Table 11.1). Some of them also had other FDA-approved indications such as bipolar disorder, behavioral problems, Tourette syndrome, hyperactivity, agitation, and anxiety (Table 11.2). Furthermore, these antipsychotics were also used "off-label" (that is, not having FDA approval) for other disorders in which psychotic symptoms, such as hallucinations, delusions, and severe thought disorder, were present.

Pharmacokinetics

First-generation antipsychotics are lipid soluble and highly bound to protein and tissue, with large volumes of distribution. Oral absorption is unpredictable, and several types of FGAs undergo first-pass metabolism in the liver, which means that oral bioavailability is low or variable. Most FGAs, however, have long half-lives of 20 to 40 hours, which allows doses to be given only once or twice a day after reaching steady-state levels. All FGAs are extensively metabolized by the liver and some have active metabolites. Metabolites of some of the phenothiazines can be detected for several months after the drug has been discontinued.

---

[4]Several possible mechanisms might account for this property. First, 5-HT is known to inhibit dopamine release in the nigrostriatal, but not the mesolimbic dopamine pathway. By blocking this action, either through 5-HT_2 receptor antagonism at the dopamine terminal or by 5-HT_{1A} antagonism at the cell body, SGAs selectively enhance dopamine release in the striatum, which mitigates neuroleptic-induced extrapyramidal symptoms. Second, clozapine and quetiapine have a low affinity for the D_2 receptor and do not attach very tightly to these binding sites. Because the natural amount of dopamine in the nigrostriatal pathway is greater than that in the mesolimbic pathway, clozapine and quetiapine may be more easily displaced from the striatal dopamine receptors by the higher concentration of the endogenous transmitter. This occurrence would normalize dopaminergic activity in the nigrostriatal system and reduce pseudoparkinsonian side effects.

TABLE 11.1 First-generation antipsychotic drugs

Generic name	Trade name	Dose equivalent (mg)[a]	Formulation[b]	Age group[c]
Chlorpromazine	Thorazine	100	PO; Sol; IM	C; A; AD
Prochlorperazine	Compazine	15	Suppository	C; A; AD
Fluphenazine	Prolixin	2	PO; Elixir; IM; Sol; LAI	AD
Trifluoperazine	Stelazine	5	PO; IM; Sol	C; AD
Perphenazine	Trilafon	8	PO	C; A; AD
Thioridazine	Mellaril	100	PO	C; A; AD
Thiothixene	Navane	4	PO	A; AD
Haloperidol	Haldol	2	PO; IM; LAI	C; A; AD
Loxapine	Loxitane	10	PO	A; AD
Molindone	Moban	10	PO	A; AD
Pimozide	Orap	2	PO	A; AD

[a]Dose equivalence: all drug doses are equated to 100 milligrams of chlorpromazine.
[b]Formulation: PO = oral, usually tablets or capsules; Sol = oral solution; Elixir = oral solution in suspension; IM = intramuscular injectable solution; LAI = long-acting injectable solution, usually one injection every 2 to 4 weeks.
[c]Age group: C = children (1–9 years old); A = adolescent (10–17 years old); AD = adult (≥18 years old).

TABLE 11.2 FDA Indications for first-generation antipsychotic drugs

Generic name	Trade name	Indications
Chlorpromazine	Thorazine	Schizophrenia; nausea; presurgical sedation; bipolar disorder, manic phase; intractable hiccups; hyperactivity; severe behavior problems
Prochlorperazine	Compazine	Schizophrenia; generalized anxiety; severe nausea and vomiting
Fluphenazine	Prolixin	Psychosis
Trifluoperazine	Stelazine	Schizophrenia; generalized anxiety disorder
Perphenazine	Trilafon	Schizophrenia; nausea and vomiting
Thioridazine	Mellaril	Schizophrenia
Thiothixene	Navane	Schizophrenia
Haloperidol	Haldol	Psychosis; Tourette syndrome; hyperactivity; severe childhood behavior problems
Loxapine	Loxitane	Schizophrenia
Molindone	Moban	Schizophrenia
Pimozide	Orap	Tourette syndrome

Pharmacological Effects

As noted earlier in this chapter, the effectiveness of the FGAs as antipsychotic agents is related to their ability to block the dopamine D_2 receptor. But, as we shall see below, blocking dopamine receptors also contributes to some of the side effects of these drugs. Other side effects occur because FGAs also block acetylcholine (muscarinic), histamine, serotonin, and norepinephrine receptors. Cholinergic blockade produces dry mouth, dilated pupils, blurred vision, cognitive impairments, constipation, urinary retention, and tachycardia. Histaminergic blockade produces sedation as well as anti-emetic effects. Blockade of the serotonin receptors is thought to be related to part of the therapeutic efficacy as well as side effects of sedation and weight gain. Nor-adrenergic blockade can result in hypotension and sedation. Lastly, through actions on the brain stem, antipsychotics suppress the centers involved in behavioral arousal, the ascending reticular activating center, and inhibit vomiting by affecting dopamine receptors in the chemoreceptor trigger zone.

All of the FGAs are equally effective in reducing the psychotic (positive) symptoms related to schizophrenia and the other disorders that can also present with psychotic symptoms, such as bipolar disorder and severe major depressive disorder. Although FGAs have been shown in the short term to reduce positive symptoms, they have not been shown to consistently reduce either the negative or cognitive symptoms of schizophrenia.

Negative Symptoms

Dopaminergic neurons of the central midbrain portion of the brain stem project to limbic structures (mesolimbic pathway), which regulate emotional expression, as well as to forebrain areas (mesocortical pathway), where emotion and cognition are integrated. It is believed that antipsychotics, by blocking dopamine D_2 receptors in the mesolimbic or mesocortical pathways, reduce the intensity of schizophrenic delusions, hallucinations, and thought disorder, that is, the *positive symptoms* of schizophrenia. Besides positive symptoms, individuals who have schizophrenia may also display negative symptoms and cognitive impairment. *Negative symptoms* of schizophrenia include deficits in communication skills, emotion, or affect; social or interpersonal skills; motivation; and psychomotor activity. It is thought that negative symptoms are related to some change in the dopamine transmission in the mesolimbic system.

Cognitive symptoms of schizophrenia include deficits in executive functions such as decision making, attention, concentration, and memory. It is thought that cognitive symptoms are related to some change in the dopamine transmission in the mesocortical system. NIMH is sponsoring an initiative to develop assessments of cognition in schizophrenia and evaluate new medications to enhance cognitive performance. This initiative, Measurement and Treatment Research to Improve Cognition in Schizophrenia (MATRICS), began around 2004 and over the last several years has refined the cognitive testing battery and set guidelines for studies of potential treatments for the cognitive impairment observed in individuals with schizophrenia (Buchanan et al., 2011; Green et al., 2014; Marder and Fenton, 2004). Several studies have been published examining a wide variety of drug agents and even transcranial direct current magnetic stimulation (TDc\MS) for their ability to improve cognition (Buchanan et al., 2011; Jarskog et al., 2013; Javitt et al., 2012; Lane et al., 2013).

Side Effects and Toxicity

To more easily describe the typical side effects associated with the FGAs, we can divide the agents into two broad categories: low-potency drugs and high-potency drugs (see Table 11.3). The low-potency FGAs are those drugs that require higher oral doses to achieve a certain level of occupancy of the dopamine receptors. The prototypical drug in this class is *chlorpromazine* (Thorazine). Drugs in the low-potency category usually require hundreds of milligrams in an oral dose to produce a therapeutic effect. By comparison, the high-potency group of antipsychotic drugs are those for which the oral dose necessary to occupy a sufficient number of receptors to produce an antipsychotic effect is in the range of tens of milligrams or less. The prototypical drug in this category is *haloperidol* (Haldol). The potency level of FGAs can be compared by establishing chlorpromazine at an oral dose of 100 milligrams as the base. Then all other drugs can be compared to this dose of chlorpromazine to determine what dose of the comparison drug will produce the same effect as 100 milligrams of chlorpromazine. For example, the dose equivalent of 100 milligrams of chlorpromazine (low potency) would be 2 milligrams of haloperidol (high potency). (Comparison tables listing the relative dose equivalents of the FGAs can be found in several publications, including Andreasen et al., 2010 and Procyshyn et al., 2015.) These dose equivalence resources are helpful to the prescriber when it becomes necessary to switch from one drug to another during treatment. The high-potency antipsychotics, such as haloperidol, are

TABLE 11.3 Side effects of the first-generation (typical) antipsychotic medications

Low-potency drugs (such as chlorpromazine)

Sedation

Anticholinergic symptoms (dry mouth, urinary retention, constipation, disorientation, confusion, memory problems)

Cardiovascular symptoms (orthostatic hypertension, arrhythmias)

Endocrine symptoms (gynecomastia, galactorrhea, weight gain, dysmenorrhea/amenorrhea)

Skin (photosensitivity reaction/pigmentation changes, sunburn)

Sexual dysfunction (anorgasmia, decreased libido, inhibition of ejaculation, retrograde ejaculation, priapism)

Ocular symptoms (retinitis pigmentosa)

High-potency drugs (such as haloperidol)

Acute dystonia

Parkinsonian symptoms (resting tremor, cogwheel-type rigidity, bradykinesia)

Akathisia

Tardive dyskinesia (TD)

Neuroleptic malignant syndrome (NMS) risk (both low- and high-potency drugs):

   Fever (>40° C [104° F])

   Severe muscle rigidity ("lead pipe" type)

   Altered consciousness (clouding of the sensorium, stupor, coma)

Autonomic changes (fluctuating blood pressure, tachypnea, diaphoresis)

no different in efficacy to the low-potency antipsychotics. All of the FGAs, regardless of their potency, effectively treat the acute positive symptoms of schizophrenia if dosed properly. For example, the response rates of individuals with schizophrenia who are treated with antipsychotic medications during their first episode ranges anywhere from 40 to 80 percent depending on the study, with an average response rate between 60 and 70 percent. The wide range of findings may be based on differences among studies in populations used, age range of subjects, inclusion and exclusion criteria, outcome measures used, doses of medication, and other variables (Agid et al., 2013; Remington et al., 2013).

The drugs in the low-potency category have an array of side effects that involve various body systems and can be associated with these drugs' action at noradrenergic, histamine, acetylcholine, and serotonin receptors. These side effects include sedation (caused by histamine, serotonin, and acetylcholine receptor blockade); dry mouth, blurred vision, urinary retention, constipation, disorientation, confusion, and memory impairment (caused by acetylcholine receptor blockade); hypotension and arrhythmias (caused by adrenergic receptor blockade); amenorrhea or disruption of the menstrual cycle, gynecomastia or breast development in males, galactorrhea or milk production in females, blockade of ovulation leading to infertility (caused by dopamine receptor blockade); and weight gain (caused by serotonin and histamine receptor blockade). Other side effects include a photosensitivity reaction to sunlight (greater risk of sunburn or skin pigmentation changes); decreased sexual libido, anorgasmia, inhibition of ejaculation; and changes in ocular function (retinitis pigmentosa, worsening of glaucoma). Since these drugs primarily block dopamine D_2 receptors, they also produce neurological side effects like extrapyramidal symptoms, akathisia, and tardive dyskinesia, which will be discussed later in conjunction with the high-potency drugs. Management of these potential side effects include: (1) starting with low doses of the medication and slowly increasing the dose over time; (2) treating the specific side effect with drugs that will counter the effect of the receptor blockade, such as giving drugs that are acetylcholine agonists to treat the effects of cholinergic receptor blockade; or (3) treating the side effect through other mechanisms, such as treating constipation with stool softeners.

There may be no other way to eliminate the side effects other than stopping (discontinuing) the offending antipsychotic drug. In this case, switching to another antipsychotic drug from a different chemical class may provide the necessary control of psychotic symptoms with less risk of unwanted side effects. The high-potency FGA drugs can produce some of the same autonomic and physiological side effects as the low-potency drugs. But the high-potency drugs are more often noted for producing an array of neurological side effects related to their blockade of dopamine receptors.

Blockade of dopamine receptors in the hypothalamic-pituitary (tuberoinfundibular) pathway cause an increase in systemic prolactin levels that can produce breast enlargement in males and lactation in females. In men, ejaculation may be blocked; in women, libido may be decreased, ovulation may be blocked, and normal menstrual cycles may be suppressed, resulting in infertility.

Blockade of dopamine receptors in the nigrostriatal pathway produces several neurological side effects including extrapyramidal symptoms; akathisia; and tardive dyskinesia. Extrapyramidal symptoms occur early in the course of treatment with antipsychotic medications and include the following types of movement disorders:

- *Dystonia* presents as involuntary muscle contractions and sustained abnormal, bizarre postures of the limbs, trunk, head, and tongue. Dystonias are the earliest of the extrapyramidal symptoms to occur. Ninety-five percent of dystonias occur within the first four days. Individuals most at risk for developing dystonia are young males. The most effective treatment for dystonia is an intramuscular (IM) injection of a cholinergic agonist such as *benztropine* (Cogentin) or *trihexyphenidyl* (Artane); the antihistamine *diphenhydramine* (Benadryl) can also be used.

- *Parkinsonian symptoms* include the classic triad of bradykinesia, tremor, and rigidity. These symptoms can appear within 5 to 30 days after the initiation of treatment. Bradykinesia is a generalized slowing of movements. The tremor is a *resting tremor*, which means that when a person engages in some voluntary movement, such as writing with a pencil or touching their finger to their nose, the tremor appears to decrease in intensity or is absent. The rigidity is what is called a *cogwheel-type rigidity*. This refers to the ratchetlike resistance an examiner can feel when they passively move the arm of a person and palpate the bicep muscle. What the examiner feels is similar to the ratcheted movement of the cogwheel of a clock. Due to the slowness and stiffness of movements, individuals can display a stiff, shuffling gait. They may also lack normal fluidity of movements such as an arm swing while walking; have a decreased blink rate; and lose a degree of postural reflexes such that they are at risk of falling. Clinicians use a standardized examination and rating scale to document the presence, type, and intensity of parkinsonian symptoms. One of the more common scales being used is the Simpson-Angus Scale (Simpson and Angus, 1970).

- *Akathisia* is a syndrome characterized by the subjective internal feeling of anxiety, manifested externally by restlessness, pacing, constant rocking back and forth, and other repetitive, purposeless, actions. These external movements are attempts by the individual to reduce the uncomfortable feeling of internal anxiety that they experience. Because it can be extremely upsetting to the patient, akathisia is a common cause of nonadherence to psychotropic treatment and may lead to an increased risk for suicide. Akathisia occurs slowly over time and is quite subtle at its outset. Many patients do not realize that they are becoming more restless until the behavioral manifestations are quite pronounced. Although its cause is not well established, a decrease in dopaminergic activity appears to be an important etiological factor. Treatments include reducing the dose of the offending antipsychotic medication, switching to a low-potency FGA, or switching to one of the newer second-generation antipsychotics with low risk for this side effect. The most effective treatment for akathisia includes either a beta-adrenergic antagonist such as *propranolol* (Inderal) or a serotonergic, 5-HT$_2$ receptor antagonist such as ritanserin or mianserine. Another option to treat akathisia is using the second-generation antidepressant drug *mirtazapine* (Remeron). Mirtazapine, in addition to its action of blocking presynaptic alpha-2 adrenergic receptors, which accounts in part for its antidepressant effect, also blocks 5-HT$_2$ receptors, which is related to its beneficial effect of reducing akathisia. Evidence suggests that the likelihood of eliciting akathisia may be increased when antipsychotic drugs—particularly the second-generation antipsychotic *aripiprazole* (Abilify) and antidepressant drugs, especially the serotonergic agents—are combined, such as in the treatment of bipolar disorder (Advokat, 2010). Akathisia is the most difficult of the early onset side effects to treat. Despite the interventions noted above, some patients may not get complete relief from this side effect. Clinicians use a standardized examination and the *Barnes Akathisia Rating Scale* (Barnes, 1989) to document the presence and intensity and functional impairment of akathisia. (For a review of the approaches to treating akathisia, see Poyurovsky, 2010.)

Tardive dyskinesia is a more serious form of movement disorder. This side effect develops later in the course of treatment, hence the name *tardive*, meaning tardy or late onset. Usually, tardive dyskinesia develops after a minimum of 6 months of continuous treatment with antipsychotic medications. But in rare situations, tardive dyskinesia can occur earlier. Victims exhibit involuntary hyperkinetic, choreiform (dancelike) movements in single or multiple locations of the body, including the head, neck, lips, tongue, jaw, arms, fingers, feet, toes, and trunk. Clinicians use a standardized examination and the *Abnormal Involuntary Movement Scale* (AIMS) to rate and document the presence, body location, and severity of tardive dyskinesia. The prevalence of tardive dyskinesia has been estimated to be 20 percent of patients who are treated with FGAs. The incidence rate is about 4 percent per year of treatment for the first 5 years. The risk of developing tardive dyskinesia depends on a number of variables, including the particular drug (such as FGA versus SGA; low potency versus high potency; oral versus depot form); the dosage; presence of any neurological brain disorder, such as traumatic brain injury (TBI) or dementia; presence of affective symptoms; gender (females are at higher risk than males); and the age of the patient (for elderly individuals, the incidence rate for developing tardive dyskinesia is about 20 to 30 percent per year of treatment).

Although the incidence of tardive dyskinesia is much less with the SGAs, it is not zero. One study found an incidence of 0.74 percent (Tenback et al., 2010), but incidence rates can be as high as 3 to 4 percent. Prevalence rates of tardive dyskinesia with the SGAs has been estimated to be about 20 percent compared to 30 percent with FGAs (Carbon et al., 2017). Options for the treatment of TD are limited. The first choice is to discontinue treatment with the offending antipsychotic agent. But this may not always be possible if it results in the reemergence of severe psychotic symptoms in that affect the health, safety, and functional capacity of the individual. Other options for treatment include switching to a drug with a lower risk of producing TD, such as an SGA. The SGA that has been shown to not only have low risk for TD but also reduces TD in patients who have it is *clozapine* (Clozaril). Tardive dyskinesia results from the long-term blockade of dopamine D_2 receptors. Although tardive dyskinesia may be controlled by increasing the dose of the antipsychotic drug, this would not be considered a useful treatment strategy. In the short run, parkinsonian symptoms may be elicited, but more importantly, eventually the TD symptoms would return and may be more severe than what they were before the antipsychotic drug dose was increased. In effect, the increased dose only masks the TD symptoms temporarily. Recently, an old drug, *tetrabenazine* (Xenazine) has been shown to reduce the severity of TD based on AIMS scores. Tetrabenzine works by blocking the vesicular monoamine transporter 2 (VMAT2), which effectively reduces or blocks the repackaging of monoamines such as dopamine into the presynaptic vesicles, thus reducing the output of dopamine from the presynaptic terminal. However, tetrabenazine has several disadvantages including a short half-life that requires TID dosing and several side effects, including sedation, depression, increased suicide risk, and, with higher doses, the possibility of producing extrapyramidal symptoms. Regardless of the treatment approach, about 20 percent of those patients who develop TD will continue to exhibit symptoms; that is, TD for those individuals is considered irreversible.

In August 2017, the FDA approved a variant of tetrabenazine, *deutetrabenazine* (Austedo), by Teva Pharmaceuticals, for the treatment of tardive dyskinesia. It was approved in April 2017 for the treatment of the movement disorder associated with Huntington's disease. Deutetrabenazine may require less frequent dosing and has a lower risk of side effects than tetrabenazine (Citrome, 2016a; Mullard, 2016). It has been shown to produce a reduction in the severity of TD symptoms based on AIMS scores. Another VMAT2-blocking drug, *valbenazine* (Ingrezza) by Neurocrine Biosciences, was approved by the FDA in April 2017 for the treatment of tardive dyskinesia. As noted with tetrabenazine, by blocking the transporter, the drug would prevent dopamine from being repackaged in the vesicles. The aim is to provide sustained, low levels of dopamine to minimize side effects associated with excessive dopamine depletion. Results of the clinical trials demonstrated a reduction in AIMS scores with treatment (Citrome, 2016b; O'Brien et al., 2015).

Although rare, one potentially lethal side effect to treatment with antipsychotic medications is neuroleptic malignant syndrome (NMS). This is an acute reaction that may occur in response to a variety of agents that increase dopaminergic transmission. The risk of developing NMS is present for any of the currently available antipsychotic medications, whether FGAs or SGAs. Its incidence in FGA-treated patients is 0.02 to 2.4 percent, and it has been reported to occur in response to the SGAs clozapine, risperidone, and olanzapine. The most common symptoms include fever; severe muscle rigidity of the "lead pipe" type; autonomic changes, such as fluctuating blood pressure; and altered consciousness that may progress to stupor or coma. The risk for developing NMS is increased by any of the following factors: presence of a neurological disorder, such as dementia; agitation; poor nutrition; dehydration; route of administration other than oral, for example, intramuscular or use of depot formulations; and the use of concurrent psychotropic agents, such as antidepressants or lithium. Eighty percent of the cases of NMS occur within the first two weeks of treatment, but it can arise at any time. NMS develops rapidly over the course of 24 to 48 hours and can last for 7 to 14 days. If NMS develops, it is considered a medical emergency, because without treatment, there is a 20 percent mortality risk. The most important aspects of effective treatment are early recognition, immediate withdrawal of the responsible agent, and initiation of supportive measures. Supportive measures include treatment with anticholinergic drugs; treatment with dopaminergic agents, such as *bromocriptine* (Parlodel), treatment with muscle relaxants, such as *dantrolene sodium* (Dantrium); and cooling the body, with ice packs among others.

Much of the art of using antipsychotic medications to treat individuals with schizophrenia lies first of all in making a correct diagnosis. Then it is important to document objectively the major symptoms being expressed. Choice of medication is based on a risk/benefit analysis, whereby an attempt is made to choose a medication that will provide the greatest benefit to the patient based on symptom reduction and functional improvement while minimizing risk-inducing side effects. This selection process should be a joint effort in which the prescriber and the patient participate as equal members of a team. Outcomes to treatment are improved when the patient feels that she or he has some control over choices and the course of treatment. The side effects of antipsychotic medications can be related to a particular drug's ability to block various transmitter receptors. Knowing this information can help the prescriber make treatment choices that will address the specific needs of a given individual while possibly avoiding unnecessary exposure to the side effects, or at least understanding what side effects to expect and then how to manage them. For example, for individuals who may be agitated or having difficulty sleeping, choosing a medication that is more sedating, like a low-potency FGA, may be desired. If anticholinergic side effects limit adherence, a high-potency FGA drug may be more appropriate, and drug-induced movement disorders, if elicited, may be controlled with anticholinergic agents.

The discovery and development of the first-generation antipsychotics was a major advance in the treatment of schizophrenia. Nevertheless, it is recognized that there are three types of unsatisfactory outcomes for schizophrenic patients treated with FGAs. The first category includes patients who are treatment resistant and refractory to medication, despite an adequate trial of an antipsychotic. The second consists of patients who have persistent negative and/or cognitive symptoms despite successful control of positive symptoms. The third consists of patients who are unable to tolerate the side effects of the antipsychotics. These three issues spurred the search for additional antipsychotic medications that perhaps would be more effective than the FGAs and could be used to treat those individuals who were refractory, would be more effective for the treatment of negative and cognitive symptoms of schizophrenia, and would produce fewer side effects compared to the FGAs.

SECOND-GENERATION ANTIPSYCHOTICS

Second-generation (or *atypical*) *antipsychotics* (SGAs) are drugs that block dopamine D_2 receptors just like the first-generation antipsychotics. The distinguishing characteristic of the SGAs is that their potency for blocking serotonin receptors—5-HT$_{1A}$ and 5-HT$_{2A}$, specifically—is as great or greater than their potency for blocking dopamine D_2 receptors. This is mechanistically different than the FGAs, whose potency for blocking dopamine receptors is greater than their potency for blocking serotonin receptors. It is believed that this ratio of 5-HT > dopamine potency and the fast dissociation of these drugs from the dopamine receptor are related to the general finding that the SGAs are less likely to produce neurological side effects, such as extrapyramidal symptoms and tardive dyskinesia, compared to the FGAs (see Kapur and Seeman, 2001; Meltzer, 2012; Newman-Tancredi and Kleven, 2011).

Table 11.4 lists the currently available second-generation antipsychotics. In general, except for *clozapine* (Clozaril) discussed below, the SGAs are as effective

TABLE 11.4 Second-generation antipsychotic drugs

Generic name	Trade name	Dose equivalence (mg)[a]	Formulation[b]	Age group[c]
Clozapine	Clozaril; Fazaclo	50–100	PO; Sol; ODT	A; AD
Risperidone	Risperdal; Consta	1–2	PO; IM; ODT; LAI	C; A; AD
Olanzapine	Zyprexa; Zydis; Relprevv	3–5	PO; IM; ODT; LAI; Combo	A; AD
Quetiapine	Seroquel	60–75	PO	C; A; AD
Ziprasidone	Geodon	50–60	PO; IM	C; A; AD
Aripiprazole	Abilify; Discmelt; Maintena	4–7	PO; Sol; IM; ODT; LAI	C; A; AD
Paliperidone	Invega; Sustenna; Trinza	1–2	PO; LAI	A; AD
Iloperidone	Fanapt	2–5	PO	AD
Asenapine	Saphris	2–5	PO-SL	A; AD
Lurasidone	Latuda	10–20	PO	A; AD
Brexpiprazole	Rexulti	1	PO	AD
Cariprazine	Vraylar	1	PO	AD

[a]Dose equivalence: All drug doses are equated to 100 milligrams of chlorpromazine.
[b]Formulation: PO = oral, usually tablets or capsules; Sol = oral solution; ODT = orally disintegrating tablet; PO-SL = oral sublingual film; Combo = combination tablet: olanzapine + fluoxetine; IM = intramuscular injectable solution; LAI = long-acting injectable solution, usually 1 injection every 2 to 4 weeks or 3 months (Trinza).
[c]Age group: C = children (1–9 years old); A = adolescent (10–17 years old); AD = adult (≥18 years old).

as the first-generation antipsychotics for treating the symptoms of schizophrenia. Also, like the FGAs, the SGAs have FDA-approved indications to treat other disorders (see Table 11.5) and can be used off-label by prescribers. (For a review of the off-label uses of the SGAs and their reported effectiveness, see Kondo and Winchell, 2016.) In general, the SGAs produce lower rates of extrapyramidal symptoms and tardive dyskinesia when compared to the FGAs, but the risk is not zero except perhaps for clozapine (Divac et al., 2014; Rummel-Kluge et al., 2012). They still can produce other physiological side effects, however, similar to those seen with the FGAs. Furthermore, many of the SGAs have been associated with a risk for producing what is known as a metabolic syndrome, which is described later in this chapter.

Although drugs such as *aripiprazole* (Abilify) and *brexpiprazole* (Rexulti) are sometimes referred to as "third-generation antipsychotics" due to their unique mechanism of action at dopamine receptors, they will be considered here for simplicity as part of the group of SGAs. We will not describe each of the SGAs in detail in this chapter, because they are similar in efficacy. Instead, in the section below, we will highlight specific aspects of some of these drugs that may be of importance when considering which drug to use for treatment.

TABLE 11.5 Indications for second-generation antipsychotic drugs

Generic name	Trade name	Indications
Clozaril	Clozapine	Schizophrenia (not first-line agent); suicide risk
Risperidone	Risperdal	Schizophrenia; BPD (mania/mixed); Tourette syndrome; irritability/aggressive behavior in autism
Olanzapine	Zyprexa	Schizophrenia; BPD (mania/depressed/mixed); treatment-resistant depression; agitation in schizophrenia or bipolar disorder
Quetiapine	Seroquel	Schizophrenia; BPD (mania/depressed/mixed)
Ziprasidone	Geodon	Schizophrenia; BPD (manic/mixed); agitation in schizophrenia or bipolar disorder; Tourette syndrome
Aripiprazole	Abilify	Schizophrenia; BPD (manic/mixed); depression; agitation in schizophrenia or bipolar disorder; irritability/aggression in autism
Paliperidone	Invega	Schizophrenia; schizoaffective disorder
Iloperidone	Fanapt	Schizophrenia
Asenapine	Saphris	Schizophrenia; BPD (manic/mixed/maintenance)
Lurasidone	Latuda	Schizophrenia; BPD (depression)
Brexpiprazole	Rexulti	Schizophrenia; MDD (adjunct)
Cariprazine	Vraylar	Schizophrenia; BPD (manic/mixed)

Clozapine

Clozapine (Clozaril) was the first atypical antipsychotic and has been demonstrated to be clinically superior to both typical and atypical antipsychotics, first, because it is effective in about one-third of patients who are resistant to conventional medications, and second, because it lacks the extrapyramidal side effects associated with the traditional neuroleptics (Meltzer, 2013; Owen et al., 2016). In fact, for patients with primary (idiopathic) parkinsonism who demonstrate psychotic symptoms (such as hallucinations and delusions), clozapine can effectively treat their psychosis without exacerbating the underlying movement disorder (Chang and Fox, 2016; Comaty and Advokat, 2001; Parkinson Study Group, 1999). And there is evidence that clozapine is the only antipsychotic drug that not only does not have a high risk of producing EPS or TD, but it can reduce or resolve TD caused by another antipsychotic drug, if the individual is switched to clozapine from that other drug (Spivak et al., 1997). Third, the FIN11 study found that clozapine compared to either FGAs or other SGAs reduced all-cause mortality rates in individuals with schizophrenia over an 11-year period and reduced suicide rates in the same population (Tiihonen et al., 2009). Evidence that clozapine reduced the risk of suicide in schizophrenia relative to other antipsychotics led to the International Suicide Prevention Trial (InterSePT) study, which compared clozapine with another SGA, olanzapine, in patients with schizophrenia or schizoaffective disorder at risk for suicide (Meltzer et al., 2003).

In this multicenter, randomized, international study, patients who were diagnosed with either schizophrenia or schizoaffective disorder and were considered high risk for suicide were treated with either clozapine or olanzapine. At the end of the two-year study period, patients treated with clozapine had fewer suicide attempts, required fewer hospitalizations to prevent suicide, and fewer of them required antidepressants or anxiolytics to address suicidal inclinations. Based on the strength of this evidence, the FDA has approved clozapine for treatment-resistant schizophrenia and the treatment of suicidal behavior in schizophrenia. Despite all of these advantages of clozapine over other antipsychotic medications, it has been underutilized clinically. In part, this may be due to the inconvenience of the required frequent blood tests for measuring levels of white blood cells and the potentially lethal side effect of agranulocytosis among other side effects that will be discussed later in this chapter.

Aripiprazole

Aripiprazole (Abilify) was approved in 2002 as perhaps the first of a new "third-generation" antipsychotic drug (Potkin et al., 2003). It has a different mechanism of action from FGAs and other SGAs. Aripiprazole is a partial agonist at D_2 and $5\text{-}HT_{1A}$ receptors as well as an antagonist at $5\text{-}HT_2$ receptors (de Bartolomeis et al., 2015; Jordan et al., 2002). This dopaminergic partial agonism is meant to stabilize the dopamine system because, although the drug binds with high affinity to D_2 receptors, it has lower intrinsic activity (less efficacy). This means that in areas of the brain where dopamine levels are normally high (for example, in the limbic and nigrostriatal systems), aripiprazole may displace dopamine from the dopamine receptor, but it will not produce as strong an effect as the natural transmitter. This effect in the limbic and nigrostriatal systems is thought to be responsible for aripiprazole's antipsychotic effect and potentially lower risk of EPS and TD. Conversely, in areas of the brain where dopamine concentration is low (for example, in the frontal lobes and/or mesocortical dopamine system), aripiprazole can produce a net increase in dopaminergic action (Lieberman, 2004; Stahl, 2002; Tamminga and Carlsson, 2002). This is thought to be related to aripiprazole's lower risk for cognitive impairment and positive effect on the negative symptoms of schizophrenia.

Aripiprazole's partial agonism at $5\text{-}HT_{1A}$ receptors confers anxiolytic or antidepressant actions. Aripiprazole has been reported to augment the effect of SSRIs in patients with depression and anxiety disorders who were only partial responders to SSRIs alone (Schwartz et al., 2007). In 2017, the FDA approved a new technology to monitor whether a person actually swallows their medication as directed. Abilify *MyCite* is a pill containing aripiprazole and a sensor that sends out an electrical signal when the pill reaches the stomach and contacts the stomach acid. The signal is transmitted to a wearable patch on the user's wrist that can link to a mobile application that allows patients to track whether they have taken their medication. The patient can also allow such information to be accessed by a caregiver or their health care provider.

Since aripiprazole has come to market, two other dopamine partial agonist (DPA) antipsychotics have been developed and approved by the FDA: *brexpiprazole* (Rexulti) and *cariprazine* (Vraylar). Cariprazine is also unique among SGAs because it has a higher affinity for D_3 receptors than D_2 receptors. It is thought that by favoring

D_3 over D_2 receptors and being a partial agonist at those receptors that cariprazine would have the necessary D_2 effects as an antipsychotic and, due to its partial agonism at D_3 receptors, it would have fewer side effects and produce less cognitive impairment (see Caccia et al., 2013). (For a comparison of the three DPA drugs, see Citrome, 2015.)

Asenapine

In 2009, *asenapine* (Saphris) was approved for the treatment of schizophrenia (5 milligrams, two times a day) and manic or mixed episodes of bipolar disorder (10 milligrams, two times a day) in adults. It received an additional indication in 2010 for the acute treatment of bipolar disorder manic or mixed episodes as an adjunct to either lithium or valproic acid. In 2015, the FDA approved asenapine for the treatment of schizophrenia and bipolar disorder in adolescents. Asenapine has a chemical structure related to the antidepressant mirtazepine. It is unique in that it must be dissolved under the tongue, with no eating or drinking for 10 minutes afterward; otherwise, it will not be adequately absorbed into the bloodstream. Bioavailability is less than 2 percent orally when simply swallowed but 35 percent sublingually when dissolved under the tongue.

Cariprazine

Cariprazine (Vraylar) was approved by the FDA in 2015 for the treatment of schizophrenia and bipolar disorder. It is reported to be a partial agonist at both D_3 and D_2 receptors. The unique aspect of this drug is that the potency of the drug is greater at the D_3 than at the D_2 receptor.

PROMINENT SIDE EFFECTS OF SECOND-GENERATION ANTIPSYCHOTICS

As noted previously, while the second-generation antipsychotic agents generally have a lower risk of producing early onset EPS and late-onset TD than the FGAs, the risk is not zero, and the SGAs can still produce EPS and TD in some proportion of the population of individuals who are treated with these agents. In addition, the SGAs can also produce many of the physiological, endocrine, and cardiovascular side effects that are associated with treatment with the FGAs. Furthermore, the SGAs are most often associated with producing an array of side effects that are collectively referred to as the *metabolic syndrome* (also see Table 11.6). This syndrome is comprised of weight gain, dyslipidemia, and glucose intolerance, which can lead to diabetes. The most characteristic side effects of specific SGAs will be described next and are summarized in Table 11.7.

Clozapine

Common side effects of clozapine include sedation, significant weight gain, decrease in seizure threshold, sialorrhea (hypersalivation), and constipation, with rare instances of agranulocytosis.

TABLE 11.6 Symptoms of metabolic syndrome

Abdominal obesity (waist circumference):
Men: >102 cm (>40 in.)
Women: >88 cm (>35 in.)
Triglyceride level (mg/dL): >150
HDL cholesterol (mg/dL):
Men: >40
Blood pressure (mm Hg): ≥130/≥85
Fasting blood glucose (mg/dL): >100

TABLE 11.7 Side effects of the second-generation (atypical) antipsychotic medications

Medication	Side effects
Clozapine	Orthostatic hypotension, anticholinergic symptoms, myocarditis, sedation, seizures, hypersalivation, neuroleptic malignant syndrome (NMS), agranulocytosis, metabolic syndrome
Risperidone	Extrapyramidal symptoms (EPS), tardive dyskinesia (TD), hyperprolactinemia, NMS
Olanzapine	Orthostatic hypotension, anticholinergic symptoms, sedation, NMS, metabolic syndrome, drug reaction with eosinophilia and systemic symptoms (DRESS), a serious dermatological reaction also affecting other internal organ systems with risk of mortality
Quetiapine	Sedation, orthostatic hypotension
Ziprasidone	Sedation, EPS, TD, increase in QT_c interval, metabolic syndrome, DRESS; Stevens-Johnson syndrome (SJS), a serious dermatological reaction with risk of mortality
Aripiprazole	Orthostatic hypotension, nausea, tremor, insomnia, headache, agitation, akathisia, risky compulsive behaviors (gambling, shopping, sexual behavior, etc.)
Paliperidone	Akathisia, EPS, tachycardia, hyperprolactinemia, QT_c prolongation
Iloperidone	Dizziness, dry mouth, fatigue, nasal congestion, somnolence, tachycardia, orthostatic hypotension, some elevation in prolactin, weight gain, hypersensitivity reactions (including anaphylaxis, angioedema, throat tightness, oropharyngeal swelling, swelling of the face, lips, mouth, and tongue, urticaria, rash, and pruritus)
Asenapine	Dizziness, EPS, TD, NMS, akathisia, oral hypoesthesia, dysgeusia, somnolence, weight gain
Lurasidone	Somnolence, akathisia, nausea, EPS, TD
Brexpiprazole	Weight gain, akathisia
Cariprazine	EPS, akathisia, TD, vomiting, dyspepsia, somnolence

Sedation, most likely stemming from the antihistaminergic action of clozapine, occurs in about 40 percent of patients. In fact, the severity of this sedation may be dose limiting and have a negative impact on adherence. Taking the drug at bedtime may help improve adherence. Weight gain is a problem for up to 80 percent of patients; it can be severe, with gains of 20 pounds or more not unusual. Of all the SGAs, clozapine is the drug most likely to cause significant weight gain (see Figure 11.2). Weight gain may also be related to an individual's BMI at the time the drug was first prescribed. Studies suggest that those individuals with higher BMIs tend to lose weight on SGAs while those with normal or low BMIs tend to gain weight (Bushe et al., 2013). (For a review of the risk of weight gain for selected antipsychotic drugs, see Musil et al., 2015.)

Seizures occur at a greater rate with clozapine than with other antipsychotics, especially at high doses (600 to 900 milligrams per day), and it has a specific warning for this adverse event. Sialorrhea (increased saliva production) occurs in one-third to one-half of patients, not only during the day but often much more extensively at night, with patients complaining of waking up with a wet pillow. The mechanism is believed to be due to an impaired ability to swallow, which causes saliva to accumulate. It may be severe and difficult to treat, although it can disappear over time. Constipation occurs in about 30 percent of patients and can be quite bothersome.

The greatest concern with clozapine is the risk of developing severe, life-threatening (although reversible) agranulocytosis, with an incidence of about 1 to 2 percent (Tschen et al., 1999). In 2015, the FDA modified the requirements that must be met to prescribe clozapine, in response to safety data that had shown that the risks of agranulocytosis were being well managed and that the fear of such a rare occurrence

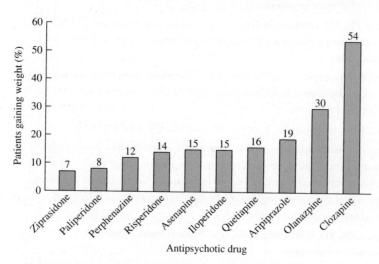

FIGURE 11.2 Percentage of patients who gained 7 percent or more of their baseline body weight while being treated with the indicated antipsychotic drugs. The 7 percent threshold is the accepted measure for determining a significant effect. [Data from Ellinger et al. (2010).]

was preventing prescribers from using clozapine in individuals for whom it could be very effective. These requirements are contained in the Clozaril Risk Evaluation and Mitigation Strategy (REMS). To ensure that signs of agranulocytosis are detected as early as possible so that it can be treated, the FDA requires that the prescriber, the pharmacy dispensing the clozapine, and the patient receiving clozapine be enrolled in the Clozaril registry. The registry tracks prescriptions and whether patients have had blood samples drawn to detect for early signs of agranulocytosis. Blood samples are assayed for the presence and number of neutrophils. There are three major types of white blood cells; granulocytes, monocytes, and lymphocytes. Granulocytes, in turn, are composed of neutrophils, eosinophils, and basophils. The neutrophils are the most abundant type of all the white blood cells in the body and also the most abundant sub-type of granulocytes. These cells are part of the body's immune system. If the number of neutrophils drops too low, the body will not be able to mount a credible defense against infection that could lead to sickness and even death. The REMS requires that absolute neutrophil counts (ANCs) must be monitored weekly for the first 6 months of therapy, then every 2 weeks for the next 6 months, and then monthly thereafter, with more frequent monitoring if the ANC decreases. If the ANC drops below a specified threshold, then clozapine must be discontinued. Other drugs that can reduce ANCs, most notably carbamazepine, should not be taken concomitantly.

Clozapine is also associated with the risk for metabolic syndrome that includes abnormalities of blood pressure, lipids, glucose utilization, and body mass index (BMI). These abnormalities contribute to an increased risk for cardiovascular disease and therefore require monitoring in those individuals who are prescribed clozapine. The American Diabetes Association and American Psychiatric Association have published suggested monitoring schedules for insulin resistance, recommending that blood glucose levels be taken at 6 months, at 1 year, and then every 5 years thereafter.

Clozapine is also highly anticholinergic, producing dry mouth, urinary retention, constipation, blurred vision, and in some individuals, cognitive impairment. Clozapine also has two black box warnings (BBWs) that are issued by the FDA and indicate the most serious risk of experiencing a side effect. One BBW is for myocarditis, which is an inflammation of the heart muscle that can cause shortness of breath, palpitations, chest pain, and lightheadedness. The other BBW is one that is associated with all antipsychotic agents, that is, increased risk of cerebrovascular events (such as stroke) when the antipsychotic is used to treat behavioral disorders, including agitation in elderly individuals with dementia.

Clozapine is the least prescribed of all the SGAs due to the need for frequent blood tests and its array of potentially serious side effects. It is, however, one of the most effective antipsychotic medications, especially for those individuals who have not responded to one or more trials of other FGA or SGA drugs. There is increasing interest in supporting the use of clozapine earlier rather than later in the course of treatment. Due to restrictions, clozapine cannot be used as a first-line agent, but some clinicians argue that it should not be the treatment of "last resort" either (Remington et al., 2013). Clozapine has been shown particularly effective in reducing mortality as noted above, specifically reducing both aggressive behavior and suicide risk (Citrome, 2009; Meltzer, 2012). It may also be beneficial in reducing smoking and use of other drugs of abuse in schizophrenic patients who have those comorbidities.

Risperidone

In addition to the side effects common to all antipsychotic drugs, risperidone, among all second-generation antipsychotics, is the one most likely to produce extrapyramidal symptoms and, by inference, tardive dyskinesia. Extrapyramidal symptoms are minimal at low doses (6 milligrams or less). The risk increases with higher doses. Further, risperidone, compared to the other SGAs, is most likely to be associated with increased prolactin levels, which can result in menstrual abnormalities, infertility, changes in libido, anorgasmia, breast enlargement, and galactorrhea (lactation) in females; and changes in libido, anorgasmia, erectile dysfunction, and gynecomastia (breast development) in males.

Olanzapine

Olanzapine is chemically similar to clozapine and both are similar to the FGA chlorpromazine. Therefore, they share a similar array of side effects. Olanzapine, of all the SGAs, has a risk of producing significant weight gain and the metabolic syndrome comparable to that seen with clozapine. Olanzapine is highly sedating and also highly

Did You Know?

There May Be a Way to Determine Which Patients Will Gain Weight When Taking Antipsychotic Medications

It is well known that one of the side effects of many antipsychotic medications is weight gain, which can be substantial. But clinicians do not currently have any reliable method of predicting in advance who would be susceptible to this common side effect. If clinicians had such a predictor, they could tailor their drug selection to agents that are least likely to produce weight gain and they also could counsel patients on proper nutrition, exercise, and weight-loss strategies. Malhotra and colleagues (2012) studied a group of individuals who had never taken antipsychotic medication previously and followed them closely for 12 weeks to make sure they took their medication as prescribed and to monitor their metabolic status. They also carried out genetic studies to identify any gene variants that might be related to those individuals within the group who gained significant weight. Their results identified markers in a gene, the melanocortin 4 receptor (MC4R), that were associated with severe weight gain in people taking second-generation antipsychotics. The MC4R region overlaps somewhat with another region previously identified as being associated with obesity in the general population. In addition, the results were replicated in three independent cohorts. Although particular gene variants were implicated, the study's sample size was small. Further research with larger samples is needed to extend the findings. Another gene of interest is the GABAA α2 receptor subunit (GABRA2), which is another candidate gene derived from genome-wide association studies. A study of 160 patients of European ancestry with schizophrenia found a marker for identifying those patients who had a propensity to gain more weight while being treated with antipsychotic medications. This finding became even more significant when the analysis was restricted to only those patients receiving clozapine or olanzapine, the two SGAs that have the highest risk for producing weight gain (Zai et al., 2015).

anticholinergic producing dry mouth, urinary retention, constipation, blurred visions, and cognitive impairment in at-risk individuals. Interestingly, despite being chemically similar to clozapine, olanzapine does not carry a risk for producing agranulocytosis and therefore does not require the blood monitoring for ANCs as is required when clozapine is being used for treatment.

A rare side effect of olanzapine has been noted in a warning to prescribers from the FDA. *Drug reaction with eosinophilia and systemic symptoms* (DRESS) may start as a rash that can spread to all parts of the body. It can include fever and swollen lymph nodes and a swollen face. It causes a higher-than-normal number of infection-fighting white blood cells called *eosinophils* that can cause inflammation or swelling. DRESS can result in injury to organs, including the liver, kidneys, lungs, heart, or pancreas. DRESS is a potentially fatal drug reaction with a mortality rate of up to 10 percent.

Another rare olanzapine side effect, with an incidence rate of 2 percent, is related only to the long-acting depot injectable form of the drug with the trade name of *Relprevv*. Postinjection delirium/sedation syndrome (PDSS) is a syndrome of intense sedation than can lead to ataxia and abrupt onset of sleep. Thus, the FDA requires that anyone who receives a Relprevv injection must stay in the clinic for a minimum of 3 hours post injection and be driven home by an escort.

Quetiapine

The most prominent side effects of quetiapine are sedation, postural hypotension, and rarely, an increase in the QT_c interval. In a normal electrocardiogram tracing, the QT interval is the time between the start of the Q wave and the end of the T wave that represents the time taken for ventricular depolarization and subsequent repolarization (Figure 11.3). The QT_c is the QT interval corrected to a standard heart rate of 60 beats per minute. An extension of the QT interval beyond 500 milliseconds increases the risk of developing a potentially fatal ventricular arrhythmia called *torsade de pointes* (see Figure 11.4). Thus, drugs like quetiapine that have the potential to increase the QT_c interval should be used with caution or not at all in individuals who have existing cardiac rhythm disturbances, who may have a condition called *congenitally long QT interval*, or in individuals who are taking other medications that could prolong the QT interval.

Ziprasidone

Ziprasidone can be sedating, but it does not produce a significant risk for weight gain. It does carry a risk of producing a metabolic syndrome and may also carry a slight risk for extending the QT_c interval. Thus, it should be used with caution in individuals who have existing cardiac disturbances, similar to what was noted for quetiapine.

Ziprasidone also carries a risk for inducing two serious and potentially fatal dermatological and systemic reactions. One, *Stevens-Johnson syndrome* (SJS), is a form of toxic epidermal necrolysis, a life-threatening skin condition, in which cell death causes

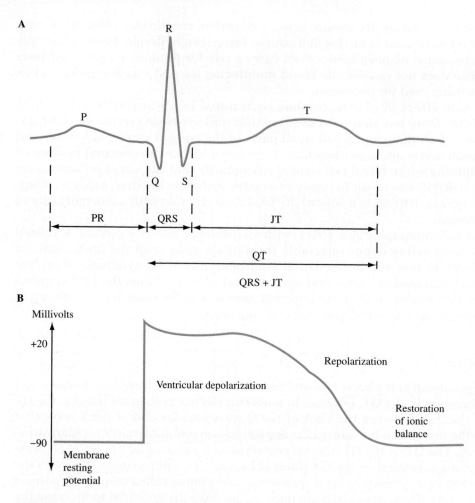

FIGURE 11.3 **A.** Normal electrocardiogram (ECG) in sinus rhythm. P wave: atrial electrical depolarization and leads to muscular contraction of the right and left ventricles. QRS complex: ventricular electrical depolarization and leads to muscular contraction of the right and left ventricles. JT: the time from the end of ventricular depolarization (QRS) to the end of ventricular repolarization. The QT interval includes both QRS and ventricular repolarization. **B.** Rapid ventricular depolarization and slower repolarization. Most of the QT interval represents ventricular repolarization.

the epidermis to separate from the dermis. This destroys the most significant barrier a person has to infection, that is, their skin. The other reaction is DRESS, described previously in the section on olanzapine. Fortunately, both SJS and DRESS are rare occurrences, but the person being treated must immediately report any development of a rash so that it can be evaluated by a medical professional (such as a dermatologist) as soon as possible. Combining drugs that each carry a risk for either SJS or DRESS (such as olanzapine and ziprasidone) increases the risk for occurrence.

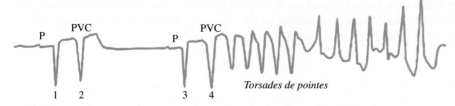

FIGURE 11.4   Characteristic development of *torsades de pointes* ventricular arrhythmia. Sinus beat with normal ventricular complex (1) followed by a premature ventricular contraction (PVC); and (2) closely coupled to the sinus beat. After a long pause (2–3), this paired complex is repeated (3–4). The second PVC initiates a bizarre ventricular arrhythmia consistent with *torsades de pointes*. This ventricular arrhythmia is accompanied by poor contraction of ventricular muscle and loss of contractility and output of blood from the heart, leading to a cardiac arrest.

Aripiprazole

Aripiprazole is relatively neutral for risk of weight gain. Its most common side effects include orthostatic hypotension, nausea, tremor, insomnia, headache, and agitation. Of all the SGAs, it is the drug most likely to produce the side effect of akathisia. In May 2016, the FDA issued a warning that aripiprazole may also produce an increased risk for pathological gambling and other compulsive behaviors, such as binge eating, and may cause hiccups.

Paliperidone

Paliperidone is one of the major metabolites of risperidone. Therefore, it can produce the same side effects as the parent drug, namely, increased risk for extrapyramidal symptoms, tardive dyskinesia, and akathisia in higher doses. Paliperidone can also increase prolactin levels, producing the same sexual side effects that were listed for risperidone above. Finally, it may rarely increase the QT_c interval.

Iloperidone

Iloperidone can produce dizziness, dry mouth, fatigue, nasal congestion, somnolence, tachycardia, orthostatic hypotension, some elevation in prolactin, and weight gain. It may also produce hypersensitivity reactions, including anaphylaxis; angioedema; throat tightness; oropharyngeal swelling; swelling of the face, lips, mouth, and tongue; urticaria; rash; and pruritus.

Asenapine

Asenapine has been reported to produce a variety of side effects, including extrapyramidal symptoms, tardive dyskinesia, akathisia, and neuroleptic malignant syndrome. It also can produce dizziness, somnolence, and weight gain. Because of its method of administration (that is, it is imbedded on a film strip that is placed under the tongue), it can produce oral hypoesthesia (numbing of the mouth and tongue) and dysgeusia (a foul, salty, rancid, or metallic taste sensation in the mouth).

Lurasidone

Lurasidone's most common side effects include somnolence, nausea, extrapyramidal symptoms, and akathisia.

Brexpiprazole

Brexpiprazole has the same side effect profile as aripiprazole discussed earlier.

Cariprazine

Similar to both aripiprazole and brexpiprazole, cariprazine's most common side effects include somnolence, dyspepsia (indigestion), vomiting, extrapyramidal symptoms, and akathisia. Cariprazine does not appear to adversely impact metabolic variables, prolactin, or the electrocardiogram (ECG) QT interval (Citrome, 2013b).

CATIE AND CUtLASS STUDIES

The Clinical Antipsychotic Trials of Intervention Effectiveness (CATIE) study was conducted in the United States between January 2001 and December 2004 at 57 clinical sites for up to 18 months or until treatment was discontinued for any reason. In the first of three phases, 1493 patients were randomly assigned to receive either one of three SGAs (olanzapine, risperidone, or quetiapine) or the FGA perphenazine under double-blind conditions. The SGA ziprasidone was added later following its FDA approval. Results showed that patients discontinued antipsychotic medications at a high rate, 64 to 82 percent across all the drugs, primarily because of lack of efficacy or intolerable side effects (extrapyramidal symptoms in the case of perphenazine and weight gain or metabolic changes from olanzapine). There was no overall difference in the rate of discontinuation between the SGAs and the FGA perphenazine (Lieberman et al., 2005).

Of the 1493 patients enrolled in the study, 1052 were eligible for phase 2. This part of the study provided two treatment pathways. The "efficacy" pathway consisted of 99 patients who had not shown optimal improvement on one of the SGAs in the first phase or who had stopped treatment for any other reason than not being able to tolerate the treatment. Patients in the efficacy pathway were offered the option of being randomly assigned to clozapine or to another SGA, other than the one they had received in phase 1. The "tolerability" pathway consisted of 444 patients who discontinued treatment in phase 1 due to intolerable side effects. These patients were offered the opportunity to receive treatment with an SGA other than the one they had previously received—excluding clozapine. The remaining 509 patients (48 percent) did not enter phase 2.

In the "efficacy" pathway, clozapine treatment was found to be more effective than the other SGAs. That is, patients receiving clozapine were less likely to discontinue therapy because of lack of therapeutic response than patients receiving any of the other newer agents. In the "tolerability" pathway, olanzapine and risperidone were more effective than quetiapine or ziprasidone in "time until discontinuation" for any reason. Neither of the phase 2 pathways included either aripiprazole or any first-generation antipsychotic (McEvoy et al., 2006; Stroup et al., 2006).

A British comparison between SGAs and FGAs—Cost Utility of the Latest Antipsychotic Drugs in Schizophrenia Studies (CUtLASS 1)—was reported in October 2006 (Jones et al., 2006). It evaluated 227 people with a diagnosis of schizophrenia who had an inadequate response or adverse reaction to their previous medication. Prescriptions for either an FGA or an SGA (excluding clozapine) were monitored for one year, with blind assessments at 12, 26, and 56 weeks. The primary outcomes measured were quality of life, symptom severity, adverse effects, participant satisfaction, and costs of care. Like the CATIE trial, the results of the CUtLASS 1 study showed that patients with schizophrenia did just as well on antipsychotic drugs from either category, with patients taking FGAs actually showing a trend toward greater improvement on the quality-of-life scale and symptom-severity scores. Participants expressed no clear preference and the costs were similar.

Although antipsychotic drugs remain the "cornerstone of treatment for schizophrenia" (Lieberman et. al., 2005), the results of the CATIE and CUtLASS 1 trials have prompted a reassessment of the perceived advantages of the second-generation antipsychotics. The initial optimism generated by second-generation antipsychotics has been tempered by evidence that they do not improve clinical outcomes as much as anticipated and are much more expensive than the older drugs. And it may be the case that FGAs and SGAs differ among themselves based on what factor is being examined. For example, one SGA may produce less extrapyramidal symptoms than a FGA, but the SGA may produce more weight gain. So, comparisons between FGAs and SGAs are not simple and may depend on a broader analysis of desired outcomes than enter into any risk/benefit analysis. Another factor in these types of analyses is the strength and/or quality of the evidence in the individual studies, which may be quite limited (see Hartling et al., 2012).

This perspective was supported by a large meta-analysis of SGAs versus FGAs (Leucht et al., 2009), which included 150 studies and more than 21,500 patients. In 95 of the 150 studies, haloperidol was the FGA compared. In this meta-analysis, amisulpride (not available in the United States), clozapine, olanzapine, and risperidone were significantly more effective at reducing overall symptom severity than the FGAs compared, whereas aripiprazole, quetiapine, sertindole, ziprasidone, and zotepine (not available in the United States) were not more effective. All SGAs produced numerically fewer extrapyramidal symptoms than haloperidol and this difference reached statistical significance. However, despite being statistically significant, the magnitude of these differences were not clinically meaningful. Zhang and colleagues (2013) published similar findings. Essentially, it is now understood that not all SGAs are the same (Komossa et al., 2009a, 2009b); they do not always produce better outcomes than FGAs, even in cases of acute toxic ingestion (Ciranni et al., 2009); and the merits of each drug have to be determined independently, taking into account side effects, costs, and benefits

(Leucht et al., 2013; Rosenheck and Sernyak, 2009). In situations where the risk of extrapyramidal symptoms may preclude the use of FGAs, such as autism, bipolar disorder, borderline personality disorder, and aggressive disorders, SGAs may be the first choice. The transition to generic status of the SGAs (reducing their cost) will most likely affect such considerations as well.[5]

IN THE PIPELINE

According to industry watchers (Fellner, 2017; Guzowski, 2016), there has been a slowdown in the number of new products for the treatment of schizophrenia entering the clinical trial phases. The ones that are in current testing seem to focus on new targets, new delivery systems, selected symptoms, or are minor improvements to existing medications. Some of these compounds have only been tested in animals (preclinical phase) while others have moved into one of the phases of clinical testing with humans. The following is a list of the compounds currently under investigation.

Compounds Targeting the Dopamine Receptor

Lundbeck Pharmaceuticals is testing a compound, Lu AF35700, which is reported to be dopamine D_1 receptor antagonist. While a previous trial of a D_1 receptor antagonist by Lundbeck was abandoned, the company thinks that Lu AF35700 will be a better drug than the one used in the previous trial and that it will be similar to clozapine without the many side effects. Since all currently marketed drugs that are effective antipsychotic agents block the D_2 dopamine receptor, it will be interesting to see if a drug with little D_2 blocking action can be an effective antipsychotic drug.

Compounds Targeting the Nicotinic Acetylcholine Receptor

Several compounds are currently being examined as possible treatments for the cognitive decline seen in Alzheimer's dementia or as an adjunctive treatment for the cognitive deficits of schizophrenia. One class of compounds being examined are the alpha-7 nicotinic acetylcholine receptor agonists. Stimulation of nicotinic receptors is thought to be related to enhanced cognitive function. Examples of compounds in this class are ABT-126 (AbbVie) and AQW051 (Novartis). A slight variation on these nicotinic agonists is a Type 1 alpha-7 nicotinic acetylcholine receptor positive allosteric modulator (PAM), AVL-3288 (Anvyl). Being an allosteric modulator, this drug will not have an immediate effect on cognitive function, but if taken consistently over time, it may enhance cognitive function in a more sustainable fashion compared to alpha-7 receptor agonists. In addition, this compound reportedly does not inhibit the upregulation of the nicotinic

---

[5]Kane and Correll (2010) provide a comprehensive summary of the history of the role of drug treatments for schizophrenia, the evolution from the FGAs to the SGAs, successes and lack of success for novel interventions, and future directions for research.

receptors that prevents receptor desensitization over time with continued use of the drug. Finally, EVP-6124/MT-4666 (Encenicline), developed by Forum Pharmaceuticals, is reported to be an alpha-7 nicotinic acetylcholine receptor partial agonist. This drug stimulates the alpha-7 nicotinic acetylcholine receptor in selected areas of the brain, like the hippocampus and cerebral cortex, and was expected to improve cognition in schizophrenia. In 2016, Forum Pharmaceuticals announced that the drug failed to meet its primary outcome targets in two phase 3 clinical trials and the drug has been sidelined.

Compounds Targeting the Glutamate System

Based on basic studies that suggest that some dysfunction in glutamate transmission may be involved with producing symptoms of schizophrenia, several pharmaceutical companies are testing drugs that modulate the activity of the glutamate receptor. ADX-1149 (JNJ-40411813), developed by Addex Therapeutics in partnership with Janssen Pharmaceuticals, functions as a metabotropic glutamatergic receptor 2 (mGlu2) selective positive allosteric modulator. NW-3509, developed by Newron Pharmaceuticals, is a voltage-gated sodium channel modulator (VGSM). NW-3509 is being tested as an adjunctive treatment to antipsychotic medications. Modulating the sodium channels reduces the hyperexcitability of neurons to bring them into the range of normal function. The company states that hyperexcitability of neurons in certain parts of the brain leads to increased activity of glutamate and relates to some of the positive symptoms of schizophrenia, such as hallucinations and delusions. Thus, regulating glutamate via sodium channel modulation is expected to reduce the expression of these positive symptoms in individuals who have schizophrenia.

Pfizer Pharmaceuticals is testing a compound, PF-04958242, which is an AMPA receptor modulator. It regulates glutamate levels through its action on AMPA receptors. Glutamate is a toxin and in high levels can kill brain cells. By acting as a neuromodulator, PF-04958242 can regulate glutamate levels and have a neuroprotective effect on brain cells involved in learning and memory. It is being tested as an adjunctive treatment to antipsychotic medication to improve cognitive deficits.

Compounds Targeting the Serotonin System

AVN-211, developed by AllaChem in partnership with Avineuro Pharmaceuticals, is a 5-HT$_6$ receptor antagonist. Blockade of the 5-HT$_6$ receptor is thought to increase glutamate and cholinergic transmission throughout the brain and elevate dopamine and norepinephrine levels in the prefrontal cortex. This compound is expected to increase cognitive abilities, especially attention, when used as an adjunctive treatment to antipsychotic drugs in individuals with schizophrenia.

Minerva Neurosciences is testing MIN-101, which is a 5-HT$_{2A}$/Sigma-2 receptor antagonist. Blockade of the 5-HT$_{2A}$ receptor is thought to improve negative symptoms and the antagonism of the Sigma-2 receptor is expected to improve motor control, learning, and memory.

Acadia Pharmaceuticals has marketed a drug, *pimavanserin* (Nuplazid), which was approved by the FDA in April 2016. Its approved indication is for the treatment of

Parkinson's disease psychosis (see further discussion in Chapter 16). The drug is a selective serotonin inverse agonist (SSIA) specifically at the 5-HT_{2A} receptor site. It is currently in trials for the adjunctive treatment of schizophrenia and psychosis associated with Alzheimer's disease. Since it is already an approved drug, prescribers can use it off-label now for the treatment of schizophrenia before it gets official FDA approval for that indication.

Compounds Targeting the Serotonin and Dopamine Systems and Other Receptors

RP-5063 (also known as RP-5000) is referred to as a *serotonin-dopamine system stabilizer* by Reviva Pharmaceuticals. It is being tested as an atypical antipsychotic agent that targets a wide variety of serotonin, dopamine, histamine, and adrenergic receptors and transporters as well. It is reported to be a partial agonist at D_2, D_3, and D_4 dopamine receptors and at 5-HT_{1A} and 5-HT_{2A} serotonin receptors. But it may also affect 5-HT_7, H_1, D_1, D_5, 5-HT_3, 5-HT_6, and alpha$_{1B}$ receptors and the serotonin transporter. Due to its complex mechanism of action, it can be assumed that in addition to acting similar to an atypical antipsychotic, it may also have an array of side effects.

Blonanserine (Lonasen) has been used in Japan and Korea and is in clinical trials here in the United States. It is an SGA with the usual dopamine/serotonin antagonist profile with some D_3 and alpha-receptor blocking activity. It has no muscarinic- or histamine-blocking effects. It is said to have the highest D_2 receptor occupancy and lowest 5-HT receptor blocking potential of all SGAs (Kishi et al., 2013).

Lumateperone (ITI-007) is a novel SGA that is reported to have 60 times more potency at blocking the 5-HT_{2A} serotonin receptor compared to its effect at dopamine receptors. It is stated to be a partial agonist at presynaptic D_2 receptors, may have activity at the serotonin transporter, and may modulate phosphorylation at the NMDA receptor. It is being referred to as a *dopamine phosphoprotein modulator*. It does not bind appreciably to histamine, 5HT_{2C}, or muscarinic receptors, indicating a favorable tolerability profile. Major side effects in current clinical trials were reported to be sedation and somnolence (Citrome, 2016b).

Compounds Targeting the Histamine System

CEP-26401 (Irdabisant), developed by Teva Pharmaceuticals, is an H_3 receptor antagonist/inverse agonist. Although this drug blocks one of the histamine receptors, it also acts as an agonist on histamine function and is reported to produce alertness and wakefulness. This drug is intended to be used with an antipsychotic agent to minimize the sedation and cognitive deficits produced by the antipsychotic drug.

Compounds Targeting the Phosphodiesterase System

Several companies are testing compounds that are inhibitors of one of the phosphodiesterase (PDE) enzyme systems. Based on animal models that purport to show that inhibition of the phosphodiesterase enzyme leads to cognitive improvement, these drugs are expected to improve cognitive deficits of individuals who have schizophrenia.

Intra-Cellular Therapies, in partnership with Takeda Pharmaceuticals, is testing an inhibitor of PDE1. Boehringer Ingelheim Pharmaceuticals is testing an inhibitor of PDE9 (BI-409306).

Omeros Corporation is testing a compound, OMS 824, which is an inhibitor of PDE10. Takeda Pharmaceuticals is testing a compound, TAK-063, which is a PDE10 inhibitor for the treatment of cognitive dysfunction in individuals with schizophrenia. Inhibition of PDE10 is expected to increase levels of cAMP and cGMP, which are thought to be associated with learning and memory. Also testing a PDE10 inhibitor are Forum Pharmaceuticals (FRM-6308), Pfizer Pharmaceuticals (PF-02545920), and Hoffmann-La Roche (RO5545965).

Compounds Affecting the Cannabinoid Receptors

McGuire and colleagues (2018) conducted a recent study that involved individuals with diagnosed schizophrenia who had been stable on their current antipsychotic medication before entry into the study. In the double-blind protocol, these patients were randomly assigned to receive either cannabidiol (CBD) or placebo along with their antipsychotic medication. After 8 weeks of treatment, the results suggested that CBD may be a useful adjunctive treatment for schizophrenia. Those individuals who had received adjunctive cannabidiol had lower positive symptom scores and greater improvement scores on standardized clinician-administered rating scales compared to individuals who received the placebo.

Compounds Pairing Antipsychotic Drugs with a Compound to Counter Certain Side Effects

ALKS-3831, developed by Alkermes Pharmaceuticals, combines an SGA, olanzapine, with a mu-opiate receptor antagonist, samidorphan. Preliminary results suggest that the samidorphan may inhibit the weight gain normally seen with olanzapine, which would reduce the risk of metabolic side effects and drug discontinuation.

Sintocinon, a synthetic oxytocin nasal spray, is being tested by Retrophin as an adjunctive agent to treatment with antipsychotics. Oxytocin is a hormone thought to be involved in mood and emotions and as such, is expected to address the negative symptom of "flat affect," that is, the lack of emotional reactivity that can occur as part of the symptom picture of schizophrenia.

Minor Modifications to Existing Drugs

ALKS-9072 (aripiprazole lauroxil), with the trade name *Aristada* and developed by Alkermes Pharmaceuticals, is a once-per-month, long-acting injectable formulation of aripiprazole. The only difference between this formulation and another once-per-month injectable formulation of aripiprazole, *Abilify Maintena*, is the site of the injection. Whereas Abilify Maintena can only be injected into the gluteal muscle, aripiprazole lauroxil can be injected into either the deltoid or gluteal muscle. This provides an alternate injection site, perhaps avoiding any local tissue irritation or pain that may develop if only one injection site is used repeatedly. Aripiprazole lauroxil (*Aristada*) was approved by the FDA in October 2015.

Reckitt Benckiser Pharmaceutical is testing a compound, RBP-7000, which is a D_2 and 5-HT_{2A} receptor antagonist. This is a long-acting depot form of risperidone that can be given once monthly. It is a slight modification of the currently approved Risperidal Consta, which is a long-acting injectable formulation of risperidone that is administered once every 2 weeks. LY03004 (Risperidone CR) is being tested by Luye America Pharmaceuticals for the treatment of schizophrenia. LY03004 is another modification of a long-acting injectable formulation of risperidone that employs microsphere technology to allow for a long-term controlled release of the drug over time.

Another controlled release (CR) formulation of risperidone is being tested by DURECT, in partnership with Zogenix, under the trade name Relday. It uses a proprietary technology, SABER, to produce a slow, controlled release of the drug over time, seeking to reduce its side effects.

RECOMMENDATIONS FOR THE TREATMENT OF SCHIZOPHRENIA

There are several sources of guidelines for the treatment of schizophrenia. Although these sources are available and periodically updated, they are not fully utilized by clinicians who treat individuals with schizophrenia. A comparison of these guidelines reveals that they are generally similar in their recommendations and, for the most part, favor the use of SGAs over FGAs. Some of these guidelines also provide recommendations for nonpharmacological treatment interventions (Kross, 2016). The most commonly cited guidelines include are published by the following:

- The National Institute for Health and Care Excellence (NICE), which last updated its guidelines for the treatment of adults in 2014 and children in 2016.

- The Patient Outcomes Research Team (PORT) recommendations for the treatment of schizophrenia, which were last updated in 2009. The PORT provides a total of 16 psychopharmacologic and 8 psychosocial treatment recommendations (Buchanan et al., 2010; Kreyenbuhl et al., 2010).

- The American Psychiatric Association (APA), which last updated its treatment guidelines in 2004 and are not considered current (Lehman et al., 2004). The APA has issued a "Guideline Watch" document published in 2009 that provides more current information, but that document still does not reflect information available since 2009 and does not represent a complete revision of the original guidelines for the treatment of individuals with schizophrenia (Dixon et al., 2009).

All the other guideline documents are old and have not seen recent revisions, including: The Expert Consensus Guidelines (McEvoy et al., 1999); The International Psychopharmacology Algorithm Project (IPAP); and the Texas Medication Algorithm Project (T-MAP) (Miller et al., 1999). The last two algorithms include consideration of the outcomes from both the CATIE and CUtLASS studies. Given the age of the existing guidelines and algorithms, there is a need to have updated information for use by both clinicians and the public. (For a comparison of some of the above guidelines, see Milner and Valenstein, 2002.)

ADDITIONAL APPLICATIONS FOR SECOND-GENERATION ANTIPSYCHOTICS

The use of SGAs in disorders that do not present with psychotic symptoms has continued to advance (Maher and Theodore, 2012). For many of these disorders, the use of SGAs is considered off-label since they have not received FDA approval (Crystal et al., 2009). Although the FGAs are also known to be efficacious in the treatment of these disorders, the more favorable neurological profile of the new agents makes the use of SGAs preferable. The Agency for Healthcare Research and Quality (AHRQ) has reviewed the literature on the off-label use of SGAs (Maglione et al., 2011) and recently updated that information (Kondo and Winchell, 2016). At present, it should be kept in mind that most of the available evidence comes from evaluations of SGAs as adjuncts to other psychotropic medication treatments, that few direct comparisons between FGAs and SGAs have been published, and that there is a growing, but not necessarily adequate body of high-quality information on the long-term safety of the SGAs. This expansion of off-label usage continues despite FDA warnings about risks concerning the use of atypical antipsychotics in certain vulnerable populations (Kuehn, 2010).

Atypical antipsychotic drugs are being used both on-label and off-label for multiple disorders, such as bipolar disorder, resistant depression, and dysthymia, as well as behavioral problems associated with dementia, autism spectrum disorders, severe treatment-resistant anxiety disorders, and borderline personality disorder. These drugs are also being used symptomatically to treat anger, aggression, and tantrums in various behavioral dyscontrol disorders.

Given the broad use of SGAs across a range of disorders that display no psychotic symptoms, it is somewhat of a misnomer to refer to them as "antipsychotic" medications. However, since "antipsychotic" is generally accepted as the class of medications in this group, we will continue to refer to them as antipsychotic drugs.

Bipolar Disorder

Except for clozapine, paliperidone, iloperidone, and brexpiprazole, all the SGAs are approved by the FDA for the treatment of some aspect of bipolar disorder, such as acute manic phase with mixed features, depressed phase, and for maintenance. In addition, these SGAs can be used as adjuncts to other medications being used as the primary treatment for bipolar disorder and some can be used alone as monotherapy. Risperidone, olanzapine, quetiapine, aripiprazole, and asenapine have been approved to treat bipolar disorder in children (6 to 10 years old) and/or adolescents (10 to 17 years old) (see Bartoli et al., 2017; Dea et al., 2016; Fornaro et al., 2016; Grande et al., 2016; Hochman et al., 2016; Shah et al., 2017).

A combination product containing the SGA olanzapine and the SSRI fluoxetine (Symbyax) was approved in 2003 for treating acute bipolar depression. Warnings and precautions for this combination drug include the same warnings and precautions that would be attached to the individual drugs. In this case, the warnings and precautions for the antipsychotic component, olanzapine, include the possible development of leukopenia; its subtype neutropenia; and agranulocytosis, that is, low white blood cell (or neutrophil) counts; risk of hypoglycemia, dyslipidemia, weight gain, and increases in prolactin levels; and risk of serotonin syndrome when combining olanzapine and/or fluoxetine with other drugs that affect serotonin levels, such as MAOIs.[6]

Unipolar Depression

Only about one-third of patients with *major depressive disorder* (MDD) who receive initial antidepressant treatment achieve remission (see STAR*D study in Chapter 12). Many agents are used to augment antidepressant treatment. Among them, the typical antipsychotic drugs, that is, the FGAs, were known to be effective, but the risk of TD and EPS discouraged their use. The first report of the use of an SGA for augmentation in MDD appeared in 1999, when eight patients with a lack of response to selective serotonin reuptake inhibitors (SSRIs) showed rapid improvement with risperidone. This was followed by the first placebo-controlled study of the olanzapine-fluoxetine combination in fluoxetine-resistant depression (Shelton et al., 2005). Currently, the SGAs are becoming widely used for the purpose of augmenting treatment with either mood stabilizers for BPD or antidepressants for BPD and/or MDD (Papakostas et al., 2004, 2005; Rapaport et al., 2006; Simon and Nemeroff, 2005; Yargic et al., 2004). At this time, only aripiprazole and brexpiprazole have an FDA indication for the treatment of major depressive disorder as adjunctive treatment to antidepressant therapy. However, any SGA can be used off-label for this purpose or as monotherapy treatment for MDD. The use of atypical antipsychotic drugs as adjunctive treatments has also become part of clinical guidelines for the treatment of individuals who have MDD and who have not responded or not responded sufficiently to treatment with antidepressant medication alone (Patkar and Pae, 2013).

Reviews of the use of different SGAs as adjunctive treatment to antidepressants for major depressive disorder report no significant differences in efficacy among them. In general, efficacy of an SGA does not appear to be affected by the duration of the trial or, in those cases where treatment resistant patients were studied, how treatment resistance was determined. However, many of the studies showed that the discontinuation rate due to side effects was significantly higher for the patients whose antidepressant treatment was augmented with an SGA compared to patients receiving a placebo as the adjunctive agent. While rates of discontinuation did not differ among the SGAs, rates of specific side effects were very different for some agents. In addition, the effect sizes of the adjunctive antipsychotic treatment were small to moderate and there was no evidence that adding an antipsychotic drug to

[6]For a review of the use of SGAs in bipolar disorder, see Fountoulakis and coworkers (2012), Buoli and coworkers (2014), and Fornaro and coworkers (2016).

the antidepressant treatment improved the individual's functional ability or quality of life (Spielmans et al., 2013; Wen et al., 2014).

The newest atypical antipsychotic drug, cariprazine, was recently shown to be an effective adjunctive treatment for MDD when added to antidepressant treatment (Durgam et al., 2016).

Dementia

Antipsychotic medications are not approved by the FDA for the treatment of neuropsychiatric symptoms, including psychosis, in the elderly with dementia. The FDA maintains a black box warning (its highest level of warning) to notify prescribers of the increased risk of death related to the use of all antipsychotic medications in the treatment of elderly patients with dementia (Maust et al., 2015).

In general, meta-analytic studies have demonstrated that there is an increased risk of death attached to the use of antipsychotic medications in individuals who have dementia and that risk seems to be dose dependent, that is, higher doses of the antipsychotic result in increased risk of mortality. Further, antipsychotic polypharmacy, that is, using two or more antipsychotics, also increases the risk of mortality compared to monotherapy (Koponen et al., 2017; Maust et al., 2015; Schneider et al., 2006; Zhai et al., 2016). Recent evidence suggests that antipsychotic medications may increase the risk for pneumonia in individuals who have Alzheimer's-type dementia compared to a matched group of elderly without dementia (Tolppanen et al., 2016). Based on these results, antipsychotic medications should be used sparingly if at all in the treatment of behavioral and psychological symptoms of dementia.

Although not approved for this indication, it will be interesting to see if pimavanserin (Nuplazid) will be used off-label to treat hallucinations and delusions in individuals who have dementia as a potentially safer alternative to the traditional antipsychotic drugs (Hunter et al., 2015).

As a result of the FDA warning and these risks, the rate of prescribing antipsychotic medications for elderly patients with dementia has declined in the Veterans Administration (VA) system (Kales et al., 2011), but is still higher than expected and continues at high rates in community-dwelling elderly (Maust et al., 2017).

There are many reasons beyond those mentioned above to be concerned about the use of antipsychotic medication in elderly patients in general and elderly patients with dementia in particular. Elderly patients are prescribed a large number of medications to treat a variety of chronic medical conditions. Adding an antipsychotic medication to what is already prescribed (1) increases the complexity of the dosing regimen; (2) makes it more difficult for the individual and their caregivers to administer the medications; and (3) increases the risk for side effects and drug–drug interactions. Furthermore, the elderly are more sensitive to the effects and side effects of medications. Some of the more relevant concerns about potential side effects include hypotension, leading to dizziness and falls; metabolic side effects of weight gain, hyperlipidemia, and glucose intolerance; anticholinergic side effects, leading to blurred vision, urinary retention, constipation, and memory impairments; and neurological side effects of extrapyramidal symptoms and tardive dyskinesia (Rothenberg and Wiechers, 2015).

There are ongoing efforts to educate both professionals and the public about the use of antipsychotic medications in the elderly, especially those with dementia. The Choosing Wisely (campaign http://www.choosingwisely.org/) is an initiative of the American Board of Internal Medicine (ABIM) Foundation in partnership with a wide variety of professional organizations. Its goal is to advance a national dialogue on avoiding wasteful or unnecessary medical tests, treatments, and procedures. This is relevant for the elderly in that the campaign intends to limit treatments to those that are supported by evidence, free from harm, and are truly necessary. This makes sense when considering the use of antipsychotics or any other psychotropic drug in the elderly. The Center for Medicare and Medicaid Services (CMS) launched National Partnership to Improve Dementia Care in Nursing Homes (http://tinyurl.com/oh3569h), an effort in 2011 to reduce the use of antipsychotic medications in nursing homes. This initiative recommends evaluating nursing home residents who are receiving antipsychotic medications to determine if they need to be continued. If antipsychotic medications are started to address indicated target neuropsychiatric or behavioral symptoms, then the medications should be discontinued after a few months and the person reevaluated to determine if further medication treatment is necessary. The American Geriatrics Society (AGS) publishes a list of drugs that would cause increased risk when used in the elderly. These lists are known as the Beers Criteria and are updated regularly by the AGS (American Geriatrics Society 2015 Beers Criteria Update Expert Panel, 2015). Finally, nonpharmacological interventions may be more useful in the long term for addressing the neuropsychiatric and behavioral symptoms of dementia, such as caregiver education, problem-solving training, behavioral interventions, and music and aroma therapies (Rothenberg and Wiechers, 2015).

In certain circumstances, it may be impossible to avoid using antipsychotic medication to treat psychotic symptoms in individuals who have dementia, especially if those symptoms are causing significant impairment in the individual's level of function or increasing the level of dangerousness to self or others. In such cases, based on the guidelines noted above, there should be an attempt to discontinue the medications after a few months unless it can be established that the person would relapse if the medications were discontinued. One symptom that predicts increased risk of relapse is the presence of hallucinations. Individuals in nursing homes who had Alzheimer's-type dementia and the presence of severe auditory hallucinations prior to receiving risperidone—and subsequently had their hallucinations reduced by the drug—were found to be at three times the risk for relapse if the drug was switched to placebo compared to those residents who continued to receive treatment with risperidone (Patel et al., 2016). It may also be the case that some elderly individuals being treated with antipsychotic medication had initiated treatment when they were younger because they were, for example, diagnosed with schizophrenia. Thus, having been continually treated with these medications as they aged, some individuals may develop dementia. There would be no strong reason to abruptly discontinue the antipsychotic medication that has been effective simply because the individual is now older and may have dementia. Since there is limited literature of high-quality, well-controlled studies pointing to the benefits of using antipsychotic medications in this population, the decision to treat elderly individuals, especially those with dementia, will always involve a thorough risk/benefit analysis based on the indications and risk of treating versus risk of not treating the individual.

Autism Spectrum Disorders, Agitation, and Aggression

According to the CDC's Autism and Developmental Disabilities Monitoring (ADDM) Network, the prevalence of *autism spectrum disorder* (ASD) is 1 in 68 children based on the most recent surveillance data of 2012. Risperidone and aripiprazole are currently approved by the FDA for the treatment of severe irritability in ASD. Compared to the literature on the use of risperidone and aripiprazole, there have been few controlled studies to support the use of other antipsychotic medications (Ji and Findling, 2015; Politte et al., 2014). But other antipsychotic medications can be used off-label for ASD. No medications have been shown to be effective in the treatment of the core symptoms of ASD, but psychotropic medications like the antipsychotics have been used to treat some of the more disruptive and co-occurring conditions, including irritability, aggression, schizophrenia, depression, and obsessive-compulsive disorder.

Concerns have been raised about the long-term safety of using antipsychotic medication in children with ASD and the studies with risperidone and aripiprazole indicated higher rates of side effects compared to children who received placebo. In particular, risperidone produced weight gain, sedation, increased appetite, increased prolactin levels, and increases in identified cases of metabolic syndrome (Politte et al., 2014; Scahill et al., 2016). Chronic prolactin elevation may exert variable effects on puberty; may reduce bone mass; and is a risk factor in infertility, breast cancer, heart disease, and prostate abnormalities (Gagliano et al., 2004). Lastly, risperidone, like other antipsychotic drugs, can produce extrapyramidal symptoms, tardive dyskinesia, and the neuroleptic malignant syndrome. Aripiprazole has been shown to produce sedation and somnolence, weight gain, increased extrapyramidal symptoms, and vomiting (Politte et al., 2014).

Posttraumatic Stress Disorder

There is evidence for the effectiveness of SGAs in treating psychotic symptoms of *posttraumatic stress disorder* (PTSD). Most of the data come from studies of combat-related PTSD in patients either unresponsive or partially responsive to antidepressants. Clinical case reports support the use of risperidone (Bartzokis et al., 2005), olanzapine (Stein et al., 2002), quetiapine (Adityanjee, 2002), ziprasidone (Siddiqui et al., 2005), and aripiprazole (Lambert, 2006) in war veterans for reducing such symptoms as hyperarousal, reexperiencing, avoidance, nightmares, and flashbacks. Similarly, risperidone monotherapy was found useful for women with a current diagnosis of PTSD as a result of domestic violence or sexual abuse. An average risperidone dose of 2.6 milligrams per day significantly reduced avoidant and hyperarousal PTSD symptoms compared with the response of the placebo group, although there were no differences between the two groups on the Hamilton Rating Scales for Anxiety or Depression (Padala et al., 2006). Several small-scale studies have suggested that risperidone in particular may have benefit for reducing the reexperience symptoms of PTSD, but the results are based on small samples and lack of control for other interventions being received at the same time. A large-scale, long-term study conducted by the VA did not find any benefit of risperidone in reducing any of the core symptoms of PTSD (Spaulding, 2012). In addition, another VA study did not find any benefit of adding risperidone as an adjunctive treatment for veterans with PTSD who failed or had only a partial response to treatment with antidepressants (Krystal et al., 2011). Based on these negative studies, the VA and Department of Defense treatment guidelines for PTSD do not recommend using antipsychotics as adjuncts to antidepressant treatment. Antipsychotic medications, however, may still be useful to treat those individuals who have posttraumatic stress disorder and are expressing psychotic symptoms (Friedman and Bernardy, 2017).

Obsessive-Compulsive Disorder

Studies have examined using risperidone, olanzapine, quetiapine, and aripiprazole to augment the clinical response of patients with *obsessive-compulsive disorder* (OCD) who were refractory to SSRI treatment. Meta-analyses of these studies offer the following findings: in general, there is limited evidence for the effectiveness of risperidone and aripiprazole and only in short-term use. Quetiapine and olanzapine are not recommended (Fineberg et al., 2015; Veale et al., 2014). Other adjunctive treatments such as the addition of cognitive-behavior therapy (CBT) or clomipramine to the SSRI have been shown to be more effective than adding an antipsychotic drug (Veale and Roberts, 2014; Veale et al., 2014) and the use of antipsychotic agents increases the risk of side effects such as weight gain, metabolic disorder, extrapyramidal symptoms, and tardive dyskinesia. And there is some evidence that some SGAs, in particular clozapine, may induce or exacerbate OCD symptoms in individuals who are receiving the SGAs for the treatment of their schizophrenia (Fonseka et al., 2014; Schirmbeck and Zink, 2012).

Borderline Personality Disorder

According to the DSM-5, *borderline personality disorder* (BoPD) affects about 1.6 to 5.9 percent of the population. Of those patients diagnosed with BoPD, about 75 percent are female, and BoPD is about five times more common among first-degree relatives of those with the disorder than in the general population. The condition is characterized by a pervasive pattern of instability of interpersonal relationships, self-image and affect, and marked impulsivity. Some individuals with BoPD may also display episodic anger, aggression (toward self and others), and even frank symptoms of psychosis.

There is no drug that has been shown to be effective in treating BoPD. Most pharmacological interventions are targeted to some of the specific symptoms of the disorder. The FGAs have been shown to improve the impulsive anger and aggression found in some individuals, but their side effects outweigh the small benefit. The SGAs, primarily olanzapine and aripiprazole, have been shown to reduce affective instability, impulsivity, psychosis, and interpersonal dysfunction (Ripoll, 2013; Rosenbluth and Sinyor, 2012). However, in two meta-analyses of pharmacotherapy for severe personality disorders, antipsychotics were found to have a very small effect, with aripiprazole being more effective than other antipsychotics (Mercer et al., 2009). A Cochrane Library review found some evidence to support the use of olanzapine, ziprasidone, and aripiprazole to treat psychosis, aggression, impulsivity, and anger, but more data is needed (Rosenbluth and Sinyor, 2012; Stoffers et al., 2010). In general, the first-line, evidence-based treatment for BoPD remains the psychotherapeutic intervention known as dialectical behavior therapy (DBT), which is a specific form of cognitive-behavior therapy (CBT) developed by Dr. Marsha Linehan.

Parkinson's Disease

Anywhere between 40 to 60 percent of individuals with Parkinson's disease develop psychotic symptoms, primarily hallucinations and delusions (Cummings et al., 2013; Gadre and Netto, 2016; Schleisman et al., 2016). Use of typical antipsychotics to treat these psychotic symptoms has not been found to be useful in that the FGAs all block D_2 receptors, which worsens the movement disorder of Parkinson's disease that is itself caused by a reduction in dopaminergic transmission within the substantia nigra system due to loss of dopamine-containing cell bodies. Studies with the SGAs, particularly risperidone and olanzapine, which also block D_2 receptors, have found that these drugs are also not useful as treatment for the psychosis seen in Parkinson's disease. Successful treatment of psychotic symptoms in Parkinson's disease would rely on use of an agent that has low to no affinity for the D_2 receptor. Two SGAs, quetiapine and clozapine, have been shown to be of some efficacy (Connolly and Lang, 2014; Schleisman et al., 2016). It has long been appreciated that clozapine can reduce psychotic reactions in patients with Parkinson's disease who are receiving dopaminergic agents. Because of clozapine's undesirable side effect profile, quetiapine has become the preferred treatment (Comaty and Advokat, 2001; Reddy et al., 2002). The efficacy of these drugs may be due to their low affinity for the dopamine receptor, which prevents interference with the treatment of Parkinson's disease.

In 2016, the FDA approved a new drug with a specific indication for the treatment of psychotic symptoms in Parkinson's disease. Pimavanserin (Nuplazid) is a $5HT_{2A}$ inverse agonist with no significant dopaminergic, histaminergic, or cholinergic activity. It has been shown in several clinical trials to be effective in reducing the severity of psychosis and caregiver burden without exacerbating the movement disorder in Parkinson's disease (Cummings et al., 2013; Gadre and Netto, 2016; Schleisman et al., 2016).

Prevention and First Episode Psychosis

It has been over 60 years since the first antipsychotic drug was brought to market. In that time, even with the development of the SGAs, we have not seen much improvement in the efficacy of antipsychotic treatment. It is still the case that when treated with antipsychotic medications, only about 50 to 70 percent of individuals with schizophrenia actually reach the level defined as response and even fewer, 40 to 50 percent, reach the level defined as remission or recovery. Since the development of the SGAs, including aripiprazole and brexpiprazole, there have not been any truly new antipsychotic agents brought to market and the pipeline for development of new agents has slowed. In light of this status, research has focused more on attempting to identify signs and symptoms that would identify individuals who are at an increased risk for developing schizophrenia and developing potential interventions that would reduce the likelihood of those individuals actually developing the disorder. Thus far, interventions that have been tested include omega-3 polyunsaturated fatty acids (PUFAs), SGAs, and several psychotherapeutic interventions. Early studies seemed to support the efficacy of PUFAs in reducing the transition of individuals who were deemed to be at high risk to actually developing schizophrenia (Amminger et al., 2010; Stafford et al., 2013). This finding, however, has not held up in more recent analyses. McGorry and coworkers (2016), in a randomized, placebo-controlled, multicenter trial of PUFAs, did not find any advantage of PUFAs over placebo in reducing the transition to schizophrenia in individuals who were identified as being at high risk. Similarly, use of SGAs risperidone or olanzapine to treat high-risk individuals did not result in any substantial reduction in the rate of transition to schizophrenia when compared to placebo (Millan et al., 2016). Furthermore, although the psychotherapeutic intervention CBT demonstrated potential to delay transition to schizophrenia early in treatment (up to 12 months), this effect was no longer evident by 18 months post intervention (Stafford et al., 2013).

In addition to the research effort to predict in advance who may develop schizophrenia and provide early interventions, another research effort has been under way to address the need for aggressive treatment of first episode psychosis (FEP). In 2008, the NIMH launched a large-scale research project to explore using early and aggressive treatment that integrated a variety of different therapeutic approaches in a coordinated system of care model. The second goal of this study was to determine the most effective way in which to have behavioral health systems adopt and implement this model of care.

The Recovery After an Initial Schizophrenia Episode (RAISE) project (http://tinyurl.com/jurx5jj) has been funded by the NIMH, with additional support from the American Recovery and Reinvestment Act (ARRA). The program continues to evolve and has published results that thus far indicate that the model can be implemented, but not all locations around the country may have the resources to provide all of the supports necessary to fully implement the program. In those areas where the program has been successfully implemented, there is evidence to show that the program has been effective in reducing the disability associated with FEP (Kane et al., 2015; Srihari et al., 2014a; Srihari et al., 2014b). More work needs to be done in both the area of prevention and aggressive treatment of FEP.

STUDY QUESTIONS

1. What are the positive and negative symptoms of schizophrenia? Why are these symptoms important in drug therapy?

2. Which neurotransmitters are most involved in the pathogenesis of schizophrenia?

3. What are the primary clinical differences between traditional and atypical antipsychotic drugs?

4. Discuss the mechanisms of action of traditional antipsychotics and atypical antipsychotics.

5. Discuss the side effects of first- and second-generation antipsychotics.

6. Name the currently available atypical antipsychotic drugs. How are they alike? How do they differ? What appears unique about ziprasidone, aripiprazole, and brexpiprazole?

7. Why might antipsychotic drugs induce weight gain and/or diabetes?

8. Compare and contrast the newer atypical antipsychotics in terms of their efficacy, diabetes potential, effect on weight gain, QT effects, and other side effects.

REFERENCES

Adityanjee, S. C. (2002). "Clinical Use of Quetiapine in Disease States Other Than Schizophrenia." *Journal of Clinical Psychiatry* 63 (Suppl. 13): 32–38.

Advokat, C. (2005). "Differential Effects of Clozapine, Compared with Other Antipsychotics, on Clinical Outcome and Dopamine Release in the Brain." *Essential Psychopharmacology* 6: 73–90.

Advokat, C. (2010). "A Brief Overview of Iatrogenic Akathisia." *Clinical Schizophrenia & Related Psychoses* 3: 226–236.

Agid, O., et al. (2013). "Meta-Regression Analysis of Placebo Response in Antipsychotic Trials, 1970–2010." *American Journal of Psychiatry* 170: 1335–1344.

American Geriatrics Society 2015 Beers Criteria Update Expert Panel. (2015). "American Geriatrics Society 2015 Updated Beers Criteria for Potentially Inappropriate Medication Use in Older Adults." *Journal of the American Geriatrics Society* 63: 2227–2246. doi: 10.1111/jgs.13702.

American Psychiatric Association. (2013). *Diagnostic and Statistical Manual of Mental Disorders*, 5th ed. [DSM-5]. *American Psychiatric Association Publishing*, Washington, D.C.

Amminger, G. P., et al. (2010). "Long-Chain Omega-3 Fatty Acids for Indicated Prevention of Psychotic Disorders: A Randomized Placebo-Controlled Trial." *Archives of General Psychiatry* 67: 146–154.

Andreasen, N. C., et al. (2010). "Antipsychotic Dose Equivalents and Dose-Years: A Standardized Method for Comparing Exposure to Different Drugs." *Biological Psychiatry* 67: 255–262.

Ban, T. A. (2007). "Fifty Years Chlorpromazine: A Historical Perspective." *Neuropsychiatric Disease and Treatment* 3: 495–500.

Barnes, T. R. E. (1989). "A Rating Scale for Drug-Induced Akathisia." *British Journal of Psychiatry* 154: 672–676.

Bartoli, F., et al. (2017). "Benefits and Harms of Low and High Second-Generation Antipsychotics Doses for Bipolar Depression: A Meta-analysis." *Journal of Psychiatric Research* 88: 38–46.

Bartzokis, G., et al. (2005). "Adjunctive Risperidone in the Treatment of Combat-Related Post-traumatic Stress Disorder." *Biological Psychiatry* 57: 474–479.

Bechtold, J., et al. (2016). "Concurrent and Sustained Cumulative Effects of Adolescent Marijuana Use on Subclinical Psychotic Symptoms." *American Journal of Psychiatry* 173: 781–789.

Buchanan, R. W., et al. (2010). "The 2009 Schizophrenia PORT Psychopharmacological Treatment Recommendations and Summary Statements." *Schizophrenia Bulletin* 36: 71–93.

Buchanan, R. W., et al. (2011). "The FDA-NIMH-MATRICS Guidelines for Clinical Trial Design of Cognitive-Enhancing Drugs: What Do We Know 5 Years Later?" *Schizophrenia Bulletin* 37: 1209–1217.

Buoli, M., et al. (2014). "Is the Combination of a Mood Stabilizer Plus an Antipsychotic More Effective than Mono-Therapies in Long-Term Treatment of Bipolar Disorder? A Systematic Review." *Journal of Affective Disorders* 152–154: 12–18.

Bushe, C. J., et al. (2013). "Weight Change by Baseline BMI from Three-year Observational Data: Findings from the Worldwide Schizophrenia Outpatient Health Outcomes Database." *Journal of Psychopharmacology* 27: 358–365.

Caccia, S., et al. (2013). "A New Generation of Antipsychotics: Pharmacology and Clinical Utility of Cariprazine in Schizophrenia." *Therapeutics and Clinical Risk Management* 9: 319–328.

Cannon, T. D., et al. (2015). "Progressive Reduction in Cortical Thickness as Psychosis Develops: A Multisite Longitudinal Neuroimaging Study of Youth at Elevated Clinical Risk." *Biological Psychiatry* 77: 147–157.

Carbon, M., et al. (2017). "Tardive Dyskinesia Prevalence in the Period of Second-Generation Antipsychotic Use: A Meta-analysis." *Journal of Clinical Psychiatry* 78: 264–278.

Chang, A., and Fox, S. H. (2016). "Psychosis in Parkinson's Disease: Epidemiology, Pathophysiology, and Management." *Drugs* 76: 1093–1118.

Ciranni, M. A., et al. (2009). "Comparing Acute Toxicity of First- and Second-Generation Antipsychotic Drugs: A 10-year, Retrospective Cohort Study." *Journal of Clinical Psychiatry* 70: 122–129.

Citrome, L. (2009). "Clozapine for Schizophrenia: Life-threatening or Life-saving Treatment?" *Current Psychiatry* 8: 57–63.

Citrome, L. (2013b). "Cariprazine in Schizophrenia: Clinical Efficacy, Tolerability, and Place in Therapy." *Advances in Therapy* 30: 114–126.

Citrome, L. (2015). "The ABC's of Dopamine Receptor Partial Agonists – Aripiprazole, Brexpiprazole and Cariprazine: the 15-min Challenge to Sort These Agents Out." *International Journal of Clinical Practice* 69: 1211–1220. doi: 10.1111/ijcp.12752.

Citrome, L. (2016a). "Breakthrough Drugs for the Interface Between Psychiatry and Neurology." *International Journal of Clinical Practice* 70: 298–299. doi: 10.1111/ijcp.12805.

Citrome, L. (2016b). "Emerging Pharmacological Therapies in Schizophrenia: What's New, What's Different, What's Next?" *CNS Spectrums* 21(S1): 4–11. doi: 10.1017/S1092852916000729.

Comaty, J. E., and Advokat, C. (2001). "Indications for the Use of Atypical Antipsychotics in the Elderly." *Journal of Clinical Geropsychology* 7: 285–309.

Connolly, B. S. and Lang, A. E. (2014). "Pharmacological Treatment of Parkinson Disease: A Review." *Journal of the American Medical Association* 311: 1670–1683.

Crystal, S., et al. (2009). "Broadened Use of Atypical Antipsychotics: Safety, Effectiveness, and Policy Challenges." *Health Affairs* 28: W770–W781.

Cummings, J., et al. (2013). "Pimavanserin for Patients with Parkinson's Disease Psychosis: A Randomised, Placebo-Controlled Phase 3 Trial." *Lancet* 383(9916): 533–540. doi: 10.1016/S0140-6736(13)62106-6.

Dea, L., et al. (2016). "Management of Bipolar Disorder." *US Pharmacist* 41: 34–37.

de Bartolomeis, A., et al. (2015). "Update on the Mechanism of Action of Aripiprazole: Translational Insights into Antipsychotic Strategies Beyond Dopamine Receptor Antagonism." *CNS Drugs* 29: 773–799.

DeLisi, L. E. (2014). "Ethical Issues in the Use of Genetic Testing of Patients with Schizophrenia and Their Families." *Current Opinion in Psychiatry* 27: 191–196.

Dhindsa, R. S., and Goldstein, D. B. (2016). "From Genetics to Physiology at Last." *Nature* 530: 162–163.

Dixon, L., et al. (2009). "Guideline Watch (September 2009): Practice Guideline for the Treatment of Patients with Schizophrenia." American Psychiatric Association. http://psychiatryonline.org/pb/assets/raw/sitewide/practice_guidelines/guidelines/schizophrenia-watch.pdf.

Divac, N., et al. (2014). "Second-Generation Antipsychotics and Extrapyramidal Adverse Effects." *BioMed Research International* 2014 (Article ID 656370): 1–6. doi: 10.1155/2014/656370.

Durgam, S., et al. (2016). "Efficacy and Safety of Adjunctive Cariprazine in Inadequate Responders to Antidepressants: A Randomized, Double-Blind, Placebo-Controlled Study in Adult Patients with Major Depressive Disorder." *Journal of Clinical Psychiatry* 77: 371–378.

Ellinger, L. K., et al. (2010). "Efficacy of Metformin and Topiramate in Prevention and Treatment of Second-generation Antipsychotic-induced Weight Gain." *Annals of Pharmacotherapy* 44: 668–679.

Fellner, C. (2017). "New Schizophrenia Treatments Address Unmet Clinical Needs." *P&T* 42: 130–134.

Fineberg, N. A., et al. (2015). "Obsessive–Compulsive Disorder (OCD): Practical Strategies for Pharmacological and Somatic Treatment in Adults." *Psychiatry Research* 227: 114–125.

Fonseka, T. M., et al. (2014). "Second Generation Antipsychotic-Induced Obsessive-Compulsive Symptoms in Schizophrenia: A Review of the Experimental Literature." *Current Psychiatry Reports* 16: 1–17.

Fornaro, M., et al. (2016). "Atypical Antipsychotics in the Treatment of Acute Bipolar Depression with Mixed Features: A Systematic Review and Exploratory Meta-Analysis of Placebo-Controlled Clinical Trials." *International Journal of Molecular Sciences* 17: 1–13.

Fountoulakis, K. N., et al. (2012). "Efficacy of Pharmacotherapy in Bipolar Disorder: A Report by the WPA Section on Pharmacopsychiatry." *European Archives of Psychiatry and Clinical Neuroscience* 262 (Suppl. 1): S1–S48.

Friedman, M. J., and Bernardy, N. C. (2017). "Considering Future Pharmacotherapy for PTSD." *Neuroscience Letters* 649: 181–185.

Gadre, P., and Netto, I. (2016). "The Efficacy of Pimavanserin in the Treatment of Parkinson's Dependent Psychosis: A Review of the Literature." *Indian Journal of Applied Research* 6: 146–149.

Gagliano, A., et al. (2004). "Risperidone Treatment of Children with Autistic Disorder: Effectiveness, Tolerability, and Pharmacokinetic Implications." *Journal of Child and Adolescent Psychopharmacology* 14: 39–47.

Geschwind, D. H., and Flint, J. (2015). "Genetics and Genomics of Psychiatric Disease." *Science* 349: 1489–1494.

Gottesman, I. I., et al. (2010). "Severe Mental Disorders in Offspring With 2 Psychiatrically Ill Parents." *JAMA Psychiatry* 67: 252–257.

Grande, I., et al. (2016). "Bipolar Disorder." *Lancet* 387: 1561–1572. doi: 10.1016/S0140-6736(15)00241-X.

Green, M. F., et al. (2014). "The MATRICS Consensus Cognitive Battery: What We Know 6 Years Later." *American Journal of Psychiatry* 171: 1151–1154.

Guzowski, S. (2016). "The Direction of the Schizophrenia Drug Pipeline." *Drug Discovery and Development Magazine*. April 14. https://www.dddmag.com/news/2016/04/direction-schizophrenia-drug-pipeline.

Hartling, L., et al. (2012). "Antipsychotics in Adults with Schizophrenia: Comparative Effectiveness of First-Generation Versus Second-Generation Medications." *Annals of Internal Medicine* 157: 498–511.

Hilker, R., et al. (2018). "Heritability of Schizophrenia and Schizophrenia Spectrum Based on the Nationwide Danish Twin Register." *Biological Psychiatry* 83:492–498. In press. doi: 10.1016/j.biopsych.2017.08.017.

Hochman, E., et al. (2016). "Antipsychotic Adjunctive Therapy to Mood Stabilizers and 1-Year Rehospitalization Rates in Bipolar Disorder: A Cohort Study." *Bipolar Disorders* 18: 684–691.

Horacek, J., et al. (2006). "Mechanism of Action of Atypical Antipsychotic Drugs and the Neurobiology of Schizophrenia." *CNS Drugs* 20: 389–409.

Howes, O., et al. (2015). "Glutamate and Dopamine in Schizophrenia: An Update for the 21st Century." *Journal of Psychopharmacology* 29: 97–115.

Hunter, N. S., et al. (2015). "Pimavanserin." *Drugs of Today* 51: 645–652.

Jarskog, L. F. et al. (2013). "Effects of Davunetide on N-acetylaspartate and Choline in Dorsolateral Prefrontal Cortex in Patients with Schizophrenia." *Neuropsychopharmacology* 38: 1245–1252.

Javitt, D. C., et al. (2012). "Has an Angel Shown the Way? Etiological and Therapeutic Implications of the PCP/NMDA Model of Schizophrenia." *Schizophrenia Bulletin* 38: 958–966.

Ji, N. Y., and Findling, R. L. (2015). "An Update on Pharmacotherapy for Autism Spectrum Disorder in Children and Adolescents." *Current Opinion in Psychiatry* 28: 91–101.

Jones, P. B., et al. (2006). "Randomized Controlled Trial of the Effect on Quality of Life of Second- vs First-Generation Antipsychotic Drugs in Schizophrenia: Cost Utility of the Latest Antipsychotic Drugs in Schizophrenia Study (CUtLASS 1)." *Archives of General Psychiatry* 63: 1079–1087.

Jordan, S., et al. (2002). "The Antipsychotic Aripiprazole Is a Potent, Partial Agonist at the Human 5-HT$_{1A}$ Receptor." *European Journal of Pharmacology* 441: 137–140.

Kales, H. C., et al. (2011). "Trends in Antipsychotic Use in Dementia 1999–2007." *Archives of General Psychiatry* 68: 190–197.

Kane, J. M., and Correll, C. U. (2010). "Past and Present Progress in the Pharmacologic Treatment of Schizophrenia." *Journal of Clinical Psychiatry* 71: 1115–1124.

Kane, J. M., et al. (2015). "Comprehensive Versus Usual Community Care for First-Episode Psychosis: 2-Year Outcomes From the NIMH RAISE Early Treatment Program." *American Journal of Psychiatry* 173: 362–372. doi: 10.1176/appi.ajp.2015.15050632.

Kantrowitz, J. T., and Javitt, D. C. (2010). "N-methyl-d-aspartate (NMDA) Receptor Dysfunction or Dysregulation: The Final Common Pathway on the Road to Schizophrenia?" *Brain Research Bulletin* 83: 108–121.

Kantrowitz, J., and Javitt, D. C. (2012). "Glutamatergic Transmission in Schizophrenia: From Basic Research to Clinical Practice." *Current Opinion in Psychiatry* 25: 96–102.

Kapur, S., and Remington, G. (2001). "Atypical Antipsychotics: New Directions and New Challenges in the Treatment of Schizophrenia." *Annual Reviews of Medicine* 52: 503–517.

Kapur, S., and Seeman, P. (2001). "Does Fast Dissociation from the Dopamine D$_2$ Receptor Explain the Action of Atypical Antipsychotics? A New Hypothesis." *American Journal of Psychiatry* 158: 360–369.

Kishi, T., et al. (2013). "Blonanserin for Schizophrenia: Systematic Review and Meta-analysis of Double-blind, Randomized, Controlled Trials." *Journal of Psychiatric Research* 47: 149–154.

Komossa, K., et al. (2009a). "Sertindole versus Other Atypical Antipsychotics for Schizophrenia." *Cochrane Database System Review* (4): CD006752. doi: 10.1002/14651858.CD006752.pub2.

Komossa, K., et al. (2009b). "Ziprasidone versus Other Atypical Antipsychotics for Schizophrenia." *Cochrane Database System Review* (4): CD006627. doi: 10.1002/14651858.CD006627.pub2.

Kondo, K., and Winchell, K. (2016). "Off-label Use of Atypical Antipsychotics: An Update." In *Comparative Effectiveness Review No. 43*. (Prepared by the Southern California Evidence-based Practice Center under Contract No. HHSA290-2007-10062-1). Rockville, MD: Agency for Healthcare Research and Quality.

Koponen, M., et al. (2017). "Risk of Mortality Associated with Antipsychotic Monotherapy and Polypharmacy Among Community-Dwelling Persons with Alzheimer's Disease." *Journal of Alzheimer's Disease* 56: 107–118.

Kreyenbuhl, J., et al. (2010). "The Schizophrenia Patient Outcomes Research Team (PORT): Updated Treatment Recommendations." *Schizophrenia Bulletin* 36: 94–103.

Krystal, J. H., et al. (2011). "Adjunctive Risperidone Treatment for Antidepressant-Resistant Symptoms of Chronic Military Service–Related PTSD: A Randomized Trial." *Journal of the American Medical Association* 306: 493–502.

Kross, J. (2016). "Current Status of Clinical Practice Guidelines in Schizophrenia." *Psychiatry Advisor*. April 18. http://www.psychiatryadvisor.com/schizophrenia-and-psychoses/clinical-practice-guidelines-in-schizophrenia-psychosis/article/490531/.

Kuehn, B. M. (2010). "Questionable Antipsychotic Prescribing Remains Common, Despite Serious Risks." *Journal of the American Medical Association* 303: 1582–1584.

Lambert, M. T. (2006). "Aripiprazole in the Management of Post-Traumatic Stress Disorder Symptoms in Returning Global War on Terrorism Veterans." *International Clinical Psychopharmacology* 21: 185–187.

Lane, H-Y., et al. (2013). "Add-on Treatment of Benzoate for Schizophrenia: A Randomized, Double-blind, Placebo-Controlled Trial of D-Amino Acid Oxidase Inhibitor." *JAMA Psychiatry* 70: 1267–1275.

Laruelle, M., et al. (2003). "Glutamate, Dopamine and Schizophrenia from Pathophysiology to Treatment." *Annals of the New York Academy of Sciences* 1003: 138–158.

Laruelle, M., and Abi-Dargham, A. (1999). "Dopamine as the Wind of the Psychotic Fire: New Evidence from Brain Imaging Studies." *Journal of Psychopharmacology* 13: 358–371.

Lehman, A. F., et al. (2004). "Practice Guideline for the Treatment of Patients with Schizophrenia, Second Edition." *American Journal of Psychiatry* 161 (2 Suppl.): 1–56.

Leucht, S., et al. (2009). "Second-Generation versus First-Generation Antipsychotic Drugs for Schizophrenia: A Meta-Analysis." *Lancet* 373: 31–41. doi: 10.1016/S0140-6736(08)61764-X.

Leucht, S., et al. (2013). "Comparative Efficacy and Tolerability of 15 Antipsychotic Drugs in Schizophrenia: A Multiple-Treatments Meta-Analysis." *Lancet* 382: 951–962. doi: 10.1016/S0140-6736(13)60733-3.

Lieberman, J. A., et al. (2001). "The Early Stages of Schizophrenia: Speculations on Pathogenesis, Pathophysiology, and Therapeutic Approaches." *Biological Psychiatry* 50: 884–897.

Lieberman, J. A. (2004). "Dopamine Partial Agonists: A New Class of Antipsychotic." *CNS Drugs* 18: 251–267.

Lieberman, J., A., et al. (2005). "Effectiveness of Antipsychotic Drugs in Patients with Chronic Schizophrenia." *New England Journal of Medicine* 353: 1209–1223.

Lopez-Munoz, F., et al. (2005). "History of the Discovery and Clinical Introduction of Chlorpromazine." *Annals of Clinical Psychiatry* 17: 113–135.

Maglione, M., et al. (2011). "Off-Label Use of Atypical Antipsychotics: An Update." *Comparative Effectiveness Review No. 43*. (Prepared by the Southern California Evidence-based Practice Center under Contract No. HHSA290-2007-10062-1). Rockville, MD: Agency for Healthcare Research and Quality.

Maher, A. R., and Theodore, G. (2012). "Summary of the Comparative Effectiveness Review on Off-Label Use of Atypical Antipsychotics." *Journal of Managed Care Pharmacy* 18 (Suppl.): S1–S20.

Malhotra, A. K., et al. (2012). "Common Variants near the Melanocortin 4 Receptor Gene Are Associated with Severe Antipsychotic Drug-induced Weight Gain." *Journal of Clinical Psychiatry* 69: 904–912.

Marder, S. R., and Fenton, W. (2004). "Measurement and Treatment Research to Improve Cognition in Schizophrenia: NIMH MATRICS Initiative to Support the Development of Agents for Improving Cognition in Schizophrenia." *Schizophrenia Research* 72: 5–9.

Maust, D. T., et al. (2015). "Antipsychotics, Other Psychotropics, and the Risk of Death in Patients with Dementia Number Needed to Harm." *JAMA Psychiatry* 72: 438–445. doi:10.1001/jamapsychiatry.2014.3018.

Maust, D. T., et al. (2017). "Psychotropic Use and Associated Neuropsychiatric Symptoms Among Patients with Dementia in the USA." *International Journal of Geriatric Psychiatry* 32: 164–174. doi: 10.1002/gps.4452.

McEvoy, J. P., et al. (1999). "The Expert Consensus Guidelines Series: Treatment of Schizophrenia." *Journal of Clinical Psychiatry* 60 (Suppl. 11): 1–80.

McEvoy, J. P., et al. (2006). "Effectiveness of Clozapine versus Olanzapine, Quetiapine and Risperidone in Patients with Chronic Schizophrenia Who Did Not Respond to Prior Atypical Antipsychotic Treatment." *American Journal of Psychiatry* 163: 600–610.

McGorry, P. D., et al. (2016). "Effect of ω-3 Polyunsaturated Fatty Acids in Young People at Ultrahigh Risk for Psychotic Disorders: The NEURAPRO Randomized Clinical Trial." *JAMA Psychiatry* 74:19–27. doi: 10.1001/jamapsychiatry.2016.2902.

McGuire, P., et al. (2018). "Cannabidiol (CBD) as an Adjunctive Therapy in Schizophrenia: A Multicenter Randomized Controlled Trial." *American Journal of Psychiatry* 175: 225–231. In press. doi: 10.1176/appi.ajp.2017.17030325.

Meltzer, H. Y. (2012). "Clozapine: Balancing Safety with Superior Antipsychotic Efficacy." *Clinical Schizophrenia & Related Psychoses* 6: 134–144.

Meltzer, H. Y. (2013). "Update on Typical and Atypical Antipsychotic Drugs." *Annual Review of Medicine* 64: 393–406.

Meltzer, H. Y., et al. (2003). "Clozapine Treatment for Suicidality in Schizophrenia: International Suicide Prevention Trial (InterSePT)." *Archives of General Psychiatry* 60: 82–91.

Mercer, D., et al. (2009). "Meta-Analyses of Mood Stabilizers, Antidepressants and Antipsychotics in the Treatment of Borderline Personality Disorder: Effectiveness for Depression and Anger Symptoms." *Journal of Personality Disorders* 23: 156–174.

Millan, M. J., et al. (2016). "Altering the Course of Schizophrenia: Progress and Perspectives." *Nature Reviews Drug Discovery* 15: 485–515.

Miller, A. L., et al. (1999). "The Texas Medication Algorithm Project (TMAP) Schizophrenia Algorithms." *Journal of Clinical Psychiatry* 60: 649–657.

Milner, K. K., and Valenstein, M. (2002). "A Comparison of Guidelines for the Treatment of Schizophrenia." *Psychiatric Services* 53: 888–890.

Mullard, A. (2016). "2015 FDA Drug Approvals." *Nature Reviews Drug Discovery* 15: 73–76.

Mulle, J. G. (2012). "Schizophrenia Genetics: Progress, At Last." *Current Opinion in Genetics & Development* 22: 238–244.

Musil, R., et al. (2015). "Weight Gain and Antipsychotics: A Drug Safety Review." *Expert Opinion on Drug Safety* 14: 73–96.

Newman-Tancredi, A., and Kleven, M. S. (2011). "Comparative Pharmacology of Antipsychotics Possessing Combined Dopamine D_2 and Serotonin 5-HT$_{1A}$ Receptor Properties." *Psychopharmacology* 216: 451–473.

O'Brien, C. F., et al. (2015). "NBI-98854, A Selective Monoamine Transport Inhibitor for the Treatment of Tardive Dyskinesia: A Randomized, Double-Blind, Placebo-Controlled Study." *Movement Disorders* 30: 1681–1687.

Owen, M. J., et al. (2016). "Schizophrenia." *Lancet* 388: 86–97. doi: 10.1016/S0140-6736(15)01121-6.

Padala, P. R., et al. (2006). "Risperidone Monotherapy for Post-Traumatic Stress Disorder Related to Sexual Assault and Domestic Abuse in Women." *International Clinical Psychopharmacology* 21: 275–280.

Papakostas, G. I., et al. (2004). "Ziprasidone Augmentation of Selective Serotonin Reuptake Inhibitors (SSRIs) for SSRI-Resistant Major Depressive Disorder." *Journal of Clinical Psychiatry* 65: 217–221.

Papakostas, G. I., et al. (2005). "Aripiprazole Augmentation of Selective Serotonin Reuptake Inhibitors for Treatment-Resistant Major Depressive Disorder." *Journal of Clinical Psychiatry* 66: 1326–1330.

Paparelli, A., et al. (2011). "Drug-induced Psychosis: How to Avoid Star Gazing in Schizophrenia Research by Looking at More Obvious Sources of Light." *Frontiers in Behavioral Neuroscience* 5: 1–9.

Parkinson Study Group. (1999). "Low-Dose Clozapine for the Treatment of Drug-Induced Psychosis in Parkinson's Disease." *New England Journal of Medicine* 340: 757–763.

Patel, A. N., et al. (2016). "Prediction of Relapse After Discontinuation of Antipsychotic Treatment in Alzheimer's Disease: The Role of Hallucinations." *American Journal of Psychiatry* 174: 362–369. doi: 10.1176/appi.ajp.2016.16020226.

Patkar, A. A., and Pae, C-U. (2013). "Atypical Antipsychotic Augmentation Strategies in the Context of Guideline-based Care for the Treatment of Major Depressive Disorder." *CNS Drugs* 27 (Suppl. 1): S29–S37.

Poels, E. M. P., et al. (2014). "Imaging Glutamate in Schizophrenia: Review of Findings and Implications for Drug Discovery." *Molecular Psychiatry* 19: 20–29.

Politte, L. C., et al. (2014). "Psychopharmacological Interventions in Autism Spectrum Disorder." *Harvard Review of Psychiatry* 22: 76–92.

Potkin, S. G., et al. (2003). "Aripiprazole, an Antipsychotic with a Novel Mechanism of Action, and Risperidone vs. Placebo in Patients with Schizophrenia and Schizoaffective Disorder." *Archives of General Psychiatry* 60: 681–690.

Poyurovsky, M. (2010). "Acute Antipsychotic-Induced Akathisia Revisited." *British Journal of Psychiatry* 196: 89–91.

Procyshyn, R. M., et al. (2015). *Clinical Handbook of Psychotropic Drugs*, 21st ed. Boston: Hogrefe.

Rapaport, M. H., et al. (2006). "Effects of Risperidone Augmentation in Patients with Treatment-Resistant Depression: Results of Open-Label Treatment Followed by Double-Blind Continuation." *Neuropsychopharmacology* 31: 2501–2513.

Reddy, S., et al. (2002). "The Effect of Quetiapine on Psychosis and Motor Function in Parkinsonian Patients with and Without Dementia." *Movement Disorders* 17: 676–681.

Remington, G., et al. (2013). "Clozapine's Role in the Treatment of First-Episode Schizophrenia." *American Journal of Psychiatry* 170: 146–151.

Ripoll, L. H. (2013). "Psychopharmacologic Treatment of Borderline Personality Disorder." *Dialogues in Clinical Neuroscience* 15: 213–224.

Rosenbluth, M., and Sinyor, M. (2012). "Off-Label Use of Atypical Antipsychotics in Personality Disorders." *Expert Opinion on Pharmacotherapy* 13: 1575–1585.

Rosenheck, R., and Sernyak, M. J. (2009). "Developing a Policy for Second-Generation Antipsychotic Drugs." *Health Affairs* 28: 782–793.

Rothenberg, K. G., and Wiechers, I. R. (2015). "Antipsychotics for Neuropsychiatric Symptoms of Dementia—Safety and Efficacy in the Context of Informed Consent." *Psychiatric Annals* 45: 348–353.

Rummel-Kluge, C., et al. (2012). "Second-Generation Antipsychotic Drugs and Extrapyramidal Side Effects: A Systematic Review and Meta-analysis of Head-to-Head Comparisons." *Schizophrenia Bulletin* 38: 167–177.

Scahill, L., et al. (2016). "Weight Gain and Metabolic Consequences of Risperidone in Young Children With Autism Spectrum Disorder." *Journal of the American Academy of Child and Adolescent Psychiatry* 55: 415–423.

Schirmbeck, F., and Zink, M. (2012). "Clozapine-Induced Obsessive-Compulsive Symptoms in Schizophrenia: A Critical Review." *Current Neuropharmacology* 10: 88–95.

Schizophrenia Working Group of the Psychiatric Genomics Consortium. (2014). "Biological Insights From 108 Schizophrenia-Associated Genetic Loci." *Nature* 511: 421–427. doi: 10.1038/nature13595.

Schleisman, A., et al. (2016). "Treatment of Parkinson's Disease Psychosis." *U.S. Pharmacist* 41: HS20–HS26.

Schneider, L. S., et al. (2006). "Effectiveness of Atypical Antipsychotic Drugs in Patients with Alzheimer's Disease." *New England Journal of Medicine* 355: 1525–1538.

Schwartz, T. L., et al. (2007). "Aripiprazole Augmentation of Selective Serotonin or Serotonin Norepinephrine Reuptake Inhibitors in the Treatment of Major Depressive Disorder." *Primary Psychiatry* 14: 67–69.

Schwartz, T. L., et al. (2012). "Genetic Data Supporting the NMDA Glutamate Receptor Hypothesis for Schizophrenia." *Current Pharmaceutical Design* 18: 1580–1592.

Sekar, A., et al. (2016). "Schizophrenia Risk from Complex Variation of Compliment Component 4." *Nature* 530: 177–183.

Shah, N., et al. (2017). "Clinical Practice Guidelines for Management of Bipolar Disorder." *Indian Journal of Psychiatry* 59: 51–56.

Siddiqui, Z., et al. (2005). "Ziprasidone Therapy for Post-Traumatic Stress Disorder." *Journal of Psychiatry & Neuroscience* 30: 430–431.

Simon, J. S., and Nemeroff, C. B. (2005). "Aripiprazole Augmentation of Antidepressants for the Treatment of Partially Responding and Nonresponding Patients with Major Depressive Disorder." *Journal of Clinical Psychiatry* 66: 1216–1220.

Simpson, G. M., and Angus, J. W. (1970). "A Rating Scale for Extrapyramidal Side Effects." *Acta Psychiatrica Scandinavica, Supplementum* 212: 11–19.

Spaulding, A. M. (2012). "A Pharmacotherapeutic Approach to the Management of Chronic Post-traumatic Stress Disorder." *Journal of Pharmacy Practice* 25: 541–551.

Spielmans, G. I., et al. (2013). "Adjunctive Atypical Antipsychotic Treatment for Major Depressive Disorder: A Meta-Analysis of Depression, Quality of Life, and Safety Outcomes." *PLOS Medicine* 10: e1001403. doi: 10.1371/journal.pmed.1001403.

Spivak, B., et al. (1997). "Clozapine Treatment for Neuroleptic-Induced Tardive Dyskinesia, Parkinsonism, and Chronic Akathisia in Schizophrenic Patients." *Journal of Clinical Psychiatry* 58: 318–322.

Srihari, V. H., et al. (2014a). "First-Episode Services for Psychotic Disorders in the U.S. Public Sector: A Pragmatic Randomized Controlled Trial." *Psychiatric Services* 66: 705–712.

Srihari, V. H., et al. (2014b). "Reducing the Duration of Untreated Psychosis and its Impact in the U.S.: The STEP-ED Study." *BMC Psychiatry* 14: 1–14. doi: 10.1186/s12888-014-0335-3.

Stafford, M. R., et al. (2013). "Early Interventions to Prevent Psychosis: Systematic Review and Meta-Analysis." *BMJ* 346: 1–13.

Stahl, S. M. (2002). "Dopamine System Stabilizers, Aripiprazole, and the Next Generation of Antipsychotics. Part 1: Goldilocks Actions at Dopamine Receptors; Part 2: Illustrating Their Mechanism of Action." *Journal of Clinical Psychiatry* 62: 841–842, 923–924.

Stein, M. B., et al. (2002). "Adjunctive Olanzapine for SSRI-Resistant Combat-Related PTSD: A Double-Blind, Placebo-Controlled Study." *American Journal of Psychiatry* 159: 1777–1779.

Stoffers, J., et al. (2010). "Pharmacological Interventions for Borderline Personality Disorder." *Cochrane Database of Systematic Reviews*, Issue 6. Art. No. CD005653. doi: 10.1002/14651858. CD005653.pub2.

Stroup, T. S., et al. (2006). "Effectiveness of Olanzapine, Quetiapine, Risperidone, and Ziprasidone in Patients with Chronic Schizophrenia Following Discontinuation of a Previous Atypical Antipsychotic." *American Journal of Psychiatry* 163: 611–622.

Taipale, H., et al., Antipsychotics and mortality in a nationwide cohort of 29,823 patients with schizophrenia, *Schizophr. Res.* (2017), https://doi.org/10.1016/j.schres.2017.12.010.

Tamminga, C. A., and Carlsson, A. (2002). "Partial Dopamine Agonists and Dopaminergic Stabilizers, in the Treatment of Psychosis." *Current Drug Targets—CNS & Neurological Disorders* 1: 141–147.

Tenback, D. E., et al. (2010). "Incidence and Persistence of Tardive Dyskinesia and Extrapyramidal Symptoms in Schizophrenia." *Journal of Psychopharmacology* 24: 1031–1035.

Tiihonen, J., et al. (2009). "11-Year Follow-up of Mortality in Patients with Schizophrenia: A Population-based Cohort Study (FIN11 study)." *Lancet* 374: 620–627.

Tolppanen, A-M., et al. (2016). "Antipsychotic Use and Risk of Hospitalisation or Death Due to Pneumonia in Persons with and Without Alzheimer's Disease." *Chest* 150: 1233–1241. doi: 10.1016/j.chest.2016.06.

Tschen, A. C., et al. (1999). "The Cytotoxicity of Clozapine Metabolites: Implications for Predicting Clozapine-Induced Agranulocytosis." *Clinical Pharmacology and Therapeutics* 65: 526–532.

van Os, J., and Kapur, S. (2009). "Schizophrenia." *Lancet* 374: 635–645.

Veale, D., and Roberts, A. (2014). "Obsessive-Compulsive Disorder." *BMJ* 348: 1–6.

Veale, D., et al. (2014). "Atypical Antipsychotic Augmentation in SSRI Treatment Refractory Obsessive-Compulsive Disorder: A Systematic Review and Meta-Analysis." *BMC Psychiatry* 14: 1–13.

Wen, X. J., et al. (2014). "Meta-Analysis on the Efficacy and Tolerability of the Augmentation of Antidepressants with Atypical Antipsychotics in Patients with Major Depressive Disorder." *Brazilian Journal of Medical and Biological Research* 47: 605–616.

Yargic, L. I., et al. (2004). "A Prospective Randomized Single-Blind, Multicenter Trial Comparing the Efficacy and Safety of Paroxetine with and Without Quetiapine Therapy in Depression Associated with Anxiety." *International Journal of Psychiatry in Clinical Practice* 8: 205–211.

Zai, C. C. H., et al. (2015). "Association Study of GABAA α2 Receptor Subunit Gene Variants in Antipsychotic-Associated Weight Gain." *Journal of Clinical Psychopharmacology* 35: 7–12.

Zhai, Y., et al. (2016). "Association Between Antipsychotic Drugs and Mortality in Older Persons with Alzheimer's Disease: A Systematic Review and Meta-Analysis." *Journal of Alzheimer's Disease* 52: 631–639.

Zhang, J-P., and Malhotra, A. K. (2013). "Genetics of Schizophrenia: What Do We Know?" *Current Psychiatry* 12: 25–33.

Zhang, J-P., et al. (2013). "Efficacy and Safety of Individual Second-Generation vs First-Generation Antipsychotics in First Episode Psychosis: A Systematic Review and Meta-analysis." *International Journal of Neuropsychopharmacology* 16: 1205–1218.

CHAPTER 12

Antidepressant Drugs

In the 65 years since antidepressant medications were first introduced into medicine, these drugs have been heavily promoted by the pharmaceutical industry and prescribed by physicians in the hope that they may:

- Alleviate the signs, symptoms, and distress associated with clinical depression
- Relieve anxiety either as a single diagnosis or as part of a simultaneous diagnosis of anxiety and depression
- Improve the lives of persons with debilitating depression
- Repair the neuronal damage associated with depression

Given these promising expectations, however, to what extent have they been accomplished?

- Depression is only modestly improved by the use of antidepressant medication. This implies these drugs have only limited efficacy.
- Side effects of the antidepressant drugs can be very bothersome and may cause individuals to prematurely discontinue their treatment.

Questions about the true efficacy of antidepressant medication have been asked almost as long as these drugs have been marketed and efficacy questions continue to this day (Cipriani et al., 2016; Holtzheimer and Mayberg, 2011; Kahn and Brown, 2015; Nierenberg, 2011). Presently, as stated by Fournier and coworkers (2010):

> The magnitude and benefit of antidepressant medication compared with placebo increases with severity of depression symptoms and may be minimal or non-existent, on average, in patients with mild to moderate symptoms. For patients with very severe depression, the benefit of medications over placebo is substantial. (47) (Figure 12.1)

Unfortunately, in patients with mild to moderate depression, antidepressants remain frequently prescribed, this despite their lack of efficacy and bothersome side effects, including sexual dysfunction, weight gain, possible adverse cognitive effects, and even increased risk for suicidal ideation. This lack of response is frequently termed *treatment-resistant depression* (TRD) and additional medications are added, usually

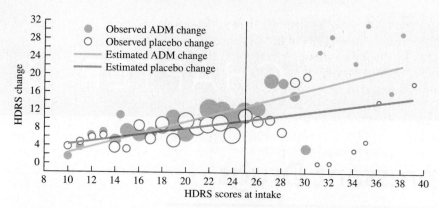

FIGURE 12.1   Efficacy of antidepressant medication and depression severity. Shown are the positive changes in the Hamilton Depression Rating Scale (HDRS, ordinate) after treatment versus the HDRS at the beginning of treatment (abscissa) in patients taking antidepressant medication (ADM, solid circles) or placebo (open circles). As illustrated, higher levels of depression at the start of treatment predicted greater medication response. The size of each circle is proportional to the number of patients at each HDRS score at intake. As illustrated, the few patients with very severe depression (HDRS scores >30) taking placebo pills exhibited wide variability in response. [Data from Fournier et al., 2010.]

producing little improvement but inducing additional side effects. There is little consensus on how to improve treatment outcomes. Combinations of antidepressants and psychotherapy differ only slightly from either alone, and alternative therapies have minimal efficacy. Perhaps "the type of treatment offered is less important than getting depressed patients involved in an active therapeutic program" (Khan, 2012).

DEPRESSION

Depression, or *major depressive disorder* (MDD) is a chronic, recurring, and potentially life-threatening illness. MDD is currently the leading cause of disability worldwide. According to the World Health Organization, depression accounts for 4.3 percent of the total worldwide burden of disease in terms of disability-adjusted life years (World Health Organization, 2013). Depression worsens the health of people with other chronic illnesses, has a tendency to recur, and is associated with increasing disability over time. About 4.7 percent of men and 8.5 percent of women experience depression in a year, and each year about 6.7 percent of the U.S. population, or approximately 16 million American adults, suffer with this illness (Substance Abuse and Mental Health Services Administration, 2016). Lifetime risk of depression has been estimated to be about 16 percent (Gartlehner et al., 2015). Depression is responsible for up to 70 percent of psychiatric hospitalizations and about 50 percent of suicides. And the number of total suicides per 100,000 population is increasing, according to the National Institute of Mental Health (NIMH). Unfortunately, the emphasis on identifying individuals who may be experiencing depression does not automatically translate into effective treatment. According to Olfson and colleagues (2016), only about one-third of those who screened positive for depression actually went on to get treatment. Holtzheimer and Mayberg (2011), as well as Olfson and colleagues, call for a rethinking of depression and its treatment.

Depression is an *affective disorder*, characterized by sometimes profound alterations of emotion or mood. Beside mood alterations, there may be decreased interest in pleasurable activities and in the ability to experience pleasure, sleep difficulties, fatigue or loss of energy, feelings of worthlessness or excessive guilt, and possible thoughts of death or suicide. Symptoms may be mild, moderate, or severe, depending on the extent of impairment in daily social and occupational functioning. Severe depression may be associated with symptoms of psychosis or loss of touch with reality. According to the DSM-5, individuals who experience ongoing symptoms of depression of any severity for a period of two years or more can be considered to have *persistent depressive disorder* (dysthymia) (American Psychiatric Association, 2013).

Symptoms of anxiety are also seen in many people with depression. Although many of the anxiety disorders have historically been treated with benzodiazepine anxiolytics (see Chapter 13), today antidepressant drugs are also used for treatment of many of the anxiety disorders. Not only are the antidepressant drugs efficacious for treating anxiety, they are less prone to induce dependence and less likely to impair learning, memory, and concentration than the benzodiazepines.[1] In addition to anxiety, individuals with depression may also frequently have co-occurring obsessive–compulsive symptoms and substance abuse (Kessler et al., 2003; Thaipisuttikul et al., 2014).

Pathophysiology of Depression

Historically, depression was conceptualized as a deficiency in the levels of various neurotransmitters, particularly the "monoamines" serotonin, norepinephrine, and dopamine. It was thought that restoring the levels of these neurotransmitters to "normal," usually by sustaining their presence in the synaptic cleft by blocking their degradation and/or presynaptic reuptake, was responsible for their efficacy in restoring a normal mood state. These proposed physiological theories of depression and the proposed effects of various antidepressants on these transmitter systems have not held up and have been largely discarded. In other words, although depression was once advertised as being the result of a "chemical imbalance" in the brain and that the antidepressants worked by correcting the imbalance, this theory has never been consistently shown to be true. In fact, one of the weaknesses of this chemical imbalance theory has been that there has been no consistent evidence to show that there is any deficiency of any of the neurotransmitters in individuals with depression compared to individuals without depression. Furthermore, studies in which the levels of these transmitters have been chemically reduced for a brief period of time have not consistently shown to produce depression in individuals (Lacasse and Leo, 2005). Another weakness of this model is that the neurotransmitter changes occur soon after drug administration, but the clinical antidepressant effect develops more slowly, often during several weeks of continuous treatment. This delay was hypothesized to be due to changes in receptor sensitivity caused by the chronic increase in synaptic levels of

---

[1]According to current diagnostic criteria, anxiety disorders include separation anxiety disorder, selective mutism, specific phobias, social anxiety disorder (social phobia), panic disorder (PD), agoraphobia, and generalized anxiety disorder (GAD).

neurotransmitter. In the past few years, however, this view has broadened, and attention has shifted to the study of the long-term actions of antidepressant treatments on intracellular processes, such as second messengers, and their functions in the neuron.

Two of these second-messenger functions are (1) to protect neurons from damage due to injury or trauma; and (2) to promote and maintain the health and stability of newly formed neurons. Research into these processes has led to a new way of thinking about depression (and the effect of antidepressant treatment) called the *neurogenic theory of depression.*

The neurogenic theory is a result of the relatively recent discovery that, contrary to what we once believed, (1) existing neurons are able to "repair" or "remodel" themselves and (2) the brain is capable of making new neurons (Andrade and Rao, 2010). In particular, it is now known that new neurons are produced throughout life in the hippocampus and the frontal cortex of several species, including humans. The birth of new neurons is called *neurogenesis.* This finding is especially relevant to understanding depressive disorders, because the hippocampus influences many functions that are impaired in a depressed person, such as attention, concentration, and memory. At the same time, we know that the hippocampus is also very vulnerable to the effects of trauma, such as hypoglycemia, lack of oxygen, toxins, infections, and especially stress, and to the hormones that are activated by stressful situations (such as corticosterone). In fact, stressful situations are known both to reduce hippocampal and frontal cortical neurogenesis and to damage existing neurons.

Among the stressful conditions that can damage the hippocampus is a state of depression—not surprising, as stress is believed to be one of the most significant causes of depression; about 50 percent of depressed patients have some abnormality in their physiological responses to stress. Moreover, hippocampal nerve cells are among the most sensitive to stress-induced damage. For example, depressed women with a history of child abuse have an 18 percent smaller left hippocampal volume than nonabused women (Grande et al., 2010). Remarkably this hippocampal shrinkage is reversible with antidepressant treatment, consistent with a role of neurotropic factors in neuronal plasticity in the hippocampus (Autry and Monteggia, 2012; Neto et al., 2011; Wainwright and Galea, 2013). Consequently, depression is now viewed as a neurodegenerative disorder (Andrade and Rao, 2010; Lucassen et al., 2010; Tripp et al., 2012). In fact, this is just one of the many theories that have been postulated to explain the development of depression. Alternative theories are the hypothalamic-pituitary-adrenal (HPA) axis dysfunction theory, the inflammation theory, and the stress generation theory (Wittenborn et al., 2016). Although each of these theories has attractive aspects to them, none of them have been shown to be sufficient to explain the complex and diverse symptom presentations of depression across individuals.

Just as a variety of stimuli can damage neurons and decrease neurogenesis, several factors are known to repair neurons and increase neurogenesis—among them, antidepressant drugs.[2] It has been proposed that the therapeutic delay in the clinical effect of antidepressants occurs because of the time required for new neurons to develop, mature, and become functional. This hypothesis is supported by the observation that the increase in neurogenesis requires chronic antidepressant administration, which is consistent with the time course for the therapeutic action of these medications. A major

---

[2] Other stimuli include electroconvulsive therapy, exercise, light therapy, and so on.

focus of current research is to identify the cellular processes in the hippocampus and frontal cortex that are responsible for the protective effects of antidepressants. Most current studies are directed toward the second-messenger systems, which are activated by the synaptic action of neurotransmitters. This action in turn stimulates production of intracellular proteins that control the expression of certain genes. (For a review of the neurobiology of depression and the significance of the influence of stress, inflammation, the immune response, and the effect of antidepressant drugs on these mechanisms, including neurogenesis, see Miller and Raison, 2016 and Wohleb et al., 2016.)

One of the intracellular targets of second-messenger systems is called *cAMP response-element-binding protein* (CREB). The fact that the amount of CREB protein increases in the hippocampus during chronic antidepressant treatment provides additional evidence for the neurogenic hypothesis. In turn, it is known that CREB activates genes that control the production of a protein called *brain-derived neurotrophic factor* (BDNF). BDNF is one of a group of substances called *neurotrophins*, produced by many brain structures, which are important for the normal development and health of the nervous system. For example, when injected into the brains of rats, BDNF not only prevents the spontaneous death of some neurons but also helps to protect neurons that have been poisoned with various toxins. Conversely, in animals, chronic stress decreases the production and amount of BDNF and other neurotrophic substances in the brain and increases cell death. As predicted by the neurogenic hypothesis, levels of BDNF and other neurotrophic substances increase in the hippocampus of rats chronically exposed to a wide range of antidepressants. Of particular significance, blood levels of BDNF are decreased in depressed patients, and some studies have found that antidepressant treatment can reverse this effect (Neto et al., 2011).

Launay and coworkers (2011) discuss the link between *fluoxetine* (Prozac), serotonin reuptake blockade, and secretion of *neurotropic factors* in the hippocampus. This mechanism may explain the synaptic action of fluoxetine and how its effect leads to the relief of depression. As stated, this appears to be the "missing link" between fluoxetine treatment and hippocampal neurogenesis; an intracellular protein (microRNA, or miR-16) sustains the hippocampal response to fluoxetine and other serotonergic agents.

If BDNF is deficient in the brains of depressed persons and if this deficiency leads to depressive symptomatology, might there be genetic influences that predispose a person to depression and perhaps offer new insights into therapy? Much has been done to elucidate candidate genes associated with major depression. Fabbri and Serretti (2015), Kupfer and coworkers (2012), Miller and Raison (2016), Mitjans and Arias (2012), Schosser and coworkers (2012), Narasimhan and Lohoff (2012), and Saveanu and Nemeroff (2012) all offer recent reviews of genetic factors in depression. Certainly, genetic variability in immune response, BDNF, as well as serotonin transporter genes appears to increase the risk of developing depressive disorders, including the risk of suicide (Miller and Raison, 2016; Sher, 2011). To date, these studies have not translated into new therapeutic drugs or into better choices of medicating depressive disorder, especially in treatment-resistant patients (Masi and Brovedani, 2011).

In summary, several lines of evidence suggest that depression is a consequence of stress, which, like any injury, disease, and physical trauma, damages the brain and weakens its ability to recover. Antidepressants relieve depressed mood by acting at the cellular level to promote neuronal survival and reverse stress-induced neuronal

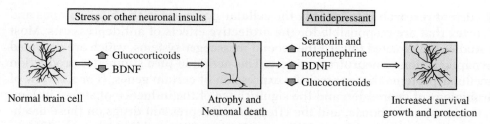

FIGURE 12.2   The figure shows a normal brain cell in the hippocampus on the left panel. In the middle panel, stress or other neuronal insults like hypoxia-ischemia, hypoglycemia, neurotoxins, and viruses can cause an increase in glucocorticoids and a decrease in the expression of BDNF. This combination causes atrophy of the brain cells in the hippocampus, which in turn leads to hippocampal shrinkage. Antidepressants and even ECT by elevating levels of serotonin and norepinephrine can increase the expression of BDNF and by reducing stress, can reduce the circulating levels of glucocorticoids, thus allowing for cell growth and increased cell survival. This leads to increased hippocampal volumes.

damage (Figure 12.2). Although the immediate effect of antidepressants is to modulate synaptic levels of neurotransmitters, their ultimate targets are the intracellular molecules responsible for maintaining neuronal health and plasticity. This reconceptualization of depressive disorder has broadened the search for new drug treatments, including agents that block the effect of stress hormones or that directly stimulate neurotrophic processes or directly block inflammatory responses (Cazorla et al., 2011; Fabbri and Serretti, 2015; Miller and Raison, 2016; Wohleb et al., 2016).

Evolution of Antidepressant Drug Development

Sixty-five years ago the antidepressant properties of the drug *imipramine* were discovered accidentally. Since then, it has been learned that imipramine and similar drugs, called *first-generation tricyclic antidepressants* (TCAs), block the presynaptic transporter protein receptors for the neurotransmitters, norepinephrine and serotonin (Table 12.1). Note that the term *tricyclic antidepressant* refers to a commonality in chemical structure, in contrast to newer antidepressants, which are defined by their mechanism of action. This is because, when the antidepressant effect of imipramine was discovered, its mechanism of action was unknown and its structural classification had to suffice, and so the classification persists to this day.

At about the same time the TCAs were discovered, another class of early antidepressant drugs, called the *first-generation monoamine oxidase inhibitors* (MAOIs), was identified. The MAOIs bind to and block the enzyme monoamine oxidase. This enzyme normally metabolizes and regulates the amount of the biogenic amine transmitters in the presynaptic nerve terminal. Therefore, the levels of these neurotransmitters increase and more transmitter is available for release when stimulated by an action potential reaching the nerve terminal. Both the TCAs and the MAOIs are effective in the treatment of major depression, but both possess adverse side effects discussed later in this chapter. Together, we refer to these two classes of drugs as *first-generation antidepressants*.

Problems with the first-generation agents prompted the search for new antidepressants that were equally effective and better tolerated, but less toxic. First was

TABLE 12.1 First-generation antidepressant drugs

Drug name: *Generic* (trade)	Sedative activity	Anticholinergic activity[a]	Reuptake inhibition		
			Norepinephrine	Serotonin	Dopamine
TRICYCLIC COMPOUNDS					
Imipramine (Tofranil)	Moderate	Moderate	+++	+++	+
Desipramine (Norpramin)	Low	Low	++++	++	+
Trimipramine (Surmontil)	High	Moderate	++	+	+
Protriptyline (Vivactil)	Moderate	Moderate	++++	++	+
Nortriptyline (Pamelor, Aventyl)	Moderate	Low	++++	++	+
Amitriptyline (Elavil)	High	High	+++	+++	+
Doxepin (Adapin, Sinequan, Silenor)	High	Moderate	+++	++	+
Clomipramine (Anafranil)	High	High	+++	++++	+
HETEROCYCLIC COMPOUNDS					
Amoxapine (Asendin)[b]	Moderate	Moderate	++++	++	+
Maprotiline (Ludiomil)	High	Moderate	++++	+	=
Trazodone (Desyrel, Oleptro)	Moderate	Low	0	++	0
MAO INHIBITORS					
Phenelzine (Nardil)	Moderate	Moderate	0	0	0
Isocarboxazid (Marplan, Enerzer)	Low	Low	0	0	0
Tranylcypromine (Parnate)	Moderate	Low	0	0	0
Selegiline (Deprenyl, Emsam)	Low	Low	0	0	0

[a]Anticholinergic activity is reflected in symptoms such as dry mouth, blurred vision, urinary retention, tachycardia, and constipation.
[b]Also has antipsychotic effects due to blockade of dopamine receptors.

the development of several drugs that were slight modifications of the basic tricyclic structure but that still exhibited antidepressant efficacy. These drugs were termed *first-generation-heterocyclic*, or *atypical antidepressants* (see Table 12.1).

During the late 1980s and continuing through to the present, newer classes of antidepressants have been developed that are grouped according to their proposed mechanism of action. These *second-generation agents* have varying degrees of monoamine uptake blocking properties as well as specific presynaptic receptor blocking properties. The first class of such second-generation drugs were the *selective serotonin reuptake inhibitors* (SSRIs), the first of which was *fluoxetine* (Prozac) (Table 12.2). Five more SSRIs were eventually marketed. Today, because of the limitations and side effects of the SSRIs, antidepressant drug research is progressing to identify compounds that act by different mechanisms. These drugs are not necessarily more clinically efficacious than the older TCAs, but they may have a more favorable profile of toxicity or side effects. The availability of the newer drugs has not yet reduced the number of treatment-resistant patients with major depression; the new drugs have only altered the profile of side effects. Three main therapeutic improvements still must be met: (1) superior efficacy, especially for treatment-resistant depression; (2) faster onset of action; and (3) improved side effect profile. The following discussion of specific antidepressant drugs is subdivided into categories according to the chronology of their introduction into medicine and the neurotransmitters on which each group is thought to act.

Did You Know?

Mystery Biography

I was born on September 2, 1948, in Shreveport, Louisiana. By the time I reached high school, I was well known for my athletic abilities—I set a national record for the javelin throw at 245 feet and was featured in *Sports Illustrated*'s Faces in the Crowd. I purposely failed my entrance exam to LSU, choosing to attend Louisiana Tech University. I was a big frat boy, pledging with Tau Kappa Epsilon. By the time 1970 rolled around, I was the first-round draft pick in the NFL, having amassed quite a record during my college years in the sport of football. In 1996, I was voted into the College Football Hall of Fame. During my time in the NFL, I started out a bit erratic, but quickly settled into my role as a team leader to four Super Bowl titles over the course of my career. I am even a key player in one of the most well-known football plays of all time. I had a 13-year football career, eventually retiring due to elbow, neck, and shoulder injuries. I was admitted into the Hall of Fame in 1989. I recently divulged to the media my corticosteroid use in the 1970s, and have been known to abuse alcohol. Specifically, following each of my divorces, I would often sink into a deep depression and have severe anxiety attacks. I attempted to self-medicate with alcohol and experienced weight loss, sleeplessness, and frequent crying episodes. I finally hit rock bottom and got myself to a psychiatrist, where I was diagnosed with clinical depression. I am currently taking Paxil CR, and feel that my depression has been well managed, though I have been living with this illness for more than 5 years. In 2001, I received a star on the Hollywood Walk of Fame, the only NFL player to achieve this accomplishment. I've written several best-selling books as well. I am living proof that one can live a successful life without being hindered by depression, as long as it is successfully treated. It took me taking that first step to ask for help in order to get myself where I am today; I am currently a spokesman for depression education programs.

Who am I? . . . Terry Bradshaw.

TABLE 12.2 Second-generation antidepressant drugs

Drug name: Generic (trade)	Sedative activity	Anticholinergic activity[a]	Reuptake inhibition		
			Norepinephrine	Serotonin	Dopamine
SELECTIVE SEROTONIN UPTAKE INHIBITORS (SSRIs)					
Fluoxetine (Prozac, Sarafem)	Low	Low	+	++++	0
Sertraline (Zoloft)	None	Low	+	+++++	++
Paroxetine (Paxil)	None	Low	+++	+++++	++
Fluvoxamine (Luvox)	None	None	++	++++	0
Citalopram (Celexa)	Moderate	Low	+	++++	0
Escitalopram (Lexapro)	Low	Low	+	++++	0
NOREPINEPHRINE + DOPAMINE REUPTAKE INHIBITORS (NDRIs)					
Bupropion (Wellbutrin, Zyban, Aplenzin, Forfivo)	Low	None	+	0	++
SEROTONIN + NOREPINEPHRINE REUPTAKE INHIBITORS (SNRIs)					
Venlafaxine (Effexor)	None	None	+	+++	+
Duloxetine (Cymbalta)	Low	Low	++++	+++++	++
Desvenlafaxine (Pristiq, Khedezla)	None	None	+	+++	+
Levomilnacipran (Fetzima)	None	None	+++	+++	0
SEROTONIN-2 ANTAGONISTS/REUPTAKE INHIBITORS (SARIs)					
Nefazodone (Serzone)	None	None	++	++	++
NORADRENERGIC/SPECIFIC SEROTONERGIC ANTIDEPRESSANTS (NASSAs)					
Mirtazapine (Remeron)	High	Moderate	+	0	0
ATYPICAL ANTIDEPRESSANTS (SSRI +)					
Vilazodone (Viibryd)	Low	Low	+++	++++	++
Vortioxetine (Trintellix)	None	None	++	++++	+

[a]Anticholinergic activity is reflected in symptoms such as dry mouth, blurred vision, urinary retention, tachycardia, and constipation.

FIRST-GENERATION ANTIDEPRESSANTS

The first two classes of antidepressants, TCAs and MAOIs (see Table 12.1), were introduced into medicine in the late 1950s and early 1960s. Drugs of both classes primarily increased the levels of norepinephrine and serotonin in the brain, which led the medical community to infer that depression resulted from a relative deficiency of these neurotransmitters. Conversely, excesses in the amounts of these transmitters were thought to lead to a state of mania. This *monoamine (receptor) hypothesis of mania and depression* did not withstand further examination because no significant deficits or excesses in the levels of norepinephrine or serotonin have been found in individuals with depression or mania, respectively. At the time, however, this concept guided the development of additional antidepressants having the same mechanism of action.

Tricyclic Antidepressants

The term *tricyclic antidepressant* describes a class of drugs that all have a characteristic three-ring molecular core. TCAs not only effectively relieve symptoms of depression; they also possess significant anxiolytic and analgesic actions. Historically, the TCAs were drugs of first choice for the treatment of major depression. The SSRIs, now being widely prescribed, are no more effective and may be considerably more expensive than TCAs. But they are less toxic, and their use is promoted by having a higher rate of patient comfort and compliance.

    Imipramine (Tofranil) is the prototype TCA, but another clinically available TCA, *desipramine* (Norpramin), is the pharmacologically active intermediate metabolite of imipramine. Likewise, *amitriptyline* (Elavil) has an active intermediate metabolite, *nortriptyline* (Pamelor, Aventyl). In fact, these two active intermediates may actually be responsible for much of the antidepressant effect of both imipramine and amitriptyline, respectively.

Mechanism of Action

TCAs exert two significant pharmacologic actions that are presumed to account for both the therapeutic effects and most side effects of these drugs:

1. They block the *presynaptic reuptake transporter* for norepinephrine and serotonin. They were therefore the first "dual action" antidepressants, decades before *venlafaxine* (Effexor) and *duloxetine* (Cymbalta).
2. TCAs block *postsynaptic receptors* for histamine and acetylcholine. Such blockade accounts for most of the side effects of this class of drugs.

    In addition to blocking receptors for histamine and acetylcholine, many of the TCAs also block alpha adrenergic receptors. Blocking alpha adrenergic receptors on peripheral blood vessels leads to dilation and a resultant drop in blood pressure, especially evident when a person transitions from a supine or seated position to standing. The subsequent abrupt drop in blood pressure can cause dizziness, increased heart rate (palpitations), and fainting (orthostatic hypotension).

    The therapeutic effects of the TCAs result from blockade of presynaptic serotonin and norepinephrine reuptake transporters. Blockade of histamine receptors results in drowsiness and sedation, an effect similar to the sedation seen after administration of the classic antihistamine *diphenhydramine* (Benadryl). Blockade of acetylcholine receptors results in confusion, memory and cognitive impairments, dry mouth, blurred vision, increased heart rate, constipation, and urinary retention.

In general, nortriptyline and desipramine are reasonable choices for initial treatment of depression when therapy with a TCA is chosen. These two TCAs cause less sedation and exert fewer anticholinergic side effects, such as cognitive impairment, than most other TCAs. Moreover, nortriptyline is known to have a therapeutic range, or window: the maximum response is most likely at blood drug concentrations between 50 and 150 nanograms per milliliter (ng/mL), which can easily be measured in clinical practice. For example, if someone is being treated with what would be considered adequate oral doses of nortriptyline and there is no apparent effect, one of the things to consider is that the blood level of the drug is below the lower end of its therapeutic window (<50 ng/mL). This could be the result of a more rapid metabolism of the drug by this individual. Similarly, if someone is experiencing several side effects, but their oral dose of the drug is relatively low, one of the possible causes is that that individual's blood level of nortriptyline is above the upper limit of the therapeutic window (>150 ng/mL). This could be the result of a slower rate of metabolism of the drug by this individual. Having the ability to use *therapeutic drug monitoring* (TDM), that is, measuring the blood levels of the drug, can assist the prescriber in making more accurate and evidence-based decisions about what steps to take next based on a person's clinical response to any drug treatment. Additionally, clinically available genomic tests advertise that they can determine if an individual may have lower or higher levels of liver enzyme activity that in turn can influence blood levels of a drug. A discussion of use of genomic tests to assist in treatment decisions is discussed in Chapter 11.

Pharmacokinetics

The TCAs are well absorbed when administered orally. Because most of them have relatively long half-lives, taking them at bedtime can reduce the impact of unwanted side effects, especially persistent sedation. These drugs are metabolized in the liver. As discussed earlier, two TCAs, imipramine and amitriptyline, are converted into pharmacologically active intermediates, that is, desmethylimipramine and nortriptyline, respectively, which are detoxified later. This combination of a pharmacologically active drug and active metabolite results in a clinical effect lasting up to four days, even longer in elderly patients, who can be adversely affected by the detrimental cognitive and other anticholinergic and sedative effects of these drugs.

TCAs readily cross the placental barrier. However, in utero exposure does not affect global IQ, language development, or behavioral development in preschool children. No fetal abnormalities from these drugs have yet been reported.

Pharmacological Effects

All the TCAs attach to and inhibit (to varying degrees) the presynaptic transporter proteins for both norepinephrine and serotonin, which is thought to account for their therapeutic efficacy. The TCAs, however, have three clinical limitations. First, TCAs in clinical practice have a slow onset of action, although overall, they seem to start acting as fast as any other antidepressant drug, provided that comparable dosage strategies can be tolerated. Second, the TCAs exert a wide variety of effects on the CNS, causing numerous adverse side effects that the SSRIs do not cause. Third, in overdose (as in suicide attempts), TCAs are cardiotoxic and potentially fatal because they can cause cardiac arrhythmias.

Because TCAs do not produce euphoria, they have no recreational or addictive liability. Therefore, abuse and psychological dependence are not concerns. The clinical choice of TCA is determined by effectiveness, tolerance of side effects, prior good response, family history of good response, and duration of action of the particular agent.

In depressed patients, TCAs elevate mood, increase physical activity, improve appetite and sleep patterns, and reduce morbid preoccupation. They are useful in treating acute episodes of major depression as well as in preventing relapses. Some patients resistant to other antidepressants respond favorably to a TCA. In addition, TCAs are clinically effective in the long-term therapy of dysthymia and in treating bipolar depression as an adjunct to a mood stabilizer, although the SSRIs are equally efficacious and better tolerated.

TCAs are effective analgesics in a variety of clinical pain syndromes, and they are consistently superior to placebo in the treatment of chronic pain. Uses include diabetes-associated peripheral neuropathies, postherpetic neuralgia, migraine headache, fibromyalgia, chronic back pain, myofascial pain, and chronic fatigue. The antidepressant action may not only provide analgesic relief but also promote well-being and improve affect as it reduces physical discomfort. One review compared the analgesic effect of three types of antidepressants and it concluded that the TCAs were slightly more efficacious than the *selective norepinephrine reuptake inhibitors* (SNRIs), which were more analgesic than the selective serotonin reuptake inhibitors (Sindrup et al., 2005).

Side Effects

Side effects follow from the anticholinergic, antihistaminic, and antiadrenergic actions that can be attributed to TCAs. In the patient on long-term TCA therapy, tolerance may develop to many of these side effects, but some will persist. Often, choosing a particular TCA with an awareness of its side effects can turn a disadvantage into a therapeutic advantage. For example, amitriptyline and *doxepin* (Silenor) are the most sedating of the TCAs, making them useful in treating people with comorbid depression and insomnia. Administering one of these drugs at bedtime would provide both the antidepressant effect and the needed sedation. Silenor is formulated in a very low dose tablet (3 or 6 milligrams), which is about 10 times the price of 10 milligram preparations of generic doxepin, and has been shown effective in older adults with insomnia, but less so in younger adults.

The effects of TCAs on memory and cognitive function are significant. The direct adverse effects on cognition are related to the anticholinergic and antihistaminic properties of the drugs, which may be partly compensated for by the improvement in mood. Relatively nonsedating compounds with minimal anticholinergic side effects cause less impairment of psychomotor or memory functions. Therefore, because the young and the elderly may be more susceptible to the anticholinergic-induced impairment of memory, patients at the extremes of age, if treated with TCAs, should probably receive a drug with low potency at blocking histaminic and cholinergic receptors.

As already noted, cardiac effects can be life-threatening when an overdose is taken, as in suicide attempts. The patient commonly exhibits excitement, delirium, and convulsions, followed by respiratory depression and coma, which can persist for several days. Cardiac arrhythmias can lead to ventricular fibrillation, cardiac arrest, and death. Thus, all TCAs can be lethal in doses that are commonly available to depressed patients. For this reason, it is unwise to dispense more than a week's supply of an antidepressant to an acutely depressed patient who is a potential suicide risk.

There have been reports of a small number of cases in the 1990s of sudden death in children receiving desipramine for the treatment of attention deficit/hyperactivity disorder (ADHD) or depression. These deaths are cause for concern when using TCAs to treat depression in children, and the therapeutic efficacy of TCAs in treating major depression in children is questionable anyway (see Chapter 15). In cases where efficacy is more demonstrable—enuresis (bedwetting), obsessive–compulsive disorder (OCD), and ADHD—use may be appropriate. However, if TCAs are used to treat children, it is wise to be cautious, especially if they are also receiving other medications that could cause sudden cardiac death, such as the stimulants for ADHD. A consult with a pediatric cardiologist may be indicated before treatment is started.

Monoamine Oxidase Inhibitors

Monoamine oxidase (MAO) is an enzyme that regulates the amount of monoamine neurotransmitters (norepinephrine, dopamine, and serotonin) in the body and the brain.[3] Drug-induced inhibition of MAO by *MAO-inhibitors* (MAOIs) allows monoamine transmitters to accumulate within the axon terminals of neurons. Such blockade of monoamine metabolism causes transmitter molecules to build up in the terminal, which means that more transmitter than usual is released into the synaptic cleft upon activation. Such accumulation results in robust antidepressant action through a different mechanism of action than the TCAs. But the efficacy of MAOIs has been limited by potentially serious, even fatal, side effects. The risk of these side effects and potential fatalities has limited the widespread clinical utility of these drugs, although they remain a very effective treatment option for individuals who do not respond to other classes of antidepressant drugs or who may present with what is termed *atypical depression*. According to DSM-5, depression with atypical features includes depressive episodes that present with mood reactivity (brief elevation in mood to positive stimuli), weight gain or increased appetite (instead of weight loss or loss of appetite), hypersomnia (instead of insomnia), and heaviness in the limbs.

Three monoamine oxidase inhibitors were developed in the mid-1950s for treating major depressive illnesses (see Table 12.1). Because of toxicity, the need for dietary

---

[3] MAO is primarily found associated with the mitochondria and metabolizes catecholamines after they are taken back up into the presynaptic neuron from the synaptic cleft. Thus, MAO prevents excess catecholamines from being repackaged into synaptic vesicles for re-release. There are two MAO isoenzymes: (1) MAO-A generally metabolizes tyramine, norepinephrine (NE), serotonin (5-HT), and dopamine (DA); and (2) MAO-B mainly metabolizes dopamine (DA). There is an anatomic distribution of the isoenzymes. MAO-B is found primarily in the brain. MAO-A is found throughout the body and especially in the gastrointestinal tract, where it may serve to limit the absorption and physiologic effect of dietary monoamines.

restrictions, and the lack of training in the use of MAOIs, they are not used very frequently in clinical practice (Shulman et al., 2013; Treviño et al., 2017).

The use of the three traditional MAOIs is limited by potentially fatal interactions when taken with certain foods and medicines. Medicines include adrenalinelike drugs found in nasal sprays, antiasthma medications, and cold medicines. Foods include those that contain tyramine, a byproduct of fermentation, such as in many aged cheeses, wines, beers, liver, and some beans. Tyramine induces release of monoamine neurotransmitters, both elevating mood[4] but also increasing blood pressure. Too much tyramine release can elevate blood pressure to extreme levels, resulting in a heart attack or rupture of an aneurysm or vascular malformation, either possibly resulting in death. Because MAO is also found in the gastrointestinal tract, inhibition of the enzyme there blocks the metabolism of dietary tyramine, resulting in increased absorption of the compound. In the absence of MAO, tyramine may modestly elevate blood pressure; in patients on MAOIs, such elevation may be extreme. Nevertheless, although they are potentially dangerous, MAOIs can be used safely with strict dietary restrictions.[5] In general practice, there have been few instances of true adrenergic crises or serotonergic crises related to use of MAOIs, so the dietary risk may be less concerning than many prescribers believe (Shulman et al., 2013). In the past decade, dietary restrictions have been revised to minimize the inconvenience of avoiding foods that have little risk of producing deleterious effects (see Flockhart, 2012 and Shulman et al., 2013).

Interest in MAOIs has remained strong because: (1) they can be as safe as SSRIs or other second-generation antidepressants; (2) they can work in many patients who respond poorly to both TCAs and second-generation antidepressants; and (3) they are particularly effective drugs for the treatment of atypical depression, masked depression (such as hypochondriasis), anorexia nervosa, bulimia, bipolar depression, dysthymia, depression in the elderly, panic disorder, and phobias (Shulman et al., 2013). They just must be used with caution.

The three classic MAOIs are irreversible in their effect, since they form a chemical bond with the MAO enzyme that cannot be broken; enzyme function returns only as new enzyme is slowly biosynthesized. For this reason, patients who need to switch from an MAOI to another type of antidepressant must still observe the dietary restrictions and other precautions for approximately 10 to 14 days, until new enzyme is produced.

A few years ago, a specific MAO-A inhibitor, *moclobemide*, was developed that was reversible in action; it did not bond as tightly to the enzyme as the classic MAOIs. When detachment occurred, MAO was again able to metabolize the tyramine and the cardiotoxic risk was minimized. Unfortunately, although this was a logical approach for developing a better MAOI, moclobemide was not a very efficacious antidepressant and is not available in the United States (Finberg and Rabey, 2016; Latufo-Neto et al., 1999).

Interest in the MAOIs has undergone recent resurgence because of the availability of a new selective, irreversible MAO-B inhibitor, *selegiline* (Eldepryl), which increases dopamine neurotransmission in the brain. Initially, selegiline was used in the treatment of

---

[4] Do we "feel better" after drinking red wine and eating tyramine-containing meats and cheeses?

[5] Multiple sites on the Web detail tyramine-free diets for use when MAOIs are prescribed.

Parkinson disease (Fabbrini et al., 2012). Selegiline then became commercially available as a transdermal patch (Emsam) that allows for slow, continuous absorption of selegiline in dosage strengths of 6, 9, and 12 milligrams. At the lowest dose of 6 milligrams, food and drug interactions were not a concern because transdermal administration bypasses the gastrointestinal tract and does not achieve blood concentrations sufficient to seriously elevate blood pressure. At doses of 9 and 12 milligrams, however, selegiline loses its specificity for MAO-B and becomes an inhibitor of both forms of MAO. This means that dietary restrictions must be followed when using the two higher dosages of the patch. As initially reported by Amsterdam (2003), selegiline, as a patch delivering 6 milligrams daily, was robustly effective in reducing moderate to severe depression, with onset of effect in only a few days. Sexual functioning was not impaired and compliance was excellent. These initial positive results were confirmed in a long-term study in which patients with major depressive disorder who responded to selegiline during acute treatment (10 weeks) were either maintained on the drug or switched to placebo. After 52 weeks, significantly fewer patients taking selegiline relapsed (16.8 percent) compared with the placebo group (30.7 percent), and they did so after a significantly longer time on the drug than those given the placebo (Amsterdam and Bodkin, 2006). Pae and coworkers (2012) stated in their analysis of selegiline that "few patients reported a hypertensive effect, and there were no objectively confirmed reports of hypertensive crisis with food at any selegiline dose" (662). Therefore, for refractory patients with severe depression, transdermal selegiline may be unique in its efficacy (see also Nandagopal and DelBello, 2009).

HETEROCYCLIC ANTIDEPRESSANTS

Efforts from the late 1970s to the mid-1980s to find structurally different agents that might overcome some of the disadvantages of the TCAs, such as slow onset of action, limited efficacy, and significant side effects, and the hypertensive crises seen in MAOIs produced the so-called heterocyclic, or *atypical*, antidepressants (see Table 12.1).

Maprotiline (Ludiomil), developed in the early 1980s, was one of the first clinically available antidepressants (other than the MAOIs) that modified the basic tricyclic structure. It has a long half-life, blocks norepinephrine reuptake, and is as efficacious as imipramine, which is considered the gold standard of TCAs. However, it offers few, if any, therapeutic advantages. A major limitation of maprotiline is that, depending on the dose, it can cause seizures in rare cases, presumably because of the accumulation of active metabolites that excite the CNS. It is generally not an antidepressant of first choice.

Amoxapine (Asendin), also introduced in the early 1980s, is the second heterocyclic antidepressant, structurally different from the TCAs. It is primarily a norepinephrine reuptake inhibitor but is also a potent blocker of serotonin 5-HT_{2A} receptors. It is clinically as effective as imipramine, although it may be slightly better at relieving accompanying anxiety and agitation. Amoxapine may produce parkinsonianlike side effects as a result of postsynaptic dopamine receptor blockade. The drug is metabolized to an active intermediate, 8-hydroxy-amoxapine, which may be responsible for the dopamine receptor blockade. As with TCAs, overdose can result in fatality. For this reason, amoxapine is also not an antidepressant of first choice.

Trazodone (Desyrel), FDA approved in 1981, is the third heterocyclic antidepressant, therapeutically as efficacious as the TCAs. However, it is not a potent reuptake blocker of either norepinephrine or serotonin, although its active metabolite, m-chlorophenyl-piperazine, is a serotonin agonist. Drowsiness is the most common side effect. This property makes this drug an attractive sleep aid for prescribers who wish to avoid the use of benzodiazepines (Chapter 13) or nonbenzodiazepine GABA receptor hypnotics (for example, "Z" drugs like zolpidem, Chapter 13). Taken at bedtime in the 25- to 100-milligram range, trazodone essentially blocks all 5-HT_{2A} receptors (at 10 milligrams), and about half of the alpha-1 adrenergic receptors and histamine receptors, producing a good night's sleep. While about 50 percent of the serotonin transporters are blocked at such doses, it is not enough for an antidepressant action. Therefore, traditional trazodone, available as a short-acting, immediate-release (IR) formulation, has often been used as a hypnotic (even though the FDA has not approved it for this indication). Its peak effect is reached and then declines relatively rapidly, and this "pulsatile" action is less likely to produce tolerance.

A new formulation of trazodone, Oleptro, an extended-release, once-daily preparation, was approved in 2010 for the treatment of major depressive disorder in adults. This formulation, in a dose of 300 milligrams, apparently provides sufficiently constant blood levels for an antidepressant effect; tolerance gradually develops to the sedation over several days. With this pharmacokinetic modification, it may be possible to regain the antidepressant benefit of trazodone. Certainly, daytime sedation may be a continuing problem with this extended-release formulation of trazodone.

Trazodone's main side effect can be serious: in rare instances, priapism (prolonged and painful penile or clitoral erection) occurs. This side effect requires prompt attention because it can lead to permanent impotence and infertility and in the case of a sustained erection, if not treated immediately, amputation due to gangrene. Any detrimental effects of an overdose of trazodone on cognitive functioning appear modest.

Clomipramine (Anafranil) is structurally a TCA, but it has a greater effect on serotonin reuptake than the classic TCAs. It is an effective antidepressant and anxiolytic. In addition, it and its active metabolite, desmethylclomipramine, also inhibit norepinephrine reuptake. Thus, it is classified as a *mixed serotonin-norepinephrine reuptake inhibitor,* similar to venlafaxine (discussed in the next sections). Clomipramine is approximately equal to the TCAs in both its efficacy and its profile of side effects.

Clomipramine has long been used to treat OCD; about 40 to 75 percent of patients with OCD respond favorably. The drug has also been used in the treatment of panic disorder and phobic disorders. Historically, it was the first antidepressant medication to be appreciated as having efficacy in the treatment of anxiety disorders, an observation later applied to the SSRI-type antidepressants.

Psychostimulants, such as the *amphetamines* and *methylphenidates*, release the neurotransmitters dopamine and norepinephrine from nerve terminals in the brain. They are occasionally examined for antidepressant efficacy (Howland, 2012). Widely used for over 60 years to treat ADHD, they promote alertness and reduce fatigue, both important features of depression. In low doses, their action is of rapid onset, and they are well tolerated with only modest side effects (see Chapter 15). However, they have to be prescribed carefully because of the potential for abuse and dependence. Despite this, psychostimulants are being reexamined for short-term use in treatment-resistant depression and perhaps in depression associated with palliative care and in the elderly (Abbasowa et al., 2013; Candy et al., 2008; Parker and Brotchie, 2010). For example, methylphenidate added to the second-generation antidepressant citalopram was shown to produce a faster onset of antidepressive effect and a higher rate of remission compared to treatment with citalopram alone or methylphenidate alone in an elderly population (Lavretsky et al., 2015).

Bupropion (Wellbutrin, Zyban) is a weak reuptake inhibitor of the neurotransmitters dopamine and norepinephrine, potentiating the synaptic effects of these transmitters. Therefore, clinically it has effects similar to those exerted by the psychostimulants, but with a lower potential for abuse. Bupropion has no effect on serotonin neurons and, therefore, does not have the side effects associated with the use of SSRIs (discussed in the next section).

Bupropion has several uses in medicine. It has been used to treat children with ADHD, although efficacy is not very robust. Under the trade name Zyban, it is FDA-approved for use in smoking-cessation programs. Bupropion is also useful for the treatment of depression as monotherapy, an add-on (augmenting) therapy in patients only partially responsive or nonresponsive to SSRIs, and in patients with difficult-to-treat bipolar depression. Like the psychostimulants, bupropion may also reduce the fatigue associated with depression. Its therapeutic efficacy is comparable to that of the SSRIs, but with a different profile of side effects (Gartlehner et al., 2011).

Bupropion is devoid of the sexual side effects frequently associated with use of the SSRIs, including loss of libido. In fact, the drug may actually enhance sexual functioning in both male and female patients. Unfortunately, when used in combination with an SSRI as augmentation therapy, this effect is less robust. Short-term treatment with long-acting bupropion (Wellbutrin SR) may result in weight loss, an advantage in patients for whom weight gain is a problem, although tolerance to this action appears to develop.

Perhaps the most bothersome side effects of bupropion include anxiety, restlessness, tremor, and insomnia. The dopaminergic actions can result in more serious anxiety disorders including the induction of psychosis de novo, similar to that seen in abusers of cocaine and methamphetamine. Seizures have been reported at higher doses and for this reason, daily doses of bupropion should not exceed 450 milligrams. Bupropion is not effective in the treatment of panic disorder and it may even exacerbate or precipitate panic in susceptible people.

Because bupropion and cocaine share similar mechanisms of action (blockade of dopamine reuptake), it is possible that bupropion exerts a reinforcing or dependency-inducing action. Although there are a few reports of snorting this drug, it does not seem to have a high abuse potential in humans, perhaps because of the occurrence of seizures (Kim and Steinhart, 2010). Lastly, since bupropion enhances dopaminergic neurotransmission, it has been tried in the treatment of abuse of other reinforcing drugs such as cocaine, methamphetamine, and especially nicotine.

SELECTIVE SEROTONIN REUPTAKE INHIBITORS

Starting with fluoxetine, *selective serotonin reuptake inhibitors* (SSRIs) have been available since 1988. The newest ones, *vilazodone* (Viibryd), was released in 2011, and *vortioxetine* (Trintellix), was released in late 2013 (see Table 12.2). These last two drugs, although blocking the reuptake of serotonin like the other SSRIs, have other effects on norepinephrine and dopamine, and thereby have a different mechanism of action compared to the earlier SSRIs. In this book, they will be discussed in their own section as being atypical "SSRI +" drugs (see Table 12.2). The earlier SSRIs include *fluoxetine* (Prozac), *paroxetine* (Paxil), *sertraline* (Zoloft), *fluvoxamine* (Luvox), *citalopram* (Celexa), and *escitalopram* (Lexapro).

These six drugs are all potent blockers of the presynaptic transporter for serotonin reuptake. The degree to which they block reuptake of other neurotransmitters, primarily norepinephrine, varies greatly, with more than a twelvefold difference between citalopram, the most selective for serotonin, and paroxetine or sertraline, the least selective for serotonin. More selectivity implies a more severe discontinuation syndrome and greater potential for inducing serotonin syndrome (both discussed later in this chapter).

These SSRIs do not block postsynaptic serotonin receptors. Therefore, the primary acute neuronal effect of SSRIs is to make more serotonin available in the synaptic cleft, which activates all of the many postsynaptic receptors for serotonin. The action of serotonin at all its postsynaptic receptors is responsible for both their therapeutic actions and their serotonergic side effects.

The current view is that increased serotonin availability at 5-HT_{1A}-type receptors is associated with antidepressant and anxiolytic effects, whereas increased serotonin availability at 5-HT_2-type and 5-HT_3-type receptors produces adverse effects. Increased 5-HT_2 receptor activity is associated with insomnia, anxiety, agitation, sexual dysfunction, and the production of a serotonin syndrome at higher doses. Increased 5-HT_3 receptor activity is responsible for the nausea that these drugs can cause. Because of their receptor selectivity, SSRIs exert few anticholinergic or antihistaminic side effects. Most importantly, these drugs are not fatal in overdose because they are devoid of the cardiac toxicity produced by TCAs.

As a general statement, the clinical differences among individual SSRIs are minimal; all are equally effective and about as effective as older antidepressants (Undurraga and Baldessarini, 2012). As noted earlier in the chapter, TCAs can be fatal in overdose and MAOIs are associated with hypertensive crises. SSRIs are not fatal in overdose. As a class, they have an efficacy of about 17 percent over placebo in clinical trials. This is not a huge improvement, but their popularity appears to be due to their perceived safety despite side effects, ease of use, and broad clinical utility for anxiety and depression, rather than to well-demonstrated superior efficacy.

It has long been recognized that if a patient fails to respond to one SSRI, another might be tried, sometimes with improved response. This suggests some differences between drugs; the six traditional SSRIs and the atypical SSRI + drugs are not necessarily interchangeable. Differences lie in individual pharmacokinetics (half-lives), receptor selectivity, and their potency at inhibiting cytochrome P450 (CYP) drug-metabolizing enzymes in the liver (Table 12.3). Different SSRIs inhibit hepatic drug-metabolizing enzymes differently, and thereby differentially affect the metabolism of other drugs the patient may be taking. For example, fluoxetine and paroxetine are potent inhibitors of CYP2D6, while fluvoxamine markedly inhibits CYP1A2 and 2C19. Citalopram and escitalopram are very weak inhibitors of drug-metabolizing enzymes and may be safer to use when a patient is on multiple medications (Spina et al., 2008).

Approved therapeutic indications for SSRI therapy include major depression, dysthymia, and all the anxiety disorders (panic disorder, OCD, GAD, PTSD, phobias),

TABLE 12.3 Ability of selective serotonin reuptake inhibitors to inhibit various subtypes of CYP liver enzymes

Drug name: *Generic* (trade)	CYP-450 1A2	CYP-450 2C9	CYP-450 2C19	CYP-450 2D6	CYP-450 3A4
Citalopram (Celexa)	0	+	+	+	0
Escitalopram (Lexapro)	0	+	+	+	0
Fluoxetine (Prozac)	++	+	++	+++	+
Paroxetine (Paxil)	+	+	++	+++	+
Sertraline (Zoloft)	+	+	+++	+	+
Fluvoxamine (Luvox)	+++	++	+++	++	+
Vilazodone (Viibryd)				+	
Vortioxetine (Trintellix)	–	–	–	–	–

although SSRIs also have benefit in other clinical situations. The conditions for which each of the newer drugs is currently FDA-approved are summarized in Table 12.4.

Before discussing individual SSRIs, we address several concerns associated with SSRI therapy:

- The treatment-resistant patient
- Serotonin syndrome
- The SSRI discontinuation syndrome
- SSRI-induced sexual dysfunction

A fifth issue, the possible effects on the fetus if the mother takes the SSRI during pregnancy or while breast-feeding, is discussed in Chapter 15.

The Treatment-Resistant Patient

Many, if not most, patients either fail to respond or only partially respond to a trial of SSRI medication. This can be due to several reasons, including inadequate dose or inadequate length of treatment. It might also be the result of administration of the drug to an individual who, based on a genetic polymorphism of their CYP liver enzymes, is considered a "rapid metabolizer," such that therapeutic blood concentrations of the drug are not achieved at normally sufficient oral dosages. Guidelines to improve the efficacy of SSRIs or any other antidepressant in partial or nonresponders include (1) increasing the dose of antidepressant; (2) switching to a different antidepressant; (3) augmenting with a non-antidepressant, such as a mood stabilizer or atypical antipsychotic drug; or (4) adding a second antidepressant to the original drug (Garcia-Toro et al., 2012). None of these strategies, however, has been found to be consistently effective and there is evidence that simply continuing treatment with the original antidepressant for a longer period of time may be more effective in the long run than switching antidepressants (Bschor et al., 2018).

TABLE 12.4 FDA-approved indications for antidepressant medication

	ADHD	MDD	GAD	OCD	Panic	PTSD	Social anxiety	Bulimia	Premenstrual dysphoria	Smoking cessation	Diabetic neuropathy	Fibromyalgia
SELECTIVE SEROTONIN REUPTAKE INHIBITORS (SSRIs)												
Fluoxetine		✓		✓	✓			✓				
Sertraline		✓		✓	✓	✓	✓		✓			
Fluvoxamine				✓			✓(CR)					
Paroxetine		✓	✓	✓	✓	✓	✓		✓(CR)			
Citalopram		✓		✓								
Escitalopram		✓	✓									
Vilazodone		✓										
Vortioxetine		✓										
SELECTIVE SEROTONIN NOREPINEPHRINE REUPTAKE INHIBITORS (SSNRIs)												
Duloxetine		✓	✓								✓	✓
Venlafaxine		✓	✓(XR)		✓(XR)		✓(XR)					
Mirtazapine		✓										
Desvenlafaxine		✓										
Milnacepran												
SELECTIVE NOREPINEPHRINE REUPTAKE INHIBITORS (SNRIs)												
Atomoxetine	✓											
NOREPINEPHRINE DOPAMINE REUPTAKE INHIBITORS (NDRIs)												
Bupropion		✓								✓		

CR = controlled-release formulation
XR = extended-release formulation

Serotonin Syndrome

High doses of an SSRI or the combination of an SSRI plus another serotonergic drug—or the combination of any drug that increases levels of serotonin, such as SNRI antidepressants—with any other drug that potentiates serotonin activity can induce the disturbing reaction termed the *serotonin syndrome*. Accumulation of serotonin leads to a cluster of responses, including cognitive disturbances, such as disorientation, confusion, and hypomania; behavioral agitation and restlessness; autonomic nervous system dysfunctions, such as fever, shivering, chills, sweating, diarrhea, hypertension, and tachycardia; and neuromuscular impairment, such as ataxia, increased reflexes, and myoclonus. Visual hallucinations have even been reported. Some of these symptoms might result from excess serotonin at 5-HT$_2$ receptors, which is the same site of action for the psychedelic drug LSD. The syndrome can even occur when SSRIs are combined with herbal substances such as St. John's wort or valerian. Once the SSRIs are discontinued, the syndrome usually resolves within 24 to 48 hours; during this time, supportive treatment for the presenting symptom(s) is indicated.

There is a positive relationship between the specificity of the SSRI, for example, in blocking the 5-HT transporter and the likelihood of producing the serotonin syndrome. Therefore, SSRIs, such as citalopram or escitalopram, which have a high degree of specificity for blocking the serotonin transporter, may pose the highest risk for causing the syndrome. But in clinical practice, any drug or combination of drugs potentiating levels of serotonin can increase the risk for producing a serotonin syndrome.

SSRI Discontinuation Syndrome

A discontinuation syndrome occurs in perhaps 60 percent of SSRI-treated patients following abrupt cessation of drug intake. This SSRI discontinuation syndrome was originally associated with abrupt cessation of paroxetine. But it can occur following discontinuation of any SSRI, although it is least likely with fluoxetine because of the drug's long half-life. Onset of the syndrome is usually within a few days and persists perhaps three to four weeks. There are six core sets of somatic signs and symptoms represented by the mnemonic FINISH (Muzina, 2010):

1. Flulike symptoms (fatigue, lethargy, myalgias, chills, headache)
2. Insomnia (sleep disturbances, vivid dreams)
3. Nausea (gastrointestinal symptoms, vomiting, diarrhea)
4. Imbalance (dizziness, vertigo, ataxia)
5. Sensory disturbances (sensation of electric shocks in the arms, legs, or head)
6. Hyperarousal (anxiety, agitation)

Other, less frequently reported symptoms of SSRI discontinuation syndrome include hyperactivity, depersonalization, depressed mood, and memory problems (confusion, decreased concentration, and slowed thinking). The dual-action antidepressants (discussed later), *venlafaxine* (Effexor) and *duloxetine* (Cymbalta), because of their serotoninergic action, can also produce this discontinuation syndrome.

Risk factors for SSRI discontinuation syndrome include abrupt termination of the antidepressant (or noncompliance or drug holidays), short half-life of the drug, long treatment duration, female gender, pregnancy, younger age, being a newborn infant of a mother who has been on serotonergic antidepressants (see Chapter 15), and vulnerability to depressive relapse.

All the somatic and psychological phenomena abate over time and obviously disappear when the SSRI is restarted. It is believed that the syndrome results from a relative deficiency of serotonin when the SSRI is stopped; however, the exact mechanism may be more complex. Therefore, tapering of all antidepressants that are being discontinued is recommended.

SSRI-Induced Sexual Dysfunction

Sexual dysfunction is often associated with major depressive disorder and SSRI medications can further compound it (Schweitzer et al., 2009). Up to 80 percent of depressed patients treated with SSRIs exhibit sexual dysfunction, including problems with orgasm, erection, sexual interest, desire, and psychological arousal. In males, ejaculatory dysfunction seems most prominent. Loss of desire and sexual dysfunction can affect medication compliance and impair interpersonal relationships. Treatment of sexual dysfunction may involve discontinuation of the SSRI and switching to an antidepressant in another class, such as bupropion, or even the newest SSRI + drugs, vortioxetine (Clayton et al., 2015; Jacobsen et al., 2015). *Sildenafil* (Viagra) and *tadalafil* (Cialis) have been found useful for some patients, including females (Nurnberg et al., 2008; Taylor et al., 2013). Furthermore, it may be the case that with successful treatment of the underlying depression with these antidepressants, the impairment in sexual function will coincidentally improve (Clayton et al., 2015).

Additional Side Effects of SSRIs

In addition to the specific issues described in the previous section, there are several other notable consequences of long-term SSRI use:

• *Suicidality.* A review of FDA trials in pediatric and adolescent patients indicated that antidepressants increased the risk of suicidal ideation and behavior. In 2005, the FDA required that manufacturers include a warning in product labeling, recommending that young patients be monitored for the occurrence of suicidality. After that, the number of prescriptions for youth fell dramatically, followed by an *increase* in adolescent suicide. In 2007, the FDA extended the suicidality warning to young adults aged 18 to 24, with the emphasis that depression itself may lead to suicide and that anyone started on antidepressants should be monitored for worsening symptoms. (The use of antidepressants in children and adolescents is discussed further in Chapter 15.) In adult and geriatric patients, however, suicidal risk lessens as depression severity decreases and so the use of antidepressants reduces suicide risk as well as the severity of depression (Figure 12.3).

• *Sleep disturbance.* SSRIs interfere with sleep function, although these difficulties vary among the agents. They may produce insomnia with sleep fragmentation (episodes of awakening).

• *Apathy.* Although uncommon, lack of motivation and apathy have been reported in children and adults treated with SSRIs.

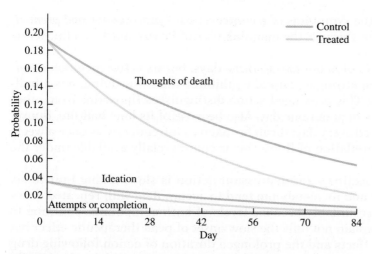

FIGURE 12.3 Probabilities of suicide risk in adult and geriatric fluoxetine and venlafaxine studies. Dark blue lines indicate estimated probabilities for control patients receiving placebo; light blue lines, estimated probabilities for treated patients; thoughts of death curves, "wishes he or she were dead or any thoughts of possible death to self" or worse; ideation curves, "suicide ideas or gestures" or worse; and attempts or completion curves, "suicide attempts or suicides." [Data from Gibbons et al., 2012.]

- *Physiological symptoms*. A variety of physiological symptoms have been reported with SSRIs. *Hyponatremia* (serum sodium concentration below 130 milliequivalents per liter) may occur within the first few weeks of treatment but will resolve after discontinuation. Symptoms include nausea, headache, lethargy, muscle cramps, seizures, coma, and possibly respiratory arrest. In adults over 50 years of age, SSRI use may slightly increase the risk of sustaining *fractures* in a fall and of osteoporosis (Eom et al., 2012). SSRIs increase the risk of gastrointestinal bleeding and easy bruising, although this is magnified by the use of certain nonsteroidal anti-inflammatory agents, such as aspirin. Both agents inhibit platelet aggregation (Bismuth-Evenzal et al., 2012). Rare cases of *cardiovascular problems*, such as arrhythmias, prolonged QTc intervals, and cardiovascular depressant effects, have been reported (Cooke and Waring, 2013). Indeed, the FDA has warned that citalopram should not be used in doses exceeding 40 milligrams daily. Vieweg and coworkers (2012), however, have refuted this statement.

Specific SSRIs

Fluoxetine

Fluoxetine (Prozac) became clinically available in the United States in 1988 as the first SSRI-type antidepressant and the first non-TCA that could be considered a first-line antidepressant. Fluoxetine's efficacy is comparable to that of the TCAs, with few or no anticholinergic or antihistaminic side effects.

Besides major depression, fluoxetine has been used in the treatment of dysthymia, bulimia, alcohol withdrawal, and virtually all the various subtypes of anxiety disorders. Specific formulations of fluoxetine, sertraline, and paroxetine have been shown to be effective in relieving the symptoms of a controversial syndrome termed *premenstrual dysphoric disorder.* For this use, the manufacturer of Prozac marketed fluoxetine under the trade name Sarafem.

Fluoxetine has a half-life of about two to three days, but its active metabolite *norfluoxetine,* which is an even stronger reuptake inhibitor than fluoxetine, has a half-life of about six to ten days. This prolonged action distinguishes fluoxetine from other SSRIs, which have half-lives of about one day. Also because of its long half-life, fluoxetine need not be administered every day; it can be taken as infrequently as once a week, and a once-weekly oral formulation of fluoxetine is commercially available under the trade name Prozac Weekly.

As with all SSRIs, fluoxetine's antidepressant action is slow, taking four to six weeks. Therefore, the drug and its metabolite tend to accumulate with repeated doses over about two months, presumably because levels of both compounds continue to increase. This action can explain not only the slow onset of peak therapeutic effect but also the late onset of side effects and the prolonged duration of action following drug discontinuation. Therapeutic trials with fluoxetine should continue for at least eight weeks before the drug is determined to be ineffective. Significant and important side effects of fluoxetine include anxiety, agitation, insomnia, and serotonin syndrome. In addition, sexual dysfunction is common.

Fluoxetine, sertraline, paroxetine, and fluvoxamine inhibit certain of the drug-metabolizing enzymes in the liver (see Table 12.3). Therefore, coadministration of any of these four drugs can increase the level of other drugs that the patient might be taking.

In 2004, the FDA approved Symbyax, a combination of fluoxetine and olanzapine, an atypical antipsychotic, for the treatment of depressive episodes associated with bipolar disorder. One review supports the benefit of this combination in treatment-resistant depression, although it produced greater increases in body weight, prolactin, and total cholesterol than either of the two agents independently or a combination of fluoxetine plus an atypical antipsychotic, such as aripiprazole, with less potential for weight gain (Bobo and Shelton, 2009). The olanzapine–fluoxetine combination drug has also been shown to enhance remission rates and promote better survival from relapse in individuals with TRD compared to treatment with fluoxetine alone (Brunner et al., 2014).

Sertraline

Sertraline (Zoloft) was the second SSRI approved for clinical use in the United States. Clinically, like all SSRIs, it is as effective as TCAs in the treatment of major depression and dysthymia, and it has fewer side effects and improved patient compliance (Ravindran et al., 2000).

Sertraline is four to five times more potent than fluoxetine in blocking serotonin reuptake but also may block the uptake of dopamine. Because of increased potency, serotonin-associated side effects (serotonin syndrome and serotonin discontinuation syndrome) may be more intense than with fluoxetine. Steady-state levels of the drug in plasma are achieved within four to seven days, and its metabolites are much less pharmacologically active. Like all SSRIs, sertraline has few anticholinergic, antihistaminic, and adverse cardiovascular effects, as well as a low risk of toxicity in overdose.

Paroxetine

Paroxetine (Paxil) was the third SSRI to become available in the United States for clinical use in treating major depression, dysthymia, various anxiety disorders, and premenstrual dysphoric disorder. The FDA has also approved paroxetine for treating *generalized anxiety disorder* (GAD), although this capability is probably shared by all SSRIs. Like sertraline, paroxetine is more potent than fluoxetine in blocking serotonin reuptake. The drug's metabolic half-life is about 24 hours and steady state is achieved in about seven days; its metabolites are relatively inactive.

Paroxetine is perhaps the SSRI most associated with serotonin syndrome. Furthermore, because it has the shortest half-life of the SSRIs, it is most associated with *serotonin discontinuation syndrome*, new onset or precipitation of psychosis, paranoid ideations, temper dyscontrol, delusions, and even visual hallucinations upon abrupt discontinuation. It is also the most likely of the SSRIs to produce an increase in prolactin levels that would increase the risk for sexual dysfunction and gynecomastia in men; and sexual dysfunction, irregular or absent menses, infertility, and galactorrhea in women. It has been reported that the use of paroxetine was associated with a small but statistically significant increase in the risk of cleft lip and palate deformities and cardiac malformations in newborns of women who took the drug during their pregnancy (Reefhuis et al., 2015). This has been confirmed through an examination of the data from the Quebec Pregnancy Cohort study (Berard et al., 2017). In December 2006, the American College of Obstetricians and Gynecologists (ACOG) published a position statement that paroxetine probably should not be used during pregnancy (see Chapter 15). Currently, ACOG continues to maintain that paroxetine should not be used during the first trimester of pregnancy. In addition, the FDA moved paroxetine from a pregnancy risk category C to category D based on the evidence of increased risk of birth defects associated with the drug.[6]

Fluvoxamine

Fluvoxamine (Luvox) is a structural derivative of fluoxetine. Like all SSRIs, fluvoxamine has well-described antidepressant properties, comparable in efficacy to the TCA imipramine, but fewer serious side effects. It has been shown effective in the treatment of all anxiety disorders. The FDA approved an extended-release formulation of this drug (Luvox CR) in 2008 for the treatment of social anxiety disorder and OCD in adult patients.

Citalopram

Citalopram (Celexa) is an SSRI available in Europe since 1989 and introduced into the United States in 1998 as the fifth SSRI. Citalopram was claimed to have a more rapid onset of action than fluoxetine, but this observation is probably overstated.

---

[6]The FDA Pregnancy Risk Categories of A, B, C, D, and X have been replaced by the Pregnancy and Lactation Labeling Rule (PLLR) as of 2015. Drugs approved after June 30, 2015, will have this new labeling information that is more detailed and provides more specific researched based information on: (1) risk in the areas of pregnancy (including labor and delivery); (2) lactation (including nursing mothers); and (3) females and males of reproductive potential. Drugs approved after 2001 will be phased in and drugs approved prior to 2001 are not included.

Efficacy was also likely overstated, with the drug being only modestly more effective than placebo treatment (Apler, 2011). Efficacy of the antidepressants, including citalopram, may in part be dependent on which depressive symptoms are being used as outcome variables. In an analysis of results from the STAR*D Study (discussed later in this chapter) to establish three symptom clusters, Chekroud and colleagues (2017) applied regression analysis to the data from the CO-MED Study (discussed later in this chapter), using those symptom clusters to see if there were any differences in the efficacy of the antidepressants used. Although there were no overall differences among the antidepressants, when symptom clusters were examined, some antidepressants were more effective against some symptoms than others. For example, in this study, citalopram was found to be more effective at treating the core emotional symptoms of depression than sleep symptoms or atypical symptoms, such as psychomotor or suicidal symptoms. As discussed earlier, high doses of citalopram have been associated with ECG irregularities and rare fatalities, but there is evidence that this risk has been overstated by the FDA (Hutton et al., 2016). It has a lower risk of inhibiting drug-metabolizing hepatic enzymes, so it might be better for patients who are taking multiple medications.

Citalopram is well absorbed orally; peak plasma levels are reached in about 4 hours. Steady state is achieved in about one week, and maximal effects are seen in about five to six weeks. The elimination half-life is about 33 hours, enabling once-per-day dosing. Older people have a reduced ability to metabolize citalopram and for this reason a 33 to 50 percent reduction in dose is necessary.

Citalopram has been reported to moderately reduce alcohol consumption in problem alcoholics. Citalopram might be expected to exert anxiolytic effects similar to those exerted by other SSRIs. Adverse effects of citalopram resemble those of other SSRIs. Citalopram has also been associated with an increased risk for musculoskeletal defects and craniosynostosis (change in skull growth pattern) if administered during the first trimester of pregnancy (Berard et al., 2017).

Escitalopram

Escitalopram (Lexapro) was released in the United States in 2002 for the treatment of major depression. It is also approved for the treatment of GAD. The drug is the therapeutically active isomer (mirror-image molecule) of citalopram. As an active isomer, the major difference is potency: escitalopram is twice as potent as citalopram, so the prescribed dose is 50 percent of the dose of citalopram. In other words, 10 milligrams of escitalopram are equivalent to 20 milligrams of citalopram. Wade and coworkers (2011) noted that while a dose of 20 milligrams (comparable to 40 milligrams of citalopram) was marginally effective in treating depression, doses to 50 milligrams were very effective in achieving remission, with 40 to 50 percent of patients eventually reaching remission over a 12-week study period. No cardiac complications were observed, even though doses were increased to as much as 50 milligrams daily.

One observation that has occurred with long-term treatment of SSRIs and other drugs that interact with the serotonin system is that over time, depressive symptoms that were once well controlled begin to re-emerge. This phenomenon has been termed the *poop-out effect*. Although this phenomenon has been thought to have evolved with the administration of the SSRIs, historically it was recognized with the first-generation antidepressants and with the MAOIs. Thus, loss of effect over time can occur with any of the currently available antidepressants. Another term used to describe this effect is *antidepressant tachyphylaxis*. Other causes for loss of antidepressant effect must be ruled out, including medication nonadherence, recurrence of symptoms of the underlying disorder related to the natural course, or use of alcohol or illicit drugs. There is no one established cause of this tachyphylaxis, but theories include pharmacokinetic, such as tolerance due to changes in absorption, distribution, metabolism, or elimination; or pharmacodynamic, such as tolerance due to changes in receptor numbers or sensitivity. One estimate of the frequency of tachyphylaxis comes from the NIMH Collaborative Depression Study, which found a rate of 25 percent of patients treated suffered loss of antidepressant effect over time (Solomon et al., 2005). It has also been reported that those individuals who experience tachyphylaxis to their initial antidepressant treatment may also be less responsive to subsequent treatments. Strategies for addressing tachyphylaxis include raising the dose of the SSRI, providing a drug holiday or decreasing the dose of the medication, switching to a different class of antidepressant drug, or augmenting treatment with another psychotropic drug, such as lithium or an antipsychotic. (For a discussion of the topic of antidepressant tachyphylaxis, see Targum, 2014.)

Norepinephrine + Dopamine Reuptake Inhibitor (NDRI)

Bupropion

Bupropion (Wellbutrin, Zyban, Forfivo, Aplenzin) blocks the reuptake of both norepinephrine and dopamine, increasing the levels of both monoamines in the synaptic cleft. It is indicated for the treatment of MDD, seasonal affective disorder (SAD), ADHD, and smoking cessation (specifically with Zyban). It has little effect on sexual function and has been used to counter the sexual dysfunction produced by treatment with the SSRIs. Depending on the dose, bupropion can lower the seizure threshold. Total daily doses should not be above 450 milligrams. Also, due to its risk of producing seizures, bupropion should not be used for treating individuals who may be in alcohol withdrawal or who may be bulimic, since these conditions, in and of themselves, increase the risk for seizures. Since it also increases levels of dopamine, bupropion also increases the risk for producing or exacerbating psychosis in individuals who present with disorders such as schizophrenia that include psychosis as a symptom. Due to its effect on norepinephrine, bupropion can also produce orthostatic hypotension and risk of falls. Slow-dose titration is recommended in susceptible individuals. There have been some reports of myocardial infarction (MI) associated with the use of Zyban for smoking cessation treatment. And as with other antidepressants, there can be some loss of antidepressant effect over time, such as poop-out or tachyphylaxis.

SEROTONIN + NOREPINEPHRINE REUPTAKE INHIBITORS

Historically, the TCAs were the first dual-action antidepressants: although they block the presynaptic reuptake of both norepinephrine and serotonin, they also block other receptors such as cholinergic and adrenergic receptors that contribute to a wide variety of side effects, thus limiting their widespread use. The unitary action of the *serotonin + norepinephrine reuptake inhibitors* (SNRIs), while associated with efficacy against a wide variety of anxiety and depressive disorders, is limited by side effects associated with serotonin overactivity. Therefore, the next variation in the mechanism of action of antidepressants targeted two different synaptic sites, which was intended to improve or maintain efficacy while limiting side effects. These next antidepressants inhibit the active presynaptic reuptake of both serotonin and norepinephrine.

Venlafaxine

Venlafaxine (Effexor) is classified as a mixed *serotonin-norepinephrine reuptake inhibitor* approved for the treatment of major depressive disorder. The serotonin blockade occurs at lower doses than does the norepinephrine blockade, and at higher doses venlafaxine also inhibits the reuptake of dopamine. Venlafaxine lacks anticholinergic or antihistaminic effects, a distinct advantage. On the other hand, it was reported that while the response and remission rates to venlafaxine XR were the same as to bupropion XL, venlafaxine produced significantly more sexual side effects (Thase et al., 2006). Some evidence also suggests that venlafaxine may be more likely than other antidepressants to trigger a manic state in people who are taking the drug as treatment for bipolar depression. This suggests a possibility that venlafaxine might precipitate agitated or aggressive behavior in some patients.

Concern was raised about venlafaxine's known association with blood pressure elevation in some 3 to 4 percent of patients using the sustained-release formulation and 2 to 13 percent of those taking the immediate-release preparation. Essentially, higher overdose fatality rates were seen according to studies using population datasets. In December 2006, the U.S. manufacturer issued a warning stating that prescriptions for venlafaxine should be written for the smallest quantity of capsules consistent with good patient management in order to reduce the risk of overdose. In 2010, however, a large population study from the United Kingdom looked at the sudden cardiac death, or near-death, rate of new users (18 to 89 years old) of several antidepressants. The results found no association of venlafaxine, used for either depression or anxiety, with increased cardiac risk over a period of 3.3 years (Martinez et al., 2010).

An extended-release formulation *venlafaxine* (Effexor XR) was approved by the FDA for the treatment of GAD as well as panic and social anxiety. Venlafaxine appears to have only minimal effects on drug-metabolizing enzymes, and drug interactions are few. Venlafaxine's primary metabolite, desvenlafaxine, is pharmacologically active; the half-lives of the parent compound and the primary metabolite are 5 hours and 11 hours, respectively.

Desvenlafaxine

In 2008, *desvenlafaxine* was approved for the treatment of major depressive disorder under the brand names Pristiq and Khedezla (Pae et al., 2009). As stated previously, desvenlafaxine is the active metabolite of venlafaxine. Therefore, it has the antidepressant efficacy, safety, and tolerability, of venlafaxine (Ferguson et al., 2012). With an 11-hour half-life, it requires only once-daily dosing. Desvenlafaxine has also been shown to reduce the frequency and severity of hot flashes in postmenopausal women, but in 2011 the FDA refused approval for this use.

Duloxetine

Duloxetine (Cymbalta) is another dual-action antidepressant that binds to and blocks the reuptake transporters for norepinephrine and serotonin. The blockade seems to be more complete than that of venlafaxine (Bymaster et al., 2005). Duloxetine seems to be mildly effective in the treatment of both depression and anxiety, and has FDA indications for major depressive disorder and generalized anxiety disorder. Cipriani and coworkers (2012), however, found evidence of superiority over other antidepressants to be underwhelming. Hellerstein and coworkers (2012) reported duloxetine useful in the acute treatment (10-week) of chronic mild depressions, including dysthymic disorder.

Duloxetine has been reported to significantly reduce physical symptoms of pain, such as backaches, headache, muscle and joint pain, and back and shoulder pain; that is, it reduces interference with daily activities as well as the time in pain while awake. This drug has been approved for the management of neuropathic pain associated with diabetic peripheral neuropathy and fibromyalgia. There is also evidence that this agent may induce a manic or hypomanic episode in patients with bipolar disorder (Peritogiannis et al., 2009).

The half-life of duloxetine is about 12 hours, allowing once-daily dosing. Nausea is the most common side effect. Weight gain and sexual dysfunction have not yet been problems with the drug (Clayton et al., 2013). Elevations in blood pressure (hypertension), theorized to be possible with duloxetine, have not yet been a major problem in clinical studies.

Levomilnacipran

Levomilnacipran (Fetzima) is another drug that blocks norepinephrine and serotonin reuptake and is approved by the FDA for the treatment of major depressive disorder. Levomilnacipran is comparable in efficacy to other antidepressants (Citrome, 2016). Its typical side effects include sexual dysfunction, tachycardia, palpitations, hypertension, and vomiting. Unlike other drugs in this class, the dose of levomilnacipran may need to be adjusted in individuals who have renal impairment (Elmaadawi et al., 2015).

All the drugs in this class, such as all serotonin-norepinephrine reuptake inhibitors, can produce sexual dysfunction, blood pressure changes, trigger a switch to mania if used alone to treat bipolar depression, and can produce tachyphylaxis (poopout) with extended treatment.

SEROTONIN-2 ANTAGONISTS/REUPTAKE INHIBITORS (SARIs)

Nefazodone

Nefazodone (Serzone) is a dual-action antidepressant that is chemically related to trazodone (see discussion aforementioned in the section on first-generation heterocyclic antidepressants), but with some important pharmacological distinctions. Nefazodone's strongest pharmacological action is 5-HT$_2$ receptor blockade, which distinguishes it from the SSRIs, and it also inhibits *both* serotonin and norepinephrine reuptake at its therapeutic dose.

Nefazodone can produce liver failure at a rate of nearly three to four times greater than that which occurs in the general population not taking the drug, resulting in death or necessitating liver transplantation. The branded drug was removed from the market in Canada and the United States, and though it is still available in generic formulations in the United States, it is seldom used because of its toxicity and the availability of many alternatives.

NORADRENERGIC/SPECIFIC SEROTONERGIC ANTIDEPRESSANT (NaSSA)

Mirtazapine

Mirtazapine (Remeron) was introduced into clinical use in the United States in 1997 and is approved for the treatment of major depressive disorder. The drug is clinically effective and its antidepressant action may be more rapid than that achieved with other antidepressants (Watanabe et al., 2011). Overall, mirtazapine is a dual-action antidepressant that increases the presynaptic release of both norepinephrine and serotonin through several actions:

- It blocks central alpha$_2$ adrenergic autoreceptors. By blocking adrenergic autoreceptors, it causes an increase in the release of norepinephrine.
- It blocks adrenergic heteroceptors located on the terminals of serotonin-releasing neurons, where they normally inhibit the release of serotonin. When these adrenergic heteroceptors are blocked, 5-HT neurons release more serotonin.
- The increased release of serotonin stimulates only 5-HT$_1$ receptors because 5-HT$_2$- and 5-HT$_3$-type receptors are specifically blocked by mirtazapine.

Although complicated, this mechanism explains how mirtazapine enhances both norepinephrine and serotonin neurotransmission. Because mirtazapine is a potent antagonist of postsynaptic 5-HT$_2$ and 5-HT$_3$ receptors, it does not produce the side effects of SSRIs, especially anxiety, insomnia, agitation, nausea, and sexual dysfunction.

Mirtazapine is also a potent blocker of histamine receptors, and drowsiness is a prominent and often therapeutically limiting side effect. Sedation may be advantageous in depressed patients with symptoms of anxiety and insomnia, a common occurrence. Because of the drowsiness, the drug is best taken at bedtime and probably should not be combined with alcohol or other CNS depressants.

Other side effects of mirtazapine include increased appetite and weight gain. The drug may therefore be advantageous in certain situations, such as in the treatment of patients with anorexia, in patients with wasting diseases such as cancer and AIDS, and in the elderly, where bedtime sedation and maintenance of body weight are a goal. The drug may produce constipation and dry mouth in some patients and changes in metabolic factors such as cholesterol and triglycerides.

Mirtazapine is rapidly absorbed orally; peak blood levels occur 2 hours after administration. The elimination half-life is 20 to 40 hours, allowing once-a-day administration, usually at bedtime to maximize sleep and minimize daytime sedation.

ATYPICAL ANTIDEPRESSANT DRUGS OR SSRI + DRUGS

Vilazodone

Vilazodone (Viibryd), approved for the treatment of major depressive disorder, is an SSRI that is also a weak stimulant at 5-HT$_{1A}$ receptors (dual serotonin action). In addition, it may also have some effect on blocking the reuptake of both norepinephrine and dopamine. Modest SSRI-like efficacy has been demonstrated, but comparative studies with any active antidepressant, such as another SSRI, have not been reported (Reinhold et al., 2012; Singh and Schwartz, 2012). Claims of more rapid onset of action and fewer sexual side effects have not been verified. Vilazodone may carry greater mortality risk compared to the other SSRIs (Nelson and Spyker, 2017). The most frequent side effects reported for vilazodone are nausea, vomiting, diarrhea, and insomnia.

To date, despite theoretical advantages and additional expense, no therapeutic advantages over preexisting older agents (for example, generics that are much less expensive) have been demonstrated (Guay, 2012).

Vortioxetine

Vortioxetine (Trintellix) is a multimodal SSRI, approved for the treatment of major depressive disorder, which exerts several different actions at various serotonin receptor subtypes. Short-term, noncomparative trials have been reported with low doses (2.5 to 5.0 milligrams daily) being ineffective (Jain et al., 2013) and higher doses (10 to 20 milligrams daily) likely effective. Like other SSRIs, vortioxetine was effective in the treatment of generalized anxiety disorder (Rothschild et al., 2012). Vortioxetine inhibits serotonin reuptake; is an agonist of the serotonin-1A (5-HT$_{1A}$) receptor; a partial agonist of the serotonin-1B (5-HT$_{1B}$) receptor; and an antagonist of 5-HT$_3$, 5-HT$_{1D}$, and 5-HT$_7$ receptors. How each action translates into antidepressant action is unknown (Stahl et al., 2013). However, it is the first antidepressant to exhibit this combination of actions at serotonin receptors. Brignone and colleagues (2016) examined studies that could be used to determine if switching from one of several other antidepressants to vortioxetine produced any additional efficacy or improvement in remission rates. They found that switching to vortioxetine produced numerically higher remission rates, but not necessarily statistically significant differences. In a double-blind, placebo-controlled study comparing vortioxetine to venlafaxine XR in Asian patients with major depressive disorder, vortioxetine was as good as but not superior to venlafaxine XR in reducing scores on a depression rating scale (Wang et al., 2015). And Citrome (2016) did not find any differences between vortioxetine and duloxetine, escitalopram, levomilnacipran, sertraline, venlafaxine, or vilazodone on the measures of *number needed to treat* (NNT), *number needed to harm* (NNH), and *likelihood to be helped or harmed* (LHH).

In some clinical studies, measures are used to communicate to clinicians how effective or harmful a drug may be when administered to individuals. Such measures include NNT, NNH, and LHH. The NNT states the number of individuals who need to be treated with a drug before one of those patients derives a benefit. Usually, an NNT below 10 is considered to be good, and the lower the number the better. Conversely, NNH is the number of individuals who are treated before one individual experiences a significant adverse effect. In this case, higher NNH numbers are better. Finally, LHH is the ratio of NNH over NNT, which gives the clinician an easy way of determining how much more benefit than harm might a person experience from treatment with a medication (Citrome and Ketter, 2013). The most likely side effects of vortioxetine are constipation, nausea, and vomiting.

STAR*D STUDY

While basic research continues to improve our understanding of the pathophysiology of depressive disorders and the mechanisms of action of antidepressants, progress has been much slower in the clinical management of depression. A nationwide clinical trial, the Sequenced Treatment Alternatives to Relieve Depression (STAR*D) study, was conducted at a cost of $35 million over a six-year period ending in 2006. The aim was to identify specific treatment strategies that would improve the long-term outcome of people with depressive disorder. The study started with almost 3000 patients at 41 clinical sites. Patients were started on citalopram at standard doses. The primary outcome was remission; patients not responding were offered a medication switch, combination, or augmentation strategies. No placebo group was included and augmentation strategies did not include the atypical antipsychotics that are today approved by the FDA for the treatment of resistant depression (olanzapine, aripiprazole, and brexpiprazole). Switch options included sertraline, bupropion-SR, or venlafaxine-XR; add-on options included either bupropion-SR or buspirone. An option for cognitive-behavior treatment was also offered. Participants who became symptom-free continued with the treatment in a follow-up period; participants who did not or who experienced intolerable side effects could continue on to other options, including mirtazapine or nortriptyline, a tricyclic antidepressant, for up to 14 weeks.

Finally, participants who had not become symptom-free were taken off all other medications and randomly switched to one of two treatments, the MAOI tranylcypromine or the combination of extended-release venlafaxine with mirtazapine.

Results

Only about 30 percent of patients placed on citalopram reached "remission," and about 10 to 15 percent more were "responders," who did not achieve remission but whose symptoms decreased to at least half of what they had been at the start of the trial. On average, it took nearly six weeks for a participant to respond and nearly seven weeks to achieve remission. With a historical response to placebo usually around 20 to 25 percent, these results were very discouraging because they documented the poor efficacy of the chosen SSRI to achieve significant therapeutic benefits.

Of the nonresponders, 51 percent agreed to switch their medication and 39 percent agreed to receive "medication augmentation"; the rest received cognitive-behavioral therapy (CBT). About 25 percent of the participants who switched became symptom-free. This result was the same for each of the three medication groups: no one drug was best, none worked more quickly than another, and there was no difference in side effects or serious problems. About one-third of the participants in the augmentation group achieved remission. Among patients who did not respond adequately to citalopram, CBT produced outcomes comparable to those of medications; antidepressant therapy was more rapidly effective than CBT, but CBT was better tolerated than were the antidepressants.

Conclusions

Over the course of all four treatment levels (a total of 48 weeks), about two-thirds of participants were able to achieve remission if they did not withdraw from the study. Dropout rates, however, were high: 21 percent after level 1, 30 percent after level 2, and 42 percent after level 3. The data show that, overall, many patients with treatment-resistant depression can get better, but the odds of remission diminish with every additional treatment strategy needed. This study illustrated for the first time what to expect with treatment changes in attempts to bring treatment-resistant patients to remission (Preskorn, 2009; Sinyor et al., 2010). Overall, there appeared to be no antidepressant that was superior to all the others, and clinical decisions currently need to be based not only on effectiveness but also on side effects, cost, and patient preference.

Another large-scale study, the Combining Medications to Enhance Depression Outcomes (CO-MED) trial, was a prospective, randomized, single-blind, multicenter, placebo-controlled trial comparing the efficacy of escitalopram monotherapy versus two-antidepressant combinations, bupropion SR plus escitalopram or venlafaxine ER plus mirtazapine, for both acute (12 weeks) and long-term (28 weeks) treatment of major depressive disorder. Rush and coworkers (2011) describe that the results of this study indicated no difference between monotherapy versus the combination therapies at either 12 weeks or 28 weeks of treatment; there was no difference among the therapies in overall quality of life or work function; and the side effect burden was greater with one of the combination therapies versus the monotherapy. The conclusion from this study was that there was no advantage in efficacy to adding another antidepressant for individuals who fail to respond fully to a single antidepressant and that the combination leads to greater risk of side effects. As discussed in a prior section, a subsequent analysis of the data from the STAR*D using symptom clusters derived from the CO-MED study found that although the overall outcomes were disappointing, that if certain drugs could be matched to certain symptom clusters, greater efficacy might be achieved (Chekroud et al., 2017).

We are still left with a continuing discussion of whether antidepressant drugs actually work. There are data and studies on both sides of this argument. Certainly, antidepressants do not work for everyone who has depression. It is more likely that the drugs work best for those who have the greater severity of symptoms or illness. Many reasons for the inability of antidepressants to separate from placebo in clinical trials have been put forth, including nonhomogenous study populations, low baseline rates of illness severity, rising rates of placebo responders in clinical studies, and shift in diagnostic inclusion criteria seen in DSM-5, among others. (For a summary of this discussion, see Bschor and Kilarski, 2017.)

Where Do We Go from Here in Antidepressant Treatment?

The STAR*D study was essentially a "shotgun" approach to treating depression: start with an SSRI and then make multiple switches or medication combinations in hopes of achieving treatment success. Overall, despite the strategy, efficacy of treatment was moderate at best and the side effect burden was high. New approaches are needed for the next decade, including the development of genetic predictability to help guide therapy, such as personalized treatment, and more effective medications with a reduced side effect burden.

Genetic Influences

As discussed already, cost-effective genetic testing is available to identify genetic deficits in drug metabolism, such as CYP enzymes, that predict drug interactions with many antidepressants. These interactions are important with many antidepressants, as they inhibit the action of these enzymes and increase the blood concentrations of other drugs. Recent interest, however, has centered on how genetic alterations may influence the clinical response—or lack of response—to these medications.

Hall-Flavin and colleagues (2012) studied polymorphisms on five genes: (1) cytochrome P450 2D6 gene, (CYP2D6); (2) cytochrome P450 2C19, (CYP2C19); (3) cytochrome P450 1A2 gene, (CYP1A2); (4) the serotonin transporter gene (SLC6A4); and (5) the serotonin 2A receptor gene (HTR2A). Using therapy guided by these results, remission of depression was significantly improved. Although expensive, some insurance is covering the cost of the testing and as genetic testing costs continue to fall, this may become a more common clinical practice.

Other genetic testing protocols also seem initially hopeful. Ellsworth and coworkers (2013) studied genetic variation of a glucocorticoid receptor protein (FKBP51) with a genotype–phenotype association between rs352428 being associated with positive responses in the STAR*D study. Adkins and colleagues (2012) studied similar genomic variations possibly involved in the side effects of citalopram, again from the STAR*D study. Singh and coworkers (2012) did much the same for dosing strategies with escitalopram. With the marketing of several genetic tests for clinical practice, the use of such testing is becoming more common not only for providing data-based decisions when initial treatments fail, but also to guide initial medication selection hopefully to maximize the probability of a good response, and avoid side effects and costly delays in recovery related to treatment failures and need for switching medications. But some of the marketing of these tests have run afoul of FDA regulations by allegedly making claims that exceeded any data to support those claims (Annas and Elias, 2014). An examination of 22 available genetic tests for clinical practice concludes that although there may be value to these tests for clinical decision making, there is a need for more research to establish reliability, validity, clinical usefulness, and cost effectiveness before such value can be established (Bousman and Hopwood, 2016; Lyman and Moses, 2016). Some of this research is being done by the companies that market the test kits (Winner and Dechairo, 2015). The Veterans Administration (VA) conducted a large-scale review of the use of genetic testing within their system and found insufficient data to support the use at the present time. The VA recommended more studies to establish reliability, validity, and cost effectiveness before recommending routine utilization for clinical practice (Dieperink et al., 2016). The *Carlat Report: Psychiatry* has reviewed the evidence for clinical utility of genetic tests for predicting response to psychiatric treatment over several years and concludes that there is still insufficient evidence to demonstrate that these tests are cost effective or valid to predict outcomes for any specific patient (Balt, 2015; Carlat, 2017; Howland, 2014). Finally, the National Academies of Sciences, Engineering, and Medicine (2017) have provided an evidence framework for assessing genetic testing.

ADDITIONAL, ALTERNATIVE, AND FUTURE APPROACHES TO TREATMENT

The history of antidepressant drugs now encompasses over 60 years. As is apparent in the descriptions of current drugs, we still seek the "perfect" antidepressant, one that is widely effective in bringing about the remission of acute episodes and preventing future relapses in the absence of significant side effects. In this section, we discuss:

- Approaches to treating individuals who do not achieve a sufficient antidepressant response from an antidepressant drug, including switching antidepressants, combining antidepressant drugs, and augmenting antidepressant treatment with other psychotropic drugs
- *Complementary and alternative medicine* (CAM) approaches to the treatment of depression
- Ketamine and other glutaminergic agonists
- Experimental agents in clinical research and trials

Treatment-Resistant Depression

In general, the response to the initial treatment with an antidepressant medication is in the range of 40 to 50 percent. Although individuals may have a reduction in symptoms, they may not reach a point in their recovery where an examination, using a standardized rating scale of the presence and severity of depressive symptoms, would indicate that they no longer meet the criteria for the diagnosis of major depressive disorder. For these individuals with *treatment-resistant depression* (TRD) a careful investigation into the reasons for lack of full response or remission is needed. Potential reasons for not achieving a good response include: (1) not receiving an adequate dose of the antidepressant drug for an adequate period of time; (2) not being given the correct diagnosis and then being treated with the wrong drug; (3) the individual, feeling that he or she is better, voluntarily stops medication and relapses; (4) or the individual is having too many uncomfortable side effects and he or she stops the medication. All these factors, if present, should be corrected before declaring that a person has TRD.

In the face of TRD, several options have been explored. One option is to simply switch to a different antidepressant medication in the same class or different class. Studies have not found great benefit in switching drugs as opposed to simply maintaining treatment for a longer period of time using the drug that was first administered. The STAR*D study did not find any significant rates of achieving remission with subsequent changes in antidepressant medication for those who did not achieve sufficient response to the first drug used. In addition, it should not be forgotten that some individuals may do best on the first-generation antidepressant drugs compared to the second-generation drugs, although the risk of side effects may be greater with the first-generation drugs.

Another approach to treatment-resistant depression is to combine antidepressant drugs. This may include combining an SSRI with an SNRI. In some small studies, combining mirtazapine with an SSRI or another antidepressant has shown some benefit. But in the CO-MED study mentioned earlier, no significant advantage was seen in combining antidepressants versus monotherapy (Haddad et al., 2015). A large-scale study using mirtazapine or placebo to augment a poor response to an SSRI or SNRI has been recently completed, but the results have not yet been published (Tallon et al., 2016).

Augmentation

Lithium has been shown to be an effective agent when combined with an antidepressant to enhance antidepressant efficacy. This is especially true for individuals who have more severe depressive symptoms and, historically, triiodothyronine (T_3) has also been used as an augmenting agent, although it has not been shown to be consistently effective in controlled studies (Haddad et al., 2015).

Certain atypical antipsychotics, including aripiprazole, olanzapine, and brexipiprazole, have been approved by the FDA for the treatment of TRD. There does seem to be some evidence for the efficacy of combining an atypical antipsychotic with an antidepressant for TRD. But this combination has been shown to increase the likelihood of side effects as well (Haddad et al., 2015). Casey and coworkers (2012) included review of three studies in patients with inadequate response to an SSRI; aripiprazole accelerated early response and this predicted maintenance of response through the end point (Figure 12.4). Richardson and colleagues (2011) noted that aripiprazole potentiated inadequate SSRI response in treating comorbid military-related PTSD and depression. Han and coworkers (2013) noted that aripiprazole potentiated escitalopram in improving both antidepressant response and reducing alcohol dependence. Similarly, *quetiapine* (Seroquel) was found to be an effective antidepressant as a sole agent (Maneeton et al., 2012) and for improving both depression and poor sleep quality (Frey et al., 2013; Sheehan et al., 2012). Finally, although not approved by the FDA for this use, *ziprasidone* (Geodon) has been shown effective for the treatment of depression (Papakostas et al., 2012a; Patkar et al., 2012). (The complete pharmacology of atypical antipsychotics is presented in Chapter 11.)

Abolfazli and colleagues (2011) demonstrated augmentation of the antidepressant action of fluoxetine by the addition of *modafinil* (Provigil), a nonstimulant wakefulness-promoting drug used to combat daytime fatigue in patients with narcolepsy. It does not produce typical psychostimulant-induced side effects and, in

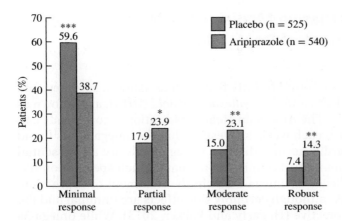

FIGURE 12.4 Percentage of 1065 patients exhibiting minimal to maximal response to aripiprazole (blue bars) or placebo (red bars) as measured by the Massachusetts General Hospital Antidepressant Treatment Response Questionnaire. Patients were classified as nonresponders to standard medication treatment and aripiprazole or placebo was added for a six-week trial of combination therapy. Asterisks indicate a statistical difference between the two treatments. [Data from Casey et al., 2012.]

narcoleptic patients, modafinil may also improve subjective well-being, reduce fatigue, and enhance cognition and concentration. Ferraro and coworkers (2013) discuss the mechanism of action of modafinil to achieve this effect. Several randomized controlled trials and a meta-analysis support the efficacy of modafinil as an augmenting agent to antidepressant treatment of unipolar depression (see Haddad et al., 2015).

Modafinil has two isomers, each of which is active. One is eliminated from the body much more quickly than the other, so essentially the activity really comes from one isomer. *Armodafinil* (Nuvigil) is the longer-acting isomer formulation of modafinil for the treatment of narcolepsy and shift-work sleep disorders. Niemegeers and colleagues (2012) reviewed the pharmacology of armodafinil and its potential use as an augmenting agent in bipolar depression.

Lamotrigine (Lamictal) is an effective anticonvulsant and mood stabilizer. Lamotrigine is unique as an anticonvulsant in that it has clearly stated antidepressant properties. Therefore, it has become a staple in the treatment of bipolar depression. However, it has not proven to be effective as an augmenting agent for the treatment of unipolar depression (see Haddad et al., 2015).

There has been some interest in examining the role of cytokines and other inflammatory markers in the evolution of depression. Studies that have attempted to use anti-inflammatory agents to augment the treatment of depression have not been dramatically successful except in the small population of individuals with depression who have elevations in laboratory indices of inflammation, and there are many risks of using anti-inflammatory agents (such as nonsteroidals) for long-term treatment (Haddad et al., 2015). For a review of the status of anti-cytokine and anti-inflammatory treatments for depression, see Kappelmann and colleagues (2018) and Raison (2017).

Complementary and Alternative Medicine (CAM) Approaches to the Treatment of Depression

Omega-3 Fatty Acids

Two types of *omega-3 fatty acids* are found in fatty fish such as salmon, sardines, and mackerel: *eicosapentaenoic acid* (EPA) and *docosahexaenoic acid* (DHA), also known as *polyunsaturated fatty acids* (PUFA). The American Heart Association recommends eating at least two servings of fatty fish each week, suggesting that the omega-3 fats found in the fish help protect against cardiovascular disease. Omega-3 oils are also essential during pregnancy for normal brain maturation in the neonate. Much speculation has developed about the potential efficacy of omega-3 oils in the treatment of depression. Here, evidence for efficacy is weak, although certainly side effects are minimal and the oils (especially EPA) are neuroprotective (Hegarty and Parker, 2013). While omega-3s may indeed improve mood (Lin et al., 2012), recent studies indicate that as sole treatments for major depressive disorder, they appear to be of minimal benefit with only some trends seen in efficacy (Bloch and Hannestad, 2012; Lesperance et al., 2011; Sublette et al., 2011). Any benefit at all has been seen only when DHA has been used as an augmenting agent with an antidepressant (Haddad et al., 2015). Considering the minimal expense, lack of side effects, and neuroprotective actions, there is little harm in a personal trial of fish oils high in DHA.

Folate

Folate is a B vitamin that occurs naturally in food and in nutritional supplements. The possible significance of folate in depressive disorder is a topic of wide discussion. Indeed, there seems to be a relationship between low folate levels in blood and depressive disorder. Thus, replacement might be a treatment for depression. The relationship between folate and antidepressants is that folate enhances the production of all three monoamines, dopamine, norepinephrine, and serotonin. Since deficiencies in these neurotransmitters are theoretically linked to depressive disorder, this might underlie the etiology of some cases of depression. It has been postulated that some people have a genetic defect in folate metabolism that might increase the risk of depression (Jamerson et al., 2013). There is ongoing controversy whether, in depressed patients with folate deficiency who have not responded to antidepressants, augmentation with a new, expensive folate metabolite, *L-methylfolate* (Deplin) or *delta methylfolate* (EnLyte), which is considered a medical food under FDA regulations, might be more effective than dietary folate.

Folate in blood is converted into dihydrofolate and then into L-methylfolate, which may be the major form of folate capable of crossing the blood–brain barrier. There, L-methylfolate helps form tetrahydrobiopterin (BH4), a cofactor in neurotransmitter production. BH4 is not entirely dependent on L-methylfolate and some folate also crosses the blood–brain barrier directly. Balt (2012) questions whether any of this is important; folate may help some persons with dietary deficiencies and depression, but whether the expense of Deplin is justified is quite unclear. (In some individuals, the genetic mutation MTHFR C677T, which is found in 22 percent of Hispanics and those of Mediterranean descent, may reduce the rate of folate to L-methylfolate conversion, which may or may not have clinical significance.)

Papakostas and coworkers (2012b) reported on two trials of L-methylfolate in depression. The substance was ineffective in one trial, but was effective in the second using a higher dose of L-methylfolate, which led them to conclude that L-methylfolate could be effective. Both trials compared L-methylfolate with placebo, but not with generic folate. A more recent double-blind, placebo-controlled study examined the effect of reduced B vitamins, including L-methylfolate, for treating depression. In individuals who had the MTHFR polymorphism and received L-methylfolate, 42 percent achieved remission of depressive symptoms by eight weeks of treatment (Mech and Farah, 2016). In patients who may have low folate levels or present with the MTHFR polymorphism, there may be benefit to adding L-methylfolate as an adjunct to antidepressant treatment (Thase, 2016).

Much of what can be said of folate can be said of vitamin D, where low vitamin D levels can be associated with depression (Hoang et al., 2011) and dietary replacement may be therapeutically effective as an adjunct to SSRI therapy (Khoraminya et al., 2013). But there are no randomized controlled trials that show that dietary supplements are of any benefit in treatment-resistant depression (Haddad et al., 2015).

S-Adenosylmethionine

S-Adenosylmethionine (SAM-e) is a naturally occurring molecule present in all body cells. It catalyzes methylating reactions, including L-methylfolate. There is some evidence for deficiency in depression with supplementation perhaps assisting to relieve mild depression, but the evidence does not support use in severely depressed persons (Carpenter, 2011). Part of this difficulty may be due to the fact that oral absorption of SAM-e is poor and less than 1 percent of the ingested drug reaches the bloodstream. Papakostas and coworkers (2012c) reviewed studies of the use of SAM-e for depression and claimed that efficacy was similar to the efficacy of tricyclic antidepressants. However, not all studies show significant effects (Nahas and Sheikh, 2011).

St. John's Wort

St. John's wort is an extract of *Hypericum perforatum*, a perennial herb. It has been used to treat depression since the initial German reports of efficacy (Linden et al., 1996; Philipp et al., 1999). In most studies, the compound was superior to placebo and equivalent to standard drugs (Apaydin et al., 2016; Nahas and Skeikh, 2011; Ng et al., 2017; Sarris et al., 2012). Mechanistically, St. John's wort mimics the neurotropic effect of BDNF in the hippocampus (Leuner et al., 2013). Most studies had significant bias. St. John's wort likely should not be combined with most other antidepressants because of its potential to induce serotonin syndrome. The drug also induces drug-metabolizing enzymes such that other drugs taken by an individual may become more toxic at usual doses (Rahimi and Abdollahi, 2012). Other side effects, such as GI distress, photodermatitis, elevated thyroid-stimulating hormones, hypertensive crisis, induction of mania, and fatigue, may further reduce its utility (Hoban et al., 2015).

Did You Know?

You—and Your Mood—Are What You Eat

There is ongoing interest and research in the area of epigenetics that focuses on the complex array of bacteria that live in our gut. Much is known about the development of the microbiome as we develop and how this microbial environment can change as a result of diet and other epigenetic factors such as stress. It has been demonstrated that the gut bacteria can influence a wide variety of physiological responses of organisms through interaction with the hypothalamic-pituitary-adrenal (HPA) axis (Chrobak et al., 2016). The gut microbiome is also important for the development of the body's immune system and participate in the body's inflammatory response reaction (Dash et al., 2015; Sharon et al., 2016).

Research in animals seems to indicate an influence of gut microbiome on certain neurotransmitter levels such as serotonin, GABA, and dopamine among others (Chroback et al., 2016). These findings from cellular and animal models showing a relationship between gut bacteria and immune, inflammatory, and neurotransmission processes naturally leads to the hypothesis that manipulation of the gut microbiome could possibly influence expression of mood and other psychiatric disorders that also involve inflammatory processes and changes in neurotransmitter levels or activity. Population studies have suggested that cultural variation in diets, such as plant-based versus animal-based protein, can produce differences in gut bacterial milieu (Dash et al., 2015). This naturally leads to the thinking that by modifying one's diet, you could influence your mood, for example. Some studies have shown the health benefits of a Mediterranean diet, including improving mood (Dash et al., 2015).

Researchers in this area are hoping to show that by observing a certain dietary regimen and using probiotics that individuals may be able to improve their mood or even prevent the onset of depression, but so far, the research is correlational and more data is needed to establish a true cause-effect relationship between gut microbiome and the central nervous system (Cepeda et al., 2017; Sharon et al., 2016).

KETAMINE AND OTHER GLUTAMINERGIC ANTAGONISTS

For over 50 years, *ketamine* (Ketalar) has been an anesthetic drug characterized by amnesia, analgesia, and out-of-body experiences. It was used for anesthesia because it was one of the only anesthetics that could produce amnesia and analgesia without perilous drops in blood pressure. Its psychedelic properties were tolerated, but because of these psychedelic side effects, ketamine and its precursor, phencyclidine (PCP), were considered drugs of abuse. In recent years, however, remarkably, low-dose intravenous infusions of ketamine have been demonstrated to produce rapid, although transient relief from depression in the majority of patients to whom it was administered. Indeed, administered in a dose of 0.5 milligrams per kilogram of body weight three times weekly over a 12-day period, response rates in TRD were about 70 percent, sustained for an average of 18 days posttreatment (Murrough et al., 2013). The response is often seen within hours and is accompanied by increases in synaptogenesis, including increased density and function of dendritic spine synapses in the prefrontal cortex. This has led to a reversal of the deficits in synaptic number and function resulting from chronic stress exposure (Duman et al., 2012). This remarkable, albeit short-lived antidepressant response is one of the more remarkable advances in recent years in the area of depression research.

The original difficulty of using ketamine for the treatment of depression was its abuse potential and that it required IV administration. Recently, the FDA has granted fast-track status to esketamine, an intranasal form of ketamine that is the S-enantiomer of ketamine and thought to be safer (Singh et al., 2016). It is currently being used off label for the treatment of depression by some prescribers. In a double-blind, placebo-controlled phase 2 clinical study, esketamine was found to be significantly more effective than placebo in rapid reduction of depressive symptoms in patients who were determined to be treatment resistant. The beneficial effects were sustained for about two months (Daly et al., 2017). Despite the appearance of so-called ketamine clinics," it should be pointed out that ketamine doses must be repeated to remain effective, since relapse occurs quickly after the injection or after the intranasal dose. It is not known how many times ketamine can be readministered over time and what long-term effects that might entail. There is the abuse liability and potential side effects, such as depersonalization, which must be addressed, and parameters for long-term administration must be developed. At present, the off-label use of ketamine is still considered experimental and concerns have been raised about such use (Harrison, 2016). Much remains to be learned in this area, but the results with ketamine are remarkable. (For more information about ketamine and its clinical application, see Fond et al., 2014; Li and Vlisides, 2016; and Newport et al., 2015.)

Other drugs that may ultimately antagonize NMDA-glutamate receptors, possibly with the psychedelic properties of ketamine, are under study (see Sos, 2016); one such agent is *rapastinel* (GLYX-13), which is discussed in the In the Pipeline section of this chapter (see Burgdorf et al., 2013). Regardless, this is further evidence of the link between deficits in brain-derived neurotropic factor and a predisposition to depressive symptomatology (Liu et al., 2012). The next several years should add considerable information to this most interesting area of research.

The success of ketamine for the treatment of depression has resulted in a resurgence of interest in research to determine if other psychedelic drugs can be useful in the treatment of psychiatric disorders like depression (Rucker et al., 2016).

EXPERIMENTAL AGENTS

At this point in time, because of economic potential, many other experimental compounds are being evaluated for use in the clinical treatment of depression or are considered as likely candidates.

Tianeptine

Tianeptine (Stablon) increases the presynaptic neuronal uptake of serotonin in the brain and thus decreases serotonin neurotransmission. However, tianeptine appears to reduce stress-induced atrophy of neuronal dendrites, exerting a neuronal protective effect against stress and restoring intracellular mechanisms adversely affected by stress and other insults.

There is some evidence to suggest it may have antidepressant properties. It does not appear to produce adverse cognitive, psychomotor, sleep, cardiovascular, body weight, or sexual side effects. Tianeptine is also effective in bipolar depression, dysthymia, and anxiety. It seems quite useful in the elderly and in patients with chronic alcoholism. This unusual compound offers both an alternative medication to standard antidepressants and new insights into the pathophysiology of depression and anxiety. Because its patent has expired, the drug has not been marketed in the United States (Deutschenbaur et al., 2016).

Agomelatine

Chapter 13 discusses *agomelatine* as an anxiolytic agent that acts as a melatonergic agonist and a serotonin 5-HT$_{2C}$ receptor antagonist, but agomelatine's potential adverse effects on the liver limit its use. Agomelatine also possesses antidepressant properties (Kasper et al., 2013), but again with the same limitation (Carney and Shelton, 2011). The drug has also been demonstrated to effectively treat *anhedonia*, which is the inability to feel pleasure, an effect that was superior to that produced by venlafaxine (Di Giannantonio and Martinotti, 2012).

IN THE PIPELINE

In addition to the substances discussed in this chapter, because of widespread need for more effective medications with fewer side effects, the pharmaceutical industry continues to investigate new agents. The list of antidepressant drugs in the pipeline was derived from *Mental Health Daily* (2015) and Dhir (2017). These experimental agents are discussed next.

Drugs That Interact with the Mu Opioid and Kappa Receptor

In this category is ALKS 5461, which has progressed to phase 3 clinical trials. ALKS 5461 is a mu receptor partial agonist and kappa receptor antagonist. It is a combination of *buprenorphine* (mu receptor partial agonist and kappa receptor antagonist) and *samidorphan* (acts as a mu receptor antagonist). It is thought that blocking kappa receptors inhibits release of dynorphins which, in turn, increases glutamate and dopamine signaling, leading to increased mood. The samidorphan blocks the euphoria and addictive potential of the buprenorphine. Unfortunately, clinical studies have shown a high rate of side effects (85 percent) with this drug and it has not been consistently shown to be effective as an antidepressant.

CERC-501 (LY-2456302) is another kappa receptor antagonist being investigated for the treatment of depression and is in the early phases of clinical trials.

Serotonin Reuptake Inhibitors and Receptor Agonists/Antagonists

DSP-1053 is a selective serotonin reuptake inhibitor (SSRI) and a serotonin 5-HT$_{1A}$ partial agonist. It is similar to vilazodone and buspirone. The company, Sunovion Pharmaceuticals, has completed phase 1 trials, but may not be moving forward with this agent.

MIN-117 is a 5-HT and dopamine reuptake inhibitor (SDRI) and an antagonist at 5-HT$_{1A}$ receptors. It also reportedly acts at 5-HT$_{2A}$, alpha$_{1A}$, and alpha$_{1B}$ receptors. This complicated mechanism of action is similar to that of vortioxetine. The company announced positive results from a phase 2a trial completed in 2016, but there are no current trials under way.

Serotonin, Norepinephrine, Dopamine Reuptake Inhibitors (SNDRIs), or Triple-Reuptake Inhibitors

Amitifadine (DOV-21,947 or EB-1010) is in this category. This drug blocks the reuptake of all three monoamines. There have been two clinical trials of the drug to treat depression. One trial was terminated in 2008 and the other was completed in 2015, but the results have not yet been published. It is more potent at blocking the uptake of 5-HT than it is at blocking uptake of norepinephrine or dopamine. The drug can be thought of as combining the effects of an SSRI with an NDRI, which suggests that it might combine the potential side effects of those types of agents. At present, Euthymics Bioscience is investigating the potential of amitifadine for treatment of alcohol use disorders and for smoking cessation. *Ansofaxine* HCl (LY03005) is another triple-reuptake inhibitor that blocks the uptake of 5-HT, norepinephrine, and dopamine. It has completed phase 1 safety and dosing studies. Another drug in this category is *tedatioxetine* (Lu AA24530), which is more potent at blocking the reuptake of 5-HT than the uptake of norepinephrine; and more potent at blocking the reuptake of norepinephrine than the uptake of dopamine. It also interacts with a number of 5-HT and adrenergic receptors. It has completed phase 2 clinical trials. Since this trial has been completed, Lundbeck and Takeda marketed vortioxetine and may not be moving forward with tedatioxetine at this time.

NMDA Receptor Agonists and Antagonists

AV-101 (4-Cl-KYN) is a prodrug that once in the body is converted to 7-chlorokynurenic acid (7-CL-KYNA), which is a potent antagonist at the NMDA receptor. This drug is similar to ketamine in that it is expected to produce a rapid resolution of depressive symptoms and the company is currently recruiting for two phase 2b clinical trials scheduled to be completed in 2019.

AVP-786 is an NMDA or sigma-1 receptor antagonist. It is a drug comprised of deuterium-modified dextromethorphan (d-DXM) and ultra-low-dose quinidine. The dextromethorphan acts as the NMDA receptor antagonist and the deuterium modification extends the half-life of the drug. The quinidine further protects the drug from metabolism by blocking CYP enzymes. Early trials have reported that the drug may cause drug-induced psychosis, so this will have to be evaluated carefully. A phase 2 clinical trial has not registered any information or updates since 2015 and Avanir Pharmaceuticals' Web site does not indicate that any current trials are being conducted for the treatment of depression.

AZD6423 is an NMDA receptor antagonist being specifically tested to ameliorate suicidal ideation. It is early in the safety phase of clinical investigation. Neurotoxicity is one of the concerning risks of repeated use of this compound.

CERC-301 is an NMDA receptor modulator being investigated as an adjunctive treatment in individuals who have refractory depression and in those individuals with suicidal ideation. The FDA granted fast-track status to this drug in 2013. It specifically interacts with the 2B subunit of the NMDA receptor. Due to this selectivity, CERC-301 is expected to avoid producing some of the significant side effects of ketamine while maintaining its rapid onset of action. Another advantage of this compound is that it can be administered orally instead of requiring IV administration.

Rapastinel (GLYX-13) is a molecule that possesses NMDA-glycine site functional partial agonistic properties. At low levels of NMDA receptor activity, rapastinel activates NMDA receptor activity, while at higher levels of NMDA receptor activity, it acts as an antagonist. Rapastinel requires IV infusion and has a rapid onset of action like ketamine, but it has not been shown to produce any psychotomimetic side effects.

NRX-1074 is an NMDA receptor partial agonist at the glycine site. This drug is similar to rapastinel, but will be marketed in both oral and IV formulations. Like rapastinel, it is fast acting and without psychotomimetic side effects. The drug has completed phase 2 clinical trials.

AXS-05, developed by Axsome Therapeutics, is a combination of *dextromethorphan*, an NMDA receptor antagonist and inhibitor of norepinephrine and serotonin transporters, and bupropion, a dopamine and norepinephrine reuptake inhibitor. AXS-05 is currently in phase 3 clinical trials to determine its efficacy for the treatment of treatment-resistant depression. Axsome Therapeutics reports that dextromethorphan is rapidly metabolized in the body, making it difficult to achieve sufficient central nervous system levels by administering it alone. Bupropion is being used to inhibit the metabolism of dextromethorphan, thus increasing dextromethorphan levels sufficiently to have a central nervous system effect.

Drugs That Affect the Glutamate System

Basimglurant (RG7090) is an mGluR5 receptor antagonist. The drug blocks glutamate's binding to its receptor and promotes neuroplasticity and increase in DA levels. The drug has completed early safety studies, but no further information is available. (For a summary of the involvement of glutamate and the NMDA receptor and clinical applications, see Deutschenbaur et al., 2016.)

Exploring Other Mechanisms for Treatment

Botox (onabotulinumtoxin A) has been in clinical trials for the treatment of depression. Injection of Botox targets the corrugator and procerus muscles within the face to paralyze them. The idea here is that facial expression can be related to how one feels. Eliminating frowning through Botox injections may lighten the facial expression and, by doing so, influence the way a person feels about themselves.

JNJ-42847922 is an orexin receptor inhibitor (OX2). *Orexin*, also called *hypocretin*, is a neuropeptide that regulates sleep, wakefulness, and appetite. This compound is being tested primarily as a sleep agent, but has gone through phase 1 clinical trials to investigate whether it might be useful to treat depressed patients who also have insomnia.

LY2940094 (now BTRX-246040), developed by BlackThorn Therapeutics, is a nociceptor-1 (NOC-1) receptor antagonist. *Nociceptin* is a neuropeptide that produces analgesia but does not act at the opiate receptors. Animal studies have suggested that the NOC-1 receptor may have downstream effects on DA and GABA neurotransmission that in turn may be involved in producing its antidepressant and antianxiety effects. Although the drug has completed some phase 2 testing, it is not clear if BlackThorn Therapeutics plans to move forward with further trials at this time.

Mifepristone (RU-486) is currently approved as an emergency abortifacient. It is a synthetic drug that binds primarily to the progesterone receptor, but also has affinity for the glucocorticoid receptor and has antiandrogenic properties. It is thought that the antiglucocorticoid effects may be responsible for improving mood and minimizing likelihood of psychosis via modulation of the hypothalamic-pituitary-adrenal (HPA) axis. Danco Laboratories, LLC is hoping to get FDA approval to treat individuals who have major depressive disorder with psychotic features. A phase 2 clinical trial was terminated because mifepristone failed to meet its primary target of reduction in psychotic symptoms compared to placebo in patients with major depressive disorder.

NSI-189 is a unique drug in that it promotes neurogenesis in the hippocampus. Other antidepressants are known to stimulate neurogenesis and expand hippocampal volume, but NSI-189 is expected to be more potent in this effect. The expansion of hippocampal volume is related to mood improvement. The drug is currently in phase 2 clinical trials.

Strada (MSI-195 or *ademetionine*) is suspected of modulating cytokines within the CNS that may influence depression, as well as indirectly altering levels of dopamine. It has also been suggested that Strada may also influence membrane fluidity and reduce neuroinflammation. The active ingredient, ademetionine, in this compound is a form of the amino acid methionine (SAMe). It is thought that individuals who have a genetic deficiency that contributes to an underactivity of the methylation process will benefit from adjunctive treatment with this drug. One phase 2 clinical trial has been completed.

STUDY QUESTIONS

1. What is the relationship between depression and the biological amine transmitters in the brain?

2. Describe the probable mechanism of both acute and ultimate effects of antidepressant drugs. What might account for the delay in clinical effect?

3. List and differentiate the major classes of antidepressants.

4. Compare and contrast imipramine and fluoxetine.

5. Discuss what happens when a patient overdoses on a tricyclic antidepressant.

6. Discuss the side effects of SSRIs. What is the serotonin syndrome? What is the SSRI discontinuation syndrome? Discuss the effects of these drugs on sexual function.

7. Which drug or class of drugs do you think is the "best" antidepressant? Why?

8. Which antidepressants are used in the treatment of anxiety disorders? Why? How do these drugs differ from the benzodiazepine-type anxiolytics?

9. Discuss the strategies being used to discover the next generation of antidepressant drugs and the types of drugs that are being developed from those approaches.

10. Discuss the role of nutraceuticals and vitamins in the treatment of depression.

REFERENCES

Abbasowa, L., et al. (2013). "Psychostimulants in Moderate to Severe Affective Disorder: A Systematic Review of Randomized Controlled Trials." *Nordic Journal of Psychiatry* 67: 369–382.

Abolfazli, R., et al. (2011). "Double-Blind, Randomized, Parallel-Group Clinical Trial of Efficacy of the Combination Fluoxetine Plus Modafinil versus Fluoxetine Plus Placebo in the Treatment of Major Depression." *Depression and Anxiety* 28: 297–302.

Adkins, D. E., et al. (2012). "Genone-Wide Pharmacogenomic Study of Citalopram-Induced Side Effects in STAR*D." *Translational Psychiatry* July 3; 2: e129.

American College of Obstetricians and Gynecologists. (2006). "Position Statement on Paroxetine." *Obstetrics and Gynecology* 108: 1601–1603.

American Psychiatric Association. (2013). *Diagnostic and Statistical Manual of Mental Disorders, 5th Edition* [DSM-5]. American Psychiatric Association, Arlington, VA.

Amsterdam, J. D. (2003). "A Double-Blind, Placebo-Controlled Trial of the Safety and Efficacy of Selegiline Transdermal System without Dietary Restrictions in Patients with Major Depressive Disorder." *Journal of Clinical Psychiatry* 64: 208–214.

Amsterdam, J. D., and Bodkin, A. (2006). "Selegiline Transdermal System in the Prevention of Relapse of Major Depressive Disorder: A 52-Week, Double-Blind, Placebo-Substitution, Parallel-Group C Clinical Trial." *Journal of Clinical Psychopharmacology* 26: 579–586.

Annas, G. J., and Elias, S. (2014). "23andMe and the FDA." *New England Journal of Medicine* 370: 985–988. doi: 10.1056/NEJMp1316367.

Andrade, C., and Rao, N. S. K. (2010). "How Antidepressant Drugs Act: A Primer on Neuroplasticity as the Eventual Mediator of Antidepressant Efficacy." *Indian Journal of Psychiatry* 52: 378–386.

Apaydin, E. A., et al. (2016). "A Systematic Review of St. John's Wort for Major Depressive Disorder." *Systematic Reviews* 5: 1.25.

Apler, A. (2011). "Citalopram for Major Depressive Disorder in Adults: A Systematic Review and Meta-Analysis of Published Placebo-Controlled Trials." *BMJ Open* 1(2): e000106.

Autry, A. E., and Monteggia, L. M. (2012). "Brain-Derived Neurotropic Factor and Neuropsychiatric Disorders." *Pharmacological Reviews* 64: 238–258.

Balt, J. (2012). "Deplin: Is It Just Folate by Another Name?" *The Carlat Psychiatry Report* 10(1): 1–8.

Balt, S. (2015). "Using Psychiatric Biomarkers in Your Practice." *The Carlat Report: Psychiatry* 13: 1–3, 6.

Berard, A., et al. (2017). "Antidepressant Use during Pregnancy and the Risk of Major Congenital Malformations in a Cohort of Depressed Pregnant Women: An Updated Analysis of the Quebec Pregnancy Cohort." *British Medical Journal Open* 7: e013372. doi: 10.1136/bmjopen-2016-013372.

Bismuth-Evenzal, Y., et al. (2012). "Decreased Serotonin Content and Reduced Agonist-Induced Aggregation in Platelets of 58 Patients Chronically Medicated with SSRI Drugs." *Journal of Affective Disorders* 136: 99–103.

Bloch, M. H., and Hannestad, J. (2012). "Omega-3 Fatty Acids for the Treatment of Depression: Systematic Review and Meta-Analysis." *Molecular Psychiatry* 17: 1272–1282.

Bobo, W. V., and Shelton, R. C. (2009). "Fluoxetine and Olanzapine Combination Therapy in Treatment-Resistant Major Depression: Review of Efficacy and Safety Data." *Expert Opinion in Pharmacotherapy* 10: 2145–2159.

Bousman, C. A., and Hopwood, M. (2016). "Commercial Pharmacogenetic-Based Decision-Support Tools in Psychiatry." *Lancet* 3: 585–590.

Brignone, M., et al. (2016). "Efficacy and Tolerability of Switching Therapy to Vortioxetine versus Other Antidepressants in Patients with Major Depressive Disorder." *Current Medical Research and Opinion* 32: 351–366.

Brunner, E., et al. (2014). "Efficacy and Safety of Olanzapine/Fluoxetine Combination vs Fluoxetine Monotherapy Following Successful Combination Therapy of Treatment-Resistant Major Depressive Disorder." *Neuropsychopharmacology* 39: 2549–2559. doi: 10.1038/npp.2014.101.

Bschor, T., et al. (2018). "Switching the Antidepressant after Nonresponse in Adults with Major Depression: A Systematic Literature Search and Meta-Analysis." *Journal of Clinical Psychiatry* 79: 11–18. In press. doi: 10.4088/JCP.16r10749.

Bschor, T., and Kilarski, L. L. (2017). "Are Antidepressants Effective? A Debate on Their Efficacy for the Treatment of Major Depression in Adults." *Expert Review of Neurotherapeutics* 16: 367–374.

Burgdorf, J., et al. (2013). "GLYX-13, an NMDA Receptor Glycine-Site Functional Partial Agonist, Induces Antidepressant-Like Effects without Ketamine-Like Side Effects." *Neuropsychopharmacology* 385: 729–742.

Bymaster, F. P., et al. (2005). "The Dual Transporter Inhibitor Duloxetine: A Review of Its Preclinical Pharmacology, Pharmacokinetic Profile, and Clinical Results in Depression." *Current Pharmaceutical Design* 11: 1475–1493.

Candy, M., et al. (2008). "Psychostimulants for Depression." *Cochrane Database of Systematic Reviews* (Issue 2): CD006722. doi: 10.1002/14651858.CD006722.pub2.

Carlat, D. (2017). "Pharmacogenetic Testing: An Update." *The Carlat Report: Psychiatry* 15: 1–3, 6, 8.

Carney, R. M., and Shelton, R. C. (2011). "Agomelatine for the Treatment of Major Depressive Disorder." *Expert Opinion on Pharmacotherapy* 12: 2411–2419.

Carpenter, D. J. (2011). "St. John's Wort and S-Adenosyl Methionine as 'Natural' Alternatives to Conventional Antidepressants in the Era of the Suicidality Boxed Warning: What Is the Evidence for Clinically Relevant Benefit." *Alternative Medicine Reviews* 16: 17–39.

Casey, D. E., et al. (2012). "Efficacy of Adjunctive Aripiprazole in Major Depressive Disorder: A Pooled Response Quartile Analysis and the Predictive Value of Week 2 Early Response." *Primary Care Companion CNS Disorders* 14(3). Pii: PCC. 11m01251.

Cazorla, M., et al. (2011). "Identification of a Low-Molecular Weight TrkB Antagonist with Anxiolytic and Antidepressant Activity in Mice." *Journal of Clinical Investigation* 121: 1846–1857.

Cepeda, M. S., et al. (2017). "Microbiome-Gut-Brain Axis: Probiotics and Their Association with Depression." *Journal of Neuropsychiatry and Clinical Neurosciences* 29: 39–44. doi: 10.1176/appi.neuropsych.15120410.

Chekroud, A. M., et al. (2017). "Reevaluating the Efficacy and Predictability of Antidepressant Treatments: A Symptom Clustering Approach." *JAMA Psychiatry* 4: 370–378. doi:10.1001/jamapsychiatry.2017.0025.

Chrobak, A. A., et al. (2016). "Interactions Between the Gut Microbiome and the Central Nervous System and Their Role in Schizophrenia, Bipolar Disorder and Depression." *Archives of Psychiatry and Psychotherapy* 2: 5–11. doi: 10.12740/APP/62962.

Cipriani, A., et al. (2012). "Duloxetine versus Other Anti-Depressive Agents for Depression." *Cochrane Database of Systematic Reviews* October 17; 10: CD006533.

Cipriani, A., et al. (2016). "Comparative Efficacy and Tolerability of Antidepressants for Major Depressive Disorder in Children and Adolescents: A Network Meta-Analysis." *Lancet* 388: 881–890.

Citrome, L. (2016). "Vortioxetine for Major Depressive Disorder: An Indirect Comparison with Duloxetine, Escitalopram, Levomilnacipran, Sertraline, Venlafaxine, and Vilazodone, Using Number Needed to Treat, Number Needed to Harm, and Likelihood to be Helped or Harmed." *Journal of Affective Disorders* 196: 225–233.

Citrome, L. and Ketter, T. A. (2013). "When Does a Difference Make a Difference? Interpretation of Number Needed to Treat, Number Needed to Harm, and Likelihood to Be Helped or Harmed." *International Journal of Clinical Practice* 67: 407–411.

Clayton, A. H., et al. (2013). "An Evaluation of Sexual Functioning in Employed Outpatients with Major Depressive Disorder Treated with Desvenlafaxine 50 mg or Placebo." *Journal of Sex Medicine* 10: 768–778.

Clayton, A. H., et al. (2015). "Sexual Dysfunction During Treatment of Major Depressive Disorder with Vilazodone, Citalopram, or Placebo: Results from a Phase IV Clinical Trial." *International Clinical Psychopharmacology* 30: 216–223.

Cooke, M. J., and Waring, W. S. (2013). "Citalopram and Cardiac Toxicity." *European Journal of Clinical Pharmacology* 69: 755–760.

Daly, E. J., et al. (2017). "Efficacy and Safety of Intranasal Esketamine Adjunctive to Oral Antidepressant Therapy in Treatment-Resistant Depression: A Randomized Clinical Trial." *Journal of Clinical Psychiatry* Published online: doi:10.1001/jamapsychiatry.2017.3739.

Dash, S., et al. (2015). "The Gut Microbiome and Diet in Psychiatry: Focus on Depression." *Current Opinion in Psychiatry* 28: 1–6. doi: 10.1097/YCO.0000000000000117.

Deutschenbaur, L., et al. (2016). "Role of Calcium, Glutamate and NMDA in Major Depression and Therapeutic Application." *Progress in Neuro-Psychopharmacology & Biological Psychiatry* 64: 325–333.

Dhir, A. (2017). "Investigational Drugs for Treating Major Depressive Disorder." *Expert Opinion on Investigational Drugs* 26: 9–24.

Dieperink, P. K., et al. (2016). *Evidence Brief: The Comparative Effectiveness, Harms, and Cost-Effectiveness of Pharmacogenomics-Guided Antidepressant Treatment versus Usual Care for Major Depressive Disorder*. Washington, DC: Department of Veterans Affairs. https://www.ncbi.nlm.nih.gov/books/NBK384610/.

Di Giannantonio, M., and Martinotti, G. (2012). "Anhedonia and Major Depression: The Role of Agomelatine." *European Neuropsychopharmacology* 22, Supplement 3: S505–S510.

Duman, R. S., et al. (2012). "Signaling Pathways Underlying the Rapid Antidepressant Actions of Ketamine." *Neuropharmacology* 62: 35–41.

Ellsworth, K. A., et al. (2013). "FKBP5 Genetic Variation: Association with Selective Serotonin Reuptake Inhibitor Treatment Outcomes in Major Depressive Disorder." *Pharmacogenetic Genomics* 23: 156–166.

Elmaadawi, A. Z., et al. (2015). "Prescribers Guide to Using 3 New Antidepressants." *Current Psychiatry* 14: 29, 32–36.

Eom, C. S., et al. (2012). "Use of Selective Serotonin Reuptake Inhibitors and Risk of Fracture: A Systematic Review and Meta-Analysis." *Journal of Bone Mineralization Research* 27: 1186–1195.

Fabbri, C., and Serretti, A. (2015). "Pharmacogenetics of Major Depressive Disorder: Top Genes and Pathways toward Clinical Applications." *Current Psychiatry Reports* 17: 1–11.

Fabbrini, G., et al. (2012). "Selegiline: A Reappraisal of Its Role in Parkinson Disease." *Clinical Neuropharmacology* 35: 134–140.

Ferguson, J. M., et al. (2012). "High-Dose Desvenlafaxine in Outpatients with Major Depressive Disorder." *CNS Spectrums* 17: 121–130.

Ferraro, L., et al. (2013). "The Vigilance Promoting Drug Modafinil Modulates Serotonin Transmission in the Rat Prefrontal Cortex and Dorsal Raphe Nucleus. Possible Relevance for Its Postulated Antidepressant Activity." *Mini-Reviews in Medicinal Chemistry* 13: 478–492.

Finberg, J. P. M., and Rabey, J. M. (2016). "Inhibitors of MAO-A and MAO-B in Psychiatry and Neurology." *Frontiers in Pharmacology* 7: 1–15.

Flockhart, D. A. (2012). "Antidepressant Medication Prescribing Practices for Treatment of Major Depressive Disorder." *Journal of Clinical Psychiatry* 73 (Suppl. 1): 17–24.

Fond, G. et al. (2014). "Ketamine Administration in Depressive Disorders: A Systematic Review and Meta-Analysis." *Psychopharmacology* 231: 3663–3676.

Fournier, J. C., et al. (2010). "Antidepressant Drug Effects and Depression Severity: A Patient-Level Meta-Analysis." *Journal of the American Medical Association* 303: 47–53.

Frey, B. N., et al. (2013). "Effects of Quetiapine Extended Release on Sleep and Quality of Life in Midlife Women with Major Depressive Disorder." *Archives of Women's Mental Health* 16: 83–85.

Garcia-Toro, M., et al. (2012). "Treatment Patterns in Major Depressive Disorder after an Inadequate Response to First-Line Antidepressant Treatment." *BMC Psychiatry* 12: 143.

Gartlehner, G., et al. (2011). "Comparative Benefits and Harms of Second-Generation Antidepressants for Treating Major Depressive Disorder: An Updated Meta-Analysis." *Annals of Internal Medicine* 155: 772–785.

Gartlehner, G., et al. (2015). *Nonpharmacological versus Pharmacological Treatments for Adult Patients with Major Depressive Disorder. Comparative Effectiveness Review No. 161*. AHRQ Publication No. 15(16)-EHC031-EF. Rockville, MD: Agency for Healthcare Research and Quality. https://www.effectivehealthcare.ahrq.gov/ehc/products/568/2155/major-depressive-disorder-report-151202.pdf.

Gibbons, R. D., et al. (2012). "Suicidal Thoughts and Behavior with Antidepressant Treatment." *Archives of General Psychiatry* 69: 580–587.

Grande, I., et al. (2010). "The Role of BDNF as a Mediator of Neuroplasticity in Bipolar Disorder." *Psychiatry Investigations* 7: 243–250.

Guay, D. R., (2012). "Vilazodone Hydrochloride: A Combined SSRI and 5-HT1A Receptor Agonist for Major Depressive Disorder." *Consulting Pharmacist* 27: 857–867.

Haddad, P. M., et al. (2015). "Managing Inadequate Antidepressant Response in Depressive Illness." *British Medical Bulletin* 115: 183–201.

Hall-Flavin, D. K., et al. (2012). "Using a Pharmacogenomic Algorithm to Guide the Treatment of Depression." *Translational Psychiatry* 2: e172.

Han, D. H., et al. (2013). "Adjunctive Aripiprazole Therapy with Escitalopram in Patients with Co-Morbid Major Depressive Disorder and Alcohol Dependence: Clinical and Neuroimaging Evidence." *Journal of Psychopharmacology* 27: 282–291.

Harrison, P. (2016). "Off Label Ketamine Prescribing: US Psychiatrists Troubled." *Medscape*, April 25. www.medscape.com/viewarticle/862386.

Hegarty, B., and Parker, G. (2013). "Fish Oil as a Management Component for Mood Disorders: An Evolving Signal." *Current Opinions in Psychiatry* 26: 33–40.

Hellerstein, D. J., et al. (2012). "A Randomized Controlled Trial of Duloxetine versus Placebo in the Treatment of Nonmajor Chronic Depression." *Journal of Clinical Psychology* 73: 984–991.

Hoang, M. T., et al. (2011). "Association Between Low Serum 25-Hydroxyvitamin D and Depression in a Large Sample of Healthy Adults: The Cooper Center Longitudinal Study." *Mayo Clinic Proceedings* 86: 1050–1055.

Hoban, C. L., et al. (2015). "A Comparison of Patterns of Spontaneous Adverse Drug Reaction Reporting with St. John's Wort and Fluoxetine During the Period 2000–2013." *Clinical and Experimental Pharmacology and Physiology* 42: 747–751.

Holtzheimer, P. E., and Mayberg, H. S. (2011). "Stuck in a Rut: Rethinking Depression and Its Treatment." *Trends in Neurosciences* 34: 1–9.

Howland, R. H. (2012). "The Use of Dopaminergic and Stimulant Drugs for the Treatment of Depression." *Journal of Psychosocial Nursing and Mental Health Services* 50: 11–14.

Howland, R. H. (2014). "Pharmacogenetic Testing in Clinical Psychiatry." *Carlat Report: Psychiatry* 12: 1–3, 8.

Hutton, L. M. J., et al. (2016). "Should We Be Worried about QTc Prolongation Using Citalopram? A Review." *Journal of Pharmacy Practice*. doi: 10.1177/0897190015624862.

Jacobsen, P. L., et al. (2015). "Effect of Vortioxetine vs. Escitalopram on Sexual Functioning in Adults with Well-Treated Major Depressive Disorder Experiencing SSRI-Induced Sexual Dysfunction." *Journal of Sexual Medicine* 12: 2036–2048.

Jain, R., et al. (2013). "A Randomized, Double-Blind, Placebo-Controlled 6-Wk Trial of the Efficacy and Tolerability of 5 mg Vortioxetine in Adults with Major Depressive Disorder." *International Journal of Neuropsychopharmacology* 16: 313–321.

Jamerson, B. D., et al. (2013). "Folate Metabolism Genes, Dietary Folate and Response to Antidepressant Medications in Late-Life Depression." *International Journal of Geriatric Psychiatry* 28: 925–932.

Kasper, S., et al. (2013). "Antidepressant Efficacy of Agomelatine versus SSRI/SNRI: Results from a Pooled Analysis of Head-to-Head Studies without a Placebo Control." *International Clinical Psychopharmacology* 28: 12–19.

Kessler, R. C., et al. (2003). "The Epidemiology of Major Depressive Disorder: Results from the National Comorbidity Survey Replication (NCS-R)." *JAMA* 289: 3095–3105.

Khan, A. (2012). "A Systematic Review of Comparative Efficacy of Treatments and Controls for Depression." *PLoS One* 7: e41778.

Khan, A., and Brown, W. A. (2015). "Antidepressants versus Placebo in Major Depression: An Overview." *World Psychiatry* 14: 294–300.

Kappelmann, N., et al. (2018). "Antidepressant Activity of Anti-Cytokine Treatment: A Systematic Review and Meta-Analysis of Clinical Trials of Chronic Inflammatory Conditions." *Molecular Psychiatry* 23: 335–343. In press. doi:10.1038/mp.2016.167.

Khoraminya, N., et al. (2013). "Therapeutic Effects of Vitamin D as Adjunctive Therapy to Fluoxetine in Patients with Major Depressive Disorder." *Australian & New Zealand Journal of Psychiatry* 47: 271–275.

Kim, D., and Steinhart, B. (2010). "Seizures Induced by Recreational Abuse of Bupropion Tablets via Nasal Insufflation." *Canadian Journal of Emergency Medicine* 12: 158–161.

Kupfer, D. J., et al. (2012). "Major Depressive Disorder: New Clinical, Neurobiological, and Treatment Perspectives." *Lancet* 379: 1045–1055.

Lacasse, J. R., and Leo, J. (2005). "Serotonin and Depression: A Disconnect Between the Advertisements and the Scientific Literature." *PLoS Medicine* 2: 1211–1216.

Latufo-Neto, F., et al. (1999). "Meta-Analysis of the Reversible Inhibitors of Monoamine Oxidase Type A Moclobemide and Brofaromine for the Treatment of Depression." *Neuropsychopharmacology* 20: 226–247.

Launay, J. M., et al. (2011). "Raphe-Mediated Signals Control the Hippocampal Response to SRI Antidepressants via miR-16." *Translational Psychiatry* 1: e56.

Lavretsky, H., et al. (2015). "Citalopram, Methylphenidate, or Their Combination in Geriatric Depression: A Randomized, Double-Blind, Placebo-Controlled Trial." *American Journal of Psychiatry* 172: 561–569.

Lesperance, F., et al. (2011). "The Efficacy of Omega-3 Supplementation for Major Depression." *Journal of Clinical Psychiatry* 72: 1054–1062.

Leuner, K., et al. (2013). "Hyperforin Modulates Dendritic Spine Morphology in Hippocampal Pyramidal Neurons by Activating Ca(2+) –Permeable TRPC6 Channels." *Hippocampus* 23: 40–52.

Li, L., and Vlisides, P. E. (2016). "Ketamine: 50 Years of Modulating the Mind." *Frontiers in Human Neuroscience* 10: 612. doi: 10.3389/fnhum.2016.00612.

Lin, P-Y, et al. (2012). "Are Omega-3 Fatty Acids Anti-Depressants or Just Mood-Improving Agents." *Molecular Psychiatry* 17: 1161–1163.

Linden, M., et al. (1996). "Psychiatric Diseases and Their Treatment in General Practice in Germany. Results of a World Health Organization (WHO) Study." *Der Nervenarzt* 67: 205–215.

Liu, C. Y., et al. (2012). "Metabotropic Glutamate Receptor 5 Antagonist 2-Methyl-6-(Phenethyl) Pyridine Produces Antidepressant Effects in Rats: Role of Brain-Derived Neurotropic Factor." *Neuroscience* 223C: 219–224.

Lucassen, P. J., et al. (2010). "Regulation of Adult Neurogenesis by Stress, Sleep Disruption, Exercise and Inflammation: Implications for Depression and Antidepressant Action." *European Neuropsychopharmacology* 20: 1–17.

Lyman, G. H., and Moses, H. L. (2016). "Biomarker Tests for Molecularly Targeted Therapies— The Key to Unlocking Precision Medicine." *New England Journal of Medicine* 375: 4–6. doi: 10.1056/NEJMp1604033.

Maneeton, N., et al. (2012). "Quetiapine Monotherapy in Acute Phase for Major Depressive Disorder: A Meta-Analysis of Randomized, Placebo-Controlled Trials." *BMC Psychiatry* 12(1): 160.

Martinez, C., et al. (2010). "Use of Venlafaxine Compared with Other Antidepressants and the Risk of Sudden Cardiac Death or Near Death: A Nested Case-Control Study." *BMJ* 340: c249. doi: 10.1136/bmj.c249.

Masi, G., and Brovedani, P. (2011). "The Hippocampus, Neurotropic Factors and Depression: Possible Implications for the Pharmacotherapy of Depression." *CNS Drugs* 25: 913–931.

Mech, A. W., and Farah, A. (2016). "Correlation of Clinical Response with Homocysteine Reduction During Therapy with Reduced B Vitamins in Patients with MDD Who Are Positive for MTHFR C677T or A1298C Polymorphism: A Randomized, Double-Blind, Placebo-Controlled Study." *Journal of Clinical Psychiatry* 77: 668–671. doi: /10.4088/JCP.15m10166.

Mental Health Daily. (2015). "20 New Antidepressants in the Pipeline (2015): Drugs in Clinical Trials." *Mental Health Blog*. Mentalhealthdaily.com/2015/09/11/new-antidepressants-in-the-pipeline-2015-drugs-in-clinical-trials/.

Miller, A. H., and Raison, C. L. (2016). "The Role of Inflammation in Depression: From Evolutionary Imperative to Modern Treatment Target." *Nature Reviews: Immunology* 16: 22–34.

Mitjans, M., and Arias, B. (2012). "The Genetics of Depression: What Information Can New Methodologic Approaches Provide?" *Actas Espanolas de Psiquitria* 40: 70–83.

Murrough, J. W., et al. (2013). "Rapid and Longer-Term Antidepressant Effects of Repeated Ketamine Infusions in Treatment-Resistant Major Depression." *Biological Psychiatry* 15: 250–256.

Muzina, D. J. (2010). "Discontinuing an Antidepressant? Tapering Tips to Ease Distressing Symptoms." *Current Psychiatry* 9: 51–61.

Nahas, R., and Sheikh, O. (2011). "Complementary and Alternative Medicine for the Treatment of Major Depressive Disorder." *Canadian Family Physician* 57: 659–663.

Nandagopal, J. J., and DelBello, M. P. (2009). "Selegiline Transdermal System: A Novel Treatment Option for Major Depressive Disorder." *Expert Opinions in Pharmacotherapy* 10: 1665–1673.

Narasimhan, S., and Lohoff, F. W. (2012). "Pharmacogenetics of Antidepressant Drugs: Current Clinical Practice and Future Directions." *Pharmacogenomics* 13: 441–464.

National Academies of Sciences, Engineering, and Medicine. (2017). *An Evidence Framework for Genetic Testing.* Washington, DC: *National Academies Press.* doi:10.17226/24632.

Newport, D. J., et al. (2015). "Ketamine and Other NMDA Antagonists: Early Clinical Trials and Possible Mechanisms in Depression." *American Journal of Psychiatry* 172: 950–966.

Niemegeers, P., et al. (2012). "Pharmacokinetic Evaluation of Armodafinil for the Treatment of Bipolar Depression." *Expert Opinion in Drug Metabolism and Toxicology* 8: 1189–1197.

Nelson, J. C., and Spyker, D. A. (2017). "Morbidity and Mortality Associated with Medications Used in the Treatment of Depression: An Analysis of Cases Reported to U.S. Poison Control Centers, 2000–2014." *American Journal of Psychiatry* 174: 438–450. doi: 10.1176/appi.ajp.2016.16050523.

Neto, F. L., et al. (2011). "Neurotropins Role in Depression Neurobiology: A Review of Basic and Clinical Evidence." *Current Neuropharmacology* 9: 530–552.

Ng, Q. X., et al. (2017). "Clinical Use of Hypericum Perforatum (St. John's Wort) in Depression: A Meta-Analysis." *Journal of Affective Disorders* 210: 211–221. doi: 10.1016/j.jad.2016.12.048.

Nierenberg, A. A. (2011). "The Current Crisis of Confidence in Antidepressants." *Journal of Clinical Psychiatry* 72: 27–33.

Nurnberg, H. G., et al. (2008). "Sildenafil Treatment of Women with Antidepressant-Associated Sexual Dysfunction: A Randomized Controlled Trial." *Journal of the American Medical Association* 300: 395–404.

Olfson, M., et al. (2016). "Treatment of Adult Depression in the United States." *JAMA Internal Medicine* 176: 1482–1491. doi: 10.1001/jamainternmed.2016.5057.

Pae, C. U., et al. (2009). "Desvenlafaxine: A New Antidepressant or Just Another One?" *Expert Opinion on Pharmacotherapy* 10: 875–887.

Pae, C. U., et al. (2012). "Safety of Selegiline Transdermal System in Clinical Practice: Analysis of Adverse Events from Postmarketing Exposures." *Journal of Clinical Psychiatry* 73: 661–668.

Papakostas, G. I., et al. (2012a). "A 12-Week, Randomized, Double-Blind, Placebo-Controlled, Sequential Parallel Comparison Trial of Ziprasidone as Monotherapy for Major Depressive Disorder." *Journal of Clinical Psychiatry* 73: 1541–1547.

Papakostas, G. I., et al. (2012b). "L-Methylfolate as Adjunctive Therapy for SSRI-Resistant Major Depression: Results of Two Randomized, Double-Blind, Parallel-Sequential Trials." *American Journal of Psychiatry* 169: 1267–1274.

Papakostas, G. I., et al. (2012c). "Folates and S-Adenosylmethionine for Major Depressive Disorder." *Canadian Journal of Psychiatry* 57: 406–413.

Parker, G., and Brotchie, H. (2010). "Do the Old Psychostimulant Drugs Have a Role in Managing Treatment-Resistant Depression?" *Acta Psychiatrica Scandinavia* 121: 308–314.

Patkar, A., et al. (2012). "A 6-Week Randomized Double-Blind Placebo-Controlled Trial of Ziprasidone for the Acute Depressive Mixed State." *PLoS One* 7: e34757. doi: 10.1371/journal.pone.0034757.

Peritogiannis, V., et al. (2009). "Duloxetine-Induced Hypomania: Case Report and Brief Review of the Literature on SNRIs-Induced Mood Switching." *Journal of Psychopharmacology* 23: 592–596.

Philipp, M., et al. (1999). "Hypericum Extract Versus Imipramine or Placebo in Patients with Moderate Depression: Randomized Multicentre Study of Treatment for Eight Weeks." *BMJ* 319: 1534–1539.

Preskorn, S. H. (2009). "Treatment Options for the Patient Who Does Not Respond Well to Initial Antidepressant Therapy." *Journal of Psychiatric Practice* 15: 202–210.

Rahimi, R., and Abdollahi, M. (2012). "An Update on the Ability of St. John's Wort to Affect the Metabolism of Other Drugs." *Expert Opinion on Drug Metabolism and Toxicology* 8: 691–708.

Raison, C. (2017). "The Promise and Limitations of Anti-Inflammatory Agents for the Treatment of Major Depressive Disorder." *Current Topics in Behavioral Neurosciences* 31: 287–302.

Ravindran, A. V., et al. (2000). "Treatment of Dysthymia with Sertraline: A Double-Blind, Placebo-Controlled Trial in Dysthymic Patients without Major Depression." *Journal of Clinical Psychiatry* 61: 821–827.

Reefhuis, J., et al. (2015). "Specific SSRIs and Birth Defects: Bayesian Analysis to Interpret New Data in the Context of Previous Reports." *BMJ* 350: h3190. doi: 10.1136/bmj.h3190.

Reinhold, J. A., et al. (2012). "Evidence for the Use of Vilazodone in the Treatment of Major Depressive Disorder." *Expert Opinions on Pharmacotherapeutics* 13: 2215–2224.

Richardson, J. D., et al. (2011). "Aripiprazole Augmentation in the Treatment of Military-Related PTSD with Major Depression: A Retrospective Chart Review." *BMC Psychiatry* 11: 86.

Rothschild, A. J., et al. (2012). "Vortioxetine (Lu AA21004) 5 mg in Generalized Anxiety Disorder: Results of an 8-Week Randomized, Double-Blind, Placebo-Controlled Clinical Trial in the United States." *European Neuropsychopharmacology* 22: 858–866.

Rucker, J. J. H., et al. (2016). "Psychedelics in the Treatment of Unipolar Mood Disorders: A Systematic Review." *Journal of Psychopharmacology* 30: 1220–1229.

Rush, A. J., et al. (2011). "Combining Medications to Enhance Depression Outcomes (CO-MED): Acute and Long-Term Outcomes of a Single-Blind Randomized Study." *American Journal of Psychiatry* 168: 689–701.

Sarris, J., et al. (2012). "St. John's Wort (*Hypericum perforatum*) versus Sertraline and Placebo in Major Depressive Disorder: Continuation Data from a 26-Week RCT." *Pharmacopsychiatry* 45: 275–278.

Saveanu, R. V., and Nemeroff, C. B. (2012). "Etiology of Depression: Genetic and Environmental Factors." *Psychiatric Clinics of North America* 35: 51–71.

Schosser, A., et al. (2012). "European Group for the Study of Resistant Depression (GSRD)—Where Have We Gone So Far?: Review of Clinical and Genetic Findings." *European Neuropsychopharmacology* 22: 453–468.

Schweitzer, I., et al. (2009). "Sexual Side-Effects of Contemporary Antidepressants: Review." *Australian and New Zealand Journal of Psychiatry* 43: 795–808.

Sharon, G., et al. (2016). "The Central Nervous System and the Gut Microbiome." *Cell* 167: 915–932. doi: 10.1016/j.cell.2016.10.027.

Sheehan, D. V., et al. (2012). "Long-Term Functioning and Sleep Quality in Patients with Major Depressive Disorder Treated with Extended-Release Quetiapine Fumarate." *International Clinical Psychopharmacology* 27: 239–248.

Sher, L. (2011). "The Role of Brain-Derived Neurotropic Factor in the Pathophysiology of Adolescent Suicidal Behavior." *International Journal of Adolescent Medicine and Health* 23: 181–185.

Shulman, K. I., et al. (2013). "Current Place of Monoamine Oxidase Inhibitors in the Treatment of Depression." *CNS Drugs* 27: 789–797. doi: 10.1007/s40263-013-0097-3.

Sindrup, S. H., et al. (2005). "Antidepressants in the Treatment of Neuropathic Pain." *Basic and Clinical Pharmacology and Toxicology* 96: 399–409.

Singh, A. B., et al. (2012). "ABCB1 Polymorphism Predicts Escitalopram Dose Needed for Remission in Major Depression." *Translational Psychiatry* 2: e198. doi: 10.1038/tp.2012.115.

Singh, J. B., et al. (2016). "Intravenous Esketamine in Adult Treatment-Resistant Depression: A Double-Blind, Double-Randomization, Placebo-Controlled Study." *Biological Psychiatry* 80: 424–431.

Singh, M., and Schwartz, T. L. (2012). "Clinical Utility of Vilazodone for the Treatment of Adults with Major Depressive Disorder and Theoretical Implications for Future Clinical Use." *Journal of Neuropsychiatric Disease and Treatment* 8: 123–130.

Sinyor, M., et al. (2010). "The Sequences Treatment Alternatives to Relieve Depression (STAR*D) Trial: A Review." *Canadian Journal of Psychiatry* 55: 126–135.

Solomon, D. A., et al. (2005). "Tachyphylaxis in Unipolar Major Depressive Disorder." *Journal of Clinical Psychiatry* 66: 283–290.

Sos, P. (2016). "Is There a Future for Other Glutamate Receptor Modulators in the Pharmacotherapy of Mood Disorders?" *Evidence Based Mental Health* 19: 95–96.

Spina, E., et al. (2008). "Clinically Relevant Pharmacokinetic Drug Interactions with Second-Generation Antidepressants: An Update." *Clinical Therapeutics* 30: 1206–1227.

Stahl, S. M., et al. (2013). "Serotonergic Drugs for Depression and Beyond." *Current Drug Targets* 14: 578–585.

Sublette, M. E., et al. (2011). "Meta-Analysis of the Effects of Eicosapentaenoic Acid (EPA) in Clinical Trials in Depression." *Journal of Clinical Psychiatry* 72: 1577–1584.

Substance Abuse and Mental Health Services Administration. (2016). *Results from the 2015 National Survey on Drug Use and Health: Detailed Tables.* Research Triangle Park, NC: RTI International. https://www.samhsa.gov/data/sites/default/files/NSDUH-DetTabs-2015/NSDUH-DetTabs-2015/NSDUH-DetTabs-2015.pdf.

Tallon, D., et al. (2016). "Mirtazapine Added to Selective Serotonin Reuptake Inhibitors for Treatment-Resistant Depression in Primary Care (MIR Trial): Study Protocol for a Randomised Controlled Trial." *Trials* 17: 66. doi: 10.1186/s13063-016-1199-2.

Targum, S. D. (2014). "Identification and Treatment of Antidepressant Tachyphylaxis." *Innovations in Clinical Neuroscience* 11: 24–28.

Taylor, M. J., et al. (2013). "Strategies for Managing Sexual Dysfunction Induced by Antidepressant Medication (Review)." *Cochrane Database of Systematic Reviews* (Issue 5): CD003382. doi: 10.1002/14651858.CD003382.pub3.

Thaipisuttikul, P., et al. (2014). "Psychiatric Comorbidities in Patients with Major Depressive Disorder." *Neuropsychiatric Disease and Treatment* 10: 2097–2103.

Thase, M. E. (2016). "Managing Medical Comorbidities in Patients with Depression to Improve Prognosis." *Journal of Clinical Psychiatry* 77 (Suppl. 1): 22–27.

Thase, M. E., et al. (2006). "A Double-Blind Comparison Between Bupropion XL and Venlafaxine XR: Sexual Functioning, Antidepressant Efficacy, and Tolerability." *Journal of Clinical Psychopharmacology* 26: 482–488.

Treviño, L. A., et al. (2017). "Antidepressant Medication Prescribing Practices for Treatment of Major Depressive Disorder." *Psychiatric Services* 68: 199–202.

Tripp, A., et al. (2012). "Brain-Derived Neurotropic Factor Signaling and Subgenual Anterior Cingulate Cortex Dysfunction in Major Depressive Disorder." *American Journal of Psychiatry* 169: 1194–1202.

Undurraga, J., and Baldessarini, R. J. (2012). "Randomized, Placebo-Controlled Trials of Antidepressants for Acute Major Depression: Thirty-Year Meta-Analytic Review." *Neuropsychopharmacology* 37: 851–864.

Vieweg, W. V., et al. (2012). "Citalopram, QTc Interval Prolongation and Torsade de Pointes. How Should We Apply the Recent FDA Ruling?" *American Journal of Medicine* 125: 859–868.

Wade, A. G., et al. (2011). "Efficacy, Safety, and Tolerability of Escitalopram in Doses up to 50 mg in Major Depressive Disorder (MDD): An Open-Label, Pilot Study." *BMC Psychiatry* 11: 42.

Wainwright, S. R., and Galea, L. A. M. (2013). "The Neural Plasticity Theory of Depression: Assessing the Roles of Adult Neurogenesis and PSA-NCAM within the Hippocampus." *Neural Plasticity* 2013: 1–14.

Wang, G., et al. (2015). "Comparison of Vortioxetine Versus Venlafaxine XR in Adults in Asia with Major Depressive Disorder: A Randomized, Double-Blind Study." *Current Medical Research and Opinion* 31: 785–794.

Watanabe, N., et al. (2011). "Mirtazapine versus Other Antidepressant Agents for Depression." *Cochrane Database of Systematic Reviews* (Issue 12): CD006528. doi: 10.1002/14651858. CD006528.pub2.

Winner, J. G., and Dechairo, B. (2015). "Combinatorial versus Individual Gene Pharmacogenomic Testing in Mental Health: A Perspective on Context and Implications on Clinical Utility." *Yale Journal of Biology and Medicine* 88: 375–382.

Wittenborn, A. K., et al. (2016). "Depression as a Systemic Syndrome: Mapping the Feedback Loops of Major Depressive Disorder." *Psychological Medicine* 46: 551–562.

Wohleb, E. S., et al. (2016). "Integrating Neuroimmune Systems in the Neurobiology of Depression." *Nature Reviews: Neuroscience* 17: 497–511.

World Health Organization. (2013). "Mental Health Action Plan 2013–2020." *World Health Organization*, Geneva, Switzerland (www.who.int).

CHAPTER 13

Anxiolytics, Sedative Hypnotics, Anesthetics, and Anticonvulsants

CLINICAL INDICATIONS

The drugs discussed in this chapter are a chemically diverse group of substances that act on the nervous system to decrease neuronal activation or increase inhibition. Clinically, they are used to treat anxiety disorders, insomnia, and seizure disorders. As such, they are usually prescribed by physicians and other medical professionals, with the exception of alcohol, which is used recreationally. Nevertheless, like alcohol, they are commonly misused, resulting in the development of a substance abuse disorder or dependence. Moreover, overdoses and withdrawal from certain of the sedative-hypnotic agents can be life-threatening.

Lower doses of these drugs usually have a calming or sedating effect, whereas higher doses have a hypnotic effect, which means they induce sleep, which is why they are often referred to as *sedative-hypnotics*. The calming effect of some of these drugs may specifically reduce anxiety, rather than induce a state of drowsiness. Such drugs are termed *anxiolytics*, *antianxiety drugs*, or *tranquilizers*. Other members of this category act specifically to suppress excessive neuronal, electrical, excitation, known as seizures, as well as the associated motor reactions, that is, convulsions; these are termed *anticonvulsants*. Some drugs, such as the barbiturates and benzodiazepines, can produce all three effects, anxiolytic, hypnotic, and anticonvulsive. Nevertheless, the three types of drug action can be differentiated because the effects may occur at different doses of the same drugs and because some drugs are highly selective for one of these effects.

Sedative-hypnotics treat the following disorders:

- *Insomnia* is defined as a condition in which the patient is unable to fall or stay asleep, even when there is ample time to do so. Insomnia can also include a feeling of dissatisfaction with the quality of sleep. The condition usually includes at least one of the following symptoms: fatigue, low energy, difficulty concentrating, mood disturbances, and decreased performance in work or at school.

- *Anxiety disorders* include several categories, not all of which are best treated with drugs. The most relevant types in regard to the sedative-hypnotics, anxiolytics, and other pharmacotherapies are the following:

  - *Generalized anxiety disorder* (GAD) is characterized by chronic, excessive worry, which could be about various aspects of life, such as money, health, and work. The emotion cannot be controlled or prevented, and is often associated with physical symptoms such as muscle tension, insomnia, problems with attention and concentration, and social withdrawal.

  - *Panic disorder* consists of repeated, spontaneous panic attacks, defined as sudden and unpredictable intervals of intense fear that can involve palpitations, pounding heart, or accelerated heart rate; sweating; trembling or shaking; sensations of shortness of breath, smothering, or choking; and a feeling of impending doom.

  - *Agoraphobia* is a complication of panic disorder, which can also be experienced without a prior panic attack. The individual fears being in places or situations that would be hard or embarrassing to escape from should a panic attack occur. Some sufferers do not even venture outside their homes.

  - *Social anxiety disorder* (also called *social phobia*) is defined as a fear of social or performance situations in which the individual expects to feel embarrassed, judged, rejected, or afraid of offending others.

  - A *phobia* is a broad category of anxiety disorder, which consists of a strong, irrational fear of something that poses minimal or no real danger. There are numerous specific phobias, including *acrophobia* (a fear of heights) and *claustrophobia* (a fear of closed-in places).

  - *Posttraumatic stress disorder* (PTSD) is a condition that develops in some people who have experienced a shocking, frightening, or dangerous event. The condition is characterized by a reexperiencing of the prior traumatic events in the form of intrusive thoughts, flashbacks, and dreams. Situations reminiscent of the trauma are avoided, and there may be numbed responsiveness to the environment, lack of interest in activities, detachment from other people or hyperarousal, hypervigilance, exaggerated startle responses, sleep disturbances, and impaired concentration.

  - *Obsessive-compulsive disorder* (OCD) was previously designated as an anxiety disorder, but is no longer in that category. OCD is a chronic disorder in which an individual has reoccurring thoughts (*obsessions*) that they cannot control, and behaviors (*compulsions*) that they have an uncontrollable urge to repeat over and over.

HISTORICAL BACKGROUND

In the mid-nineteenth century, *bromide* and *chloral hydrate* became available as sleep-inducing agents and used as alternatives to alcohol and opium. In 1912, *phenobarbital* was introduced as a sedative drug, the first of the structurally classified

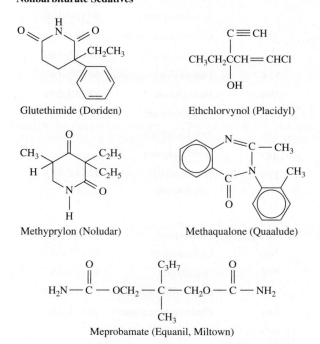

Nonbarbiturate Sedatives

FIGURE 13.1 Chemical structures of classical sedatives. Barbiturates are defined by containing the barbiturate nucleus. Nonbarbiturate sedatives do not have this basic structure.

group of drugs called *barbiturates* (Figure 13.1). Between 1912 and 1950, about 50 different barbiturate formulations were commercially marketed. As the dangers of death from barbiturate overdose became recognized, several other sedatives, including *meprobamate* (Equanil) and *carisoprodol* (Soma), were marketed as potentially safer alternatives. While overdose lethality may have been reduced, other dangers remained, including dependence and addiction.

In 1960, *chlordiazepoxide* (Librium) was marketed as the first of a new structural class of anxiolytic and sedating drugs called *benzodiazepines;* the primary ones are listed in Table 13.1. The benzodiazepines had one major advantage over the barbiturates: unless they were combined with alcohol or opioids, benzodiazepines were rarely, if ever, fatal in cases of overdose. Because of this improved safety, the benzodiazepine tranquilizers became a popular choice among physicians for the treatment of anxiety and insomnia.

TABLE 13.1 Benzodiazepines

Drug name		Dosage form		Active metabolite	Active compounds in blood	Mean elimination half-life (hours and range)
Generic	Trade	Oral	Parenteral			
LONG-ACTING AGENTS						
Diazepam	Valium	X	X	Yes	Diazepam	24 (20–50)
					Nordiazepam	60 (50–100)
Chlordiazepoxide	Librium	X		Yes	Chlordiazepoxide	10 (8–24)
					Nordiazepam	60 (50–100)
Flurazepam	Dalmane	X		Yes	Desalkylflurazepam	80 (70–160)
Halazepam	Paxipam	X		Yes	Halazepam	14 (10–20)
					Nordiazepam	
Prazepam	Centrax	X		Yes	Nordiazepam	
Chlorazepate	Tranxene	X		Yes	Nordiazepam	
Clobazam	Onfi	X		Yes	N-desmethyl clobazam	32 (12–42)
INTERMEDIATE-ACTING AGENTS						
Lorazepam	Ativan	X	X	No	Lorazepam	15 (10–24)
Clonazepam	Klonopin	X		No	Clonazepam	30 (18–50)
Quazepam	Dormalin	X		Yes	Quazepam	35 (25–50)
					Desalkylflurazepam	80 (70–160)
Estazolam	ProSom	X		Yes	Hydroxyestazolam	18 (13–35)
SHORT-ACTING AGENTS						
Midazolam	Versed		X	No	Midazolam	2.5 (1.5–4.5)
Oxazepam	Serax	X		No	Oxazepam	8 (5–15)
Temazepam	Restoril	X		No	Temazepam	12 (8–35)
Triazolam	Halcion	X		No	Triazolam	2.5 (1.5–5)
Alprazolam	Xanax	X		No	Alprazolam	12 (11–18)

Today, we are in the midst of an epidemic of deaths from drug overdoses. In 2013, an estimated 22,767 people in the United States died as the result of an overdose involving prescription drugs; benzodiazepines were involved in about 31percent of these fatal overdoses (Bachhuber et al., 2016). Most of these overdoses involved combining a benzodiazepine with alcohol or opioids. In September 2016, the FDA drew attention to the potentially fatal interaction between benzodiazepines and opioid analgesics and serious risks of extreme sleepiness, respiratory depression, coma, and death. The FDA now requires its strongest black box warnings on all opioid and benzodiazepine packaging advising of the risks of combining drugs from these two classes (Hawkins et al., 2016; Horsfall and Sprague, 2016; McCarthy, 2016; Stein et al., 2016).

SITES AND MECHANISMS OF ACTION

Initially, the barbiturates were thought to produce their sedative-hypnotic, anxiolytic, anticonvulsant, and general anesthetic actions by a nonselective neuronal depression throughout the brain. Brainstem depression was presumed to increase as dosage increased, accounting for the deep coma, cessation of respiration, and death that can follow barbiturate overdose. Today, we have a much better understanding of specific receptor–drug interactions that mediate the actions of barbiturates.

In our current era of drug development, we name new drugs not so much by their structure, as in the case of barbiturates and benzodiazepines, but by the receptors to which they bind or which underlie their major clinical action, such as a selective serotonin reuptake inhibitor, a serotonin 1A receptor agonist, a dopamine$_2$ blocker, and so on. If discovered today, a barbiturate or a benzodiazepine would be called a *GABA receptor agonist*. Because of what is now known of GABA receptors and because specific binding sites for both barbiturates and benzodiazepines on the GABA receptor have been identified (Figure 13.2), these and related drugs are called *benzodiazepine receptor agonists* (BZRAs). This term includes both the benzodiazepines and several

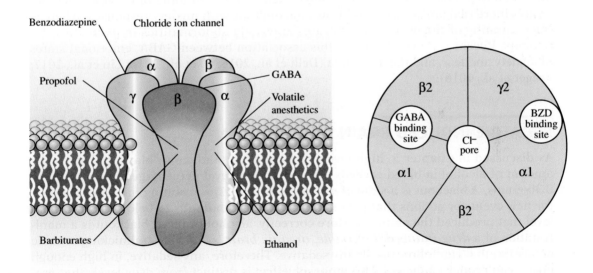

FIGURE 13.2 The GABA$_A$ receptor complex. This complex consists of several protein subunits, with each comprised further of subunit families. Different drugs bind at different sites on this complex. GABA is the normal transmitter. Benzodiazepines potentiate the influence of GABA. Other drugs, such as propofol and barbiturates, not only potentiate GABA, but can also open the channel directly. The inset is a schematic cross section of the receptor complex.

newer nonbenzodiazepines that are widely prescribed to improve the quality of sleep in the clinical management of insomnia.

Benzodiazepines facilitate the binding of GABA to its receptor. They do not directly stimulate the GABA receptor; rather, they bind to a site adjacent to the GABA receptor, producing a three-dimensional conformational change in the receptor structure that, in turn, increases the affinity of GABA for the receptor. That effect, in turn, increases the inhibitory synaptic action of GABA, facilitating the influx of chloride ions, causing hyperpolarization of the postsynaptic neuron and depressing its excitability.

Barbiturates also act at the GABA receptor, but in a slightly different manner. Whereas benzodiazepines increase the *frequency* of the chloride ion channel opening at the $GABA_A$ receptor, the main pharmacological effect of barbiturates is an increase in the duration of chloride ion channel opening at the $GABA_A$ receptor. This direct action of opening the chloride ion channel is why barbiturates are more toxic compared to benzodiazepines in cases of overdose.

Benzodiazepines exert their anxiolytic properties by acting on GABA neurons at limbic centers. Their actions at other regions, such as the cerebral cortex and brain stem, produce side effects such as sedation, increased seizure threshold, cognitive impairment, amnesia, and muscle relaxation. The amygdala, orbitofrontal cortex, and insula are the neuroanatomical structures most associated with the production of behavioral fear reactions and the mediation of anxiety and panic in the central nervous system. Electrical stimulation of these structures evokes behavioral and physiological responses that are associated with fear and anxiety. Electrical lesions of the amygdala in animals result in an anxiolytic effect. PET scanning of the brain demonstrates increased amygdala blood flow concomitant with anxiety responses, whereas MRI scanning of the brain demonstrates amygdala abnormalities in panic disorder patients. Recent reviews document this association between GABA, emotional states of anxiety and fear, and the amygdala (Delli et al., 2016; Di et al., 2016; Liu et al., 2017; Prager et al., 2016).

SEDATIVE-INDUCED BRAIN DYSFUNCTION

As discussed in Chapter 5, high levels of alcohol can induce a "blackout" when the amount of alcohol in blood exceeds a blood alcohol level percentage of about 0.25 to 0.30 grams. A blackout is a state of *anterograde amnesia*, resulting in loss of memory for new events or actions that persist until blood alcohol falls to below the threshold level that produced the amnesia. More correctly, alcohol-induced blackout is a manifestation of a *drug-induced, reversible, organic brain syndrome* (mimicking organic dementia) that can follow use of any sedative. Therefore, any sedative, in high enough doses, can produce amnesia. This amnestic effect is distinct from drug levels that produce loss of consciousness, as a person can be in a blackout and still be awake and capable of performing behavioral activities. Indeed, sedative-hypnotic medications now carry an FDA warning concerning a potential for inducing *complex sleep-related behaviors*, which may include driving a motor vehicle ("sleep driving"), making phone calls, preparing and eating food, and similar activities, all while having no memory of having done so.

Stemming from their amnestic effect, some sedative drugs are sometimes called "date rape" drugs. A person who takes the drug does not remember what happened during the period of intoxication, despite being in a state of wakefulness and able to be an active participant in sexual activity. In medicine, this is seen when medical professionals induce a state of *conscious sedation*, where the patient may be awake and cooperative yet does not remember the medical procedure. One example is the administration of the short-acting benzodiazepine *midazolam* (Versed) so the patient does not remember a colonoscopy, despite having been awake during the procedure.

People who already have some natural loss of nerve cell function, such as the elderly, are more likely to be adversely affected by these drugs. They experience increased disorientation and further clouding of consciousness. Frequently, these people exhibit a state of drug-induced paradoxical excitement, which is characterized by a labile personality with marked anger, delusions, hallucinations, and confabulations, that is, unconscious fabrication of information to fill memory gaps. Treating drug-induced memory loss requires that administration of the sedative drug (or alcohol) be stopped.

BARBITURATES

As mentioned, barbiturates are among the earliest sedative-hypnotic drugs. During their decades of use, barbiturates were associated with thousands of suicides, deaths from accidental ingestion, widespread dependency and abuse, and many serious interactions with other drugs and alcohol. They are now rarely used; however, they remain the classic prototype of sedative-hypnotic drugs.

Pharmacokinetics

All barbiturates are similar in structure. They are classified by their individual pharmacokinetics. Their half-lives can be quite short, such as the 3-minute redistribution half-life for thiopental, or as long as several days, as in the case of phenobarbital (discussed below). The hypnotic action of ultrashort-acting barbiturates such as thiopental is terminated by redistribution, while the action of other barbiturates is determined by their rate of metabolism by enzymes in the liver.

Barbiturates are well absorbed orally and well distributed to most body tissues. The ultrashort-acting barbiturates are exceedingly lipid soluble, cross the blood-brain barrier rapidly, and induce sleep within seconds following their intravenous injection. Because the longer-acting barbiturates are more water soluble, they are slower to penetrate the central nervous system (CNS). Sleep induction with these compounds, therefore, is delayed for 20 to 30 minutes, and residual hangover is prominent since the plasma half-lives of most barbiturates are longer than that needed for 8 hours of sleep.

Pharmacological Effects

Barbiturates have a low degree of selectivity, and it is not possible to achieve anxiolysis without evidence of sedation. Barbiturates are not analgesic; they cannot be relied on to produce sedation or sleep in the presence of even moderate pain. Sleep patterns are decidedly affected by barbiturates; rapid eye movement (REM) sleep is markedly suppressed. Because dreaming occurs during REM sleep, barbiturates suppress dreaming. During drug withdrawal, dreaming becomes vivid and excessive. This increase in dreaming during withdrawal, termed *REM rebound*, is one example of a withdrawal effect following prolonged periods of barbiturate ingestion. The vivid nature of the dreams can lead to insomnia, which can be clinically relieved by restarting the drug, terminating the withdrawal response.

Since barbiturates depress memory functioning, they are *cognitive inhibitors*. Drowsiness and more subtle alterations of judgment, cognitive functioning, motor skills, physical coordination, and behavior may persist for hours or days until the barbiturate is completely metabolized and eliminated. Sedative doses of barbiturates have minimal effect on respiration, but overdoses, or combinations of barbiturates and alcohol, can result in death.

Barbiturates exert few significant effects on the cardiovascular system, the gastrointestinal tract, the kidneys, or other organs until toxic doses are reached. In the liver, barbiturates stimulate the synthesis of enzymes that metabolize other drugs, as well as the barbiturates themselves, which produces significant tolerance to the drugs.

Psychological Effects

The behavioral, motor, and cognitive inhibitions caused by barbiturates are similar to those caused by alcohol. A person may respond to low doses either with relief from anxiety (the expected effect) or with social withdrawal, emotional depression, or aggressive and violent behavior. Higher doses lead to more general behavioral depression and sleep. Mental set and physical or social setting can determine whether relief from anxiety, mental depression, aggression, or another unexpected or unpredictable response is experienced. Driving skills, judgment, insight, and memory all become severely impaired during the period of intoxication.

Clinical Uses

Use of barbiturates has declined rapidly for several reasons: (1) they are lethal in overdose; (2) they have a narrow therapeutic-to-toxic range; (3) they have a high potential for inducing tolerance, dependence, and abuse; and (4) they interact dangerously with many other drugs, sometimes fatally. Because of these disadvantages, barbiturates have largely been replaced by benzodiazepines. Occasionally, barbiturates, such as butalbital, are found in combination with other medications, such as aspirin or acetaminophen combined with caffeine in Fiorinol or Fioricet, for the treatment of migraine headache. They are also used as part of a lethal cocktail in those jurisdictions in the United States where physician-associated suicide is allowed.

Adverse Reactions

Drowsiness is an inescapable accompaniment to the anxiolytic effect and is often the effect sought if the drug is intended to produce either daytime sedation or nighttime sleep. Barbiturates as cognitive inhibitors significantly impair motor and intellectual performance and judgment. It should be emphasized that all sedatives are equivalent to alcohol in their effects and when used with alcohol, their effects are additive and persist longer than might be predicted. There are no specific antidotes with which one can treat barbiturate overdose. Treatment is aimed at supporting the respiratory and cardiovascular system until the drug is metabolized and eliminated.

Tolerance

Barbiturates can induce tolerance by either of two mechanisms: (1) the induction of drug-metabolizing enzymes in the liver; or (2) the adaptation of neurons in the brain to the presence of the drug. With the latter mechanism, tolerance develops primarily to the sedative effects and much less to the brain-stem depressant effects on respiration. Thus, the margin of safety for the person who uses the drug decreases as they need to use more of the drug to achieve the desired sedative effect, leading to increasing respiratory depression.

Physical Dependence

Normal clinical doses of barbiturates can induce a degree of physical dependence, usually manifested by sleep difficulties during attempts at withdrawal. Withdrawal from high doses of barbiturates may result in hallucinations, restlessness, disorientation, and even life-threatening convulsions.

NONBARBITURATE SEDATIVE-HYPNOTIC DRUGS

Paraldehyde, introduced into medicine before the barbiturates, is a polymer of acetaldehyde, an intermediate byproduct in the body's metabolism of ethyl alcohol. Administered either rectally or orally, paraldehyde was historically used to treat delirium tremens, the severe alcohol withdrawal symptoms experienced by alcoholics undergoing detoxification. Paraldehyde is rapidly absorbed from both rectal and oral routes and sleep ensues within 10 to 15 minutes after hypnotic doses. Most of the drug is metabolized in the liver to acetaldehyde, although some is eliminated through the lungs, producing a characteristic unpleasant breath odor.

 Chloral hydrate (Noctec) is yet another drug of historical interest, having been available clinically since the late 1800s. It is rapidly metabolized to *trichlorethanol*, a derivative of ethyl alcohol, which is a nonselective CNS depressant and the active form of chloral hydrate. The drug is an effective sedative-hypnotic, with a plasma half-life of about 4 to 8 hours. Next-day hangover is less likely to occur than with compounds having longer half-lives. Withdrawal of the drug may be associated with disrupted sleep and intense nightmares. The combination of chloral hydrate with alcohol can produce increased intoxication, stupor, and amnesia. This mixture, called a *Mickey Finn*, was an early example of a date rape drug combination.

In the early 1950s, several "nonbarbiturate" sedatives, such as *glutethimide* (Doriden), *ethchlorvynol* (Placidyl), and *methyprylon* (Noludar), were introduced as anxiolytics, daytime sedatives, and hypnotics. They somewhat resembled the barbiturates (see Figure 13.1), but they did not have the exact barbiturate nucleus and could not legally be called barbiturates, despite being pharmacologically interchangeable. These drugs offered no advantages over the barbiturates. Now considered obsolete for use in medicine, they are occasionally encountered as drugs of abuse.

Meprobamate (Equanil, Miltown) was marketed in 1955 as an alternative to the barbiturates for daytime sedation and anxiolysis. The term *tranquilizer* was used to describe it in a marketing attempt to distinguish it from the barbiturates, a distinction that was not borne out in clinical practice. Like barbiturates, meprobamate produces long-lasting daytime sedation, mild euphoria, and relief from anxiety. Meprobamate is a less potent respiratory depressant than the barbiturates and attempted suicides from overdose are seldom successful unless the drug is mixed with opioid narcotics such as morphine or oxycodone. Despite a continuing reduction in clinical use, abuse and dependency continue and are difficult to treat. There is a possibility that use of meprobamate during pregnancy may be associated with an increased frequency of congenital malformations.

Carisoprodol (Soma) is a precursor compound to meprobamate; after it is absorbed, it is rapidly metabolized to meprobamate, which is the active form of the drug. For some reason, it continues to be prescribed by physicians. As an intoxicant, Soma is increasingly encountered as a drug of abuse.

Methaqualone (Quaalude) is another nonbarbiturate sedative that has little clinical reason to justify its previously widespread use. During the late 1970s, its popularity and level of abuse rivaled that of marijuana and alcohol. The attention was due to an undeserved reputation as an aphrodisiac. Indeed, being a sedative, methaqualone was actually an *anaphrodisiac*, much like alcohol. However, methaqualone was a date rape drug, because its amnestic effect occurred at doses lower than that required to produce incapacitation or unconsciousness. Extensive illicit use and numerous deaths led to its being banned in the United States in 1984, although illicit supplies occasionally emerge as a drug of abuse.

Gamma hydroxybutyrate (GHB, Xyrem) is interesting because it is an endogenous neurotransmitter, synthesized from glutamate, exhibiting binding to GHB receptors present on both pre- and postsynaptic neurons, inhibiting GABA release. In overdose, GHB acts both directly as a partial $GABA_B$ receptor agonist and indirectly through its metabolism to GABA. Absalom and coworkers (2012) discuss the complicated mechanisms of action of GHB in greater detail.

GHB has a rapid onset of about 15 minutes and a short half-life of about 30 minutes. The drug is rapidly metabolized to carbon dioxide and water. It is detectable in urine for only very brief periods of time. Overdoses are characterized by stupor, delirium, unconsciousness, coma, and death. Combined with alcohol, the drug's toxic potential is greatly magnified. Acute withdrawal in a GHB-dependent person results in rapid onset of insomnia, anxiety, hallucinations, tremors, agitation, and other signs (Schep et al., 2012). Withdrawal symptoms usually resolve in about 3 to 10 days.

GHB was synthesized and developed in 1960 as a short-acting anesthetic. It later achieved popularity as a recreational drug and a nutritional supplement marketed to bodybuilders. (GHB is thought to promote a deep sleep and, because growth hormone is produced during sleep, the drug allegedly increases levels of growth hormone.) As a drug of abuse, it was classified in 1990 as a Schedule I drug in the United States and sales were banned.[1] However, it and its precursors, gamma butyrolactone (GBL) and 1,4-butanediol (1,4-BD), remain available on the Internet. In 2002, *sodium oxybate* (Xrem, a formulation of GHB) was approved by the FDA for the treatment of narcolepsy and was classified as a Schedule III drug. In January 2017, the FDA approved the first generic version of *Xyrem* (sodium oxybate) oral solution to treat cataplexy and excessive daytime sleepiness in patients with narcolepsy.

The drug is administered twice nightly as a hypnotic, promoting improved sleep. This tends to decrease daytime sleepiness and also reduce the number of sudden short attacks of weak or paralyzed muscles, known as *cataplexy*, which can occur in patients with narcolepsy. Interestingly, this was the first and thus far only time a single drug was classified in two schedules by the FDA, depending on its intended use.[2]

Besides approved use in the treatment of narcolepsy, there has been some interest in the use of GHB in the treatment of alcohol withdrawal (Keating, 2014). As a sedative, GHB has been abused as a purported aphrodisiac and a euphoriant. It has been sold illicitly under such names as "RenewTrient," "Revivarant," "Blue Nitro," "Remiforce," "GH Revitalize," and "Gamma G." It has been called "nature's Quaalude" and "Liquid Ecstasy" among a variety of other names. As a date rape drug, it produces alcohollike disinhibition and amnesia, although the victim is not necessarily asleep or unconscious.

Did You Know?

Detecting Spiked Drinks

Two new technological advances have been developed to determine whether a date rape drug has been surreptitiously slipped into a drink. The first is *Personal Drink ID* (PdID), designed by scientist David Wilson from Toronto, Canada. This thumb drive-sized device contains a mechanism that detects drugs and will indicate whether or not an unknown chemical has been introduced into a drink. Just dip the PdID into the liquid and the LED display will flash a warning. The second item is even more discreet. Developed by four North Carolina State University undergraduate students—Ankesh Madan, Stephen Gray, Tasso Von Windheim, and Tyler Confrey-Maloney, this clever method uses chemicals that react when exposed to rohypnol and GHB. The chemicals are ingredients in nail polish, called "Undercover Colors." When the polish is brushed on the nail, it serves as a "test strip," which changes color when it interacts with the date rape drugs. This product can warn you about a potentially dangerous drink and it never runs out of power. Even if you think it is sufficient never to leave your drink unattended, it should be kept in mind that even the bartender who mixes the drink or the server who brings it to you might not be trustworthy.

---

[1] An FDA Schedule I classification means that the drug has a high potential for abuse with no therapeutic use. Schedules II through V allow for therapeutic use under varying degrees of prescription regulation.

[2] This might provide a model for classification of marijuana, where recreational use might remain as Schedule I, while medical use might be classified as Schedule II or III.

BENZODIAZEPINES

In the 1960s, the benzodiazepines replaced the barbiturates and quickly became the most widely used class of psychotherapeutic drugs. The terms *tranquilizer* and *anxiolytic* rapidly became synonymous with the *benzodiazepines*.

These drugs are still popular. In one survey (Olfson et al., 2014), the percentage of the population receiving any benzodiazepine ranged from 2.6 percent in the youngest group (age range 18 to 26) to 8.7 percent in the oldest group (age range 65 to 80). Of those who filled at least one benzodiazepine prescription (estimated at 75 million nationally), 15 percent of the youngest age group and 31percent of the oldest group continued the medication for at least 120 days—even though there are no FDA indications for the use of benzodiazepines for more than 2 to 4 weeks of use—and 24 percent of users overall took long-acting benzodiazepines. Nonpsychiatric providers wrote most benzodiazepine prescriptions, especially long-term prescriptions generally and long-acting benzodiazepine prescriptions for older patients.

Benzodiazepines are often used or misused by opioid-dependent persons to self-medicate opioid withdrawal and anxiety, to intensify the effects of methadone by reducing its metabolism, or to ameliorate the adverse effects of cocaine and methamphetamine. An FDA-conducted study showed that from 2002 to 2014, the proportion of people taking an opioid analgesic and receiving an overlapping benzodiazepine prescription increased by 41 percent. In 2014, 2.5 million more opioid analgesic users received concomitant benzodiazepines, compared with 2002. Prescribing benzodiazepines concurrently with opioid analgesics has been shown to raise the risk for fatal overdose. New research documents the risk of fatal overdose to be four times that of opioids taken alone, even at low doses. In United States veterans receiving opioid analgesics, 27 percent also received benzodiazepines. In this study, about 50 percent of the overdose deaths occurred when both of these drug types were prescribed concurrently to veterans (Park et al., 2015). These data are all the more sobering in light of the fact that benzodiazepines do not adequately treat patients with posttraumatic stress disorder.

Pharmacokinetics

Sixteen benzodiazepine derivatives remain available for prescription (see Table 13.1). They differ from one another mainly in their pharmacokinetic parameters and the routes through which they are administered. Pharmacokinetic differences include rates of metabolism to pharmacologically active intermediates and plasma half-lives of both the parent drug and any active metabolites. Thirteen of the benzodiazepines are commercially available in the United States; ten are available in dosage forms intended only for oral ingestion, two (diazepam and lorazepam) are available for both oral use and use by injection, and one (midazolam) is available only in injectable formulation.

Absorption and Distribution

Benzodiazepines are well absorbed when they are taken orally; peak plasma concentrations are achieved in about one hour. Some, such as oxazepam and lorazepam, are absorbed more slowly, while others, such as triazolam, are absorbed more rapidly. Clorazepate is metabolized in gastric juice to an active metabolite nordiazepam, which is completely absorbed.

Metabolism and Excretion

Psychoactive drugs are usually metabolized to pharmacologically inactive products, which are then excreted in urine. Although some benzodiazepines behave this way, several are first metabolized to pharmacologically active intermediates; these products, in turn, are detoxified by further metabolism before they are excreted (Figure 13.3). As can be seen from Table 13.1 and Figure 13.3, several benzodiazepines are metabolized into a long-lasting, pharmacologically active metabolite nordiazepam, the half-life of which is about 60 hours, much longer in the elderly. Thus, the long-acting benzodiazepines are long acting primarily because of the long half-life of a pharmacologically active metabolite. In contrast, the short-acting benzodiazepines are short acting because they are metabolized directly into inactive products that are then excreted in the urine.

Benzodiazepines in the Elderly

The elderly have a reduced ability to metabolize long-acting benzodiazepines and their active metabolites. In this population, the elimination half-life for diazepam and its active metabolite is about 7 to 10 days. Since it takes about six half-lives to rid the body completely of a drug, it may take an elderly patient 6 to 10 weeks to become drug-free after stopping the drug. With short-acting benzodiazepines, such as midazolam, pharmacokinetics are not so drastically altered, but the dose necessary to achieve effect is reduced by about 50 percent.

Because all benzodiazepines can produce cognitive dysfunction, elderly patients can become clinically demented as a result. In general, benzodiazepines should likely be avoided in the elderly. Rang and Dale (1991) stated some years ago:

> At the age of 91, the grandmother of one of the authors was growing increasingly forgetful and mildly dotty, having been taking nitrazepam for insomnia regularly for years. To the author's lasting shame, it took a canny general practitioner to diagnose the problem. Cancellation of the nitrazepam prescription produced a dramatic improvement. (637)

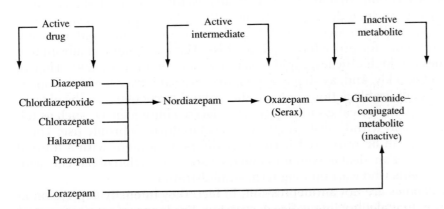

FIGURE 13.3 Metabolism of benzodiazepines. The intermediate metabolite nordiazepam is formed from many agents. Oxazepam (Serax) is commercially available and is also an active metabolite in the metabolism of nordiazepam to its inactive products.

Paterniti and coworkers (2002) followed over 130 benzodiazepine-using elderly people for up to 4 years. Even periodic use was associated with prolonged decreases in cognitive performance, compared with non-drug-taking elderly. Elderly adults who suffer from chronic obstructive pulmonary disease are also at increased risk of untoward respiratory effects from benzodiazepine use (Vozoris et al., 2014). Increases in the incidence of falls and bone fractures constitute another significant problem with benzodiazepines in the elderly (Nurmi-Luthje et al., 2006).

Pharmacological Effects

All benzodiazepines are termed *pure GABA agonists* because they facilitate GABA binding at GABA receptors. When GABA attaches to $GABA_A$ receptors, it causes them to open chloride ion channels, slowing down neurotransmission. Benzodiazepines bind to a specific benzodiazepine modulatory site next to the $GABA_A$ receptor (see Figure 13.2) and enhance the opening of the ion channel, increasing the efficacy of endogenous GABA. This increased inhibitory influence in the brain presumably leads to antianxiety and sedative effects.

Low doses of benzodiazepines moderate anxiety, agitation, and fear by their actions on receptors located in the amygdala, orbitofrontal cortex, and insula. Mental confusion and amnesia follow action on GABA neurons located in the cerebral cortex and the hippocampus. The mild muscle relaxant effects of the benzodiazepines are probably caused both by their anxiolytic actions and by effects on GABA receptors located in the spinal cord, cerebellum, and brain stem. The antiepileptic actions seem to follow from actions on GABA receptors located in the cerebellum and the hippocampus. The behavioral rewarding effects, drug abuse potential, and psychological dependency probably result from actions on GABA receptors that modulate the discharge of neurons located in the ventral tegmentum and the nucleus accumbens.

Clinical Uses and Limitations

Benzodiazepines have actions that are therapeutically useful as hypnotics; anxiolytics for GAD, panic disorders, including agoraphobia, other phobias, and social anxiety; anticonvulsants, especially for alcohol withdrawal; muscle relaxants; and amnesics as adjuncts to anesthetics for procedural memory loss. The major clinical advantages of benzodiazepines are high efficacy, rapid onset of action, and low toxicity. That is, they work, they act quickly, and, as single agents, they are safe. Psychomotor impairment is one of the undesirable actions of benzodiazepines, particularly in the elderly. Sometimes there is a paradoxical excitatory effect. Adverse consequences, such as tolerance, dependence, and withdrawal symptoms, develop during chronic use. These symptoms, however, can be mitigated with lower doses, treatment with a limited duration—4 weeks being an ideal maximum—and the careful selection of patients with the exception of patients who warrant long-term administration.

The benzodiazepines are not antidepressant; in fact, they intensify depression in much the same way that alcohol intensifies depression. For longer-term treatment of such disorders as insomnia, generalized anxiety, phobias, and panic disorder, behavioral treatments and antidepressant drugs are now preferred over benzodiazepine therapy. In instances where a combination of CBTs and benzodiazepines are used to treat anxiety, the benzodiazepines have the potential to interfere with the cognitive therapy, perhaps significantly reducing its efficacy. A cognitive inhibitor could certainly be predicted to block cognitive-based psychological therapies.[3]

They should be avoided in situations requiring fine motor or cognitive skills or mental alertness, or in situations where alcohol or other CNS depressants are used. They should be used only with great caution in the elderly, in children or adolescents, and in anyone with a history of drug misuse or ongoing abuse. Because of long half-lives, evening use is no guarantee that one will be drug-free the next day.

One possible indication for benzodiazepine therapy is for the short-term treatment of anxiety that is so debilitating that the patient's life-style, work, and interpersonal relationships are severely hampered. A benzodiazepine may alleviate the symptoms of nervousness, dysphoria, and psychological distress.

Because they are sedating, benzodiazepines can be used as hypnotics for the treatment of insomnia. Agents with rapid onset, a 2- to 3-hour half-life, and no active metabolites may be preferred to minimize daytime sedation (note that few benzodiazepines fit this profile; Table 13.1). Use in treating insomnia is also limited by the development of tolerance and dependence, as reflected by rebound increases in insomnia upon drug discontinuation.

The benzodiazepines have been used as muscle relaxants, both to directly reduce states associated with increased muscle tension and to reduce the psychological distress that can predispose to muscle tension. But they do not directly relax muscles. They relieve only the distress associated with muscle tension (much like alcohol). Of all benzodiazepines, only diazepam is approved by the FDA for treating spasticity and muscle spasms (Fudin and Raouf, 2016).

Benzodiazepines are exceedingly effective in producing anterograde amnesia, that is, amnesia that starts at the time of drug administration and ends when the blood level of drug has decreased to a point where memory function is regained. For this use, two injectable benzodiazepines are available—lorazepam, when long-lasting amnesia is desirable, and midazolam, when shorter periods of amnesia are desirable.

Often, however, an amnestic effect is undesirable. For example, concern has been expressed about an illegally imported date rape drug, which turned out to be a benzodiazepine that is commercially marketed outside the United States. This drug, *flunitrazepam* (Rohypnol), is very similar to triazolam; it produces anxiolysis, sedation, and amnesia, especially when taken with alcohol. When an unknowing victim ingests the drug and alcohol, the effect closely resembles the effect of a Mickey Finn (chloral hydrate in alcohol), and amnesia is achieved without loss of consciousness.[4]

Panic attacks and phobias can be treated with benzodiazepines such as *alprazolam* (Xanax), although the efficacy of benzodiazepines may be less than that of the

---

[3] A patient is often unaware of this interaction since the long half-lives of benzodiazepines imply that a patient is seldom, if ever, free of the drug. Neither the patient nor the therapist knows the patient's cognitive ability in the absence of a benzodiazepine drug.

[4] Rohypnol intoxication and the amnesia it causes can begin within about 30 minutes, peak within 2 hours, and persist for up to 8 hours. With a combination of Rohypnol and alcohol, the amnestic and intoxicating effects can last 8 to 18 hours. Disinhibition is another widely reported effect of Rohypnol when it is ingested alone or in combination with alcohol.

serotonin-type antidepressants (Moylan et al., 2012). Unlike with the benzodiazepines, SSRIs do not cause impairments in psychomotor performance, do not impair learning and cognition, do not reduce alertness, and have little or no potential for dependence and abuse. Alternatives to benzodiazepines for the treatment of generalized anxiety and panic disorders include SSRIs, dual-action antidepressants such as venlafaxine, and mood-stabilizing anticonvulsants such as pregabalin (Rickels et al., 2012). Panic disorder can be effectively treated with either a benzodiazepine or a selective serotonin reuptake inhibitor, or both. But relapse may occur in the majority of patients, even after long-term therapy. However, resumption of therapy with either drug or with a different medication can be successful in preventing or reducing the incidence of additional attacks in nearly all patients (Osterweil, 2014).

It should be noted, however, that the efficacy of antidepressants for anxiety may be weaker than previously reported. In a review of 57 premarketing trials presented to the FDA, regarding 9 second-generation antidepressants used to treat anxiety disorders, some 41, or 72 percent, of the trials were considered positive. Yet 43 of the 45 articles that went on to be published, or 96 percent, had positive conclusions. That is, trials considered positive were 5 times more likely to be published than trials not considered positive (Roest et al., 2015).

Because benzodiazepines can substitute for alcohol, they are used both in treating acute alcohol withdrawal and in long-term therapy to reduce the rate of relapse to previous drinking habits. Today, however, certain of the antiepileptic mood stabilizers are viable alternatives. Finally, all benzodiazepines exert antiepileptic actions because they raise the threshold for generating seizures. In general, however, benzodiazepines are used as secondary drugs or as adjuvants to other, more specific anticonvulsants.

Side Effects and Toxicity

Common acute side effects associated with benzodiazepine therapy are usually dose-related extensions of the intended actions, including sedation, drowsiness, ataxia, lethargy, mental confusion, motor and cognitive impairments, disorientation, slurred speech, amnesia, and induction or extension of the symptoms of dementia. At higher doses, mental and psychomotor dysfunction progress to hypnosis. Used for the treatment of insomnia, benzodiazepines can cause the expected sedation, or they can induce paradoxical agitation, such as anxiety, aggression, hostility, and behavioral disinhibition. In addition, cessation of use results in rebound increases in insomnia (REM rebound) and anxiety. It has been reported that regardless of age, patients with delirium also had a greater mortality if treated with benzodiazepines than if they were not given benzodiazepines (Serna et al., 2015).

Impairment of motor abilities—especially a person's ability to drive an automobile— is common. In monograph form, Baselt (2014) reviews the literature on specific drugs and their side effects, including references for blood concentrations associated with driving impairments.[5] In general, when viewed as a group, all benzodiazepines are capable of impairing driving, even at therapeutic concentrations (Papoutsis et al., 2016).

---

[5] Impairment was measured by the standard deviation of lateral position (that is, tracking of the vehicle while driving on a city street).

By far, the most contentious issues concern the long-term effects of benzodiaze-pines on dementia and mortality. With regard to dementia, Yaffe and Boustani (2014) report that taking benzodiazepines for three months or more increased the risk of Alzheimer's disease up to 51 percent. Longer exposure and long-acting agents were more likely to increase the risk. Treating symptoms that might signal the beginning of dementia, such as anxiety, depression, or sleep disorders, did not change the outcome. In 2012, the list of inappropriate drugs for the elderly was updated by the American Geriatrics Society, which added benzodiazepines, specifically because of the adverse cognitive impairment. Nevertheless, these drugs are still used by nearly 50 percent of older adults (Billioti de Gage et al., 2014). In contrast, another analysis concluded that there is no "causal association between benzodiazepine use and dementia" (Gray et al., 2016), and a meta-analysis of recent reviews noted that among 11 studies published on benzodiazepines and risk of dementia, 9 of them found that the drugs have a harmful effect, one study concluded that benzodiazepines have protective effects, and the most recently published study said that benzodiazepines have no effect on risk of dementia (Pariente et al., 2016). Most recently, in persons with Alzheimer's disease, the use of benzodiazepines and benzodiazepinelike drugs was reported to be associated with a 20 percent increased risk of stroke (Taipale et al., 2017).

With regard to mortality, the use of benzodiazepines, nonbenzodiazepines, and other anxiolytic and hypnotic drugs was associated with elevated risk for death during the first year after they were prescribed; higher drug doses were associated with a higher risk of death (Weich et al., 2014). It was pointed out that many patients in this study were prescribed drugs from more than one class (for example, 18 per-cent were prescribed both benzodiazepines and nonbenzodiazepines). Although it is possible that the outcome could be confounded by multiple prescriptions or other variables, results of this study support the admonition that these drugs should be used carefully.

Tolerance and Dependence

When benzodiazepines are taken for prolonged periods of time, dependence can develop. An unusual aspect of these drugs is that dependence can develop in the absence of tolerance (Soyka, 2017). Early withdrawal signs include a return and possi-ble intensification of the anxiety state for which the drug was originally given. Rebound increases in insomnia, restlessness, agitation, irritability, and unpleasant dreams grad-ually appear. In rare instances, hallucinations, psychoses, and seizures have been reported. Most of these withdrawal symptoms subside within one to four weeks. There are, however, effective methods for discontinuing benzodiazepine administration that are less likely to produce these symptoms (Thirtala et al., 2013; Vicens et al., 2014). It is generally agreed that discontinuation of benzodiazepines should occur gradually over several weeks, with weekly dose reductions of 50 percent or so, or, in severe cases, to 10 to 25 percent biweekly. Soyka (2017) provides a comprehensive review of the clin-ical use and treatment for benzodiazepine dependence. Hadley and coworkers (2012) discuss a protocol for gradual tapering of benzodiazepines with replacement with *pre-gabalin* (Lyrica) as a safe and effective method for discontinuing long-term benzodiaz-epine therapy and dependence.

Effects in Pregnancy

Benzodiazepines are commonly used by women of reproductive age, and hence many women are exposed to them (Enato et al., 2011). *Diazepam* (Valium) is one of the most frequently prescribed drugs in pregnancy, taken by up to 33 percent of pregnant women. During pregnancy, all benzodiazepines freely cross the placenta and accumulate in the fetal circulation. Benzodiazepines administered during the first trimester of pregnancy do not seem to be associated with an increased risk of congenital malformations (Bellantuono et al., 2013); during the entire pregnancy, the odds ratio of having any form of malformation is 1.07 (95 percent confidence limits = 0.91 to 1.25), mostly accounted for by a slight risk of oral cleft malformations.

Near the time of delivery, if a mother is taking high doses of benzodiazepines, a fetus can develop benzodiazepine dependence or even a "floppy-infant syndrome," followed after delivery by signs of withdrawal. Because benzodiazepines are excreted in breast milk and because they can accumulate in nursing infants, taking benzodiazepines while breast-feeding is not recommended.

FLUMAZENIL: A BENZODIAZEPINE RECEPTOR ANTAGONIST

Flumazenil (Romazicon) is a benzodiazepine that binds with high affinity to benzodiazepine receptors on the $GABA_A$ complex, but after binding, it exhibits no intrinsic activity. As a consequence, it competitively blocks the access of pharmacologically active benzodiazepines to the receptor, effectively reversing the antianxiety and sedative effects of any benzodiazepines administered before flumazenil.

Flumazenil is metabolized quite rapidly in the liver and has a short half-life of about 1 hour. Because this half-life is much shorter than that of most benzodiazepines, the benzodiazepine effects can reappear as flumazenil is eliminated, thus necessitating reinjection. Flumazenil is utilized as an antidote, which is administered by intravenous injection when benzodiazepine overdose is suspected, although such use is fairly rare due to fear of precipitating withdrawal seizures.

NEW APPROACHES FOR THE TREATMENT OF ANXIETY

Given the prevalence of anxiety disorders, and the adverse side effects or modest efficacy of current medications, there is significant interest in developing better drugs. Here we summarize some of these agents, several of which are discussed elsewhere in this book.

1. In preclinical animal testing, the experimental compound 2-262 showed anxiolytic action with reduced sedation, adverse memory impairments, and reduced abuse liability (Yoshimura et al., 2014). This agent is a non-alpha-selective GABA receptor agonist that is selective for the beta-2/3-subunit of the receptor.
2. The noradrenergic beta-receptor antagonist *propranolol*, commonly called a *beta-blocker*, has been effective against a variety of anxiety disorders, particularly

phobias (see Steenen et al., 2016, for references). Propranolol is widely used to treat various heart conditions by acting at peripheral noradrenergic sites to reduce hypertension, coronary artery disease, and cardiac arrhythmias (especially rapid heart rates). Because of these beneficial effects, propranolol can have a calming action against performance anxiety or "stage fright," test anxiety, and so forth. Essentially, the individual feels less nervous because the cardiovascular system is less active. Propranolol seems to reduce the emotional reaction when a "fear memory" is reactivated. This use suggests that propranolol might be useful in treating anxiety disorders based on disturbing memories, such as PTSD. In a review of such potential use against PTSD-induced sleep disruptions, nightmares, global functioning, and other associated symptoms, Steenen and coworkers (2016) concluded that there is insufficient evidence of efficacy to justify use for PTSD or any of the anxiety disorders. Interestingly, this guarded opinion is contraindicated by a study in which propranolol appeared to reduce emotional fear in healthy persons suffering from arachnophobia (fear of spiders) (Soeter and Kindt, 2015).

3. Stein and coworkers (2014) analyzed data from 45 clinical centers worldwide testing whether 25 to 50 milligrams per day of the melatonin agonist *agomelanine* would be effective in the treatment of patients with PTSD. Agomelanine reduced the mean total scores on the main measure (the Hamilton Anxiety Rating Scale) and produced fewer adverse effects than a comparative group that received the SSRI-antidepressant *escitalopram* (Lexapro).

4. Pregabalin (Lyrica) has been favorably tried as a treatment for generalized anxiety disorder (Baldwin et al., 2015; Frampton, 2014). Pregabalin acts to reduce presynaptic calcium influx into neurons. This action serves to reduce excitatory neurotransmission. Pregabalin is approved by the FDA to treat epilepsy, fibromyalgia, and neuropathic pain. Clinical efficacy usually takes only a few days and improvements are maintained long term with continued use. Pregabalin can be effective for several anxiety disorders including, but not limited to, elderly patients with GAD, patients with severe anxiety, and as an adjunct to standard antidepressants in resistant depression. Unfortunately, pregabalin may have adverse teratogenic effects when taken by a pregnant female (Winterfeld et al., 2016).

5. The *serotoninergic antidepressants* may have efficacy in treating PTSD (Lancaster et al., 2016), improving reexperiencing, avoidance, numbing, hyperarousal, and quality of life. Sertraline and paroxetine are approved by the FDA for use in PTSD, while fluvoxamine and citalopram have also been found effective. A recent antidepressant reportedly effective in PTSD is vilazodone (Durgam et al., 2016).

6. Clinical trials have reported the efficacy of *prazosin* (Minipress) for PTSD-related sleep disruptions, nightmares, global functioning, and other PTSD symptoms (Singh et al., 2016). Prazosin is somewhat related to propranolol. In one study of veterans, prazosin was reported to be not very effective; doses were low and there were many who discontinued the drug (Alexander et al., 2015). Higher doses might be more effective (Koola et al., 2014). Prazosin may be more effective in patients with higher baseline blood pressure (Raskind et al., 2016). Finally, a related drug, *doxazosin* (Cardura) was only modestly effective (Amos et al., 2014; Rodgman et al., 2016).

DRUGS INTENDED FOR THE TREATMENT OF INSOMNIA

Pharmacologic therapy of insomnia in the United States includes the following drugs approved by the FDA:

- Benzodiazepine receptor agonist (BZRAs) hypnotics, such as triazolam, estazolam, temazepam, flurazepam, and quazepam
- Nonbenzodiazepine hypnotics, such as zaleplon, zolpidem, and eszopiclone
- Ramelteon, a melatonin receptor agonist
- *Doxepin*, an antidepressant
- *Suvorexant*, the recently approved orexin receptor antagonist (Table 13.2)

Drugs that have been used off label include other antidepressants, antihistamines, antipsychotics (see Table 13.4), and melatonin. Complementary and alternative treatments have also been tried as therapy for insomnia, including acupuncture and Chinese herbal medicine (Qaseem et al., 2016).

Benzodiazepine Receptor Agonist Hypnotics

Chronic insomnia can manifest itself as difficulty falling asleep, difficulty staying asleep, waking up too early, or waking in the morning without feeling "refreshed." About 10 percent of people experience chronic insomnia. Roughly 50 percent of

TABLE 13.2 Hypnotics approved by the FDA for insomnia

Drug class	Generic name	Trade name	Dose (mg)	Elimination half-life (hour range)	Tmax (hours)	Indication[a]	DEA class
Benzodiazepines	*Estrazolam*	Prosom	1, 2	10–24	1.5–2	SOI, SMI	IV
	Flurazepam	Dalmane	15, 30	48–120	1.5–4.5	SOI, SMI	IV
	Quazepam	Doral	7.5, 15	48–120	2–3	SOI, SMI	IV
	Temazepam	Restoril	7.5, 15	8–22	1–2	SOI, SMI	IV
	Triazolam	Halcion	0.125, 0.25	2–4	2–6	SOI	IV
Benzodiazepine agonists	*Zaleplon*	Sonata	5, 10, 20	1	1	SOI	IV
	Zolpidem	Ambien	5, 10	2.5	1.6	SOI	IV
	Zolpidem CR	Ambien CR	6.25, 12.5	2.8	1.5	SOI, SMI	IV
	Eszopiclone	Lunesta	1, 2, 3	6	1	SOI, SMI	IV
Melatonin agonist	*Ramelteon*	Rozerem	8	1–2.6	0.75	SOI	None
H. antagnoist	*Doxepin*	Silenor	3, 6	15.3	3.5	SMI	None
Orexin antagonist	*Suvorexant*	Belsomra	5–20	12	2	SOI, SMI	IV

[a] SOI (sleep onset insomnia); SMI (sleep maintenance insomnia).
[Data from Asnis et al., 2016.]

people with other medical or psychological conditions complain of insomnia. Consequences of insomnia include daytime fatigue, lack of energy, poor concentration and memory, moodiness and irritability, and difficulty completing tasks. Treatments can be either psychological or pharmacological. Of the psychological therapies, *cognitive-behavioral therapies for insomnia* (CBT-I) have been found very effective (Trauer et al., 2015). Advantages of CBT-I include lack of drug side effects, no dependence or withdrawal issues, and safety for use in the pregnant patient. Unfortunately, CBT-I is expensive, has a delayed onset of effect, and is not readily available.

In contrast, pharmacotherapies with BZRAs are rapidly effective, inexpensive, and readily available. Disadvantages of medication include next-day impairment, dependence, and withdrawal issues.

As noted earlier, all benzodiazepines exhibit hypnotic properties and five of them, namely flurazepam, estazolam, quazepam, temazepam, and triazolam, are specifically approved by the FDA for the treatment of insomnia (Table 13.3), although others, such as alprazolam, are widely used and similarly effective for this purpose. Triazolam has the shortest half-life, 2 to 4 hours, and is associated with the least daytime sedation. It may not provide adequate sedation through the night. Conversely, the others have longer half-lives and increase sleep maintenance, but they may have adverse cognitive consequences the next day. Tolerance and dependence are also potentially harmful. Benzodiazepines may be useful in patients with comorbid anxiety disorders.

Complex Sleep-Related Behavior

In March 2007, the FDA released an advisory requesting that all manufacturers of sedative-hypnotic products for the treatment of various *complex sleep-related behaviors* (CSBs), which are used to induce or maintain sleep, strengthen their product labeling to include risks of "sleep driving" and "sleep-related activities" (Inagaki et al., 2010; Zammit, 2009). Thirteen products were listed on the FDA advisory. These included the barbiturates Butisol, Carbrital, and Seconal; the benzodiazepines Dalmane, Halcion, ProSom, and Restoril; the nonbenzodiazepine BZRAs Ambien, Sonata, and Lunesta; the melatonin agonist Rozerem (discussed in next section); and two miscellaneous agents, Doral and Placidyl. This advisory is not all-inclusive, as all benzodiazepines are associated with the same risks of sleep driving and sleep-related activities. Originally thought to be rare events, the incidence has been increasing, likely due to improved awareness and reporting. Chen and coworkers (2014) noted that 24 percent of adults and 17 percent of elderly patients reported experiencing some sort of adverse sleep-related effect of zolpidem. Such effects appear to be somewhat related to doses and their resultant blood concentrations. For example, adults reporting sleep-related effects ingested an average dose of 15 milligrams while persons without adverse effects ingested an average dose of 6.8 milligrams. Elderly patients with sleep-related behaviors did not use a higher dose than persons without such effects (12 milligrams average for each group).

TABLE 13.3 Adverse effects of benzodiazepines, nonbenzodiazepine hypnotics, sedating antidepressants, melatonin agonists, and potential adverse effects of orexin antagonists

Adverse Effects[b]	Benzodiazepines (for example, clonazepam, lorazepam)	Nonbenzodiazepines (for example, zolpidem, zaleplon)	Sedating antidepressants (for example, trazodone, doxepin)	Melatonin agonists[a] (for example, ramelteon)	Orexin antagonists (for example, suvorexant)
Morning sedation	+	+	+	–	+
Hypnagogic hallucinations, sleep paralysis	–	–	–	–	+
Unsteady gait, falls	++	+	+	–	+/–
Confusion	++	+	–	–	–
Amnesia	+	+	–	–	–
Dependence and abuse	+	+/–	–	–	–
Rebound insomnia	+	+	–	–	–
Respiratory depression	+	+/–	–	–	–
Orthostasis	–	–	+	–	–
Anticholinergic effects	–	–	++/+	–	–

[a] Melatonin side effects differ from these symptoms; see text.
[b] Some effects such as morning sedation may depend on the particular compound's pharmacokinetics.
[Data from Scammell and Winrow, 2011.]
Note: Frequency indicated by the following symbols: ++, common; +, occasional; –, rare.

Did You Know?

Snails to Treat Sleep Disorders

Over the last 50 years, science has benefited greatly from studying venomous cone snails. Compounds isolated from these marine predators have been shown to block pain and protect against heart attacks. Now, the latest group of chemicals isolated from a cone snail has been found to put mice to sleep. In their normal environment, the snails use these substances, called *conotoxins*, to capture prey. In a study published in the journal *Toxicon*, researchers Franklin and Rajesh (2015) describe 14 new peptide toxins they isolated and sequenced from the venom of the cobweb cone (*Conus araneosus*). When five of these compounds were injected into mice, four had no effect, but one put the animals to sleep for several hours. This finding provides new avenues for investigating drugs that might be helpful for treating sleep disorders.

Nonbenzodiazepine Hypnotics

The *nonbenzodiazepines* (NBZRAs) were developed in an effort to improve the safety and side effect profile of benzodiazepines. The approach was to design drugs that had more selective effects at the subunits of the $GABA_A$ receptor. The benzodiazepines bind to the alpha subunit of the $GABA_A$ receptor diffusely, with a nonselective action at the $\alpha1$, $\alpha2$, $\alpha3$, and $\alpha5$ subtypes. In contrast, the first NBZRA, zolpidem, approved by the FDA in 1993, and another, zaleplon, selectively attach to the $\alpha1$ subtype, while the third NBZRA, eszopiclone, is predominantly selective for the $\alpha2$ and $\alpha3$ subtypes, relative to the $\alpha1$ subtype. Because these three hypnotic agents all start with the letter Z, they are sometimes referred to as the *Z drugs* (Figure 13.4). The preferential selectivity of the NBZRAs, and the fact that their half-lives are short (8 hours or less) are presumed to be responsible for less motor and neuropsychological impairment, and less dependence, withdrawal, and abuse, relative to the benzodiazepines. They are also safe in regard to overdoses, but whether or not they produce less next-day fatigue than benzodiazepines is still debated. Cimolai (2017) in fact, argues that adverse reactions to these drugs may be as common and serious as to the classic benzodiazepines. Currently, there are only three FDA-approved NBZRAs and four preparations of zolpidem available: zaleplon, eszopiclone, zolpidem and zolpidem-extended release, zolpidem sublingual high dose (Edluar), zolpidem sublingual low dose (Intermezzo), and zolpidem oral spray (Zolpimist) (Asnis, 2016).

Zolpidem

Zolpidem (Ambien, Ambien CR, Edluar, and Intermezzo) is marketed for the treatment of insomnia. Binding to the alpha-1 subunit of the $GABA_A$ receptor, it exhibits primarily a hypnotic rather than an anxiolytic effect. With a half-life of about 2.0 to 2.5 hours, zolpidem is often compared to *triazolam* (Halcion), a benzodiazepine with similar pharmacokinetics; at comparable doses, there appears to be little to differentiate the two drugs. A controlled-release formulation of zolpidem (Ambien CR) is available as a sublingual tablet (Edluar). Also, a new formulation, Intermezzo, is a low-dose formulation of zolpidem (1.75 milligrams for women and 3.5 milligrams for men) intended to be taken when one wakens in the middle of the night and cannot get back to sleep.[6]

---

[6] But only when one still has at least 4 hours of bedtime left.

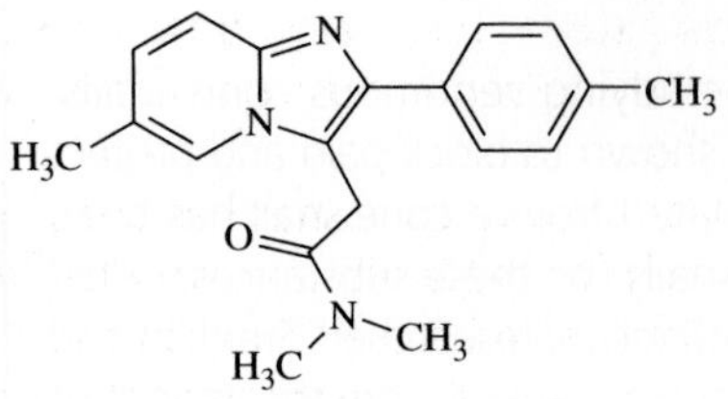

Zolpidem (Ambien)

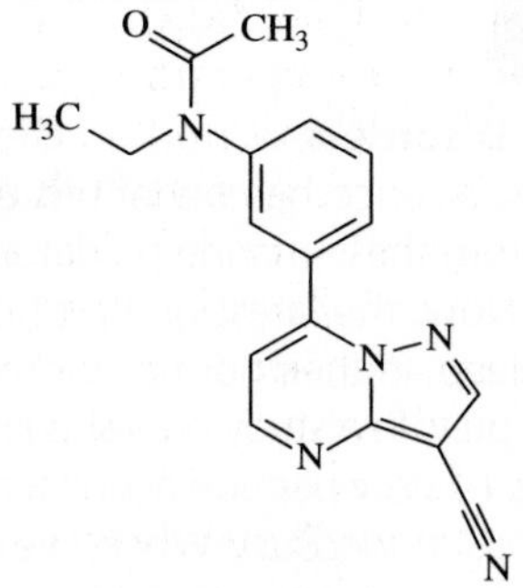

Zaleplon (Sonata)

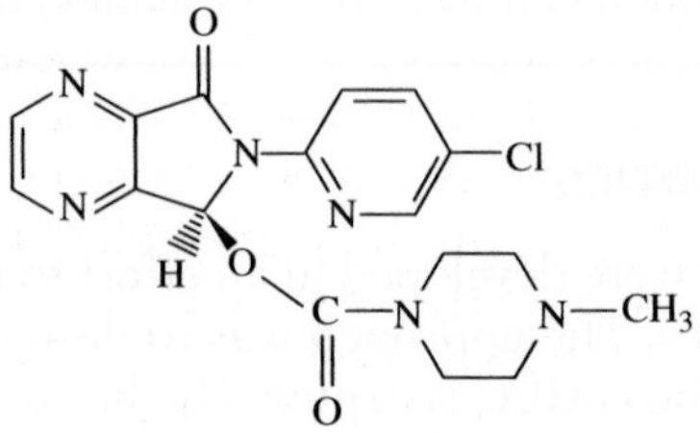

Eszopiclone (Lunesta)

FIGURE 13.4 Structural formulas of zolpidem (Ambien), zaleplon (Sonata), and eszopiclone (Lunesta). Note the close (but dissimilar) relationship of their basic three-ring structures to the benzodiazepine nucleus. Thus, these three compounds are nonbenzodiazepines despite similar GABAergic actions and clinical effects.

At doses of 5 to 10 milligrams, zolpidem produces sedation and promotes a physiological pattern of sleep in the absence of anxiolytic, anticonvulsant, or muscle relaxant effects. Memory is adversely affected as it is by benzodiazepines, and drug-induced blackouts and sleep-related activities are common.

Dose-related adverse effects of zolpidem include drowsiness, dizziness, and nausea. In doses of 5 milligrams, zolpidem exhibits minimal next-day effects on memory or psychomotor performance, such as driving; however, doses of 10 to 20 milligrams significantly impair performance and memory even 4 hours after taking the drug. In January 2013, the FDA informed the manufacturers that the recommended dosage of zolpidem for women should be lowered from 10 to 5 milligrams for immediate-release products (Ambien, Edluar, and Zolpimist) and either 6.25 or 12.5 milligrams for men. For extended-release products (Ambien CR), the FDA recommended lowering the dosage from 12.5 to 6.25 milligrams for women and to either 6.25 or 12.5 milligrams for men. Further, the FDA informed the manufacturers that the labeling should recommend that health care professionals prescribe the lowest effective dose.

According to a Substance Abuse and Mental Health Services Administration report released on August 2014, women accounted for two-thirds of visits to the emergency department involving zolpidem overmedication in 2010. The largest age bracket involved were patients ages 45 to 54. Overdoses of 40 times the therapeutic dose

(400 milligrams) have not been fatal. In the elderly, as with BZRAs, confusion, falls, memory loss, and psychotic reactions have been reported. For example, one study found zolpidem users had about double the hip fracture rate as nonusers. Rates were 21 times higher in older users (age ≥65) than in younger users and two times higher in elderly users than in elderly nonusers (Lin et al., 2014).

Interestingly, results of a randomized trial (Perliss et al., 2015) show that people who suffer from chronic insomnia do not need to take zolpidem (Ambien) every night for it to continue to be effective. The trial included 56 patients who responded to four weeks of nightly zolpidem at 10 milligrams. These patients were then assigned to one of three maintenance schedules: nightly dosing; intermittent dosing, in which the drug was taken 3 to 5 nights per week according to patient preference; and partial rein-forcement dosing, in which capsules were taken every night, but half of the doses were placebos. An analysis performed on the data of the 41 compliant patients showed that after 1 month, the three dosing schedules were statistically indistinguishable on sev-eral sleep measures such as sleep latency and waking after sleep onset. The researchers interpreted these results to mean that (1) on the nights when there is no medication, patients are exhibiting a conditioned response; (2) on the nights when medication is taken, the capsule serves as a conditioned stimulus for that physiologic response. Pre-sumably this approach would be effective for other sedative-hypnotics and, perhaps, other response systems as well.

Finally, zolpidem is the hypnotic agent most associated with inducing complex sleep-related behaviors, resulting in thousands of legal cases. Wong and coworkers (2017) concluded that there is "a significant association between zolpidem and the induction of these bizarre sleep-related behaviors."

Zaleplon

Zaleplon (Sonata) is a second nonbenzodiazepine agonist that binds to the alpha-1 subunit of the GABA$_A$ receptor. In general, it exerts actions similar to those of zol-pidem as a hypnotic agent. The half-life of zaleplon is very short (about 1 hour), and only about 30 percent of the dose reaches the bloodstream; most undergoes first-pass metabolism in the liver. Because zaleplon is poorly absorbed and short acting, it does not require predicting that insomnia will occur on a particular night. Instead, if unable to fall asleep and stay asleep without pharmacological assistance, the person has the option of taking this very short-acting agent without fear of detrimental effects the next morning.

Sleep is quite rapidly induced with zaleplon at doses of 5 to 10 milligrams, and sleep quality is improved without rebound insomnia. Zaleplon appears particularly noteworthy in its lack of deleterious effects on psychomotor function and driving abil-ity the morning following use. Allowing at least 4 hours from drug intake to driving results in few adverse effects. In fact, at 4 hours after oral administration, most of the drug has been eliminated from the body. Dependence is unlikely to develop because of the short half-life: by morning, the drug is metabolized. In essence, a person taking the drug withdraws daily, and drug does not persist in the body. At extremely high doses (25 to 75 milligrams), an abuse potential comparable to that seen for triazolam (Halcion) is seen.

Eszopiclone

Eszopiclone (Lunesta) is the third NBZRA approved for the treatment of insomnia. It is the active isomer of *zopiclone* (Immovane), which has been used outside the United States for many years. Eszopiclone shares all the actions of zolpidem and traditional benzodiazepines. Because of a half-life of about 6 hours, eszopiclone has the most prolonged action of the NBZRAs. Therefore, it might be preferable to the others for improving both sleep latency and sleep maintenance. But this benefit is offset by increased risk of next-day sedation. At its highest dose level of 3 milligrams, next-day memory impairments and poor performance on measures of psychomotor performance have been reported. In April 2014, the generic formulation of eszoplicone was approved by the FDA. In May 2014, the FDA recommended that the starting dose be lowered from 2 to 1 milligram after a study found that patients taking higher doses were at increased risk for severe psychomotor and memory impairment the next morning. The agency noted that the dose can be increased to 2 or 3 milligrams as needed, but it cautions people who take 3 milligrams against driving or doing other activities that require their full attention the next day.

In spite of their proven efficacy for reducing insomnia, the benzodiazepines and associated Z-drugs cannot be expected to produce remission. In a real-world study of patients, mostly with comorbid medical and psychiatric disorders, sleep disturbances were not eliminated in those using BZRAs and NBZRAs (Pillai et al., 2017).

Partial Agonists at GABA$_A$ Receptors

"Full" BZRA agonists are effective anxiolytics and sedatives; however, their use is limited by rebound anxiety on discontinuation, physical dependence, abuse potential, and side effects that include ataxia, sedation, memory impairments, and cognitive disturbances. For many years, attempts have been made to identify "partial" agonists of GABA receptors, that is, *partial BZRAs*, in the hope of providing anxiolytics that may be equally effective without the side effects that limit the use of the benzodiazepines. To date, several have been examined, although none are currently available. Alpidem was briefly marketed for the treatment of anxiety, but was withdrawn because of liver toxicity (Skolnick, 2012). EVT-201 is a modulator of the GABA-A receptor and has shown efficacy in older patients with insomnia (Zisapel, 2015). Extracts of valerian are partial GABA-A and serotonin-5-A receptor agonists (Dietz et al., 2005) and are useful in treating insomnia as over-the-counter products.

Melatonin Receptor Agonists for Insomnia

Melatonin, or 5-methoxy-N-acetyltryptamine, is a naturally occurring hormone produced from the amino acid tryptophan, the precursor to serotonin, and secreted by the pineal gland in a circadian rhythm. Neurons in the anterior hypothalamus, within the suprachiasmatic nucleus (SCN), coordinate the timing of this circadian system by controlling the production of melatonin in the pineal gland in response to the environmental light–dark cycle. Light activates receptors in the retina, which project to the SCN, and neurons in the SCN release norepinephrine in a circadian rhythm, which regulates the production of melatonin in the pineal gland. This physiological system increases melatonin levels as bedtime approaches; hormonal levels plateau during the night, and decrease as sleep ends in the morning. Nocturnal plasma melatonin concentrations can be as much as tenfold higher than daytime concentrations. Normally, the SCN is reset daily by light coming from the retina during the day and melatonin during the night. These anterior hypothalamic neurons contain a high concentration of two high-affinity G protein–coupled receptors, MT_1 and MT_2.

Melatonin itself remains available as an over-the-counter compound promoted for the treatment of insomnia. It has a short half-life and limited efficacy, except perhaps in people with disrupted sleep–wake cycles, such as shift workers and people with "jet lag" (Sadeghniiat-Haghighi et al., 2016). Wade and coworkers (2007) reported several years ago that prolonged-release melatonin may have significant and clinically meaningful efficacy in persons aged 55 years and older.

Several melatonin receptor agonists have recently become available for the treatment of insomnia, depression, and circadian rhythms sleep–wake disorders and are described in the following sections.

Ramelteon

Ramelteon (Rozerem), approved in 2005, was the first commercially available dual agonist of melatonin receptors. It promotes drowsiness via MT1 receptor stimulation and synchronization of the circadian clock via MT2 receptor stimulation. It is approved by the FDA for the treatment of insomnia characterized by difficulty with sleep onset. The drug is thought to be nonaddicting and therefore devoid of abuse potential. Rebound insomnia following a period of nightly drug use has not been reported. In an available 8 milligram dose, it is taken 30 minutes before going to bed. A half-life of about 1.5 to 3 hours (quite variable) is thought to leave little morning drowsiness, although next morning driving performance has been reported as being impaired (Mets et al., 2011). In controlled trials, efficacy was quite modest, with sleep onset occurring only about 10 or 15 minutes earlier than after taking placebo and with total sleep time little affected (Liu and Wang, 2012). In an updated review (Kuriyama et al., 2014), ramelteon improved some sleep parameters in adults with insomnia with short-term use, but it had an overall modest clinical impact. Comparisons with established anti-insomnia drugs, including the NBZRAs, have not been reported. Therefore, its efficacy relative to other therapeutic options cannot be estimated at this time. Norris and coworkers (2013) studied ramelteon as an adjunct to regular psychiatric medications in patients with euthymic bipolar disorder. The authors reported that patients were only about half as likely to relapse, compared with placebo-treated patients. Brower and coworkers (2011), in a study of five alcohol-dependent patients, noted improved insomnia scores and total sleep time, and a shorter time to fall asleep. Given its lack of abuse potential, ramelteon deserves further study in this population. Hatta and coworkers (2014) report that ramelteon, like melatonin, reduces the risk of delirium in patients at risk for this condition.

Circadin

Circadin is a prolonged-release melatonin formulation that matches the physiological profile of melatonin secretion. It is reported to improve sleep quality and latency, and daytime function, in elderly insomnia patients. The clinical use of Circadin does not impair memory or decrease vigilance and is stated to have no significant withdrawal symptoms.

Agomelatine

Agomelatine is a weak melatonin-1 and melatonin-2 receptor agonist and a weak serotonin-2c antagonist. It seems to have some efficacy as an antidepressant (Taylor et al., 2014) as well as improving sleep behaviors with minimal daytime somnolence. A reversible increase in liver enzymes has been reported (Perlemuter et al., 2016).

Tasimelteon

In January 2014, *tasimelteon* was approved by the FDA for non-24-hour sleep–wake disorder for those who are totally blind and cannot perceive enough light to establish a normal sleep schedule (Leger et al., 2015). It is a melatonin-1 and melatonin-2 receptor agonist with greater binding to the melatonin-2 receptor. There is currently no other treatment for the condition, and the FDA estimates that as many as 100,000 patients in the United States have this sleep–wake disorder. Drug interactions can be significant, including a manifold increase in blood concentrations in patients also taking antidepressants, such as fluvoxamine, that inhibit CYP1A2 and CYP3A4/5 enzymes (Ogilivie et al., 2015). The most common side effects with the drug included headache, elevated liver enzymes, nightmares or unusual dreams, disturbed sleep, upper respiratory or urinary tract infection, and drowsiness.

An experimental agent, TK-301 is another agonist for the melatonin receptors MT_1 and MT_2 that is under development for the treatment of insomnia and other sleep disorders. It is in the same class of melatonin receptor agonists as ramelteon and tasimelteon. Clinical studies have not yet been published.

Several reviews of melatonin receptor agonists for the treatment of insomnia are available (Emet et al., 2016; Laudon and Frydman-Marom, 2014; Liu et al., 2016; Williams et al., 2016).

Orexin Receptor Antagonists for Insomnia

Because the GABAergic and melatonergic systems enhance inhibitory processes, drugs developed for insomnia that act through these systems are agonists. But another potential approach for enhancing sleep is to block activity in wake-promoting systems. This would include antagonism of histamine, serotonin, norepinephrine, dopamine, and acetylcholine pathways. Agents that block these receptors have been around for many years, including antidepressants, antipsychotics, and antihistamines (see Tables 13.2 and 13.4). Many of these agents, however, are nonselective and their mechanisms of action on wake-promoting systems are not well understood.

The orexin system, first described in 1998, has a key role in supporting and maintaining wakefulness. The *orexin* neuropeptide transmitters, named *orexin-A* and *orexin-B*, were originally thought to promote feeding behaviors (*orexis* in Greek means appetite). It has since been realized that while orexin effects on feeding are less pronounced than originally thought, their effects on arousal and sleep are profound. The regulation of sleep and wakefulness is mediated by the interaction of multiple nuclei within the hypothalamus. Orexin neuropeptides seem to regulate the transition between wakefulness and sleep and aid the transition towards wakefulness by activating neural pathways of the ascending arousal system (Kumar et al., 2016). The perifornical-lateral hypothalamic region is the origin of orexigenic neurons that project broadly in the CNS with especially dense connections with wake-promoting cholinergic, serotonergic, noradrenergic, and histaminergic neurons. The precursor is prepro-orexin peptide, which is split into the two orexin neurotransmitters (orexin-A and orexin-B). These bind with two G-protein-coupled receptors (OX1R and OX2R) that have both common and distinct distributions.

In 2014, the FDA approved *suvorexant* (Belsomra), the first *orexin receptor antagonist* for the treatment of insomnia with sleep onset or sleep maintenance difficulties (see Table 13.2). Suvorexant is very selective, with comparable antagonistic affinity for both OX1R and OX2R receptors. Essentially, suvorexant promotes sleep by reducing the arousing wake drive.

Suvorexant should only be taken once per night, within 30 minutes of retiring, with at least 7 hours available before the individual expects to wake up. The dose range is 10 to 20 milligrams per day with a half-life of 12 hours, and the total dose should not be greater than 20 milligrams once daily. There are no active metabolites. In trials of up to 1 year in duration, withdrawal or rebound effects were not seen when the drug was stopped (Asnis et al., 2016). Efficacy appears good (Herring et al., 2016; Norman and Anderson, 2016). Belsomra was not compared to other drugs indicated for insomnia, so its safety or effectiveness relative to other insomnia medications is unknown. Belsomra shares the risk seen with other hypnotics of sleep driving and other complex behaviors while not being fully awake. So far, orexin antagonists have only been studied in clinical trials. Therefore, it is too early to know if it will be sufficiently effective and safe in the real world to be a first-line insomnia treatment or only reserved for those who have failed other treatments. Suvorexant was well tolerated, with the most common adverse event, somnolence, reported in 13 percent of participants. Although suvorexant is the only orexin receptor antagonist with current FDA approval for the treatment of insomnia, other agents in development have shown similar results for improving sleep efficiency. (For a summary of the common side effects of drugs used to treat insomnia, see Table 13.3.)

"Off-Label" Treatment for Insomnia

Several other medications are widely used "off label" for the treatment of insomnia (Table 13.4). These include several sedating antidepressants such as trazodone and amitriptyline (Chapter 12), and the antihistamine *diphenhydramine* (Benadryl).

TABLE 13.4 Off-label medications for insomnia

Drug class	Generic name	Trade name	Dose (mg)	Elimination half life (h)	T_{max} (h)
Sedating Antidepressants	*Trazodone*	Desyrel[a]	25–150	9 (7–15)	1–2
	Amitriptyline	Elavil[a]	10–100	30 (5–45)	2–5
Sedating antipsychotics	*Quetiapine*	Seroquel	25–100	6	1–2
Antihistamines	*Diphenhydramine*	Benadryl	25–50	4–8	1–4
Anticonvusants	*Gabapentin*	Neurontin	100–900	5–9	1.6–3

[a] These trade names are no longer available in the United States.
[Data from Asnis et al., 2016.]

Interestingly, in 2010, the first *antihistamine and tricyclic antidepressant* (TCA), *doxepin* (Silenor) for insomnia, was approved by the FDA. At low doses of 3 and 6 milligrams, doxepin preferentially blocks the histaminic H1 receptor, which is thought to mediate its effect on insomnia, because the antidepressant dose is 150 to 300 milligrams per day. Doxepin was effective for maintenance sleep problems with minimal side effects in both younger and older populations for up to 3 to 6 months. The observation that it is ineffective for sleep-onset problems is probably related to the fact that it takes about 3.5 hours to reach maximum levels.

The antipsychotic drug *quetiapine* (Chapter 11) has been used for insomnia, but according to new recommendations issued by leading Canadian psychiatric organizations, antipsychotics should not be routinely used to treat primary insomnia.

GENERAL ANESTHETICS

All sedatives in sufficient doses can produce amnesia and loss of consciousness. General anesthetics are drugs that produce these effects for the performance of surgical procedures. The two types of general anesthetics are (1) those administered by inhalation through the lungs and (2) those injected directly into a vein. Inhalation anesthetics in current use include one gas, nitrous oxide, and five volatile liquids, namely isoflurane, halothane, desflurane, enflurane, and sevoflurane. These drugs produce a dose-related depression of all functions of the CNS—an initial period of sedation followed by the onset of sleep. As anesthesia deepens, both amnesia and unconsciousness are induced. Adding an opioid narcotic such as morphine to a volatile anesthetic adds analgesic action to this state of unconsciousness.

The inhaled anesthetic agents are subject to misuse. *Nitrous oxide,* a gas of low anesthetic potency, is an example. Currently used in anesthesia as well as a carrier gas in whipped cream charger cans called *whippets,* nitrous oxide induces a state of behavioral disinhibition, analgesia, and mild euphoria. Since the inhalation of nitrous oxide dilutes the air that a person is breathing, extreme caution must be exercised to prevent hypoxia. If the nitrous oxide is mixed only with room air, hypoxia results, which could produce irreversible brain damage. (Other forms of inhalant abuse are discussed in Chapter 5.)

Several injectable anesthetics are available. *Thiopental* (Pentothal) and *methohexital* (Brevital) are ultrashort-acting barbiturates. *Propofol* (Diprovan) and *etomidate* (Amidate) are structurally unique; propofol structurally resembles the neurotransmitter GABA. Because propofol and etomidate are now generically available, more expensive preparations have been marketed. *Fospropofol* (Lusedra) is a prodrug and is rapidly converted to propofol, its active form (Bengalorkar et al., 2011). *Desmedetomidine* (Precedex) is structurally related to etomidate and likely works with identical efficacy (Mizrak et al., 2010). It is an alpha-2 agonist at the adrenergic receptor and is available commercially for sedation procedures in medicine.

ANTIEPILEPTIC DRUGS

Sedative-hypnotic drugs used for the treatment of epilepsy have been called *anticonvulsants* or *antiepileptic drugs*. The number of these drugs commercially available has more than doubled in the last 15 years. Currently 27 anticonvulsants are available, and of these, 9 have become available since 2009 (Table 13.5). Sirven and coworkers (2012) present an introduction to understanding how these drugs work to control brain excitability and epileptic seizures.

In recent years, their uses have been expanded to treatment of bipolar disorder; treatment of aggressive and explosive behavioral disorders in children, adolescents, and adults; management of alcohol withdrawal and cravings; treatment of chronic pain; and management of certain anxiety disorders such as posttraumatic stress disorder, generalized anxiety disorder, and even certain components of borderline personality disorder. These nonepileptic uses necessitate the terms *mood stabilizer* to cover this multitude of actions. In this section, the original indication of these drugs, as antiepileptic agents or anticonvulsants, are discussed. The currently available antiepileptic drugs are listed in Table 13.5.

TABLE 13.5 Antiepileptic drugs currently approved by the FDA

Before 1993	1993–2005	2009–2016
Carbamazepine	Felbamate	Vigabatrin
Clonazepam	Gabapentin	Rufinamide
Diazepam	Lamotrigine	Lacosamide
Ethosuximide	Levetiracetam	Clobazam
Lorazepam	Oxcarbazepine	Ezogabine
Phenobarbital	Pregabalin	Perampanel
Phenytoin	Tiagabine	Stiripentol
Primidone	Topiramate	Eslicarbazepine
Valproic acid	Zonisamide	Brivaracetam

[Data from Sirven et al., 2012.]

    Phenobarbital, a barbiturate (Figure 13.5), was the first widely effective antiepileptic drug. This and other barbiturates, because of their sedative and adverse cognitive depressant effects, are today rarely used; equally effective, more specific, and less sedating antiepileptic agents are now available.

    Phenytoin (Dilantin), introduced into medicine in 1938, remains a commonly used *hydantoin* anticonvulsant, producing less sedation than do the barbiturates. Phenytoin

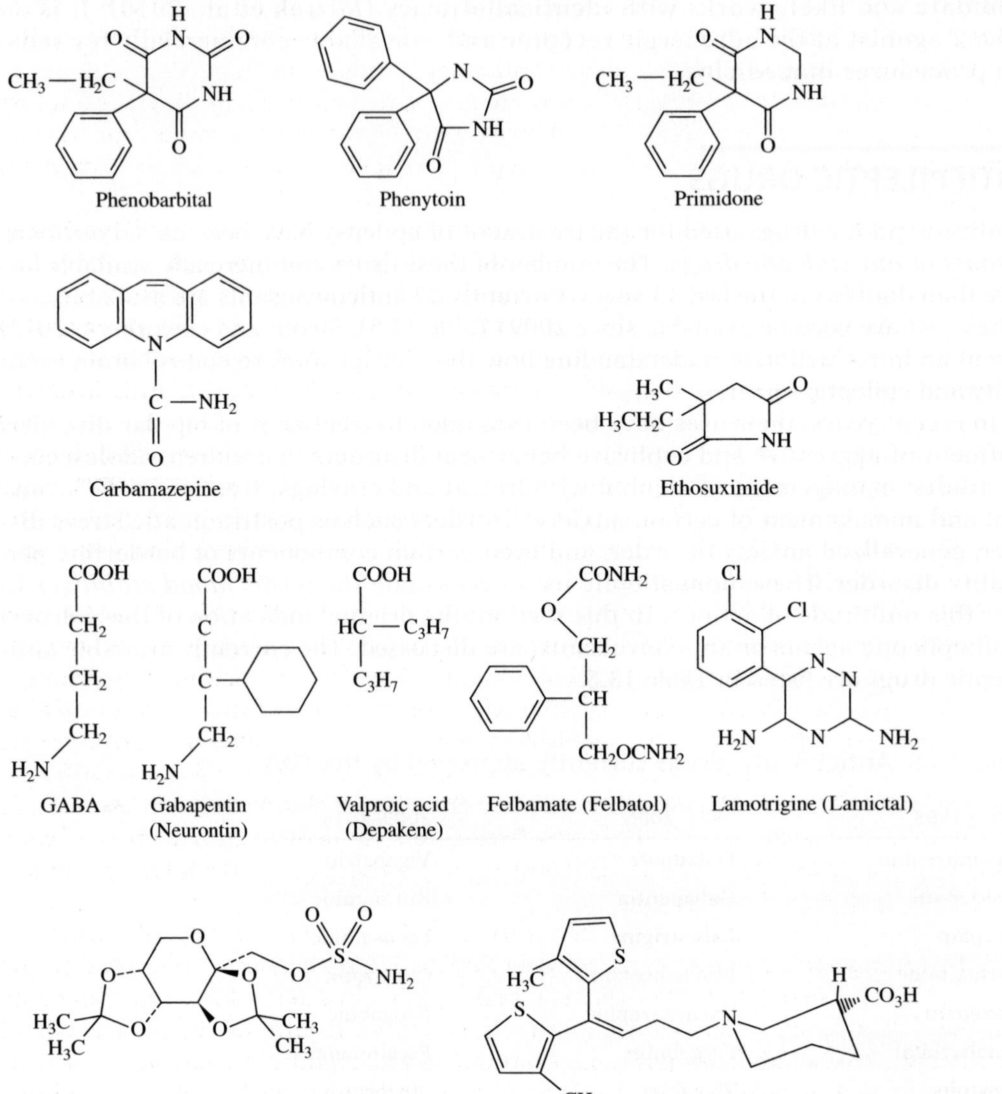

FIGURE 13.5 Chemical structures of older antiepileptic medications.

has a half-life of about 24 hours; thus, daytime sedation can be minimized if the patient takes the full daily dose at bedtime. Many bothersome side effects limit its use in favor of newer, less toxic agents. Other, older anticonvulsants include *primidone* and *ethosuximide*, both introduced in the late 1950s.

Valproic acid (Divalproex, Depakene, Depakote), introduced in 1974, is effective in treating *petit mal* seizure disorders in children. It acts by augmenting the postsynaptic action of GABA. Valproic acid has a short half-life of about 6 to 12 hours; it must therefore be administered two or three times a day. Common side effects include sedation and cognitive impairments. Serious side effects are rare, but liver failure has been reported. Like many of the newer anticonvulsants, valproic acid is effective in people with bipolar disorder, posttraumatic stress disorder, borderline personality disorder, aggressive behaviors, schizophrenia, and alcohol and cocaine dependence. A long-acting, slow-release formulation (Depakote-ER) is approved for the treatment of migraine headache.

Carbamazepine (Tegretol, Equitro), introduced in 1963, is an antiepileptic drug with a sedative effect that is perhaps less intense than that of the other antiepileptic agents. The primary limitations of carbamazepine include serious alterations in the cellular composition of blood (reduced numbers of white blood cells), presumably secondary to a depressant effect on bone marrow. Carbamazepine also increases the production of drug-metabolizing enzymes in the liver, such that both itself (*autoinduction*) as well as other drugs metabolized by the same enzymes are metabolized much faster than would normally be expected and these drugs become clinically "less effective" due to lower-than-expected blood concentrations. Often, the dose of these drugs needs to be doubled to compensate. For nonepileptic use, carbamazepine has been used in the treatment of bipolar disorder, explosive behavioral disorders, pain syndromes, and alcohol withdrawal.

Gabapentin (Neurontin), introduced in 1993, is a structural analog of GABA, and was synthesized as a specific GABA-mimetic antiepileptic drug. Gabapentin is effective in treating both an anxiety disorder (phobia) and pain (reflex sympathetic dystrophy). Since then, gabapentin has been used in a wide variety of chronic pain states. Gabapentin can be effective in treating alcohol withdrawal and for prevention of relapse. A related drug, *pregabalin* (Lyrica), was introduced as an anticonvulsant in 2004 for adult patients with partial-onset seizures, that is, seizures that do not encompass the whole brain. Like gabapentin, pregabalin is used to treat several pain disorders, such as diabetic peripheral neuropathy, fibromyalgia, postherpetic neuralgia, and neuropathic pain from spinal cord injury.

Lamotrigine (Lamictal), introduced into medicine in 1995, acts by inhibiting ion fluxes through sodium channels, stabilizing neuronal membranes, and inhibiting the presynaptic release of neurotransmitters, principally glutamate. First introduced as an antiepileptic drug, it has beneficial effects on mood, mental alertness, and social interactions in some epilepsy patients. An unusual and significant advantage of lamotrigine is that it improves cognitive functioning and exerts antidepressant actions. Clinically, it has been used for the treatment of resistant depression as well as the depressive phase in bipolar disorder. It does not appear to cause a "manic flip" in such patients.

Oxcarbazepine (Trileptal) is a structural derivative of carbamazepine. It differs in two ways: (1) it is rapidly metabolized by a process called *reduction* to an active molecule; and (2) it has not been associated with the white blood cell toxicity associated with carbamazepine. Oxcarbazepine is being increasingly used to treat bipolar illness and other disorders for which carbamazepine is also effective.

Tiagabine (Gabitril) became clinically available in 1998 as another antiepileptic drug. The drug acts by inhibiting neuronal and glial uptake of GABA, secondary to its irreversibly inhibiting one of the GABA reuptake transporters located on the presynaptic nerve terminals of GABA-releasing neurons. This action serves to prolong GABA's synaptic action. Tiagabine appears to be less useful in the treatment of bipolar illness than other antiepileptic drugs. It has shown modest efficacy in the treatment of generalized anxiety disorder (Pollack et al., 2008).

Several other antiepileptic drugs introduced between 1993 and 2005 have found use in the treatment of bipolar illness: *topiramate* (Topamax), *levetiracetam* (Keppra), and *zonisamide* (Zonegran). Topiramate is discussed in Chapter 5 for its use in treating alcoholism. Zonisamide has been shown to be effective as an antiobesity agent when combined with a balanced low-calorie diet. It has also been used to treat binge-eating disorder.

Levetiracetam (Keppra) is effective in treating partial-onset seizures, the most common form of epilepsy. It has a unique mechanism of action (Yan et al., 2013) making it suitable for add-on therapy of epilepsy in both adults and children with refractory seizures.

Lacosamide (Vimpat) is an anticonvulsant, introduced in 2008, that appears to act in a different way than other anticonvulsants such as phenytoin. Traditional anticonvulsants affect a "fast action potential generation," while lacosamide interacts with sodium channels without effecting fast inactivation. It is a "novel sodium channel modulator" useful in the treatment of partial-onset (focal) seizures (McGinnis and Kessler, 2016; Vossler et al., 2016). It may exert fewer cognitive-depressing side effects than other anticonvulsants (Lancman et al., 2016).

Vigabatrin (Sabril), long available in Europe, was introduced into the United States in 2010. Despite serious side effects, it is indicated for two forms of severe epilepsy: (1) infantile spasms and (2) as adjunctive therapy for refractory partial epilepsy in adults who have not responded to other agents. Because its use is associated with loss of peripheral vision and can even produce permanent loss of vision, it is available only through a single national pharmacy and with requirements for formal ophthalmologic evaluation with continuing follow-up.

Rufinamide (Banzel) is another new antiepileptic agent, structurally different from other anticonvulsants. It is approved by the FDA for a specific type of epilepsy, namely Lennox-Gastaut syndrome (McMurray and Striano, 2016). It is also effective in refractory partial seizures; it seems to have no adverse effects on cognitive functioning.

Clobazam (Onfi) is a benzodiazepine approved in the United States in 2011 for the treatment of seizures associated with Lennox-Gastaut syndrome. It is also indicated as therapy for refractory epilepsy and for the short-term treatment of severe anxiety and agitation as seen in psychotic disorders. Like all benzodiazepines, adverse sedation and cognitive deficits are common. Interestingly, the active metabolite of clobazam,

N-desmethylclobazam, has some preferential binding to the alpha-2 subunit of the benzodiazepine receptor and as a result may have analgesic activity in contrast to other benzodiazepines (Raivenius et al., 2016)

Ezogabine (Potiga) appears to act by opening potassium channels in the brain. Such action is unique among anticonvulsants. Dizziness, somnolence, fatigue, and confusional states have been reported with its use.

Stiripentol (Diacomit) is another new antiepileptic drug that acts by increasing GABA transmission and by limiting GABA synaptic uptake, prolonging GABA activity. It has a specific use in treating severe myoclonic epilepsy in infants. It strongly inhibits the metabolism of other drugs, making other drugs both more effective—but possibly toxic too. As a result, dose reductions of other medications are usually required. The drug has not been approved by the FDA in the United States; however, it may be legally imported under an "orphan drug" status with the FDA on a "compassionate-use basis." It appears effective in a rare childhood genetic form of epilepsy, Dravet syndrome (DeLiso et al., 2016).

Perampanel (Fycompa) was approved by the FDA in 2012. It is unique as a blocker of the AMPA subtype of glutamate receptors, giving it a wide spectrum of anticonvulsant usefulness. Labeling contains a black box warning of adverse effects including "aggression, hostility, irritability, anger, and homicidal ideation." Other adverse effects that have been reported include suicidal thoughts and behavior, dizziness, gait disturbances, somnolence, and fatigue.

In 2013, the FDA approved *eslicarbazepine* (Aptiom) as an ancillary medication to treat partial seizures. Eslicarbazepine is a prodrug to oxcarbazepine (Trileptal). Eslicarbazene, therefore, shares the actions of oxcarbazepine, including potential to treat not only epilepsy but bipolar disorder and certain pain syndromes (Johannessen et al., 2016). Eslicarbazene is also claimed to be effective in drug-resistant patients who experience fewer side effects and drug interactions with a beneficial effect on quality of life and alertness (Schmid et al., 2016).

In early 2016, the FDA approved *brivaracetam* (Briviact) to treat partial and major motor seizures. While efficacy has been demonstrated (Ben-Menachem et al., 2016; Moseley et al., 2016), its efficacy does not seem to surpass that of levetiracetam (Keppra) (Zhang et al., 2016).

Antiepileptic Drugs in Pregnancy

Approximately 1 million women with epilepsy in the United States are in their active reproductive years. Most require anticonvulsant medication during pregnancy, and many anticonvulsants have adverse fetal outcomes. However, most women with epilepsy will have a normal pregnancy and a favorable outcome (Klein, 2011). Antiepileptic medications are also used to treat an expanding range of medical conditions including bipolar disorder, migraine headache, and chronic pain syndromes, which increases the overall risk to the fetus of a congenital malformation. Statistically, women who took an anticonvulsant during a prior pregnancy and delivered a normal infant were not at risk of delivering an infant with a congenital malformation during a subsequent pregnancy. However, if an infant was delivered with a malformation during the prior pregnancy, there was a twofold to threefold increased risk of a fetal malformation in their next pregnancy (Vajda et al., 2017). When multiple anticonvulsants are prescribed during pregnancy, the risk is tripled, especially when valproic acid (Depakote) is included (Nadebaum et al., 2012). Use of valproic acid during pregnancy is especially problematic. In June 2011, the FDA issued a safety announcement on the adverse impact of valproic acid on cognitive impairments in offspring of mothers who took valproic acid during pregnancy. Several recent reviews relevant to antiepileptic drugs during pregnancy are available (Bromley, 2016; de Jong et al., 2016; Ferri et al., 2016; Martinez et al., 2016; Patel and Pennell, 2016; Pennell, 2016).

Antiepileptic Drugs and Risk of Suicidal Thoughts and Behavior

In December 2008, the FDA issued a warning that the use of antiepileptic drugs as a class may increase the risk of suicidal thoughts and behaviors. The medical community received this warning with skepticism (Kanner, 2011). Specifically, the skepticism stemmed from the understanding that multiple other factors may be involved in the increased rate of suicidality in patients taking anticonvulsants for depression, epilepsy, surgery, bipolar disorder, substance abuse, and anxiety disorders. Patients later diagnosed with epilepsy had a pretreatment incidence of a suicide attempt almost twofold to threefold before any diagnosis (Hesdorffer et al., 2016). Since anticonvulsant medications had not yet been prescribed, any increase was not due to medication. Likely increases were caused by comorbid disorders such as depression or bipolar disorder (Ferrer et al., 2014).

Regardless, patients taking antiepileptic drugs should be carefully monitored for behavioral changes that could be precursors to emerging suicidality, including drug-induced anxiety, agitation, hostility, and mania or hypomania (Mula and Sander, 2015). This warning applies whether anticonvulsants are used to treat seizures, psychiatric disorders, pain, migraine headaches, or other conditions.

STUDY QUESTIONS

1. Describe the mechanism action of benzodiazepines and how it differs from that of barbiturates.
2. Describe the structure and function of the benzodiazepine receptor.
3. List some of the clinical uses of benzodiazepines.
4. What is the difference between benzodiazepines and the so-called "Z-drugs"?
5. Discuss the melatonergic and orexigenic hypnotic drugs.
6. What are the most common anesthetic drugs and their mechanisms of action?
7. Discuss the anticonvulsant drugs; what are their indications, how do their mechanisms of action differ, and what are the most important side effects?

REFERENCES

Absalom, N., et al. (2012). "Alpha-4/Beta-o GABA(A) Receptors Are High-Affinity Targets for Gamma-Hydroxybutyric Acid (GHB)." *Proceedings of the National Academy of Sciences USA* 109: 13404–13409.

Alexander, B., et al. (2015). "Early Discontinuation and Suboptimal Dosing of Prazosin: A Potential Missed Opportunity for Veterans with Posttraumatic Stress Disorder." *Journal of Clinical Psychiatry* 76: e639–e644.

Amos, T., et. al. (2014). "Pharmacological Interventions for Preventing Post-Traumatic Stress Disorder (PTSD)." *Cochrane Database Systematic Review* 7: CD006239. doi: 10.1002/14651858. CD006239.pub2.

Asnis, G. M., et al. (2016). "Pharmacotherapy Treatment Options for Insomnia: A Primer for Clinicians." *International Journal of Molecular Sciences* 17: 50. doi: 10.3390/ijms17010050.

Bachhuber, M. A., et al. (2016). "Increasing Benzodiazepine Prescriptions and Overdose Mortality in the United States, 1996–2013." *American Journal of Public Health* 106: 686–688.

Baldwin, D. S., et al. (2015). "Efficacy and Safety of Pregabalin in Generalised Anxiety Disorder: A Critical Review of the Literature." *Journal of Psychopharmacology* 29: 1047–1060.

Baselt, R. (2014). *Disposition of Toxic Drugs and Chemicals in Man*, 10th ed. Seal Beach, CA: Biomedical Publications.

Bellantuono, C., et al. (2013). "Benzodiazepine Exposure in Pregnancy and Risk of Major Malformations: A Critical Overview." *General Hospital Psychiatry* 35: 3–8.

Bengalorkar, G. M., et al. (2011). "Fospropofol: Clinical Pharmacology." *Journal of Anaesthesiology and Clinical Pharmacology* 27: 79–83.

Ben-Menachem, E., et al. (2016). "Efficacy and Safety of Brivaracetam for Partial-Onset Seizures in 3 Pooled Clinical Studies." *Neurology* 87: 314–323.

Billioti de Gage, S., et al. (2014). "Benzodiazepine Use and Risk of Alzheimer's Disease: Case-Control Study." *BMJ* 349: g5205. doi: 10.1136/bmj.g5205.

Bromley, R. (2016). "The Treatment of Epilepsy in Pregnancy: The Neurodevelopmental Risks Associated with Exposure to Antiepileptic Drugs." *Reproduction Toxicology* 64: 203–210.

Brower, K. J., et al. (2011). "Ramelteon and Improved Insomnia in Alcohol-Dependent Patients: A Case Series." *Journal of Clinical Sleep Medicine* 7: 274–275.

Chen, C. S., et al. (2014). "Clinical Correlates of Zolpidem-Associated Complex Sleep-Related Behaviors: Age Effect." *Journal of Clinical Psychiatry* 75: e1314–e1318.

Cimolai, N. (2017). "Safety with Zopiclone Use: Contemporary Issues." *Current Psychopharmacology* 6: 43–50.

de Jong, J., et al. (2016). "The Risk of Specific Congenital Anomalies in Relation to Newer Antiepileptc Drugs: A Literature Review." *Drugs—Real World Outcomes* 24: 131–143.

DeLiso, P., et al. (2016). "Patients with Dravet Syndrome in the Era of Stiripentol: A French Cohort Cross-Sectional Study." *Epilepsy Research* 125: 42–46.

Delli, P. S., et al. (2016). "GABA Content within the Ventromedial Prefrontal Cortex is Related to Trait Anxiety." *Social Cognitive & Affective Neuroscience* 11: 758–766.

Di, S., et al. (2016). "Acute Stress Suppresses Synaptic Inhibition and Increases Anxiety via Endocannabinoid Release in the Basolateral Amygdala." *Journal of Neuroscience* 36: 8461–8470.

Dietz, B. M., et al. (2005). "Valerian Extract and Valerenic Acid are Partial Agonists of the 5HT-5a Receptor in vitro." *Brain Research Molecular Brain Research* 18: 191–197.

Durgam, S., et al. (2016). "Efficacy and Safety of Vilazodone in Patients with Generalized Anxiety Disorder: A Randomized, Double-Blind, Placebo-Controlled, Flexible-Dose Trial." *Journal of Clinical Psychiatry* 77:1687–1694. doi: 10.4088/JCP.15m09885.

Emet, M., et al. (2016). "A Review of Melatonin, its Receptors and Drugs." *Eurasian Journal of Medicine* 48: 135–141.

Enato, E., et al. (2011). "The Fetal Safety of Benzodiazepines: An Updated Meta-Analysis." *Journal of Obstetrics and Gynaecology Canada* 33: 46–48.

Ferrer, P., et al. (2014). "Antiepileptic Drugs and Suicide: A Systematic Review of Adverse Effects." *Neuroepidemiology* 42: 107–120.

Frampton, J. (2014). "Pregabalin: A Review of its Use in Adults with Generalized Anxiety Disorder." *CNS Drugs* 28: 835–854.

Franklin, J.B., and Rajesh, R.P. (2015). "A sleep-inducing peptide from the venom of the Indian cone snail Conus araneosus" *Toxicon* Sep;103:39–47.

Fudin, J., and Raouf, M. (2016). "A Review of Skeletal Muscle Relaxants for Pain Management: Spasticity and Spasm: 2 Distinct Reactions to Motor Neurons that Require Unique and Sometimes Complementary Therapies." *Practical Pain Management.* June 1. https://www.practicalpainmanagement.com/treatments/pharmacological/non-opioids/review-skeletal-muscle-relaxants-pain-management.

Gray, S. L., et al. (2016). "Benzodiazepine Use and the Risk of Incident Dementia or Cognitive Decline: Prospective Population Based Study." *BMJ* 352: i90. doi: http://dx.doi.org/10.1136/bmj.i90.

Hadley, S. J., et al. (2012). "Switching from Long-Term Benzodiazepine Therapy to Pregabalin in Patients with Generalized Anxiety Disorder: A Double-Blind, Placebo-Controlled Trial." *Journal of Psychopharmacology* 26: 461–470.

Hatta, K., et al. (2014). "Preventive Effects of Ramelteon on Delirium: A Randomized Placebo-Controlled Trial." *JAMA Psychiatry* 71:397–403. doi: 10.1001/jamapsychiatry.2013.3320.

Hawkins, E. J., et al. (2016). "Survey of Primary Care and Mental Health Prescribers' Perspectives on Reducing Opioid and Benzodiazepine Co-Prescribing Among Veterans." *Pain Medicine* 18:454–467. doi: 10.1093/pm/pnw140.

Herring, W. J., et al. (2016). "Suvorexant in Patients with Insomnia: Pooled Analysis of Three-Month Data from Phase-3 Randomized Controlled Clinical Trials." *Journal of Clinical Sleep Medicine* 12: 1215–1225.

Hesdorffer, D. C., et al. (2016). "Occurrence and Recurrence of Attempted Suicide Among People with Epilepsy." *JAMA Psychiatry* 73: 80–86.

Horsfall, J. T., and Sprague, J. E. (2016). "The Pharmacology and Toxicology of the 'Holy Trinity'." *Basic & Clinical Pharmacology & Toxicology* 120: 115–119. doi: 10.1111/bcpt.12655.

Inagaki, T., et al. (2010). "Adverse Reactions to Zolpidem: Case Reports and a Review of the Literature." *The Primary Care Companion* 12: PCC09r00849. doi: 10.4088/PCC.09r00849bro.

Johannessen, L. C., et al. (2016). "The Impact of Pharmacokinetic Interactions with Eslicarbazepine Acetate versus Oxcarbazepine and Carbamazepine in Clinical Practice." *Therapeutic Drug Monitoring* 38: 499–505.

Kanner, A. M. (2011). "Are Antiepileptic Drugs used in the Treatment of Migraine Associated with an Increased Risk of Suicidality?" *Current Pain and Headache Reports* 15: 164–169.

Keating, G. M. (2014). "Sodium Oxybate: A Review of its Use in Alcohol Withdrawal Syndrome and in the Maintenance of Abstinence in Alcohol Dependence." *Clinical Drug Investigations* 34: 63–80.

Klein, A. M. (2011). "Epilepsy Cases in Pregnant and Postpartum Women: A Practical Approach." *Seminars in Neurology* 31: 392–396.

Koola, M. M., et al. (2014). "High-Dose Prazosin for the Treatment of Post-Traumatic Stress Disorder." *Therapeutic Advances in Psychopharmacology* 4: 43–47. doi: 10.1177/2045125313500982.

Kumar, A., et al. (2016). "Emerging Role of Orexin Antagonists in Insomnia Therapeutics: An Update on SORAs and DORAs." *Pharmacology Reports* 68: 231–242.

Kuriyama, A., et al. (2014). "Ramelteon for the Treatment of Insomnia in Adults: A Systematic Review and Meta-Analysis." *Sleep Medicine* 15: 385–392. doi: 10.1016/j.sleep.2013.11.788.

Lancaster, C. L., et al. (2016). "Posttraumatic Stress Disorder: Overview of Evidence-Based Assessment and Treatment." *Journal of Clinical Medicine* 5: 105. doi: 10.3390/jcm5110105.

Lancman, M. E., et al. (2016). "The Effects of Lacosamide on Cognition, Quality-of-Life Measures, and Quality of Life in Patients with Refractory Partial Epilepsy." *Epilepsy & Behavior* 61: 27–33.

Laudon, M., and Frydman-Marom, A. (2014). "Therapeutic Effects of Melatonin Receptor Agonists on Sleep and Comorbid Disorders." *International Journal of Molecular Sciences* 15: 15924–15950.

Leger, D., et al. (2015). "Safety Profile of Tasimelteon, a Melatonin MT1 and MT2 Receptor Agonist: Pooled Safety Analysis from Six Clinical Studies." *Expert Opinions on Drug Safety* 14: 1673–1685.

Lin, F-Y, et al. (2014). "Retrospective Population Cohort Study on Hip Fracture Risk Associated with Zolpidem Medication." *Sleep* 37: 673–679. doi: 10.5665/sleep.3566.

Liu, J., and Wang, L. N. (2012). "Ramelteon in the Treatment of Chronic Insomnia: Systematic Review and Meta-Analysis." *International Journal of Clinical Practice* 66: 867–873.

Liu, J., et al. (2016). "MT1 and MT2 Melatonin Receptors: A Therapeutic Perspective." *Annual Reviews of Pharmacology and Toxicology* 56: 361–383.

Liu, Z. P. et al. (2017). "Delta Subunit-Containing Gamma-Aminobutyric Acid-A Receptor Disinhibits Lateral Amygdala and Facilitates Fear Expression in Mice." *Biological Psychiatry* 81: 990–1002. doi: 10.1016/j.biopsych.2016.06.022.

Martinez, F. M., et al. (2018). "Comparative Study of Antiepileptic Drug Use during Pregnancy over a period of 12 years in Spain. Efficacy of the Newer Antiepileptic Drugs Lamotrigine, Levetiracetam, and Oxcarbazepine." *Neurologica* 33: 78–84. In press. doi: 10.1016/j.nrl.2016.05.004.

McCarthy, M. (2016). "US Drug Labels to Warn of Risks of Combining Opioids and Benzodiazepines." *BMJ* 354: i4784. doi: 10.1136/bmj.i4784.

McGinnis, E., and Kessler, S. K. (2016). "Lacosamide Use in Children with Epilepsy: Retention Rate and Effect of Concomitant Sodium Channel Blockers in a Large Cohort." *Epilepsia* 57: 1416–1425.

McMurray, R., and Striano, P. (2016). "Treatment of Adults with Lennox-Gastaut Syndrome: Further Analysis of Efficacy and Safety/Tolerability of Rufinamide." *Neurology and Therapeutics* 5: 35–43.

Mets, M. A., et al. (2011). "Next-Day Effects of Ramelteon (8 mg), Zopiclone (7.5 mg), and Placebo on Highway Driving Performance, Memory Functioning, Psychomotor Performance, and Mood in Healthy Adult Subjects." *Sleep* 34: 1327–1334.

Mizrak, A., et al. (2010). "Pretreatment with Desmedetomidine or Thiopental Decreases Myoclonus After Etomidate: A Randomized, Double-Blind Controlled Trial." *Journal of Surgical Research* 159: e11–e16.

Moseley, B. D., et al. (2016). "Efficacy, Safety, and Tolerability of Adjunctive Brivaracetam for Secondarily Generalized Tonic-Clonic Seizures: Pooled Results from Three Phase III Studies." *Epilepsy Research* 127: 179–185.

Moylan, S., et al. (2012). "The Role of Alprazolam for the Treatment of Panic Disorder in Australia." *Australia and New Zealand Journal of Psychiatry* 46: 212–224.

Mula, M., and Sander, J. W. (2015). "Suicide and Epilepsy: Do Antiepileptic Drugs Increase the Risk?" *Expert Opinions on Drug Safety* 14: 553–558.

Nadebaum, C., et al. (2012). "Neurobehavioral Consequences of Prenatal Antiepileptic Drug Exposure." *Developmental Neuropsychology* 37: 1–29.

Norman, J. L., and Anderson, S. L. (2016). "Novel Class of Medications, Orexin Receptor Antagonists, in the Treatment of Insomnia – Critical Appraisal of Suvorexant." *Nature and Science of Sleep* 14: 239–247.

Norris, E. R., et al. (2013). "A Double-Blind, Randomized, Placebo-Controlled Trial of Adjunctive Ramelteon for the Treatment of Insomnia and Mood Stability in Patients with Euthymic Bipolar Disorder." *Journal of Affective Disorders* 144: 141–147.

Nurmi-Luthje, I., et al. (2006). "Use of Benzodiazepines and Benzodiazepine-Related Drugs Among 223 Patients with an Acute Hip Fracture in Finland: Comparison of Benzodiazepine Findings in Medical Records and Laboratory Assays." *Drugs and Aging* 23: 27–37.

Ogilvie, B. W., et al. (2015). "Clinical Assessment of Drug-Drug Interactions of Tasimeltion, a Novel Melatonin Receptor Agonist." *Journal of Clinical Pharmacology* 55: 1004–1011.

Olfson, M., et al. (2014). "Benzodiazepine use in the United States." *JAMA Psychiatry* 72: 136–142. doi: 10.1001/jamapsychiatry.2014.1763.

Osterweil, N. (2014). "Panic Attacks Return after Drugs Stop, but Yield to Retreatment." *Clinical Psychiatry News.* May 6. http://www.mdedge.com/clinicalpsychiatrynews/article/82156/anxiety-disorders/panic-attacks-return-after-drugs-stop-yield.

Papoutsis, I., et al. (2016). "Benzodiazepines and Driving: Pharmacological and Legal Aspects." *European Journal of Forensic Sciences* 3: 26–34.

Pariente, A., et al. (2016). "The Benzodiazepine-Dementia Disorders Link: Current State of Knowledge." *CNS Drugs* 30: 1–7.

Park, T. W., et al. (2015). "Benzodiazepine Prescribing Patterns and Deaths from Drug Overdose Among US Veterans Receiving Opioid Analgesics: Case-Cohort Study." *BMJ* 350: h2698. doi: http://dx.doi.org/10.1136/bmj.h2698.

Patel, S. I., and Pennell, P. B. (2016). "Management of Epilepsy during Pregnancy: An Update." *Therapeutic Advances in Neurological Disorders* 9: 118–129.

Paterniti, S., et al. (2002). "Long-Term Benzodiazepine Use and Cognitive Decline in the Elderly: The Epidemiology of Vascular Aging Study." *Journal of Clinical Psychopharmacology* 22: 285–293.

Pennell, P. B. (2016). "Use of Antiepileptic Drugs during Pregnancy: Evolving Concepts." *Neurotherapeutics* 13: 811–820. doi: 10.1007/s13311-016-0464-0.

Perlemuter, G., et al. (2016). "Characterisation of Agomelanine-Induced Increase in Liver Enzymes: Frequency and Risk Factors Determined from a Pooled Analysis of 7605 Treated Patients." *CNS Drugs* 30: 877–888.

Perlis, M., et al. (2015). "Durability of Treatment Response to Zolpidem with Three Different Maintenance Regimens: A Preliminary Study." *Sleep Medicine* 16: 1160–1168. doi: 10.1016/j.sleep.2015.06.015.

Pillai, V., et al. (2017). "Effectiveness of Benzodiazepine Receptor Agonists in the Treatment of Insomnia: An Examination of Response and Remission Rates." *Sleep* 40(2). doi: 10.1093/sleep/zsw044.

Pollack, M., et al. (2008). "Tiagabine in Adult Patients with Generalized Anxiety Disorder: Results from 3 Randomized, Double-Blind, Placebo-Controlled, Parallel-Group Studies." *Journal of Clinical Psychopharmacology* 28: 308–316.

Prager, E. M., et al. (2016). "The Basolateral Amygdala Gamma-aminobutyric Acidergic System in Health and Disease." *Journal of Neuroscience Research* 94: 548–567.

Qaseem, A., et al (2016). "Management of Chronic Insomnia Disorder in Adults: A Clinical Practice Guideline from the American College of Physicians." *Annals of Internal Medicine* 165: 125–133. doi: 10.7326/M15-2175.

Raivenius, W. T., et al. (2016). "The Clobazam Metabolite N-desmethyl Clobazam Is an Alpha2 Preferring Benzodiazepine with an Improved Therapeutic Window for Antihyperalgesia." *Neuropharmacology* 109: 366–375.

Rang, H. P., and Dale, M. M. (1991). *Pharmacology,* 2nd ed. Edinburgh: Churchill Livingstone.

Raskind, M. A., et al. (2016). "Higher Pretreatment Blood Pressure Is Associated with Greater Posttraumatic Stress Disorder Symptom Reduction in Soldiers Treated with Prazosin." *Biological Psychiatry* 80: 736–742.

Rickels, K., et al. (2012). "Adjunctive Therapy with Pregabalin in Generalized Anxiety Disorder Patients with Partial Response to SSRI or SNRI Treatment." *International Clinical Psychopharmacology* 27: 142–150.

Rodgman, C., et al., (2016). "Doxazosin XL Reduces Symptoms of Posttraumatic Stress Disorder in Veterans with PTSD: A Pilot Clinical Trial." *Journal of Clinical Psychiatry* 77: e561–e565.

Roest, A. M., et al. (2015). "Reporting Bias in Clinical Trials Investigating the Efficacy of Second-Generation Antidepressants in the Treatment of Anxiety Disorders: A Report of 2 Meta-analyses." *JAMA Psychiatry* 72: 500–510. doi: 10.1001/jamapsychiatry.2015.15.

Sadeghniiat-Haghighi, K., et al., (2016). "Melatonin Therapy in Shift Workers with Difficulty Falling Asleep: A Randomized, Double-Blind, Placebo-Controlled Crossover Field Study." *Work* 55: 225–230. doi: 10.3233/WOR-162376.

Scammell, T.E. and Winrow, C. (2011). "Orexin Receptors: Pharmacology and Therapeutic Opportunities." *Annual Review of Pharmacology and Toxicology* 51: 243–266. doi: 10.1146/annurev-pharmtox-010510-100528

Schep, L. J., et al. (2012). "The Clinical Toxicology of gamma-Hydroxybutyrate, gamma-butyrate, and 1,4-Butanediol." *Clinical Toxicology* 50: 458–470.

Schmid, E., et al. (2016). "Overnight Switching from Oxcarbazepine to Eslicarbazepine Acetate: An Observational Study." *Acta Neurologica Scandinavica* 135: 449–453. doi: 10.1111/ane.12645.

Serna, M., et al. (2015). "Benzodiazepines and Drugs with Anticholinergic Activity Increase Mortality in Patients with Delirium." Annual Meeting of the American Psychiatric Association. Abstract P2–85. https://www.researchgate.net/profile/Joachim_Raese/publication/275652291_Benzodiazepines_and_drugs_with_anticholinergic_activity_increase_mortality_in_delirium/links/5542d1d00cf234bdb21a2e34.pdf.

Singh, B., et al. (2016). "Efficacy of Prazosin in Posttraumatic Stress Disorder: A Systematic Review and Meta-Analysis." *Primary Care Companion CNS Disorders* 18. doi: 10.4088/PCC.16r01943.

Sirven, J. I., et al. (2012). "Antiepileptic Drugs 2012: Recent Advances and Trends." *Mayo Clinic Proceedings* 87: 879–889.

Skolnick, P. (2012). "Anxioselective Anxiolytics: On a Quest for the Holy Grail." *Trends in Pharmacological Sciences* 33: 611–620.

Soeter, M., and Kindt, M. (2015). "An Abrupt Transformation of Phobic Behavior after a Post-Retrieval Amnesic Agent." *Biological Psychiatry* 78: 880–886.

Soyka, M. (2017). "Treatment of Benzodiazepine Dependence." *New England Journal of Medicine* 376: 1147–1157. doi: 10.1056/NEJMra1611832.

Steenen, S. A., et al. (2016). "Propranolol for the Treatment of Anxiety Disorders: Systematic Review and Meta-Analysis." *Journal of Psychopharmacology* 30: 128–139. doi: 10.1177/0269881115612236.

Stein, B. D., et al. (2016). "Opioid Analgesic and Benzodiazepine Prescribing among Medicaid-Enrollees with Opioid Use Disorders: The Influence of Provider Communities." *Journal of Addiction Disorders* 36: 14–22. doi: 10.1080/10550887.2016.1211784.

Stein, D. J., et al. (2014). "Agomelatine in Generalized Anxiety Disorder: An Active Comparator and Placebo-Controlled Study." *Journal of Clinical Psychiatry* 75: 362–368.

Taipale, H., et al. (2017). "Use of Benzodiazepines and Related Drugs is Associated with a Risk of Stroke among Persons with Alzheimers Disease." *International Clinical Psychopharmacology* 32: 135–141.

Taylor, D., et al. (2014). "Antidepressant Efficacy of Agomelatine: Meta-Analysis of Published and Unpublished Studies." *BMJ* 348: g1888. doi: 10.1136/bmj.g1888.

Thirtala, T., et al. (2013). "Consider This Slow-Taper Program for Benzodiazepines." *Current Psychiatry* 12: 55–56.

Trauer, J. M., et al. (2015). "Cognitive-Behavioral Therapy for Chronic Insomnia: A Systematic Review and Meta-Analysis." *Annals of Internal Medicine* 163: 191–204.

Vajda, F. J., et al. (2017). "Antiepileptic Drugs, Foetal Malformations and Spontaneous Abortions." *Acta Neurologic Scandinavica* 135(3): 360–365. doi: 10.1111/ane.12672.

Verster, J. C., and Roth, T. (2013). "Blood Drug Concentrations of Benzodiazepines Correlate Poorly with Actual Driving Impairment." *Sleep Medicine Review* 17: 153–159.

Vicens, C., et al. (2014). "Comparative Efficacy of Two Interventions to Discontinue Long-Term Benzodiazepine Use: Cluster Randomised Controlled Trial in Primary Care." *British Journal of Psychiatry* 204: 471–479.

Vindenes, V., et al. (2012). "Impairment Based Legislative Limits for Driving Under the Influence of Non-Alcohol Drugs in Norway." *Forensic Science International* 219: 1–11.

Vossler, D. G., et al. (2016). "Long-Term Exposure and Safety of Lacosamide Monotherapy for the Treatment of Partial-Onset (focal) Seizures: Results from a Multicenter, Open-Label Trial." *Epilepsia* 57: 1625–1633. doi: 10.1111/epi.13502.

Vozoris, N. T., et al. (2014). "Benzodiazepine Drug Use and Adverse Respiratory Outcomes among Older Adults with COPD." *European Respiratory Journal* 44: 332–340. doi: 10.1183/09031936.00008014.

Wade, A. G., et al. (2007). "Efficacy of Prolonged Release Melatonin in Insomnia Patients aged 55–80 Years: Quality of Sleep and next-Day Alertness Outcomes." *Current Medical Research Opinions* 23: 2597–2605.

Weich, S., et al. (2014). "Effect of Anxiolytic and Hypnotic Drug Prescriptions on Mortality Hazards: Retrospective Cohort Study." *BMJ* 348: g1996. doi: 10.1136/bmj.g1996.

Williams, W. P., et al. (2016). "Comparative Review of Approved Melatonin Agonists for the Treatment of Circadian Rhythm Sleep-Wake Disorders." *Pharmacotherapy* 36: 1028–1041.

Winterfeld, U., et al. (2016). "Pregnancy Outcome Following Maternal Exposure to Pregabalin May Call for Concern." *Neurology* 86: 2251–2257.

Wong, C. K., et al. (2017). "Spontaneous Adverse Event Reports Associated with Zolpidem in the United States 2003–2012." *Journal of Clinical Sleep Medicine* 13: 223–234. doi: 10.5664/jcsm.6452.

Yaffe, K., and Boustani, M. (2014). "Benzodiazepines and Risk of Alzheimer's Disease." *BMJ* 349: g5312. doi: 10.1136/bmj.g5312.

Yan, H. D., et al. (2013). "Inhibitory Effects of Levetiracetam on the High-Voltage-Activated L-Type Ca(2+) Channels in Hippocampal CA3 Neurons of Spontaneously Epileptic Rat (SER)." *Brain Research Bulletin* 90: 142–148.

Yoshimura, R. F., et al. (2014). "Limited Central Side Effects of a β-Subunit Subtype-Selective $GABA_A$ Receptor Allosteric Modulator." *Journal of Psychopharmacology* 28: 472–478. doi: 10.1177/0269881113507643.

Zammit, G. (2009). "Comparative Tolerability of Newer Agents for Insomnia." *Drug Safety* 32: 735–748.

Zhang, L., et al. (2016). "Levetiracetam vs. Brivaracetam for Adults with Refractory Focal Seizures: A Meta-Analysis and Indirect Comparison." *Seizure* 39: 28–33.

Zisapel, N. (2015). "Current Phase II Investigational Therapies for Insomnia." *Expert Opinions on Investigational Drugs* 24: 401–411.

CHAPTER 14

Drugs Used to Treat Bipolar Disorder

BIPOLAR DISORDER

Bipolar disorder, also known as *manic-depressive disorder*, is one of the ten most disabling conditions in the world, with a lifetime prevalence of about 1 percent across all populations, regardless of nationality, race, or socioeconomic status (Grande et al., 2016; Merikangas et al., 2011). People who have the disorder lose many years of healthy functioning, in which their livelihood, marriage, social relationships, and even lives may be destroyed. The illness is episodic, with alternating periods of mania or depression nearly a third of the time and intervening periods of at least some degree of recovery and sometimes remission (Figure 14.1). Although it may appear in childhood or adolescence, the diagnosis is difficult and it is still being debated (Chapter 15). The main problems in diagnosis are that mania or hypomania may be underreported, that symptoms of unipolar and bipolar depression overlap, and that there is a high degree of comorbidity with many other psychiatric conditions (Hirschfeld, 2009). Generally, onset is between the second and third decade of life or later, often with a significant delay between the appearance of symptoms and a correct diagnosis and treatment. In fact, estimates of the delay between onset of symptoms and correct diagnosis and appropriate treatment range from six years in one meta-analytic study (Dagani et al., 2016) to ten years in epidemiological studies (Dodd et al., 2007). Some of the delay is related to the difficulty in making a diagnosis of bipolar disorder. In one study, after careful assessment by skilled clinicians who diagnosed bipolar disorder, it was subsequently found on reevaluation that 20 percent of those individuals were rediagnosed with a different disorder (Ruggero et al., 2010); and up to one-fifth of individuals who are initially diagnosed with unipolar depression turn out subsequently to have a bipolar disorder (Goldberg et al., 2001; Smith et al., 2011). The Bipolar Disorder: Improving Diagnosis, Guidance, and Education (BRIDGE) study found that almost one-half of patients presenting with a depressive episode were mistakenly diagnosed with unipolar depression when in fact they had bipolar disorder that was detected after a more comprehensive evaluation (Angst et al., 2011). The differences in the proportion of misdiagnosed patients seen in the studies by Smith (2011), Angst (2011), and their colleagues can be attributed to differences in methodology, diagnostic criteria, and statistical design between the two studies. The key point in these and other similar studies is that it is relatively common to misdiagnose someone as having a unipolar depression when, in fact, that depressive episode may be part of a bipolar cycle. Most patients experience several episodes during the course of their lives. The risk of recurrence has been reported to be 24 percent by six months, 36 percent by one year, and 61 percent by four years (Baldassano, 2009). Grande and coworkers (2016) present a review of the epidemiology and treatment of bipolar disorder.

There are several subtypes of the disorder. The traditional subtype, *bipolar I* (BP-I) *disorder*, includes at least one episode of full-blown mania with or without an episode of major depression. The disorder is classified as *bipolar II* (BP-II) if the manic episode is less severe, or "hypomanic," and episodes of major depression also occur. A patient is said to be a "rapid cycler" if at least four illness episodes occur in a 12-month period. Several other bipolar subtypes have been described, exhibiting varying degrees of severity in recurrent mood swings. For example, DSM-5 lists ten specifiers that can be attached to a bipolar disorder diagnosis to further define the presenting symptoms and characteristics of the disorder. Together, the variants bring the prevalence of all bipolar disorders to 3.9 to 4.4 percent of U.S. residents (Merikangas et al., 2011; National Institute of Mental Health, 2005).

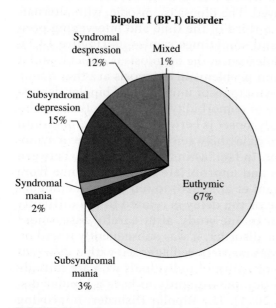

FIGURE 14.1 Percentage of time spent in each mood state for individuals who have bipolar I disorder. Two-thirds of the time they have no symptoms and they are depressed (subsyndromal or syndromal) more than three times more frequently than they are manic (subsyndromal and syndromal mania) during the course of the disorder. [Data from Parikh et al., 2015.]

Despite intensive care and treatment, outpatients with bipolar disorder have a considerable degree of illness-related morbidity and variability in illness cycles, including a three- to sixfold greater amount of time spent depressed than time spent manic (Jann, 2014; Post et al., 2005) (see also Figure 14.1). Those patients who have residual subsyndromal depressive symptoms following a manic episode may have a poorer outcome and more difficulty reaching functional recovery over their lifetimes (Gitlin et al., 2011). Furthermore, patients who have mixed episodes, that is, symptoms of both mania and depression during the same episode (Swann et al., 2013), have been shown to have an earlier age of onset of bipolar disorder; have more frequent hospitalizations; and have episodes of illness as observed in a ten-year prospective study (Gonzalez-Pinto et al., 2011). Moreover, there is a high rate of mortality (Kupfer, 2005); one of every four or five untreated or inadequately treated patients commits suicide during the course of the illness, a rate ten times that of the general population. Other predictors of mortality in bipolar patients include male gender, history of alcoholism, and poor occupational status before the index episode, as well as a history of previous episodes, psychotic features, mixed episodes, and residual affective symptoms between episodes. This speaks to the need for aggressive treatment of bipolar disorder with a goal of reaching full remission from each episode, if possible.

DIAGNOSTIC AND TREATMENT ISSUES

Bipolar versus Unipolar Depression

Similar to unipolar depression, the symptoms of bipolar depression, as described by patients, include, in decreasing order of prevalence, sadness, insomnia, feelings of worthlessness, loss of energy and ability to concentrate, inability to enjoy everyday activities, thoughts of death and suicide, and an inability to function. Manic symptoms include various aspects of behavioral and physiological hyperactivity, such as erratic sleep, increased sexual interest, emotional elation and racing thoughts, increased physical activity, impulsiveness, poor judgment, and reckless and aggressive behavior. And up to 75 percent of individuals presenting with mania will have psychotic symptoms, such as delusions of grandeur and hallucinations (Grande et al., 2016).

Comorbid substance abuse affects at least 60 percent of bipolar I and 50 percent of bipolar II patients, with reported rates for alcohol (82 percent), cocaine (30 percent), marijuana (29 percent), sedatives or amphetamines (21 percent), and opioids (13 percent). It may, at least initially, represent an attempt at self-medication for the symptoms accompanying the affective disorder. Unfortunately, substance abuse is associated with a greater risk of "switching" or "flipping" from a depressive episode to one of mania, hypomania, or a mixed mood state (Ostacher et al., 2010).

Although a patient with bipolar disorder may present initially with either mania or depression, most patients seek treatment for depression (Jann, 2014). As a result, many are incorrectly diagnosed with unipolar depression and consequently receive inappropriate treatment with antidepressants alone. Unfortunately, while antidepressants can be effective against depressive symptomatology, they may induce or trigger a manic episode flip, which results in serious adverse consequences for the patient (Goldberg, 2010; Patel et al., 2015; Vieta et al., 2010). The risk of such an event is apparently greater if patients have more severe manic symptoms at baseline before addition of the antidepressant and if the antidepressant is maintained for longer periods of time (Frye et al., 2009; McGirr et al., 2016). Because of this risk, administration or addition of a mood stabilizer (MS) or an atypical antipsychotic medication is the most commonly recommended pharmacological treatment for bipolar depression (Bauer and Mitchner, 2004; Grande et al., 2016; Jann, 2014; Mundo et al., 2006).

Unfortunately, even combinations of antidepressants and mood stabilizers may not completely prevent the risk of a manic episode, and the risk varies depending on which antidepressants and mood stabilizers are combined (Goldberg, 2010; Leverich et al., 2006). Long-term treatment with antidepressant and mood stabilizer combinations may even worsen manic symptom severity (Goldberg et al., 2007) or increase the likelihood of a manic episode in patients (McGirr et al., 2016). Given that maintenance treatment with antidepressants, along with the mood stabilizer, may not prevent depressive relapses, weaning patients off antidepressants 6 to 12 months after remission of the depressive episode, and continuing the mood stabilizer has been advised (Goodwin et al., 2016; Yatham et al., 2013).

Obviously, because of these significant differences in recommended pharmacological treatments, it is important to be able to differentiate between unipolar and bipolar depression. Although the distinction is not always easy to make, some clinical features have been proposed to help (Leonpacher et al., 2015; Perlis et al., 2006a). Unipolar depression usually develops after the age of 25 years and may be preceded by an extended period of gradually worsening symptoms. Unipolar patients usually have no history of mania or hypomania. In contrast, bipolar depression typically occurs before the age of 25 years, with a more abrupt onset of hours or days, and may be periodic or seasonal.

Bipolar disorder is highly heritable and may run in families, which makes a thorough family history a crucial component of the diagnosis. Similarly, a personal history of disruptive behavioral patterns or evidence of mania, hypomania, increased energy, or decreased need for sleep may suggest a bipolar diagnosis, as would treatment-emergent mania or hypomania during antidepressant monotherapy. In addition, the presence of severe psychomotor retardation, high risk of suicidal behavior, presence of psychotic symptoms, more "atypical" depressive symptoms, such as hypersomnia and weight gain, and a greater degree of functional disruption point more toward bipolar than unipolar depression (Leonpacher et al., 2015). It has recently been proposed that postpartum depression may also be misdiagnosed as major depressive disorder when, in fact, more than half of the patients who received a referral diagnosis of postpartum depression were later found to have bipolar disorder (Sharma et al., 2009).

Research is under way to determine if techniques such as neuroimaging can help identify epigenetic biomarkers that can reliably predict if individuals who present in a depressed state are likely to have unipolar or bipolar depression. Such biomarkers would help the clinician determine which pharmacotherapeutic strategy has the best chance of success without risking a switch to mania (Buoli et al., 2016; de Almeida et al., 2013; Özerdem et al., 2016; Sigitova et al., 2017).

Overview of Pharmacotherapy

Medications are currently available to treat acute manic as well as mixed states, acute bipolar depression, and for the prophylactic prevention of recurrent episodes. However, the quality of evidence for efficacy in each of these phases differs among the putative mood stabilizers. Table 14.1 summarizes the relative effectiveness of the available agents for each phase (see also Bartoli et al., 2017; Bauer, 2005; Goldberg, 2010; Lindström et al., 2017; McGirr et al., 2016; and Muneer, 2016). These drugs include the lithium ion, several anticonvulsant "neuromodulators," and second-generation antipsychotics (SGAs).

TABLE 14.1 Comparison of the efficacy of drugs for the treatment of bipolar I disorder[a]

Drug	Acute mania/ mixed	Acute bipolar depression	Mood stabilizer prophylaxis
Lithium	++++	++	+++
Valproic acid	+++	++	+
Carbamazepine	+++	++	+
Oxcarbazepine	+++	+	+
Lamotrigine	0	+++	+++
Gabapentin	0	0	0
Topiramate	0	0	0/+
Aripiprazole	+++	0	0
Haloperidol	+++	0	0
Olanzapine	+++	++	+++
Risperidone	+++	0	+++
Paliperidone	++	?	++
Quetiapine	+++	+++	+++
Ziprasidone	+++	0	0
Asenapine	+++	0	?
Lurasidone	+	+++	?
Cariprazine	+++	++	?

[a]Key
++++ = Highly effective
+++ = Substantially effective
++ = Effective
+ = Possibly effective
0 = Not effective
? = Not enough information
Note: It should be noted that most antipsychotic medications can be used to treat acute mania in bipolar disorders either alone or in combination with a mood stabilizer. Antipsychotic medications can also be used as adjunctive treatment with mood stabilizers to treat bipolar depression and combined with mood stabilizers for ongoing maintenance treatment of bipolar disorder. The combination drug olanzapine–fluoxetine is indicated for and is effective for the treatment of acute bipolar depression and for maintenance therapy.
[Data based on author's review of the literature.]

The classic mood stabilizer is *lithium* (Eskalith, Lithobid). Although lithium may effectively control manic symptoms and reduce the recurrence of both manic and depressive episodes, its bothersome and potentially serious side effects have necessitated a search for equally effective, safer, and more tolerable agents. Today, it is recognized that combination treatment with two or more medications is often required, preferably with adjunctive psychosocial interventions.

Historically, there have been many guidelines that have been published by various organizations and groups to provide assistance to prescribers when making decisions about how best to treat individuals with bipolar disorder. In 1996, the American Psychiatric Association (APA) published its first clinical practice guideline for the treatment of patients with bipolar disorder. The APA published a revision in 2002, emphasizing that the major objectives of intervention are to treat acute manic episodes and to reduce their frequency of recurrence. Another update, the Texas Implementation of Medical Algorithms (TIMA), was the result of a consensus conference in May 2004 convened by the Texas Department of State Health Services, which reinforced the general treatment goals of (1) symptomatic remission, (2) full return of psychosocial functioning, and (3) prevention of relapses and recurrences (Suppes et al., 2005). Since the APA had not formally updated their clinical practice guideline since the last revision in 2002, they instead issued a "Guideline Watch" in November 2005 to provide further information to prescribers (Hirschfeld, 2005). The International Society for Bipolar Disorders (ISBD) issued guidelines in 2009 for monitoring the safety of drug treatments in bipolar disorder that recognized the challenging side effect burden of many of these drugs, as described below (Ng et al., 2009). The APA then published a second edition of their Practice Guideline for the treatment of bipolar disorder in 2010 (Hirschfeld et al., 2010); and the Veterans Administration (VA) in collaboration with the Department of Defense (DoD) published their Clinical Practice Guideline for the management of adults with bipolar disorder within their system in 2010 (Management of Bipolar Disorder Working Group, 2010). In addition, there are others that have been published as well as articles critiquing the existing guidelines based on developing information and research.

For acute manic episodes, first-line treatment according to most current research includes the use of one of the mood stabilizing drugs, most commonly valproic acid (VPA) and an SGA, most notably risperidone, olanzapine, or quetiapine (Grande et al., 2016; Jann, 2014; Muneer, 2016; Shah et al., 2017). Lithium is also considered a first-line agent and although monotherapy is the ideal, lithium is not rapid in onset and has many side effects that may be intolerable to many individuals (Gitlin, 2016; Jann, 2014; Lindström et al., 2017). For those who can tolerate lithium, however, it can be combined with another mood stabilizer or an SGA to gain as rapid control over acute manic symptoms as possible. Once stabilized, an attempt may be made to withdraw the SGA or mood stabilizer to see if lithium monotherapy can sustain stability.

Mixed episodes, presenting with both depressive and manic symptoms, are relatively frequent in bipolar disorder. As many as 40 percent of cases present with this combination of symptoms and individuals who present with mixed features may have more severe pathology, higher frequency of comorbidities, higher rates of suicide, and poorer outcomes. Treatment for individuals with mixed features can include lithium and other mood stabilizers, such as VPA. However, some have reported that these agents may be less efficacious than they are in treating purely manic symptoms. More research needs to be done to make a more definitive statement about their efficacy. But some recent studies suggest that for individuals who present with mixed features, that the SGAs, particularly olanzapine, lurasidone, an olanzapine-fluoxetine combination, or asenapine may be effective treatment agents (Jann, 2014; Rosenblat and McIntyre, 2016).

For the special situation of patients who have a pattern of rapid cycling, a recent review of the literature concludes that rapid-cycling patients have worse outcomes than patients without rapid cycling, have a high risk for suicide, and have high comorbidity with substance use and anxiety disorders. The literature suggests the following:

1. There is still uncertainty of any difference in acute response to treatment between rapid cyclers and nonrapid cyclers.
2. In contrast to earlier beliefs, lithium and anticonvulsants have comparable, but relatively low, efficacies in rapid cyclers.
3. No consistent evidence supports combinations of anticonvulsants being better than monotherapy for rapid cycling.
4. The atypical antipsychotics risperidone, aripiprazole, olanzapine, asenapine, lurasidone, and quetiapine are effective in acute episodes of rapid cyclers and appear promising for response maintenance.
5. Olanzapine is equally effective to anticonvulsants during acute treatment.
6. There is an association between antidepressant use and the presence of rapid cycling, although a causal relationship cannot yet be established (Fountoulakis et al., 2013; Muneer, 2017).

In addition, combinations of mood stabilizers, such as the antiepileptic drugs (AEDs) and SGAs, are the rule rather than the exception for the treatment of mixed states of bipolar disorder (Muneer, 2017; Shah et al., 2017).

First-line treatment of acute bipolar depression is monotherapy with the third-generation neuromodulator anticonvulsant lamotrigine, including the addition of an antimanic agent if there is a history of severe mania. Other guidelines indicate that lithium may not be as effective as other treatments for bipolar depression. However, lithium can be used in combination with SGAs, particularly quetiapine, for the treatment of bipolar depression. Antidepressants should not be used alone to treat bipolar depression, but may be considered in combination with a mood stabilizer or SGA. The olanzapine-fluoxetine combination drug was designed to target bipolar depression using the antipsychotic drug olanzapine to protect against possible switch to mania that can be induced by the antidepressant fluoxetine. Antiepileptic drugs found useful for the treatment of bipolar depression include carbamazepine, oxcarbazepine, and valproic acid. Antipsychotic drugs found to be useful for the treatment of bipolar depression include olanzapine, quetiapine, lurasidone, aripiprazole, and cariprazine (Bartoli et al., 2017; Grande et al., 2016; Jann, 2014; Lindström et al., 2017; Muneer, 2016; Shah et al., 2017).

For maintenance treatment, regardless of whether the most recent episode was manic, depressed, or mixed, it is acceptable to stay on the acute-phase medication if it is well tolerated. If the most recent or predominant phase is manic, the medications with the most research support for maintenance treatment include lithium, valproic acid, olanzapine, quetiapine, ziprasidone, aripiprazole, asenapine, clozapine, paliperidone long-acting injectable (LAI), and risperidone LAI. If the most recent or predominant phase is depressed, the medications with the most research support include lithium, lamotrigine, valproic acid, olanzapine, quetiapine, and possibly paliperidone LAI and risperidone LAI (Grande et al., 2016; Jann, 2014; Shah et al., 2017). Lastly, in many cases, some aforementioned combination may be necessary to achieve long-term stability.

Pathophysiology and Mechanisms of Drug Action

Identifying the therapeutic action of mood stabilizers in the treatment of bipolar disorder has been particularly challenging and, as yet, there is no unifying hypothesis. It is difficult to understand how any single drug class can reduce symptoms of both mania and depression. Furthermore, it has proven difficult to find a mechanism among the relevant drug classes that would account for this dual therapeutic efficacy.

Mood stabilizers may have some neurobiological actions in common with antidepressants. This conclusion comes from growing evidence of similarities between the damaging effects of depression and bipolar disorder on the brain. As discussed in Chapter 12, severe depression is associated with an increase in neuronal vulnerability to injury or trauma, including stress, which may damage neural structures and produce functional impairment. Imaging and postmortem studies have shown similar types of structural changes in the brains of patients diagnosed with bipolar disorder. As in major depressive disorder, reductions in the volume of the prefrontal cortex and hippocampus are significant (Bertolino et al., 2003); the number of neurons and glial cells in the prefrontal cortex is decreased; and levels of the neurochemical N-acetyl-aspartate, which is considered a marker of neuronal "health," are lower (Zarate et al., 2005). However, more recent studies have cast doubt on these findings. These studies have not found consistent evidence of any gray or white matter changes being associated with bipolar disorder (Özerdem et al., 2016).

Like antidepressants, mood stabilizers may reverse some of the impairments in brain structure and levels of brain-derived neurotrophic factor (BDNF), reversals that could be relevant to the therapeutic benefit of mood stabilizers in bipolar disorder (Cunha et al., 2006; Yasuda et al., 2009). In laboratory models, lithium was found to protect neurons against a variety of toxic agents and to promote the growth of neuronal processes; in the human brain, lithium increases levels of N-acetyl-aspartate and gray matter volume. But in spite of their common neuroprotective effects, no universal mechanism has yet been identified to account for the therapeutic and neurobiological similarities between antidepressants and mood stabilizers. While antidepressants and antipsychotics have some common effects on neurotransmitter receptors in the brain, which could be relevant to their common antidepressant efficacy (Yatham et al., 2005), neither lithium nor the neuromodulatory anticonvulsants share these mechanisms of action. That is, unlike antidepressants and antipsychotics, lithium and many of the anticonvulsants do not exert their primary effect at neuronal synapses. Instead, these drugs seem to act intracellularly to produce changes that "stabilize" neuronal membranes.

Currently, the most extensively studied putative mechanisms of mood stabilizers are the second- and third-messenger systems, that is, the intracellular biochemical processes produced by activation of G-protein-coupled receptors. It has already been established that lithium, valproic acid, and carbamazepine interact with various enzymes involved in these intracellular signaling pathways, especially involving glutamate neural transmission in the hippocampus (Schloesser et al., 2012). Although individual drugs may interact at different sites within the neurochemical systems, they may all ultimately produce some final common effect that is responsible for their clinical efficacy in bipolar disorder (Gould et al., 2004; Rapoport et al., 2009).[1] For example, valproic acid inactivates voltage-gated sodium channels; lamotrigine blocks both voltage-gated sodium channels and certain calcium channels; and valproic acid and lamotrigine act on presynaptic transporters to enhance clearance of glutamate and so indirectly reduce excitatory neurotransmission (Schloesser et al., 2012). The target sites of the hippocampus and its connections with the prefrontal cortex and amygdala make these actions relevant for understanding some of the effects of these drugs on behaviors associated with bipolar disorder, including decreased executive function or impulsivity; changes in mood polarity; and changes in cognition and memory function. Finally, there is increasing evidence of the impact of circulating glucocorticoids on mood disorders. Hypercortisolemia can produce mood changes, may occur in bipolar disorder patients, and has deleterious effects on the brain. Cortisol elevation can be reversed by chronic treatment with lithium and valproic acid, suggesting new targets for drug development (Schloesser et al., 2012).

Examining more recent literature has not provided any further clarity to understanding the pathophysiology of bipolar disorder or to understanding how such a wide variety of drugs with such varied mechanisms of action can be effective for the treatment of manic, depressed, mixed, and rapid-cycling phases of the disorder. The mechanisms postulated to be involved in the etiology of bipolar disorder include circadian dysregulation; genetic mutations; immunological, endocrine, neurophysiological, and structural alterations; neuroinflammation; oxidative stress; and changes in calcium signaling and membrane and vesicular transport (Ashok et al., 2017; Buoli et al., 2016; Muneer, 2017; Özerdem et al., 2016; Sigitova et al., 2017). The drugs used to treat bipolar disorder have been theorized to affect a wide range of receptors, proteins, transporters, and intracellular transcription processes in an effort to explain how these drugs work in bipolar disorder. For example, lithium is thought to affect glutamate transmission, as do valproic acid and lamotrigine; affect up- or downregulation of various monoamine receptors; increase serotonin release; inhibit phosphorylating enzymes that regulate the body's molecular clock located in the hypothalamus; and, among other theories, interact with cyclic AMP. (For a detailed discussion of how these mechanisms relate to the efficacy of lithium as a mood stabilizer, see Oruch et al., 2014; and Vosahlikova and Svoboda, 2016. Future targets for potential agents to treat bipolar disorder are discussed in Brady and Keshavan, 2015.)

STEP-BD STUDY

To provide therapeutic guidelines for practitioners, a large-scale, federally funded trial, the STEP-BD study, compared pharmacological treatments for bipolar disorder in a semicontrolled, real-world environment. STEP-BD stands for Systematic Treatment Enhancement Program for Bipolar Disorder and was one of several studies funded by

---

[1]One possibility is suggested by the fact that lithium and valproic acid, like antidepressants, increase the levels of proteins, such as the *cAMP response element-binding protein* (CREB), that activates genes that produce additional proteins (bcl-2) and a neurotrophic factor (BDNF), which is known to protect neurons from the toxic effects of injury or trauma. Because of this, the two drugs are sometimes referred to as "neuroprotective" agents.

the National Institute of Mental Health (NIMH) designed to determine the real-world effectiveness of the major psychiatric drug classes. Like its companion studies for depression (the STAR*D trial, Chapter 12) and schizophrenia (the CATIE trial, Chapter 11), STEP-BD (completed in 2005) involved large numbers of typical patients and used few exclusion criteria in an effort to make the results more generalizable for treatment in standard clinical practice.

The nature, scope, and overall design of the STEP-BD study is described in Sachs and coworkers (2003) and a summary of the initial results is described in Bowden and colleagues (2012a). The data from STEP-BD continue to be analyzed and multiple studies are published yearly based on these subsequent analyses. In brief, Perlis and coworkers (2006b) found that only 58.4 percent (858 patients) of a subset of 1469 patients who participated for at least two years achieved recovery, defined as having only two symptoms of the disorder for at least eight weeks; almost half of this group, 48.5 percent, or 416 patients, had a recurrence at some point, most commonly to a depressive episode (72 percent); recurrence was most likely in those who had residual symptoms at recovery or had an additional psychiatric illness. Unfortunately, Sachs and coworkers (2007) found no benefit from adding an antidepressant to a mood stabilizer; patients who were treatment resistant could choose to enter the last portion of the program; the 66 participants who agreed were randomly assigned one of three additional agents: (1) the anticonvulsant *lamotrigine* (Lamictal); (2) the antipsychotic *risperidone* (Risperdal); or (3) inositol, a sugar, which is an isomer of glucose and is normally a component of one of the second-messenger pathways. Recovery rates were 23.8 percent, 4.6 percent, and 17.4 percent, respectively. These were not statistically different from one another, perhaps because of the small number of subjects; however, the relatively poor effect of the antipsychotic was unexpected (Nierenberg et al., 2006).

One particularly important finding of the STEP-BD study was the confirmation that valproic acid may increase the risk of *polycystic ovarian syndrome* (PCOS). PCOS symptoms, including menstrual irregularities, acne, male-pattern hair loss, elevated testosterone, and excessive body hair, were found in 9 of 86 women (10.5 percent) on VPA compared to only 2 of 144 women on another agent (1.4 percent) (Joffe et al., 2006). Valproic acid also increases the risk of certain birth defects and is not recommended for women who are pregnant (see Chapter 15).

Peters and colleagues (2011) noted five main lessons from the STEP-BD study that could inform clinical practice:

1. Antidepressants added to mood stabilizers are no more effective than placebo for treatment of bipolar depression.

2. Antidepressants did not induce mania more frequently than placebo in bipolar depressed patients receiving mood stabilizers who had no history of antidepressant induced mania.

3. Patients with an acute depressive episode who also had subsyndromal manic symptoms did not recover any faster with the addition of antidepressants to their mood stabilizers compared to similar patients who did not receive add-on antidepressants. If anything, those who received the antidepressants were more likely to relapse or have an exacerbation of their manic symptoms.

4. Lamotrigine showed benefit for treatment-resistant bipolar depression.

5. Intensive psychosocial treatments provided more rapid recovery, improved social functioning, and greater life satisfaction compared to simple collaborative care.

   More recent examination of the data from the STEP-BD study identified several interesting aspects of bipolar disorder and use of certain medications for treatment. El-Mallakh and coworkers (2015) determined that use of antidepressants to treat bipolar disorder, even with mood stabilizers on board, tended to increase the rate of rapid cycling in patients who were identified as rapid cyclers. This subpopulation of individuals experienced more frequent episodes of depression rather than mania, especially during the first year of follow-up. The authors noted that the mood stabilizer medications were not protective against the increased rate of depressive episodes and that bupropion was the only antidepressant that did not seem to induce a worsening of rapid cycling. This supports concern for use of antidepressants to treat bipolar depression, even when mood stabilizers are present.

   Even though the original findings of the STEP-BD study failed to identify any advantage of adding an antidepressant to mood stabilizers to treat bipolar depression, Tada and colleagues (2015) suggest that for a few very selective types of patients, using higher doses of antidepressants may produce a more durable level of recovery. The use of high-dose antidepressants may only be effective for those patients who did not exhibit any mood destabilization or any manic symptoms or adverse events during the early phase of treatment.

   Examining specific symptoms of bipolar disorder and monitoring their change with treatment may help a prescriber determine which patients will achieve a more durable improvement and also potentially identify those depressed patients who may be at risk for a switch to mania. Of all the symptoms of bipolar disorder listed in the DSM-5, Mizushima and coworkers (2017) found that (1) improvement in rating scale scores for self-esteem and loss of energy within 2 weeks of starting treatment predicted a more sustained period of recovery; and that (2) improvement in scores measuring psychomotor retardation predicted a potential risk to switch to mania. They suggest that when treating bipolar patients, it is important to monitor certain key symptoms rather than relying on total rating scale scores as measures of improvement and for identifying potential risks.

MOOD STABILIZERS

Lithium

Lithium has historically been the drug of first choice for treating bipolar disorder and reducing its rate of relapse.[2] It remains the "gold standard" for the treatment of the classic presentation of bipolar mania. Unfortunately, its clinical effectiveness is less than that predicted by clinical trials and relapse often occurs because of patient

---

[2]For a historical overview of lithium therapy and commentaries on lithium, see four related letters in Schou (1997).

nonadherence to therapy. This problem needs to be recognized during treatment and alternative agents should be considered.

Lithium (Li^+) is the lightest of the alkali metals and shares some characteristics with sodium (Na^+). In nature, lithium is abundant in some alkaline mineral spring waters. Devoid of psychotropic effects in normal people, lithium is effective in treating 60 to 80 percent of acute manic and hypomanic episodes, although in the past few years, its use has declined because of toxicity, side effects, nonadherence, and resulting relapse as well as the availability of alternatives.

The discovery—and "rediscovery" of lithium—as a drug has a long history (Shorter, 2009). The modern era begins with the Australian physician John Cade, who noted that when lithium was administered to guinea pigs (lithium was used as a solvent in which to dissolve the injectable drugs he was studying), the animals became lethargic. Taking an intuitive leap, Cade administered lithium to patients with acute mania and noted remarkable improvement. However, because of the earlier problems with lithium as a salt substitute that had resulted in some deaths, the medical community took more than 20 years to accept this agent as an effective treatment for mania. Fortunately, research in the 1970s found lithium to be clearly superior to placebo in the prophylaxis of bipolar disorder; less than a third of lithium-treated patients relapsed, compared with 80 percent of placebo-treated patients.

Many controlled studies demonstrate lithium's efficacy for acute mania, acute depressive episodes, and maintenance treatment for relapse prevention (Geddes et al., 2010). Baldessarini and Tondo (2000) recommended lithium as a drug of first choice for both the treatment of acute manic attacks and the long-term management of bipolar disorder. Indeed, they concluded that "no other proposed mood-stabilizing treatment has such substantial research evidence of long-term efficacy in both type I and type II bipolar disorders, as well as yielding a substantial reduction of mortality risk" (190).

Despite being the "gold standard" of bipolar treatment, real-world experience indicates that lithium is utilized far less often now than are anticonvulsants or antipsychotic medications. It has been argued that lithium is less effective than these other agents due to findings indicating that lithium may be most effective for a subpopulation of individuals with bipolar disorder (Can et al., 2014); that requirements for routine periodic blood tests to measure lithium levels may make it inconvenient and costly for some patients; and that its spectrum of side effects may limit its choice for some patients. In addition, there may be some evidence to suggest that lithium may work best for those individuals whose genotype has four single-nucleotide polymorphisms (SNPs) located in a region of chromosome 21 (Hou et al., 2016), perhaps further explaining the observed limited effectiveness of lithium for some bipolar patients. Despite these disadvantages, reviews of the historical effectiveness of lithium support its stature as a first-line treatment for individuals with the more "classic" presentation of bipolar disorder (Gershon et al., 2009; Vosahlikova and Svoboda, 2016) (Table 14.2). When used properly in accurately diagnosed patients, lithium has the greatest efficacy compared to other drugs, reducing suicidal risk and self-harm rates (Hayes et al., 2016; Toffol et al., 2015) (Figure 14.2). Also, lithium can enhance the effectiveness of antidepressants (Grof et al., 2009); and lithium is an effective agent for maintenance treatment (Coryell, 2009). Moreover, a recent study suggests that certain stem cell electrophysiological characteristics may be able to be used to predict which bipolar

TABLE 14.2 Signature of a lithium responder[a]

Essential features
Recurrent mood disorder
Episodic course of illness with distinct mood periods
Remission is complete between episodes
Pattern of mania, then depression sequence
Later age of onset
Indicative features
Absence of rapid-cycling pattern
Family member who is lithium responder
Episodic course in another family member
No significant psychiatric comorbidity

[a]The features tabulated can be broadly regarded as a "signature" of potential lithium response, and although not predictive in an absolute manner, are suggestive of an increased likelihood of a response to treatment with lithium. However, when determining treatment choice, the overall clinical profile of the patient needs to be considered along with tolerability and patient preference.
[Data from Gershon et al., (2009), Grof (2006), and Rybakowski (2014).]

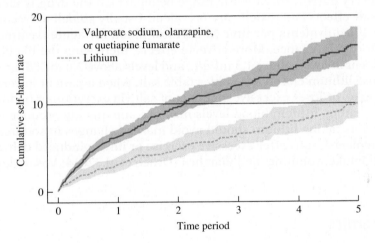

Valproate, olanzapine, or quetiapine	4523	2482	1561	1026	708	493
Lithium	2148	1458	1066	804	649	509

FIGURE 14.2 Cumulative rates of individuals who were seen either in an emergency department or in primary care after attempting to harm themselves intentionally over a five-year period. The top curve represents individuals who had been receiving either valproate, olanzapine, or quetiapine; the lower curve represents individuals who had been receiving lithium. At each time point, individuals receiving lithium had lower rates of self-harm than individuals receiving any of the other drugs listed. The table below the graph indicates the total number of individuals in both groups who were at risk for self-harm at each time point. Total number in the group at time point 0 was 6671 (4523 were receiving valproate, olanzapine, or quetiapine; and 2148 were receiving lithium). [Data from Hayes et al., 2016.]

patients will be most responsive to lithium (Stern et al., 2017), although this procedure is not ready for clinical application at this time. But this is an example of some of the research being done to identify biological markers of disorders to improve the reliability of diagnosis and treatment selection.

Pharmacokinetics

The therapeutic efficacy of lithium is directly correlated with its blood level. Peak blood levels of lithium are reached within 3 hours of oral administration, with complete absorption within 8 hours. The drug crosses the blood–brain barrier slowly and incompletely. Although the clinical significance of this observation is unclear, there can be a twofold variation in the concentration of lithium in the brain compared with its concentration in plasma.

Lithium is not metabolized and is excreted unchanged by the kidneys, with only small amounts excreted through the skin. About half an oral dose is eliminated within 18 to 24 hours and the rest, which is taken up by the cells of the body, is excreted over the next 1 to two weeks. Thus, when therapy is initiated, lithium slowly accumulates over about two weeks until a steady state is reached, making once-daily dosing possible for many patients.

Lithium has a very narrow therapeutic range below which the drug is ineffective and above which side effects and toxicity are prevalent. Usually guidelines recommend about 0.8 to 1.2 milliequivalents per liter (mEq/L) of blood for acute treatment and 0.6 to 0.8 mEq/L for maintenance. More adverse effects, increasing the likelihood of discontinuation, occur at levels above 1.5 mEq/L, and levels above 2.0 mEq/L are potentially lethal. Because lithium closely resembles table salt, when a patient lowers his or her normal salt intake, or loses excessive amounts of salt via excretion of bodily fluids such as through sweating, lithium blood levels may rise and quickly produce toxicity. Consequently, patients taking lithium should avoid marked changes in sodium intake or excretion, and replenish salts after excessive exercise or illness-induced dehydration via decreased fluid intake, vomiting, and diarrhea (Oruch et al., 2014; Vosahlikova and Svoboda, 2016).

Pharmacodynamics

In therapeutic concentrations, lithium has almost no discernible psychotropic effect in normal persons and, unlike many psychoactive drugs, does not produce sedation, depression, or euphoria. Although the mechanism of action has not been proved, lithium, valproic acid, and lamotrigine are all known to inhibit the intracellular enzyme glycogen synthase kinase-3 (GSK-3). One consequence is an increase in the level of a protein, b-catenin, which promotes cell survival and stimulates axonal growth. Lithium's effect on GSK-3, in animal and tissue models, has been shown to be related to effects on neurotransmitter systems, several signaling pathways, and levels of BDNF, among other physiological effects (Can et al., 2014; Oruch et al., 2014; Vosahlikova and Svoboda, 2016). Based on the wide array of effects listed earlier, it is difficult to pinpoint exactly how lithium works and through what mechanisms.

Cui and coworkers (2007) and Vosahlikova and Svoboda (2016) found that lithium and valproic acid protected neurons in the brains of rats (in culture) from damage due to oxidative stress. Oxidative stress occurs when intracellular enzymes cannot sufficiently reduce the levels of toxic substances produced by metabolic activity. In this environment, lithium and valproic acid increased the amount of the antioxidant enzyme glutathione, which plays an important role in reducing oxidative damage. Chronic treatment with lamotrigine and carbamazepine had similar effects. Valproic acid also influences DNA to alter genetic processes in ways that could protect cells from injury or toxic agents. The interaction of valproic acid with DNA is believed to increase levels of cellular protective proteins, such as CREB and *bcl-2* and other neurotrophic substances, such as BDNF (Can et al., 2014; Einat and Manji, 2006; Vosahlikova and Svoboda, 2016; Zarate et al., 2006).

Another study found that the volume of gray matter in the brains of patients with bipolar disorder who were taking lithium was as much as 15 percent larger in areas that are critical for paying attention and controlling emotions, compared to the brain volume of people without the disorder and of patients with bipolar disorder who were not taking lithium (Bearden et al., 2007; Oruch et al., 2014; Vosahlikova and Svoboda, 2016). (For a thorough discussion of the proposed mechanisms of action of lithium derived from biochemical, neurological, physiological, genetic, and clinical models and how these results may apply to lithium's effect in clinical pathology, see Can et al., 2014; Oruch et al., 2014; and Vosahlikova and Svoboda, 2016.)

Side Effects and Toxicity

Because of lithium's extremely narrow therapeutic range, lithium blood levels must be closely monitored. The occurrence and intensity of side effects and toxic reactions are usually related to plasma drug concentrations and involve the nervous system, gastrointestinal (GI) tract, kidneys, thyroid, cardiovascular system, and skin.

Early signs of lithium toxicity include ataxia, dysarthria, and a slight impairment in coordination. These effects can be seen at plasma levels below but approaching 1.5 mEq/L. In addition, lithium-induced tremor is very common, and more than 30 percent of patients report this reaction even at therapeutic blood levels of 0.6 to 1.2 mEq/L. At plasma levels of 1.5 to 2.0 mEq/L, patients may experience listlessness, nausea, slurring of speech, diarrhea, nystagmus (uncontrollable, jerky eye movements in any direction), and the appearance of a coarse tremor. Weight gain may be substantial during long-term therapy—up to 30 percent of patients become obese, a prevalence three times greater than in the general population that can profoundly affect adherence (Can et al., 2014; Gitlin, 2016; Murru et al., 2015; Oruch et al., 2014). At plasma levels of 2.0 to 2.5 mEq/L, patients experience further coarsening of the tremor, confusion, delirium, and pronounced ataxia (Gitlin, 2016; Murru et al., 2015). Lastly, at plasma levels of 2.5 mEq/L and above, patients experience significant alterations of consciousness, hyperextension of the extremities, choreoathetosis, seizures, and possibly death. Fortunately, the mortality rate of lithium overdose or toxicity is less than 1 percent (Gitlin, 2016).

In addition to the plasma level–related side effects noted earlier, lithium may elicit a variety of dermatological reactions. These include rashes, acne, psoriasis, hair and nail disorders, lesions of the mucosal tissue, and like conditions (Gitlin, 2016; Jafferany, 2008; Murru et al., 2015). As many as 60 percent of patients on lithium may experience increased thirst and water intake (*polydipsia*), and urine output (*polyuria*) due to an impairment of renal concentrating ability, which can lead to a nephrogenic diabetes insipidus. Kidney function should be assessed periodically to identify those individuals who may be developing kidney dysfunction. Lithium does lead to a small decrease in glomerular filtration rate, that is not functionally significant. And permanent kidney damage is rare, occurring in about 1 percent of patients taking lithium continuously for 15 years (Clos et al., 2015; Gitlin, 2016; McKnight et al., 2012; Murru et al., 2015; Shine et al., 2015).

A hypothyroid condition may develop, and enlargement of the gland, such as hypertrophy or goiter, can occur at normal doses along with effects on the parathyroid gland (Gitlin, 2016; Murru et al., 2015; Shine et al., 2015). Adverse effects on memory and cognition are common, and patients often complain of memory problems. Consistent with these effects, some researchers found improvements in motor performance, cognition, and creative ability after lithium withdrawal. Severe cognitive deficits are seen with lithium toxicity (Gitlin, 2016; Murru et al., 2015). Lithium can also produce sexual dysfunction (Gitlin, 2016).

Treatment of poisoning or overdose is nonspecific; there is no antidote to lithium. Usually drug administration is stopped and sodium-containing fluids are infused immediately. If toxic signs are serious, hemodialysis, gastric lavage, diuretic therapy, antiepileptic medication, and other supports may be needed. Complete recovery may be prolonged, with full return of renal and neurological function taking weeks or months. See Li (2011), Gitlin (2016), and Murru and colleagues (2015) for a summary of how to use lithium most effectively for clinical treatment of bipolar disorder as well as how to reduce the risk of lithium-induced side effects and to manage side effects when they occur.

Effects in Pregnancy

There is concern about the use of lithium during pregnancy, particularly in the first trimester, as there is a risk of fetal malformation of the cardiovascular system involving the tricuspid valve, *Ebstein's anomaly*, but this is rare (Murru et al., 2015). Furthermore, the defect can be detected on radiographic examination and is surgically correctable preterm or following delivery. The risk of not treating bipolar disorder, however, is greater when considering the health and welfare of both the mother and the child. In addition, it is necessary to compare the risk of this teratogenic effect from lithium with the risk of using other drugs, such as antiepileptic agents or even antipsychotics during pregnancy (Gentile, 2012; Hogan and Freeman, 2016). When a pregnant woman is on lithium therapy, the drug should be discontinued several days before delivery because (1) when the water breaks, acute dehydration will quickly increase lithium to toxic levels; and (2) the newborn will have difficulty excreting the drug. However, it is important for the mother to restart her lithium within 24 hours of delivery to reduce the risk of relapse. Breast-feeding is also a consideration during lithium therapy because lithium passes easily into breast milk and the level in breast milk is about 50 percent of the level in the mother's blood. When considering all the risks and benefits to treatment, most guidelines consider lithium generally the safest choice among the class of mood-stabilizing drugs for use in pregnancy. (For a summary of the approaches to treating women with bipolar disorder before, during, and after pregnancy, see Grande et al., 2016; Grover and Avasthi, 2015; Hogan and Freeman, 2016; Khan et al., 2016; Novosolov, 2012; and Wichman, 2016.)

Nonadherence

Nonadherence is associated with significant morbidity, recurrent episodes, and greatly increased suicide risk. Nevertheless, up to 50 percent of patients on lithium stop taking the drug against medical advice. Some years ago it was felt that discontinuation of lithium treatment would result in treatment resistance when therapy was resumed, but this does not appear to be the case.

Nonadherence seems to result primarily from intolerance of side effects, particularly memory impairment and cognitive slowing, weight gain, and the subjective feeling of reduced energy and productivity. Other reasons include missing the manic "highs," belief that the disorder has resolved and the drug is unnecessary, and feelings of stigmatism in having a psychiatric illness.

Lithium therapy reduces suicidal behaviors in bipolar patients. Unfortunately, when patients stopped taking the drug, the rate of suicide attempts increased fourteenfold and the rate of completed suicides thirteenfold. The prophylactic effect of lithium on mortality and morbidity was confirmed by Cipriani and coworkers (2005), who reported that lithium was effective in the prevention of suicide, deliberate self-harm, and death from all causes in patients with mood disorders. It should be appreciated that reduction of suicidal behavior occurs independently of lithium's effect on mood. There is growing evidence for the effectiveness of lithium as an antisuicide agent, even when used as an adjunct medication, in any situation in which suicide is a concern (Baldessarini et al., 2006; Hayes et al., 2016).

Combination Therapy

Combination therapy—often lithium plus an antiepileptic or antipsychotic drug—can provide both greater therapeutic efficacy and better protection against relapse than lithium therapy alone. In fact, combination therapy has become the rule rather than the exception (Geddes et al., 2004; Grande et al., 2016; Shah et al., 2017), with lithium most effective for mania, augmenting antidepressant efficacy in refractory patients, and maintenance. Furthermore, an anticonvulsant such as lamotrigine is often helpful against bipolar depression (Goodwin et al., 2004; Jann, 2014).

LiTMUS Study

Sponsored by the NIMH, the Lithium Treatment Moderate-Dose Use Study (LiTMUS) was designed using the STAR*D model for antidepressant treatment (see Chapter 12). LiTMUS was intended to answer the question of whether combining lithium with other mood stabilizers or SGAs resulted in any greater benefit, relative to the additional side effect risk, than just using the mood stabilizers or SGAs alone. Patients with either bipolar I or bipolar II disorders who were at least mildly ill and had not previously been treated with adjunctive lithium were eligible to be randomized to one of two groups and followed for six months. The two groups were: (1) optimized personalized treatment (OPT), which was based on the Texas Implementation of Medication Algorithm, a decision tree approach to making medication decisions based on objective assessment of patient outcomes at each treatment visit; and (2) OPT plus adjunctive lithium. LiTMUS was a naturalistic study that allowed for a broader range of participants, including those with substance abuse and other comorbid conditions. In fact, the few exclusion criteria were a contraindication to the use of lithium, pregnancy, age less than 18 years, and unwillingness to comply with study requirements (Nierenberg et al., 2009).

The overall finding of LiTMUS was that there was no difference between the two treatment groups in the primary outcome measure of change in psychiatric symptoms as measured by a variety of symptom rating scales. That is, adding lithium to OPT did not improve outcomes. But a secondary finding revealed that the OPT + lithium group was less likely to be treated with SGAs than the OPT only group, suggesting that the lithium add-on permitted less exposure to SGAs, thus avoiding their potential side effects. The authors offered several possible reasons for the apparent lack of effectiveness of added lithium, including the fact that the lithium doses used produced blood levels below 0.6 mEq/L (normal maintenance range would be 0.6 to 0.8 mEq/L), which suggested that prescribers were not being aggressive enough with the lithium treatment despite following the study protocol (Nierenberg et al., 2013).

The BALANCE Study

The Bipolar Affective disorder: Lithium/ANtiConvulsant Evaluation (BALANCE) study recruited individuals with bipolar disorder from 41 sites in the United States, United Kingdom, Italy, and France who required maintenance medication treatment. Recruitment took place between May 2001 and February 2007. BALANCE was a randomized, open-label, three-group trial of maintenance therapy, with up to 24 months of follow-up. The study was designed to determine if the combination treatment of lithium plus valproic acid was better than either drug alone in preventing relapse into an episode of bipolar I disorder during the two-year follow-up period. The results of the study found that individuals who received the combination treatment had fewer relapses than those who received valproic acid alone. Although the sample sizes were too small to make definitive determinations, it appeared that lithium monotherapy was slightly more effective than valproic acid monotherapy. The differences were small, the lithium dose was lower than recommended for clinical effectiveness, and many of the individuals receiving combination therapy also needed additional treatment medications during follow-up. The general recommendation from the BALANCE study is that individuals with bipolar disorder who require maintenance treatment would do better with a combination treatment using lithium plus valproic acid rather than being treated with either drug alone (Geddes et al., 2010).

MOOD STABILIZERS: ANTIEPILEPTIC DRUGS

Only about 60 to 70 percent of patients with bipolar disorder can be adequately helped by lithium alone, both for maintenance and for relapse prevention; and lithium is even less effective in controlling episodes of rapid-cycling mania. Therefore, there is a need for alternative agents in patients who are treatment refractory, nonadherent, or intolerant of lithium's side effects. One alternative is anticonvulsants, that is, antiepileptic drugs (AEDs). The variety of disorders for which these drugs are now used is much broader than their original indication for epilepsy. Chapter 5 describes their use in alcohol detoxification and relapse prevention. Chapter 13 describes their use in the treatment of anxiety disorders and the control of emotional outbursts in such disorders as posttraumatic stress disorder (PTSD). Lastly, Chapter 15 describes their use in treating aggressive and explosive behavioral disorders in children and adolescents.

First-generation AEDs included phenobarbital, as well as other kinds of barbiturates, and phenytoin and its derivatives, none of which, however, proved useful in treating bipolar illness.[3] Second-generation AEDs included *valproic acid* (Divalproex, Depakote) and *carbamazepine* (Tegretol, Equetro), which have significant side effects that limit their use.

In particular, many of the AEDs produce birth defects, but there is great variability among reports. This variability may be because the baseline rate of all major congenital anomalies in newborns in the U.S. population is between 2 and 4 percent (Montouris, 2005) and because epilepsy per se is associated with an increased risk of such anomalies (Perucca, 2005). There is also agreement that the magnitude of the risk increases in offspring exposed to polypharmacy (Perucca, 2005). The most common congenital malformations from AEDs are the same as the malformations in the general population, such as heart defects, clubfoot, and cleft palate.

In addition to these concerns, the FDA issued a warning in 2008 about increased suicidal behavior related to use of AEDs. Despite studies questioning the increased suicide risk (Gibbons et al., 2009), the FDA warning has been supported by an analysis of individual medications based on a large dataset of more than 250,000 patients (Patorno et al., 2010). Although not all AEDs were associated with an increased risk, the results showed that the class-wide warning was warranted and remains in effect.

Carbamazepine

Studies conducted in the early 1990s indicated that carbamazepine (Tegretol, Equetro) might be as effective as lithium in preventing the recurrence of mania (Dea et al., 2016; Muneer et al., 2016; Shah et al., 2017). Equetro is an extended-release form of carbamazepine approved by the FDA in 2005 for the treatment of manic and mixed episodes of bipolar disorder. In bipolar patients not previously treated with mood stabilizers, lithium is superior to carbamazepine in prophylactic efficacy (Grande et al., 2016; Hartong et al., 2003). Because of the correlation between therapeutic effectiveness and

---

[3]Phenytoin was never widely used as a mood stabilizer, although there are some positive reports (Bersudsky, 2005; Mishory et al., 2000).

plasma level, one reason patients may fail to respond to carbamazepine is inadequate blood levels. The therapeutic level for epilepsy and for bipolar disorder is estimated to be the same, between 4 and 12 micrograms per milliliter.

Several possible mechanisms have been proposed to explain carbamazepine's action in treating epilepsy and bipolar disorder. Its anticonvulsant effects may occur because it reduces neuronal excitation by blocking sodium channels and thus the ability of sodium to initiate action potentials. Its benefit for bipolar disorder may be related to the fact that carbamazepine, like lithium, inhibits enzyme activity in intracellular second-messenger systems. In the treatment of bipolar disorder, carbamazepine is useful as a prophylaxis for reducing the frequency of episodes, and it may be the better choice for episodes of mixed mania and rapid cycling.

Adverse effects of carbamazepine include GI upset, sedation, ataxia, tremors, visual disturbances, and rare but life-threatening dermatological reactions, namely *Stevens-Johnson syndrome* (SJS) and *toxic epidermal necrolysis* (TENS), which may be caused by a metabolite, carbamazepine-epoxide. While the risk of the skin reactions is 1 to 6 per 10,000 new Caucasian users of the drug, the risk is estimated to be about 10 times higher for those of Asian ancestry. Therefore, an FDA requirement stipulates that manufacturers add a recommendation to the labeling of this drug that patients of Asian ancestry get a genetic blood test that would indicate whether they were in the population at risk. Although impairment of higher-order cognitive functioning is modest, some patients may be particularly sensitive to this side effect. More serious reactions involve the blood and range from a relatively benign reduction in white blood cell count (*leucopenia*) to, on rare occasions, a severe reduction in white blood cell count (*agranulocytosis*). For this reason, carbamazepine received an FDA black box warning and a recommendation for periodic blood tests.

Drug interactions involving carbamazepine are common and result from drug-induced stimulation of drug-metabolizing enzymes, especially CYP-3A4 in the liver. As a result, acute blood levels may decrease, which may require increasing the dose by up to 100 percent to maintain a therapeutic blood level. This effect also extends to other drugs metabolized by the same enzyme family when combined with carbamazepine. For example, aripiprazole and valproic acid blood levels are reduced when combined with carbamazepine such that it may be necessary to increase the dose of these drugs to compensate if carbamazepine is added.

As stated, because carbamazepine is potentially teratogenic, affecting neural tube development and causing spina bifida, heart defects, decreased head circumference, and delayed development (Hogan and Freeman, 2016), it should not be administered during pregnancy if at all possible. Thus, carbamazepine is considered a second- or even third-line drug for the treatment of bipolar disorder.

Oxcarbazepine

Oxcarbazepine (Trileptal) can be considered a safer carbamazepine, capable of replacing carbamazepine for all its uses with comparable efficacy and greatly improved safety. Oxcarbazepine is essentially carbamazepine with an oxygen molecule attached to one of the rings. The liver can thus easily metabolize the drug by a process called *hydroxylation.* In fact, this process occurs within 5 minutes after drug absorption, and the monohydroxy derivative is the active form of the drug; oxcarbazepine is, therefore, an inactive prodrug. Because of this easy metabolic process, there is no enzyme induction, no alteration in liver enzymes, no white blood cell problems, no required blood monitoring, and few drug interactions.

Oxcarbazepine is approved for use in epilepsy and can be used off-label to treat bipolar disorder and other disorders treatable with carbamazepine. It may be superior to placebo in the treatment of acute mania in adults but less effective when compared to lithium, valproic acid, and the antipsychotics.

While oxcarbazepine is considered a second- or third-line agent for the treatment of bipolar disorder, it can cause tiredness, headache, dizziness and ataxia, and some allergic reactions. Teratogenic effects are also likely. Like carbamazepine, prescribers should check the genetic profile of individuals of Asian ancestry to determine if they carry a particular allele that would increase their risk of developing the serious and potentially lethal dermatological skin reactions SJS or TENS when treated with oxcarbazepine.

Valproic Acid

Valproic acid (Divalproex, Depakene, Depacon, Depakote) is the second anticonvulsant that was systematically studied for treatment of bipolar illness and has been used for this disorder since 1994. In 2008, the FDA approved a delayed-release valproic acid therapy in a softgel capsule (Stavzor) for bipolar disorder, epilepsy, and migraine headache. In 2009, the FDA approved a generic version of Depakote extended-release (ER) tablets.

Several actions of valproic acid have been identified. First, it binds to and inhibits GABA transaminase, the enzyme that breaks down GABA. Therefore, the drug's anticonvulsant activity may be related to increased brain concentrations of GABA. Second, valproic acid may increase GABA by blocking its reuptake into glia and nerve endings. Third, valproic acid may also work by suppressing repetitive neuronal firing through inhibition of voltage-sensitive sodium channels. A fourth mechanism was proposed by Chen and coworkers (1999), who observed an effect of valproic acid on enzymes associated with the cellular organization of DNA. By influencing these enzymes and altering DNA function, valproic acid may be involved in gene transcription.

Valproic acid is particularly effective in the treatment of acute mania, mixed states, schizoaffective disorder, and rapid-cycling bipolar disorder. It may be more effective than other agents in treating lithium-resistant patients, producing a positive response in up to 71 percent of patients. The combination of valproic acid and lithium may be more effective than either agent alone. The BALANCE Study, discussed earlier, found that the combination of lithium and valproic acid seemed to be most effective in preventing manic episodes and lithium alone to be most effective in preventing depressive episodes. Although the study had no placebo group, it was a real-world design and argues for greater use of lithium (Geddes et al., 2010).

Valproic acid has traditionally been administered in divided doses through the day. An ER preparation allows once-daily dosing, usually at bedtime, to improve adherence and help alleviate daytime sedation and memory impairment. Depakene comes in capsules and as a syrup; Depacon is the intravenous solution; and Depakote comes in the form of either immediate release or ER tablets. Effective dose levels are determined by blood levels (as with lithium) and normal therapeutic blood levels should be between 50 and 150 micrograms per milliliter.

Side effects associated with valproic acid include GI upset, sedation, lethargy, weight gain, hand tremor, alopecia (hair loss), and some metabolic changes in the liver. In females, the drug has been associated with an 8 percent prevalence of marked obesity, polycystic ovaries, menstrual disturbances, and markedly increased levels of serum androgens (increased testosterone levels). Valproic acid may increase serum lipid levels and also carries a risk of producing SJS. Therefore, valproic acid should not be combined with any other drug that also has a risk of producing SJS or TENS, such as lamotrigine, carbamazepine, or oxcarbazepine. Lastly, valproic acid may be slightly more detrimental to cognitive function than carbamazepine.

Like lithium and carbamazepine, valproic acid can be teratogenic, increasing the risk of spina bifida, neural tube defects, craniofacial and cardiovascular defects, and developmental deficits in the infant, including reductions in IQ levels. It has been suggested that this property may be related to its interaction with DNA. Withdrawal symptoms, including irritability, jitteriness, abnormal tone, feeding difficulties, and seizures, have been described in infants whose mothers took valproic acid during pregnancy. Consequently, caution must be exercised in using valproic acid in women who may become pregnant during drug therapy. Other serious side effects of valproic acid, which have resulted in an FDA black box warning, include hepatotoxicity (liver damage) and pancreatitis (inflammation of the pancreas).

An analog of valproic acid, *valnoctamide*, has been used in Europe but is not available in the United States. Valnoctamide does not go through the same metabolic pathway and its chemical structure is sufficiently different from valproic acid such that it is much less teratogenic. It has been tested in one controlled trial as an add-on to risperidone and compared to placebo add-on. Valnoctamide was found to be significantly more effective than placebo on all measures (Mathews et al., 2012).

Lamotrigine

A third-generation AED, lamotrigine (Lamictal), was found to be equal to lithium in preventing relapse to any manic episode and better than lithium in preventing relapse to a depressive episode (Amann et al., 2011; Bowden et al., 2003; Dea et al., 2016; Grande et al., 2016). Furthermore, lamotrigine is less likely to cause a manic shift compared with the conventional antidepressants (Goldberg et al., 2009; Keck et al., 2003). Conversely, it is not useful for acute mania, and in five different studies lamotrigine performed no better than placebo against acute bipolar depression.

In 2003, lamotrigine was approved for the long-term maintenance of adults with bipolar I disorder, that is, for delaying the time to relapse to depressive and manic symptoms. This benefit is most evident if patients respond acutely to lamotrigine. Generic lamotrigine tablets were approved by the FDA in 2008 and the chewable tablet formulation in 2009. That same year the FDA also approved Lamictal ODT, an orally disintegrating lamotrigine tablet, for long-term treatment of bipolar I disorder.

In some studies lamotrigine was shown to be less effective than lithium in long-term maintenance (Kessing et al., 2012), as add-on medication (Kemp et al., 2012), and for bipolar depression (Bowden et al., 2012b). Some of the more recent negative findings may be due to the fact that adding lamotrigine to other drugs may increase adverse reactions or that lamotrigine is simply not effective in refractory patients. Regardless of the reason, lamotrigine's inconsistent history, specifically for bipolar depression, has been reflected in the recommendations of various clinical treatment guidelines about where it should be placed—that is, as a first-line, second-line, mono-therapy, or add-on-only treatment option (Tränkner et al., 2013).

Lamotrigine's major mechanism of action is the blockade of voltage-dependent sodium channel conductance, which inhibits depolarization of the glutaminergic pre-synaptic membrane and reduces glutamate release, particularly in the cortex and hip-pocampus. This decrease in neuronal excitability may account for its antiepileptic, mood-stabilizing, and analgesic effects (Ketter et al., 2003), and it may also have some neuroprotective effects in people who suffer traumatic brain injuries (Pachet et al., 2003).

After oral administration, lamotrigine is rapidly and completely absorbed, reaching peak plasma concentrations in 1 to 5 hours. It is metabolized before excretion, with a half-life of 26 hours, which can decrease to about 7.4 hours when used with phenytoin or carbamazepine, requiring increased doses of lamotrigine, or the half-life can increase to 60 hours when used with valproic acid, requiring decreased doses of lamotrigine (Hurley, 2002). No therapeutic blood levels are necessary to adjust oral doses.

Side effects associated with lamotrigine include dizziness, tremor, blurred vision, somnolence, headache, nausea, constipation, increased liver enzymes, menstrual dis-turbances, and rash. The most serious side effect is SJS, which conceivably may be severe enough to require hospitalization and prove fatal. Adolescents are believed to be more prone to this reaction, so the drug is not indicated for patients younger than 16 years of age. The incidence of SJS is currently about 1 in 500, which may be reduced by a slow titration of dose over about 6 weeks (Calabrese et al., 2002; Dea et al., 2016; Jann, 2014; Murru et al., 2015; Shah et al., 2017). In marked contrast to other antiepileptic agents, lamotrigine can improve cognitive functioning or at least has not been shown to produce any cognitive dysfunction (Khan et al., 2004; Murru et al., 2015).

Of all the antiepileptic drugs, lamotrigine has been found to be the safest to use in pregnancy compared to other AEDs. There has been no evidence of increased fetal mal-formations (Hogan and Freeman, 2016; Moore et al., 2012; Vajda et al., 2013; Wichman, 2016). Blood levels of lamotrigine are affected by changes in hormone levels. When a woman who takes lamotrigine wishes to get pregnant and stops her oral contracep-tives, her lamotrigine levels may rise and she may be at greater risk for experiencing adverse effects. To reduce the risk, the lamotrigine dose should be lowered. During pregnancy, lamotrigine levels tend to drop due to hormonal influences on the drug's metabolism, which may entail a need to increase the lamotrigine dose to compensate. Then, postpartum, when hormonal levels again drop, there may again be a need to readjust the lamotrigine dose (Hogan and Freeman, 2016; Wichman, 2016). Lastly, lamotrigine is considered relatively safe with careful monitoring if a woman wishes to breastfeed (Grover and Avasthi, 2015; Hogan and Freeman, 2016; Khan et al., 2016).

Gabapentin and Pregabalin

Introduced in the United States in 1993 as an anticonvulsant for the treatment of partial complex seizures, *gabapentin* (Neurontin, Gralise) is also used for the treatment of anxiety, neuropathic pain, substance dependency, and behavioral dyscontrol. Mechanistically, it is a GABA analogue, but it has little or no action on the GABA receptor. Although it increases GABA levels, it is not clear how much the increase contributes to its efficacy. A derivative of gabapentin, *pregabalin* (Lyrica), was approved for use in the United States in 2005 for the treatment of pain states, such as diabetic peripheral neuropathy and postherpetic neuralgia, and as adjunctive therapy in the treatment of partial seizures in adults (Beydoun et al., 2005). In June 2007, the FDA approved Lyrica for the treatment of fibromyalgia.

Since both of these drugs have antiepileptic effects, it was thought that like other AEDs they might have usefulness for the treatment of bipolar disorder. Some open-label studies have suggested that these drugs might be useful as adjunctive treatment for individuals who do not derive full benefit from treatment with other mood stabilizers or who may be presenting with anxiety or agitation along with symptoms of bipolar disorder (Muneer, 2016). Gabapentin and pregabalin, however, are not effective as monotherapy for bipolar disorder.

Topiramate

Topiramate (Topamax, Topiragen, Trokendi XR, Qsymia, Qudexy XR), discussed in Chapter 5 as an antiepileptic drug used to prevent relapse in people with alcoholism, is a very potent anticonvulsant and has been approved by the FDA for the treatment of migraine headaches. Structurally different from other agents in this group, it is derived from the sugar D-fructose and was initially developed as an antidiabetic drug. Topiramate has multiple mechanisms of action. It inhibits sodium conductance, decreasing the duration of spontaneous bursts and the frequency of generated action potentials; it enhances GABA by unknown mechanisms; and it blocks the AMPA subtype glutamate receptor.

The initial positive results of open-label studies of the drug to treat bipolar disorder were not supported by four clinical trials showing topiramate monotherapy to be ineffective in acute mania (Kushner et al., 2006). In addition, topiramate was no different than placebo when combined with either valproic acid or lithium for the treatment of bipolar I disorder (Chengappa et al., 2006). The main advantage of topiramate is that it is associated with weight loss rather than weight gain. This characteristic may make the drug useful as an adjunctive agent to offset the weight gain associated with other antimanic drugs (Muneer, 2016). Due to the side effects of topiramate noted in the following text, however, *metformin* (Glucophage), an antidiabetic drug that promotes weight loss, may be a better choice in this regard (Ellinger et al., 2010; Mahmoudi-Gharaei et al., 2012).

Unfortunately, the cognitive impairment, including word-finding difficulties, concentration and attention deficits, confusion, and memory problems induced by topiramate is greater than that produced by other anticonvulsants, although impairment may occur more frequently at higher doses and with rapid dose increases. Other side effects include tingling in the extremities, irritability, anxiety, somnolence, ataxia, dizziness, impaired or slurred speech, fatigue, and depression.

Studies of pregnant women taking topiramate indicated a significantly higher rate of fetal malformations, particularly oral cleft and cardiac defects (Wichman, 2016). As a result, the FDA changed topiramate's pregnancy classification to category D, that is, evidence of teratogenicity in humans; however, the drug may be used if its benefit outweighs its risk (Nonacs, 2012).

Topiramate is excreted unchanged and is less likely to be involved in drug interactions mediated by the liver. However, this drug has the potential to increase plasma levels of other drugs excreted by the kidneys, such as lithium. It may also increase the incidence of kidney stones.

ATYPICAL ANTIPSYCHOTICS FOR BIPOLAR DISORDER

Acute Mania

For decades, predating the use of lithium by 20 years, traditional antipsychotic drugs were used to help control the symptoms of acute mania. The fact that the antimanic potency of the typical antipsychotics was positively associated with their affinity for D_2 receptors supported a "dopamine blockade" hypothesis (Harrison-Read, 2009) consistent with the possibility that schizophrenia and bipolar disorder share some common genetic origin (Lichtenstein et al., 2009). The relationship of dopamine receptor activity to emotional presentations of either mania or depression is still being evaluated and according to some authors, there is sufficient pharmacological and imaging evidence to continue to pursue this line of thinking (Ashok et al., 2017).

First- and second-generation antipsychotics have efficacy either as monotherapy or as adjunctive agents for the treatment of acute mania. The earliest example of combined treatment for acute mania was the use of lithium with chlorpromazine. In their meta-analysis, Scherk and coworkers (2007) concluded:

> SGAs as add-on medication to mood stabilizers are superior to mood stabilizers alone for acute manic symptoms, as indicated by greater reductions in mania scores, higher response rates, and fewer dropouts due to inefficacy. . . . Combination treatment with a second-generation atypical antipsychotic and a mood stabilizer should be the treatment of choice, in particular for severe manic episodes. (442)

Recently, clozapine was also found to have the same benefit (Nielsen et al., 2012).

Among the antipsychotic drugs, one meta-analysis showed the three most effective were haloperidol, risperidone, and olanzapine; when dropout rates were considered, olanzapine, risperidone, and quetiapine were better than haloperidol. Taken together, given their effectiveness and acceptability, olanzapine and risperidone were considered superior to all other drugs. Cipriani and coworkers (2011), however, note that this finding only applies to the short-term acute treatment of manic symptoms and not to the long-term maintenance treatment of either bipolar mania or depression. For maintenance, lithium remains one of the most effective drugs (Yildiz et al., 2011). Other studies of the use of antipsychotics for the treatment of acute mania indicate that aripiprazole, asenapine, haloperidol, olanzapine, and quetiapine have the greatest efficacy, followed by chlorpromazine and ziprasidone (Geddes and Miklowitz, 2013; Grande et al.,

2016; Shah et al., 2017). Also, a consensus guideline on the use of aripiprazole for the treatment of mania was published in the United Kingdom (Aitchison et al., 2009).

Bipolar Depression

Olanzapine has been reported to be as effective for bipolar depression as the antidepressant fluoxetine alone or in combination with fluoxetine as the approved drug Symbyax (Amsterdam and Shults, 2005; Corya et al., 2006). Both Symbyax and lamotrigine had an equally low risk of inducing mania, which is a serious concern when using an antidepressant for the treatment of bipolar depression. Studies have examined the relative risk of three other antidepressants—sertraline, bupropion, and venlafaxine—for producing a manic switch when used as adjuncts to mood stabilizers. Overall, the rate was higher for individuals with bipolar I disorder (30.8 percent) than for individuals with bipolar II disorder (18.6 percent), although eventually only 23.3 percent of patients did not switch. However, venlafaxine was reported to be more likely than the other two antidepressants to produce a switch (Leverich et al., 2006; Post et al., 2006). These results suggest that people with bipolar II disorder might be less vulnerable to an antidepressant-induced switch. This suggestion is supported by Altshuler and coworkers (2006), who found less switching with adjunctive selective serotonergic reuptake inhibitors (SSRIs) in bipolar II than in bipolar I patients; and by Parker and coworkers (2006), who successfully treated depressed bipolar II patients for nine months with SSRIs, without any worsening of symptoms. More recent reviews of this subject find that the risk of manic switch, when using antidepressant drugs along with a mood stabilizer or antipsychotic, is not as high as previously thought. However, these latter studies seemed to indicate that the switch to mania was more likely to occur when treating bipolar II disorders or in high-risk individuals who present with evidence of hypomanic or frank manic symptoms. Thus, the relative risk for manic switch when using antidepressants to treat someone with bipolar II disorder is still an unanswered question. Using SSRIs (except paroxetine, which was found to be ineffective) and bupropion has been shown to be effective in the treatment of bipolar depression if used with a mood stabilizer or antipsychotic agent (Geddes and Miklowitz, 2013; Jann, 2014; Shah et al., 2017; Tada et al., 2015).

Several studies have supported the use of quetiapine in treating bipolar depression, including a retrospective chart review (Shajahan and Taylor, 2010), two clinical trials (McElroy et al., 2010; Young et al., 2010), and an open-label study (Jeong et al., 2013). In 2009, *quetiapine fumarate* (Seroquel XR) extended-release tablets were approved by the FDA for acute treatment for depressive, manic, and mixed bipolar disorder episodes and for maintenance therapy as adjunctive treatment to lithium or valproic acid.

One of the newer antipsychotic agents, *asenapine* (Saphris), has been shown to be effective in the short term (three weeks) in reducing manic symptoms compared to placebo as monotherapy. Furthermore, asenapine was also found to be equal to olanzapine in an extension study at reducing both manic and depressive symptoms and, when added to either lithium or valproic acid, was more effective than placebo at reducing manic symptoms (Chwieduk et al., 2011).

De Fruyt and colleagues (2012) performed a meta-analysis of studies that examined the effectiveness of SGAs in the treatment of acute bipolar depression. Of the SGAs examined, quetiapine and, to a lesser extent, olanzapine (but not aripiprazole) demonstrated significant improvement (see also Tsai et al., 2011). But the authors point out that adverse events like weight gain, akathisia, and sedation produced by the SGAs may have reduced overall effectiveness. Also, the number of total studies used in the analysis was small and demonstrated clinical heterogeneity, making interpretation and generalizability of the results difficult.

Although the SGAs may be less likely to elicit movement disorders than the older drugs in schizophrenic patients, there is evidence that patients with bipolar disorder may be more susceptible to these side effects (Ghaemi et al., 2006). One meta-analysis (Gao et al., 2008) concluded that patients with bipolar disorder were approximately twice as likely as patients with schizophrenia to suffer movement disorders, such as extrapyramidal symptoms and akathisia, and require an increase in the use of anticholinergic drugs to treat these symptoms. Olanzapine, however, did not increase EPS when compared to placebo in patients with bipolar disorder, but did increase the risk in patients with schizophrenia, while aripiprazole was more likely to cause akathisia in patients with bipolar disorder, but not patients with schizophrenia.

Although considered a first-generation antipsychotic (FGA) drug, *loxapine* (Loxitane) more closely resembles SGAs in its activity profile. A new formulation of this drug, Adasuve, has been approved for the treatment of agitation in adults with schizophrenia or bipolar disorder. This formulation of loxapine is a powder that is aerosolized and administered via inhalation. In clinical trials, the drug reduced agitation within 10 minutes. Due to the risk of causing bronchospasm, the drug can only be used under specified procedural restrictions dictated by the FDA's *risk evaluation and mitigation strategy* (REMS) and only in facilities that are capable of providing immediate treatment for acute bronchospasm. This drug should not be used in anyone with a compromised respiratory system, such as patients with *chronic obstructive pulmonary disease* (COPD).

Nivoli and colleagues (2011) reviewed the available guidelines for the treatment of bipolar depression and found it difficult to make comparisons. They noted that antidepressants for bipolar depression should be avoided in the absence of mood stabilizers and they saw that SGA monotherapy was becoming more recognized as first-line treatment. One of the findings from the STEP-BD study was that using more than one SGA in the treatment of bipolar disorder does not improve response to treatment and, in fact, may reduce clinical outcomes (Brooks et al., 2011). More recent reviews of the treatments for bipolar disorder indicate that of the atypical antipsychotics, lurasidone, quetiapine, and the olanzapine-fluoxetine combination drug have the best evidence for efficacy in the treatment of bipolar depression—and cariprazine, which is new to the market, may also be efficacious as early studies suggest (Bartoli et al., 2017; Dea et al., 2016; Grande et al., 2016; Jann, 2014; Muneer et al., 2016; Shah et al., 2017). (For a review of the use of mood stabilizers and antipsychotic agents as treatments for bipolar disorder, see Bourin et al., 2013.)

Maintenance of Remission

Risperidone has been found effective in extension trials as monotherapy or as adjunctive treatment in sustaining remission from mania while not inducing depression (Hirschfeld et al., 2006; Rendell et al., 2006). Macfadden and coworkers (2011) administered long-acting risperidone in depot form (Risperdal Consta) to patients who were rapid cyclers. By the end of the 16-week study, 61.3 percent of those who completed the study qualified for remission. Olanzapine (Tohen et al., 2006), quetiapine (Calabrese et al., 2005), aripiprazole (Keck et al., 2006, 2007), and ziprasidone (Bowden et al., 2010) have all been found more effective than placebo for maintenance treatment, and olanzapine was reported comparable to lithium (Tohen et al., 2005). Quetiapine was as effective as lithium at delaying onset of subsequent mood symptoms in bipolar patients who had been previously stabilized on quetiapine. Patients maintained on quetiapine, or who were switched to lithium, had more time free of any subsequent mood symptoms compared to patients on placebo (Weisler et al., 2011). More recent evidence finds that quetiapine is the most effective agent for maintenance treatment of bipolar disorder, followed by aripiprazole, clozapine, olanzapine, ziprasidone, paliperidone LAI, and risperidone LAI (Dea et al., 2016; Grande et al., 2016).

When using antipsychotic drugs as monotherapy or as adjunctive agents in the treatment of bipolar disorders, the prescriber must also be aware of what risks they pose when used during pregnancy and in the postnatal period. Several studies have examined the antipsychotics for potential malformation risks, risks to the baby as a result of breast-feeding, and on development. The results vary and there does not seem to be consistency in determining the risk for use of antipsychotics. Some studies find increased risks for malformations, cardiac defects, preterm delivery, low birth weight, and small for gestational age (Wichman, 2016). Other studies do not find significant evidence for concern (Hogan and Freeman, 2016). As with any other medication to be used during pregnancy, it is important to carefully weigh the benefits versus the risks to mother and fetus and postnatal risks to the baby. Careful monitoring of treatment and mother's and baby's response is also crucial. More research in this area is needed. Grover and Avasthi (2015), Hogan and Freeman (2016), Khan and colleagues (2016), and Wichman (2016) review recent studies on use of antipsychotics during pregnancy and during the postnatal period.

In summary, monotherapy, with either lithium or valproic acid, is considered the first line of treatment for all phases of bipolar disorder; and some of the SGAs can also be used as monotherapy. If that approach is ineffective, the next step usually involves combining two agents or substituting an SGA (if one was not used as a first-line treatment) in place of one of the mood stabilizers, or adding lamotrigine or one of the SGAs (if not used during first-line treatment) to the monotherapy agent if the primary phase of illness is depression. Indeed, on average, most patients with bipolar disorder receive three or more medications (Thase, 2012). Table 14.3 summarizes the current treatments approved by the FDA for bipolar disorder in adults.

It should be noted that there has been continued interest in nutraceuticals for the treatment of psychiatric disorders. There is a long history of exploring the efficacy of omega-3 fatty acids which are *polyunsaturated fatty acids* (PUFAs) in a wide variety of disorders, including schizophrenia, major depression, and bipolar disorder. Some studies are able to demonstrate variances in levels of PUFAs in humans and that deficiencies in PUFAs may be related to a risk for mood disorders. However, randomized controlled trials of the efficacy of PUFAs for the treatment of bipolar disorder have shown no evidence of effectiveness for the treatment of mania and only suggestive evidence of efficacy for bipolar depression when used as an adjunct to mood stabilizer treatment. There is insufficient evidence to suggest PUFAs would be of value for

TABLE 14.3 FDA approved treatments for bipolar disorder in adults

Generic name	Mania	Depression	Mixed	Maintenance
Lithium	X			X
Carbamazepine[a]	X		X	
Divalproex	X			
Lamotrigine				X
Olanzapine/fluoxetine		X		
Aripiprazole[b]	X		X	
Quetiapine[b]	X	X	X	X
Risperidone[b]	X		X	X[c]
Olanzapine[b]	X		X	X
Ziprasidone[b]	X		X	X
Asenapine[b]	X		X	X
Lurasidone[b]		X		

[a]Equetro XR version.
[b]Monotherapy or as adjunct agent.
[c]As the long-acting injection (LAI) formulation.

the treatment of bipolar disorders at this time (Messamore et al., 2017; Saunders et al., 2016).

Also, *ketamine* (Ketalar), a noncompetitive NMDA antagonist, has been evaluated in subanesthetic doses in individuals with bipolar disorder. In a double-blind, randomized, placebo-controlled crossover study, a single IV infusion of ketamine to individuals receiving lithium or valproic acid improved depressive symptoms compared to placebo. Although the onset of the effect was within 40 minutes, the duration of the effect was short (up to three days). Despite the impressive results, the use of ketamine is not currently practical given the need for IV administration, the short duration of action, and the side effects associated with it being a general anesthetic (Diazgranados et al., 2010). But as noted in Chapter 12 on antidepressants, ketamine has been formulated into a version that can be inhaled. It has been used clinically off label for the treatment of depression and can also be used to rapidly treat the depression of bipolar disorder. But there are risks and there is insufficient evidence to support ketamine's use in this way.

IN THE PIPELINE

The following classes of drugs may soon be used in the future to treat bipolar disorder:

- *Serotonin receptor antagonists.* Intra-Cellular Therapies is evaluating ITI-007 for the treatment of bipolar depression. ITI-007 is primarily a potent inhibitor of the 5-HT$_{2A}$ receptor and is in phase III trials.

- *Serotonin and dopamine partial agonist.* Reviva Pharmaceuticals is testing RP-5063, which they refer to as a dopamine-serotonin stabilizer. It is similar to the current atypical antipsychotic drugs and has completed phase I trials.

- *Serotonin 1A receptor agonist.* SK Biopharmaceuticals is testing SKL-PSY/FZ-016, which has completed preclinical trials and is preparing for phase I testing.

- *Antiepileptic drugs.* SK Biopharmaceuticals is also testing YKP-3089 (Cenobamate), a new antiepileptic drug in phase II trials.

PSYCHOTHERAPEUTIC AND PSYCHOSOCIAL TREATMENTS

Bipolar disorder is one of the most difficult psychiatric conditions to treat and due to a variety of factors, including lack of adherence to treatment, the relapse rate, psychological impact, and social impact is high. Patients with bipolar disorder suffer from the psychosocial consequences of past episodes, the ongoing vulnerability to future episodes, and the burden of adhering to a long-term treatment plan that may involve some unpleasant side effects. In addition, many patients have clinically significant mood instability between episodes.

Successful treatment involves a social network primed to recognize the early symptoms of an episode, to seek help for patients who lack insight into their condition, and to assist with recognition of side effects and toxicities, hopefully improving adherence to the treatment plan. According to Geddes and Miklowitz (2013), the common objectives for psychosocial interventions for bipolar disorder include:

- The ability to identify warning signs of impending illness and provide early intervention
- Helping the individual accept the reality of their illness
- Providing support that would enable the individual to adhere to their medication treatment
- Providing the individual with better coping skills to mitigate the effect of life stressors that had previously triggered an episode of illness
- Helping the individual establish regular daily routines including meals, exercise, and sleep-wake cycles
- Assisting the individual to reengage with family and friends, and find or keep employment
- Teaching families how to have conversations with the individual to avoid conflicts and withdrawal
- Reducing the influence of any drug or alcohol misuse

It is also important to ensure that the manic state is not being caused by medications, such as antidepressants, caffeine, herbals containing ephedrine, behavioral stimulants, including illegal drugs such as cocaine, corticosteroids (cortisone), anabolic steroids, antiparkinsonian drugs, over-the-counter cough and cold preparations, and diet aids. Also, a good physical examination is important in order to rule out an underlying medical condition, such as hyperthyroidism, that could trigger or exacerbate a manic episode.

Psychotherapy with pharmacotherapy is associated with 30 to 40 percent reduction in relapse rates over 12 to 30 months (Miklowitz, 2008). Evidence, based psychotherapeutic and psychosocial treatments when combined with medication treatment have been shown to produce improved outcomes compared to medication alone. For example, *family-focused therapy* (FFT) teaches families about the disorder, how to recognize signs of episodes, how to support the individual's efforts to manage the illness through adherence to the treatment plan, how to avoid negative communication styles that exacerbate or trigger episodes, and other skills. FFT has been shown to reduce the frequency of relapse and rehospitalization, improve medication adherence, reduce symptom severity, and reduce frequency of depressive episodes.

Interpersonal and social rhythm therapy (IPSRT) stresses the importance of establishing and maintaining a regular life schedule and teaching the individual and their family problem-solving skills that will improve the individual's satisfaction within social situations. IPSRT has been shown to reduce illness recurrence.

Cognitive-behavioral therapy (CBT) teaches the individual about their illness, how to recognize signs and symptoms of episodes, and cognitive coping strategies. CBT has been shown to reduce the rate of rehospitalization, improve social functioning, and reduce severity of symptoms within episodes. Psychoeducational interventions have been shown to decrease recurrence rates and improve functional outcomes.

Geddes and Miklowitz (2013), Hollon and colleagues (2010), and Shah and colleagues (2017) all review evidence-based psychotherapeutic and psychosocial interventions for bipolar disorder and their efficacy. Finally, it is important to understand that these same treatments are not just effective when combined with medication for the treatment of bipolar disorder. They are also effective when combined with medication for the treatment of individuals with schizophrenia, major depression, and other psychiatric disorders.

STUDY QUESTIONS

1. Discuss the symptomatology of bipolar disorder, including the subtypes and the issue of unipolar versus bipolar depression. Why is it important to try to differentiate them?

2. What are the major pharmacological drug categories useful in the treatment of bipolar disorder and the major drugs in each category?

3. Compare and contrast the anticonvulsants that have some efficacy in treating bipolar disorder with those that do not.

4. Which antipsychotics have been found useful for treatment of bipolar disorder?

5. What are the difficulties in using mood stabilizers for pregnant women?

6. What are the major side effects associated with the drugs in each of the classes of medications used to treat bipolar disorders?

7. What are the most effective psychotherapeutic interventions for the treatment of bipolar disorder and how do they improve treatment outcomes?

REFERENCES

Aitchison, K. J., et al. (2009). "A UK Consensus on the Administration of Aripirazole for the Treatment of Mania." *Journal of Psychopharmacology* 23: 231–240.

Altshuler, L. L., et al. (2006). "Lower Switch Rate in Depressed Patients with Bipolar II than Bipolar I Disorder Treated Adjunctively with Second-Generation Antidepressants." *American Journal of Psychiatry* 163: 313–315.

Amann, B., et al. (2011). "Lamotrigine: When and Where Does It Act in Affective Disorders? A Systematic Review." *Journal of Psychopharmacology* 25: 1289–1294.

American Psychiatric Association. (2002). "Practice Guideline for the Treatment of Patients with Bipolar Disorder (Revision)." *American Journal of Psychiatry* 159 (Suppl. 4): 1–50.

Amsterdam, J. D., and Shults, J. (2005). "Comparison of Fluoxetine, Olanzapine, and Combined Fluoxetine Plus Olanzapine Initial Therapy of Bipolar Type I and Type II Major Depression—Lack of Manic Induction." *Journal of Affective Disorders* 87: 121–130.

Angst, J., et al. (2011). "Prevalence and Characteristics of Undiagnosed Bipolar Disorders in Patients with a Major Depressive Episode: The BRIDGE Study." *Archives of General Psychiatry* 68: 791–799.

Ashok, A. H., et al. (2017). "The Dopamine Hypothesis of Bipolar Affective Disorder: The State of the Art and Implications for Treatment." *Molecular Psychiatry* 22: 666–679. doi: 10.1038/mp.2017.16.

Baldassano, C. F. (2009). "Promoting Wellness in Patients with Bipolar Disorder: Strategies to Move beyond Maintaining Stability and Minimizing Adverse Events in Effective Long-Term Management." *Current Psychiatry* 8 (Suppl. 10): S12–S18.

Baldessarini, R. J., and Tondo, L. (2000). "Does Lithium Treatment Still Work? Evidence of Stable Responses over Three Decades." *Archives of General Psychiatry* 57: 187–190.

Baldessarini, R. J., et al. (2006). "Decreased Risk of Suicides and Attempts During Long-Term Lithium Treatment: A Meta-Analytic Review." *Bipolar Disorders* 8: 625–639.

Bartoli, F., et al. (2017). "Benefits and Harms of Low and High Second-Generation Antipsychotics Doses for Bipolar Depression: A Meta-Analysis." *Journal of Psychiatric Research* 88: 38–46.

Bauer, M. S. (2005). "How Solid Is the Evidence for the Efficacy of Mood Stabilizers in Bipolar Disorder?" *Essential Psychopharmacology* 6: 301–318.

Bauer, M. S., and Mitchner, L. (2004). "What Is a 'Mood Stabilizer'? An Evidence-Based Response." *American Journal of Psychiatry* 161: 3–18.

Bearden, C. E., et al. (2007). "Greater Cortical Gray Matter Density in Lithium-Treated Patients with Bipolar Disorder." *Biological Psychiatry* 62: 7–16.

Bersudsky, Y. (2005). "Phenytoin: An Anti-Bipolar Anticonvulsant?" *International Journal of Neuropsychopharmacology* 9: 479–484.

Bertolino, A., et al. (2003). "Neuronal Pathology in the Hippocampal Area of Patients with Bipolar Disorder: A Study with Proton Magnetic Resonance Spectroscopic Imaging." *Biological Psychiatry* 53: 906–913.

Beydoun, A., et al. (2005). "Safety and Efficacy of Two Pregabalin Regimens for Add-On Treatment of Partial Epilepsy." *Neurology* 64: 475–480.

Bourin, M., et al. (2013). "How to Assess Drugs in the Treatment of Acute Bipolar Mania?" *Frontiers in Pharmacology* 4: 4. doi: 10.3389/fphar.2013.00004.

Bowden, C. L., et al. (2003). "A Placebo-Controlled 18-Month Trial of Lamotrigine and Lithium Maintenance Treatment in Recently Manic or Hypomanic Patients with Bipolar I Disorder." *Archives of General Psychiatry* 60: 392–400.

Bowden, C. L., et al. (2010). "Ziprasidone Plus a Mood Stabilizer in Subjects with Bipolar I Disorder: A 6-Month, Randomized, Placebo-Controlled, Double-Blind Trial." *Journal of Clinical Psychiatry* 71: 130–137.

Bowden, C. L., et al. (2012a). "Aims and Results of the NIMH Systematic Treatment Enhancement Program for Bipolar Disorder (STEP-BD)." *CNS Neuroscience & Therapeutics* 18: 243–249. doi: 10.1111/j.1755-5949.2011.00257.x.

Bowden, C. L., et al. (2012b). "Lamotrigine (Lamictal IR) for the Treatment of Bipolar Disorder." *Expert Opinion on Pharmacotherapy* 13: 2565–2571.

Brady, R. O., and Keshavan, M. (2015). "Emergent Treatments Based on the Pathophysiology of Bipolar Disorder: A Selective Review." *Asian Journal of Psychiatry* 18: 15–21.

Brooks, J. O., et al. (2011). "Safety and Tolerability Associated with Second-Generation Antipsychotic Polytherapy in Bipolar Disorder: Findings from the Systematic Treatment Enhancement Program for Bipolar Disorder." *Journal of Clinical Psychiatry* 72: 240–247.

Brown, E. B., et al. (2006). "A 7-Week, Randomized Double-Blind Trial of Olanzapine/Fluoxetine Combination versus Lamotrigine in the Treatment of Bipolar I Depression." *Journal of Clinical Psychiatry* 67: 1025–1033.

Buoli, M., et al. (2016). "Biological Aspects and Candidate Biomarkers for Psychotic Bipolar Disorder: A Systematic Review." *Psychiatry and Clinical Neurosciences* 70: 227–244.

Calabrese, J. R., et al. (2002). "Rash in Multicenter Trials of Lamotrigine in Mood Disorders: Clinical Relevance and Management." *Journal of Clinical Psychiatry* 63: 1012–1019.

Calabrese, J. R., et al. (2005). "A Randomized, Double-Blind, Placebo-Controlled Trial of Quetiapine in the Treatment of Bipolar I or II Depression." *American Journal of Psychiatry* 162: 1351–1360.

Can, A., et al. (2014). "Molecular Actions and Clinical Pharmacogenetics of Lithium Therapy." *Pharmacology, Biochemistry and Behavior* 123: 3–16.

Chen, G., et al. (1999). "Valproate Robustly Enhances AP-1 Mediated Gene Expression." *Brain Research: Molecular Brain Research* 64: 52–58.

Chengappa, R., et al. (2006). "Adjunctive Topiramate Therapy in Patients Receiving a Mood Stabilizer for Bipolar I Disorder: A Randomized, Placebo-Controlled Trial." *Journal of Clinical Psychiatry* 67: 1698–1706.

Chwieduk, C. M., et al. (2011). "Asenapine: A Review of Its Use in the Management of Mania in Adults with Bipolar I Disorder." *CNS Drugs* 25: 251–267.

Cipriani, A., et al. (2005). "Lithium in the Prevention of Suicidal Behavior and All-Cause Mortality in Patients with Mood Disorders: A Systematic Review of Randomized Trials." *American Journal of Psychiatry* 162: 1805–1819.

Cipriani, A., et al. (2011). "Comparative Efficacy and Acceptability of Antimanic Drugs in Acute Mania: A Multiple-Treatments Meta-Analysis." *Lancet* 378: 1306–1315.

Clos, S., et al. (2015). "Long-Term Effect of Lithium Maintenance Therapy on Estimated Glomerular Filtration Rate in Patients with Affective Disorders: A Population-Based Cohort Study." *Lancet Psychiatry* 2: 1075–1083. doi: 10.1016/S2215-0366(15)00316-8.

Corya, S. A., et al. (2006). "A 24-Week Open-Label Extension Study of Olanzapine-Fluoxetine Combination and Olanzapine Monotherapy in the Treatment of Bipolar Depression." *Journal of Clinical Psychiatry* 67: 798–806.

Coryell, W. (2009). "Maintenance Treatment in Bipolar Disorder: A Reassessment of Lithium as the First Choice." *Bipolar Disorders* 11 (Suppl. 2): 77–83.

Cui, J., et al. (2007). "Role of Glutathione in Neuroprotective Effects of Mood Stabilizing Drugs Lithium and Valproate." *Neuroscience* 144: 1447–1453.

Cunha, A. B. M., et al. (2006). "Serum Brain-Derived Neurotrophic Factor Is Decreased in Bipolar Disorder During Depressive and Manic Episodes." *Neuroscience Letters* 398: 215–219.

Dagani, J., et al. (2016). "Meta-Analysis of the Interval between the Onset and Management of Bipolar Disorder." *Canadian Journal of Psychiatry* 62: 247–258. doi: 10.1177/0706743716656607.

Dea, L., et al. (2016). "Management of Bipolar Disorder." *U.S. Pharmacist* 41: 34–37.

De Almeida, J., et al. (2013). "Distinguishing Between Unipolar Depression and Bipolar Depression: Current and Future Clinical and Neuroimaging Perspectives." *Biological Psychiatry* 73: 111–118.

De Fruyt, J., et al. (2012). "Second Generation Antipsychotics in the Treatment of Bipolar Depression: A Systematic Review and Meta-Analysis." *Journal of Psychopharmacology* 26: 603–617.

Diazgranados, N., et al. (2010). "A Randomized Add-On Trial of an N-Methyl-D-Aspartate Anatagonist in Treatment-Resistant Bipolar Depression." *Archives of General Psychiatry* 67: 793–802.

Dodd, B. M., et al. (2007). "History of Illness Prior to a Diagnosis of Bipolar Disorder or Schizoaffective Disorder." *Journal of Affective Disorders* 103: 181–186.

Einat, H., and Manji, H. K. (2006). "Cellular Plasticity Cascades: Genes-to-Behavior Pathways in Animal Models of Bipolar Disorder." *Biological Psychiatry* 59: 1160–1171.

Ellinger, L. K., et al. (2010). "Efficacy of Metformin and Topiramate in Prevention and Treatment of Second-Generation Antipsychotic-Induced Weight Gain." *Annals of Pharmacotherapy* 44: 668–679.

El-Mallakh, R. S., et al. (2015). "Antidepressants Worsen Rapid-Cycling Course in Bipolar Depression: A STEP-BD Randomized Clinical Trial." *Journal of Affective Disorders* 184: 318–321.

Fountoulakis, K. N., et al. (2013). "A Systematic Review of the Evidence on the Treatment of Rapid Cycling Bipolar Disorder." *Bipolar Disorders* 15: 115–137.

Frye, M., et al. (2009). "Correlates of Treatment-Emergent Mania Associated with Antidepressant Treatment in Bipolar Depression." *American Journal of Psychiatry* 166: 164–172.

Gao, K., et al. (2008). "Antipsychotic-Induced Extrapyramidal Side Effects in Bipolar Disorder and Schizophrenia: A Systematic Review." *Journal of Clinical Psychopharmacology* 28: 203–209.

Geddes, J. R. and Miklowitz, D. J. (2013). "Treatment of Bipolar Disorder." *Lancet* 381: 1-20.

Geddes, J. R., et al. (2004). "Long-Term Lithium Therapy for Bipolar Disorder: Systematic Review and Meta-Analysis of Randomized Controlled Trials." *American Journal of Psychiatry* 161: 217–222.

Geddes, J. R., et al. (2010). "Lithium Plus Valproate Combination Therapy versus Monotherapy for Relapse Prevention in Bipolar I Disorder (BALANCE): A Randomized Open-Label Trial." *Lancet* 375: 385–395. doi: 10.1016/S0140-6736(09)61828-6.

Gentile, S. (2012). "Lithium in Pregnancy: The Need to Treat, the Duty to Ensure Safety." *Expert Opinion on Drug Safety* 11: 425–437.

Gershon, S., et al. (2009). "Lithium Specificity in Bipolar Illness: A Classic Agent for the Classic Disorder." *Bipolar Disorders* 11 (suppl. 2): 34–44.

Ghaemi, S. N., et al. (2006). "Extrapyramidal Side Effects with Atypical Neuroleptics in Bipolar Disorder." *Progress in Neuro-Psychopharmacology & Biological Psychiatry* 30: 209–213.

Gibbons, R., et al. (2009). "Relationship between Antiepileptic Drugs and Suicide Attempts in Patients with Bipolar Disorder." *Archives of General Psychiatry* 66: 1354–1360.

Gitlin, M. (2016). "Lithium Side Effects and Toxicity: Prevalence and Management Strategies." *International Journal of Bipolar Disorders* 4: 1–10. doi: 10.1186/s40345-016-0068-y.

Gitlin, M. J., et al. (2011). "Subsyndromal Depressive Symptoms after Symptomatic Recovery from Mania Are Associated with Delayed Functional Recovery." *Journal of Clinical Psychiatry* 72: 692–697.

Goldberg, J. F. (2010). "Antidepressants in Bipolar Disorder: 7 Myths and Realities." *Current Psychiatry* 9: 41–48.

Goldberg, J. F., et al. (2001). "Risk for Bipolar Illness in Patients Initially Hospitalized for Unipolar Depression." *American Journal of Psychiatry* 158: 1265–1270.

Goldberg, J. F., et al. (2007). "Adjunctive Antidepressant Use and Symptomatic Recovery among Bipolar Depressed Patients with Concomitant Manic Symptoms: Findings from the STEP-BD." *American Journal of Psychiatry* 164: 1348–1355.

Goldberg, J. F., et al. (2009). "Mood Stabilization and Destabilization During Acute and Continuation Phase Treatment for Bipolar I Disorder with Lamotrigine or Placebo." *Journal of Clinical Psychiatry* 70: 1273–1280.

Gonzalez-Pinto, A., et al. (2011). "Poor Long-Term Prognosis in Mixed Bipolar Patients: 10-year Outcomes in the Vitoria Prospective Naturalistic Study in Spain." *Journal of Clinical Psychiatry* 72: 671–676.

Goodwin, G. M., et al. (2004). "A Pooled Analysis of Two Placebo-Controlled 18-Month Trials of Lamotrigine and Lithium Maintenance in Bipolar I Disorder." *Journal of Clinical Psychiatry* 64: 432–441.

Goodwin, G. M., et al. (2016). "Evidence-Based Guidelines for Treating Bipolar Disorder: Revised Third Edition Recommendations from the British Association for Psychopharmacology." *Journal of Psychopharmacology* 30: 495–453. doi: 10.1177/0269881116636545.

Gould, T. D., et al. (2004). "Emerging Experimental Therapeutics for Bipolar Disorder: Insights from the Molecular and Cellular Actions of Current Mood Stabilizers." *Molecular Psychiatry* 9: 734–755.

Grande, I., et al. (2016). "Bipolar Disorder." *Lancet* 387: 1561–1572.

Grof, P., et al. (2009). "A Critical Appraisal of Lithium's Efficacy and Effectiveness: The Last 60 Years." *Bipolar Disorders* 11 (Suppl. 2): 10–19.

Grover, S., and Avasthi, A. (2015). "Mood Stabilizers in Pregnancy and Lactation." *Indian Journal of Psychiatry* 57 (Suppl. 2): S308–S323. doi: 10.4103/0019-5545.161498.

Harrison-Read, P. E. (2009). "Antimanic Potency of Typical Neuroleptic Drugs and Affinity for Dopamine D2 and Serotonin 5-HT2A Receptors—A New Analysis of Data from the Archives and Implications for Improved Antimanic Treatments." *Journal of Psychopharmacology* 23: 899–907.

Hartong, E. G., et al. (2003). "Prophylactic Efficacy of Lithium versus Carbamazepine in Treatment-Naïve Bipolar Patients." *Journal of Clinical Psychiatry* 64: 144–151.

Hayes, J. F., et al. (2016). "Self-Harm, Unintentional Injury, and Suicide in Bipolar Disorder during Maintenance Mood Stabilizer Treatment: A UK Population-Based Electronic Health Records Study." *JAMA Psychiatry* 73: 630–637.

Hirschfeld, R. (2005). *Guideline Watch: Practice Guideline for the Treatment of Patients with Bipolar Disorder, 2nd edition.* Arlington, VA: American Psychiatric Association. http://psychiatryonline.org/pb/assets/raw/sitewide/practice_guidelines/guidelines/bipolar-watch.pdf.

Hirschfeld, R. (2009). "Making Efficacious Choices: The Integration of Pharmacotherapy and Nonpharmacologic Approaches to the Treatment of Patients with Bipolar Disorder." *Current Psychiatry* 8 (Suppl. 10): S6–S11.

Hirschfeld, R., et al. (2006). "An Open-Label Extension Trial of Risperidone Monotherapy in the Treatment of Bipolar I Disorder." *International Journal of Clinical Psychopharmacology* 21: 11–20.

Hirschfeld, R., et al. (2010). *Practice Guideline for the Treatment of Patients with Bipolar Disorder,* 2nd ed. Arlington, VA: American Psychiatric Association. https://psychiatryonline.org/pb/assets/raw/sitewide/practice_guidelines/guidelines/bipolar.pdf.

Hogan, C. S., and Freeman, M. P. (2016). "Adverse Effects in the Pharmacologic Management of Bipolar Disorder During Pregnancy." *Psychiatric Clinics of North America* 39: 465–475.

Hollon, S. D., et al. (2010). "A Review of Empirically Supported Psychological Therapies for Mood Disorders in Adults." *Depression and Anxiety* 27: 891–932.

Hou, L., et al. (2016). "Genetic Variants Associated with Response to Lithium Treatment in Bipolar Disorder: A Genome-Wide Association Study." *Lancet* 387: 1085–1093.

Hurley, S. C. (2002). "Lamotrigine Update and Its Use in Bipolar Disorders." *Annals of Pharmacotherapy* 36: 860–873.

Jafferany, M. (2008). "Lithium and Skin: Dermatologic Manifestations of Lithium Therapy." *International Journal of Dermatology* 47: 1101–1111.

Jann, M. W. (2014). "Diagnosis and Treatment of Bipolar Disorders in Adults: A Review of the Evidence on Pharmacologic Treatments." *American Health and Drug Benefits* 7: 489–499.

Jeong, J-H., et al. (2013). "Efficacy of Quetiapine in Patients with Bipolar I and II Depression: A Multicenter, Prospective, Open-Label, Observational Study." *Neuropsychiatric Disease and Treatment* 9: 197–204.

Joffe, H., et al. (2006). "Valproate Is Associated with New-Onset Oligoamenorrhea with Hyperandrogenism in Women with Bipolar Disorder." *Biological Psychiatry* 59: 1078–1086.

Keck, P. E., et al. (2003). "Advances in the Pharmacological Treatment of Bipolar Depression." *Biological Psychiatry* 53: 671–679.

Keck, P. E., et al. (2006). "A Randomized, Double-Blind, Placebo-Controlled 26-Week Trial of Aripiprazole in Recently Manic Patients with Bipolar I Disorder." *Journal of Clinical Psychiatry* 67: 626–637.

Keck, P. E., et al. (2007). "Aripirazole Monotherapy for Maintenance Therapy in Bipolar I Disorder: A 100 Week, Double-Blind Study versus Placebo." *Journal of Clinical Psychiatry* 68: 1480–1491.

Kemp, D. E., et al. (2012). "Lamotrigine as Add-On Treatment to Lithium and Divalproex: Lessons Learned from a Double-Blind, Placebo-Controlled Trial in Rapid-Cycling Bipolar Disorder." *Bipolar Disorders* 14: 780–789.

Kessing, L. V., et al. (2012). "An Observational Nationwide Register Based Cohort Study on Lamotrigine versus Lithium in Bipolar Disorder." *Journal of Psychopharmacology* 26: 644–652.

Ketter, T. A., et al. (2003). "Potential Mechanisms of Action of Lamotrigine in the Treatment of Bipolar Disorders." *Journal of Clinical Psychopharmacology* 23: 484–495.

Khan, S. J., et al. (2016). "Bipolar Disorder in Pregnancy and Postpartum: Principles of Management." *Current Psychiatry Reports* 18: 1–11.

Kupfer, D. J. (2005). "The Increasing Medical Burden in Bipolar Disorder." *Journal of the American Medical Association* 293: 2528–2530.

Kushner, S. F., et al. (2006). "Topiramate Monotherapy in the Management of Acute Mania: Results of Four Double-Blind Placebo-Controlled Trials." *Bipolar Disorders* 8: 15–27.

Leonpacher, A. K., et al. (2015). "Distinguishing Bipolar from Unipolar Depression: The Importance of Clinical Symptoms and Illness Features." *Psychological Medicine* 45: 2437–2446. doi: 10.1017/S0033291715000446.

Leverich, G. S., et al. (2006). "Risk of Switch in Mood Polarity to Hypomania or Mania in Patients with Bipolar Depression during Acute and Continuation Trials of Venlafaxine, Sertraline, and Bupropion as Adjuncts to Mood Stabilizers." *American Journal of Psychiatry* 163: 232–239.

Li, D. (2011). "Using Lithium in Bipolar Disorder: A Primer." *Carlat Psychiatry Report* 9: 1–3.

Lichtenstein, P., et al. (2009). "Common Genetic Determinants of Schizophrenia and Bipolar Disorder in Swedish Families: A Population-Based Study." *Lancet* 373: 234–239.

Lindström, L., et al. (2017). "Maintenance Therapy with Second Generation Antipsychotics for Bipolar Disorder: A Systematic Review and Meta-Analysis." *Journal of Affective Disorders* 213: 138–150.

Macfadden, W., et al. (2011). "Adjunctive Long-Acting Risperidone in Patients with Bipolar Disorder Who Relapse Frequently and Have Active Mood Symptoms." *Biomed Central Psychiatry* 11: 171.

Mahmoudi-Gharaei, J., et al. (2012). "Topiramate versus Valproate Sodium as Adjunctive Therapies to a Combination of Lithium and Risperidone for Adolescents with Bipolar I Disorder: Effects on Weight and Serum Lipid Profiles." *Iranian Journal of Psychiatry* 7: 1–10.

The Management of Bipolar Disorder Working Group. (2010). *VA/DoD Clinical Practice Guideline for Management of Bipolar Disorder in Adults*. Washington, D.C.: Department of Veterans Affairs/ Department of Defense. http://www.healthquality.va.gov/bipolar/bd_306_sum.pdf.

Mathews, D. C., et al. (2012). "New Drug Developments for Bipolar Mania." *Psychiatric Times* 29 (Issue 12). http://www.psychiatrictimes.com/bipolar-disorder/new-drug-developments-bipolar-mania.

McElroy, S. L., et al. (2010). "A Double-Blind Placebo-Controlled Study of Quetiapine and Paroxetine as Monotherapy in Adults with Bipolar Depression (EMBOLDEN II)." *Journal of Clinical Psychiatry* 71: 163–174.

McGirr, A., et al. (2016). "Safety and Efficacy of Adjunctive Second-Generation Antidepressant Therapy with a Mood Stabiliser or an Atypical Antipsychotic in Acute Bipolar Depression: A Systematic Review and Meta-Analysis of Randomised Placebo-Controlled Trials." *Lancet* 3: 1138–1146.

McKnight, R. F., et al. (2012). "Lithium Toxicity Profile: A Systematic Review and Meta-Analysis." *Lancet* 379: 721–728.

Merikangas, K. R., et al. (2011). "Prevalence and Correlates of Bipolar Spectrum Disorder in the World Mental Health Survey Initiative." *Archives of General Psychiatry* 68: 241–251.

Messamore, E., et al. (2017). "Polyunsaturated Fatty Acids and Recurrent Mood Disorders: Phenomenology, Mechanisms, and Clinical Application." *Progress in Lipid Research* 66: 1–13.

Miklowitz, D. J. (2008). "Adjunctive Psychotherapy for Bipolar Disorder: State of the Evidence." *American Journal of Psychiatry* 165: 1408–1419.

Mishory, A., et al. (2000). "Phenytoin as an Antimanic Anticonvulsant: A Controlled Study." *American Journal of Psychiatry* 157: 463–465.

Mizushima, J., et al. (2017). "Early Improvement in Specific Symptoms Predicts Subsequent Recovery in Bipolar Depression: Reanalysis of the Systematic Treatment Enhancement Program for Bipolar Disorder (STEP-BD) Data." *Journal of Clinical Psychiatry* 78: e146–e151.

Montouris, G. (2005). "Safety of the Newer Antiepileptic Drug Oxcarbazepine during Pregnancy." *Current Medical Research Opinion* 21: 693–701.

Moore, J. L., et al. (2012). "Lamotrigine Use in Pregnancy." *Expert Opinion on Pharmacotherapy* 13: 1213–1216.

Mundo, E., et al. (2006). "Clinical Variables Related to Antidepressant-Induced Mania in Bipolar Disorder." *Journal of Affective Disorders* 92: 227–230.

Muneer, A. (2016). "Pharmacotherapy of Acute Bipolar Depression in Adults: An Evidence Based Approach." *Korean Journal of Family Medicine* 37: 137–148.

Muneer, A. (2017). "Mixed States in Bipolar Disorder: Etiology, Pathogenesis and Treatment." *Chonnam Medical Journal* 53: 1–13.

Murru, A., et al. (2015). "Management of Adverse Effects of Mood Stabilizers." *Current Psychiatry Reports* 17(8): 1–10.

National Institute of Mental Health. (2005). *Bipolar Disorder among Adults*. www.nimh.nih.gov/ health/statistics/prevalence/bipolar-disorder-among-adults.shtml. (Note: Statistics based on three 2005 studies.)

Ng, F., et al. (2009). "The International Society for Bipolar Disorders (ISBD) Consensus Guidelines for the Safety Monitoring of Bipolar Disorder Treatments." *Bipolar Disorders* 11: 559–595.

Nielsen, J., et al. (2012). "Real-World Effectiveness of Clozapine in Patients with Bipolar Disorder: Results From a 2-Year Mirror-Image Study." *Bipolar Disorders* 14: 863–869.

Nierenberg, A. A., et al. (2006). "Treatment-Resistant Bipolar Depression: A STEP-BD Equipoise Randomized Effectiveness Trial of Antidepressant Augmentation with Lamotrigine, Inositol, or Risperidone." *American Journal of Psychiatry* 163: 210–216.

Nierenberg, A. A., et al. (2009). "Lithium Treatment—Moderate Dose Use Study (LiTMUS) for Bipolar Disorder: Rationale and Design." *Clinical Trials* 6: 637–648. doi: 10.1177/1740774509347399.

Nierenberg, A. A., et al. (2013). "Lithium Treatment Moderate-Dose Use Study (LiTMUS) for Bipolar Disorder: A Randomized Comparative Effectiveness Trial of Optimized Personalized Treatment with and without Lithium." *American Journal of Psychiatry* 170: 102–110. doi: 10.1176/appi.ajp.2012.12060751.

Nivoli, A. M. A., et al. (2011). "New Treatment Guidelines for Acute Bipolar Depression: A Systematic Review." *Journal of Affective Disorders* 129: 14–26.

Novosolov, F. (2012). "Treating Bipolar Disorder during Pregnancy and Lactation." *Carlat Report-Psychiatry* 10: 1–2, 4–5.

Nonacs, R. (2012). "Topiramate (Topamax) Associated with an Increased Risk of Oral Clefts." *Massachusetts Center for Women's Mental Health*. February 8. http://www.womensmentalhealth.org/posts/topiramate-topamax-associated-with-an-increased-risk-of-oral-clefts/.

Ostacher, M. J., et al. (2010). "Impact of Substance Use Disorders on Recovery from Episodes of Depression in Bipolar Disorder Patients: Prospective Data from the Systematic Treatment Enhancement Program for Bipolar Disorder (STEP-BD)." *American Journal of Psychiatry* 167: 289–297.

Özerdem, A., et al. (2016). "Neurobiology of Risk for Bipolar Disorder." *Current Treatment Options in Psychiatry* 3: 315–329.

Oruch, R., et al. (2014). "Lithium: A Review of Pharmacology, Clinical Uses, and Toxicity." *European Journal of Pharmacology* 740: 464–473.

Pachet, A., et al. (2003). "Beneficial Behavioural Effects of Lamotrigine in Traumatic Brain Injury." *Brain Injury* 17: 715–722.

Parikh, S. V., et al. (2015). "Combined Treatment: Impact of Optimal Psychotherapy and Medication in Bipolar Disorder." *Bipolar Disorders* 17: 86–96.

Parker, G., et al. (2006). "SSRIs as Mood Stabilizers for Bipolar II Disorder? A Proof of Concept Study." *Journal of Affective Disorders* 92: 205–214.

Patel, R., et al. (2015). "Do Antidepressants Increase the Risk of Mania and Bipolar Disorder in People With Depression? A Retrospective Electronic Case Register Cohort Study." *BMJ Open* 5: e008341. doi: 10.1136/bmjopen-2015-008341.

Patorno, E., et al. (2010). "Anticonvulsant Medications and the Risk of Suicide, Attempted Suicide, or Violent Death." *JAMA* 303: 1401–1409.

Perlis, R. H., et al. (2006a). "Clinical Features of Bipolar Depression versus Major Depressive Disorder in Large Multicenter Trials." *American Journal of Psychiatry* 163: 225–231.

Perlis, R. H., et al. (2006b). "Predictors of Recurrence in Bipolar Disorder: Primary Outcomes from the Systematic Treatment Enhancement Program for Bipolar Disorder (STEP-BD)." *American Journal of Psychiatry* 163: 217–224.

Perucca, E. (2005). "Birth Defects after Prenatal Exposure to Antiepileptic Drugs." *Lancet Neurology* 4: 781–786.

Peters, A. T., et al. (2011). "Stepping Back to Step Forward: Lessons from the Systematic Treatment Enhancement Program for Bipolar Disorder (STEP-BD)." *Journal of Clinical Psychiatry* 72: 1429–1431.

Post, R. M., et al. (2005). "The Impact of Bipolar Depression." *Journal of Clinical Psychiatry* 66 (Suppl. 5): 5–10.

Post, R. M., et al. (2006). "Mood Switch in Bipolar Depression: Comparison of Adjunctive Venlafaxine, Bupropion and Sertraline." *British Journal of Psychiatry* 189: 124–131.

Rapoport, S. I., et al. (2009). "Bipolar Disorder and Mechanisms of Action of Mood Stabilizers." *Brain Research Reviews* 61: 185–209.

Rendell, J. M., et al. (2006). "Risperidone Alone or in Combination for Acute Mania." *Cochrane Database of Systematic Reviews* (January 25): CD004043.

Rosenblat, J. D., and McIntyre, R. S. (2016). "Treatment of Mixed Features in Bipolar Disorder." *CNS Spectrums* 22: 141–146. doi: 10.1017/S1092852916000547.

Ruggero, C. J., et al. (2010). "Ten-Year Diagnostic Consistency of Bipolar Disorder in a First-Admission Sample." *Bipolar Disorders* 12: 21–31.

Rybakowski, J. K. (2014). "Response to Lithium in Bipolar Disorder: Clinical and Genetic Findings." *ACS Chemical Neuroscience* 5: 413–421.

Sachs, G. S., et al. (2003). "Rationale, Design, and Methods of the Systematic Treatment Enhancement Program for Bipolar Disorder (STEP-BD)." *Journal of Clinical Psychiatry* 53: 1028–1042.

Sachs, G. S., et al. (2007). "Effectiveness of Adjunctive Antidepressant Treatment for Bipolar Depression." *New England Journal of Medicine* 356: 1711–1722.

Saunders, E. F. H., et al. (2016). "Omega-3 and Omega-6 Polyunsaturated Fatty Acids in Bipolar Disorder: A Review of Biomarker and Treatment Studies." *Journal of Clinical Psychiatry* 77: e1301–e1308.

Scherk, H., et al. (2007). "Second-Generation Antipsychotic Agents in the Treatment of Acute Mania." *Archives of General Psychiatry* 64: 442–455.

Schloesser, R. J., et al. (2012). "Mood-Stabilizing Drugs: Mechanisms of Action." *Trends in Neuroscience* 35: 36–46. doi: 10.1016/j.tins.2011.11.009.

Schou, M. (1997). "Forty Years of Lithium Treatment." *Archives of General Psychiatry* 54: 9–23.

Shah, N., et al. (2017). "Clinical Practice Guidelines for Management of Bipolar Disorder." *Indian Journal of Psychiatry* 59: 51–66.

Shajahan, P., and Taylor, M. (2010). "The Uses and Outcomes of Quetiapine in Depressive and Bipolar Mood Disorders in Clinical Practice." *Journal of Psychopharmacology* 24: 565–572.

Sharma V., et al. (2009). "Bipolar II Postpartum Depression: Detection, Diagnosis, and Treatment." *American Journal of Psychiatry* 166: 1217–1221.

Shine, B., et al. (2015). "Long-Term Effects of Lithium on Renal, Thyroid, and Parathyroid Function: A Retrospective Analysis of Laboratory Data." *Lancet* 386: 461–468. doi: 10.1016/S0140-6736(14)61842-0.

Shorter, E. (2009). "The History of Lithium Therapy." *Bipolar Disorders* 11 (Suppl. 2): 4–9.

Sigitova, E., et al. (2017). "Biological Hypotheses and Biomarkers of Bipolar Disorder." *Psychiatry and Clinical Neurosciences* 71: 77–103.

Smith, D. J., et al. (2011). "Unrecognised Bipolar Disorder in Primary Care Patients with Depression." *British Journal of Psychiatry* 199: 49–56.

Stern, S., et al. (2017). "Neurons Derived from Patients with Bipolar Disorder Divide into Intrinsically Different Sub-Populations of Neurons, Predicting the Patients' Responsiveness to Lithium." *Molecular Psychiatry*. In press. doi: 10.1038/mp.2016.260.

Suppes, T., et al. (2005). "The Texas Implementation of Medication Algorithms: Update to the Algorithms for Treatment of Bipolar I Disorder." *Journal of Clinical Psychiatry* 66: 870–886.

Swann, A. C., et al. (2013). "Bipolar Mixed States: An International Society for Bipolar Disorders Task Force Report of Symptom Structure, Course of Illness, and Diagnosis." *American Journal of Psychiatry* 170: 31–42.

Tada, M., et al. (2015). "Antidepressant Dose and Treatment Response in Bipolar Depression: Reanalysis of the Systematic Treatment Enhancement Program for Bipolar Disorder (STEP-BD) Data." *Journal of Psychiatric Research* 68: 151–156.

Thase, M. E. (2012). "Bipolar Disorder Maintenance Treatment: Monitoring Effectiveness and Safety." *Journal of Clinical Psychiatry* 73: e15. doi: 10.4088/JCP.10060tx4cc.

Toffol, E., et al. (2015). "Lithium is Associated with Decrease in All-cause and Suicide Mortality in High-risk Bipolar Patients: A Nationwide Registry-based Prospective Cohort Study." *Journal of Affective Disorders* 183: 159–165.

Tohen, M., et al. (2005). "Olanzapine versus Lithium in the Maintenance Treatment of Bipolar Disorder: A 12-Month, Randomized, Double-Blind, Controlled Clinical Trial." *American Journal of Psychiatry* 162: 1281–1290.

Tohen, M., et al. (2006). "Randomized, Placebo-Controlled Trial of Olanzapine as Maintenance Therapy in Patients with Bipolar I Disorder Responding to Acute Treatment with Olanzapine." *American Journal of Psychiatry* 163: 247–256.

Tränkner, A., et al. (2013). "A Critical Review of the Recent Literature and Selected Therapy Guidelines since 2006 on the Use of Lamotrigine in Bipolar Disorder." *Neuropsychiatric Disease and Treatment* 9: 101–111.

Tsai, A. C., et al. (2011). "Aripiprazole in the Maintenance Treatment of Bipolar Disorder: A Critical Review of the Evidence and Its Dissemination into the Scientific Literature." *PLoS Medicine* 8: e1000434. doi: 10.1371/journal.pmed.1000434.

Vajda, F., et al. (2013). "Lamotrigine in Epilepsy, Pregnancy and Psychiatry – A Drug for All Seasons?" *Journal of Clinical Neuroscience* 20: 13–16. doi: 10.1016/j.jocn.2012.05.024.

Vieta, E., et al. (2010). "Treatment Options for Bipolar Depression: A Systematic Review of Randomized, Controlled Trials." *Journal of Clinical Psychopharmacology* 30: 579–590.

Vosahlikova, M., and Svoboda, P. (2016). "Lithium – Therapeutic Tool Endowed with Multiple Beneficiary Effects Caused by Multiple Mechanisms." *Acta Neurobiologiae Experimentalis* 76: 1–19.

Weisler, R. H., et al. (2011). "Continuation of Quetiapine versus Switching to Placebo or Lithium for Maintenance Treatment of Bipolar I Disorder (Trial 144: A Randomized Controlled Study)." *Journal of Clinical Psychiatry* 72: 1462–1464.

Wichman, C. L. (2016). "Managing Your Own Mood Lability: Use of Mood Stabilizers and Antipsychotics in Pregnancy." *Current Psychiatry Reports* 18: 1–5.

Yasuda, S., et al. (2009). "The Mood Stabilizers Lithium and Valproate Selectively Activate the Promoter IV of Brain-Derived Neurotrophic Factor in Neurons." *Molecular Psychiatry* 14: 51–59.

Yatham, L. N., et al. (2005). "Atypical Antipsychotics in Bipolar Depression: Potential Mechanisms of Action." *Journal of Clinical Psychiatry* 66 (Suppl. 5): 40–48.

Yatham, L. N., et al. (2013). "Canadian Network for Mood and Anxiety Treatments (CANMAT) and International Society for Bipolar Disorders (ISBD) Collaborative Update of CANMAT Guidelines for the Management of Patients with Bipolar Disorder: Update 2013." *Bipolar Disorders* 15: 1–44. doi: 10.1111/bdi.12025.

Yildiz, A., et al. (2011). "Efficacy of Antimanic Treatments: Meta-Analysis of Randomized, Controlled Trials." *Neuropsychopharmacology* 36: 375–389.

Young, A. H., et al. (2010). "A Double-Blind, Placebo-Controlled Study of Quetiapine and Lithium Monotherapy in Adults in the Acute Phase of Bipolar Depression (EMBOLDEN I)." *Journal of Clinical Psychiatry* 71: 150–162.

Zarate, C. A., et al. (2005). "Molecular Mechanisms of Bipolar Disorder." *Drug Discovery Today: Disease Mechanisms* 2: 435–445.

Zarate, C. A., et al. (2006). "Cellular Plasticity Cascades: Targets for the Development of Novel Therapeutics for Bipolar Disorder." *Biological Psychiatry* 59: 1006–1020.

PART 4

Special Populations and Integration

Part 4 continues the discussion about the use of addictive and psychotropic drugs presented in Parts 2 and 3 as they apply to the special populations of children and adolescents (Chapter 15) and the elderly (Chapter 16). It is important to understand how the effects of drugs and treatment approaches vary based on the consideration of age and the associated physiological changes that occur with aging.

Chapter 15 examines the drug treatment of mental disorders during pregnancy. Then the discussion turns to the very young and the use of psychotropic medications, which is becoming more prevalent, even among preschool-age children. It is important to understand the risks of this exposure versus the evidence of benefit for disorders detected at this age. The continuing use of stimulants for the treatment of attentional disorders, not only in children and adolescents, but also in adults, is an ongoing area of research.

In Chapter 16, the authors discuss the use of psychotropic medications in the elderly and how changing physiology, natural course of mental disorders, and response to these agents have an impact on approaches to treatment.

Finally, in Chapter 17, a variety of trends are discussed that have a significant influence on how psychotropic medications are used—and whether they should be used. Policy changes at the federal, state, and local levels of government can affect access to medications, and budgetary decisions can determine utilization. Changes in nosology influence indications for medications and the implementation of the new DSM-5 will be discussed in that regard. There is also continuing concern about the difficulty of demonstrating that the newer psychotropic drugs are any better than older drugs, including evidence that in many trials, new drugs fail to exceed the effects of placebo. Shifting priorities influence drug development in new areas as well, such as treatments for dementia. At the same time, the pipeline for development of new drugs in all psychotropic classes has been declining over the last several years. Lastly, it is important to recognize that drug treatment alone rarely produces remission or can maintain recovery. Most studies show that the combination of pharmacotherapy and evidence-based psychotherapy not only promotes a greater chance of reaching remission, but also increases the probability that an individual will sustain recovery over a longer period of time.

CHAPTER 15

Child and Adolescent Psychopharmacology

PREGNANCY AND PSYCHOTROPIC DRUGS

The baseline rate of congenital malformations in the United States is approximately 3 percent of all pregnancies. In most cases, the causes are unknown. In 1979, with the intent of making clear a drug's possible risk for producing birth defects if taken during pregnancy, the FDA (Food and Drug Administration) established five risk categories, ettered A, B, C, D, and X. These categories were constructed by evaluating the reliability of information and the risk to benefit ratio of a drug. Detrimental effects of drugs and their metabolites in breast milk, however, were not considered.

In 2015, the letter categories for pregnancy risk were revised in an effort to make them more relevant for patients as well as medical personnel. According to the FDA, several developments prompted this reassessment. First, most women take at least one medication during pregnancy and the use of four or more medications during pregnancy has more than doubled over the last 30 years. Second, many pregnant women have chronic conditions, such as asthma, high blood pressure, depression, and diabetes, requiring them to continue taking medications they took before pregnancy. Furthermore, new health problems may begin or old ones may get worse during pregnancy, requiring treatment. Lastly, a woman's body changes throughout her pregnancy, which may affect the medication dose she needs.

The new legislation, the Pregnancy and Lactation Labeling Final Rule (PLLR), went into effect on June 30, 2015. But the implementation schedule for including this information on the package inserts varies. The labeling information on drugs approved after this date is meant to be more detailed and include data based on specific research regarding (1) the risk of taking drugs during pregnancy, labor and delivery, (2) the risk of using the drugs during lactation, and (3) a new section on females and males of reproductive potential concerning the need for pregnancy testing, recommendations for contraception, and information about infertility in regard to the drug.

Although an improvement from the previous version, the new labeling still does not give a definitive "yes or no" answer on whether a drug is safe for a specific patient in the majority of cases. Moreover, some drugs, especially if they were approved before 2001, may still carry the old designation, while drugs approved after 2001 will be phased in. (For more information on the changes to the labeling system, see Freeman, 2015; additional updates can be accessed at the FDA website.)

The FDA's concerns are intended to address the ongoing issue of maternal psychotropics. If the mother takes psychoactive medicines with frequency, is there a potential for such medication to injure the fetus, resulting in birth defects or, later in life, in developmental problems? Conversely, are there fetal developmental problems that might follow from the mother experiencing untreated mental health disorders?

By definition, a psychoactive medication crosses the blood–brain barrier and reaches the brain. The blood–brain barrier is the most resistant of all physiological barriers to drug distribution. In contrast, the placental barrier is the easiest to cross, which means that, as a general rule, *a fetus will have about the same blood level of drug as does the mother*. Therefore, risks of using medication during pregnancy include:

- Risk of potential teratogenic (birth defect, usually structural) damage to the fetus (See Table 15.1 for select drugs and their teratogenic effects)
- Risk of postnatal behavioral abnormalities in the child exposed to medication in utero
- Risk of perinatal syndromes (that is, within several weeks immediately before or after birth) or neonatal toxicity in the child if the mother continues medications while breast-feeding

On the other hand, untreated maternal mental illness may result in:

- Poor compliance with prenatal care
- Inadequate nutrition
- Exposure to undesired drugs, medications, or herbals
- Increased alcohol, caffeine, and tobacco use
- Deficits in mother-infant bonding
- Neglect of proper postnatal infant care
- Disruptions in the family environment

Pregnancy and Substances of Abuse

Nicotine

It is well established that women who smoke have a harder time becoming pregnant. Smoking during pregnancy is also linked to preterm delivery, low birth weight, and sudden infant death syndrome (SIDS), among other adverse effects. Unfortunately, women who smoke during pregnancy may not acknowledge the extent of their habit, which means that the degree of fetal exposure to nicotine from pregnant smokers and

TABLE 15.1 Select drugs and their teratogenic effect

Drug	Trimester	Effect
Amphetamines	All	Suspected abnormal developmental patterns, impaired school performance
Antidepressants, tricyclic	Third	Neonatal withdrawal symptoms have been reported in a few cases with clomipramine, desipramine, and imipramine
Barbiturates	All	Chronic use can lead to neonatal dependence
Carbamazepine	First	Neural tube defects
Clomipramine	All	Prolonged symptomatic neonatal hypoglycemia
Cocaine	All	Increased risk of spontaneous abruption of placenta and premature labor, neonatal cerebral infarction, abnormal development, and decreased school performance
Diazepam	All	Chronic use may lead to neonatal dependence
Alcohol	All	Risk of fetal alcohol syndrome and alcohol-related neurodevelopmental defects
Heroin	All	Chronic use leads to neonatal dependence
Lithium	First and third	Ebstein's anomaly (cardiac malformation), neonatal toxicity after third trimester
Methadone	All	Chronic use may lead to neonatal abstinence syndrome

SOURCE: G. Koren, Special Aspects of Perinatal & Pediatric Pharmacology, Chapter 59 in B. G. Katzung, *Basic and Clinical Pharmacology*, 14 ed. (New York: McGraw-Hill Education).

secondhand smoke is not easily determined (Hall et al., 2016; Hyland et al., 2015). Interestingly, the nicotine half-life in infants and young children is similar to that of adults and is influenced by CYP2A6 genotype, but not independently by age, sex, or race (Dempsey et al., 2013). This implies that the ability to metabolize nicotine occurs early in development. Unfortunately, "heavy" maternal nicotine has been reported to increase the odds of the offspring developing schizophrenia by 38 percent (Niemelä et al., 2016), and to lead to other nervous system anomalies (Marroun et al., 2014).

Alcohol

While the damaging effect of heavy drinking on the fetus has also been well established, there is still no consensus on the impact of low amounts of alcohol. In the United States, the surgeon general has advised women against drinking alcohol during pregnancy. Nevertheless, according to a federal government survey, 1 in 10 pregnant women in the United States drink alcohol, and 1 in 30 binge drink. Unmarried pregnant women were nearly five times more likely to binge drink than were married pregnant women (Tan et al., 2015). Nearly 3 of 5 (59 percent) pregnant teens in the United States reported having used one or more substances in the previous 12 months, a rate that is nearly two times as great as that of nonpregnant teens (35 percent), and the most commonly used substance was alcohol, at 16 percent (Salas-Wright et al., 2015). Alcohol use during pregnancy is common in many countries and as such, fetal alcohol syndrome (FAS) is a relatively prevalent alcohol-related birth defect. The global prevalence of alcohol use during pregnancy was recently estimated to be 9.8 percent and the estimated prevalence of FAS in the general population was estimated to be 14.6 per 10,000 people. Popova and colleagues (2017) concluded that 1 in every 67 women who consumed alcohol during pregnancy would deliver a child with FAS, which translates to about 119,000 children born with FAS in the world every year. (See Chapter 5 for more information about FAS. Updated guidelines for diagnosing fetal alcohol spectrum disorders (FASD) have been published; see Hoyme et al., 2016.)

Cannabis

Cannabis, typically in the form of marijuana, is the most common illicit substance used by pregnant women, with prevalence as high as 30 percent in some communities. With the advent of marijuana's legalization in several U.S. states, the American College of Obstetricians and Gynecologists (ACOG) has published its position on use of this agent during pregnancy and breast-feeding, essentially recommending that the use of marijuana, even for medicinal purposes, should be discouraged during pregnancy and lactation (American College of Obstetricians and Gynecologists Committee on Obstetric Practice, 2015). A systematic review of research on maternal, fetal, and neonatal outcomes up to 6 weeks postpartum after exposure to cannabis reported that infants exposed to cannabis in utero had decreased birth weight and were more likely to need placement in the neonatal intensive care unit compared with infants whose mothers did not use cannabis during pregnancy. However, it was difficult to determine specific consequences of maternal cannabis use because the various studies used different measures, the researchers had to rely on participant self-report of cannabis use, and participants often used other substances besides cannabis (Gunn et al., 2016).

Stimulants

Sowell and coworkers (2010) described the neonatal toxicity associated with maternal use of methamphetamine. Kousik and coworkers (2012) and Kiyatkin (2013) review the effects of psychostimulants, such as methamphetamine, Ecstasy, cocaine, and nicotine, on blood–brain barrier structure, accounting for much of the neurotoxicity of these drugs, an effect that presumably can also occur in utero. Current information does not link stimulants to major congenital malformations, but it is too soon to draw any conclusions about possible behavioral teratogenicity produced by short- or long-term exposure. Because of a lack of comprehensive data on use or misuse of these drugs, it is difficult to determine their reproductive safety. One study has shown that exposure to psychostimulants and to serotonergic-noradrenergic antidepressants, such as venlafaxine, after the twentieth week of gestation carried considerable risk of hypertension in the pregnant woman (Newport et al., 2016). The data suggest a potential impact on fetal growth rather than a risk of teratogenicity.

In one review of attention deficit/hyperactivity disorder (ADHD), and pregnancy (Freeman 2014), the medications most commonly used were methylphenidate (82.4 percent), risperidone (29.4 percent), selective serotonin reuptake inhibitors (SSRIs) (16.4 percent), and imipramine (4.6 percent). The most frequent delivery complication was neonatal hypoxia (15.6 percent). The most frequent side effect occurring during pregnancy was decreased maternal appetite (34.9 percent).

The timing of stimulant exposure may determine the impact on fetal growth. In a large prospective study in which 237 pregnant women were treated with dextroamphetamine to prevent excessive weight gain, discontinuation of the drug before 28 weeks of gestation did not affect birth weights, but later discontinuation resulted in birth weights that were 4 percent lower. Neonatal length and head circumference were not affected, and there was no association with any type of malformation (Freeman, 2014). A subsequent study suggests that methylphenidate does not seem to increase the risk for major malformations. Further studies are required to establish its safety in pregnancy and its possible association with miscarriages (Diav-Citrin et al., 2016).

Did You Know?

Pregnancy Criminalization Laws

A new report in 2017 from the organization Amnesty International describes the effect of what they term pregnancy criminalization laws in the United States, which punish women for engaging in behaviors that could damage a fetus. Currently, laws that make fetuses potential crime victims have been enacted in 38 states. In 23 of those states, the fetal age is irrelevant, meaning it could just have been conceived. Most of the time, the laws are applied to women who have abused drugs during their pregnancy, but the reach may be much broader. Punishments have been meted out to women for falling down stairs, not putting on seat belts when riding in cars, attempting suicide, and declining medical treatment. Unfortunately, the outcome may produce some unintended consequences, such as abortions or child abandonment, to avoid potential criminal punishment. Moreover, pregnant women struggling with drug abuse or mental problems may not seek help because they fear prosecution. The report argues for more support, assistance, and access to treatment services, rather than criminalization and incarceration in such situations.

Antidepressants in the Pregnant Female and Neonatal Outcomes

Perhaps no topic in psychopharmacology is as controversial as the use of antidepressants in pregnancy. Concerns have been raised that antidepressants administered during pregnancy promote miscarriage, congenital malformations, persistent pulmonary hypertension of the newborn, autism spectrum disorder, or long-term neurocognitive deficits. While some research concludes that antidepressants cause fetal and neonatal abnormalities, other data show that such risks are no greater than the baseline for congenital outcomes seen in 1 to 3 percent of the overall population. In addition, maternal depression can also cause problems during pregnancy as a consequence of drug abuse, malnutrition, suicidal ideation or premature birth. Some data suggest that anti-irritability and anti-anxiety actions of several SSRIs may help mothers regain their capacity to better listen and respond to their children, and that the children are likely to respond accordingly (Weissman et al., 2015).

Considerations about the risk–benefit relationship must take into account the consequences of treating maternal depression compared with the consequences of not addressing the condition (Robinson, 2015). The literature is replete with contradictory findings, concerns about whether pregnant women adhere to the medications, questions about whether all drugs have the same risks, or the extent to which the mothers' lifestyle contributes to the outcomes (Gentile, 2015). As recently as 2014, one review concluded that there was not sufficient evidence to make informed decisions about treatment with antidepressants during pregnancy (McDonagh et al., 2014). Since then, more evidence has been published, although decisions about whether to treat pregnant women with antidepressants may not be any less difficult.

Bérard and colleagues have reported that several SSRI and non-SSRI antidepressants used during pregnancy were associated with major cardiac and other congenital malformations in the offspring (Bérard et al., 2015; 2016; 2017). This is supported by Jordan and colleagues (2016), who concluded that women who took SSRIs 3 months before or after becoming pregnant had a small but significantly increased risk of having a baby with major congenital anomalies or being stillborn. Wemakor and colleagues (2015) also report an increase in several specific congenital anomalies, including cardiac heart disorders, with prenatal SSRI exposure. Nörby and colleagues (2016) found maternal use of antidepressants during pregnancy was associated with increased neonatal morbidity and a higher rate of admissions to the neonatal intensive care unit, but the absolute risk for severe disease was low.

Chiari type I malformation is a condition in which the brain tissue in the cerebellum extends into the spinal canal. Researchers identified Chiari type I malformations in 18 percent of children whose mothers took SSRIs for depression. Just 3 percent of children whose mothers had no history of depression were identified with Chiari type I malformations (Knickmeyer et al., 2014). Some data show that antidepressant exposure late in pregnancy slightly increases the likelihood of persistent pulmonary hypertension of the newborn (Grigoriadis et al., 2014; Huybrechts et al., 2015). Other studies report more spontaneous abortions (Andrade, 2014), perhaps related to the increased risk of postpartum hemorrhage (Grzeskowiak, 2015). A higher risk of preterm birth was found by Huybrechts and colleagues (2014), but no increase in cardiac malformations. In contrast, Malm and colleagues (2015) found that women treated with SSRIs while pregnant had a lower risk of preterm birth and cesarean delivery but a higher risk of babies with neonatal complications than women with psychiatric disorders who did not take SSRIs.

In contrast to the previously noted studies, Petersen and colleagues (2016b) did not find that congenital heart anomalies occurred in children born of mothers that were simply exposed to various antidepressant treatments. Rather, such birth defects were more likely to occur in offspring of older women, women with diabetes, a body mass index above 30 BMI, or a history of substance abuse, regardless of antidepressant use.

Another possible variable influencing the relationship between SSRI treatment and congenital heart defects in the offspring is the presence of several as yet unidentified genetic variants, in either the mother or the offspring (Nembhard et al., 2017).

Research within the last few years has repeatedly shown that there is no long-term neurodevelopmental impairment of children exposed in utero to antidepressants, even if some short-term deficits occur (Andrade, 2016; Grzeskowiak et al., 2015; Nulman et al.,

2015; Salisbury et al., 2015; Santucci et al., 2014; Suri et al., 2014). But disorders of motor, speech, and language might be greater in children whose mothers filled at least two SSRI prescriptions while pregnant (Brown et al., 2016).

One concern that has recently received substantial attention is the use of antidepressants during pregnancy and the risk of autism in the offspring (see King, 2017 for a discussion of one recent positive report). Although some evidence supported a relation (Rais and Rais, 2014), the preponderance of the data does not indicate that antidepressants in gestation are a significant risk for autism in the offspring (Brown et al., 2017; Clements et al., 2015; Hviid et al., 2013; Mezzacappa et al., 2017; Oberlander and Zwaigenbaum, 2017; Sujan et al., 2017). In children of mothers who did not take antidepressants during pregnancy, the rates of autism across these studies were low, ranging around 1 to 2 percent. Women who did use antidepressants during pregnancy were approximately twice as likely to have children with a diagnosis of autism spectrum disorder. But even with this increase, the rate of autism was low. Furthermore, even this association was often reduced by statistical adjustments for numerous confounding variables. As a result, it is not clear that the antidepressants are the cause of the autism increase. The most compelling evidence against a causal effect was provided by Sujan and colleagues (2017). This group compared families in which one child was exposed to antidepressants in utero, while a sibling was not exposed. If antidepressants were responsible for causing autism, there would be a higher rate of autism in the exposed sibling, but there was no such relationship. This suggests that genetic and shared environmental factors might be responsible for both the increase in antidepressant use and autism. In summary, although the incidence of autism in the offspring is increased if antidepressants are taken by the mother during pregnancy, the likelihood is still low, it may not be directly caused by the drug, and the consequences of not taking antidepressants need to be considered.

Antipsychotics in the Pregnant Female and Neonatal Outcomes

The increased use of antipsychotic drugs by pregnant women during the last decade is largely due to the overall greater use of more tolerable atypical antipsychotics in bipolar disorder and major depression as well as schizophrenia. Atypical antipsychotic drugs may also be prescribed for other mental health disorders, many of which occur in women of childbearing age (Toh et al., 2013). Clinicians need to balance several competing interests when managing episodes of major psychiatric illness during the prenatal period. Pregnant mothers with bipolar disorder or schizophrenia who abruptly terminate treatment have a high risk of relapse. Schizophrenia is associated with a high risk of obstetric complications for the mothers, and both bipolar disorder and schizophrenia increase such risks for the newborn. These two disorders, if untreated, represent risk factors for birth defects in their own right (Tosato et al., 2017).

Kulkarni and colleagues (2014) found that administration of mood stabilizers or high doses of antipsychotics to pregnant women resulted in 43 percent—three times the national rate—of babies requiring a special care nursery or a neonatal intensive care unit. Additionally, 18 percent were born prematurely, 37 percent developed respiratory distress, and 15 percent exhibited withdrawal symptoms (In 2011, the FDA issued an advisory concerning the possibility of extrapyramidal [motor] movements and discontinuation symptoms in newborns whose mothers took antipsychotics during pregnancy.) But Vigod and colleagues (2015) report that although users of antipsychotics had higher base rates of outcome events than the general population, they had no increased incidence of gestational diabetes, hypertension disorders of pregnancy, or thromboembolism, and no increased rates of adverse short-term perinatal outcomes, such as preterm delivery, low birth weight, delivery complications, or congenital anomalies. This may be surprising, because atypical antipsychotics cause high rates of excessive weight gain. Habermann and colleagues (2013) found no teratogenic risk in atypical antipsychotics, but postnatal disorders occurred significantly more often in infants exposed prenatally to both atypical and nonatypical antipsychotics compared to untreated control patients, that is, 15.6, 21.6, and 4.2 percent, respectively.

Sadowski and coworkers (2013) found that in utero exposure to monotherapy of atypical antipsychotics resulted in little risk to the fetus, whereas polydrug therapy was associated with adverse outcomes for both the mother and the child. Similarly, Peng and coworkers (2013) found only minor effects in women exposed only to atypical antipsychotics during pregnancy and, by 1 year of age, even these had dissipated. The findings of Cohen and colleagues (2016) show only a possibly modest, increased absolute risk of congenital malformations—an increase that, if it exists, might be due to other factors, particularly polypharmacy. The results of Petersen and colleagues (2016a) also support the conclusion that antipsychotic medications in pregnancy produce only modest danger of adverse reactions and birth outcomes as long as adjustments are made in regard to health and lifestyle. In general, current evidence suggests that patients with major psychiatric disorders responding well to atypical antipsychotics are best served by continuing their medications during pregnancy.

Mood Stabilizers in the Pregnant Female and Neonatal Outcomes

Untreated bipolar disorder in the pregnant female is associated with relapse to drug and alcohol abuse, manic episodes, interpersonal life disruptions, and early postpartum mania, depression, and psychosis (DiFlorio et al., 2013). Medication-free patients with bipolar disorder were at much greater relapse risk than those receiving prophylactic medication during pregnancy (66 percent compared to 23 percent) or in the postpartum period (65 compared to 29 percent) (Wesseloo et al., 2016). The clinical features of perinatal women with bipolar disorder are much more severe than those of women seeking care for other psychiatric conditions, including greater history of suicidal behavior and substance abuse, and more difficulties during childbirth and while breast-feeding (Battle et al., 2014).

Lithium is recognized as a modest teratogen, with a potential for fetal cardiac malformations greater than that in the general population (Nguyen et al., 2009). In a large study comparing pregnant women who were treated with lithium to those who were not, Diav-Citrin and colleagues (2014) found that the lithium-treated group had more miscarriages, terminations, and preterm births than the nonlithium group. Even after accounting for confounding variables, such as smoking, birth order, and bipolar disorder, lithium increased cardiovascular risk to the fetus. If lithium is absolutely necessary during pregnancy, doses should be minimized and the fetus closely monitored. The serum concentration of maternal lithium declines during pregnancy, which may require dose increases of as much as 50 percent during the third trimester (Westin et al., 2017). During periods of breast-feeding, some lithium is transferred to the infant. However, the amount of lithium was small and produced no untoward adverse effects in the nursing infants. According to Viguera and coworkers (2007), "[m]aternal serum, breast milk, and infant concentrations of lithium averaged 0.76, 0.35, and 0.16 mEq/L [milliequivalents per liter] respectively, each lithium level lower than the preceding level by approximately one-half" (p. 342).

Valproic acid (Depakote) is associated with the highest rate of major congenital malformations, with a relative risk estimated to be up to 16 percent compared to about 2.9 percent in nonmedicated females (Nguyen et al., 2009; Tomson and Battino, 2009). In addition, use of valproic acid during pregnancy has been associated with impaired cognitive functioning at 3 years of age in offspring with an IQ that is (1) 9 points lower than children exposed to lamotrigine; (2) 7 points lower than those exposed to phenytoin; and (3) 6 points lower than children exposed to carbamazepine (Banach et al., 2010; Meador et al., 2013). Finally, evidence has been reported that fetal exposure to valproic acid may increase the risk for autism spectrum disorders (Bromley et al., 2008; Christensen et al., 2013). Incidence rates for autism spectrum disorders ranged from less than 1 percent in control children to 2 percent with lamotrigine monotherapy and 6 percent with valproic acid monotherapy. The FDA has concluded that women of childbearing potential should only use valproic acid if it is essential to manage their medical condition and only if they have been adequately warned of its potential for causing harm.

Carbamazepine (Tegretol, Equitro) is considered to be slightly teratogenic, increasing the incidence of adverse fetal outcomes by about 3 percent over unmedicated females. Interestingly, abnormal effects on postnatal growth and development have not been reported by its close structural derivative, oxcarbazepine.

Lamotrigine (Lamictal) is not considered to be a major teratogen, although a slightly increased incidence of cleft lips and cleft palates has been reported. The mean lamotrigine concentration in breast milk was 41 percent of the maternal level; the mean fetal blood concentration was 18 percent of the maternal level and about 50 percent of the concentration in breast milk. No adverse events were observed in breast-fed infants (Newport et al., 2008).

Topiramate (Topamax), used in the treatment of epilepsy, bipolar disorder, borderline personality disorder, and migraine headache, has been associated with an increase in major congenital malformations, although the numbers of pregnancies studied is small (Hunt et al., 2008). Oral clefts and penile malformations in male infants occurred at a rate of about 11 times the control rate. Larger sample numbers are needed before more definitive interpretations can be made.

In one review, prenatal exposure to antiepileptic drugs was associated with an increased risk of being born with a low Apgar score, but the absolute risk of a low Apgar score was over 2 percent. The increased risk is not a class effect, but such risk may be particularly high with carbamazepine, valproic acid, and topiramate (Christensen et al., 2015).

In a study of breast-feeding women with epilepsy who take an antiepileptic drug as monotherapy, Meador and colleagues (2014) found that cognition and verbal abilities in their children assessed at age 6 years were not negatively affected. Limitations of this study include the absence of data on drug dosage during gestation and breast-feeding and on concentrations in breast milk and children's serum.

In general, infants exposed to psychotropic drugs during pregnancy have poorer outcomes than unexposed infants and should be considered a high-risk population (Sutter-Dalley et al., 2015). Jones and colleagues (2014) provide a comprehensive review of bipolar disorder, affective psychosis, and schizophrenia in pregnancy and the postpartum period.

DRUGS OF ABUSE IN CHILDREN AND ADOLESCENTS

Drug abuse is a significant contributor to three of the leading causes of death among adolescents—vehicular accidents, homicide, and suicide—and increases risk-taking behaviors while the youths are under the influence, including driving while impaired, unsafe sexual activity, and violence. It is also associated with low educational achievement.

Fortunately, according to the most recent results from the NIH-funded Monitoring the Future annual survey, fewer adolescents are using drugs than in the past. The 2016 survey of over 45,000 junior high and high school students found that the use of prescription opioids, cigarettes, e-cigarettes, and alcohol declined, while past-month marijuana use was fairly steady among twelfth graders. Perhaps not surprisingly, states with medical marijuana laws had higher rates of past-year marijuana and marijuana edible use among twelfth graders than states without such laws.

Common Addictive Substances

The following sections summarize major developments regarding the use of the most common addictive substances in children and adolescents.

Nicotine

Compared with nonusers, teenage e-cigarette users were more than four times as likely to later start using cigarettes or other smokeable tobacco products, according to the results of a longitudinal 12-month study of California high school students. Leventhal and colleagues (2015) also found that e-cigarette users at baseline had a more than twofold risk of smoking cigarettes versus teens who had never used e-cigarettes. Another small survey showed that the most common reasons teens gave for initially trying e-cigarettes were curiosity, the "cool" factor, and peer pressure. But 6 months later, none of those reasons were significant predictors of continued e-cigarette use. Smoking cessation was the only reason that was significantly associated with continued e-cigarette use after 6 months. At that point, however, 80 percent of teens who said they used e-cigarettes in order to quit smoking were still smoking traditional cigarettes

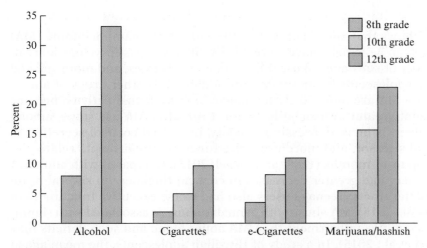

FIGURE 15.1   Percent of 8th, 10th and 12th Grade Students That Used Alcohol, Cigarettes, E-Cigarettes or Marijuana/Hashish, in the Past Month. Data from Johnston, L.D., et al. Monitoring the Future national survey results on drug use: 1975–2017: Overview, key findings on adolescent drug use.

(Bold et al., 2016). The use of e-cigarettes, in addition to regular cigarettes, seems to be related to the fact that 24 to 48 percent of U.S. middle and high school nonsmoking students are exposed to secondhand smoke (Agaku et al., 2016; Wang, 2017). As of January 1, 2016, Hawaii became the first state to prohibit anyone under the age of 21 from purchasing any type of cigarette (see Figure 15.1 for prevalence of e-cigarettes in 8th, 10th and 12th grade students.).

Alcohol

Siqueira and colleagues (2015) cited survey results indicating that children start to think positively about alcohol between ages 9 and 13; that 4.5 percent of 14- and 15-year-olds reported binge drinking, that is, depending on age and sex, 3 or more to 5 or more drinks on one occasion; and nearly two-thirds of high school students reported binge drinking on more than one occasion in the past 30 days. Although high socioeconomic status was associated with a greater risk of binge drinking, the greatest risk of extreme binge drinking was associated with lower socioeconomic status and with living in rural areas. Extreme binge drinkers, that is, 15 or more drinks on one occasion, were more likely to be young white men from rural areas. In fact, in rural primary care clinics, Clark and colleagues (2016) found 10 percent of youth over age 14 years met the criteria for a DSM-5 alcohol use disorder in the past year. The developing adolescent brain is more vulnerable to brain damage caused by alcohol as well as cognitive impairment versus the adult brain. In a longitudinal study, heavy-drinking teens lost more gray matter and gained less white matter over time than their peers who did not drink (Squeglia et al., 2015). The differences, seen on sequential magnetic resonance imaging, were similar regardless of sex.

Stimulants

Current literature shows that adolescents in treatment for methamphetamine (MA) abuse are more likely to be female, have a greater likelihood of past psychiatric treatment, a family history of substance abuse, higher depression rates, and more suicidal ideation relative to adolescents being treated for addiction to other drugs of abuse. Adolescents who use MA are more likely to engage in risky sexual activity, become pregnant, and exhibit greater antisocial behavior. Even after MA use stops, among former MA users there is more depression, anxiety, increased cortisol secretion in response to a social stressor, and more executive function impairments relative to non-MA users for up to 11 months (Buck and Siegel, 2015). Compared with adult MA users, adolescent users had greater decreases in cortical thickness in several brain areas and white matter tracts. Teenage users also had worse executive function than adult users (Lyoo et al., 2015). MA abuse with cannabis abuse is associated with significantly more neurocognitive impairment than MA abuse alone and such deficits may be enduring (Cuzen et al., 2015). In a study of Brazilian adolescents, the mean age at which they had started using cocaine was between 13 and 14 years, usually after two and a quarter years of using tobacco, alcohol, or cannabis. Comorbid conduct disorder, oppositional defiant disorder, and ADHD were diagnosed significantly more in users than in nonusers (Pianca et al., 2016).

Cannabis

As noted in Chapter 9, as of December 2016, 28 states and the District of Columbia have laws legalizing marijuana for medicinal purposes. Currently, seven of these states and the District of Columbia have also adopted laws legalizing marijuana for recreational use; three of these states, California, Massachusetts, and Nevada, passed measures in November 2016. The effect of such changes on public health are already being recognized. Investigators reviewed data from the American Association of Poison Control Centers National Poison Data System from 2005 to 2011 to determine if reports of unintentional exposures in children aged 9 years and younger were more common in states that had decriminalized marijuana. During the entire study period, across all states, there were only 985 reports of unintentional marijuana exposures in this age group. No deaths or long-term morbidity were reported. Call frequency increased by 30 percent per year in states that had decriminalized the drug before 2005, by 12 percent per year in states that had decriminalized between 2005 and 2011, and did not change in states that had not decriminalized (Wang et al., 2014). A study from Colorado found a small but substantial portion of young children admitted to the hospital for bronchiolitis had evidence of marijuana in their systems. Using a new assay developed by the Centers for Disease Control and Prevention (CDC), Wilson and colleagues (2016), reported that 7 out of 43 children (16 percent) younger than 2 years of age with bronchiolitis had marijuana metabolites (COOH-THC) in their urine at levels of 0.04 to 1.5 nanograms per milliliter.

Stronger strains and formulations of cannabis pose a risk to the developing brains of adolescents. Given the realities of medicalization, decriminalization, and legalization, as well as widespread recreational use, there is increased interest in minimizing adverse effects, particularly on youth (Smith, 2016).

As noted in Chapter 9, cannabis use in adolescence is associated with an increased risk of developing affective and psychotic disorders, including schizophrenia, in young adulthood (Bechtold et al., 2016; Manseau and Goff, 2015; Richter et al., 2016). The association is strongest in vulnerable youth, such as those who have suffered child abuse or have a family history of schizophrenia, and may not be a concern in less susceptible populations. This conclusion is borne out by a long-term study focused on 408 boys in the Pittsburgh Youth Study who were followed over the course of 20 years. Participants were categorized into one of four groups determined by their patterns of marijuana use from age 15 to 26: (1) early-onset chronic users, (2) late increasing users, (3) adolescence-limited users, and (4) low or nonusers. At age 36, participants were questioned about their current physical and mental health issues. Researchers found no significant differences among the four groups on indicators of physical health, which included asthma, allergies, headaches, high blood pressure, having a health condition that limited activity, having a serious injury in the past year, or having a history of concussion. Similarly, they found no group differences on mental health indicators that included a lifetime diagnosis of anxiety disorders, mood disorders, or psychotic disorders (Bechtold et al., 2015).

Nevertheless, there is also evidence that early-onset marijuana use has long-lasting consequences on physical and mental status. Moreover, adolescents are now using e-cigarettes to "smoke" pot. Roughly 18 percent of e-cigarette users and of cannabis users in one study reported using e-cigarettes to vaporize cannabis (Morean et al., 2015). Swedish researchers reported that men who had used marijuana heavily at ages 18 and 19 were 40 percent more likely to die by age 60 compared to men who had not used the drug (Manrique-Garcia et al., 2016). Heavy marijuana smoking was associated with smaller body size in adolescent boys relative to their peers. Individuals identified as "marijuana addicts" during childhood were 4.6 inches shorter and 4 kilograms lighter than nonsmokers by the age of 20 (Jabeen et al., 2015).

In young males, early and heavy use has been associated with deficiencies in brain structure, including cerebral cortical maturation and thickness (French et al., 2015; Ganzer et al., 2016), dopaminergic alterations (Renard et al., 2016), and thalamic connectivity (Buchy et al., 2015). Several years of daily marijuana use in young adults was associated with an abnormally shaped hippocampus and deficits on long-term memory tests relative to their nonusing peers (Smith et al., 2015). Other functional impairments include amygdalar hypersensitivity to threat (Spechler et al., 2015); impaired decision-making capabilities (Gonzalez et al., 2015); poor intelligence test performance (Camchong et al., 2017; Castellanos and Gralnik, 2016); and poorer academic performance (Meier et al., 2015).

All these outcomes imply long-term problems with societal achievement. Young people who were daily marijuana users before age 17 and followed up to age 30 had much worse outcomes than infrequent or nonusers. In analyses that controlled for key social confounding factors, including parental and peer variables, a dose-response relationship was found between use frequency and dropping out of high school, failure to get a college degree, marijuana dependence, use of illicit drugs, and suicide attempts (Silins et al., 2014). A study that followed nearly 950 people from birth through midlife has found a link between regular marijuana use and negative job prospects as adults. As compared to their parents, those involved in the study were more likely to face financial difficulties, including food insecurity and debt, if they were heavy marijuana users (Cerdá et al., 2016).

There has also been concern about the increase in availability of medical marijuana in regard to abuse of the drug. Interestingly, the data suggest that availability of medical marijuana does not cause a surge in pot smoking among teens. Researchers looked at 24 years of survey data from the Monitoring the Future study, which included 1,098,270 adolescents who lived in the 48 contiguous states and attended more than 400 schools from 1991 to 2014. The teens were surveyed during eighth, tenth, and twelfth grades. In 23 states and the District of Columbia, some form of medical marijuana is permitted. In those states where medical marijuana was in some way legal, 15.87 percent of adolescents had consumed marijuana in the past 30 days compared with 13.27 percent of those in states with no medical marijuana permissions (Hasin et al., 2015), a nonsignificant difference. Moreover, the data indicated that states with a medical marijuana law had an increased prevalence of marijuana use even before the law was passed.

The use of synthetic cannabinoids (SCs) perhaps warrants greater concern. In the first prospective study of SCs, researchers have found that symptoms of depression, drinking alcohol, and using marijuana were linked to an increased risk of SC use one year later (Ninnemann et al., 2017). Depressive symptoms, but not anxiety or impulsivity, were predictive of later SC use. Clayton and colleagues (2017) reported that when compared to students who used marijuana only, students who used synthetic cannabinoids were more likely to engage in substance use and sexually risky behavior and to engage in more aggressive behaviors if they (1) used the drug before the age of 13 years or (2) used the drug more than 20 times in the last 30 days.

In new recommendations, the American Academy of Pediatrics (AAP) opposes outright marijuana legalization but supports decriminalization for those 21 and younger (Ammerman et al., 2015).

Guidelines for Prevention, Diagnosis and Treatment of Substance Abuse in Adolescents

The U.S. Preventive Services Task Force (USPSTF), a voluntary organization that is independent of government and industry and funded by the Agency for Healthcare Research and Quality, reviews medical evidence and makes recommendations about specific preventive care services. In developing their most recent guideline (Moyer et al., 2014), the USPSTF found only six fair or good studies of four different primary care interventions to prevent children and adolescents from using illicit drugs or misusing prescription drugs. The four interventions were face-to-face counseling, videos, print materials, and interactive computer-based tools. The six studies yielded practically no evidence of significant improvements in health outcomes.

The USPSTF noted that more adolescents use illicit drugs or intentionally misuse prescription drugs than use tobacco (see Figures 15.2 and 15.3). Currently, the AAP recommends that clinicians screen all adolescents for alcohol and drug use, and based on those results, provide guidance, appropriate counseling interventions,

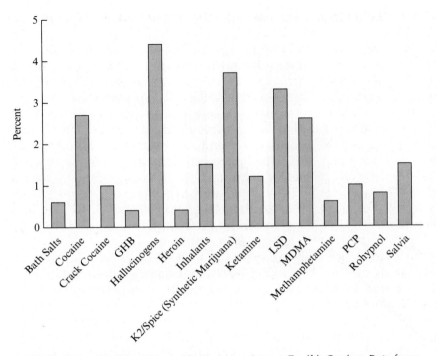

FIGURE 15.2 Illegal Drug Use In The Past Year Among Twelfth Graders. Data from Johnston, L.D., et al. Monitoring the Future national survey results on drug use: 1975–2017: Overview, key findings on adolescent drug use.

and, if necessary, referrals for treatment. The behavioral health screening tool recommended by the AAP's Committee on Substance Abuse, CRAFFT (Car, Relax, Alone, Forget, Friends, Trouble), consists of six questions designed to screen adolescents simultaneously for high-risk alcohol and other drug disorders. It can be administered in less than 2 minutes as either an interview or by self-report. The CRAFFT is meant to determine whether a more extensive discussion about drug use may be warranted.

In fact, a screening tool based on only a single question can accurately identify substance use disorders among teens. Levy and colleagues (2014) assessed some 200 adolescents aged 12 to 17 with an electronic screening tool that began with, "In the past year, how many times have you used [x]?" Use of eight substances, including alcohol, marijuana, and illegal drugs, was evaluated. Participants who reported some use were asked follow-up questions based on their frequency of use. The screening took an average of 32 seconds to complete, had excellent validity, and was similarly accurate whether self- or staff-administered. All participants also completed a structured diagnostic interview as the gold standard.

Lastly, the significant public health consequences of substance abuse by adolescents prompted the development of Substance use screening, Brief Intervention, and Referral to Treatment (SBIRT). In 2011, a policy statement on SBIRT from the AAP introduced the concepts and described the available options for guiding adolescent screening and treatment. The document has since been updated and simplified,

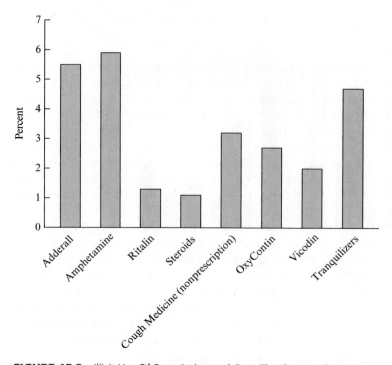

FIGURE 15.3 Illicit Use Of Prescription and Over-The-Counter Drugs In The Past Year Among Twelfth Graders. Data from Johnston, L.D., et al. Monitoring the Future national survey results on drug use: 1975–2017: Overview, key findings on adolescent drug use.

and provides advice for pediatricians in efforts to prevent, detect, assess, and intervene in dealing with substance abuse in all venues relevant to adolescents (Levy et al., 2016).

The Adolescent Brain Cognitive Development Study

Following the 2012 legalization of marijuana in Colorado and Washington, the head of NIDA responded to this change in policy by initiating an ambitious effort to follow 10,000 U.S. adolescents for 10 years to try to find out if marijuana, alcohol, and nicotine use produced changes in brain function and behavior. This study, the Adolescent Brain Cognitive Development (ABCD) Study (ABCDStudy.org), is the largest long-term study of brain development and child health in the United States. The ABCD Research Consortium consists of a coordinating center, a data informatics and analysis center, and 21 research sites across the country, with the goal of recruiting approximately 10,000 children ages 9–10 and following them into early adulthood. The objective is to integrate information on structural and functional brain imaging with data on genetics, neuropsychological, behavioral, and other health assessments so that the various influences on a young person's life course will be better understood. The study will emphasize the effect of drugs, including polydrug use and frequency of use, on all aspects of development. The Consortium was funded in 2015 and information on the progress of the study can be found on the Web site. As of January 31, 2018, enrollment totaled 7440 participants.

Psychopharmacology of Child and Adolescent Mental Health Disorders

Mental health problems of adults are commonly reported to occur before age 24. The proactive study by Patton and colleagues (2014) confirms that most disorders of anxiety and depression in adults start in adolescence. In this study, a large community sample of adolescents was followed up at several time points over a 14-year period from mid adolescence into their late 20s. Depression and anxiety were common during adolescence, affecting 29 percent of boys and 54 percent of girls. Almost 60 percent of participants who had an episode during adolescence reported a further episode as a young adult. By the late 20s, however, the prevalence of disorder had decreased and many of the participants who had an adolescent episode did not have another episode as a young adult. Several characteristics predicted ongoing disorder into adulthood, namely, longer duration of adolescent disorder, parental separation or divorce, and being of the female gender. Because the risk for persistence into adulthood is greater for adolescents with more than one episode, prompt recognition and treatment of the first episode might lead to fewer cases after age 21. While these results are encouraging, the consequences of childhood psychiatric disorders are still severe. Copeland and colleagues (2015) found that such adults who had a childhood psychiatric disorder were more than three times as likely to have health, legal, financial, and social problems as adults, even if they had never received a formal psychiatric diagnosis.

ANTIDEPRESSANTS IN CHILDHOOD AND ADOLESCENCE

Perhaps the greatest controversy in child and adolescent psychopharmacology is that surrounding the use of antidepressant medication to treat major depressive disorders in children and adolescents. Do these medications work? Do they increase the risk of suicide? Is their cost-benefit ratio worth the risks involved? These and other questions plague prescribers, let alone parents and patients. In essence, controversy surrounds the balance between expected benefits and effectiveness in relieving depression versus potential risks, especially the risk of suicide.

Research conducted in the late 1990s and early 2000s demonstrated several important points:

- There was a high prevalence of suicidal ideation and completed suicides among untreated children and adolescents with depressive disorders.
- Sixty-two percent of children with depression had experienced childhood adversity, with traumatic events (35 percent) and bullying victimization (29 percent) most commonly reported (Tunnard et al., 2014).
- Not only does depression exist in adolescence, but adolescence is the period of highest risk for onset of depression.
- Adolescent depression has a protracted, longitudinal course with persistence into adult life (adolescents do not "grow out of it"), which results in ongoing disruption of interpersonal relationships, risk for substance abuse, early pregnancy, low educational achievement, poor occupational functioning, unemployment, and continued risk of suicide.

- Untreated childhood and adolescent depression is associated with later development of serious personality disorders in early adulthood; dependent, antisocial, passive-aggressive, substance abuse, and histrionic personality disorders.

Emslie and coworkers (1997) demonstrated that *fluoxetine* (Prozac) was superior to placebo treatment in lowering scores on the Children's Depression Rating Scale—Revised. This led to widespread off-label use of fluoxetine for child and adolescent depression, culminating in the NIMH-funded Treatment for Adolescents with Depression Study (TADS), the first phase of which was published in 2004 (Treatment for Adolescents with Depression Study [TADS] Team, 2004). The 12-week TADS study compared usual clinical management with fluoxetine (10 to 40 milligrams per day) alone, cognitive behavioral therapy (CBT) alone, or the combination of CBT and fluoxetine. Response to combination treatment (71 percent) was significantly greater than to fluoxetine alone (61 percent), CBT alone (43 percent), and placebo (usual clinical management, 35 percent). Fluoxetine monotherapy was superior to placebo and to CBT alone. This study set the standard that the best treatment of child and adolescent depression is a combination of fluoxetine and CBT.

Results of longer-term phases of the TADS study have supported the initial conclusion. In general, the combination therapy of CBT plus fluoxetine has emerged as therapy of choice for child and adolescent depression. The landmark Treatment of Resistant Depression in Adolescents (TORDIA) study showed very clearly that combining both treatments is more effective than using medication alone. Published in 2008, the study remains a key piece of clinical evidence for helping youngsters with treatment-resistant depression (Brent et al., 2008). It included about 300 teens who were unresponsive to their initial 8-week SSRI therapy. They were then randomized to 12 weeks of either switching to a different SSRI alone; switching to venlafaxine alone; or switching to either of the drugs plus CBT. Adding CBT to either medication showed a higher response rate (55 percent) than did the medication alone (40 percent). The new drugs alone were equally effective (new SSRI, 47 percent; venlafaxine, 48 percent). More recently, Kennard and colleagues (2014) confirmed that adding 6 months of CBT to the medication management of children and adolescents with major depressive disorder reduced the likelihood of depression relapse. The study involved 200 participants, ages 8 to 17, with major depression. During the 6 months studied, participants who received medication management plus CBT had a 9 percent relapse rate compared to a 26.5 percent relapse rate for participants who received medication alone. Zhou and colleagues (2014) also concluded that SSRI therapy plus CBT was significantly more effective than SSRI therapy alone. In addition, the superiority of fluoxetine is supported by the results of Le Noury and colleagues (2015), who showed that neither paroxetine nor high-dose imipramine showed efficacy for major depression in adolescents, and that there was an increase in harms with both drugs. A larger review of 34 trials including 5260 participants and 14 antidepressant treatments (Cipriani et al., 2016) also found that only fluoxetine was statistically significantly more effective than placebo. Fluoxetine was also better tolerated than duloxetine and imipramine. Discontinuations resulting from adverse events were more common in patients given imipramine, venlafaxine, and duloxetine than in those given placebo.

Fluoxetine appears to be the best choice in regard to the risk–benefit profile of anti-depressants in the acute pharmacological treatment of major depressive disorder in childhood and adolescence.

Currently, fluoxetine is approved by the FDA for treatment of depression in children as young as 6 years and older, and duloxetine is approved for children as young as 7 years and older. In 2009, the FDA gave approval for the use of *escitalopram* (Lexapro) for the treatment of depression in adolescents ages 12 to 17 years. This approval was based on three studies on citalopram and escitalopram, the last study reporting that scores on the Child Depression Rating Scale were reduced by 22 points compared with a 19-point reduction in the placebo-treated group (Emslie et al., 2009).

Antidepressants and Suicide in Children and Adolescents

In 2002, 264 children and adolescents ages 5 to 14 years died by suicide in the United States, the fifth leading cause of death in this age group. An FDA report linked many of these deaths to SSRI treatment. Based on this finding, regarding SSRI use and the possibility of drug-caused increases in suicidal ideation (Gibbons et al., 2007) the FDA published a warning in 2003 and required a black box warning for children in 2005 and for adults 18 to 24 in 2007. The association of antidepressant use with a doubling of suicidality risk and aggression in children, but not adults, has recently been replicated (Sharma et al., 2016).

Within 2 years after the FDA advisory was issued, antidepressant use plunged 31 percent among adolescents and 24 percent among young adults. Unexpectedly, the reduction in antidepressant use as a result of FDA warnings resulted not only in reduced SSRI prescriptions, but an increase in suicide attempts and possibly suicides (Gibbons et al., 2007; Lu et al., 2014). This indicated that perhaps SSRI therapy was indeed effective in the long-term treatment of depression and an overall reduction in suicides.

Vitiello and coworkers (2009) noted that the primary precursors for suicidal events were persistent and severe suicidal ideation and depression, as opposed to the stimulatory effects of medication. Consistent with this view, researchers (Rahn et al., 2015) found that while SSRIs made children more impulsive during the first month of treatment, they did not create thoughts of suicide where such thoughts did not previously exist. They suggested dosing regimens similar to those used for adults when they experience negative side effects: start with half the typical initial SSRI dose, then slowly increase it to therapeutic level. Lowering the dose during initiation of treatment had also been advised by Brent and Gibbons (2014) and Miller and colleagues (2014), who found the rate of self-harm was greatest in the 3 months after initiating higher versus modal doses. In fact, lower doses have been prescribed significantly more since the FDA warning (Bushnell et al., 2015). Cousins and Goodyear (2015) argue that according to current data, SSRIs do not pose a danger to human adolescent brain development and that there is insufficient information to confirm or deny that depressed adolescents given SSRIs are at risk of developing suicidal side effects. In their opinion, while the decision requires medical judgment, the benefits of SSRI medication outweigh the risks and provide an important option for moderate to severe adolescent depression.

ANTIPSYCHOTICS IN CHILDREN AND ADOLESCENTS

Schizophrenia and its related conditions are considered quite rare in children, and when it occurs it presents significant clinical challenges. The American Academy of Pediatrics, the American Academy of Child and Adolescent Psychiatry, and the American Academy of Neurology have no guidelines or position statements regarding the use of antidepressants and antipsychotics in children younger than 3. Nevertheless, early detection and treatment of young persons at risk for psychosis is regarded as a promising strategy in fighting the devastating consequences of psychotic disorders (Schimmelmann et al., 2013). About one in three patients with schizophrenia develops symptoms of psychosis between the ages of 10 and 20 years. Since childhood and adolescent schizophrenia are generally associated with a poor long-term outcome, effective treatments are needed for children and adolescents with psychotic disorders or, more hopefully, who are in a prodromal phase, that is, the phase between initial symptoms and first-episode psychosis.

Atypical antipsychotics are currently first-line treatments for early onset psychosis and schizophrenia spectrum disorders. Recently, there has been an increase in the use of antipsychotics in children and adolescents for neurodevelopmental, behavioral, and psychiatric disorders, while at the same time, the age of prescription has decreased (see Tables 11.1 and 11.4).

Unfortunately, we do not know much about the safety of these medications in this group of patients (Memarzia et al., 2014; Schneider et al., 2014). According to information from the prescription data company IMS Health, almost 20,000 prescriptions for *risperidone* (Risperdal), *quetiapine* (Seroquel), and other antipsychotic medications were written in 2014 for children 2 and younger, representing a 50 percent increase from 13,000 in the previous year (Schwarz, 2015).

Although the FDA has approved the use of several atypical antipsychotics for use in children and adolescents, their serious side effects are the same as in adult patients, namely, extrapyramidal symptoms, tardive dyskinesia, weight gain, metabolic syndrome, and symptoms of hyperprolactinemia (Shapiro et al., 2014).

Between 2006 and 2010, prescription rates decreased among young and older children, but increased among adolescents and young adults. Rates were highest for males, mostly for disruptive disorders. Almost all prescriptions were for off-label use (over 60 percent) and antipsychotics were the only psychotropic prescribed in 15 to 28 percent of cases (Olfson et al., 2015). In looking at clinical diagnoses, researchers found that ADHD and disruptive behavior disorders were the most common diagnoses among boys ages 1 to 18 years receiving antipsychotics, suggesting clinicians are prescribing the drugs off-label. Boys ages 1 to 6 years were more than twice as likely as girls the same age to receive an antipsychotic prescription (0.16 compared to 0.06 percent). The pattern continued for boys and girls ages 7 to 12 years, but the gender gap narrowed in adolescence, and by young adulthood, rates were comparable between the sexes, with 0.88 percent of young men receiving a prescription compared to 0.81 percent of young women.

Because the use of second-generation antipsychotics increases the risk for weight gain, elevated glucose, insulin resistance, hyperlipidemia, and development of type 2 diabetes, monitoring is recommended (Delate et al., 2014). Only one of the 1023 pediatric patients included in a study of SGAs by Delate and colleagues received all baseline and follow-up metabolic monitoring. By 2011, only 60.5 percent had at least one baseline monitoring and only 55.3 percent had at least one follow-up monitoring. The most frequently reported adverse events were weight gain and elevated triglyceride levels.

Besides their FDA-approved indications, these agents are also prescribed for a variety of off-label conditions, including depression, anxiety, mood dysregulation, and aggressive behavior. In one meta-analysis, Galling and colleagues found that the mean age of study participants who had taken antipsychotics (Galling et al., 2016) was 14.1 years and that 60 percent of these participants were male. The mean age of the participants who had not taken antipsychotics was 13.2 years, 55.7 percent of whom were male. In the antipsychotic group, about 47 percent had a disruptive behavior disorder, attention deficit/hyperactivity disorder, or a mood spectrum disorder. The risk of diabetes did not significantly vary by baseline antipsychotic dosage in the analysis, but it did increase with cumulative dose of antipsychotics. In a recent meta-analysis of 41 studies ($n = 518,919$, mean age = 12.8 years, males = 65.7 percent), Cervesi and coworkers (2017) found that there was a significant increase in diagnoses of mood disorder among youth treated with antipsychotics due to an increase in those with bipolar spectrum disorders.

Although data are scarce, long-acting injectable (LAI) use in youth appear to be effective, with adverse reactions comparable to those of oral preparations (Lytle et al., 2017). No controlled trials were found. Most patients (80.6 percent) were boys. Primary diagnoses included bipolar I disorder, schizophrenia, and bipolar spectrum disorders. The LAIs used were mostly risperidone long-acting injection (66.7 percent), paliperidone palmitate, fluphenazine decanoate, aripiprazole extended-release injectable, zuclopenthixol decanoate, and olanzapine extended release. The medication was well tolerated by 82.4 percent with clinical improvement described in most cases. The most common side effects were weight gain (mean 5.7 percent at ±4.1 kilograms in the open-label trial), tremor (5.6 percent), and oculogyric crisis (5.6 percent).

A recent review by Pillay and colleagues (2017) summarized the overall clinical outcomes of atypical antipsychotics, that is, second-generation antipsychotics (SGAs) in this population, relative to placebo:

- The SGAs have a slight positive effect in schizophrenia, increasing response rates with clinically insignificant effects for negative and positive symptoms, but an overall functional improvement. The evidence for many drug comparison outcomes was often insufficient. Quetiapine was not effective at either high or low doses.

- In bipolar disorder, the SGAs may reduce manic and depressive symptoms, and slightly improve overall functioning. Aripiprazole alone and SGAs may improve response and remission rates for manic or mixed states, while quetiapine has no benefit for depression.

- In regard to autism spectrum disorders, SGAs and especially risperidone and aripiprazole may decrease irritability, and also reduce lethargy/social withdrawal, stereotypy, and inappropriate speech.

- For attention deficit/hyperactivity disorder and disruptive, impulse-control, and conduct disorders, SGAs as a group (and risperidone individually) may decrease some behavior problems and aggression. In children who have a diagnosis of conduct disorder or ADHD that does not respond to stimulants, risperidone by itself may reduce hyperactivity.

ANXIOLYTICS IN CHILDREN AND ADOLESCENTS

The prevalence of anxiety disorders in children ranges from 10 to 20 percent (Piacentini et al., 2014), although they are often misdiagnosed as ADHD or depression. It is now generally agreed that psychotherapy and pharmacotherapy are effective in treating anxiety disorders and maintaining improvements (Kodish et al., 2011; Rynn et al., 2011). SSRIs and CBT are evidence-based treatments. Recommended starting doses for SSRI treatment of childhood anxiety are fluvoxamine, 25 milligrams per day; fluoxetine, 10 milligrams per day; and sertraline, 25 milligrams per day. Lower starting doses can be used and doses can be increased as needed and tolerated. Continuation treatment is recommended for about 1 year following remission in symptoms, as some symptoms of anxiety persist, even among those children showing improvement after 12 weeks of treatment (Ginsburg et al., 2011). If symptoms return, medication reinitiation should be seriously considered.

The largest randomized, controlled treatment study of anxiety in children and youth, the Child/Adolescent Anxiety Multimodal Study, included 488 patients (74 percent less than 12 years old) with disorders of separation anxiety, generalized anxiety, or social phobia. After 12 weeks, a combination therapy of sertraline and CBT was associated with a significantly higher response rate (81 percent) than CBT alone (60 percent), sertraline alone (55 percent), or placebo (28 percent), based on a standardized clinician rating of severity of illness (Walkup et al., 2008). During maintenance treatment, 412 responders in the 3 active treatment groups continued their assigned treatments for an additional 6 months; 325 completed the extended treatment study. Overall, more than 80 percent of acute (within 12 weeks) responders maintained positive outcomes at 24 and 36 weeks (Piacentini et al., 2014). Long-term outcomes were assessed in a follow-up study with in-person or telephone interviews of children and parents at an average of 6 years after the study began (Ginsburg et al., 2014). Defined as a lack of any of the three study diagnoses—separation anxiety, generalized anxiety disorder, or social phobia—remission was found in 46.5 percent with no significant differences by original treatment assignment or interim treatment type. From a large number of variables analyzed, only male sex and higher family functioning significantly predicted remission.

Obsessive-Compulsive Disorder

There is little research on obsessive-compulsive disorder (OCD) in preschoolers. However, OCD may emerge in preschool children as early as 2 years of age, being more common in males (Coskun et al., 2012). As stated in a recent Pediatric OCD Treatment Study (POTSII), partial response to SSRIs is the norm and augmentation with short-term OCD-specific CBT provides additional benefit (Franklin et al., 2011). Study results revealed that 68 percent of OCD youths receiving medication management plus CBT strategy were considered responders, which was superior to 34 percent in the CBT group and 30 percent in the medication-only group.

Even so, nearly 30 percent of all young people diagnosed with OCD are resistant to SSRI plus CBT. Augmentation strategies include atypical antipsychotics. In a study by Masi and coworkers (2010), 39 adolescents (mean age 12 years) were titrated to a final dose of 12 milligrams of aripiprazole per day and the drug was effective in more than 50 percent of patients resistant to continuing SSRI therapy. (For further analyses, see the Brown University Child & Adolescent Psychopharmacology Update, 2011; Pessina et al., 2009.) D-cycloserine (DCS), a partial agonist at the glycine site of the N-methyl-D-aspartate receptor, enhanced fear extinction in preclinical studies. Fear extinction is a laboratory procedure in animals that is believed to be a model for assessing anxiety reduction. For this reason, Storch and coworkers (2016) tested DCS in children diagnosed with OCD. In an 8-week double-blind study, 142 children with OCD (mean age, 12.7; range, 7 to 17) received 10 sessions of family-based CBT and were randomized to augmentation with DCS or placebo. Both groups improved, with posttreatment response rates of 72 percent for placebo and 83 percent for DCS, but with no significant difference between them. Antidepressant use was unrelated to outcome.

Posttraumatic Stress Disorder

Strawn and coworkers (2010) in a meta-analysis of published literature noted that the data do not support the use of SSRIs as first-line treatments for posttraumatic stress disorder (PTSD) in children and adolescents. For example, *sertraline* (Zoloft) was ineffective in a placebo-controlled study in 131 youths (6 to 17 years) with PTSD (Robb et al., 2010). Limited evidence notes that atypical antipsychotics and several mood stabilizers may attenuate some symptoms, such as intrusive thoughts. Antiadrenergic agents, such as clonidine, guanfacine, and prazosin, can reduce symptoms such as hyperarousal, intrusive thoughts, and impulsivity. Other medications may be needed to target various associated PTSD symptoms such as depression, affect instability, disruptive behavior, and dysregulated attachment.

Cognitive inhibitors are not indicated for use in children and adolescents. This greatly limits the use of benzodiazepines, lithium, and tricyclic antidepressants. Currently, it is thought that prolonged exposure therapy and CBT are more effective in treating PTSD than is an SSRI or no treatment (Rothbaum et al., 2012).

MEDICATIONS FOR THE TREATMENT OF BIPOLAR DISORDER

It is commonly agreed that juvenile bipolar disorder is probably overdiagnosed, with other disorders such as ADHD, conduct disorder, oppositional defiant disorder, severe mood dysregulation or disruptive mood dysregulation disorder, and temper dysregulation disorder with dysphoria all frequently misdiagnosed as bipolar disorder (Hauser and Correll, 2013). In preschoolers, irritability, not elevated mood, seems to be the core feature (Parry and Levin, 2012). Studies have reported the efficacy of aripiprazole (Findling et al., 2012) and quetiapine (Joshi et al., 2012) in preschool-onset bipolar disorder. Seida and coworkers (2012) reviewed the safety and efficacy of second-generation antipsychotic medications in children and young adults. Luby and Navsaria (2010) discuss bipolar prodromal symptoms and early markers for the eventual development of the disorder. More than half of children with bipolar disorder experienced a prodromal period of greater than 1 year, and another 44 percent demonstrated a short-lasting, subacute prodrome (duration of between 1 month and 1 year). Symptoms included agitation, anxiety, appearing stubborn, bold and bossy behavior, decreased concentration, changes in sleep and mood, excitability, grandiosity, high energy, mood lability, and somatic complaints.

It is rarely a decision whether to treat or not to treat; when a youth is manic, the question is which medication to use rather than whether to use a medication (Goldstein, 2012). Geller and coworkers (2012), in a multicenter study, compared lithium, valproic acid, and risperidone in a trial termed Treatment of Early Age Mania (TEAM). The response rate for risperidone (68 percent) was significantly higher than the rate for lithium (36 percent) or valproic acid (24 percent). Quetiapine and aripiprazole, from other studies, are at least as effective as risperidone. These newer antipsychotic drugs differ mainly in their respective side effect profiles, particularly weight gain and metabolic abnormalities. Risperidone, aripiprazole, quetiapine, and olanzapine are all approved by the FDA for the treatment of bipolar youth as well as for the treatment of disruptive and aggressive behaviors. Doey (2012) reviewed clinical trials with aripiprazole (Abilify) and concluded that it was effective in youth with schizophrenia and bipolar disorder, as well as in populations with mixed symptoms. Findling and coworkers (2013) published the results of a 26-week study of aripiprazole in 210 youths aged 10 to 17 years old diagnosed with bipolar I with or without psychotic features. Doses of 10 and 30 milligrams per day were significantly more effective on all measures than placebo, although the rates of completing the study were low in all groups. Joshi and coworkers (2013) reported on the efficacy of paliperidone in a small, 8-week, open-label (not blinded) trial of bipolar youth. Doses of 3 and 6 milligrams per day significantly improved mania scores, but weight gain was substantial. Pathak and coworkers (2013) reported on the efficacy of quetiapine in a 3-week study in bipolar youth. The drug was more effective than placebo in improving manic symptoms.

While the use of valproic acid has been decreasing in youth with bipolar disorder, the use of *lamotrigine* (Lamictal) has been increasing (Tran et al., 2012). Biederman and coworkers (2010) demonstrated the efficacy of lamotrigine in a 12-week, open study in 39 children with bipolar disorder. Skin rashes did occur in some children, but the rashes resolved with cessation of drug treatment. Interestingly, lamotrigine use in pediatric bipolar disorder is associated with cognitive improvements, especially in the areas of working and verbal memory (Pavuluri et al., 2010). Egunsola and colleagues (2015) confirmed that rash was the most commonly reported adverse drug reaction (ADR), occurring in 7.3 percent of the pediatric patients. Stevens-Johnson syndrome was rarely reported, with a risk of 0.09 per 100 patients. Discontinuation due to an ADR was recorded in 72 children, that is, 1.9 percent of all treated patients.

Findling and coworkers (2015) conducted a multicenter, randomized, double-blind, placebo-controlled study of pediatric participants aged 7 to 17 years diagnosed with bipolar I with manic or mixed episodes, and compared lithium ($n = 53$) versus placebo ($n = 28$) for up to 8 weeks. Lithium was superior to placebo in reducing manic symptoms, with 47 percent either very much or much improved compared with placebo (21 percent very much or much improved). Not only was lithium generally well tolerated, it did not produce weight gain, which differs from other medications normally indicated for adolescents with bipolar disorder.

SSRI antidepressant therapy is generally discouraged in pediatric bipolar disorder. Occasionally an SSRI might be used, following mood stabilization with a mood stabilizer and if depression persists.

MEDICATIONS FOR TREATING AUTISM SPECTRUM DISORDERS

Autism is a pervasive developmental disorder characterized by severe impairment in several areas of development, including deficits in social interactions and communication skills, and the presence of stereotyped behavior, interests, and activities. Autism must present before age 3 and this is true of the many other disorders that are collectively called *autism spectrum disorders* (ASDs), such Asperger's syndrome. Medications do not cure ASDs, but may be effective in treating various behavioral symptoms that interfere with daily life and may cause impairment or distress (Kumar et al., 2012). Physical aggression and self-injurious behaviors are especially problematic in adolescents, whose large size and physical strength create additional danger. Medications can be quite useful in reducing the intensity and frequency of these behaviors (Propper and Orlik, 2011).

Historically, antidepressants were used in attempts to reduce the anxiety, agitation, and compulsiveness associated with autism (Doyle and McDougle, 2012), but lack of efficacy and a high incidence of side effects, such as behavioral activation and agitation, limit their use. Clomipramine may have some efficacy for the treatment of repetitive behaviors, stereotypies, and obsessiveness in some persons with an ASD.

Atypical antipsychotic drugs are clinically the most effective drugs for reducing aggression, irritability, and severe tantrums in youth with autism (Doyle and McDougle, 2012). Risperidone and aripiprazole are currently considered first-line therapy in child and adolescent autism, and are approved by the FDA for the treatment of irritability, aggression, and self-injurious behaviors. Paliperidone, the active metabolite of risperidone, has also been shown to be effective (Stigler et al., 2012). Weight gain, glucose intolerance, prolactin increases, and hyperlipidemia are limiting and are serious considerations in children and adolescents. Relevant reviews include Marcus et al. (2011), Ching and Pringsheim (2012), Elbe and Lalani (2012), Kirino (2012), and Pringsheim and Gorman (2012).

In the treatment of hyperactivity, impulsiveness, and attention deficit associated with ASD, traditional anti-ADHD medications, including methylphenidate, atomoxetine, and guanfacine (Scahill et al., 2015), and clonidine (Doyle and McDougle, 2012) have demonstrated modest efficacy. Side effects, mostly irritability, often limit therapeutic use.

MEDICATIONS FOR TREATING BEHAVIORAL OR AGGRESSIVE DISORDERS

Severe childhood aggression is one of the most challenging disorders to treat. Belden and coworkers (2012) noted that preschoolers diagnosed with psychiatric disorders were three times as likely as healthy preschoolers to be classified as aggressors, victims, and aggressive victims; children diagnosed with preschool-onset disruptive, depressive, and anxiety disorders were at least six times more likely to become aggressive victims during elementary school as are normal preschoolers. Nevels and coworkers (2010) discuss medication use in children, including treatment of aggression comorbid with ADHD.

Nonpharmacological treatments have advantages over medication treatment, but efficacy is variable. Once nonpharmacological approaches have been tried and found inadequate, the second choice is medication. Disruptive behavioral disorders include conduct disorder, oppositional defiant disorder, and disruptive behavior not otherwise specified (NOS). About 50 percent of youth with behavioral disruptive disorders progress to antisocial personality disorder as adults suggesting that their externalizing disruptive symptoms in childhood can be a marker for more pervasive psychopathology as adults.

Psychostimulants such as methylphenidate and amphetamine products, which are commonly used to treat ADHD, may ameliorate aggression, but comorbidity with conduct disorder is less responsive. *Mood stabilizers,* such as lithium, and anticonvulsants, such as lamotrigine and valproic acid, reduce aggressive behaviors in children with explosive tempers and mood lability (Pappadopulos et al., 2011). Requirements for frequent blood testing with some of these drugs may be unappealing to many patients and providers. *Atypical antipsychotic* medications are currently the mainstay in the treatment of aggressive disorders in children and adolescents. Risperidone and olanzapine (see Farmer et al., 2011) have been used to target aggressive behaviors, but they tend to cause weight gain and other adverse metabolic effects. Aripiprazole can be used and has a better side effect profile (Ercan et al., 2012).

To study polypharmacy, the NIH funded a multisite study, Treatment of Severe Child Aggression (TOSCA) (Farmer et al., 2011). This study began by administering the stimulant medication methylphenidate for 9 weeks to children 6 to 12 years old with ADHD and comorbid aggression, that is, oppositional defiant disorder or conduct disorder, while their parents received training in behavior management procedures. Children whose behaviors were not normalized received a second medication, either risperidone or placebo, by random assignment. The study results showed that the group that received methylphenidate and risperidone, showed significant improvement on average with moderately better behavior in anger, irritability, and aggression, according to parents, than children who received only methylphenidate. Parents also reported that children receiving both drugs were less likely to be impaired socially or academically by their anger and irritability than children receiving only the methylphenidate therapy (Gadow et al., 2014). McQuire and colleagues (2015) have confirmed that in the short-term, antipsychotics such as risperidone and aripiprazole can reduce some behavioral difficulties in children with intellectual disabilities. Unfortunately, the side effects of increased prolactin and weight gain were problematic. Efficacy of anticonvulsants and antioxidants for reducing challenging behavior was inconclusive. All evidence was of low quality and there was no information from long-term follow-up studies.

ANALGESICS IN CHILDHOOD AND ADOLESCENCE

Perhaps prompted by the ongoing prescription opiate epidemic, several recent studies have reviewed the epidemiology of pain and surveyed the use of opiate drugs in children and adolescents. Liossi and Howard (2016) report that in children and adolescents, the median prevalence of idiopathic pain is 11 to 38 percent. The highest rates are associated with headaches (23 to 51 percent), functional abdominal pain (2 to 41 percent), back pain (14 to 24 percent), and musculoskeletal pain (4 to 40 percent). High rates are also reported in children with organic diseases, such as sickle cell disease, and with persistent postoperative pain after major surgery. An annual survey of high school seniors between 1976 and 2015 compared the medical and nonmedical use of opiates (McCabe et al., 2017). Medical rates ranged from 13 to 20 percent and were higher than nonmedical use, which ranged from 6 to 13 percent. But the two were consistently and strongly correlated over time, especially among male adolescents, with medical use preceding nonmedical in those who reported both; and both uses declined between 2013 and 2015. Allen and colleagues (2017) compared opiate exposures of children and adolescents between 2000 and 2015. Most exposures occurred among children aged less than 5 years old (60 percent) and were unintentional (56 percent), whereas among adolescents (72 percent), exposures were intentional, including suspected suicide, abuse, and misuse. Consequently, it is not surprising that adolescents were more likely than other age groups to be admitted to a health care facility or have a serious outcome. Moreno (2015) found that nearly all accidental ingestions of opioids by children are due to family members leaving their medication in accessible locations in the home. Half of the adolescents who misused prescription opioids got them from past prescriptions that belonged to them, a family member, or a friend, and 8 percent shared these prescriptions with others.

Efforts have been made to address concerns raised by opiate misuse in youth. As reported by Budnitz and colleagues (2016), between 2008 and 2015, there was a threefold increase, from over 3 to over 9 million, in the number of buprenorphine and naloxone prescriptions dispensed. When prescriptions were dispensed as unit-dose tablet packages or film strips from 2013 to 2015, as opposed to multidose bottles from 2008 to 2010, there was a nearly two-thirds reduction in the rate of emergency room visits by children for buprenorphine or naloxone ingestion. An obvious conclusion is that modifications in packaging and formulation might prevent pediatric ingestions.

In April 2017, the FDA published a contraindication warning on codeine and tramadol drug labels stating that codeine should not be used to treat pain or cough, and that tramadol should not be used to treat pain in children younger than 12 years or to treat children younger than 18 years for pain after surgery to remove tonsils and adenoids. An additional warning recommended against the use of these two drugs in adolescents between 12 and 18 years who have conditions that may impair breathing, such as obesity, obstructive sleep apnea, or severe lung disease. Breast-feeding mothers were also warned not to take codeine or tramadol.

Unlike the warning in regard to codeine and tramadol, the opiate analgesic Oxycontin was approved by the FDA in August 2015 for a specific group of children who are 11 years or older who are in severe pain and have been prescribed an opioid for 5 days or more. In other words, Oxycontin is not meant to be administered to children as a first-line option or for a brief, acute pain reaction that might occur, such as the extraction of wisdom teeth. However, for years, this potent, long-acting drug has been used off-label to treat very sick children suffering pain from cancer or spinal fusion surgery. To guard against pediatric misuse, the FDA required postapproval studies from the manufacturer, Purdue Pharma. In one study, adverse events such as respiratory depression, overdoses, and accidental exposure must be reported for patients ages 11 to 17. Side effects and medication errors must be comprehensively analyzed.

In addition, Purdue will have to provide a national summary of the prescription volume for Oxycontin in children younger than 17, as well as the types of providers and the conditions for which it is prescribed (Saint-Louis, 2015).

Graudins and colleagues (2014) published the results of a double-blind, randomized, controlled trial comparing intranasal fentanyl and ketamine in children aged 3 to 13 years and weighing less than 110 pounds. Both drugs were associated with similar pain reduction (79 and 82 percent reduction in pain, respectively) in children with moderate to severe pain from limb injury, although ketamine was associated with more minor adverse events.

ATTENTION DEFICIT/HYPERACTIVITY DISORDER

Issues associated with attention deficit/hyperactivity disorder (ADHD) have generated much controversy. Current criteria for ADHD require that the symptoms of inattention and/or hyperactivity and impulsivity must be present before 12 years of age (DSM-5) and that they must be sufficiently severe to impair the individual's life functions. Emotional dysregulation has also been proposed as an additional category of impairment (Shaw et al., 2014). Although ADHD is commonly presented as the most common neurodevelopmental childhood disorder, conflicts abound, such as the question of whether it can be reliably diagnosed in preschool children, the role and side effects of medications in treatment, and the degree to which the childhood disorder persists or occurs de novo (for the first time) in adulthood. There is also some argument as to whether the condition actually exists as a real behavioral disorder or, if it does exist, whether it is overdiagnosed (Furey and Furey, 2014). To this end, some recent physiological measures have been proposed to make diagnoses more accurate (Fried et al., 2014; Helgadóttir et al., 2015).

During the past few years, a sharp increase in the rates and diagnoses of ADHD has been noted (Fairman et al., 2017), although whether that reflects a true increase in prevalence or other factors, such as methodological differences in diagnoses or the addition of adult patients, is also an ongoing issue (Polanczyk et al., 2014). It has been reported that 7 years after an initial diagnosis of ADHD in children between the ages of 3 and 6 years old, about 30 percent no longer met the criteria for the disorder, but were determined to have anxiety, autism, or a learning disorder, while about 12 percent had no behavioral disorder (Law et al., 2014).

Recent reviews (Chan et al., 2016; Feldman and Reiff, 2014) state that ADHD affects about 9.5 percent of U.S. children aged 3 to 17 years old. The current consensus is that one-third of those affected by ADHD in childhood continue to be affected into adulthood, with an estimated adult prevalence of 4.4 percent. In 2013, revised diagnostic criteria were included in the DSM-5, specifically regarding individuals aged 17 years or older, incorporating recent research supporting the long-term aspects of the disorder.

Medications for Treating ADHD

Medical treatment of ADHD is not new. Amphetamines such as Benzedrine and dextroamphetamine were used to treat ADHD as early as 1937; *methylphenidate* (Ritalin) was introduced in the United States in 1955 and formally approved by the

FDA for use in children in 1961. Since then, multiple formulations of stimulants have been marketed and nonstimulant products have appeared (See the Psychostimulant Table in Chapter 17).

Stimulant agents are still the first-line drug treatments of ADHD. They include the various short- and long-term formulations of methylphenidate and amphetamine. Second-tier drugs that have shown benefit are nonstimulants, such as atomoxetine and alpha-adrenergic agonists. Most clinical trials have compared the ADHD medications with placebo; there are few trials directly comparing ADHD medications to each other. Efforts to compare the stimulant and nonstimulant drugs through meta-analyses are inconsistent, sometimes but not always indicating that stimulants are more effective than nonstimulants (Bellino et al., 2014; Chan et al., 2016). There is some evidence that early recognition of the disorder and treatment during childhood will result in a better long-term adult outcome (Fredriksena et al., 2013). Guidelines and reviews for the pharmacological treatment of ADHD are available and generally support the use of current medications across the life span. One difference among countries is that drug treatment of preschool children and those with mild symptoms are more likely to be accepted in the United States compared to Europe (Chan et al., 2016; Bolea-Alamañac et al., 2014; Thapar and Cooper, 2016).

Methylphenidate

Because it is so widely used and because no one dosage regimen is ideal, multiple different dosage forms and methods of delivering methylphenidate to the bloodstream have been devised. *Methylphenidate* (Ritalin) is of rapid onset and short duration and must be administered two or three times daily—but not in the evening—to permit the blood level to drop and allow for normal sleep. The short half-life is a problem in some children who experience an end-of-dose rebound in dysfunctional behavior.

Dependable extended-release preparations have become available. The prototype is Concerta, an osmotic-release preparation that delays absorption and extends duration up to 12 hours. The product is prepared with 22 percent of the drug in a coating on the outside of the capsule for immediate release of the drug and 78 percent delivered by an "osmotic pump" that releases the drug over a 10-hour period in gradually increasing serum concentrations. One daily dose of Concerta yields about the same plasma concentrations as three daily doses of immediate-release methylphenidate and with essentially equal efficacy. Other new formulations of methylphenidate for oral administration are of two types:

1. Single-pulse, sustained-release formulations, such as Ritalin-SR, Metadate ER, and Methylin CD, use a wax matrix to prolong release. Their duration of action is about 8 hours, but may be unreliable compared with other preparations.

2. Beaded, double-pulse products, such as Ritalin LA, Focalin XR, and Metadate CD, use an extended release formulation with bimodal release. Ritalin LA and Focalin XR are composed of 50 percent of an immediate release formulation and 50 percent of enteric-coated, delayed-release beads. Metadate CD is composed of 30 percent immediate release beads and 70 percent delayed release beads that are released 4 hours later, eliminating the dose normally taken at midday with lunch.

In 2007, a transdermal methylphenidate delivery system, that is, a skin patch, sold under the trade name Daytrana, was introduced. The patch is applied daily, has a clinical onset of effect within 2 hours, and is worn for a maximum of 9 hours. Following removal, the effects of the methylphenidate continue for another 3 hours. Patches containing 10, 15, 20, and 30 milligrams are available. If removed before 9 hours, less drug is absorbed and the duration of action is decreased. In June 2015, the FDA warned that Daytrana may cause loss of skin color. The skin condition, chemical leukoderma, is not physically harmful, but the results are permanent. Patients and caregivers should notify their clinicians immediately if they observe new areas of lightened skin. The reported areas of pigmentation loss have included the area under the patch itself and spanned up to 8 inches in diameter.

A liquid suspension formulation of methylphenidate (Quillivant XR) is also approved by the FDA for ADHD. Efficacy was reported by Wigal and colleagues (2013) in a study of 45 children aged 6 to 12 years old. ADHD symptoms were reduced beginning at 45 minutes and continuing for 12 hours postdose.

Also, commercially available is *dexmethylphenidate* (d-methylphenidate or Focalin), the active D-isomer of methylphenidate. This isomer has twice the potency of methylphenidate, so the dose of dexmethylphenidate is one-half the dose of methylphenidate. Focalin is available in an extended-release formulation (Focalin XR).

Amphetamines

Amphetamines have been used for the treatment of ADHD since 1937. Safer (2016) reviewed recent trends in stimulant medication and found that the use of amphetamines has now surpassed methylphenidate, that total stimulant prescription sales to adults are now greater than those for youth, and that more adult women are prescribed stimulants than adult men.

Available amphetamines include *dextroamphetamine* (Dexedrine), *mixed amphetamine salts* (Adderall), an *extended-release formulation of Adderall* (Adderall XR), and *lisdexamfetamine* (Vyvanse). A transdermal amphetamine preparation is currently under development. In lisdexamfetamine, a molecule of dextroamphetamine is bonded to L-lysine, a naturally occurring amino acid, resulting in a molecule lacking biological activity, that is, a prodrug. When taken orally, the bond is broken by gastrointestinal enzymes and releasing the amphetamine, which is then absorbed. If crushed and injected, the bond is only slowly broken and theoretically, diversion to nonmedical use, that is, abuse, may be reduced. Doses of 10, 30, and 70 milligrams of lisdexamfetamine result in bioavailability of about 5 to 30 milligrams of dextroamphetamine (Goodman, 2010; Faraone et al., 2012). In 2015, the FDA approved lisdexamfetamine to treat binge-eating disorder, the first product to be approved for the condition.

New Formulations

Evekeo is a short-term immediate-release amphetamine similar to Adderall, except that it is composed of 50 percent of the 2 isomers, d- and l- amphetamine, whereas Adderall is 75 percent d-amphetamine and 25 percent l-amphetamine. It was approved in 2014 for the treatment of ADHD in patients 3 years of age and older; for narcolepsy, and as a short-term obesity treatment, when indicated, for patients 12 years of age or older.

In 2015, two new stimulant formulations were approved for the treatment of ADHD: QuilliChew ER and Dyanavel XR. Quillichew ER is a long-acting methylphenidate chewable tablet that allows once-daily dosing. It contains approximately 30 percent immediate release and 70 percent extended release methylphenidate. Methylin CT, approved in 2003, is also a methylphenidate formulation already available as a chewable tablet. The difference is that Methylin CT is a short-acting formulation, while QuilliChew ER offers the advantage of once-daily dosing.

Dyanavel XR is an extended-release oral suspension, a liquid formulation that contains a 3.2:1 ratio of the d- to l-amphetamine isomer (see Chapter 3), with immediate-release and extended-release components. It is the only extended-release liquid formulation for children 6 years and older. There are now liquid formulations available for both methylphenidate, Quillivant XR, and amphetamine, Dyanavel XR.

In January 2016, Adzenys, an extended-release amphetamine, was approved by the FDA for patients 6 years and older as the first extended-release drug for ADHD that dissolves in the mouth. That is, the drug is an orally disintegrating tablet, a longer-acting version of amphetamine. It is also the first to come in a blister pack, not a pill bottle, which makes it very portable and convenient.

In February 2016, the FDA approved a generic version of Adderall XR.

Did You Know?

New Drug Formulation Helps ADHD-Diagnosed Students Get Ready for School

A new formulation of long-acting methylphenidate for ADHD-diagnosed children and adolescents is under FDA review. The drug HLD200 was developed to provide stimulant exposure during the early morning hours, when children or adolescents usually wake up to prepare for school. Although current methylphenidate agents are given in the morning and can control symptoms for up to 12 hours, it may take 2 hours before they become active. As a result, in order for blood levels of the stimulant to be effective during the early morning hours, parents must wake their children up at 4 A.M. to administer the drug, and then both the child and the parent have to get back to sleep. The new pill is coated with two layers of a compound that prevents release of the drug until it has reached the colon. This means that, when given once at night, blood levels do not begin to increase until 8 hours after the drug is taken. The drug effectively improved morning routines such as being quiet; following directions; not being too distracted, hyperactive, talkative, or forgetful; and being more organized in dressing and getting to school. The results suggest that by early morning the blood levels are already sufficient to reduce the difficulties of preparing ADHD-diagnosed children for school (Pliszka et al., 2017).

Alternative Medications for Treating ADHD

About 10 to 30 percent of ADHD patients do not respond adequately to stimulants and are considered to be treatment-resistant. In addition, some children and their parents may desire that stimulants not be used. Therefore, there is a need for treatment alternatives for patients with ADHD and the three reviewed in this section are now approved for use by the FDA.

In 2003, the FDA approved *atomoxetine* (Strattera) for the acute treatment of child and adult ADHD. In 2008, the FDA expanded its approval to include indication for the maintenance treatment of ADHD in children and adolescents. That is, the drug has been demonstrated to continue to be effective for long-term treatment, not just for the immediate reduction of symptoms. This is the first selective norepinephrine reuptake inhibitor (SNRI) antidepressant approved for use in treating ADHD in children 6 years of age and older as well as in adults. At a daily dose of about 1.4 to 1.8 milligrams per kilogram of body weight, the drug is effective in reducing ADHD symptoms (Bushe and Savill, 2014; Kratochvil et al., 2011). A U.K. study of 201 children with ADHD reported that atomoxetine was more effective in treatment-naive patients than in patients who had been previously treated with stimulant medication (Prasad et al., 2007), suggesting that it might be beneficial for patients to try a trial of atomoxetine prior to initiation of stimulants. It may take up to 4 weeks for atomoxetine to be effective and 12 weeks for maximum efficacy (Bushe and Savill, 2014). Abuse potential appears to be minimal (Upadhyaya et al., 2013). Schwartz and Correll (2014) review, and confirm, the safety and effectiveness of atomoxetine as monotherapy for pediatric ADHD and Asherson et al. (2014) and Camporeale and their colleagues (2015) review its use in adults. However, in children and adolescents who had an inadequate response to methylphenidate, atomoxetine was found to be less therapeutically effective than lisdexamfetamine (Nagy et al., 2016).

Two CNS-acting antihypertensive (blood pressure-lowering) alpha-2 agonists in extended release formulation—*clonidine* (Kapvay) and *guanfacine* (Intuniv)—are approved by the FDA for the treatment of ADHD, either as monotherapy or used concomitantly with a stimulant. Bukstein and Head (2012) report that guanfacine-ER works better as an adjunct to stimulants rather than as a sole agent. Jain et al. (2011) detailed the efficacy of extended-release clonidine with a daily dosage of 0.2 and 0.4 milligrams in reducing inattention scores and hyperactivity and impulsivity scores. These two drugs are, however, generally considered to be second-line medications. Sedation and fatigue are common side effects, but these side effects are not limiting and decrease with the duration of treatment (Faraone and Glatt, 2010). Guanfacine has modest efficacy at a dose of 2 to 4 milligrams per day, a longer half-life than clonidine, and is less sedating.

Newcorn and colleagues (2016) have reported a long-term efficacy study of guanfacine extended-release, showing that patients who continued on the drug were less likely to have a relapse of their ADHD symptoms compared to patients who were withdrawn from the drug. Hirota and colleagues (2014) reviewed the use of the two alpha-2 agonists for ADHD in youth, as both monotherapy or as an add-on to stimulant therapy. Results were modest, with more hypotension, bradycardia, and QTc prolongation than placebo.

Although not approved for the treatment of ADHD, tricyclic antidepressants (especially nortriptyline; see Chapter 12) have been studied and have occasionally been reported to be effective. However, cognitive impairments, limited efficacy, and rare cases of potentially fatal cardiac toxicities associated with tricyclic antidepressant use in children and adolescents pose considerable limitations (Otasowie et al., 2014).

Clinical Trial Outcomes

The Preschool ADHD Treatment Study (PATS) first demonstrated the potential utility of methylphenidate for treating ADHD in preschoolers (Greenhill et al., 2006). At an average daily dose of 14 milligrams, immediate-release methylphenidate, with a range of 7.5 to 30 milligrams divided into three daily increments, produced significant reduction on scores of ADHD symptom scales, although efficacy was less than that cited for school-age children (Abikoff et al., 2009). In a 10-month continuation phase of the PATS study, with gradual dose increases, efficacy could be maintained, but significant variability was observed, with many subjects dropping out of the study due to adverse drug effects or worsening behaviors (Vitiello et al., 2007).

Riddle and coworkers (2013) reported on a 6-year follow-up of the original PATS participants. Symptom severity initially decreased from baseline to year 3, but then remained relatively stable and in the moderate-to-severe range through year 6 of treatment. Overall, 89 percent met ADHD symptoms and impairment criteria. The authors conclude that the "course (of ADHD over 6 years) is generally chronic, with high symptom severity and impairment, in very young children with moderate-to-severe ADHD, despite treatment with medication" (264).

As noted above, aggressive behavior in children has been treated with antipsychotics as well as stimulants. This is consistent with a study by Aman and colleagues (2014). In a group of 168 patients aged 6 to 12 years old and diagnosed with ADHD and either conduct disorder or oppositional defiant disorder, they reported that risperidone combined with a stimulant produced better scores on aggression ratings than the stimulant alone.

The classic Multimodal Treatment Study of Children with Attention-Deficit/Hyperactivity Disorder (MTA Cooperative Group, 1999) included a cohort of 579 children with ADHD assigned to 14 months of (1) medication management; (2) intensive behavior treatment; (3) combined medication and CBT treatment; or (4) standard community care. Carefully structured medication management resulted in a better outcome than did intensive CBT treatment. Combined treatment yielded an outcome that was better than the outcome of CBT treatment, but equivalent to the outcome of medication management. A 24-month follow-up of the MTA study (MTA Cooperative Group, 2004) showed that cessation of drug therapy was associated with clinical deterioration; continued drug therapy was associated with only mild deterioration; and stimulant initiation in the group not receiving stimulants in the early study was associated with clinical improvements.

At 8 years, 33 percent of the original participants were still receiving medication, usually stimulants (83 percent) (Molina et al., 2009). While improvements seen at the end of the 14-month study were generally maintained, MTA participants were not "normalized," with 30 percent still meeting the criteria for ADHD. Clinically significant antisocial behavior was present in 25 to 30 percent of MTA participants; 25 percent met criteria for oppositional defiant disorder or conduct disorder; 27 percent had been arrested at least one time; and 30 percent reportedly had moderate to serious delinquent behavior. Academically, medicated children with ADHD had significant improvements in mathematics and reading scores over untreated children with ADHD, but these improvements were insufficient to eliminate the test score gap between children with ADHD and those without (Barnard-Brak and Brak, 2011).

The MTA trial became a long-term observational study that included 515 of the original study participants as well as 289 individuals from the same schools, recruited to provide a local normal comparison group. Follow-up data in adulthood were available for 92.4 percent of the ADHD group and for 93.4 percent of the non-ADHD comparison group who started the observational phase. After they had reached adulthood, the participants completed the Conners Adult ADHD Rating Scale to determine symptom persistence. The results showed that those who continued to receive medications showed no differences in symptom severity in comparison to those who took treatment holidays or who stopped treatment altogether. That is, there was still a significant difference in symptom severity between the overall ADHD group and the comparison group. Furthermore, the outcome was the same whether the ADHD medication was used consistently, inconsistently, or minimally (Swanson and the MTA Cooperative Group, 2017).

In addition to the results of this classic longitudinal study, two other significant reviews have recently questioned the benefit of stimulant treatment for ADHD in children and adolescents. Punja et al. (2016) summarized the data for amphetamines in patients aged 3 to 17 years. The latter group found that the total ADHD core symptom severity scores were improved by amphetamines, according to the ratings of parents, teachers, and clinicians, and that the proportion of those who improved was higher when children were taking amphetamines. The most commonly reported adverse events were reduced appetite, insomnia, trouble sleeping, abdominal pain, nausea, vomiting, headaches, and anxiety. Punja and colleagues, however, stated that most of the included studies were at high risk of bias and they criticized the overall quality of the evidence as being low to very low on most outcomes. The methylphenidate analysis of Storebø and colleagues (2015) was even more negative. While the results did suggest that methylphenidate improved "teacher-reported ADHD symptoms, teacher-reported general behavior, and parent-reported quality of life among children and adolescents diagnosed with ADHD" (2), the authors severely criticized the poor quality of the evidence. This negative conclusion elicited a strong rebuttal from Banaschewski and colleagues (2016), who argue that "the study selection is flawed and undertaken without sufficient scientific justification resulting in an underestimation of effect sizes, which, furthermore, are inadmissibly clinically interpreted. The methodology of the assessment of bias and quality is not objective and cannot be substantiated by the data" (307).

Perhaps one way of understanding this extensive literature on the effectiveness of the stimulant medications for ADHD is to acknowledge that the drugs do not influence the underlying symptomatology, but rather, modulate the expression of the affected behavior. In addition, age alone may modify the severity of the disorder and the need for medications may decrease with maturity.

ADHD in Adults

Although classically considered a disorder of childhood, the last decade has seen evidence showing that ADHD continues to impair function into adulthood and that it responds to pharmacotherapy. Research studies have suggested that 30 to 70 percent of children with ADHD continue to have symptoms of the disorder when they become adults. The DSM-5 criteria require that adults must have had multidimensional ADHD symptoms before the age of 12. In addition to identification of a childhood disorder that might have been ADHD, an adult diagnosis also also (1) must document at least five ongoing, significant symptoms of either inattention or hyperactivity and impulsivity; (2) must show significant behavioral or functional impairment in at least two settings, such as home, work, school, or social, that are due to the ADHD symptoms; and (3) the symptoms must be interpreted best as ADHD rather than some other condition.

Several studies have now provided evidence that ADHD not only can continue into adulthood, but that there is also a late-onset variation of the disorder without a childhood diagnosis (Agnew-Blaise et al., 2016; Caye et al., 2016). One of these studies even concluded that 90 percent of participants with adult ADHD did not have a history of childhood ADHD (Moffitt et al., 2015).

With regard to medications, Lensing and colleagues (2015) reported that most adults aged 50 and above with ADHD reported regular pharmacotherapy for ADHD, that their attention was improved by the drugs, and that employment was associated with more favorable outcomes. Grebla and colleagues (2016) found that in total, 56.9 percent of adults with ADHD used long-acting monotherapy, 30.7 percent used short-acting monotherapy, and 12.5 percent combined different ADHD medications. Bushe and colleagues (2016) reported that the efficacy of atomoxetine and OROS methylphenidate in adults does not differ significantly. Modafinil was reasonably tolerated by adults with ADHD, but it did not demonstrate a benefit for symptoms (Arnold et al., 2014). Rucklidge and colleagues (2014) have even seen benefits from a micronutrient formula containing all vitamins (except K) and 16 minerals at 2 to 400 times the recommended daily allowance.

Side Effects of Stimulant Medications

Common side effects of stimulant medications include insomnia, elevations in blood pressure and heart rate, reduction in appetite, and possible growth suppression. There have been some conflicting data with regard to this last side effect, with one review reporting reduced height in adults diagnosed in childhood (Swanson et al., 2017) and another study finding no difference in ultimate height, albeit with a developmental delay in ADHD-treated youth (Harstad et al., 2014). The difference may be due to the extent of long-term (including current) stimulant use and mitigation by drug holidays (Ibrahim and Donyai, 2015).

Other potential side effects include adverse psychiatric problems, including new or worsening behavioral and thought problems, new or worsening bipolar illness, new or worsening aggressive or hostility problems, and in children and teenagers, new psychiatric symptoms, including hearing voices, believing things that are not true, increased suspiciousness, or new manic symptoms, especially if there is a familial predisposition

(MacKenzie et al., 2015). All these effects are predictable consequences seen in some people using any psychostimulant, whether for therapeutic purposes or for abuse purposes.

Stimulants may delay growth initially, but a rebound may occur in later adolescence, producing a BMI greater than that in children without a history of ADHD or stimulant use, which has significant implications (Schwartz et al., 2014).

As long ago as the 1990s, case reports of sudden, unexplained deaths in children raised concerns about stimulant use. The FDA ultimately requested in 2006 that a warning be added to the package inserts of these drugs, noting that the medications should not be prescribed for children or adolescents with known heart problems, such as cardiomyopathy or rhythm disturbances, which could increase the likelihood of adverse cardiac reactions. Furthermore, Dalsgaard and coworkers (2014) found an increase in overall cardiovascular events in stimulant users, whether ADHD patients or not, although the total risk was low (see also Kelly et al., 2014). Shin and coworkers (2016) report an increased risk of arrhythmias—but not stroke or myocardial infarction—from methylphenidate, with the highest risk soon after the start of treatment.

An important concern with ADHD medication is whether exposure to stimulants might increase future stimulant abuse. ADHD itself has been associated with an increased likelihood of substance abuse (Kolla et al., 2016; Sundquista et al., 2014). However, stimulant medication appears either to reduce this association (Davis et al., 2015; McCabe et al., 2016) or, at least, not increase the probability (Humphreys et al., 2013). ADHD patients who receive consistent stimulant treatment are also less likely to start smoking (Schoenfelder et al., 2014). Drug abuse co-occurring with ADHD is associated with other behavioral problems, such as antisocial behavior (Muld et al., 2013), and represents a difficult psychiatric situation (Cunill et al., 2015). A related concern, which has received extensive attention, is the issue of nonmedical stimulant use, particularly among college students. Most reviews confirm that such nonmedical use is primarily to improve academic performance rather than recreational. (For a thorough discussion of this problem, see Benson et al., 2015; Cassidy et al., 2015; and Wilens et al., 2016.)

Although side effects are normally considered to be a negative consequence of drug treatments, there are numerous positive effects of stimulant drugs on the behavior of children and adults that might not be typically appreciated. Lisdexamfetamine has been shown to improve "emotional lability" in children diagnosed with ADHD (Childress et al., 2014). Other medications have reportedly reduced the risk for new-onset depression (Chang et al., 2016), suicidality (Chen et al., 2014) and trauma and injury (Dalsgaard et al., 2015a; Man et al., 2015), including vehicular accidents (Chang et al., 2017), in persons with ADHD who have more than double the risk for premature death from unnatural and accidental causes compared to those without ADHD (Dalsgaard et al., 2015b). Stimulants also do not increase the risk of tics (muscle spasms) (Cohen et al., 2015). This is an important finding, because about half of patients with tics have comorbid ADHD and about 20 percent of ADHD patients have tic disorders. Waxmonsky and colleagues (2014) have even found that parent–child interactions improved when adults with ADHD were treated with medication. Specifically, parents praised their children more and engaged in less negative talk.

In the Pipeline

EB-1020 is an experimental dopamine-norepinephrine reuptake inhibitor shown to be effective in an animal model of ADHD (Bymaster et al., 2012). This drug may have both antidepressant and anti-ADHD activity.

Mazindol is a known imidazoisoindole derivative and not related to amphetamines or metabolized to an amphetaminelike compound. It blocks dopamine and norepinephrine reuptake similarly to amphetamine. According to data from one preliminary study, mazindol could be an efficacious ADHD medication that is well tolerated and of long duration, that is, over 8 hours, in children (Konofal et al., 2014).

Dasotraline—(1R,4S)-4-(3,4-Dichlorophenyl)-1,2,3,4-tetrahydronaphthalen-1-amine—is a novel compound that acts as a potent inhibitor of human dopamine transporters, norepinephrine transporters, and a weaker inhibitor of human serotonin transporters. One study (Koblan et al., 2015) provided preliminary evidence that once-daily dosing may be a safe and efficacious treatment for adult ADHD. Sunovion Pharmaceuticals announced that dasotraline significantly improved symptoms of ADHD in children for up to 24 hours in a phase III study. Results were presented at the 6th World Congress on ADHD in 2017. In November 2017, the FDA agreed to review the New Drug Application for dasotraline submitted by the Sunovion company.

STUDY QUESTIONS

1. Discuss the designated categories of risk for drugs administered during pregnancy.

2. What are the consequences of various drugs of abuse on the fetus?

3. What are the congenital effects of antidepressants?

4. How does the drug treatment of depression in children and adolescents differ from that of adults?

5. What types of drugs are used to address disruptive behaviors in autism spectrum disorders and aggressive behavior in children generally?

6. Which psychotropic drug category appears to be the safest in regard to birth defects?

7. Which psychotropic drug category is associated with the greatest likelihood of birth defects?

8. Describe the use of analgesics in children.

9. Compare the characteristics of ADHD in children versus adults. Do they differ? Do the treatments differ?

10. What new drugs are being developed for treatment of ADHD?

REFERENCES

Abikoff, H., et al., (2009). "Effects of MPH-OROS on the Organizational, Time Management, and Planning Behaviors of Children With ADHD." *Journal of the American Academy of Child & Adolescent Psychiatry* 48: 166–175.

Agaku, I. T., et al. (2016). "Prevalence and Determinants of Secondhand Smoke Exposure Among Middle and High School Students." *Pediatrics* 137: 1–9. doi: 10.1542/peds.2015-1985.

Agnew-Blais, J. C., et al. (2016). "Evaluation of the Persistence, Remission, and Emergence of Attention-Deficit/Hyperactivity Disorder in Young Adulthood." *JAMA Psychiatry* 73: 713–720. doi: 10.1001/jamapsychiatry.2016.0465.

Allen, J. D., et al. (2017). "Prescription Opioid Exposures Among Children and Adolescents in the United States: 2000–2015." *Pediatrics* 139: 110. doi: 10.1542/peds/2016-3382.

Aman, M. G., et al. (2014). "What Does Risperidone Add to Parent Training and Stimulant for Severe Aggression in Child Attention-Deficit/Hyperactivity Disorder?" *Journal of the American Academy of Child and Adolescent Psychiatry* 53: 47–60. doi: 10.1016/j/jaac.213.09.022.

American College of Obstetricians and Gynecologists Committee on Obstetric Practice. (2015). "Committee Opinion No. 637: Marijuana Use during Pregnancy and Lactation." *Obstetrics and Gynecology* 26: 234–238. doi: 10.1097/01.AOG.0000467192.89321.a6.

Ammerman, S., et al. (2015). "The Impact of Marijuana Policies on Youth: Clinical, Research, and Legal Update." *Pediatrics* 135: e769–e785. doi: 10.1542/peds.2014-4147.

Amnesty International. (2017). "Criminalizing pregnancy: Policing pregnant women who use drugs in the USA." Index number: AMR 51/6435/2017. Retrieved from: https://www.amnesty.org/en/documents/amr51/6435/2017/en/

Andrade, C. (2014). "The Safety of Duloxetine during Pregnancy and Lactation." *Journal of Clinical Psychiatry* 75: e1423–e1427.

Andrade, C. (2016). "Adverse Outcomes Following Serotonin Reuptake Inhibitor Exposure During Pregnancy." *Journal of Clinical Psychiatry* 77: e199–e200.

Arnold, V. K., et al. (2014). "A 9-Week, Randomized, Double-Blind, Placebo-Controlled, Parallel-Group, Dose-Finding Study to Evaluate the Efficacy and Safety of Modafinil as Treatment for Adults With ADHD." *Journal of Attention Disorders* 18: 133–144.

Asherson, P., et al. (2014). "Efficacy of Atomoxetine in Adults with Attention Deficit Hyperactivity Disorder: An Integrated Analysis of the Complete Database of Multicenter Placebo-Controlled Trials." *Journal of Psychopharmacology* 28: 837–846. doi: 10.1177/0269881114542453.

Banach, R., et al. (2010). "Long-Term Developmental Outcome of Children of Women with Epilepsy, Unexposed or Exposed Prenatally to Antiepileptic Drugs: A Meta-Analysis of Cohort Studies." *Drug Safety* 33: 73–79.

Banaschewski, T., et al. (2016). "Trust, but Verify. The Errors and Misinterpretations in the Cochrane Analysis by O. J. Storebo and Colleagues on the Efficacy and Safety of Methylphenidate for the Treatment of Children and Adolescents with ADHD." *Zeitschrift für Kinder- und Jugendpsychiatrie und Psychotherapie* 44: 307–314. doi: 10.1024/1422-4917/a000433.

Barnard-Brak, L., and Brak, V. (2011). "Pharmacotherapy and Academic Achievement among Children with Attention-Deficit Hyperactivity Disorder." *Journal of Child & Adolescent Psychopharmacology* 21: 597–603.

Battle, C. L., et al. (2014). "Clinical Correlates of Perinatal Bipolar Disorder in an Interdisciplinary Obstetrical Hospital Setting." *Journal of Affective Disorders* 158: 97–100.

Bechtold, J., et al. (2015). "Chronic Adolescent Marijuana Use as a Risk Factor for Physical and Mental Health Problems in Young Adult Men." *Psychology of Addictive Behaviors* 29: 552–563. doi: 10.1037/adb0000103.

Bechtold, J., et al. (2016). "Concurrent and Sustained Cumulative Effects of Adolescent Marijuana Use on Subclinical Psychotic Symptoms." *American Journal of Psychiatry* 173: 781–789. doi: 10.1176/appi.ajp.2016.15070878.

Belden, A. C., et al. (2012). "Relational Aggression in Children with Preschool-Onset Psychiatric Disorders." *Journal of the American Academy of Child and Adolescent Psychiatry* 51: 889–901.

Bellino, S., et al. (2014). "Pharmacological Treatment of Attention Deficit Hyperactivity Disorder (ADHD): A Systematic Review of Recent Data." *Current Psychopharmacology* 3: 93–107

Benson, K., et al. (2015). "Misuse of Stimulant Medication among College Students: A Comprehensive Review and Meta-analysis" *Clinical Child and Family Psychology Review* 18: 50–76. doi: 10.1007/s10567–014–0177-z.

Bérard, A., et al. (2015). "Sertraline use During Pregnancy and the Risk of Major Malformations." *American Journal of Obstetrics and Gynecology* 212: 795.e1–795.e12. doi: 10.1016/j. ajog.2015.01.034. PMID: 25637841.

Bérard, A., et al. (2016). "The Risk of Major Cardiac Malformations Associated with Paroxetine Use During the First Trimester Of Pregnancy: A Systematic Review And Meta-Analysis." *British Journal of Pharmacology* 81: 589–604. doi: 10.1111/bcp.12849.

Bérard, A., et al. (2017). "Antidepressant use During Pregnancy and the Risk of Major Congenital Malformations in a Cohort of Depressed Pregnant Women: An Updated Analysis of the Quebec Pregnancy Cohort." *BMJ Open* 7: e013372.

Biederman, J., et al. (2010). "A Prospective Open-Label Trial of Lamotrigine Monotherapy in Children and Adolescents with Bipolar Disorder." *CNS Neuroscience & Therapeutics* 16: 91–102.

Bold, K. W., et al. (2016). "Reasons for Trying E-Cigarettes and Risk of Continued Use." *Pediatrics* 139: 1–8. doi: 10.1542/pediatrics.2016–0895.

Bolea-Alamañac, B., et al. (2014). "Evidence-Based Guidelines for the Pharmacological Management of Attention Deficit Hyperactivity Disorder: Update on Recommendations from the British Association for Psychopharmacology." *Journal of Psychopharmacology* 28: 179–203. doi: 10.1177/0269881113519509.

Brent, D. A., et al. (2008). "Switching to Another SSRI or to Venlafaxine with or without Cognitive Behavioral Therapy for Adolescents with SSRI-Resistant Depression." *JAMA* 299: 901–913.

Brent, D. A., and Gibbons, R. (2014). "Initial Dose of Antidepressant and Suicidal Behavior in Youth: Start Low, Go Slow." *JAMA Internal Medicine* 74: 909–111. doi: 10.1001/ jamainternmed.2013.14016.

Bromley, R. L., et al. (2008). "Autism Spectrum Disorders Following *in utero* Exposure to Antiepileptic Drugs." *Neurology* 71: 1923–1924.

Brown University Child & Adolescent Psychopharmacology Update. (2011). "Adding Full CBT Shows Best Response in Pediatric SRI-Partial Responders with OCD." *Brown University Child & Adolescent Psychopharmacology Update* 13: 1–4.

Brown, A. S., et al. (2016). "Association of Selective Serotonin Reuptake Inhibitor Exposure During Pregnancy with Speech, Scholastic, and Motor Disorders in Offspring." *JAMA Psychiatry* 73: 1163–1170. doi: 10.1001/jamapsychiatry.2016.2594.

Brown, H. K., et al. (2017). "Association Between Serotonergic Antidepressant Use During Pregnancy and Autism Spectrum Disorder in Children." *JAMA.* 317: 1544–1552. doi: 10.1001/ jama.2017.3415.

Buchy, L., et al. (2015). "Evaluating the Impact of Cannabis Use on Thalamic Connectivity in Youth at Clinical High Risk of Psychosis." *BMC Psychiatry* 15: 276.

Buck, J. M., and Siegel, J. A. (2015). "The Effects of Adolescent Methamphetamine Exposure." *Frontiers in Neuroscience* 9: 151. doi: 10.3389/fnins.2015.00151.

Budnitz, D. S., et al. (2016). *Notes from the Field:* Pediatric Emergency Department Visits for Buprenorphine/Naloxone Ingestion—United States, 2008–2015. MMWR Morbidity and Mortality Weekly Reports 65: 1148–1149.

Bukstein, O. G., and Head, J. (2012). "Guanfacine ER for the Treatment of Adolescent Attention-Deficit Hyperactivity Disorder." *Expert Opinion on Pharmacotherapy* 13: 2207–2213.

Bushe, C., et al. (2016). "A Network Meta-Analysis of Atomoxetine and Osmotic Release Oral System Methylphenidate in the Treatment Of Attention Deficit/Hyperactivity Disorder in Adult Patients." *Journal of Psychopharmacology* 30: 444–458. doi: 10.1177/0269881116636105.

Bushe, C. J., and Savill, N. C. (2014). "Systematic Review of Atomoxetine Data in Childhood and Adolescent Attention-Deficit Hyperactivity Disorder 2009–2011: Focus on Clinical Efficacy and Safety." *Journal of Psychopharmacology* 28: 204–211. doi: 10.1177/0269881113478475.

Bushnell, G. A., et al. (2015). "Dosing of Selective Serotonin Reuptake Inhibitors among Children and Adults Before and After the FDA Black-Box Warning." *Psychiatric Services* (Washington, D.C.) 67: 302–309. doi: 10.1176/appi.ps.201500088.

Bymaster, F. P., et al. (2012). "Pharmacological Characterization of the Norepinephrine and Dopamine Reuptake Inhibitor EB-1020: Implications for Treatment of Attention-Deficit/Hyperactivity Disorder." *Synapse* 66: 522–532.

Camchong, J., et al. (2017). "Adverse Effects of Cannabis on Adolescent Brain Development: A Longitudinal Study." *Cerebral Cortex* 27: 1922–1930. doi: 10.1093/cercor/bhw015.

Camporeale, A., et al. (2015). "Safety and Tolerability of Atomoxetine in Treatment of Attention Deficit Hyperactivity Disorder in Adult Patients: An Integrated Analysis of 15 Clinical Trials." *Journal of Psychopharmacology* 29: 3–14.

Cassidy, T. A., et al. (2015). "Nonmedical Use and Diversion of ADHD Stimulants Among U.S. Adults Ages 18–49 A National Internet Survey." *Journal of Attention Disorders* 19: 630–640.

Castellanos, D., and Gralnik, L. M. (2016). "Synthetic Cannabinoids 2015: An Update for Pediatricians in Clinical Practice." *World Journal of Clinical Pediatrics* 5: 16–24.

Caye, A., et al. (2016). "Attention-Deficit/Hyperactivity Disorder Trajectories from Childhood to Young Adulthood: Evidence from a Birth Cohort Supporting a Late-Onset Syndrome." *JAMA Psychiatry* 73: 705–712. doi: 10.1001/jamapsychiatry.2016.0383.

Cerdá, M., et al. (2016) "Persistent Cannabis Dependence and Alcohol Dependence Represent Risks for Midlife Economic and Social Problems: A Longitudinal Cohort Study." *Clinical Psychological Science* 4: 1028–1046. doi: 10.1177/2167702616630958.

Cervesi, C., et al. (2017). "Extent, Time Course, and Moderators of Antipsychotic Treatment in Youth with Mood Disorders: Results of a Meta-Analysis and Meta-Regression Analyses." *Journal of Clinical Psychiatry* 78: 347–357. doi: 10.4088/JCP.15r10435.

Chan, E., et. al. (2016). "Treatment of Attention-Deficit/Hyperactivity Disorder in Adolescents: A Systematic Review." *JAMA* 315: 1997–2008. doi: 10.1001/jama.2016.5453.

Chang, Z., et al. (2016). "Medication for Attention-Deficit/Hyperactivity Disorder and Risk for Depression: A Nationwide Longitudinal Cohort Study." *Biological Psychiatry* 80: 916–922.

Chang, Z., et al. (2017). "Association Between Medication Use for Attention-Deficit/ Hyperactivity Disorder and Risk of Motor Vehicle Crashes." *JAMA Psychiatry* 74: 597–603. doi: 10.1001/jamapsychiatry.2017.0659.

Chen, Q., et al. (2014). "Drug Treatment for Attention-Deficit/Hyperactivity Disorder and Suicidal Behaviour: Register Based Study." *BMJ* 18: 348: g3769. doi: 10.1136/bmj.g3769.

Childress, A. C., et al. (2014). "The Effects of Lisdexamfetamine Dimesylate on Emotional Lability in Children 6 to 12 Years of Age with ADHD in a Double-Blind Placebo-Controlled Trial." *Journal of Attention Disorders* 18: 123–132.

Ching, H. and Pringsheim, T. (2012). "Aripiprazole for Autism Spectrum Disorders (ASD)." *Cochrane Database of Systematic Reviews* 16: CD009043.

Christensen, J., et al. (2013). "Prenatal Valproate Exposure and Risk of Autism Spectrum Disorders and Childhood Autism." *JAMA* 309: 1696–703. doi: 10.1001/jama.2013.2270.

Christensen, J., et al. (2015). "Apgar-Score in Children Prenatally Exposed to Antiepileptic Drugs: A Population-Based Cohort Study." *BMJ Open* 5: e007425. doi: 10.1136/bmjopen-2014–007425.

Cipriani, A., et al. (2016). "Comparative Efficacy and Tolerability of Antidepressants for Major Depressive Disorder in Children and Adolescents: A Network Meta-Analysis." *Lancet* 388: 881–890. doi: 10.1016/S0140-6736(16)30385-3.

Clark, D. B., et al. (2016). "Screening for Underage Drinking and *Diagnostic and Statistical Manual of Mental Disorders*, 5th Edition Alcohol Use Disorder in Rural Primary Care Practice." *Journal of Pediatrics* 173: 214–220. doi: 10.1016/j.jpeds.2016.02.047.

Clayton, H. B., et al. (2017). "Health Risk Behaviors with Synthetic Cannabinoids Versus Marijuana." *Pediatrics* 139: e20162675. doi: 10.1542/peds.2016–2675.

Clements, C. C., et al. (2015). "Prenatal Antidepressant Exposure is Associated with Risk for Attention-Deficit Hyperactivity Disorder but Not Autism Spectrum Disorder in a Large Health System." *Molecular Psychiatry* 20: 727–734. doi: 10.1038/mp.2014.90.

Cohen, S. C., et al. (2015). "Meta-Analysis: Risk of Tics Associated with Psychostimulant Use in Randomized, Placebo-Controlled Trials." *Journal of the American Academy of Child and Adolescent Psychiatry* 54: 728–736. doi: 10.1016/j.jaac.2015.06.011.

Cohen, L. S., et al. (2016). "Reproductive Safety of Second-Generation Antipsychotics: Current Data from the Massachusetts General Hospital National Pregnancy Registry for Atypical Antipsychotics." *American Journal of Psychiatry* 173: 263–270. doi: 10.1176/appi.ajp.2015.15040506.

Copeland, W. E., et al. (2015). "Adult Functional Outcomes of Common Childhood Psychiatric Problems: A Prospective Longitudinal Study." *JAMA Psychiatry* 72: 892–899. doi: 10.1001/jamapsychiatry.2015.0730.

Coskun, M., et al. (2012). "Phenomenology, Psychiatric Comorbidity and Family History in Referred Preschool Children with Obsessive-Compulsive Disorder." *Child & Adolescent Psychiatry and Mental Health* 6: 36–44.

Cunill, R., et al. (2015). "Pharmacological Treatment of Attention Deficit Hyperactivity Disorder with Co-Morbid Drug Dependence." *Journal of Psychopharmacology* 29:15–23. doi: 10.1177/0269881114544777.

Cousins, L., and Goodyer, I. M. (2015). "Antidepressants and the Adolescent Brain." *Journal of Psychopharmacology* 29: 545–555.

Cuzen, N. L., et al. (2015). "Methamphetamine and Cannabis Abuse in Adolescence: A Quasiexperimental Study on Specific and Long-Term Neurocognitive Effects." *BMJ Open* 5: e005833. doi: 10.1136/bmjopen-2014- 005833.

Dalsgaard, S., et al. (2014). "Cardiovascular Safety of Stimulants in Children with Attention-Deficit/Hyperactivity Disorder: A Nationwide Prospective Cohort Study." *Journal of Child and Adolescent Psychopharmacology* 24: 302–310. doi: 10.1089/cap.2014.0020.

Dalsgaard, S., et al. (2015a). "Effect of Drugs on The Risk of Injuries in Children with Attention Deficit Hyperactivity Disorder: A Prospective Cohort Study." *Lancet Psychiatry* 2: 702–709. doi: 10.1016/S2215–0366(15)00271–0.

Dalsgaard, S., et al. (2015b). "Mortality in Children, Adolescents, and Adults with Attention Deficit Hyperactivity Disorder: A Nationwide Cohort Study." *Lancet* 385: 2190–2196. doi: 10.1016/S0140-6736(14)61684-6.

Daughton, J. M., and C. J. Kratochvil. (2009). "Review of ADHD Pharmacotherapies: Advantages, Disadvantages, and Clinical Pearls." *Journal of the American Academy of Child and Adolescent Psychiatry* 48: 243–244.

Davis, C., et al. (2015). "Attention-Deficit/Hyperactivity Disorder in Relation to Addictive Behaviors: A Moderated-Mediation Analysis of Personality-Risk Factors and Sex." *Frontiers in Psychiatry.* 6: 47.

Delate, T., et al. (2014). "Metabolic Monitoring in Commercially Insured Pediatric Patients Newly Initiated to Take a Second-Generation Antipsychotic." *JAMA Pediatrics* 168: 679–681. doi: 10.1001/jamapediatrics.2014.224.

Dempsey, D. A., et al. (2013). "CYP2A6 Genotype but not Age Determines Cotinine Half-life in Infants and Children." *Clinical Pharmacology and Therapeutics* 94: 400–406. doi:10.1038/clpt.2013.114.

Di Florio, A., et al. (2013). "Perinatal Episodes Across the Mood Disorder Spectrum." *JAMA Psychiatry* 70: 168–175.

Diav-Citrin, O., et al. (2014). "Pregnancy Outcome Following in Utero Exposure to Lithium: A Prospective, Comparative, Observational study." *American Journal of Psychiatry* 171: 785–794. doi: 10.1176/appi.ajp.2014.12111402.

Diav-Citrin, O., et al. (2016). "Methylphenidate in Pregnancy: A Multicenter, Prospective, Comparative, Observational Study." *Journal of Clinical Psychiatry* 77: 1176–1181. doi: 10.4088/JCP.15m10083.

Doey, T. (2012). "Aripiprazole in Pediatric Psychosis and Bipolar Disorder: A Clinical Review." *Journal of Affective Disorders* 138 (Suppl.): S15–S21.

Doyle, C. A., and McDougle, C. J. (2012). "Pharmacologic Treatments for the Behavioral Symptoms Associated with Autism Spectrum Disorders across the Lifespan." *Dialogues in Clinical Neuroscience* 14: 263–279.

Egunsola, O., et al. (2015). "Pharmacology and Therapeutics Safety of Lamotrigine in Paediatrics: A Systematic Review." *BMJ Open* 5: e007711. doi: 10.1136/bmjopen-2015–007711.

Elbe, D., and Lalani, Z. (2012). "Review of the Pharmacotherapy of Irritability of Autism." *Journal of the Canadian Academy of Child & Adolescent Psychiatry* 21: 130–146.

Emslie, G. J., et al. (1997). "A Double-Blind, Randomized, Placebo-Controlled Trial of Fluoxetine in Children and Adolescents with Depression." *Archives of General Psychiatry* 54: 1031–1037.

Emslie, G., et al. (2009). "Escitalopram in the Treatment of Adolescent Depression: A Randomized, Placebo-Controlled Multisite Trial." *Journal of the American Academy of Child & Adolescent Psychiatry* 48: 721–729.

Ercan, E. S., et al. (2012). "Aripiprazole in Children and Adolescents with Conduct Disorder: A Single-Center, Open-Label Study." *Pharmacopsychiatry* 45: 13–19.

Farmer, C. A., et al. (2011). "The Treatment of Severe Child Aggression (TOSCA) Study: Design Challenges." *Child and Adolescent Psychiatry and Mental Health* 5: 36–47.

Fairman, K. A., et al. (2017). "Diagnosis and Treatment of ADHD in the United States: Update by Gender and Race." *Journal of Attention Disorders.* In press. doi: 10.1177/1087054716688534.

Faraone, S. V., et al. (2012). "Dose Response Effects of Lisdexamfetamine Dimesylate Treatment in Adults with ADHD: An Exploratory Study." *Journal of Attention Disorders* 16: 118–127.

Faraone, S. V., and Glatt, S. J. (2010). "Effects of Extended-Release Guanfacine on ADHD Symptoms and Sedation-Related Events in Children with ADHD." *Journal of Attention Disorders* 13: 532–538.

Feldman, H., and Reiff, M. I. (2014). "Attention Deficit–Hyperactivity Disorder in Children and Adolescents." *New England Journal of Medicine* 370:838–846. doi: 10.1056/NEJMcp1307215.

Findling, R. L., et al. (2012). "Double-Blind, Randomized, Placebo-Controlled, Long-Term Maintenance Study of Aripiprazole in Children with Bipolar Disorder." *Journal of Clinical Psychiatry* 73: 57–63.

Findling, R. L., et al. (2013). "Aripiprazole for the Treatment of Pediatric Bipolar Disorder: A 30-Week Randomized, Placebo-Controlled Study." *Bipolar Disorder* 15: 138–149.

Findling, R. L., et al. (2015). "Lithium in the Acute Treatment of Bipolar I Disorder: A Double-Blind, Placebo-Controlled Study." *Pediatrics* 136: 885–894. doi: 10.1542/peds.2015-0743.

Franklin, M. E., et al. (2011). "Cognitive Behavior Therapy Augmentation of Pharmacotherapy in Pediatric Obsessive-Compulsive Disorder: The Pediatric OCD Treatment Study II (POTS II) Randomized Controlled Trial." *JAMA* 306: 1224–1232.

Fredriksena, M., et al. (2013). "Long-Term Efficacy and Safety of Treatment with Stimulants and Atomoxetine in Adult ADHD: A Review of Controlled and Naturalistic Studies." *European Neuropsychopharmacology* 23: 508–527.

Freeman, M. P. (2014). "ADHD and Pregnancy." *American Journal of Psychiatry* 171: 723–728.

Freeman, M. P. (2015). "Psychotropic Medication Use During Pregnancy: Changes to the Labeling System and the Importance of Exposure Registries." *Journal of Clinical Psychiatry* 76: 990–991.

French, L., et al. (2015). "Early Cannabis Use, Polygenic Risk Score for Schizophrenia and Brain Maturation in Adolescents." *JAMA Psychiatry* 72: 1002–1011.

Fried, M., et al. (2014). "ADHD Subjects Fail to Suppress Eye Blinks and Microsaccades while Anticipating Visual Stimuli but Recover with Medication." *Vision Research* 101: 62–72. doi: 10.1016/j.visres.2014.05.004.

Furey, R., and Furey, C. (2014). "The Economics of Inattention: A Review of The ADHD Explosion: Myths, Medication, Money, and Today's Push for Performance by Stephen P. Hinshaw and Richard M. Scheffler." *New PsycCRITIQUES* 59(40). doi: 10.1037/a0037889.

Gadow, K. D., et al. (2014). "Risperidone Added to Parent Training and Stimulant Medication: Effects on Attention-Deficit/Hyperactivity Disorder, Oppositional Defiant Disorder, Conduct Disorder, and Peer Aggression" *Journal of the American Academy of Child and Adolescent Psychiatry* 53: 948–959.e1. doi: 10.1016/j.jaac.2014.05.008.

Galling, B., et al. (2016). "Type 2 Diabetes Mellitus in Youth Exposed to Antipsychotics: A Systematic Review and Metaanalysis." *JAMA Psychiatry* 73: 247–259. doi: 10.1001/jamapsychiatry.2015.2923.

Ganzer, F., et al. (2016). "Weighing the Evidence: A Systematic Review on Long-Term Neurocognitive Effects of Cannabis Use in Abstinent Adolescents and Adults." *Neuropsychological Reviews* 26: 186–222. doi: 10.1007/s11065-016-9316-2.

Gentile, E. S. (2015). "Managing Antidepressant Treatment in Pregnancy and Puerperium. Careful with that axe, Eugene." *Expert Opinion in Drug Safety* 14: 1011–1014. doi: 10.1517/14740338.2015.1037273.

Geller, B., et al. (2012). "A Randomized Controlled Trial of Risperidone, Lithium, or Divalproex Sodium for Initial Treatment of Bipolar I Disorder, Manic or Mixed Phase, in Children and Adolescents." *Archives of General Psychiatry* 69: 515–528.

Gibbons, R. D., et al. (2007). "Relationship Between Antidepressants and Suicide Attempts: An Analysis of the Veterans Health Administration Data Sets." *American Journal of Psychiatry* 164: 1044–1049.

Ginsburg, G. S., et al. (2011). "Remission after Acute Treatment in Children and Adolescents with Anxiety Disorders: Findings from the CAMS." *Journal of Consulting and Clinical Psychology* 79: 806–813.

Ginsburg, G. S., et al. (2014). "Naturalistic Follow-Up of Youths Treated for Pediatric Anxiety Disorders." *JAMA Psychiatry* 71: 310–318. doi: 10.1001/jamapsychiatry.2013.4186.

Goldstein, B. I. (2012). "Pharmacologic Treatment of Youth with Bipolar Disorder: Where to Next?" *Carlat Report: Child Psychiatry.* https://thecarlatchildreport.com/free_articles/pharmacologic-treatment-youth-bipolar-disorder-where-next-free-article.

Gonzalez, R., et al. (2015). "The Role of Decision-Making in Cannabis-Related Problems Among Young Adults." *Drug & Alcohol Dependence* 154: 214–221.

Goodman, D. W. (2010). "Lisdexamfetamine Dimesylate (Vyvanse), a Prodrug Stimulant for Attention-Deficit Hyperactivity Disorder." *Pharmacy & Therapeutics* 35: 273–287.

Goodman, D. W., et al. (2016). "Clinical Presentation, Diagnosis and Treatment of Attention-Deficit Hyperactivity Disorder (ADHD) in Older Adults: A Review of the Evidence and Its Implications for Clinical Care." *Drugs & Aging* 33: 27–36. doi: 10.1007/s40266-015-0327-0.

Graudins, A., et al. (2014). "The PICHFORK (Pain in Children Fentanyl or Ketamine) Trial: A Randomized Controlled Trial Comparing Intranasal Ketamine and Fentanyl for the Relief of Moderate to Severe Pain in Children with Limb Injuries." *Annals of Emergency Medicine* 65: 248–254.e1. doi: 10.1016/j.annemergmed. 2014.09.024.

Grebla, R., et al. (2016). Medication Use among Commercially-Insured Adults with Attention-Deficit/Hyperactivity Disorder (ADHD) in the U.S. American Psychiatric Association Annual Meeting, May 14–18, Atlanta, Georgia.

Greenhill, L. L., et al. (2006). "Efficacy and Safety of Immediate-Release Methylphenidate Treatment for Preschoolers with ADHD." *Journal of the American Academy of Child & Adolescent Psychiatry* 45: 1284–1293.

Grigoriadis, S., et al. (2014). "Prenatal Exposure to Antidepressants and Persistent Pulmonary Hypertension of the Newborn: Systematic Review and Meta-Analysis." *BMJ* 348: f6932 doi: 10.1136/bmj.f6932.

Grzeskowiak, L. E., et al. (2015). "Prenatal Antidepressant Exposure and Child Behavioural Outcomes at 7 Years of Age: A Study Within the Danish National Birth Cohort." *BJOG: An International Journal of Obstetrics & Gynaecology* 123: 1919–1928. doi: 10.1111/1471–0528.13611.

Grzeskowiak, L. E. (2015). "Antidepressant use in late Gestation and Risk of Postpartum Haemorrhage: A Retrospective Cohort Study." *BJOG: An International Journal of Obstetrics & Gynaecology* 123: 1929–1936. doi: 10.1111/1471–0528.13612.

Gunn, J. K. L., et al. (2016). "Prenatal Exposure to Cannabis and Maternal and Child Health Outcomes: A Systematic Review and Meta-Analysis." *BMJ Open* 6: e009986. doi:10.1136/bmjopen-2015-009986

Habermann, F., et al. (2013). "Atypical Antipsychotic Drugs and Pregnancy Outcome: A Prospective, Cohort Study." *Journal of Clinical Psychopharmacology* 33: 453–462. doi: 10.1097/JCP.0b013e318295fe12.

Hall, E. S., et al. (2016). "Self-Reported and Laboratory Evaluation of Late Pregnancy Nicotine Exposure and Drugs of Abuse," *Journal of Perinatology* 36: 814–818. doi:10.1038/jp.2016.100.

Harstad, E. B., et al. (2014). "ADHD, Stimulant Treatment, and Growth: A Longitudinal Study." *Pediatrics* 134: e935–e944. doi: 10.1542/peds.2014–0428.

Hasin, D. S., et al. (2015). "Medical Marijuana Laws and Adolescent Marijuana Use in the USA from 1991 to 2014: Results from Annual, Repeated Cross-Sectional Surveys." *Lancet Psychiatry* 2: 601–608. doi: 10.1016/S2215–0366(15)00217–5.

Hauser, M., and Correll, C. U. (2013). "The Significance of At-Risk or Prodromal Symptoms for Bipolar I Disorder in Children and Adolescents." *Canadian Journal of Psychiatry* 58: 22–31.

Helgadóttir, H., et al. (2015). "Electroencephalography as a Clinical Tool for Diagnosing and Monitoring Attention Deficit Hyperactivity Disorder: A Cross-Sectional Study." *BMJ Open* 5: e005500. doi: 10.1136/bmjopen-2014–005500.

Hirota, T, et al. (2014). "Alpha-2 Agonists for Attention-Deficit/Hyperactivity Disorder in Youth: A Systematic Review and Meta-Analysis of Monotherapy and Add-On Trials to Stimulant Therapy." *Journal of the American Academy of Child and Adolescent Psychiatry* 53: 153–173. doi: 10.1016/j.jaac.2013.11.009

Hoyme, H. E., et al. (2016). "Updated Clinical Guidelines for Diagnosing Fetal Alcohol Spectrum Disorders." *Pediatrics* 138. pii: e20154256. doi: 10.1542/peds.2015–4256.

Humphreys, K. L., et al. (2013). "Stimulant Medication and Substance Use Outcomes: A Meta-Analysis." *JAMA Psychiatry* 70: 740–749.

Hunt, S., et al. (2008). "Topiramate in Pregnancy: Preliminary Experience from the UK Epilepsy and Pregnancy Register." *Neurology* 71: 272–276.

Huybrechts, K. F., et al. (2014). "Preterm Birth and Antidepressant Medication Use during Pregnancy: A Systematic Review and Meta-Analysis." *PLOS One* 9: e92778. doi: 10.1371/journal.pone.0092778

Huybrechts, K. F., et al. (2015). "Antidepressant Use Late in Pregnancy and Risk of Persistent Pulmonary Hypertension of the Newborn." *JAMA* 313: 2142–2151. doi: 10.1001/jama.2015.5605.

Hviid, A., et al. (2013). "Use of Selective Serotonin Reuptake Inhibitors during Pregnancy and Risk of Autism." *New England Journal of Medicine* 369: 2406–2415. doi: 10.1056/NEJMoa1301449.

Hyland, A., et al. (2015). "Associations of Lifetime Active and Passive Smoking with Spontaneous Abortion, Stillbirth and Tubal Ectopic Pregnancy: A Cross-Sectional Analysis of Historical Data From the Women's Health Initiative." *Tobacco Control* 24: 328–335.

Ibrahim, K., and Donyai, P. (2015). "Drug Holidays from ADHD Medication: International Experience Over the Past Four Decades." *Journal of Attention Disorders* 19: 551–568.

Jabeen, S., et al. (2015). "Evidence of Stimulation of Pubertal Development and Suppression of Growth Rate in Boys Smoking Marijuana Cigarettes." *Endocrine Abstracts* GP.08.08. doi: 10.1530/endoabs.37.GP.08.08.

Jain, R., et al. (2011). "Clonidine Extended-Release Tablets for Pediatric Patients with Attention-Deficit/Hyperactivity Disorder." *Journal of the American Academy of Child & Adolescent Psychiatry* 50: 171–179.

Jones, I., et al. (2014). "Bipolar Disorder, Affective Psychosis, and Schizophrenia in Pregnancy and the Post-Partum Period." *Lancet* 384: 1789–99. doi: 10.1016/S0140-6736(14)61278-2.

Jordan, S., et al. (2016). "Selective Serotonin Reuptake Inhibitor (SSRI) Antidepressants in Pregnancy and Congenital Anomalies: Analysis of Linked Databases in Wales, Norway and Funen, Denmark." *PLOS One* 11: e0165122. doi: 10.1371/journal.pone.0165122.

Joshi, G., et al. (2012). "A Prospective Open-Label Trial of Quetiapine Monotherapy in Preschool and School Age Children with Bipolar Spectrum Disorder." *Journal of Affective Disorders* 136: 1143–1153.

Joshi, G., et al. (2013). "A Prospective Open-Label Trial of Paliperidone Monotherapy for the Treatment of Bipolar Spectrum Disorders in Children and Adolescents." *Psychopharmacology* 227: 449–458.

Johnston, L. D., Miech, R. A., O'Malley, P. M., Bachman, J. G., Schulenberg, J. E., & Patrick, M. E. (2018). Monitoring the Future national survey results on drug use: 1975–2017: Overview, key findings on adolescent drug use. Ann Arbor: Institute for Social Research, The University of Michigan.

Kelly, A. S., et al. (2014). "Cardiac Autonomic Dysfunction and Arterial Stiffness among Children and Adolescents with Attention Deficit Hyperactivity Disorder Treated with Stimulants." *Journal of Pediatrics* 165: 755–759. doi: 10.1016/j.jpeds.2014.05.043.

Kennard, B. D., et al. (2014). "Sequential Treatment with Fluoxetine and Relapse-Prevention CBT to Improve Outcomes in Pediatric Depression." *American Journal of Psychiatry* 171: 1083–1090. doi: 10.1176/appi.ajp.2014.13111460.

Kiyatkin, E. A. (2013). "The Hidden Side of Drug Action: Brain Temperature Changes Induced By Neuroactive Drugs." *Psychopharmacology (Berl)*. 225: 765–780. doi: 10.1007/s00213-012-2957-9.

King, B. H. (2017). "Association between Maternal Use of SSRI Medications and Autism in Their Children." *JAMA* 317: 1568–1569. doi: 10.1001/jama.2016.20614.

Kirino, E. (2012). "Efficacy and Safety of Aripiprazole in Child and Adolescent Patients." *European Child and Adolescent Psychiatry* 21: 361–368.

Knickmeyer, R. C., et al. (2014). "Rate of Chiari I Malformation in Children of Mothers with Depression with and without Prenatal SSRI Exposure." *Neuropsychopharmacology* 39: 2611–2621. doi: 10.1038/npp.2014.114.

Koblan, K. S., et al. (2015). "Dasotraline for the Treatment of Attention-Deficit/Hyperactivity Disorder: A Randomized, Double-Blind, Placebo-Controlled, Proof-of-Concept Trial in Adults." *Neuropsychopharmacology* 40: 2745–2752. doi: 10.1038/npp.2015.124.

Kodish, I., et al. (2011). "Pharmacotherapy for Anxiety Disorders in Children and Adolescents." *Pediatric Clinics of North America* 58: 55–72.

Kollins, S. K., et al. (2014). "A Pilot Study of Lis-Dexamfetamine Dimesylate (LDX/SPD489) to Facilitate Smoking Cessation in Nicotine-Dependent Adults with ADHD." *Journal of Attention Disorders* 18: 158–168.

Kolla, N. J., et al. (2016). "Adult Attention Deficit Hyperactivity Disorder Symptom Profiles and Concurrent Problems with Alcohol and Cannabis: Sex Differences in a Representative, Population Survey." *BMC Psychiatry* 16: 50. doi: 10.1186/s12888-016-0746-4.

Konofal, E., et al. (2014). "Pilot Phase II Study of Mazindol in Children with Attention Deficit/ Hyperactivity Disorder." *Drug Design, Development and Therapy* 8: 2321–2332.

Kousik, S. M., et al. (2012). "The Effects of Psychostimulant Drugs on Blood Brain Barrier Function and Neuroinflammation." *Frontiers in Pharmacology* 3: 121 doi: 10.3389/fphar.2012.00121.

Kratochvil, C. J., et al. (2011). "A Double-Blind, Placebo-Controlled Study of Atomoxetine in Young Children with ADHD." *Pediatrics* 127: e862–e868.

Kulkarni, J., et al. (2014). "A Prospective Cohort Study of Antipsychotic Medications in Pregnancy: The First 147 Pregnancies and 100 One Year Old Babies." *PLOS One* 9: e94788. doi: 10.1371/journal.pone.0094788.

Kumar, B., et al. (2012). "Drug Therapy in Autism: A Present and Future Perspective." *Pharmacological Reviews* 64: 1291–1304.

Law, E. C., et al. (2014). "Attention-Deficit/Hyperactivity Disorder in Young Children: Predictors of Diagnostic Stability." *Pediatrics* 133: 659–667. doi: 10.1542/peds.2013-3433.

Le Noury, J., et al. (2015). "Restoring Study 329: Efficacy and Harms Of Paroxetine and Imipramine in Treatment Of Major Depression in Adolescence." *BMJ* 351: h4320.

Lensing, M. B., et al. (2015). "Psychopharmacological Treatment of ADHD in Adults Aged 50+: An Empirical Study." *Journal of Attention Disorders* 19: 380–389.

Leventhal, A. M., et al. (2015). "Association of Electronic Cigarette Use with Initiation of Combustible Tobacco Product Smoking in Early Adolescence." *JAMA* 31: 700–707. doi: 10.1001/jama.2015.8950.

Levy, S., et al. (2014). "An Electronic Screen for Triaging Adolescent Substance Use by Risk Levels." *JAMA Pediatrics* 168: 822–828. doi: 10.1001/jamapediatrics.2014.774.

Levy, S. J., et al. (2016). "Substance Use Screening, Brief Intervention, and Referral to Treatment." *Pediatrics* 138: e20161211. doi: 10.1542/peds.2016-1211.

Liossi, C., and Howard, R. F. (2016). "A Biopsychosocial Framework for Assessing and Managing Chronic Pain in Children." *Pediatrics* 138: 1–11. doi: 10.1542/peds.2016-0331.

Lu, C., et al. (2014). "Changes in Antidepressant Use by Young People and Suicidal Behavior after FDA Warnings and Media Coverage: Quasi-Experimental Study." *BMJ* 348: g3596.

Luby, J. L., and Navsaria, N. (2010). "Pediatric Bipolar Disorder: Evidence for Prodromal States and Early Markers." *Journal of Child Psychology and Psychiatry* 51: 459–471.

Lyoo, I. K., et al. (2015). "Predisposition to and Effects of Methamphetamine Use on the Adolescent Brain." *Molecular Psychiatry* 20: 1516–1524. doi: 10.1038/mp.2014.191.

Lytle, S., et al. (2017). "Long-Acting Injectable Antipsychotics in Children and Adolescents." *Journal of Child and Adolescent Psychopharmacology* 27: 2–9. doi: 10.1089/cap.2016.0055.

MacKenzie, L. E., et al. (2015). "Stimulant Medication and Psychotic Symptoms in Offspring of Parents with Mental Illness." *Pediatrics* 137: 1–10. doi: 10.1542/peds.2015-2486.

Malm, H., et al. (2015). "Pregnancy Complications Following Prenatal Exposure to SSRIs or Maternal Psychiatric Disorders: Results from Population-Based National Register Data." *American Journal of Psychiatry* 172: 124–1232. doi: 10.1176/appi.ajp.2015.14121575.

Man, K. K., et al. (2015). "Methylphenidate and the Risk of Trauma." *Pediatrics* 135: 40–48. doi: 10.1542/peds.2014-1738.

Manrique-Garcia, E., et al. (2016). "Cannabis, Psychosis, and Mortality: A Cohort Study of 50,373 Swedish Men." *American Journal of Psychiatry* 73: 790–798. doi: 10.1176/appi.ajp.2016.14050637.

Manseau, M. W., and Goff, D. C. (2015). "Cannabinoids and Schizophrenia: Risks and Therapeutic Potential." *Neurotherapeutics* 12: 816–824.

Marcus, R. N., et al. (2011). "Safety and Tolerability of Aripiprazole for Irritability in Pediatric Patients with Autistic Disorder: A 52-Week, Open-Label, Multicenter Study." *Journal of Clinical Psychiatry* 72: 1270–1276.

Marroun, H. E. et al. (2014). "Prenatal Tobacco Exposure and Brain Morphology: A Prospective Study in Young Children." *Neuropsychopharmacology* 39: 792–800. doi: 10.1038/npp.2013.273.

Masi, G., et al. (2010). "Aripiprazole Augmentation in 39 Adolescents with Medication-Resistant Obsessive-Compulsive Disorder." *Journal of Clinical Psychopharmacology* 30, 688–693.

McCabe, S. E., et al. (2016). "Age of Onset, Duration, and Type of Medication Therapy for Attention-Deficit/Hyperactivity Disorder (ADHD) and Substance Use during Adolescence: A Multi-Cohort National Study." *Journal of the American Academy of Child & Adolescent Psychiatry* 55: 479–486.

McCabe, S. E., et al. (2017). "Trends in Medical and Nonmedical Use of Prescription Opioids among US Adolescents: 1976–2015." *Pediatrics* 139: 1–9. doi: 10.1542/peds.2016-2387.

McDonagh, M. S., et al. (2014). "Depression Drug Treatment Outcomes in Pregnancy and the Postpartum Period: A Systematic Review and Meta-Analysis." *Obstetrics and Gynecology* 124: 526–534. doi: 10.1097/AOG.0000000000000410.

McQuire, C., et al. (2015). "Pharmacological Interventions for Challenging Behaviour in Children with Intellectual Disabilities: A Systematic Review and Meta-Analysis." *BMC Psychiatry* 15: 303. doi: 10.1186/s12888-015-0688-2.

Meador, K. J. (2013). "Fetal Antiepileptic Drug Exposure and Cognitive Outcomes at Age 6 Years (NEAD Study): A Prospective Observational Study." *Lancet Neurology* 12: 244–52. doi: 10.1016/S1474-4422(12)70323-X.

Meier, M. H., et al. (2015). "Associations of Adolescent Cannabis Use with Academic Performance and Mental Health: A Longitudinal Study of Upper Middle Class Youth." *Drug & Alcohol Dependence* 156: 207–212.

Meador, K. J., et al. (2014). "Breastfeeding in Children of Women Taking Antiepileptic Drugs: Cognitive Outcomes at Age 6 Years." *JAMA Pediatrics* 168: 729–736. doi: 10.1001/jamapediatrics.2014.118.

Memarzia, J., et al. (2014). "The Use of Antipsychotics in Preschoolers: A Veto or A Sensible Last Option?" *Journal of Psychopharmacology* 28: 303–19. doi: 10.1177/0269881113519506.

Mezzacappa, A., et al. (2017). "Risk for Autism Spectrum Disorders According to Period of Prenatal Antidepressant Exposure: A Systematic Review and Meta-analysis." *JAMA Pediatrics* 171: 555–563. doi: 10.1001/jamapediatrics.2017.0124.

Miller, M., et al. (2014). "Antidepressant Dose, Age, and the Risk of Deliberate Self-Harm." *JAMA Internal Medicine* 174: 899–909.

Moffitt, T. E., et al. (2015). "Is Adult ADHD a Childhood-Onset Neurodevelopmental Disorder? Evidence from a Four-Decade Longitudinal Cohort Study." *American Journal of Psychiatry* 172: 967–977. doi: 10.1176/appi.ajp.2015.14101266.

Morean, M. E., et al. (2015). "High School Students' Use of Electronic Cigarettes to Vaporize Cannabis." *Pediatrics* 136: 1–6. doi: 10.1542/peds.2015-1727.

Moreno, M. A. (2015). "The Misuse of Prescription Pain Medicine Among Children and Teens." *JAMA Pediatrics* 169: 512.

Moyer, V., et al. (2014). "Primary Care Behavioral Interventions to Reduce Illicit Drug and Non-medical Pharmaceutical Use in Children and Adolescents: U.S. Preventive Services Task Force Recommendation Statement." *Annals of Internal Medicine* 160: 634–639.

Molina, B. S., et al. (2009). "The MTA at 8 Years: Prospective Follow-Up of Children Treated for Combined-Type ADHD in a Multisite Study." *Journal of the American Academy of Child & Adolescent Psychiatry* 48: 484–500.

MTA Cooperative Group (1999). "A 14-Month Randomized Clinical Trial of Treatment Strategies for Attention-Deficit/Hyperactivity Disorder." *Archives of General Psychiatry* 56: 1073–1086.

MTA Cooperative Group (2004). "National Institute of Mental Health Multimodal Treatment Study of ADHD Follow-Up: Changes in Effectiveness and Growth after the End of Treatment." *Pediatrics* 113: 762–769.

Muld, B. B., et al. (2013). "Attention Deficit/Hyperactivity Disorders with Co-Existing Substance Use Disorder Is Characterized by Early Antisocial Behaviour and Poor Cognitive Skills." *BMC Psychiatry* 13: 336, doi: 10.1186/1471-244X-13-336.

Nagy, P., et al. (2016). "Functional Outcomes from a Head-to-Head, Randomized, Double-Blind Trial of Lisdexamfetamine Dimesylate and Atomoxetine in Children and Adolescents with Attention-Deficit/Hyperactivity Disorder and an Inadequate Response to Methylphenidate." *European Child & Adolescent Psychiatry* 25: 141–149. doi: 10.1007/s00787-015-0718-0.

Nembhard, W. N., et al. (2017). "Maternal and Infant Genetic Variants, Maternal Periconceptional Use of Selective Serotonin Reuptake Inhibitors, and Risk of Congenital Heart Defects in Offspring: Population Based Study." *BMJ* 356: j832. doi: 10.1136/bmj.j832.

Nevels, R. M., et al. (2010). "Psychopharmacology of Aggression in Children and Adolescents with Primary Neuropsychiatric Disorders: A Review of Current and Potentially Promising Treatment Options." *Experimental and Clinical Psychopharmacology* 18: 184–201.

Newcorn, J. H., et al. (2016). "Extended-Release Guanfacine Hydrochloride In 6–17-Year Olds with ADHD: A Randomised-Withdrawal Maintenance of Efficacy Study." *Journal of Child Psychology and Psychiatry and Allied Disciplines* 57: 717–728. doi: 10.1111/jcpp.12492.

Newport, D. J., et al. (2008). "Lamotrigine in Breast Milk and Nursing Infants: Determination of Exposure." *Pediatrics* 122: e223–e231.

Newport, D. J., et al. (2016). "Prenatal Psychostimulant and Antidepressant Exposure and Risk of Hypertensive Disorders of Pregnancy." *Journal of Clinical Psychiatry* 77: 1538–1545.

Nguyen, H. T. T., et al. (2009). "Teratogenesis Associated with Antibipolar Agents." *Advances in Therapy* 26: 281-294. doi: 10.1007/s12325-009-0011-z.

Ninnemann, A. L., et al. (2017). "Longitudinal Predictors of Synthetic Cannabinoid Use in Adolescents." *Pediatrics* 138: 1–7. doi: 10.1542/peds.2016-3009.

Nörby, U., et al. (2016). "Neonatal Morbidity after Maternal Use of Antidepressant Drugs during Pregnancy." *Pediatrics* 138: 1–10. doi: 10.1542/peds.2016-0181.

Nulman, I., et al. (2015). "Neurodevelopment of Children Prenatally Exposed to Selective Reuptake Inhibitor Antidepressants: Toronto Sibling Study." *Journal of Clinical Psychiatry* 76: e842–e847.

Oberlander, T. F., and Zwaigenbaum, L. (2017). "Disentangling Maternal Depression and Antidepressant Use During Pregnancy as Risks for Autism in Children." *JAMA* 317: 1533–1534. doi: 10.1001/jama.2017.3414.

Olfson, M., et al. (2015). "Treatment of Young People with Antipsychotic Medications in the United States." *JAMA Psychiatry* 72: 867–874. doi: 10.1001/jamapsychiatry.2015.0500.

Otasowie, J., et al. (2014). "Tricyclic Antidepressants for Attention Deficit Hyperactivity Disorder (ADHD) in Children and Adolescents." *Cochrane Database Systemic Review* 9: CD006997. doi: 10.1002/14651858.CD006997.pub2.

Pappadopulos, E., et al. (2011). "Experts' Recommendations for Treating Maladaptive Aggression in Youth." *Journal of Child and Adolescent Psychopharmacology* 21: 505–515.

Parry, P. I., and Levin, E. C. (2012). "Pediatric Bipolar Disorder in an Era of 'Mindless Psychiatry.'" *Journal of Trauma & Dissociation* 13: 51–68.

Pathak, S., et al. (2013). "Efficacy and Safety of Quetiapine in Children and Adolescents with Mania Associated with Bipolar I Disorder: A 3-Week, Double-Blind, Placebo-Controlled Trial." *Journal of Clinical Psychiatry* 74: e100–e109.

Patton, G. C., et al. (2014). "The Prognosis of Common Mental Disorders in Adolescents: A 14-Year Prospective Cohort Study." *Lancet* 383: 1404–1411. doi: 10.1016/S0140-6736(13)62116-9.

Pavuluri, M. N., et al. (2010). "Enhanced Working and Verbal Memory after Lamotrigine Treatment in Pediatric Bipolar Disorder." *Bipolar Disorder* 12: 213–220.

Peng, M., et al. (2013). "Effects of Prenatal Exposure to Atypical Antipsychotics on Postnatal Development and Growth of Infants: A Case-Controlled, Prospective Study." *Psychopharmacology* 228: 577–584.

Pessina, E., et al. (2009). "Aripiprazole Augmentation of Serotonin Reuptake Inhibitors in Treatment-Resistant Obsessive-Compulsive Disorder: A 12-Week, Open-Label Preliminary Study." *International Clinical Psychopharmacology* 24: 265–269.

Petersen, I., et al. (2016a). "Risks Associated with Antipsychotic Treatment in Pregnancy: Comparative Cohort Studies Based on Electronic Health Records." *Schizophrenia Research* 176: 349–356. doi: 10.1016/j.schres.2016.07.023.

Petersen, I., et al. (2016b). "Selective Serotonin Reuptake Inhibitors and Congenital Heart Anomalies: Comparative Cohort Studies of Women Treated Before and during Pregnancy and Their Children." *Journal of Clinical Psychiatry*. 77: e36–4e2. doi: 10.4088/JCP.14m09241.

Piacentini, J., et al. (2014). "24- and 36-week outcomes for Child/Adolescent Anxiety Multimodal Study (CAMS)." *Journal of the American Academy of Child and Adolescent Psychiatry* 53: 297–310. doi: 10.1016/j.jaac.2013.11.010.

Pianca, T. G., et al. (2016). "Crack Cocaine Use in Adolescents: Clinical Characteristics and Predictors of Early Initiation." *Journal of Clinical Psychiatry* 77: e1205–e1210.

Pillay, J., et al. (2017). "First- and Second-Generation Antipsychotics in Children and Young Adults: Systematic Review Update." *Comparative Effectiveness Review* 184: 1–567.

Pliszka, S. R., et al. (2017). "Efficacy and Safety of HLD200, Delayed-Release and Extended-Release Methylphenidate, in Children with Attention-Deficit/Hyperactivity Disorder." *Journal of Child and Adolescent Psychopharmacology* 27: 474–482. doi: 10.1089/cap.2017.0084

Polanczyk, G. V., et al. (2014). "ADHD Prevalence Estimates across Three Decades: An Updated Systematic Review and Meta-Regression Analysis." *International Journal of Epidemiology* 43: 434–442.

Popova, S., et al. (2017). "Prevalence of alcohol consumption during pregnancy and Fetal Alcohol Spectrum Disorders among the general and Aboriginal populations in Canada and the United States." *European Journal of Medical Genetics* 60: 32–48. doi: 10.1016/j.ejmg.2016.09.010.

Prasad, S., et al. (2007). "A Multi-Centre, Randomized, Open-Label Study of Atomoxetine Compared with Standard Current Therapy in UK Children and Adolescents with Attention-Deficit/Hyperactivity Disorder." *Current Medical Research and Opinion* 23: 379–394.

Pringsheim, T., and Gorman, D. (2012). "Second-Generation Antipsychotics for the Treatment of Disruptive Behavior Disorders in Children: A Systematic Review." *Canadian Journal of Psychiatry* 57: 722–727.

Propper, L., and Orlik, H. (2011). "Pharmacotherapy of Severe Disruptive Behavioral Symptoms Associated with Autism." *Child & Adolescent Psychopharmacology News* 16: 1–8.

Punja, S., et al. (2016). "Amphetamines for Attention Deficit Hyperactivity Disorder (ADHD) in Children and Adolescents." *Cochrane Database Systematic Review* 2: CD009996. doi: 10.1002/14651858.CD009996.pub2.

Rahn, K. A., et al. (2015). "The Role of 5-HT1A Receptors in Mediating Acute Negative Effects of Antidepressants: Implications in Pediatric Depression." *Translational Psychiatry* 5: e563. doi: 10.1038/tp.2015.57.

Rais, T. B., and Rais, A. (2014). "Association Between Antidepressants Use During Pregnancy and Autistic Spectrum Disorders: A Meta-Analysis." *Innovation in Clinical Neuroscience* 11: 18–22.

Renard, J., et al. (2016). "Adolescent Cannabinoid Exposure Induces a Persistent Sub-Cortical Hyper-Dopaminergic State and Associated Molecular Adaptations in the Prefrontal Cortex." *Cerebral Cortex* 27: 1297–1310. doi: 10.1093/cercor/bhv335.

Richter, L., et al. (2016). "Assessing the Risk of Marijuana Use Disorder among Adolescents and Adults who use Marijuana." *American Journal of Drug and Alcohol Abuse* 13: 1–14.

Riddle, M. A., et al. (2013). "The Preschool Attention-Deficit/Hyperactivity Disorder Treatment Study (PATS) 6-Year Follow-Up." *Journal of the American Academy of Child & Adolescent Psychiatry* 52: 264–278.

Robb, A. S., et al. (2010). "Sertraline Treatment of Children and Adolescents with Posttraumatic Stress Disorder: A Double-Blind, Placebo-Controlled Trial." *Journal of Child and Adolescent Psychopharmacology* 20: 463–471.

Robinson, G. E. (2015). "Controversies about the Use of Antidepressants in Pregnancy." *Journal of Nervous and Mental Disease* 203: 159–163.

Rothbaum, B. O., et al. (2012). "Early Intervention May Prevent the Development of Posttraumatic Stress Disorder: A Randomized Pilot Civilian Study with Modified Prolonged Exposure." *Biological Psychiatry* 72: 957–963.

Rucklidge, J. J., et al. (2014). "Vitamin-Mineral Treatment of Attention-Deficit Hyperactivity Disorder in Adults: Double-Blind Randomised Placebo-Controlled Trial." *British Journal of Psychiatry* 204: 306–315. doi: 10.1192/bjp.bp.113.132126.

Rynn, M., et al. (2011). "Advances in Pharmacotherapy for Pediatric Anxiety Disorders." *Depression and Anxiety* 28: 76–87.

Sadowski, A., et al. (2013). "Pregnancy Outcomes Following Maternal Exposure to Second-Generation Antipsychotics Given with Other Psychotropic Drugs: A Cohort Study." *BMJ Open* 3: e003062. doi: 10.1136/bmjopen-2013-003062.

Safer, D. J. (2016). "Recent Trends in Stimulant Usage." *Journal of Attention Disorders* 20: 471–477.

Saint-Louis, C. (2015). "F.D.A. Approval of OxyContin Use for Children Continues to Draw Scrutiny." *New York Times*. October 8. https://www.nytimes.com/2015/10/09/health/fda-approval-of-oxycontin-for-children-continues-to-draw-scrutiny.html.

Salas-Wright, C. P., et al. (2015). "Substance Use and Teen Pregnancy in the United States: Evidence from the NSDUH 2002-2012." *Addictive Behaviors* 45: 218–225.

Salisbury, A. L., et al. (2015). "The Roles of Maternal Depression, Serotonin Reuptake Inhibitor Treatment, and Concomitant Benzodiazepine use on Infant Neurobehavioral Functioning Over the First Postnatal Month." *American Journal of Psychiatry* 173: 147–157. doi: 10.1176/appi.ajp.2015.14080989.

Santucci, A. K., et al. (2014). "Impact of Prenatal Exposure to Serotonin Reuptake Inhibitors or Maternal Major Depressive Disorder on Infant Developmental Outcomes." *Journal of Clinical Psychiatry* 75: 1088–1095.

Scahill, L., et al. (2015). "Extended-Release Guanfacine for Hyperactivity in Children with Autism Spectrum Disorder." *American Journal of Psychiatry* 172: 1197–1206. doi: 10.1176/appi.ajp.2015.15010055.

Seida, J. C., et al. (2012). "Antipsychotics for Children and Young Adults: A Comparative Effectiveness Review." *Pediatrics* 129: e771–e784. doi: 10.1542/peds.2011-2158.

Shapiro, M., et al. (2014). "Safety Profile of the Use of Second Generation Antipsychotics in the Child and Adolescent Population." *Current Psychopharmacology* 3: 146–150.

Schimmelmann, B. G., et al. (2013). "The Significance of At-Risk Symptoms for Psychosis in Children and Adolescents." *Canadian Journal of Psychiatry* 58: 32–40.

Schneider, C., et al. (2014). "Antipsychotics Use in Children and Adolescents: An On-Going Challenge in Clinical Practice." *Journal of Psychopharmacology* 28: 615–623. doi: 10.1177/0269881114533599.

Schoenfelder, E. N., et al. (2014). "Stimulant Treatment of ADHD and Cigarette Smoking: A Meta-Analysis." *Pediatrics* 133: 1070–1080.

Schwarz, A. (2015). "Still in a Crib, Yet Being Given Antipsychotics." *New York Times*. December 10. https://www.nytimes.com/2015/12/11/us/psychiatric-drugs-are-being-prescribed-to-infants.html.

Schwartz, B. S., et al. (2014). "Attention Deficit Disorder, Stimulant Use, and Childhood Body Mass Index Trajectory." *Pediatrics* 133: 668–676. doi: 10.1542/peds.2013-3427.

Schwartz, S., and Correll, C. U. (2014). "Efficacy and Safety of Atomoxetine in Children and Adolescents with Attention-Deficit/Hyperactivity Disorder: Results from a Comprehensive Meta-Analysis and Metaregression." *Journal of the American Academy of Child and Adolescent Psychiatry* 53: 174–187. doi: http://dx.doi.org/10.1016/j.jaac.2013.11.005.

Sharma, T., et al. (2016). "Suicidality and Aggression during Antidepressant Treatment: Systematic Review and Meta-Analyses Based on Clinical Study Reports." *BMJ* 352: doi: https://doi.org/10.1136/bmj.i65.

Shaw, P., et al. (2014). "Emotion Dysregulation in Attention Deficit Hyperactivity Disorder." *American Journal of Psychiatry* 171: 276–293.

Shin, J.-Y., et al. (2016). "Cardiovascular Safety of Methylphenidate among Children and Young People with Attention-Deficit/Hyperactivity Disorder(ADHD) Nationwide Self-Controlled Case Series Study." *BMJ* 353: i2550. doi: 10.1136/bmj.i2550.

Silins, E., et al. (2014). "Young Adult Sequelae of Adolescent Cannabis Use: An Integrative Analysis." *Lancet Psychiatry* 1: 286–293. doi: 10.1016/S2215-0366(14)70307-4.

Siqueira, L., et al. (2015). "Clinical Report: Binge Drinking." *Pediatrics* 136: e718–e726. doi: 10.1542/peds.2015-2337.

Smith, M. J., et al. (2015). "Cannabis-Related Episodic Memory Deficits and Hippocampal Morphological Differences in Healthy Individuals and Schizophrenia Subjects." *Hippocampus* 25: 1042–1051. doi: 10.1002/hipo.22427.

Smith, D. E. (2016). "Marijuana: A Fifty-Year Personal Addiction Medicine Perspective." *Journal of Psychoactive Drugs* 48: 3–10.

Sowell, E. R., et al. (2010). "Differentiating Prenatal Exposure to Methamphetamine and Alcohol versus Alcohol and Not Methamphetamine using Tensor-Bases Brain Morphometry and Discriminant Analysis." *Journal of Neuroscience* 30: 3876–3885.

Spechler, P. A., et al. (2015). "Cannabis Use in Early Adolescence: Evidence of Amygdala Hypersensitivity to Signals of Threat." *Developmental Cognitive Neuroscience* 16: 63–70.

Squeglia, L. M., et al. (2015). "Brain Development in Heavy-Drinking Adolescents." *American Journal of Psychiatry* 172: 531–542. doi: 10.1176/appi.ajp.2015.14101249.

Stigler, K. A., et al. (2012). "Paliperidone for Irritability in Adolescents and Young Adults with Autistic Disorder." *Psychopharmacology* 223: 237–245.

Storch, E. A., et al. (2016). "Efficacy of Augmentation of Cognitive Behavior Therapy with Weight-Adjusted d-Cycloserine vs Placebo in Pediatric Obsessive-Compulsive Disorder: A Randomized Clinical Trial." *JAMA Psychiatry* 73: 779–788. doi: 10.1001/jamapsychiatry.2016.1128.

Storebø, O. J., et al. (2015). "Methylphenidate for Attention-Deficit/Hyperactivity Disorder in Children and Adolescents: Cochrane Systematic Review with Meta-Analyses and Trial Sequential Analyses of Randomised Clinical Trials." *BMJ* 351 doi: https://doi.org/10.1136/bmj.h5203.

Strawn, J. R., et al. (2010). "Psychopharmacological Treatment of Posttraumatic Stress Disorder in Children and Adolescents: A Review." *Journal of Clinical Psychiatry* 71: 932–941.

Sujan, A. C., et al. (2017). "Associations of Maternal Antidepressant Use during the First Trimester of Pregnancy with Preterm Birth, Small for Gestational Age, Autism Spectrum Disorder, and Attention-Deficit/Hyperactivity Disorder in Offspring." *JAMA* 317: 1553–1562. doi: 10.1001/jama.2017.3413.

Sundquista, J., et al. (2014). "Attention-Deficit/Hyperactivity Disorder and Risk for Drug Use Disorder: A Population-Based Follow-Up and Co-Relative Study." *Psychological Medicine* 45: 977–983. doi: 10.1017/S0033291714001986.

Suri, R., et al. (2014). "Acute and Long-Term Behavioral Outcome of Infants and Children Exposed in Utero to Either Maternal Depression or Antidepressants: A Review of the Literature." *Journal of Clinical Psychiatry* 75: e1142–e1152.

Sutter-Dallay, A.-L., et al. (2015). "Impact of Prenatal Exposure to Psychotropic Drugs on Neonatal Outcome in Infants of Mothers with Serious Psychiatric Illnesses." *Journal of Clinical Psychiatry* 76: 967–973. doi: 10.4088/JCP.14m09070.

Swanson, J. M., and for the MTA Cooperative Group (2017). "Young Adult Outcomes in the Follow-Up of the Multimodal Treatment Study of Attention-Deficit/Hyperactivity Disorder: Symptom Persistence, Source Discrepancy, and Height Suppression." *Journal of Child Psychology and Psychiatry and Allied Disciplines* 58: 663–678. doi: 10.1111/jcpp.12684.

Swanson, J. M., et al. (2017). "Young Adult Outcomes in the Follow-Up of The Multimodal Treatment Study of Attention-Deficit/Hyperactivity Disorder: Symptom Persistence, Source Discrepancy, and Height Suppression." *The Journal of Child Psychology and Psychiatry* 58: 663–678. doi: 10.1111/jcpp.12684.

Tan, C. H., et al. (2015). "Alcohol Use and Binge Drinking Among Women of Childbearing Age — United States, 2011–2013." *Morbidity and Mortality Weekly Report* (MMWR) 64: 1042–1046.

Thapar, A. and Cooper, M. (2016). "Attention Deficit Hyperactivity Disorder." *Lancet* 387: 1240–1250. doi: 10.1016/S0140-6736(15)00238-X.

Toh, S., et al. (2013). "Prevalence and Trends in the Use of Antipsychotic Medications During Pregnancy in the U.S., 2001–2007: A Population-Based Study of 585,615 Deliveries." *Archives of Women's Mental Health* 16: 149–157.

Tomson, T. and Battino, D. (2009). "Teratogenic Effects of Antiepileptic Medications." *Neurology Clinics* 27: 993–1002.

Tosato, S., et al. (2017). "A Systematized Review of Atypical Antipsychotics in Pregnant Women: Balancing Between Risks of Untreated Illness and Risks of Drug-Related Adverse Effects." *Journal of Clinical Psychiatry* 78: e477–e489. doi: 10.4088/JCP.15r10483.

Tran, A. R., et al. (2012). "National Trends in Pediatric Use of Anticonvulsants." *Psychiatric Services* (Washington D.C.) 63: 1095–1101. doi: 10.1176/appi.ps.201100547.

Treatment for Adolescents with Depression Study (TADS) Team (2004). "Fluoxetine, Cognitive-Behavioral Therapy, and Their Combination for Adolescents with Depression: Treatment for Adolescents with Depression Study (TADS) Randomized Controlled Trial." *JAMA* 292: 807–820.

Tunnard, C., et al. (2014). "The Impact of Childhood Adversity on Suicidality and Clinical Course in Treatment-Resistant Depression." *Journal of Affective Disorders* 152: 122–130.

Upadhyaya, H. P., et al. (2013). "A Review of the Abuse Potential Assessment of Atomoxetine: A Nonstimulant Medication for Attention-Deficit Hyperactivity Disorder." *Psychopharmacology* 226: 189–200.

Vigod, S. N., et al. (2015). "Antipsychotic Drug Use in Pregnancy: High Dimensional, Propensity Matched, Population-Based Cohort Study." *BMJ* 350: h2298. doi: 10.1136/bmj.h2298.

Viguera, A. C., et al. (2007). "Lithium in Breast Milk and Nursing Infants: Clinical Implications." *American Journal of Psychiatry* 164: 342–345.

Vitiello, B., et al. (2007). "Effectiveness of Methylphenidate in the 10-Month Continuation Phase of the Preschoolers with Attention-Deficit/Hyperactivity Disorder Treatment Study (PATS)." *Journal of Child & Adolescent Psychopharmacology* 17: 593–604.

Vitiello, B., et al. (2009). "Suicidal Events in the Treatment of Adolescents with Depression Study (TADS)." *Journal of Clinical Psychiatry* 70: 741–747.

Walkup, J. T., et al. (2008). "Cognitive Behavioral Therapy, Sertraline, or a Combination in Childhood Anxiety." *New England Journal of Medicine* 359: 2753–2766.

Wang, G. S., et al. (2014). "Association of Unintentional Pediatric Exposures with Decriminalization of Marijuana in the United States." *Annals of Emergency Medicine* 63: 684–689. doi: 10.1016/j.annemergmed.2014.01.017.

Wang, T. W. (2017). "Secondhand Exposure to Electronic Cigarette Aerosol Among US Youths." *JAMA Pediatrics* 171: 490–492. doi: 10.1001/jamapediatrics.2016.4973.

Waxmonsky, J. G., et al. (2014). "Does Pharmacological Treatment of ADHD in Adults Enhance Parenting Performance? Results of a Double-Blind Randomized Trial." *CNS Drugs* 28: 665–677.

Weissman, M. M., et al. (2015). "Treatment of Maternal Depression in a Medication Clinical Trial and its Effect on Children." *American Journal of Psychiatry* 172: 450–459. doi: 10.1176/appi.ajp.2014.13121679.

Wemakor, A., et al. (2015). "Selective Serotonin Reuptake Inhibitor Antidepressant Use in First Trimester Pregnancy and Risk of Specific Congenital Anomalies: A European Register-Based Study." *European Journal of Epidemiology* 11: 1187–1198. doi: 10.1007/s10654-015-0065-y.

Wesseloo, R., et al. (2016). "Risk of Postpartum Relapse in Bipolar Disorder and Postpartum Psychosis: A Systematic Review and Meta-Analysis." *American Journal of Psychiatry* 173: 117–127. doi: 10.1176/appi.ajp.2015.15010124.

Westin, A. A., et al. (2017). "Changes in Drug Disposition of Lithium During Pregnancy: A Retrospective Observational Study of Patient Data from Two Routine Therapeutic Drug Monitoring Services in Norway." *BMJ Open* 7: e015738. doi: 10.1136/bmjopen-2016–015738.

Wilens, T., et al. (2016). "Nonmedical Stimulant Use in College Students: Association with Attention-Deficit/Hyperactivity Disorder and Other Disorders." *Journal of Clinical Psychiatry* 77: 940–947.

Wilson, K. M., et al. (2016). "Marijuana Exposure in Children Hospitalized for Bronchiolitis." *Pediatric Academic Societies*. Abstract 4460.8.

Zhou, X., et al. (2014). "Systematic Review of Management for Treatment-Resistant Depression in Adolescents." *BMC Psychiatry* 14: 340. doi: 10.1186/s12888-014-0340-6.

CHAPTER 16

Geriatric Psychopharmacology

This chapter reviews how the drugs discussed in earlier chapters are applied in geriatric populations to treat disorders and disruptive behavior, including depression, anxiety disorders, behavioral agitation and aggression, Parkinson's disease, and Alzheimer's disease. First, however, we present several general principles concerning the actions and effects of psychoactive drugs administered to elderly patients:

- Lower doses of medication are often as effective in the elderly as higher doses in younger people.
- When initiating drug therapy in the elderly, it is wise to "start low and go slow."
- Elimination half-lives are often prolonged in the elderly, sometimes to about twice as long as half-lives in younger people due to pharmacokinetic changes that occur with aging, such as decreased liver enzyme activity. These physiological changes require adjustment of total daily doses and frequency of dosing of many medications.
- Sedative-hypnotic drugs, especially the long-half-life benzodiazepines, can be quite "dementing" in the elderly, causing marked and often prolonged cognitive impairment presenting as memory deficiencies and possibly even leading to a misdiagnosis of dementia.
- Sedative-hypnotic drugs can also induce psychomotor incoordination, resulting in an increased incidence of falls, altered driving behaviors, and so on.
- Depression and comorbid anxiety are common in the elderly and need to be addressed and treated.
- Psychological therapies can be used effectively to treat anxiety disorders, sleep disorders, and other psychological disorders for which drugs are often prescribed.
- Inappropriate drug use in the elderly is a common problem with potentially tragic consequences.
- Substance abuse in the elderly often goes undetected and therefore untreated, leading to broader psychological, psychiatric, and physiological morbidities.
- About half of elderly patients experience chronic or persistent pain and pain is often missed, misdiagnosed, or undertreated in the elderly (Atkinson et al., 2013; Dentino et al., 2017; Paladini et al., 2015).

INAPPROPRIATE DRUG USE IN THE ELDERLY

The elderly are frequently prescribed medication that they do not need or that cause them significant problems, either because of extensions of expected pharmacological effects or through adverse interactions with other medications. Inappropriate medication use in the elderly is a major functional and safety issue and may cause a substantial proportion of drug-related hospital or care-center admissions (Charlesworth et al., 2015; Maust et al., 2017a, 2017b). While only 14 percent of Americans are aged 65 years or older, this group represents the largest per capita consumers of prescription medications. Studies of community-dwelling adults have found that 39 percent take five or more prescription medications, 38 percent at least one or more over-the-counter medications, and 64 percent at least one or more dietary supplements (Charlesworth et al., 2015; Page et al., 2010; Qato et al., 2016). And this trend of geriatric polypharmacy has been rising. To help bring attention to the inappropriate drug use in the elderly, M. H. Beers in 1997 developed specific criteria for inappropriate use, which included a list of drugs that were either ineffective or posed unnecessarily high risks for people over 65 years of age. This list is updated periodically and the most recent version (2015) can be found on the American Geriatrics Society Web site (http://www.americangeriatrics.org).

In addition, workers in different health care systems have developed modifications of the Beers criteria designed to fit their specific population. The National Committee for Quality Assurance (NCQA) publishes the Healthcare Effectiveness Data and Information Set (HEDIS) and incorporates the Beers criteria into one of its quality measures: Potentially Harmful Drug-Disease Interactions in the Elderly. This quality measure is updated in concert with updates in the Beers criteria and can be found on the NCQA Web site (http://www.ncqa.org). There is also the Zhan modification of the Beers criteria for community-dwelling elderly (Barnett et al., 2006); the Improved Prescribing in the Elderly Tool (Ryan et al., 2009); and the Medication Appropriateness Index (Steinman et al., 2006). All of these tools attempt to identify medicines commonly considered of more risk than benefit to the elderly.

The extent of inappropriate prescription use is common, with a rate between 20 and 40 percent. In elderly patients taking eight or more medications, the incidence of inappropriate drug use rises to well over 60 percent. Among the psychoactive medicines, long-acting benzodiazepines are most commonly inappropriately prescribed, followed by drugs with anticholinergic side effects, such as tricyclic antidepressants, then antihistamines, skeletal muscle relaxants, and opioid narcotics. There remains a question about the risk for dementia from use of benzodiazepines in the elderly. Some studies have found that continued use of these agents can increase the subsequent risk of dementia by 50 percent (Billioti de Gage et al., 2010; Billioti de Gage et al., 2014). A newer study, however, failed to find any association between benzodiazepine use and subsequent increase in dementia (Gray et al., 2016). Another study points to an increased risk for pneumonia in dementia patients who are treated with benzodiazepines (Taipale et al., 2017). Another type of inappropriate drug use scenario in the elderly is the concomitant use of two or more psychotropic medicines of the same therapeutic class.

Inappropriate drug use can lead to suboptimal care that is not consistent with evidence-based clinical practice (Maust et al., 2017b). All the lists that identify inappropriate drug use in the elderly recommend avoiding drugs that produce (1) *cognitive inhibition*, with drug-induced dementia as the most severe manifestation, (2) *unwanted sedation,* leading to falls and hip fractures, or (3) *bizarre behaviors* and/or *drug-induced delirium*. Tricyclic antidepressants or other drugs with anticholinergic properties and sedating antihistamines are particular drugs of concern, along with the benzodiazepines and opiates (Tannenbaum et al., 2012). Indeed, discontinuing such medications can lead to improvements in psychomotor and cognitive functioning, including memory and attention (Nishtala et al., 2009; Carnahan, 2010; Tsunoda et al., 2010).

CONTROL OF AGITATED AND AGGRESSIVE BEHAVIORS IN THE ELDERLY

Atypical antipsychotic medications (Chapter 11) had become the standard of care for *behavioral and psychological symptoms of dementia* (BPSD). These medicines were thought to control agitated and aggressive behaviors in the elderly, especially residents of care centers. In 2005, however, the Food and Drug Administration (FDA) issued a public health advisory warning indicating a 1.7-fold risk of all-cause mortality from these medicines compared to placebo. The FDA subsequently issued a black box warning on the use of any first-, second-, or third-generation antipsychotic for the treatment of agitation and psychosis in dementia patients. This advisory has been controversial because some studies have failed to verify any increased risk of death (Simoni-Wastila et al., 2009; Elie et al., 2009). But other studies confirm some degree of increased risk of mortality in individuals with dementia who are treated with antipsychotic medication (Farlow and Shamliyan, 2017; Koponen et al., 2017; Meeks, 2010; Zhai et al., 2016). The risk may vary depending on the drug used (greater for haloperidol and least for quetiapine (Huybrechts et al., 2012; Kales et al., 2012)). For dementia patients treated with antipsychotic drugs, the risk for myocardial infarction (MI) was found to be double that of the rate in individuals not receiving antipsychotics (Pariente et al., 2012). And antipsychotics have been shown to increase morbidity risk, including pneumonia (Tolppanen et al., 2016).

Despite the FDA advisory and controversy, the use of atypical antipsychotics to treat elderly persons with BPSD continues, especially in long-term-care settings (Connelly et al., 2009; Olfson et al., 2015). However, Dorsey and coworkers (2010) reported that this use of atypical antipsychotic medicines is decreasing in the elderly with dementia. This has been confirmed through additional studies that attribute the decline to the FDA's initial health care warning followed by the black box warning (Kales et al., 2011; Ventimiglia et al., 2010). In a national survey of prescriptions within nursing home facilities, Briesacher and colleagues (2013) found that during 2009 to 2010, 22 percent of residents received at least one antipsychotic medication during their stay; of the antipsychotics prescribed, the two most frequently administered were quetiapine and risperidone, accounting for 55.5 percent of all of the antipsychotics prescribed. The 22 percent figure is a decrease from 2006 statistics

TABLE 16.1 Most commonly prescribed antipsychotic medications in nursing homes

Generic drug name	Number of residents prescribed drug	Percent of all antipsychotic medication prescribed
Quetiapine fumarate	1,356,223	31.1
Risperidone	1,061,897	24.4
Olanzapine	570,453	13.1
Haloperidol	402,077	9.2
Aripiprazole	347,900	8.0
Clozapine	232,125	5.3
Ziprasidone	138,881	3.2
Chlorpromazine	65,159	1.5
Fluphenazine	54,867	1.3
All others	109,141	2.9

indicating that 29 percent of nursing facility residents received at least one antipsychotic medication (see Chen et al., 2010).

Certain interventions can have a positive effect on reducing use of antipsychotic medications for individuals with dementia. Pharmacological medication reviews have been shown to reduce unnecessary antipsychotic utilization, but may not be as effective if there is no access to or utilization of evidence-based behavioral interventions to reduce the incidence of psychological and behavioral disorders (Ballard et al., 2016). (See Table 16.1 for the most commonly prescribed antipsychotics in nursing homes.) An initiative by the federal Centers for Medicare and Medicaid Services (CMS) to target excessive use of these drugs in the absence of an appropriate diagnosis or documentation of medical necessity is an example of these types of interventions. This initiative, the Partnership to Improve Dementia Care, began in May 2012 and (1) involves special training for nursing facility staff on humane methods for addressing BPSD; (2) publishing data on use of antipsychotics on the Nursing Home Compare public Web site; (3) revising staffing patterns, activities, and pain management detection and treatment; and (4) including information on the use of antipsychotics as part of the CMS quality review of nursing facilities. Regulations associated with this initiative also stress the limited duration for use of antipsychotic medications for nursing home residents and periodic review of antipsychotic usage to determine if the medication should be continued. The goal for this program initially was to reduce the use of antipsychotic medication in nursing facilities by 15 percent. By the end of 2013, that goal was actually exceeded and the program set new goals of reducing antipsychotic medication use by 25 percent by the end of 2015 and by 30 percent by the end of 2016 (Ellis et al., 2015). According to CMS, as of the third quarter of 2015, use of antipsychotic medication in nursing facilities had decreased by 27 percent close to the program's target goal of 30 percent by the end of 2016.

Another initiative to reduce inappropriate use of antipsychotic medication in the elderly, the Choosing Wisely Campaign, is a joint effort by the American Geriatric Society (AGS) and the American Psychiatric Association (APA). The mission of this program is to promote conversations between clinicians and patients by helping patients choose care that is "supported by evidence; not duplicative of other tests or procedures already received; free from harm; and truly necessary" (http://www.choosingwisely.org/our-mission/).

The antipsychotic drugs have also been used to relieve various core symptoms that arise in the course of dementia (Farlow and Shamliyan, 2017; Olfson et al., 2015; Omelan, 2006), specifically:

- Agitation, such as pacing, wandering, restlessness, or the inability to sit long enough to eat
- Aggression, either verbal or physical, which might be directed at staff or other residents
- Physical resistance and noncompliance with care
- Psychosis marked by hallucinations or delusions
- Depressive symptoms, such as apathy or lack of interest
- Inappropriate sexual behaviors that are verbal or physical
- Sleep disturbances, such as day–night reversal

In some cases, although agitation and aggression apparently may be reduced by administering an atypical antipsychotic drug, there is little evidence of drug efficacy against the core symptoms of dementia. According to Omelan (2006) and Rothenberg and Wiechers (2015), certain behaviors should not be expected to improve, such as wandering, pacing, entering rooms uninvited, and disruptive vocalizations.

Initially, when the second-generation antipsychotic medications first came to market, *risperidone* (Risperdal) and *olanzapine* (Zyprexa) were used most frequently in this population, but *quetiapine* (Seroquel) has rapidly gained favor, perhaps because quetiapine seems to cause less undesired weight gain and has less propensity to induce type 2 diabetes. Unfortunately, Paleacu and coworkers (2008) reported results from a six-week, double-blind, placebo-controlled study of 44 patients with dementia and BPSD showing that quetiapine in quite large doses was only modestly more effective than placebo in reducing behavioral symptoms. A few patients, however, showed a positive and sustained response. In another study of risperidone in the treatment of agitation and psychosis in patients with Alzheimer's disease, Devanand et al. (2012) found that some patients had a modest reduction in target symptoms, but this was not maintained and some patients did not respond. Those that responded after 16 weeks of treatment were randomized into three groups: the first group continued treatment with risperidone for 32 weeks; the second group continued treatment with risperidone for 16 weeks and was then switched to placebo for 16 weeks; the third group was switched to placebo for 32 weeks. The results indicated that for those patients who derived some benefit from risperidone, there was an increase in relapse rates for those switched to placebo compared to those continuing with risperidone treatment, indicating that the risperidone was of some benefit.

Streim and coworkers (2008) reported on the efficacy of *aripiprazole* (Abilify) in the treatment of psychosis in nursing home patients with Alzheimer's disease. The drug did not confer specific benefits for the treatment of psychotic symptoms, but BPSD symptoms—including agitation, anxiety, and depression—were significantly improved, with a low risk of side effects. De Deyn and colleagues (2013) also found some efficacy of aripiprazole for treatment of psychosis and agitation in patients with Alzheimer's disease; although the effect was modest and the drug produced a high degree of sedation. They recommend using the drug only in selected patient populations that are resistant to nonpharmacological treatment and/or have persistent, severe psychotic symptoms and/ or agitation leading to significant morbidity. Although aripiprazole is capable of reducing anxiety and agitation, it can also produce these same symptoms as side effects in about 8 to 10 percent of patients at doses of about 10 milligrams per day (Coley et al., 2009).

Despite these positive findings of the efficacy of second-generation antipsychotics (SGAs) on BPSD, not all studies have shown them to be beneficial. Jin and colleagues (2013) conducted a study in which the subjects and their treatment providers could choose to be assigned to one of several SGAs; despite this flexibility in choosing treatments, they found a high discontinuation rate of SGAs when used to treat older individuals with dementia and that one-half of the patients remained on the study medication for less than 6 months. In addition, there was a high incidence of metabolic syndrome (36 percent), and serious (24 percent) and nonserious (51 percent) adverse events; and there was no improvement in psychotic symptoms. The authors point out that the overall risk–benefit ratio for the atypical antipsychotics in patients over age 40 was not favorable, regardless of diagnosis or drug; but they caution that the results do not suggest that SGAs should not be used in older patients with psychosis, only that there are no safe and effective treatment alternatives and short-term use may be necessary for controlling severe psychotic symptoms in some patients.

Therefore, at this point, despite the FDA's public health advisory, an atypical antipsychotic remains a cautious optional choice for the treatment of severe BPSD in the elderly with dementia. However, the use of SGAs for BPSD must be weighed against the risk not only of increased mortality for which the FDA has issued its black box warning, but also against the increased morbidity of worsening cognitive decline. One of the findings from the 36-week Clinical Antipsychotic Trials of Intervention Effectiveness-Alzheimer's Disease (CATIE-AD) indicated that, compared to placebo, use of SGAs such as olanzapine, risperidone, or quetiapine "are associated with greater rates of decline in cognitive function in Alzheimer's patients with psychotic or aggressive behavior and that the magnitude of this additional decline is clinically relevant, reaching at least as great a magnitude as the effect of cholinesterase inhibitors but in the negative direction" (Vigen et al., 2011, 837). In the Dementia Antipsychotic Withdrawal Trial (DART-AD), long-term-care residents with Alzheimer's disease were randomized to continue their antipsychotic regimen or to be switched to placebo and then followed for 12 months; the authors found no significant difference between groups on level of cognitive symptoms or neuropsychiatric symptoms, both of which worsened (Ballard et al., 2008; see also Meeks, 2010).

In agitated, aggressive, anxious elderly with dementia, the benefits of behavioral improvement, if it occurs, may allow the patient to remain in a less structured and less confining environment than otherwise would be possible. Thus, the humanitarian benefits of trying antipsychotic medications may outweigh any increase in risk in some patients. But given the current literature suggesting minimal to weak effects, these agents should be used with discretion, close monitoring, and only as part of a nonpharmacological, environmental, and behavioral intervention package (Omelan, 2006; Porsteinssona and Antonsdottir, 2017). In addition, when these drugs are used, they should be for the short term and discontinued when no longer needed, because the target behaviors may decrease or subside naturally. In some cases, however, drug treatment may need to be continued, as discontinuation may cause an individual to relapse and symptoms such as hallucinations to re-emerge. One possible predictor of increased risk for relapse upon discontinuation is the presence of severe levels of hallucinations present before initiation of treatment (Patel et al., 2017).

UNDERTREATMENT OF THE ELDERLY: FOCUS ON DEPRESSION

Untreated depression in the elderly can seriously reduce both the quality and length of life. However, depression in the elderly remains underdiagnosed and often poorly or inadequately treated. According to 2014 statistics from the CDC, the highest rate of suicide deaths for males and females combined is in the 45 to 54 age group at 20.2 deaths per 100,000 population; next highest is in the 85 and over age group at 19.3 deaths per 100,000 population. Males in all age groups have higher rates of death compared to females and the highest rate is in males who are 85 years of age or older; their rate is 49.9 deaths per 100,000 population. Adults 65 years of age and older have a rate of death by suicide of 16.6 per 100,000 population, which is higher than the national average of 13.0 deaths per 100,000 population. In addition, based on three national surveys conducted between 2001 and 2003, it has been observed that of the individuals with some mental health disorder, about 41 percent perceive the need for help and seek it and about 16 percent seek it from a mental health professional. The problem is that most older adults with mental health issues do not perceive the need for help, such that less than 8 percent of those who are 65 years or older sought help in the previous year of this study (Mackenzie et al., 2010). Subsequent studies continue to find that the 65+ age group has the highest rates of not receiving mental health treatment and the lowest rate of perceived need for treatment (Choi et al., 2014). Factors that may be related to this age group's underutilization of mental health services are discussed by Kessler et al. (2015).

Although most older adults prefer to receive their mental health services from their primary care provider, that may not be the most effective intervention for this population. It has been suggested that a team approach to treating depression in the elderly can be quite successful. For example, Van Leeuwen and coworkers (2009) present the results of one team approach program, IMPACT, for Improving Mood: Promoting Access to Collaborative Treatment, which involves a team comprised of a depression case manager, such as a psychologist, social worker or a nurse; a primary care physician; and a consulting psychiatrist. In assessing and endorsing this program, Hunkeler and coworkers (2006) state:

> Tailored collaborative care actively engages older adults in treatment for depression and delivers substantial and persistent long-term benefits. Benefits included less depression, better physical functioning, and an enhanced quality of life. The IMPACT model may show the way to less depression and healthier lives for older adults. (259)

Further analysis of the data from the IMPACT trial found that elderly depressed patients had lower risk of subsequent cardiovascular disease (CVD) than elderly depressed patients not receiving integrated care (Stewart et al., 2014). Penkunas and Hahn-Smith (2015) confirmed that using an evidence-based collaborative treatment model such as IMPACT can produce improved outcomes for elderly individuals who suffer from late-life depression.

In support of this collaborative care model, Reynolds and coworkers (2006) studied 116 patients over the age of 70 who had been diagnosed with major depression. Here, they compared the efficacy of placebo medication, medication alone, psychological therapy alone, and combined medication and psychological therapy. The medication chosen was *paroxetine* (Paxil); the psychological therapy chosen was weekly interpersonal psychotherapy (IPT). Combination therapy improved the percentage of patients achieving remission from 35 percent with either therapy alone to 58 percent, a remarkable improvement. Results indicated that depression in the elderly is best treated by a combination of antidepressant medication and psychological interventions. But not all studies have found that communication between mental health professionals and primary care providers is a necessary component for the effectiveness of collaborative care interventions for the treatment of depression in the elderly (Chang-Quan et al., 2009).

Antidepressants to Treat Depression in the Elderly

Paroxetine was effective in the Reynolds study as well as in a study by Dombrovski and coworkers (2007). Kasper and coworkers (2006) demonstrated the efficacy of *escitalopram* (Lexapro) in the elderly (mean age 74 years; 82 percent female) for the treatment of depression; escitalopram was later noted to be less efficacious for the treatment of generalized anxiety disorder in the elderly (Lenze et al., 2009). Nelson and coworkers (2006) reported results on the use of *mirtazepine* (Remeron) to treat major depression in 50 patients aged 85 and older residing in nursing homes. In 45 percent of patients, mirtazepine (average dose 18 milligrams per day) was effective in decreasing the average Hamilton Rating Scale for Depression score from 17 at baseline to 7 at end point. Sedation and weight gain were prominent side effects. Administering the drug at bedtime took advantage of sedation as a sleep aid. Weight gain was also seen as a positive effect in this age group, where maintaining adequate body weight is often a concern. Concern is always present when using sedative medication at bedtime in the elderly. In this study, the incidence of falls did not seem to increase; however, a control (placebo) group was not employed, so the incidence of falls could not be determined with certainty. Kok et al. (2011) analyzed the results of eight double-blind, randomized controlled trials of antidepressant continuation treatment of depression in the elderly using relapse as an outcome indicator. They found that continuation of antidepressant treatment resulted in fewer relapses when compared to placebo, suggesting that continued treatment with antidepressants is efficacious in maintaining recovery from depression in the elderly. There was no difference in effectiveness between first- and second-generation antidepressants, but there is still concern about the use of antidepressants in the elderly. Some of the concerns include the low rate of response to antidepressant treatment by the elderly and increased risk for morbidity and mortality, including stroke, myocardial infarction, increased risk of suicide, seizures, and falls (Coupland et al., 2011). Other authors have also found that use of SSRIs in treating depression in the elderly with dementia led to a significant increase in falls; the risk of falling was related to the dose of the SSRI (Sterke et al., 2012a).

The presence of an anxiety disorder comorbid with a depressive disorder correlates with poorer outcome for depression treatment (Lenze et al., 2005). Similarly, a high pretreatment level of anxiety increases the risk of nonresponse to antidepressant treatment as well as the risk of recurrence in the first 2 years of maintenance treatment (Andreescu et al., 2007). These results indicate that depressed elderly patients should be screened for anxiety disorders and treated for them, if they are present, as aggressively as for the depressive disorder.

In a small study of older patients with unipolar depression that was resistant to selective serotonin reuptake inhibitors (SSRIs), Rutherford and coworkers (2007) reported that *aripiprazole* (Abilify) augmentation of therapy with the SSRI citalopram resulted in a 50 percent rate of remission in formerly resistant elderly. This outcome was verified by Lenze and coworkers (2008), who also noted that remission was sustained in all 24 patients during 6 months of continuation treatment. The authors added:

> Incomplete response in the treatment of late-life depression is a large public health challenge: at least 50 percent of older people fail to respond adequately to first-line antidepressant pharmacotherapy, even under optimal treatment conditions. Treatment-resistant late-life depression increases risk for early relapse, undermines adherence to treatment for coexisting medical disorders, amplifies disability and cognitive impairment, imposes greater burden on family caregivers, and increases the risk for early mortality, including suicide. (419)

Despite the lack of conclusive evidence that antidepressants or adjunctive use of antipsychotics will consistently improve depressive illness in the elderly, it is important to carefully evaluate the elderly for not only depression but also other comorbid disorders that can influence psychological presentation and functional ability. Collaborative care models that integrate primary care treatment with specialty behavioral health treatment are demonstrating advantages over traditional forms of health care service delivery. This includes the appropriate use of medications in combination with evidence-based psychotherapies for the elderly (Hall and Reynolds, 2014). If late-life depression is overlooked or not adequately treated, there is some evidence moderate to severe symptoms of depression may increase the risk for subsequent development of dementia (Kaup et al., 2016).

PARKINSON'S DISEASE

Parkinson's disease (PD) is the second most common neurodegenerative disease after Alzheimer's disease. According to the Parkinson's Disease Foundation, about 1 million Americans and 10 million people worldwide are currently living with PD. More than 60,000 new cases are diagnosed in the United States each year. Although the cause of Parkinson's disease remains unknown, its symptoms are thought to follow from a deficiency in the number and function of dopamine-secreting neurons located primarily in the substantia nigra, a subthalamic area of the brain. Progressive loss of these neurons is a feature of normal aging; however, most people do not lose the huge number of dopamine neurons required to cause PD symptoms.

Chapter 11 discussed the first-generation, or traditional, antipsychotic agents, such as haloperidol and other high, potency agents, used to treat schizophrenia. The most prominent side effects of those drugs are movement disorders that resemble those seen in idiopathic Parkinson's disease. Mechanistically, these side effects result from drug-induced blockade of dopamine-2 receptors, resulting in a hypodopaminergic state. PD is similarly associated with a hypodopaminergic state, but characterized by a progressive loss of dopamine neurons. Currently, there are no effective neuroprotective therapies. Patients are currently treated with a combination of the dopamine replacement therapies discussed here or receive deep brain electrical stimulation to combat behavioral symptoms (Williams et al., 2010). The ideal candidate therapy would be one that prevents neurodegeneration of dopamine neurons in the brain, and specific neurotropic factors are being researched. Transplantation of dopaminergic stem cells into the brains of persons with PD has not yet met with success (Olanow et al., 2009a). The most common approach to therapy of PD is through dopamine replacement interventions designed to maintain dopaminergic function and slow the effect of the loss of dopamine neurons.

Current research suggests that Parkinson's disease is not only a motor disorder, but also presents with nonmotor symptoms that may actually precede the onset of observable motor deficits by a period of 5 to 20 years. Some candidate nonmotor signs include olfactory, bowel, sleep, and mood disorders (Sauerbier et al., 2016). It is considered a multisystemic disorder with multiple phenotypic presentations, each of which may have a unique etiology that includes specific gene variants combined with environmental influences (Delamarre et al., 2017; Ferreira and Massano, 2017). Regardless of the etiology of neuronal loss in Parkinson's disease, the clinical features emerge when about 80 percent of dopamine neurons are lost. The clinical syndrome of Parkinson's disease has several cardinal features:

- Bradykinesia (slowness and poverty of movement)
- Muscle rigidity (especially a "cogwheel" rigidity)
- Resting tremor, which usually abates during voluntary movement
- Impairment of postural balance, leading to disturbances of gait and falling
- Without treatment, progression over 5 to 10 years to a state of severe rigidity and loss of movement in which patients cannot care for themselves. (The 1990 film *Awakenings* depicts this feature of Parkinson's disease.)

The availability of effective treatments for PD symptoms has radically altered the prognosis of this disease. In most cases, good functional mobility can be maintained for many years and the life expectancy of an affected person has been greatly extended. Replacement of the dopamine or the administration of either dopaminergic agonists or inhibitors of dopamine breakdown can restore function and ameliorate much of the symptomatology. These three approaches—dopamine replacement therapy, administration of a dopaminergic agonist, and administration of dopamine breakdown inhibitors—underlie much of today's treatment of the disease. Increasing dopamine in the brain, however, does bring with it some untoward effects, including impulse control disorders such as pathological gambling, binge eating, reckless driving, and hypersexuality (Abler et al., 2009; Weintraub et al., 2010), as well as dyskinetic movement disorders.

Levodopa

Levodopa, a precursor drug to dopamine, continues to be the mainstay of therapy for Parkinson's disease, although today it is usually used in combination with other medications. Because a loss of dopamine is the primary problem in PD patients, replacement of the dopamine would be expected to ameliorate the symptoms of the disease. It does, but not by itself, because dopamine poorly crosses the blood–brain barrier from plasma into the central nervous system (CNS). The precursor compound in the biosynthesis of dopamine from the amino acid tyramine, *dihydroxyphenylalanine*, or *dopa*, crosses the blood–brain barrier and in the CNS, is converted into dopamine, replacing the dopamine that is absent. Therefore, today levodopa—the *levo* isomer being more active than the *dextro* isomer—is the most effective treatment for motor disability. Many practitioners consider an initial beneficial response an important criterion for the diagnosis of parkinsonism.

Mechanism of Action

Administered orally, levodopa is rapidly absorbed into the bloodstream, where most of it (about 95 percent) is converted to dopamine in the plasma. Although only a small amount (about 1 to 5 percent) of levodopa crosses the blood–brain barrier and is converted to dopamine in the brain, it is enough to alleviate the symptoms of PD. In the CNS, levodopa is converted to dopamine, primarily within the presynaptic terminals of dopaminergic neurons in the basal ganglia.

One problem with this therapy is that, when levodopa is administered by itself, it is converted to dopamine in the body, resulting in undesirable side effects such as nausea. One approach to solving the problem is to reduce the high levels of dopamine in the systemic circulation while maintaining sufficient quantities in the brain. To do so, the biosynthetic pathway that leads to dopamine (see Figure 16.1) must be examined. Since the enzyme *dopa decarboxylase* is responsible for converting dopa to dopamine by inhibiting this enzyme in the systemic circulation but not in the brain, systemic biotransformation of the drug should be reduced, with a concomitant reduction in blood levels of dopamine and therefore, in side effects. The drug needed a unique characteristic: it would have to be active in the body, but not cross the blood–brain barrier into the brain. Thus, the metabolic conversion would occur in the CNS but not in the periphery.

An example of such a drug is *carbidopa* in combination with levodopa (Sinemet). The combination is also marketed as a rapidly dissolving tablet (Parcopa); a controlled release version (Sinemet CR); an extended-release version (Rytary);

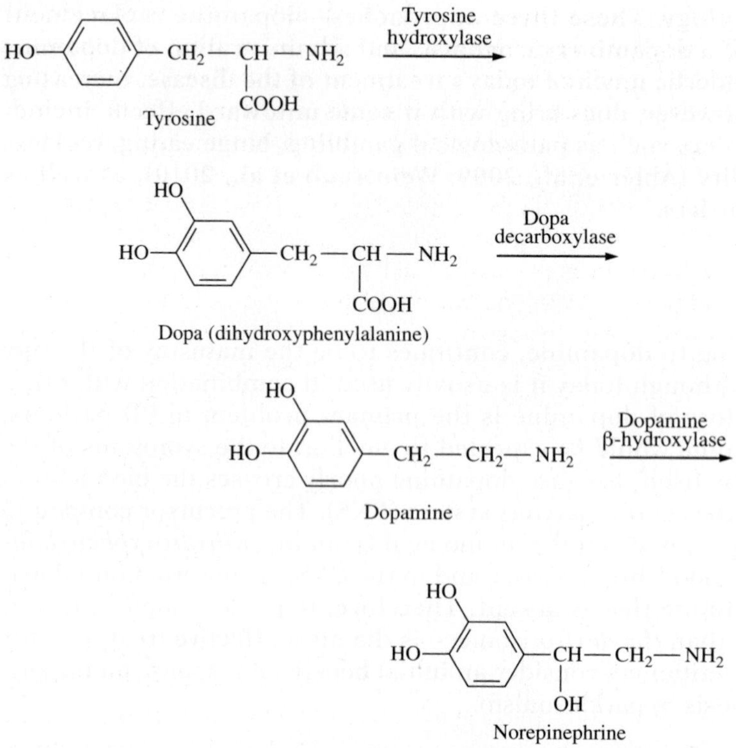

FIGURE 16.1 Synthesis of dopamine from tyrosine.

a carbidopa-levodopa-entacapone combination (Stalevo); and as a gel (Duopa) that can be infused directly into the small intestine via a surgically implanted tube. The entacapone in Stalevo selectively inhibits an enzyme called *catechol-o-methyltransferase* (COMT) in the periphery, which further protects the levodopa from peripheral degradation and enhances central bioavailability. By combining entacapone and/or carbidopa with levodopa, the dose of levodopa is reduced by 75 percent, with a concomitant reduction in side effects and no loss of CNS therapeutic effect. (Entacapone and COMT inhibitors will be discussed in more detail in the next section.) The current treatment of Parkinson's disease relies heavily on the use of Sinemet. The combination of levodopa and carbidopa provides near-maximal therapeutic benefit with the fewest side effects.

Limitations of Levodopa Therapy

Unfortunately, as time goes on, each dose of levodopa may become less effective and the patient's symptoms fluctuate dramatically between doses, eventually developing into the "on-off" phenomenon. During the "on" phase, symptoms are under good control, but as the medication effect "wears off" between doses, symptoms become more evident; this is referred to as the "off" phase. Part of the phenomenon is due to the short half-life of levodopa and can be minimized by increasing the dose and/or by decreasing the interval between doses. This adjustment, however, risks the development of levodopa-induced movement disorders (dyskinesia), which can be as uncomfortable and disabling as the rigidity and akinesia of parkinsonism. Indeed, within about 5 years after initiating levodopa treatment, over 50 percent of patients develop these disabling motor disorders. An alternative to using COMT inhibitors to reduce "off" periods is treatment with *rasagiline* (Azilect), which has been shown to increase "on" times and decrease "off" periods when combined with carbidopa or levodopa (Giugni and Okun, 2014). Rasagiline is a centrally acting selective inhibitor of MAO-B that is thought to increase extracellular dopamine in the striatum.

The most common side effects of levodopa include hypotension, nausea, dry mouth, dizziness, sedation, and headache early in the course of treatment. Motor symptoms, such as dyskinesias, can develop as the disease progresses. Still later and as the patient ages, confusion, delusions, hallucinations, and agitation may be seen. Although psychotic symptoms in other disorders, such as schizophrenia, are treated with antipsychotic medication, using such drugs for patients with Parkinson's disease is problematic, since the drugs block dopamine receptors and would be expected to worsen the core symptoms of the disorder and block the effects of the drugs used to enhance dopamine activity.

Clozapine has been shown to be effective in reducing psychotic symptoms in individuals with Parkinson's disease, but clozapine requires regular blood drawing to monitor for signs of agranulocytosis.[1] An alternative would be quetiapine, but it may be much weaker than clozapine (Giugni and Okun, 2014). A new drug has been approved by the FDA specifically to treat psychosis in Parkinson's disease. *Pimavanserin* (Nuplazid) is an atypical antipsychotic drug that is an inverse agonist at 5-HT$_{2A}$ receptors, thus reducing serotoneric activity (Howland, 2016). It is effective in reducing hallucinations and delusions without causing a worsening of parkinsonian symptoms (Bozymski et al., 2017; Kianirad and Simuni, 2017; Mathis et al., 2017).

Does levodopa therapy adversely accelerate the course of PD? According to most experts, there is no reason to be concerned about advancing the disorder by appropriate use of levodopa, which does not lose its effectiveness over time. But after about 5 years of treatment, motor complications such as dyskinesias and the "on-off" effect develop as the brain continues to lose dopamine-producing neurons and the remaining neurons make less dopamine. Therefore, it is important to have a comprehensive discussion with patients, spouses, families, and caregivers about the available options and when to start treatment. Although starting treatment early can reduce symptoms, the efficacy may be time limited. Furthermore, waiting too long to start treatment can subject the patient and their loved ones to a significantly reduced quality of life and rising risks of other forms of morbidity, like falling.

COMT Inhibitors

As mentioned earlier, another target for the PD therapeutic regimen involves an enzyme called catechol-o-methyltransferase (COMT). Even with the Sinemet combination, much of an oral dose of levodopa is wasted. COMT in the vasculature of the gastrointestinal (GI)

---

[1] Agranulocytosis occurs when the body does not produce enough white blood cells to fight off infections. For additional information, see the discussion of agranulocytosis related to clozapine in Chapter 11.

tract and liver converts levodopa to an inactive metabolite with no clinical benefit. The half-life and clinical effects of Sinemet can be increased with the addition of a COMT-inhibitory drug. In 1998, the first of these drugs, *tolcapone* (Tasmar), was introduced; it blocks the COMT enzyme, increasing the half-life of levodopa and prolonging its effect. Unfortunately, tolcapone caused a few cases of serious liver toxicity, so in late 1998, it was withdrawn from the market in Canada and in Europe. In the United States, its use is restricted to cases where all other adjunctive therapies have failed, and close monitoring of liver function is required.

A second COMT inhibitor, *entacapone* (Comtan), became available in 2001 and has not yet been associated with liver toxicity. Like tolcapone, entacapone inhibits peripheral COMT, but does not alter central COMT. Inhibition of peripheral degradation of levodopa increases central levodopa and therefore, central dopamine concentrations. Co-administration of entacapone with levodopa plus carbidopa potentiates the effects of levodopa in patients with PD and reduces the "off" periods, but use of the COMT inhibitor has also resulted in an increased risk for producing dyskinesias (Giugni and Okun, 2014). In 15 to 20 percent of patients, the "on-off" phenomenon may be extreme and disabling; doses of levodopa that originally were effective for 8 hours last for only 1 or 2 hours.

In 2004, the FDA approved a fixed combination product, Stalevo, containing levodopa, carbidopa, and entacapone. The combination provides more dopamine to the brain for a longer period of time, providing more "on" time and less "off" time associated with each dose of levodopa (Giugni and Okun, 2014; Hauser, 2009). The most common side effects associated with the use of COMT inhibitors like entacapone include dyskinesia, hallucinations, confusion, nausea, diarrhea, orange discoloration of the urine, and low blood pressure after standing up. In fact, in the randomized controlled trial, Stalevo Reduction in Dyskinesia Evaluation in Parkinson's Disease (STRIDE-PD), it was found that adding entacapone did indeed reduce the frequency of the "on-off" episodes, but it also increased the frequency of dyskinesias. The results also indicated that there was an increase in the frequency of cardiovascular events such as myocardial infarction and stroke (Stocchi et al., 2010). Thus, there was some concern about using Stalevo. But a later analysis of the data from the STRIDE-PD study focusing specifically on the occurrences of cardiovascular events did not find any increase in myocardial infarctions, stroke, or death in Parkinson's patients who were treated with Stalevo versus those treated with Sinement (Graham et al., 2013).

Dopamine Receptor Agonists

Between 1 and 5 years after the start of levodopa therapy, most patients gradually become less responsive. One hypothesis for this effect is that the progression of PD may be associated with an increasing inability of dopamine neurons to synthesize and store dopamine. To relieve this problem, attempts have been made to identify drugs that directly stimulate postsynaptic dopamine receptors in the basal ganglia. These drugs do not depend on the ability of existing dopaminergic neurons to synthesize dopamine. As a result, they are increasingly being advocated for use in early stages of Parkinson's disease, especially in patients younger than about 65. These drugs might also be effective in the later stages of Parkinson's disease, when dopamine neurons are largely absent or nonfunctional.

Several dopamine receptor agonists are available in the United States for the treatment of PD: *bromocriptine* (Parlodel), *pramipexole* (Mirapex), transdermal *rotigotine* (Neupro), and *ropinirole* (Requip). *Apomorphine* (Apokyn) is an old drug that can be used as an adjunctive treatment for the sudden appearance of the "off" phase. It is injected and its effects last about 30 minutes. It is usually used as a "rescue" medication when the levodopa effect wears off between doses. Clinicians must be trained in its administration and it causes significant nausea and must be taken with antinausea medication.

Bromocriptine has been available since 1978 and has a structure that closely resembles that of dopamine. Pramipexole and ropinirole were marketed in 1997. They are indicated for use in early-onset Parkinson's disease; their efficacy and safety profile is much better than that of bromocriptine. Both can increase quality of life in the early stages of the disease by improving motor problems and decreasing fluctuations in response to levodopa. Pramipexole also exerts a beneficial antidepressant effect (Fernandez and Merello, 2010). Their long half-lives may at least partially explain the reduction in the "on-off" phenomenon of levodopa therapy. Side effects of dopamine agonists include somnolence, dizziness and orthostatic hypotension, nausea and vomiting, hallucinations, confusion, swelling of the legs and feet, insomnia, dyskinesias, and impulse control disorders such as compulsive gambling, buying sprees, overeating, reckless driving, and hypersexuality (see Weintraub et al., 2010 and references therein). Pramipexole and probably ropinirole cause what is known as "sleep attacks." These are unpredictable sudden onset episodes of extreme sedation or drowsiness. Thus, patients must be warned about driving and the increased risk of attack if using other drugs that cause sedation or have other disorders of sleep regulation.

Selective Monoamine Oxidase-B Inhibitors

Selegiline (Eldepryl and, as a rapidly dissolving tablet, Zelapar) reduces PD symptoms through a unique mechanism.[2] The enzyme *monoamine oxidase* (MAO) exists in two isoenzyme forms: MAO-A and MAO-B. Although both are present in the brain, MAO-B is the more predominant enzyme, while MAO-A is more predominant in the periphery, especially in the GI tract; MAO-A is more closely involved with tyramine, norepinephrine, serotonin, and to some extent, dopamine nerve terminals, while MAO-B has preferential affinity for dopamine neurons located in the substantia nigra. Selegiline selectively and irreversibly inhibits MAO-B. As a result, selegiline inhibits the local breakdown of dopamine, thus preserving the small amounts of dopamine that are present. Both actions enhance the therapeutic effect of levodopa. Unlike the older

---

[2] In Chapter 12, selegiline is discussed as the antidepressant transdermal skin patch Emsam.

nonselective MAO inhibitors used as clinical antidepressants (Chapter 12), selegiline does not inhibit peripheral metabolism of levodopa; thus, it can safely be taken with levodopa. Selegiline also exhibits fewer drug-food interactions, at least at the lowest dose commercially available of 6 milligrams daily. Unfortunately, in Parkinson's disease, selegiline's usefulness is limited.

Approved by the FDA in May 2006, rasagiline (Azilect) is the second selective MAO-B inhibitor for Parkinson's disease. Olanow and coworkers (2009b) reported a possibly beneficial effect of the early use of rasagiline at a dose of 1 milligram per day, but negative findings at a dose of 2 milligrams per day. Rasagiline may also possess a potential neuroprotective effect against the progression of Parkinson's disease (Malaty and Fernandez, 2009; Naoi and Maruyama, 2009). Other studies have been consistent showing a small beneficial effect of rasagiline in PD treatment (Leegwater-Kim and Bortan, 2010; Lew et al., 2010) and some authors suggest that MAO-B drugs should be used as the initial treatment for Parkinson's disease due to their safety profile. By using them first, providers can save the use of L-dopa until PD symptoms become more severe and disabling (Löhle and Reichmann, 2011). Side effects associated with the selective MAO-B inhibitors include agitation, dizziness, nausea, headache, back pain, and difficulty falling asleep, especially with selegiline. Thus, selegiline should not be given after 1:00 PM. In older adults with Parkinson disease, selegiline often causes confusion, which may prevent it from being useful in this group. Combining MAO-B inhibitors with drugs that increase dopaminergic activity can sometimes produce dyskinesias, hallucinations, and hypertension.

Muscarinic Receptor Antagonists

Although widely used before the introduction of levodopa, certain anticholinergic (anti-ACh) agents, such as muscarinic antagonists, are now used much less and are considered second-tier agents for the treatment of PD symptoms. The use of these drugs was based on an understanding of the control of fine motor movements through the nigrostriatal system. The normal control of movement requires a "balance" between dopamine and acetylcholine transmission within this system, hence the so-called *dopamine-acetylcholine balance theory* of movement disorders. Any shift in this balance through an increase or decrease in one neurotransmitter relative to the other results in hypo- or hyperkinetic movement disorders. In Parkinson's disease, the dopamine-producing cell bodies in the substantial nigra are being destroyed and dopamine output is decreasing, producing a functional imbalance in the dopamine-acetylcholine transmission in favor of acetylcholine. To restore balance, you can either (1) increase the dopamine transmission by using one of the methods described earlier, such as replacement, postsynaptic stimulation, or inhibition of breakdown; or (2) decrease the effect of acetylcholine by using anti-ACh drugs.

Occasionally, anticholinergic drugs are used as an adjunct to L-dopa in patients with tremors that are difficult to control. Anticholinergic drugs relieve tremor in about 50 percent of patients, but they do not reduce rigidity or motor slowing. Anti-ACh drugs, however, can produce cognitive dysfunction that limits their use, especially in the elderly, who may already have an underlying cognitive disorder. Representative agents include *trihexyphenidyl* (Artane), *biperiden* (Akineton), and *benztropine* (Cogentin). Occasionally, the antihistaminic drug *diphenhydramine* (Benadryl) is also used, because Benadryl has significant anticholinergic properties. Typical side effects of anticholinergic drugs include dry mouth, blurred vision, constipation, urinary retention, and the already mentioned potential for cognitive impairment.

Amantadine and Memantine

Amantadine (Symmetrel) is an antiviral agent used to treat viral influenza with modest antiparkinsonian actions. Its mechanism of action in Parkinson's disease is unclear; it may alter dopamine release or reuptake, or it may have anticholinergic properties. Its effect is mainly to reduce dyskinesias, but this may only be temporary. Side effects include dry mouth, constipation, urinary retention, swelling of the ankles, confusion, possible visual hallucinations, and a blotchy, purplish skin rash on the extremities (levido reticularis). Amantadine and a related drug, *memantine*, are active at NMDA-type glutaminergic receptors; this action perhaps offers a degree of "brain protection" that may contribute to its effects. Memantine is used to treat the cognitive and behavioral effects of dementia. Side effects include diarrhea, dizziness, weakness, sleepiness or trouble sleeping, and nausea.

In the Pipeline

Research continues to look for better treatments for Parkinson's disease, especially for interventions that could arrest or even reverse the damage being done to the dopamine cell bodies. Some of the more recent approaches include:

Therapeutic Agents:

- Gene therapies that modify cells other than dopamine neurons to produce dopamine.
- Variations on existing levodopa-carbidopa formulations. Examples include IPX203, which is an updated version of Rytary.
- COMT inhibitors.
- Dopamine agonists.
- New formulations of levodopa. An example is CVT-301, which is an inhaled version of levodopa that is used as a "rescue" medication for "off" periods; and NDO612H, which is a formulation of levodopa that can be continuously infused subcutaneously to even out fluctuations in symptom control.
- New formulations of apomorphine. An example is APL-130277, which is a sublingual formulation to be used as a "rescue" medication for "off" periods.
- Adenosine$_{2A}$ (A2A) receptor antagonists, which will attempt to reduce "off" times and suppress dyskinesias. Examples include *istradefylline* and *tozadenant*. The A2A receptor is expressed in the brain and has a role in the regulation of glutamate and dopamine, making it an interesting target for the treatment of PD.

Neuroprotective Agents:

- Gene therapies targeted to boost brain levels of GDNF (glial cell line, derived neurotrophic factor), a naturally occurring protein that protects dopamine neurons in the brain.
- Immunotherapies and drug therapies intended to either eliminate or stabilize alpha-synuclein, a protein whose buildup in the brain and its misfolding is thought to be related to PD.
- Herbals, including ECGC, which is found in green tea, that stops alpha-synuclein clumps from forming in the brain; and *inosine*, a nutritional supplement that converts to urate, which is a naturally occurring antioxidant.
- *Isradipine* (Prescal), a calcium channel blocker currently in phase III trials; and *nilotinib* (Tasigna), a drug used to treat blood cancers that is being tested for safety due to side effects.

ALZHEIMER'S DISEASE

Alzheimer's disease (AD) is the most common neurodegenerative disease and accounts for the majority of all cases of dementia. Alzheimer's disease is a progressive disease that results in the irreversible loss of cholinergic neurons, particularly in the cerebral cortex and hippocampus. Onset occurs generally after 60 years of age, but is being increasingly reported in people younger than 60. Upwards of 10 million Americans who are part of the baby-boom demographic will develop Alzheimer's disease unless science finds a way to effectively treat and prevent this debilitating and tragic disease. By 2025, the number of people age 65 and older with Alzheimer's disease is estimated to reach 7.1 million—a 35 percent increase from the 5.3 million aged 65 and older currently affected in 2017. By 2050, the number of people aged 65 and older with Alzheimer's disease may almost triple, from 5.3 million to a projected 13.8 million, barring the development of medical breakthroughs to prevent, slow, or stop the disease. Although there was some recent data to suggest that rates of new cases of Alzheimer's disease was trending downward, this may be an expression of the normal variation in the rate of onset of the disorder seen in different epidemiological studies (Jones and Greene, 2016; Larson and Langa, 2017). In addition to the slightly more than 5 million Americans living with Alzheimer's disease, there are about another 200,000 Americans younger than age 65 who have either early-onset Alzheimer's disease or another form of dementia. In 2017, Alzheimer's cost the nation $259 billion. This number is expected to rise to $1.1 trillion by 2050 (Alzheimer's Association, 2017).

Time between symptom onset and death may span 4 to 8 years. Alzheimer's disease is the sixth leading cause of death in the United States. (See Did You Know: Alzheimer's Disease Death Rate Per 100,000 Population by U.S. State, 2015.) The gradual and continuous decline caused by Alzheimer's disease is characterized by cognitive deterioration, changes in behavior, loss of functional independence, and increasing requirements for care. Hallmarks of Alzheimer's disease include progressive

Did You Know?

Alzheimer's Disease Death Rate Per 100,000 Population by U.S. State, 2015

As of 2015, South Carolina had the highest age-adjusted average annual death rate from Alzheimer's disease in the United States at 46.2 per 100,000 population. Rounding out the top 10 U.S. states for 2015, age-adjusted death rates per 100,000 population after South Carolina are Washington (44.4), Mississippi (44.1), Tennessee (43.4), Louisiana (42.5), Georgia (42.4), Alabama (41.8), Arkansas (41.5), Utah (40.7), and Texas (38.2). The CDC states the most closely correlated risk factors for Alzheimer's disease are age and genetics. However, high blood pressure, high cholesterol, and diabetes may also contribute.

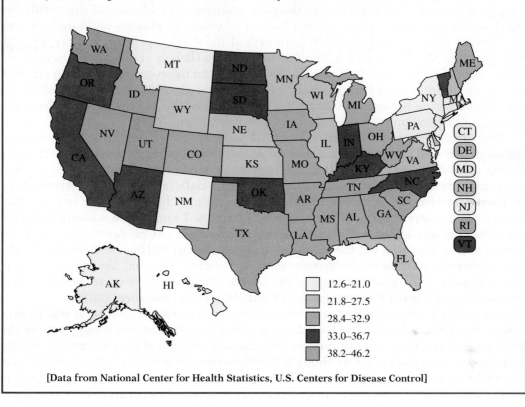

	12.6–21.0
	21.8–27.5
	28.4–32.9
	33.0–36.7
	38.2–46.2

[Data from National Center for Health Statistics, U.S. Centers for Disease Control]

impairment in memory, judgment, decision making, orientation to physical surroundings, and language. *Dementia*, defined as cognitive impairment with the inability to form new memory, is the critical feature of Alzheimer's disease. Diagnosis is based on neurological examination and the exclusion of other causes of dementia. A combined workgroup from the National Institute on Aging (NIA) and the Alzheimer's Association has established guidelines for an AD diagnosis (Jack et al., 2011; McKhann et al., 2011). These diagnostic guidelines are a revision of the original guidelines published in 1984 (McKhann et al., 1984). The new guidelines have added two modifications to the original 1984 guidelines: (1) the incorporation of biomarker tests[3] and (2) the identification of three stages of the disease. These three stages include: (1) a preclinical stage in which biomarker changes may signal the presence of the disease before any cognitive or behavioral signs or symptoms appear. This is currently only a research tool since no reliable biomarkers have been established; (2) mild cognitive impairment (MCI), which is a stage of the disorder that presents with mild cognitive changes that do not necessarily impair daily functioning or always progress to definitive Alzheimer's disease; and (3) Alzheimer's disease with all of the recognized signs and symptoms (Karlawish et al., 2017; McKhann et al., 2011). A definitive diagnosis can be made only at autopsy, where neuronal loss and accumulation of deposits of protein plaques (amyloid-β) and neurofibrillatory tangles, composed of abnormal microtubules (tau), are observed. It is currently not known whether the plaques and tangles cause Alzheimer's disease, are inactive by-products of the disease process, or may actually be protective. Much research is devoted to this area (Briggs et al., 2016; Rhein et al., 2009), but the results thus far from studies of potential interventions affecting amyloid have been disappointing (Briggs et al., 2016; Green et al., 2009; Rosenblum, 2014). In fact, in the period between 2002 and 2012, only one of the 244 drugs for Alzheimer's disease actually completed clinical trials (Karlawish et al., 2017).

The drugs currently used for treating AD patients act on brain neurotransmitters, although it is well recognized that they do not alter the course of the disease. The fact that some of the symptoms of AD are thought to be due to a deficiency of acetylcholine neurotransmission has given rise to a cholinergic-deficiency theory of Alzheimer's disease. Therefore, reinforcing cholinergic function by inhibiting the enzyme that breaks down acetylcholine in the synapse (Chapters 2 and 3) is a widespread therapy. These drugs, called *acetyl-cholinesterase inhibitors* (AChE-Is), do not alter the course of the dementia, but they attempt to slow cognitive decline. As Alzheimer's disease progresses and fewer cholinergic neurons remain functional, the effects of these drugs diminish. The pharmacology of the four available cholinesterase inhibitors was reviewed by Bishara and coworkers (2015) and Shah and coworkers (2010).

Memantine, discussed earlier in the section on Parkinson's disease, is not an acetylcholinesterase inhibitor, but it is also used for AD treatment and is approved by the FDA for this use. Furthermore, memantine may act through effects exerted at specific subtypes of glutamate neurons thought be important for memory formation. Neither the AChE-Is nor memantine attack the root cause of Alzheimer's disease, which is believed to involve brain proteins and peptides rather than neurotransmitters. Thus, they may forestall further functional decline for a limited time, but they have not been shown to slow the disease progression or avoid the ultimate outcome.

Cognitive Impairments and Treatment

Alzheimer's disease is associated not only with cognitive impairments, but with a myriad of bothersome mood alterations and behavioral symptoms that pose further challenges to treatment.

---

[3] *Biomarker tests* are clinical tests that can measure some biological change in the body or brain that can be reliably associated with the presence of the disease.

Depression and Apathy

Depression associated with Alzheimer's disease is common. Some estimates are that between 30 and 50 percent of AD patients have comorbid depression (Aboukhatwa et al., 2010; Zhao et al., 2016). Depression in this population should be treated with antidepressant medications that lack anticholinergic side effects. Thus, SSRIs are most commonly used rather than the tricyclic agents (Chapter 12) because they are better tolerated and produce fewer adverse cognitive effects; in addition, SSRIs can be combined with drugs used to treat Alzheimer's disease with few adverse interactions (Aboukhatwa et al., 2010; Khundakar and Thomas, 2015). There is, however, some suggestion that some antidepressants including SSRIs may actually increase the risk of dementia in the elderly, so they should be used with caution (Wang et al., 2016a).

Apathy may be a prominent behavioral feature of Alzheimer's disease that could be mistaken for depression. Approaches to treatment for this symptom include use of the psychostimulants, the antidepressant bupropion, the dopamine receptor agonist bromocriptine, and the antiparkinsonian agents amantadine and memantine.

Behavioral Disturbances and Dementia

Psychosis, agitation, and other behavioral disturbances may require treatment with a newer atypical antipsychotic agent discussed earlier for behavioral and psychological symptoms of dementia. But the use of these agents have their own risk of side effects including oversedation; metabolic syndrome, including exacerbation or onset of diabetes; movement disorders; akathisia; and falls (Maust et al., 2015; Sterke et al., 2012b). Pimavanserin, mentioned above, is currently in clinical trials to determine its efficacy and safety for the treatment of agitation and aggression in AD patients.

For behavioral and psychiatric symptoms of dementia, it is important to first consider nonpharmacological interventions, such as behavioral approaches. If behavioral approaches have not been successful, then consider only those medications that have (1) the lowest potential for causing adverse effects in individuals with dementia; (2) the lowest effective dose; and (3) the shortest time needed to resolve the identified problem. Based on the BEERS criteria, the Centers for Medicare and Medicaid Services (CMS) use the National Committee for Quality Assurance (NCQA) and Pharmacy Quality Alliance (PQA) quality measure *Use of High-Risk Medications in the Elderly* (HRM) to monitor and evaluate the quality of care provided to Medicare beneficiaries. The HRM measure requires prescribers to justify using drugs such as antipsychotics to manage behavioral disorders in elderly individuals, particularly those with dementia, and to reevaluate the need to continue those drugs at specified time periods. In addition, there are recommendations for alternative drugs that are safer to use than these risky medications for treating a variety of disorders in elderly individuals (see Hanlon et al., 2015). These recommendations are supported by other studies that indicate little benefit with high risks of adverse events for drugs such as antipsychotics, anticonvulsants, and anticholinesterase inhibitors (Farlow and Shamliyan, 2017; Maust et al., 2015; Porsteinssona and Antonsdottir, 2017; Seitz et al., 2013).

Omega-3 Fatty Acids.   Early studies on the effects of diet rich in fish oils, such as the omega-3 fatty acids *decosahexaenoic acid* (DHA) and *eicosapentaenoic acid* (EPA), reported a 47 percent reduction in the incidence of Alzheimer's disease in a large population of British elderly (Schaefer et al., 2006). Low blood levels of DHA were thought to increase the risk for Alzheimer's disease (Pauwels et al., 2009). In addition, DHA was found to have beneficial effects against age-related cognitive decline (Yurko-Mauro et al., 2010). Based on these early findings, it was thought that taking omega-3 fatty acid supplements or eating foods rich in omega-3s might be a good prophylactic intervention for Alzheimer's disease. Subsequent studies, however, have not replicated these earlier findings. There is no strong evidence that taking EPA and DHA supplements or eating fish and other omega-3 rich foods on a regular basis has any beneficial effect for individuals who currently suffer from dementia, nor are these approaches a useful means of protecting against the development of dementia (Dangour et al., 2010; Quinn et al., 2010; Thomas et al., 2015; Wu et al., 2015).

Acetylcholinesterase Inhibitors

As discussed earlier, deficits in the functioning of acetylcholine-secreting neurons (cholinergic deficits) are correlated with the cognitive impairments of Alzheimer's disease. Consistent with this idea is the observation that patients with severe Alzheimer's disease show ACh and AChE levels that are 60 to 85 percent lower than normal, which implies very little residual AChE in the cortex—a condition that is still compatible with life, but no longer optimal for brain function. In addition, drugs that block the actions of acetylcholine, such as scopolamine, are intense cognitive inhibitors. Therefore, drugs that increase acetylcholine levels might be cognitive enhancers and slow the rate of progression of cognitive decline seen in Alzheimer's disease.

The most successful effort to increase cholinergic functioning has targeted the AChE enzyme, inhibition of which increases levels of acetylcholine in the brain. Four AChE-I medications have been approved by the FDA for AD treatment: *tacrine* (Cognex), *donepezil* (Aricept), *rivastigmine* (Exelon), and *galantamine* (Razadyne). Each improves cholinergic neurotransmission by preventing the synaptic breakdown of acetylcholine in the brain. These drugs can produce only modest improvements in cognition and activities of daily living, but their side effects include nausea, diarrhea, abdominal cramping, and anorexia. The side effects result from inhibition of AChE in the periphery, not from the elevations of acetylcholine in the brain. In small numbers of patients receiving AChE-I medication, drug-induced increases in aggressive behaviors may be seen (Coco and Cannizaro, 2010); these behaviors are reversible with drug discontinuation or dosage reductions, and treatment with antipsychotic drugs without stopping the AChE-I may be sometimes helpful. The modest efficacy combined with these side effects tends to limit the therapeutic usefulness of these agents.

Tacrine was the first of these agents to be approved; it is now the least used of the four, primarily because it needs frequent administration and can cause a reversible toxicity to the liver. Liver toxicity has not been associated with donepezil, rivastigmine, or galantamine.

Donepezil appears to be selective for AChE in the brain more than in the periphery. It has a long half-life and produces fewer gastrointestinal side effects. It is much more tolerable than tacrine. Petersen and coworkers (2005) reported that donepezil may slow the progression of cognitive decline in early AD, but that the protective effect was lost after 18 months of treatment. Winblad and coworkers (2006) reported that donepezil improved cognitive ability and helped preserve patient functioning. Burns and coworkers (2007) reported that over 24 weeks of treatment, donepezil produced positive effects on cognition, but that effect was lost over 132 weeks of study. Furthermore, if treatment was discontinued, benefits were not regained after treatment restart. Finally, Doody and coworkers (2009) reported that in a 48-week study, donepezil was no better than placebo in elderly patients with MCI. Persons with such MCIs are expected to progress to AD within about 6 years. In 2010, the FDA approved a new 23-milligram dose of donepezil for moderate to severe Alzheimer's disease. There has been controversy over this approval because the data on which it was based did not show any clinically meaningful difference between the 23-milligram dose and the original 5-milligram or 10-milligram tablets. But side effects were much greater with the 23-milligram tablet, indicating a greater risk for little to no additional benefit for the higher dose. In summary, donepezil can provide minimal to moderate stability in cognitive function and behavioral improvement for some AD patients. Maybe about one-third of individuals will derive some benefit and one-fifth will demonstrate much more definitive benefit. The effect is temporary, lasting anywhere from 6 months to about 1 year on average, and it will not affect the progression of the disease. Some studies, however, suggest that beneficial effects, especially on behavioral symptoms, can last much longer. The current recommendations for treatment indicate that individuals receiving these drugs should be re-evaluated regularly and a risk-to-benefit analysis be conducted to determine if any benefits seen outweigh any distress experienced by the individual due to the side effects of these drugs. There is no recommendation to stop treatment arbitrarily at any time point because the decline in cognitive function may occur quickly and the individual may not respond as well to the readministration of the drug. It is recommended that as long as some benefit to the individual and their caretakers can be demonstrated and the individual is not suffering any significant distress from side effects, the treatment can be continued (Bishara et al., 2015; Briggs et al., 2015; Campos et al., 2016; Ferreira-Vieira et al., 2016).

Rivastigmine is clinically effective, producing modest improvements in cognitive functioning and activities of daily living (Olin et al., 2010). It is better tolerated than tacrine, but somewhat less so than donepezil. In contrast to the other three agents, rivastigmine causes a very slow reversible inhibition of AChE, prolonging its therapeutic action. Also available is a rivastigmine transdermal patch (Exelon Patch). Oral administration of cholinesterase inhibitors is limited by wide fluctuations in blood concentrations. With the patch, 24-hour concentrations remain relatively stable. Several articles attest to the superiority of the patch over oral administration of capsules (Darreh-Shori and Jelic, 2010; Grossberg et al., 2009; Sadowsky et al., 2010). Caregivers prefer the patch to the capsule (Grossberg et al., 2009); however, to avoid toxicity, only one patch should be used at a time. As discussed for donepezil, use of rivistigmine depends on a risk-to-benefit determination. Like all anticholinesterase inhibitors, it provide only temporary and minimal to moderate effects on cognition and does not alter disease progression (Bishara et al., 2015; Briggs et al., 2015; Campos et al., 2016; Ferreira-Vieira et al., 2016).

Galantamine appears to have a safety and efficacy profile similar to that of rivastigmine in measures of both cognitive functioning and functional ability. In a study of quite elderly patients (average age 84 years) with severe Alzheimer's disease,

Burns and coworkers (2009) reported that galantamine moderately improved cognitive functioning, but failed to significantly improve measures of overall activities of daily living.

These data imply that cholinesterase inhibitors have modest but positive effects compared with placebo in AD treatment, affecting cognition, function, and behavioral outcomes. They are effective in mild to moderate Alzheimer's disease, and data with galantamine suggest that this effect can also be seen in severe Alzheimer's disease as well.

There are limitations to these medications, however, because although stabilization occurs, there is typically only a modest improvement from baseline. Additionally, the effects are not sustained indefinitely and the disease continues to progress even while patients are receiving treatment with cholinesterase inhibitors. Adverse effects are manageable and, with careful titration, patients can tolerate increases quite well. However, side effects can include diarrhea, nausea, vomiting, dyspepsia, asthenia, dizziness, headache, weight loss, and even anorexia—sometimes to such an extreme that patients must discontinue treatment (Bishara et al., 2015; Briggs et al., 2015; Campos et al., 2016; Ferreira-Vieira et al., 2016). The patch delivery system may reduce some of these side effects. Additional AD therapies need to be developed that include highly tolerable agents with alternative mechanisms of action and broader efficacy to delay disease onset, arrest the disease, and even reverse the progression of the disease entirely. Until these new therapies are developed, the cholinesterase inhibitors will remain important AD treatments.

A naturally occurring AChE-I, *huperzine A*, has been studied as a treatment for Alzheimer's disease. This substance, derived from the moss *Huperzia serrata*, has been used for centuries as a Chinese folk medicine. It has modest AChE-I activity and it may be useful as an alternative medication for the treatment of AD (Li et al., 2008; Desilets et al., 2009; Wang et al., 2016b). But not all evidence supports a benefit of huperzine for the treatment of AD (Rafii et al., 2011).

Memantine

As discussed in Chapters 2 and 3, *glutamate* is the principal excitatory neurotransmitter in the brain. Glutaminergic overactivity may result in neuronal damage, a phenomenon termed *excitotoxicity*. Excitotoxicity ultimately leads to neuronal calcium overload and has been implicated in neurodegenerative disorders. In addition, glutaminergic NMDA receptor activity appears to be important in memory processes, dementia, and the pathogenesis of Alzheimer's disease. Glutaminergic overstimulation at NMDA receptors is thought to be toxic to neurons and prevention of this neurotoxicity affords a degree of brain protection to limit further deterioration.

Memantine (Namenda; Namenda XR) is a moderate-affinity noncompetitive NMDA receptor antagonist that has been shown to reduce clinical deterioration in patients with moderate to severe Alzheimer's disease, a phase associated with significant distress for patients and caregivers alike and for which no other treatments are available (Aarsland et al., 2009; Campos et al., 2016). Its efficacy is modest and as with the acetylcholinesterase inhibitors, its beneficial effect is temporary and it does not alter the course of the underlying disorder (Briggs et al., 2016). It appears to have therapeutic potential without the undesirable side effects associated with high-affinity NMDA antagonists such as ketamine (Chapter 8). The side effects of memantine include dizziness, somnolence, headache, constipation, and hypertension. Some studies have found that it delays clinical worsening in moderate to severe Alzheimer's disease (Hellweg et al., 2012), but other studies have not found strong evidence of any benefit from memantine in mild Alzheimer's disease (Briggs et al., 2016; Campos et al., 2016) and only meager evidence for efficacy in moderate Alzheimer's disease (Matsunaga et al., 2015; Schneider et al., 2011). It has not been shown to be effective in reducing agitation associated with AD (Fox et al., 2012; Herrmann et al., 2013).

Tariot (2006) and Cummings and coworkers (2006) all reported improved cognition, patient functioning, and behaviors, as well as amelioration of agitation and other negative behaviors, in AD patients treated with a combination of an AChE-I and memantine. It is thought that the combination may delay nursing home placement, a step that can be exceedingly distressing to AD patients and their caregivers (Rountree et al., 2013; see also Atri et al., 2013; Gauthiera and Molinuevo, 2013; and Zhu et al., 2013 for the effects of combining AChE-Is with memantine).

In 2014, the FDA approved Namzaric, a single, pill combination of memantine extended release and donepezil. This combination pill allows for administering an acetylcholinesterase inhibitor plus memantine together, rather than having to administer the two medications individually, as had been done by prescribers prior to 2014. Namzaric simplifies administration and according to research, improves the efficacy on cognitive deficits and other symptoms in moderate to severe Alzheimer's disease over either of the medications alone (Atri et al., 2015; Greig, 2015), although not all studies find that adding a second AD drug produces any additional benefit or the additional effects are minimal over either drug alone (Campos et al., 2016; Howard et al., 2012).

As with other NMDA antagonists, high brain concentrations of memantine can inhibit glutaminergic mechanisms of synaptic plasticity that are believed to underlie learning and memory. In other words, at high doses, memantine can produce the same amnestic effects as ketamine. At lower, clinically relevant doses, however, memantine seems to promote cellular plasticity, can preserve or enhance memory, and can protect against the excitotoxic destruction of cholinergic neurons. As a "weak" NMDA antagonist, memantine may reduce overactive NMDA receptor activity that would be neurotoxic while sparing the synaptic responsiveness required for normal behavioral functioning, cognition, and memory.

Although there may be some evidence for the use of AchE-Is and memantine in the treatment of the cognitive decline associated with AD dementia, it should be noted that there is no evidence that they are of any clinical value in the treatment of cognitive decline associated with other types of dementia, such as Lewy body, vascular, and frontotemporal, or reducing the risk of developing dementia in patients with mild cognitive impairment (Bishara et al., 2015; O'Brien and Burns, 2011). In fact, a Cochran review of the literature concludes that there is little evidence that AchE-Is affect progression to dementia in MCI, and this weak evidence is overshadowed by the greater risk of adverse events, particularly in the GI tract. Therefore, AchE-Is are not recommended for MCI (Campos et al., 2016; Russ and Morling, 2012).

In the Pipeline

The following list includes not only drugs that show promise, but also drugs that have thus far been tried and proved ineffective or harmful and which are no longer in contention for the treatment of Alzheimer's disease. It is important to include the failures as evidence of the effort being made to find a drug that can be effective in treating Alzheimer's disease.

The experimental approaches listed below comprise two major categories: (1) those interventions designed to reduce the severity of symptoms of Alzheimer's disease and (2) those interventions designed to actually modify disease progression or even prevent the development of the disease.

- Drugs that target amyloid-β formation, *bapineuzumab* and *solanezumab*, both failed in large clinical trials. A third drug, *crenezumab*, is being tested in a large Colombian family that has a rare form of Alzheimer's disease, which develops in a high proportion of family members by middle age (Callaway, 2012). Other drugs and compounds that limit amyloid-β formation by blocking β-secretase activity are still under investigation (Folch et al., 2016). Similar drugs, such as *semagacestat* and *avagacestat*, that inhibit the γ-secretase enzyme, which contributes to the formation of amyloid-β, have not shown any benefit in Alzheimer's disease. In some cases, these drugs have accelerated the cognitive and functional deterioration and increased the risk of skin cancer, and studies have ceased (Bishara et al., 2015).

- Other trials have focused on preventing the development of amyloid plaques. For example, *tramiprosate* and *tarenflurbil* are two such drugs designed to target plaque formation. Neither of these experimental medicines has demonstrated sufficient efficacy (Sabbagh, 2009). However, in a preliminary one-year study, Wilcock and coworkers (2008) reported positive effects of tarenflurbil on global functioning and activities of daily living in patients with mild Alzheimer's disease, but not in patients with moderate Alzheimer's disease. The drug had no significant effect on cognitive functioning. In fact, one drug company has discontinued all trials with gamma secretase inhibitors such as tarenflurbil due to lack of efficacy and the increased risk of skin cancer (British Association for Psychopharmacology, 2011).

- Heavy metal chelators to dissolve amyloid plaques are being examined based on the fact that metals like zinc and copper have been implicated in the formation of plaques (Bishara et al., 2015).

- *Latrepirdine* (Dimebon), an old antihistamine drug used in Russia, was assessed in several trials of individuals with mild to moderate Alzheimer's disease. The trials were considered failed and the drug did not separate from placebo. For this reason, obviously, latrepirdine was never approved for use in the United States. Antihistamine H$_3$ receptor blocking drugs have also been examined in clinical trials and have not been successful thus far (Godyń et al., 2016).

- Anti-inflammatory drugs, such as NSAIDS and COX-2 inhibitors, have been disappointing in controlled trials (Bishara et al., 2015; Folch et al., 2016).

- Statins, which are drugs used to treat high cholesterol, have not shown any benefit in treating Alzheimer's disease or preventing the onset of the disorder (Bishara et al., 2015).

- PBT2, developed by Prana Biotechnology, is a drug that is proposed to work by preventing the interaction of synaptic zinc and copper with amyloid-β to prevent the amyloid-β from becoming toxic. PBT2 continues in clinical trials.

- Intravenous immunoglobulin (IVIG) has been tried in mild to moderate Alzheimer's disease. IVIG contains antibodies to amyloid-β protein. This study found that the growth rate of ventricular space showed less ventricular expansion, that is, less brain shrinkage, compared to a placebo group. The study was not designed as an effectiveness study, however, so no conclusions about the results on cognitive function can be made. A rash and hemolytic anemia developed in 21 percent of the study patients. IVIG clinical trials are ongoing. Trials of other vaccines, such as AN1792, were stopped due to significant brain inflammation. But studies of vaccines with less risk for inflammation are ongoing, despite negative outcomes from all prior studies thus far (Godyń et al., 2016).

- Selective alpha-7 nicotinic receptor agonists are being studied in individuals with mild to moderate Alzheimer's disease.

- Based on a finding of zinc deficiency in AD patients (Unzeta et al., 2016), clinical trials are being conducted with dietary supplements of oral zinc cysteine. Hippocampal zinc modulates the NMDA receptor and in absence of this modulation by zinc, excess neuroexcitation can lead to cell death. The administration of zinc would be expected to maintain the modulation of the NMDA receptor activity. The outcomes examine zinc and copper levels and performance on cognitive tests.

- Antioxidants that also prevent aggregation, neurotoxicity, and deposition of amyloid-β are in clinical trials for treating AD patients (Folch et al., 2016).

- Drugs that regulate glucose and lipid metabolism but also suppress inflammation are being tested. Two such agents, *pioglitazone* (Actos) and *rosiglitazone* (Avandia), are used to treat diabetes and are being studied for their efficacy in Alzheimer's disease. So far, results have been unimpressive. Another diabetes drug being studied in this regard is *metformin* (Glucophage). Insulin itself is being tested as an agent to suppress the expression of amyloid precursor protein (APP), from which amyloid-β is derived (Folch et al., 2016). Glucagonlike peptide 1 (GLP-1) receptor antagonists, such as liraglutide, have been examined and thus far have not shown any benefit in the treatment of Alzheimer's disease (Godyń et al., 2016).

- Drugs that block the formation of tumor necrosis factor (TNF) and reduce inflammation are being studied as neuroprotective agents that prevent the onset of Alzheimer's disease. Anti-TNF drugs are normally used to treat rheumatoid arthritis (RA), but other drugs used to treat RA, such as prednisone, sulfasalazine, and rituximab, have not been associated with lower AD risk.

- Cotinine, a compound derived from tobacco that is nontoxic and longer lasting than nicotine, is being studied in AD animal models. In mice, cotinine reduced the deposits of amyloid plaques and seemed to block their formation.

- Orcein, a red dye that is derived from lichens and used to color fabrics and food, has been shown to reduce small toxic protein aggregates in Alzheimer's disease. Orcein binds to small amyloid aggregates that are toxic and converts them into large, mature plaques that are considered nontoxic to neuronal cells (Lam et al., 2016).

Another dye, methylene blue, is also being clinically tested in Alzheimer's disease based on the same mechanism of action.

- *Bexarotene* (Targretin), a drug approved for the treatment of cancer, is being studied in AD animal models. *Apolipoprotein E* (ApoE), the main cholesterol carrier in the brain, facilitates clearance of amyloid-β from the brain. Bexarotene increases ApoE expression, which also increases the removal of amyloid-β from the brain. ApoE has been shown in mice to not only arrest the progression of memory deficits, but in some cases reverse the AD pathology (Cramer et al., 2012). Recently, however, four other labs reported they could not replicate this finding (see Fitz et al., 2013; Price et al., 2013; Tesseur et al., 2013; Veeraraghavalu et al., 2013). But other cancer drugs, such as *erlotinib* (Tarceva) and *fefitinib* (Iressa), are being studied in fruit flies based on their ability to block the epidermal growth factor receptor (EGFR), which is active in many cancers. It is thought that EGFR activation also exacerbates memory loss and amyloid-β formation. For this reason, drugs that block EGFR should improve memory and block amyloid-β formation.

- Studies of a nutrient "cocktail," Souvenaid, showed limited improvement on one neuropsychological test while failing to demonstrate any improvement on a host of secondary measures of neuropsychological function. Souvenaid consists of omega-3 fatty acids, uridine, choline, selenium, folic acid, and the vitamins B6, B12, C, and E. This combination of nutrients was believed to promote the formation of new nerve synapses (Olde Rikkert et al., 2015).

- Clinical studies have been conducted with a selective $5HT_6$ receptor antagonist as an adjunctive agent to ongoing treatment with an AChE-I. The initial positive results support moving forward with additional studies. Studies using the $5HT_6$ receptor antagonist alone did not show any benefit. For this reason, drugs in this category, such as *idalopirdine*, may best be suited as an adjunctive treatment with acetylcholinesterase-blocking drugs, such as donepezil (Goydń et al., 2016). However, the results of three recent clinical trials failed to find any benefit of adding idalopirdine to cholinesterase inhibitors on cognitive function during 24 weeks of treatment (Atri et al., 2018).

- Peptides related to angiotensin IV, a blood pressure modulator, were observed to reverse learning deficits in animal models of dementia. To prevent it from rapid metabolism in the periphery, scientists have produced a smaller molecule, named *Dihexa*, that can cross the blood–brain barrier. The developers have stated that this compound is seven times more potent than brain-derived neurotrophic factor (BDNF), which is a growth-promoting protein associated with brain development and stimulation of neuronal connections. Clinical trials will be some time down the road, as basic safety of the compound must be demonstrated first (Wright and Harding, 2016).

- Clinical trials are being conducted using a formulation of caprylic triglyceride, a medium, chain triglyceride and fatty acid, designed to improve cognitive function in mild to moderate Alzheimer's disease.

- A novel alpha-2_c adrenoreceptor antagonist has shown initial positive results in a clinical trial of AD patients as an add-on therapy to existing treatment with AChE-Is. The alpha-2_c adrenoreceptor is thought to regulate dopamine and serotonin activity in the brain.

- *Sodium phenylbutyrate* (Buphenyl) is approved by the FDA to treat elevated ammonium levels. Buphenyl is now being studied as a stimulator of neuronal growth and as a neuroprotective agent.

- Drugs are being tested that target tau. These include (1) tau kinase inhibitors, such as lithium, to prevent tangles from forming and (2) tau aggregation inhibitors, such as TRX-0237, to dissolve tau tangles (Bishara et al., 2015).

- Two compounds found in cinnamon are being examined for their ability to reduce tau tangles and act as antioxidants. The first compound, *cinnamaldehyde*, can reduce tau tangles. The other compound, *epicatechin*, serves as an antioxidant. The same properties are also found in blueberries. Also, *curcumin*, an extract of turmeric, is being studied for its antioxidant and anti-inflammatory properties (Bishara et al., 2015).

To target disease prevention or modification, there is a need to identify a reliable relationship between amyloid formation, for example, and cognitive decline. Panza and coworkers (2009) and Frisardi and coworkers (2010) have reviewed research targeting antiamyloid drugs as disease-modifying agents in Alzheimer's disease. However, as described earlier in this section, none of these approaches has proven to be effective. Why? Some research indicates that the amyloid deposition has already occurred and reached a plateau well before even mild cognitive impairment or frank dementia can be detected, making pharmacological intervention at this point ineffective for reducing the progressive rate of cognitive decline (Chetelat et al., 2010). This finding speaks to the need to discover valid and reliable biological markers for the disorder so that individuals with a high risk for AD can be treated as soon as possible, well before incident symptoms occur (Selkoe, 2011).

Some work is being done to find these biological markers. Roe and colleagues (2013) used a range of available biomarkers for Alzheimer's disease to predict which individuals would develop AD symptoms. After following these individuals for several years, they were able to predict with a fair degree of accuracy who would develop the disorder and they found that any of the biomarkers were as good as any other for this prediction. They found that by combining the biomarker data with certain demographic information from the patients, they could enhance the predictive value.

Despite some of the more positive findings on biomarkers, the FDA has been concerned about the reliance on the use of biomarkers and imaging as outcome indicators for trials of AD treatment drugs. They have issued a guidance document that identifies what elements the FDA considers relevant for determining whether a proposed biomarker will be accepted as a measure of risk for Alzheimer's disease in clinical trials. This Biomarker Qualification Program (BQP) allows researchers to register proposed biomarkers that meet the FDA's criteria to be used in testing potential drugs (Amur et al., 2015).

Another problem for researchers in this area is identifying the underlying cause of or trigger for the reduction in cholinergic activity seen in individuals with dementia. As discussed earlier in this chapter, there is no definitive answer to the question of whether the plaques and tangles seen in the brains of individuals with Alzheimer's disease at autopsy are the result of or related to the cause of the disorder. There are multiple theories about the cause of Alzheimer's disease, including the amyloid cascade hypothesis, the cholinergic hypothesis, the dendritic hypothesis, the mitochondrial cascade hypothesis, the metabolic hypothesis, the neuroinflammatory hypothesis, and so on (Folch et al., 2016). The drug trials discussed in this section aim to address the deficiencies in neuronal structure and function that are believed to be caused by factors related to one of these theories.

Nehls (2016) has suggested that focusing on just one factor as the target for therapeutic interventions may not be the most fruitful. His argument is that Alzheimer's disease is multifactorial, involving genetic, behavioral, environmental, neuronal, and physiological causes, among others. He offers his *Unified Theory of Alzheimer's Disease* (UTAD) to integrate all of these potential causative factors as a rational strategy for approaching potential treatments. (For a summary of the current status of prevention studies, treatment studies, and rational strategies for ongoing research, see Briggs et al., 2016; de Souza Cazarim et al., 2016; Folch et al., 2016; Gandy and Dekosky, 2013; Kumar and Ekavali, 2015; Kumar et al., 2016; McHardy et al., 2017; and Scheltens et al., 2016.)

Principles of Care for Patients with Alzheimer's Disease

In 2008, the American College of Physicians and the American Academy of Family Physicians published clinical practice guidelines for the pharmacological treatment of dementia (Qaseem et al., 2008; Raina et al., 2008). These guidelines were reaffirmed in 2013.

In 2006, the American Association for Geriatric Psychiatry outlined minimal care standards and principles for AD patients and their caregivers. The association issued a position statement calling on clinicians to treat Alzheimer's disease as part of their typical practice (Lyketsos et al., 2006). The statement focuses on the following five important areas of therapy:

- AD therapies targeting aspects of the current pathophysiological understanding of the disease
- Symptomatic therapies for cognitive symptoms
- Symptomatic therapies for other neuropsychiatric symptoms
- Interventions targeted at and the provision of supportive care for patients
- Interventions targeted at and the provision of supportive care for caregivers

These principles still apply today. Disease therapies include therapies aimed at preventing deposits of amyloid plaques and preventing excitotoxic neuronal damage. Therapies for cognitive symptoms include the use of AChE-I drugs and memantine, and involve methodologies for maintaining adherence to treatments (Campbell et al., 2017). Therapies for other symptoms might include treatments for depression, agitation, aggression, and delusions, among other symptoms; and these therapies can be both nonpharmacological and pharmacological.

Supportive care for patients and caregivers should be tailored to the condition, circumstances, and progression of functional and cognitive decline. Caregivers need to be educated about Alzheimer's disease and how their services are essential. They especially need to be given emotional support and respite.

STUDY QUESTIONS

1. What is Parkinson's disease?
2. List the various ways that dopaminergic action in the brain might be augmented or potentiated.
3. Explain how carbidopa potentiates the action of levodopa.
4. Explain how a COMT inhibitor potentiates the action of levodopa.
5. Differentiate the newer from the older dopamine receptor agonists.
6. How does selegiline work in the treatment of Parkinson's disease?
7. Besides treatment with drugs, how might parkinsonism be managed? List the nonpharmacological options.
8. What are some of the current hypotheses for the genesis of Alzheimer's disease?
9. What are the currently available medications used to treat Alzheimer's disease?
10. What are some of the reasons that there is no effective treatment for Alzheimer's disease despite years of research?
11. Differentiate cholinesterase inhibitors from one another and from memantine.

REFERENCES

Aarsland, D., et al. (2009). "Memantine in Patients with Parkinson's Disease Dementia or Dementia with Lewy Bodies: A Double-Blind, Placebo-Controlled, Multicentre Trial." *Lancet Neurology* 8: 613–618.

Abler, B., et al. (2009). "At-Risk for Pathological Gambling: Imaging Neural Reward Processing Under Chronic Dopamine Agonists." *Brain* 132: 2396–2402.

Aboukhatwa, M., et al. (2010). "Antidepressants Are a Rational Complementary Therapy for the Treatment of Alzheimer's Disease." *Molecular Neurodegeneration* 5: 10. doi: 10.1186/1750-1326-5-10.

Alzheimer's Association. (2017). *2017 Alzheimer's Disease Facts and Figures*. https://www.alz.org/facts/.

Amur, S., et al. (2015). "Biomarker Qualification: Toward a Multiple Stakeholder Framework for Biomarker Development, Regulatory Acceptance, and Utilization." *State of the Art* 98: 34–46.

Andreescu, C., et al. (2007). "Effect of Comorbid Anxiety on Treatment Response and Relapse Risk in Late-Life Depression: Controlled Study." *British Journal of Psychiatry* 190: 344–349.

Atkinson, T. J., et al. (2013). "Medication Pain Management in the Elderly: Unique and Underutilized Analgesic Treatment Options." *Clinical Therapeutics* 35: 1669–1689.

Atri, A., et al. (2013). "Memantine in Patients with Alzheimer's Disease Receiving Donepezil: New Analyses of Efficacy and Safety for Combination Therapy." *Alzheimers Research & Therapy* 5: 6. doi: 10.1186/alzrt160.

Atri, A., et al. (2015). "Cumulative, Additive Benefits of Memantine Donepezil Combination Over Component Monotherapies in Moderate to Severe Alzheimer's Dementia: A Pooled Area Under the Curve Analysis." *Alzheimer's Research & Therapy* 7: 1–12.

Atri, A., et al. (2018). "Effect of Idalopirdine as Adjunct to Cholinesterase Inhibitors on Change in Cognition in Patients with Alzheimer Disease: Three Randomized Clinical Trials." *JAMA* 319: 130–142.

Ballard, C., et al. (2008). "A Randomised, Blinded, Placebo-controlled Trial in Dementia Patients Continuing or Stopping Neuroleptics (The DART-AD Trial)." *PLOS One Medicine* 5(4): e76. doi: 10.1371/journal.pmed.0050076.

Ballard, C., et al. (2016). "Impact of Antipsychotic Review and Nonpharmacological Intervention on Antipsychotic Use, Neuropsychiatric Symptoms, and Mortality in People with Dementia Living in Nursing Homes: A Factorial Cluster-Randomized Controlled Trial by the Well-Being and Health for People with Dementia (WHELD) Program." *American Journal of Psychiatry* 173: 252–262.

Barnett, M. J., et al. (2006). "Comparison of Rates of Potentially Inappropriate Medication Use According to the Zhan Criteria for VA versus Private Sector Medicare HMOs." *Journal of Managed Care Pharmacy* 12: 362–370.

Billioti de Gage, S., et al. (2010). "Benzodiazepine Use and Risk of Dementia: Prospective Population Based Study." *BMJ* 345: e6231. doi: 10.1136/bmj.e6231.

Billioti de Gage, S., et al. (2014). "Benzodiazepine Use and Risk of Alzheimer's Disease: Case-Control Study." *BMJ* 349: 1–10: doi: 10.1136/bmj.g5205.

Bishara, D., et al. (2015). "The Pharmacological Management of Alzheimer's Disease." *Progress in Neurology and Psychiatry* 19(4): 9–16. 10.1002/pnp.387.

Bozymski, K. M., et al. (2017). "Pimavanserin: A Novel Antipsychotic for Parkinson's Disease Psychosis." *Annals of Pharmacotherapy* 51: 479–487.

Briesacher, B. A., et al. (2013). "Antipsychotic Use Among Nursing Home Residents." *JAMA* 309: 440–442.

Briggs, R., et al. (2016). "Drug Treatments in Alzheimer's Disease." *Clinical Medicine* 16: 247–253.

British Association for Psychopharmacology. (2011). "Updated Consensus Statement on Antidementia Drugs in Clinical Practice." *The Brown University Psychopharmacology Update* 22: 1, 6–7.

Burns, A., et al. (2007). "Efficacy and Safety of Donepezil over 3 Years: An Open-Label, Multicentre Study in Patients with Alzheimer's Disease." *International Journal of Geriatric Psychiatry* 22: 806–812.

Burns, A., et al. (2009). "Safety and Efficacy of Galantamine (Reminyl) in Severe Alzheimer's Disease (the SERAD Study): A Randomized, Placebo-Controlled, Double-Blind Trial." *Lancet Neurology* 8: 39–47.

Callaway, E. (2012). "Alzheimer's Drugs Take a New Tack." *Nature* 489: 13–14.

Campbell, N. L., et al. (2017). "Adherence and Tolerability of Alzheimer's Disease Medications: A Pragmatic Randomized Trial." *Journal of the American Geriatric Society* 65: 1497–1504. doi: 10.1111/jgs.14827.

Campos, C., et al. (2016). "Treatment of Cognitive Deficits in Alzheimer's Disease: A Psychopharmacological Review." *Psychiatria Danubina* 28: 2–12.

Carnahan, R. M. (2010). "How to Manage Your Patient's Dementia by Discontinuing Medications." *Current Psychiatry* 9: 34–37.

Chang-Quan, H., et al. (2009). "Collaborative Care Interventions for Depression in the Elderly: A Systematic Review of Randomized Controlled Trials." *Journal of Investigative Medicine* 57: 446–455.

Charlesworth, C. J., et al. (2015). "Polypharmacy Among Adults Aged 65 Years and Older in the United States: 1988–2010." *Journals of Gerontology: Medical Sciences* 70: 989–995.

Chen, Y., et al. (2010). "Unexplained Variation across US Nursing Homes in Antipsychotic Prescribing Rates." *Archives of Internal Medicine* 170: 89–95. doi: 10.1001/archinternmed.2009.469.

Chetelat, G., et al. (2010). "Relationship Between Atrophy and β-amyloid Deposition in Alzheimer Disease." *Annals of Neurology* 67: 317–324.

Choi, N. G. et al. (2014). "Treatment Use, Perceived Need, and Barriers to Seeking Treatment for Substance Abuse and Mental Health Problems among Older Adults Compared to Younger Adults." *Drug and Alcohol Dependence* 145: 113–120.

Coco, D. L., and Cannizaro, E. (2010). "Inappropriate Sexual Behaviors Associated with Donepezil Treatment: A Case Report." *Journal of Clinical Psychopharmacology* 30: 221–222.

Coley, K. C., et al. (2009). "Aripiprazole Prescribing Patterns and Side Effects in Elderly Psychiatric Inpatients." *Journal of Psychiatric Practice* 15: 150–153.

Connelly, P. J., et al. (2009). "Fifteen Year Comparison of Antipsychotic Use in People with Dementia Within Hospital and Nursing Home Settings: Sequential Cross-Sectional Study." *International Journal of Geriatric Psychiatry* 25: 160–165.

Coupland, C. A. C., et al. (2011). "A Study of the Safety and Harms of Antidepressant Drugs for Older People: A Cohort Study Using a Large Primary Care Database." *Health Technology Assessment* 15: 1–202; i–xii: doi: 10.3310/hta15280.

Cramer, P. E., et al. (2012). "ApoE-Directed Therapeutics Rapidly Clear β-Amyloid and Reverse Deficits in AD Mouse Models." *Science* 335: 1503–1506.

Cummings, J. L., et al. (2006). "Behavioral Effects of Memantine in Alzheimer's Disease Patients Receiving Donepezil Treatment." *Neurology* 67: 57–63.

Dangour, A. D., et al. (2010). "Effect of 2-y n-3 Long-chain Polyunsaturated Fatty Acid Supplementation on Cognitive Function in Older People: A Randomized, Double-blind, Controlled Trial." *American Journal of Clinical Nutrition* 91: 1725–1732.

Darreh-Shori, T., and Jelic, V. (2010). "Safety and Tolerability of Transdermal and Oral Rivastigmine in Alzheimer's Disease and Parkinson's Disease Dementia." *Expert Opinion on Drug Safety* 9: 167–176.

De Deyn, P. P., et al. (2013). "Aripiprazole in the Treatment of Alzheimer's Disease." *Expert Opinion on Pharmacotherapy* 14: 459–474.

Delamarre, A., and Meissner, W. G. (2017). "Epidemiology, Environmental Risk Factors and Genetics of Parkinson's Disease." *Presse Médicale* 46: 175–181.

Dentino, A., et al. (2017). "Pain in the Elderly: Identification, Evaluation, and Management of Older Adults with Pain Complaints and Pain-related Symptoms." *Primary Care Clinical Office Practice* 44: 519–528.

Desilets, A. R., et al. (2009). "Role of Huperzine-A in the Treatment of Alzheimer's Disease." *Annals of Pharmacotherapeutics* 43(2, Pt. 1): 514–518. doi: 10.1016/j.lpm.2017.01.001.

de Souza Cazarim, M., et al. (2016). "Perspectives for Treating Alzheimer's Disease: A Review on Promising Pharmacological Substances." *Sao Paulo Medical Journal* 134: 342–354.

Devanand, D. P., et al. (2012). "Relapse Risk after Discontinuation of Risperidone in Alzheimer's Disease." *New England Journal of Medicine* 367: 1497–1507.

Dombrovski, A. Y., et al. (2007). "Maintenance Treatment for Old-Age Depression Preserves Health-Related Quality of Life: A Randomized, Controlled Trial of Paroxetine and Interpersonal Psychotherapy." *Journal of the American Geriatrics Society* 55: 1325–1332.

Doody, R. S., et al. (2009). "Donepezil Treatment of Patients with MCI: A 48-Week Randomized, Placebo-Controlled Trial." *Neurology* 72: 1555–1561.

Dorsey, E. R., et al. (2010). "Impact of FDA Black Box Advisory on Antipsychotic Medication Use." *Archives of Internal Medicine* 170: 96–103.

Elie, M., et al. (2009). "A Retrospective, Exploratory, Secondary Analysis of the Association between Antipsychotic Use and Mortality in Elderly Patients with Delirium." *International Psychogeriatrics* 21: 588–592.

Ellis, M. L., et al. (2015). "Assessing Approaches and Barriers to Reduce Antipsychotic Drug Use in Florida Nursing Homes." *Aging & Mental Health* 19: 507–516.

Farlow, M. R., and Shamliyan, T. A. (2017). "Benefits and Harms of Atypical Antipsychotics for Agitation in Adults with Dementia." *European Neuropsychopharmacology* 27: 217–231. doi: 10.1016/j.euroneuro.2017.01.002.

Fernandez, H. H., and Merello, M. (2010). "Pramipexole for the Treatment of Depressive Symptoms in Patients with Parkinson's Disease: Can We Kill Two Birds with One Stone?" *Lancet Neurology,* 9: 556–557.

Ferreira, M., and Massano, J. (2017). "An Updated Review of Parkinson's Disease Genetics and Clinicopathological Correlations." *Acta Neurological Scandinavica* 135: 273–284. doi: 10.1111/ane.12616.

Ferreira-Vieira, T. H., et al. (2016). "Alzheimer's Disease: Targeting the Cholinergic System." *Current Neuropharmacology* 14: 101–115.

Fitz, N. F., et al. (2013). "Comment on "ApoE-Directed Therapeutics Rapidly Clear β-Amyloid and Reverse Deficits in AD Mouse Models"." *Science* 340: 924.

Folch, J., et al. (2016). "Current Research Therapeutic Strategies for Alzheimer's Disease Treatment." *Neural Plasticity* 2016: Article ID 8501693. doi: 10.1155/2016/8501693.

Fox, C., et al. (2012). "Efficacy of Memantine for Agitation in Alzheimer's Dementia: A Randomized Double-blind Placebo Controlled Trial." *PLOS One* 7: e35185; doi: 10.1371/journal.pone.0035185.

Frisardi, V., et al. (2010). "Towards Disease-Modifying Treatment of Alzheimer's Disease: Drugs Targeting Beta-Amyloid." *Current Alzheimer's Research* 7: 40–55.

Gandy, S., and Dekosky, S. T. (2013). "Toward the Treatment and Prevention of Alzheimer's Disease: Rational Strategies and Recent Progress." *Annual Review of Medicine* 64: 367–383.

Gauthiera, S., and Molinuevo, J. L. (2013). "Benefits of Combined Cholinesterase Inhibitor and Memantine Treatment in Moderate–Severe Alzheimer's Disease." *Alzheimer's & Dementia* 9: 326–331.

Godyń, J., et al. (2016). "Therapeutic Strategies For Alzheimer's Disease In Clinical Trials." *Pharmacological Reports* 68: 127–138.

Graham, D. J., et al. (2013). "Cardiovascular and Mortality Risks in Parkinson's Disease Patients Treated with Entacapone." *Movement Disorders* 28: 490–497.

Gray, S. L., et al. (2016). "Benzodiazepine Use and Risk of Incident Dementia or Cognitive Decline: Prospective Population Based Study." *BMJ* 352: 1–9: doi: 10.1136/bmj.i90.

Green, R. C., et al. (2009). "Effect of Tarenflurbil on Cognitive Decline and Activities of Daily Living in Patients with Mild Alzheimer Disease." *JAMA* 302: 2557–2564.

Greig, S. L. (2015). "Memantine ER/Donepezil: A Review in Alzheimer's Disease." *CNS Drugs* 29: 963–970.

Grossberg, G., et al. (2009). "Safety and Tolerability of the Rivastigmine Patch: Results of a 28-Week Open-Label Extension." *Alzheimer Disease & Associated Disorders* 23: 158–164.

Giugni, J. C., and Okun, M. S. (2014). "Treatment of Advanced Parkinson's Disease." *Current Opinion in Neurology* 27: 450–460.

Hall, C. A., and Reynolds, C. F. (2014). "Late-Life Depression in the Primary Care Setting: Challenges, Collaborative Care, and Prevention." *Maturitas* 79: 147–152.

Hanlon, J. T., et al. (2015). "Alternative Medications for Medications in the Use of High-Risk Medications in the Elderly and Potentially Harmful Drug–Disease Interactions in the Elderly Quality Measures." *Journal of the American Geriatric Society* 63: e8–e18.

Hauser, R. A. (2009). "Levodopa: Past, Present, and Future." *European Neurology* 62: 1–8.

Hellweg, R., et al. (2012). "Efficacy of Memantine in Delaying Clinical Worsening in Alzheimer's Disease (AD): Responder Analyses of Nine Clinical Trials with Patients with Moderate to Severe AD." *International Journal of Geriatric Psychiatry* 27: 651–656.

Herrmann, N., et al. (2013). "A Randomized, Double-blind, Placebo-controlled Trial of Memantine in a Behaviorally Enriched Sample of Patients with Moderate-to-Severe Alzheimer's Disease." *International Psychogeriatrics* 25: 919–927.

Howard, R., et al. (2012). "Donepezil and Memantine for Moderate-to-Severe Alzheimer's Disease." *New England Journal of Medicine* 366: 893–903.

Howland, R. H. (2016). "Antidepressant, Antipsychotic, and Hallucinogen Drugs for the Treatment of Psychiatric Disorders: A Convergence at the Serotonin-2A Receptor." *Journal of Psychosocial Nursing* 54: 21–24.

Hunkeler, E. M., et al. (2006). "Long-Term Outcomes from the IMPACT Randomized Trial for Depressed Elderly Patients in Primary Care." *BMJ* 332: 259–263.

Huybrechts, K. F., et al. (2012). "Differential Risk of Death in Older Residents in Nursing Homes Prescribed Specific Antipsychotic Drugs: Population Based Cohort Study." *BMJ* 344: e977 doi: 10.1136/bmj.e977.

Jack, C. R., et al. (2011). "Introduction to the Recommendations From the National Institute on Aging-Alzheimer's Association Workgroups on Diagnostic Guidelines for Alzheimer's Disease." *Alzheimer's & Dementia* 7: 257–262.

Jin, H., et al. (2013). "Comparison of Longer-term Safety and Effectiveness of 4 Atypical Antipsychotics in Patients Over Age 40: A Trial Using Equipoise-stratified Randomization." *Journal of Clinical Psychiatry* 74: 10–18.

Jones, D. S., and Greene, J. A. (2016). "Is Dementia in Decline? Historical Trends and Future Trajectories." *New England Journal of Medicine* 37: 507–509.

Kales, H. C., et al. (2011). "Trends in Antipsychotic Use in Dementia 1999–2007." *Archives of General Psychiatry* 68: 190–197.

Kales, H. C., et al. (2012). "Risk of Mortality among Individual Antipsychotics in Patients with Dementia." *American Journal of Psychiatry* 169: 71–7 9.

Karlawish, J., et al. (2017). "Alzheimer's Disease: The Next Frontier – Special Report 2017." *Alzheimer's & Dementia* 13: 374–380. doi: 10.1016/j.jalz.2017.02.006.

Kasper, S., et al. (2006). "Escitalopram in the Long-Term Treatment of Major Depressive Disorder in Elderly Patients." *Neuropsychobiology* 54: 152–159.

Kaup, A. R., et al. (2016). "Trajectories of Depressive Symptoms in Older Adults and Risk of Dementia." *JAMA: Psychiatry* 73:525–531. doi:10.1001/jamapsychiatry.2016.0004.

Kessler, E-M., et al. (2015). "Attitudes towards Seeking Mental Health Services Among Older Adults: Personal and Contextual Correlates." *Aging & Mental Health* 19: 182–191.

Khundakar, A. A., and Thomas, A. J. (2015). "Neuropathology of Depression in Alzheimer's Disease: Current Knowledge and the Potential for New Treatments." *Journal of Alzheimer's Disease* 44: 27–41.

Kianirad, Y., and Simuni, T. (2017). "Pimavanserin, A Novel Antipsychotic For Management of Parkinson's Disease Psychosis." *Expert Review of Clinical Pharmacology* 10: 1161–1168. doi: 10.1080/17512433.2017.1369405.

Kok, R. M., et al. (2011). "Continuing Treatment of Depression in the Elderly: A Systematic Review and Meta-analysis of Double-blinded Randomized Controlled Trials with Antidepressants." *American Journal of Geriatric Psychiatry* 19: 249–255.

Koponen, M., et al. (2017). "Risk of Mortality Associated with Antipsychotic Monotherapy and Polypharmacy among Community-Dwelling Persons with Alzheimer's Disease." *Journal of Alzheimer's Disease* 56:107–18. doi: 10.3233/JAD-160671.

Kumar, A., and Ekavali, A. S. (2015). "A Review on Alzheimer's Disease Pathophysiology and its Management: An Update." *Pharmacological Reports* 67: 195–203.

Kumar, A., et al. (2016). "Current and Novel Therapeutic Molecules and Targets in Alzheimer's Disease." *Journal of the Formosan Medical Association* 115: 3–10.

Lam, H. T., et al. (2016). "Stabilization of α-Synuclein Fibril Clusters Prevents Fragmentation and Reduces Seeding Activity and Toxicity." *Biochemistry* 55: 675–685.

Larson, E. B., and Langa, K. M. (2017). "What's the 'Take Home' from Research on Dementia Trends?" *PLOS Med* 14(3): e1002236. doi:10.1371/journal.pmed.1002236.

Leegwater-Kim, J., and Bortan, E. (2010). "The Role of Rasagiline in the Treatment of Parkinson's Disease." *Clinical Interventions in Aging* 5: 149–156.

Lenze, E. J., et al. (2005). "Efficacy and Tolerability of Citalopram in the Treatment of Late-Life Anxiety Disorders: Results from an 8-Week, Randomized, Placebo-Controlled Trial." *American Journal of Psychiatry* 162: 145–150.

Lenze, E. J., et al. (2008). "Incomplete Response in Later-Life Depression: Getting to Remission." *Dialogues in Clinical Neurosciences* 10: 419–430.

Lenze, E. J., et al. (2009). "Escitalopram for Older Adults with Generalized Anxiety Disorder." *JAMA* 301: 295–303.

Lew, M. F., et al. (2010). "Long-Term Efficacy of Rasagiline in Early Parkinson's Disease." *International Journal of Neuroscience* 120: 404–408.

Li, J., et al. (2008). "Huperzine A for Alzheimer's Disease." *Cochrane Datebase of Systematic Reviews* 16: CD005592.

Löhle, M., and Reichmann, H. (2011). "Controversies in Neurology: Why Monoamine Oxidase B Inhibitors Could Be a Good Choice For the Initial Treatment of Parkinson's Disease." *BMC Neurology* 11: 1–7: http://www.biomedcentral.com/1471-2377/11/112.

Lyketsos, C. G., et al. (2006). "Position Statement of the American Association for Geriatric Psychiatry Regarding Principles for Care of Patients with Dementia Resulting from Alzheimer's Disease." *American Journal of Geriatric Psychiatry* 14: 561–572.

Mackenzie, C. S., et al. (2010). "Correlates of Perceived Need for and Use of Mental Health Services by Older Adults in the Collaborative Psychiatric Epidemiology Surveys." *American Journal of Geriatric Psychiatry* 18: 1103–1115.

Malaty, I. A., and Fernandez, H. H. (2009). "Role of Rasagiline in Treating Parkinson's Disease: Effect on Disease Progression." *Therapeutics and Clinical Risk Management* 5: 413–419.

Mathis, M. V., et al. (2017). "The US Food and Drug Administration's Perspective on the New Antipsychotic Pimavanserin." *Journal of Clinical Psychiatry* 78: e668–e673.

Matsunaga, S., et al. (2015). "Memantine Monotherapy for Alzheimer's Disease: A Systematic Review and Meta-Analysis." *PLOS One*, 10(4): e0123289. doi:10.1371/journal.pone.0123289.

Maust, D. T., et al. (2015). "Antipsychotics, Other Psychotropics, and the Risk of Death in Patients With Dementia: Number Needed to Harm." *JAMA: Psychiatry* 72: 438–445.

Maust, D. T., et al. (2017a). "Antidepressant Prescribing in Primary Care to Older Adults without Major Depression." *Psychiatric Services* 68: 449–455. doi: 10.1176/appi.ps.201600197.

Maust, D. T., et al. (2017b). "Trends in Central Nervous System-Active Polypharmacy Among Older Adults Seen in Outpatient Care in the United States." *JAMA: Internal Medicine* 177: 583–585. doi: 10.1001/jamainternmed.2016.9225.

McHardy, S. F., et al. (2017). "Recent Advances in Acetylcholinesterase Inhibitors and Reactivators: An Update on the Patent Literature (2012–2015)." *Expert Opinion on Therapeutic Patents* 27: 455–476. doi: 10.1080/13543776.2017.1272571.

McKhann, G., et al. (1984). "Clinical Diagnosis of Alzheimer's Disease: Report of The NINCDS-ADRDA Work Group under the Auspices of Department of Health and Human Services Task Force on Alzheimer's Disease." *Neurology* 34: 939–944.

McKhann, G. M., et al. (2011). "The Diagnosis of Dementia Due to Alzheimer's Disease: Recommendations from the National Institute on Aging-Alzheimer's Association Workgroups on Diagnostic Guidelines for Alzheimer's Disease." *Alzheimer's & Dementia* 7: 263–269.

Meeks, T. (2010). "Drugs, Death, and Disconcerting Dilemmas." *Psychiatric Times* 27: 1–7.

National Center for Health Statistics, U.S. Centers for Disease Control, retrieved at https://www.cdc.gov/nchs/pressroom/sosmap/alzheimers_mortality/alzheimers_disease.htm.

Naoi, M., and Maruyama, W. (2009). "Functional Mechanism of Neuroprotection by Inhibitors of Type B Monoamine Oxidase in Parkinson's Disease." *Expert Reviews in Neurotherapeutics* 9: 1233–1250.

Nehls, M. (2016). "Unified Theory of Alzheimer's Disease (UTAD): Implications For Prevention and Curative Therapy." *Journal of Molecular Psychiatry* 4: 1–52. doi: 10.1186/s40303-016-0018-8.

Nelson, J. C., et al. (2006). "Mirtazepine Orally Disintegrating Tablets in Depressed Nursing Home Residents 85 Years of Age and Older." *International Journal of Geriatric Psychiatry* 21: 898–901.

Nishtala, P. S., et al. (2009). "Anticholinergic Activity of Commonly Prescribed Medications and Psychiatric Adverse Effects in Older People." *Journal of Clinical Pharmacology* 49: 1176–1184.

O'Brien, J. T., and Burns, A. (2011). "Clinical Practice with Anti-dementia Drugs: A Revised (Second) Consensus Statement from the British Association for Psychopharmacology." *Journal of Psychopharmacology* 25: 997–1019.

Olanow, C. W., et al. (2009a). "Dopaminergic Transplantation for Parkinson's Disease: Current Status and Future Prospects." *Annals of Neurology* 66: 591–596.

Olanow, C. W., et al. (2009b). "A Double-Blind, Delayed-Start Trial of Rasagiline in Parkinson's Disease." *New England Journal of Medicine* 361: 1268–1278.

Olde Rikkert, M. G. M., et al. (2015). "Tolerability and Safety of Souvenaid in Patients with Mild Alzheimer's Disease: Results of Multi-Center, 24-Week, Open-Label Extension Study." *Journal of Alzheimer's Disease* 44: 471–480.

Olfson, M., et al. (2015). "Antipsychotic Treatment of Adults in the United States." *Journal of Clinical Psychiatry* 76: 1346–1353.

Olin, J. T., et al. (2010). "Rivastigmine in the Treatment of Dementia Associated with Parkinson's Disease: Effects on Activities of Daily Living." *Dementia and Geriatric Cognitive Disorders* 29: 510–515.

Omelan, C. (2006). "Approaches to Managing Behavioural Disturbances in Dementia." *Canadian Family Physician* 52: 191–199.

Page, R. L., et al. (2010). "Inappropriate Prescribing in the Hospitalized Elderly Patient: Defining the Problem, Evaluation Tools, and Possible Solutions." *Clinical Interventions in Aging* 5: 75–87.

Paladini, A., et al. (2015). "Chronic Pain in the Elderly: The Case for New Therapeutic Strategies." *Pain Physician* 18: E863–E876.

Paleacu, D., et al. (2008). "Quetiapine Treatment for Behavioural and Psychological Symptoms of Dementia in Alzheimer's Disease Patients: A 6-Week, Double-Blind, Placebo-Controlled Study." *International Journal of Geriatric Psychiatry* 23: 393–400.

Panza, F., et al. (2009). "Disease-Modifying Approach to the Treatment of Alzheimer's Disease: From Alpha-Secretase Activators to Gamma-Secretase Inhibitors and Modulators." *Drugs and Aging* 26: 537–555.

Pariente, A., et al. (2012). "Antipsychotic Use and Myocardial Infarction in Older Patients with Treated Dementia." *Archives of Internal Medicine* 172: 648–653.

Patel, A. N., et al. (2017). "Prediction of Relapse after Discontinuation of Antipsychotic Treatment in Alzheimer's Disease: The Role of Hallucinations." *American Journal of Psychiatry* 174: 362–369.

Pauwels, E. K., et al. (2009). "Fatty Acid Facts, Part IV: Docosahexaenoic Acid and Alzheimer's Disease. A Story of Mice, Men and Fish." *Drug News and Perspectives* 22: 205–213.

Penkunas, M. J., and Hahn-Smith, S. (2015). "An Evaluation of IMPACT for the Treatment of Late-Life Depression in a Public Mental Health System." *Journal of Behavioral Health Services & Research* 42: 334–345.

Petersen, R., et al. (2005). "Vitamin E and Donepezil for the Treatment of Mild Cognitive Impairment." *New England Journal of Medicine* 352: 2379–2388.

Porsteinssona, A. P., and Antonsdottir, I. M. (2017). "An Update on the Advancements in the Treatment of Agitation in Alzheimer's Disease." *Expert Opinion on Pharmacotherapy* 18: 611–620. doi: 10.1080/14656566.2017.1307340.

Price, A. R., et al. (2013). "Comment on "ApoE-Directed Therapeutics Rapidly Clear β-Amyloid and Reverse Deficits in AD Mouse Models"." *Science* 340: 924.

Qaseem, A., et al. (2008). "Current Pharmacologic Treatment of Dementia: A Clinical Practice Guideline from the American College of Physicians and the American Academy of Family Physicians." *Annals of Internal Medicine* 148: 370–378.

Qato, D. M., et al. (2016). "Changes in Prescription and Over-the-Counter Medication and Dietary Supplement Use Among Older Adults in the United States, 2005 vs 2011." *JAMA: Internal Medicine* 176: 473–482. doi: 10.1001/jamainternmed.2015.8581.

Quinn, J. F., et al. (2010). "Docosahexaenoic Acid Supplementation and Cognitive Decline in Alzheimer Disease." *JAMA* 304:1903–1911. doi: 10.1001/jama.2010.1510.

Rafii, M. S., et al. (2011). "A Phase II Trial of Huperzine A in Mild to Moderate Alzheimer Disease." *Neurology* 76: 1389–1394.

Raina, P., et al. (2008). "Effectiveness of Cholinesterase Inhibitors and Memantine for Treating Dementia: Evidence Review for a Clinical Practice Guideline." *Annals of Internal Medicine* 148: 379–397.

Reynolds, C. F., et al. (2006). "Maintenance Treatment of Major Depression in Old Age." *New England Journal of Medicine* 354: 1130–1138.

Rhein, V., et al. (2009). "Amyloid-Beta and Tau Synergistically Impair the Oxidative Phosphorylation System in Triple Transgenic Alzheimer's Disease Mice." *Proceedings of the National Academy of Science* 106: 20057–20062.

Roe, C. M., et al. (2013). "Amyloid Imaging and CSF Biomarkers in Predicting Cognitive Impairment Up to 7.5 Years Later." *Neurology* 80:1784–1791.

Rosenblum, W. I. (2014). "Why Alzheimer Trials Fail: Removing Soluble Oligomeric Beta Amyloid Is Essential, Inconsistent, And Difficult." *Neurobiology of Aging* 35: 969–974.

Rothenberg, K. G., and Weichers, I. R. (2015). "Antipsychotics for Neuropsychiatric Symptoms of Dementia—Safety and Efficacy in the Context of Informed Consent." *Psychiatric Annuals* 45: 348–353.

Rountree, S. D., et al. (2013). "Effectiveness of Antidementia Drugs in Delaying Alzheimer's Disease Progression." *Alzheimer's & Dementia* 9: 338–345.

Russ, T. C., and Morling, J. R. (2012). "Cholinesterase Inhibitors for Mild Cognitive Impairment." *Cochrane Database of Systematic Reviews* 12(9): CD009132. doi: 10.1002/14651858.CD009132.pub2.

Rutherford, B., et al. (2007). "An Open Trial of Aripiprazole Augmentation for SSRI Non-Remitters with Late-Life Depression." *International Journal of Geriatric Psychiatry* 22: 986–991.

Ryan, C., et al. (2009). "Appropriate Prescribing in the Elderly: An Investigation of Two Screening Tools, Beers Criteria Considering Diagnosis and Independent of Diagnosis and Improved Prescribing in the Elderly Tool to Identify Inappropriate Use of Medicines in the Elderly in Primary Care in Ireland." *Journal of Clinical Pharmacy and Therapeutics* 34: 369–376.

Sabbagh, M. N. (2009). "Drug Development for Alzheimer's Disease: Where Are We Now, and Where Are We Headed?" *American Journal of Geriatric Pharmacotherapy* 7: 167–185.

Sadowsky, C. H., et al. (2010). "Safety and Tolerability of Rivastigmine Transdermal Patch Compared with Rivastigmine Capsules in Patients Switched from Donepezil: Data from Three Clinical Trials." *International Journal of Clinical Practice* 64: 188–193.

Sauerbier, A., et al. (2016). "New Concepts in The Pathogenesis and Presentation of Parkinson's Disease." *Clinical Medicine* 16: 365–370. doi: 10.7861/clinmedicine.16-4-365.

Schaefer, E. J., et al. (2006). "Plasma Phosphatidylcholine Docosahexaenoic Acid Content and Risk of Dementia and Alzheimer's Disease." *Archives of Neurology* 63: 1545–1550.

Scheltens, P., et al. (2016). "Alzheimer's Disease." *Lancet* 388: 505–517.

Schneider, L. S., et al. (2011). "Lack of Evidence for the Efficacy of Memantine in Mild Alzheimer Disease." *Archives of Neurology* 68: 991–998.

Seitz, D. P., et al. (2013). "Pharmacological Treatments for Neuropsychiatric Symptoms of Dementia in Long-term Care: A Systematic Review." *International Psychogeriatrics* 25: 185–203.

Selkoe, D. J. (2011). "Resolving Controversies on the Path to Alzheimer's Therapeutics." *Nature Medicine* 17: 1060–1065.

Shah, D., et al. (2010). "Medications for Treating Alzheimer's Dementia." *Carlat Psychiatry Report* 8(4): 1–3.

Simoni-Wastila, L., et al. (2009). "Association of Antipsychotic Use with Hospital Events and Mortality Among Medicare Beneficiaries Residing in Long-Term Care Facilities." *American Journal of Geriatric Psychiatry* 17: 417–427.

Steinman, M. A., et al. (2006). "Polypharmacy and Prescribing Quality in Older People." *Journal of the American Geriatric Society* 54: 1516–1523.

Sterke, C. S., et al. (2012a). "Dose–response Relationship between Selective Serotonin Re-uptake Inhibitors and Injurious Falls: A Study in Nursing Home Residents With Dementia." *British Journal of Clinical Pharmacology* 73: 812–820.

Sterke, C. S., et al. (2012b). "New Insights: Dose-Response Relationship between Psychotropic Drugs and Falls: A Study in Nursing Home Residents with Dementia." *Journal of Clinical Pharmacology* 52: 947–955.

Stewart, J. C., et al. (2014). "Effect of Collaborative Care for Depression on Risk of Cardiovascular Events: Data from the IMPACT Randomized Controlled Trial." *Psychosomatic Medicine* 76: 29–37.

Stocchi, F., et al. (2010). "Initiating Levodopa/Carbidopa Therapy with and Without Entacapone in Early Parkinson Disease: The STRIDE-PD Study." *Annals of Neurology* 68: 18–27.

Streim, J. E., et al. (2008). "A Randomized, Double-Blind, Placebo-Controlled Study of Aripiprazole for the Treatment of Psychosis in Nursing Home Patients with Alzheimer Disease." *American Journal of Geriatric Psychiatry* 16: 537–550.

Taipale, H., et al. (2017). "Risk of Pneumonia Associated with Incident Benzodiazepine Use among Community Dwelling Adults with Alzheimer Disease." *Canadian Medical Association Journal* 189: E519–E529.

Tannenbaum, C., et al. (2012). "A Systematic Review of Amnestic and Non-Amnestic Mild Cognitive Impairment Induced by Anticholinergic, Antihistamine, GABAergic and Opioid Drugs." *Drugs & Aging* 29: 639–658.

Tariot, P. N. (2006). "Contemporary Issues in the Treatment of Alzheimer's Disease: Tangible Benefits of Current Therapies." *Journal of Clinical Psychiatry* 67, Supplement 3: 15–22.

Tesseur, I., et al. (2013). "Comment on "ApoE-Directed Therapeutics Rapidly Clear β-Amyloid and Reverse Deficits in AD Mouse Models"." *Science* 340: 924.

Thomas, J., et al. (2015). "Omega-3 Fatty Acids in Early Prevention of Inflammatory Neurodegenerative Disease: A Focus on Alzheimer's Disease." *Biomed Research International* 2015: Article ID 172801. doi: 10.1155/2015/172801.

Tolppanen, A-M., et al. (2016). "Antipsychotic Use and Risk of Hospitalization or Death Due to Pneumonia in Persons with and Those without Alzheimer Disease." *Chest* 150: 1233–1241.

Tsunoda, K., et al. (2010). "Effects of Discontinuing Benzodiazepine-Derivative Hypnotics on Postural Sway and Cognitive Functions in the Elderly." *International Journal of Geriatric Psychiatry* 25: 1259–1265. doi: 10.1002/gps.2465.

Unzeta, M., et al. (2016). "Multi-Target Directed Donepezil-Like Ligands for Alzheimer's Disease." *Frontiers in Neuroscience* 10: 1–24.

Van Leeuwen, W. E., et al. (2009). "Collaborative Depression Care for the Old-Old: Findings from the IMPACT Trial." *American Journal of Geriatric Psychiatry* 17: 1040–1049.

Veeraraghavalu, K., et al. (2013). "Comment on "ApoE-Directed Therapeutics Rapidly Clear β-Amyloid and Reverse Deficits in AD Mouse Models"." *Science* 340: 924.

Ventimiglia, J., et al. (2010). "An Analysis of the Intended Use of Atypical Antipsychotics in Dementia." *Psychiatry (Edgemont)* 7(11): 14–17.

Vigen, C. L. P., et al. (2011). "Cognitive Effects of Atypical Antipsychotic Medications in Patients with Alzheimer's Disease: Outcomes From CATIE-AD." *American Journal of Psychiatry* 168: 831–839.

Wang, C., et al. (2016a). "Antidepressant Use in the Elderly Is Associated with an Increased Risk of Dementia." *Journal of Alzheimer's Disease and Related Disorders* 30: 99–104.

Wang, Z-Y., et al. (2016b). "Pharmacological Effects of Active Components of Chinese Herbal Medicine in the Treatment of Alzheimer's Disease: A Review." *American Journal of Chinese Medicine* 44: 1525–1541.

Weintraub, D., et al. (2010). "Impulse Control Disorders in Parkinson's Disease: A Cross-Sectional Study of 3,090 Patients." *Archives of Neurology* 67: 589–595.

Wilcock, G. K., et al. (2008). "Efficacy and Safety of Tarenflurbil in Mild to Moderate Alzheimer's Disease: A Randomized Phase II Trial." *Lancet Neurology* 7: 483–493.

Williams, A., et al. (2010). "Deep Brain Stimulation Plus Best Medical Therapy versus Best Medical Therapy Alone for Advanced Parkinson's Disease (PD SURG Trial): A Randomized, Open-Label Trial." *Lancet Neurology,* 9: 681–681.

Winblad, B., et al. (2006). "Donepezil in Patients with Severe Alzheimer's Disease: Double-Blind, Parallel-Group, Placebo-Controlled Study." *Lancet* 367: 1057–1065.

Wright, J. W., and Harding, J. W. (2016). "Small Molecule AngIV-based Analogs to Treat Alzheimer's Disease." *International Journal of Drug Development and Research* 8: 21–27.

Wu, S., et al. (2015). "Omega-3 Fatty Acids Intake and Risks Of Dementia and Alzheimer's Disease: A Meta-Analysis." *Neuroscience and Biobehavioral Reviews* 48: 1–9.

Yurko-Mauro, K., et al. (2010). "Beneficial Effects of Docosahexaenoic Acid on Cognition in Age-related Cognitive Decline." *Alzheimer's & Dementia* 6: 456–464.

Zhai, Y., et al. (2016). "Association Between Antipsychotic Drugs and Mortality in Older Persons with Alzheimer's Disease: A Systematic Review and Meta-Analysis." *Journal of Alzheimer's Disease* 52: 631–639.

Zhao, Q-F., et al. (2016). "The Prevalence of Neuropsychiatric Symptoms in Alzheimer's Disease: Systematic Review and Meta-Analysis." *Journal of Affective Disorders* 190: 264–271.

Zhu, C. W., et al. (2013). "Long-term Associations Between Cholinesterase Inhibitors and Memantine Use and Health Outcomes Among Patients with Alzheimer's Disease." *Alzheimer's & Dementia* 9: 733–740.

CHAPTER 17

Challenging Times
for Mental Health

In the last edition—the thirteenth—the following paragraph summarized the situation in regard to the psychopharmacological treatment of mental disorders:

> During the last 30 years no new fundamentally novel drugs for mental illness have been developed, and the usefulness of even current medications is being challenged. Efforts to develop an effective drug for Alzheimer's disease have not been successful. Even the criteria by which psychiatric disorders are diagnosed have been revised. Many pharmaceutical companies are abandoning their psychotropic research programs. And all of this is occurring at a time of diminished public resources when the economy has suffered a severe downturn.

Unfortunately, there has not been much progress. There are still no fundamentally new drugs for mental illness or Alzheimer's disease and the benefits of current drug treatment continue to be questioned. Pharmaceutical research into mental illness has not rebounded and although the economy as a whole has gradually recovered, it is not clear if that will be sustained. The need for mental health treatment is still critical, especially for substance use disorders, and particularly for the abuse of opioid prescriptions and "new pharmacological substances." The revision of diagnostic categories has been called inadequate for practical application to real-world difficulties.

These ongoing problems have prompted several responses. First, the limitations of traditional psychopharmacological treatment have reactivated interest and support for nonpharmacological approaches to mental illness, particularly psychotherapy, but also somatic treatments, such as transcranial therapy for depression. Second, the scope of pharmacological research is being extended to include a deeper understanding of basic neurophysiology, such as the circuitry of fear, rather than specific clinical syndromes, such as anxiety symptoms. Third, there has been a renewal of national investment in research and increased public support for better therapy and treatment of mental illness.

EPIDEMIOLOGY OF MENTAL ILLNESS

According to Substance Abuse and Mental Health Services Administration's (2016; SAMHSA) National Survey on Drug Use and Health (NSDUH), an estimated 43.4 million (17.9 percent) of Americans ages 18 and up experienced some form of mental illness in 2015. In 2015, over 27 million people in the United States reported current use of illicit drugs or misuse of prescription drugs and over 66 million people—nearly a *quarter of the adult and adolescent population*—reported binge drinking in the past month. Among these, 7.9 million people had both a mental disorder and substance use disorder, that is, a co-occurring mental *and* substance use disorder.

Serious mental illness (SMI), defined by the SAMHSA as resulting in serious functional impairment, affects nearly 10 million American adults each year. According to the National Survey on Drug Use and Health (NSDUH), in 2015, there were an estimated 9.8 million adults aged 18 or older in the United States with SMI within the past year. This number represented 4.0 percent of all U.S. adults.

Consistent with previous reports, Walker and colleagues (2015) summarized data from 148 studies and found that individuals suffering from mental illness had a relative risk of mortality that was 2.22 times higher than the comparison population. Furthermore, they estimate that about 8 million deaths were related to mental disorders every year with a potential median of a decade of lost life. The likelihood of homicide was more than seven times greater among those with any mental disorder than in the general population, according to one analysis (Crump et al., 2013), and for those with substance abuse disorders, the risk was 16 times greater. People with mental illness are also four times more likely to be victimized in nonlethal violent incidents than people in the general population.

How does this situation compare with previous estimates? It has been proposed that we are in the middle of a mental health crisis. The number of psychiatric beds in state hospitals has dropped to a historic low from 558,922 in 1955 (337 per 100,000) to 37,679 in 2016 (11.7 per 100,000) (Fuller et al., 2016). Between 2003 and 2013, there was a 10.2 percent decrease in the number of psychiatrists per 100,000 people in surveyed locations. During the same time, there was an increase in the numbers of primary care physicians and neurologists (Bishop et al., 2016). The decline in psychiatrists has been attributed to poor reimbursement, lack of coverage (such as when psychiatric diagnoses are not considered a "medical" condition), or problems qualifying for disability.

The existence of an epidemic in mental illness has also been refuted (Pies, 2015). First, it has been argued that the increase in the incidence and prevalence of mental disorders was not estimated correctly because these values were calculated from rates of medication prescriptions, diagnoses and treatment rates made in offices, or "putative" assessments of disability assumed to be due to mental illness. These indirect measures are not synonymous with a true increase in prevalence. Second, epidemiological surveys found that in 2013, the rate of SMI in U.S. adults was 4.2, while in 2010 the number was 5.0 and in 2009, 4.8 percent. The SMI rate was estimated at 8.3 percent in 2002 and 5.4 percent in 1990. Although estimates may vary, depending on the data source, the demographic data do not show a current epidemic of serious mental illness. Similar outcomes are seen in specific disorders with no evidence of significant increases in the proportion of adults with depression or schizophrenia. This is also true for children and adolescents with SMI.

Nevertheless, a substantial number of individuals continue to suffer from the burden of mental health disorders. The World Health Organization estimates that one in four people will have an episode of mental illness in their lifetime, and that mental and behavioral problems are the biggest single cause of disability on the planet (World Health Organization, 2001). Unfortunately, most people with behavioral problems do not receive therapy. Surveys report that as few as 35 percent of people with severe symptoms of depression were seen by a mental health therapist in the past year (Pratt and Brody, 2014). A survey by SAMHSA found that the reasons people gave for not seeking care included the expense, not having mental health insurance, the stigma of a mental illness diagnosis, fear of losing a job, and privacy concerns. Such views inhibit people from getting help. In one study, 93 percent of individuals with schizophrenia, depression, or bipolar disorder anticipated discrimination—and 87 percent experienced it—in at least one area of life, such as in their social life, education, housing, work, and so on (Farrelly et al., 2014). This perspective seems consistent with results of a global survey about mental illness in which responses were obtained from more than 1 million people and 229 sites. While nearly half of those surveyed from developed nations believed that mental illness and physical illness were similar, only 7 percent of this same group felt that mental illness could be overcome (Seeman et al., 2016).

Unfortunately, there have been no significant improvements in the pharmacological treatment of mental disorders. After the development of Prozac and the newer antipsychotic drugs decades ago, psychiatric researchers attempted to maintain these successes and to address the stigmatization of the mentally ill by focusing on the medical model, that is, by emphasizing that mental illness is a brain disease (Makari, 2015). But the newest drugs, while safer and with fewer side effects, target the same transmitter systems as the older ones and do not improve outcomes (Friedman, 2015). Acknowledgement of this situation prompted a reassessment of the approach to diagnosis, research, and treatment of mental illness.

Diagnostic Revisions

Publication of the fifth edition of the *Diagnostic and Statistical Manual of Mental Disorders* (DSM-5) in May 2013 was a significant development in the mental health profession. In general, there was an overall effort to improve what is known about the relationship between behavioral and psychological disorders—as well as their relationships to conditions covered by other applicable medical specialties—and move toward a more global system. Another important change was that the new manual was more compatible with the *International Classification of Diseases* (ICD) *System*, which is used by the rest of the world outside of North America. That is, the revisions of the DSM-5 are now more aligned with the structure of the disorders in the ICD (Clay, 2013). A third difference is the use of a continuum of symptoms rather than discrete diagnostic boundaries. Fourth, the "multiaxial" system, which used five different axes for psychiatric diagnoses, comorbid medical conditions, nonmedical factors, and other disabilities, was discontinued. In general, intellectual and personality disorders were given more equality with other diagnoses (Kupfer et al., 2013).

Research Domain Criteria: A Research Framework for New Ways of Studying Mental Disorders

The current diagnostic system of the DSM tried to apply a scientific basis for the distinction between those who were sick and those who were well. But the National Institute for Mental Health recently rejected this approach and stated that it was not producing useful research (Luhrmann, 2015). In 2013, its director, Thomas R. Insel, stated that no unique neurophysiological processes had been discovered by psychiatric research that could explain specific diagnoses. The DSM criteria had not kept up with developments in genetics, neuroscience, and behavioral science. The system for reviewing research grant applications had been based on DSM-defined disorders, but researchers increasingly wanted to study certain mechanisms, such as working memory, that cut across disorders.

Research into the neurobiology of mental disorders showed similar neuronal substrates across diagnostic categories. It was concluded that diagnoses were not useful or accurate for understanding the brain and would no longer be used to guide research. The institute eliminated the tradition in which research was guided by diagnoses, for example, a scientist who would identify as a "depression" researcher.

A new program was developed called *Research Domain Criteria* (RDoC). Under this scheme, all research protocols must have a neuroscientific basis in some biological structure, such as genes, cells, or circuits, that cuts across behavioral, cognitive, and social domains, such as acute fear, loss, or arousal. Since 2014, in order to receive the institute's support, clinical researchers must explicitly focus on a target such as a biomarker or neural circuit. To use an example from the program's Web site, psychiatric researchers will no longer study people with anxiety; instead they will study *fear circuitry*.

The RDoC is not a new distinct diagnostic nosology, but rather a research paradigm about psychopathology intended to build a research literature based on genetics, neuroscience, and behavioral science (Cuthbert, 2014). It is a four-dimensional matrix. The first dimension is divided into five major domains of functioning. They include:

1. Aversive properties, that is, those systems that respond to aversive or negative situations
2. Appetitive properties, or a "positive valence," such as working toward rewards
3. Cognitive systems
4. Systems for social processes
5. Arousal and regulatory systems

The second dimension includes what are called "units of analysis." These are different ways in which one can study the functional domains of the first dimension. They include genetics; molecular processes and cellular processes; measures of circuits; physiological measures, such as heart rate, skin conductance, or serum cortisol; behavioral measures, such as an assessment battery; and self-reports, which are defined to include questionnaires as well as structured diagnostic interviews. The aim is to acquire a comprehensive understanding of how a particular concept, such as "working memory," works at multiple levels.

The third dimension is neurodevelopment. This is important because psychiatric disorders are now understood to be developmental disorders. Therefore, it is vital to understand how the functional domains and the units of analysis described earlier evolve with the maturing organism.

The fourth dimension is environmental influences. When something happens in the environment at a certain stage of neurodevelopment, it can influence the functioning of all of the above dimensions. Over all, the emphasis is on broader research to identify etiology and find better targets.

Resurgence of Nonpharmacological Therapies

Neurobiological mechanisms mediate all of our human experience, and it is certainly worthwhile to learn as much as possible about how the brain works. But that is not the same as assuming that our experiences of low mood or psychosis, for example, should be labeled as an illness. It is being increasingly appreciated that even severe mental disorders are not simply due to genetic anomalies or impaired brain substrates. The role of experience is being realized as an important contribution to our mental state, and that even severe mental problems may be the result of traumatic life events that alter our interaction with the world. The ultimate benefit of psychiatric medications is being questioned, relative to that of psychological and behavioral therapies (Kinderman, 2014).

This is illustrated by a study by Leucht and colleagues, who performed a meta-analytical review of the effectiveness of medication and psychotherapy for major psychiatric conditions (see Huhn et al., 2014). They organized 61 meta-analyses on 21 disorders, which included 137,126 patients, into 3 comparisons: pharmacotherapy (33 meta-analyses) or psychotherapy (17 meta-analyses) compared with placebo or no treatment; head-to-head comparisons of pharmaco- and psychotherapies (7 meta-analyses); and combinations of both treatments (12 meta-analyses). Direct comparisons showed that psychotherapy had a slight edge in regard to preventing a relapse into depression and bulimia; pharmacotherapy was more effective for dysthymic disorder and schizophrenia. Therapeutic combinations were more effective than either therapy alone, except for posttraumatic stress disorder and psychodynamic therapy for schizophrenia.

Although pills are cheaper and faster, it is not uncommon for patients to prefer psychotherapy. In their meta-analysis of the literature, McHugh and coworkers (2013) provided an estimate of the proportion of patients that preferred psychotherapeutic approaches as opposed to medications for treatment of psychiatric disorders. Overall, they reported a "threefold preference for psychological treatment relative to medication" (p. 595). This was most evident in younger patients and in women. Moreover, many problems are social and environmental, for which there is no quick biological cure. Furthermore, some disorders, such as borderline and narcissistic personality disorders, are known not to have drug treatments, but can respond to therapy (Friedman, 2015). See discussion by Boggs, 2014.

Davey (2014) expressed this perspective as a summary of the shortcomings of (current) drug treatments for mental illness, which include:

1. Drugs alone are not good enough, may promote relapse, and are more effective when combined with psychotherapy.
2. Drugs may unnecessarily turn a short-term problem into a lifetime concern.
3. Drugs may give the message that mental problems are purely a medical issue and "out of the hands" of the patient.
4. Diagnostic criteria are all or none, not dimensional; but symptoms may vary in intensity.
5. Drugs are being promoted for normal difficulties of life.
6. Side effects of drugs, especially psychological, may cause people to stop taking them or diminish their benefit.
7. There are publication biases for reporting the positive effects of drugs.
8. Drugs do not help change the way people think or their socioeconomic environments.
9. Poorly trained practitioners make it easier to use drugs.
10. Drug companies have more clout than psychotherapy groups.

On the other hand, the alternative of psychotherapy is not always available; it may not be covered by insurance; it can be expensive; and it may take much longer to be effective than some drug treatments, for example, to alleviate anxiety. Nevertheless, many medications, such as drugs for the treatment of psychosis and bipolar disorder, may take weeks to show improvement, and it may take more than one trial to determine the optimum dose regimen. During that time, psychological support is, understandably, crucial to maintain the best outcome for the patient. Unfortunately, the overall success rate of psychiatric medications has remained relatively constant at only about 66 percent.

Policy Developments

In December 2016, President Barack Obama signed the 21st Century Cures Act after it sailed through the House of Representatives and was passed by the Senate 94 to 5. Although the Act has been acclaimed for its provisions to accelerate drug discovery, it also contains sections meant to improve mental health treatment and to fight the opioid epidemic. Continued support for the latter objective was provided when President Trump declared the opioid epidemic a "national public health emergency" in October 2017. Supporters have proposed that it is the most important piece of legislation concerning mental health since the 2008 law requiring parity of insurance coverage for mental and physical health.

There is strong support for science in this new legislation. Federal agencies are urged to fund only those initiatives with significant research backing and to determine if patients truly benefit. Laws that mandated parity for mental and physical therapies are strengthened. Furthermore, there are provisions for increasing the number of psychiatrists and psychologists to alleviate the current shortage.

In addition, the law synthesizes ideas from several legislators and urges the states to offer early intervention for psychosis, an approach that is considered to have great potential for improving mental health.

The bill was crafted with input from many stakeholders, including patients, researchers, and industry representatives. Most provisions are noncontroversial, such as proposals for a strategic plan, initiatives for specific research efforts, sharing of data, and promoting reproducibility of research outcomes. Billions of dollars are designated for individual projects, such as Vice President Biden's cancer "moonshot," and $30 million are earmarked for regenerative medicine research using adult stem cells.

Clinical Examples

The following examples illustrate clinical applications of current understanding of best practices in psychopharmacology. Clients L (Thomas et al., 2012), M (Ostermann et al., 2013), and N (Doellinger et al., 2016) are taken from the clinical literature and describe real-life case presentations.[1]

Client A was a 45-year-old male who was prescribed lithium for a diagnosis of bipolar II disorder. He presented with complaints of an 80-pound weight gain and an inability to remember names. Recognizing these problems as side effects of lithium therapy, the therapists noted a study on the efficacy of valproic acid for bipolar II and decided to make that medication switch. Thereafter, Client A lost about 40 pounds and his memory function improved, allowing him to continue working.

Five years later, Client A presented with complaints of listlessness, lack of energy, and sexual dysfunction. It was discovered that the client had been diagnosed with

---

[1]Another real case was presented in the *New York Times Magazine* of February 17, 2013. The patient was a 55-year-old man who suffered from depression and alcoholism and was admitted to the hospital after a fall down a flight of stairs in his home. Because he had not been found for a few days, his condition was extremely serious and it took five weeks of medical treatment before he was able to transfer to a rehabilitation facility. After two weeks in rehabilitation, the patient began to have hallucinations and started talking to people who were not there, but whom he feared were going to hurt him. Even after his sleeping medication was changed (which was thought to be the source of the symptoms), the hallucinations continued. He also had a fever, racing heart rate, high blood pressure, and hyperreflexia. Fortunately, the attending physician noted that the patient had been prescribed a second antidepressant during the last two days of his rehabilitation treatment, as well as a heartburn medication, all of which raised his serotonin level. Within 24 hours after being put on a drug that blocks serotonin, the patient was alert and talking, his hallucinations were gone, his heart rate and blood pressure were normal, and the tremors were resolving. This real-life incident illustrates the importance of communication as part of the collaboration among all medical personnel associated with patient care.

depression and had been prescribed *escitalopram* (Lexapro) in addition to the valproic acid. Escitalopram and valproic acid were discontinued and the initiation of *aripiprazole* (Abilify) and *lamotrigine* (Lamictal) was recommended, either alone or in combination. Valproic acid and escitalopram were replaced with aripiprazole. Two weeks later, the client reported that the new drug was "intolerable" and complained of aches, myalgias, flulike symptoms, and electric shocks in his head. The psychologist determined that the client had serotonin discontinuation syndrome rather than side effects of aripiprazole and counseled the client about serotonin discontinuation syndrome. Three weeks later, the symptoms had ceased, the client was more energized, sexual function was improving, and no bipolar symptoms were reported. Continual progress was made over the next few months.

Client B, a man in his late twenties, was referred by a physician for evaluation of cognitive difficulties. Neuropsychological testing was performed and diagnosis was made of notable cognitive dysfunction, with the greatest difficulty being word finding. Medication review revealed that the client had recently been prescribed *topiramate* (Topamax) for anxiety and posttraumatic stress disorder (PTSD). Replacement of the topiramate with *pregabalin* (Lyrica) led to rapid resolution of the cognitive difficulties.

Client C was a 48-year-old woman diagnosed with depression and anxiety. She was prescribed *sertraline* (Zoloft) and showed some improvement, but she gradually developed a panic disorder. Further history taking revealed that she had recently undergone surgery for breast lesions that were diagnosed as benign breast cysts. It turned out that Client C was a heavy coffee drinker. Sertraline interferes with the metabolism of caffeine, which resulted doubling her blood level of caffeine. Caffeinism is associated with increasing anxiety, panic disorder, and the development of benign breast cysts. Cessation of caffeine drinking, which included drinking smaller amounts of caffeinated and eventually only drinking decaffeinated coffee, led to resolution of the panic disorder.

Client D was a 28-year-old Gulf War veteran with severe PTSD, presenting with nighttime terrors and threatening actions toward his wife. Moreover, he was amnestic for these episodes. Medication review revealed a prescription for *zolpidem* (Ambien) for sleep. It was determined that the Ambien might be causing the amnesia. Replacement of Ambien with gabapentin at bedtime improved PTSD symptoms and the amnestic episodes were resolved.

Client E was an 88-year-old female care center resident whose family took her to therapy for increasing dementia. Medication review revealed that she had been receiving *imipramine* (Tofranil) for depression and *diazepam* (Valium) for anxiety and sleep difficulties. Because tricyclic antidepressants have anticholinergic difficulties, they can cause cognitive impairments. Benzodiazepines are widely known to worsen dementias. Cessation of these medicines and replacement with *quetiapine* (Seroquel) and *mirtazapine* (Remeron) at bedtime led to cognitive improvements, reductions in anxiety, better sleep patterns, and improvements in appetite.

Client F was a 5-year-old girl presenting with rages and aggressive behaviors made worse by psychostimulants and antidepressants. She was prescribed *valproic acid* (Depakote) and showed marked improvement in behavior. When she was referred to a psychologist, it was decided that with behavioral improvement, family therapy could be instituted to address problems underlying the client's behaviors. The possibility was also raised that, with effective family therapy, the valproic acid might eventually be stopped.

Client G, a 69-year-old female, was brought to the emergency department confused and disoriented—she did not know where she was—and suffering from delusions—stating that she was a movie star and the hospital a movie studio. She experienced a fluctuating course of agitation, had not slept in days, and was aggressive and disruptive. She had no history of mental illness and there was no evidence of illegal drug or alcohol use. The medical examination revealed a systemic infection; laboratory tests also indicated an elevation in her serum glucose levels. The psychologist determined that the patient was in a state of delirium possibly caused by her systemic infection. The goal was to stabilize her behaviorally and to treat the source of the infection. It was important to reduce her level of agitation, provide treatment for her delusion, improve her orientation, and provide something that allowed her to sleep.

The recommendation was to use the second-generation antipsychotic drug risperidone rather than the alternate option of a benzodiazepine, because in elderly patients and those with delirium, a benzodiazepine has the potential to paradoxically increase agitation and worsen the delirium, an idiosyncratic response. There was a need for an antipsychotic that could be given by intramuscular injection to reduce the agitation quickly and facilitate sleep. Afterwards, the drug could be given orally on a regular dosing schedule to maintain stability. Several antipsychotics have acute intramuscular formulations, including haloperidol, risperidone, olanzapine, and aripiprazole. Haloperidol was excluded because of the concern for producing extrapyramidal side effects, which are more likely in the elderly, and when the drug is given by intramuscular injection. The hospital formulary did not include aripiprazole; olanzapine was excluded because its high anticholinergic effect would tend to worsen the delirium. In addition, olanzapine has a risk of producing metabolic side effects that include insulin resistance and can worsen diabetes. Since this patient had increased blood glucose levels, olanzapine would not be the best choice. It was felt that risperidone was the least risky and would provide the most benefit. Risperidone was given in small doses, that is, 0.5 milligram via intramuscular injection on an as-needed basis and then orally in low doses, starting with 0.5 milligram twice per day. With this regimen, the patient was able to sleep, her delusion subsided, and she became calm and regained her orientation to place. She was able to be discharged after two days with a referral to an outpatient psychiatrist who could follow her for ongoing treatment as needed.

Client H was a 55-year-old diabetic man with mild hypertension and painful diabetic neuropathy who suffered previous depressive episodes and one suicide attempt. He met the current criteria for a major depressive episode with some anxiety. He had been treated with paroxetine, sertraline, and bupropion. His depression improved slightly with each of these medications, but it never remitted. With the diagnosis of major depressive disorder with anxious features confirmed, the goal was to reduce the depressive symptoms, anxiety, and possibly his neuropathic pain. Assuming that his previous trials had been adequately treated, a dual reuptake inhibitor was recommended because he had not achieved remission with two selective serotonin reuptake inhibitors. Given his mild hypertension, venlafaxine was not chosen. Although tricyclic antidepressants can help with neuropathic pain and depression, they are not a good choice, given their side effect profile and lethality in overdose. Duloxetine has an indication for neuropathic pain, depression, and anxiety, and was successfully prescribed. Because duloxetine is a CYP2D6 and CPY1A2 inhibitor and has potential drug–drug interactions, the patient was instructed to tell his physician if he took any other medications or supplements.

Client I was a 33-year-old woman hospitalized with her first episode of mania. She had no previous history of a depressive episode, no drug or alcohol history, and no medical issues. Because her first presentation was a manic episode, she was prescribed lithium. Prior to starting that drug, however, she was given a pregnancy test, and her baseline serum creatinine and thyroid hormone levels were obtained. Her choice of a birth control method was discussed and documented. She was prescribed the average starting dose of 300 milligrams twice a day, but after one week, she complained of stomach irritation and some diarrhea. Because gastrointestinal irritation and diarrhea are common, particularly early in treatment, she was encouraged to drink adequate fluid. Then the dose of 300 milligrams twice a day was maintained to see if the side effects resolved.

Client J was a 27-year-old male admitted secondary to a manic episode. He had five to six manic or depressive episodes a year and struggled on and off with alcohol abuse. Valproic acid treatment was started because the patient was a rapid cycler, with four or more depressive or manic episodes per year, and because of his comorbid alcohol abuse. He started on 250 milligrams twice a day, which was increased to 500 milligrams twice a day. His valproic acid blood level was low and it turned out that his liver enzymes had doubled. While it is not unusual for patients on anticonvulsants to experience an increase in liver enzymes, as long as their dosage is not tripled, no change in therapy is indicated. Nevertheless, the patient should be monitored.

Client K, a 21-year-old male with symptoms consistent with schizophrenia, was admitted because of profound psychotic behavior. He was treatment naive and an antipsychotic was recommended. His fasting lipid profile showed that the patient had mildly elevated total cholesterol and a low HDL—a so-called good cholesterol—for his age. Because of the increased risk of dyslipidemia, olanzapine and quetiapine were ruled out, and risperidone, ziprasidone, and aripiprazole were recommended. But when risperidone was started and increased to 3 milligrams twice a day, which is a high average dose, the patient complained that he felt "uncomfortable" in his skin, like "I can't sit still." Given his descriptions, he was likely experiencing akathisia, which is not uncommon with risperidone. Because akathisia is associated with an increased risk for suicide, it needs to be addressed, although current options are often unsatisfactory. For client K, the dose of risperidone was reduced, but then the psychosis worsened. A low, 15-milligram dose of the 5HT2 serotoninergic antagonist mirtazapine was added and the patient's akathisia decreased. The goal was to eventually reduce the risperidone dose so that the adjunct mirtazapine would effectively suppress the akathisia.

Client L was a 20-year-old unmarried healthy male without a previous psychiatric diagnosis or therapy. He was brought to the emergency department by police in a condition of acute agitation, confusion, suicidal thoughts, and self-inflicted injury as a result of smoking the synthetic cannabinoid drug, K2. The symptoms were consistent with known psychiatric effects of K2. In addition to the agitation and significant abrasions, the patient's respiratory rate was 30. After the patient was stabilized, he was transferred for monitoring to the inpatient psychiatric unit. The next day, the psychiatric evaluation concluded that there was complete resolution of his symptoms. The patient was discharged to his home, as he maintained his denial of any prior psychiatric history.

Client M was a 49-year-old male admitted with a diagnosis of a first-time severe, major depression as a result of discontinuation of 8 years of daily triptan use. Triptans are indicated for acute migraine treatment. Their mechanisms of action include high-affinity serotonin 5-HT(1B/D) receptor agonism with less potent 5-HT(1A) receptor affinity. Major depression has been reported to occur as a result of both migraine headaches as well as triptan administration. Previous treatment with serotonergic antidepressants were ineffective for client M. His depressive symptoms, however, were successfully resolved with a nonserotonergic medication. This is the first demonstration that abrupt termination of chronic extensive triptan use may elicit severe major depression. The symptoms were most likely be due to long-term serotonergic changes, such as downregulation and desensitization of 5-HT(1) receptors. The current case suggests that nonserotonergic medications may be a useful alternative for this condition.

Client N, a 53-year-old woman diagnosed with recurrent major depression, was admitted to the psychiatry department suffering from a severe depressive episode lasting six weeks, which was accompanied by psychotic symptoms. Her current medications were 200 milligrams of sertraline per day and 2 milligrams of risperidone per day. For eight weeks, she was treated with the same sertraline dose, 4 milligrams of risperidone and slow-release bupropion titrated to 300 milligrams per day. When this regimen did not produce any improvement, a course of eight to ten electroconvulsive therapy (ECT) sessions were started. Two days after the first session, the patient had 3 generalized tonic–clonic seizures within 6 hours. After phenytoin and valproic acid were added to the daily medications, there were no more seizures. Two days later, following clinical consultation, phenytoin and bupropion were withdrawn and ECT resumed. There were no more seizures, and the patient was eventually discharged after substantial improvement and recovery from depressive symptoms. This case describes the occurrence of post-ECT spontaneous seizures that might have been induced by the addition of bupropion, which can have proconvulsive effects, although convulsive thresholds may also be reduced by both sertraline and risperidone.

What do these cases have in common? First, all clients had been prescribed reasonable medications as therapy. Second, while efficacious, all the medications had significant side effects that limited optimal life functioning. Third, suggestions were made for reasonable modifications in therapy that often resulted in improved compliance, better life functioning, or amenability to the institution of psychological therapies.

To make specific suggestions for a client, it is important to be aware of three important factors that may affect patient compliance:

1. *Can the client afford the prescribed medication?* Patients and physicians alike are susceptible to ads for heavily promoted, expensive, brand-name medications. New medicines may have significant advantages over older medicines, but they also have their own constellation of side effects. Fortunately, in the past couple of years, numerous psychotherapeutic drugs have become available in less-expensive generic forms.

2. *Can the client tolerate any degree of weight gain?* Some clients can tolerate a degree of weight gain, while undesirable weight gain might lead to noncompliance in others. In choosing an antidepressant, for example, *mirtazapine* (Remeron) might be appropriate for a client who can tolerate weight gain, while *duloxetine* (Cymbalta) or *bupropion* (Wellbutrin) might be appropriate for a client who wants to lose weight. The same considerations apply in the treatment of bipolar disorder and behavioral disorders associated with anger, agitation, and aggressive behaviors.

3. *Can the client tolerate any degree of cognitive dysfunction?* Many psychotherapeutic drugs are associated with drug-induced cognitive dysfunction; among them are benzodiazepines, tricyclic antidepressants, lithium, some anticonvulsant mood stabilizers, and some antipsychotic drugs. The young, the elderly, and people suffering from traumatic brain injury (for example) might not tolerate agents that can be detrimental to cognitive functioning. Others, however, might be able to tolerate some degree of cognitive slowing if the therapeutic benefit seems to outweigh the side effects. If these agents are prescribed, dysfunction may interfere not only with the efficacy of cognitive therapies, but also with overall life functioning.

Understandably, it is not easy for practitioners to keep up with new developments. One major development is that indications for the psychoactive drugs have increased to include broader applications. This raises concerns about possibly dangerous interactions. But there are several ways in which the often overwhelming complexity of current drug treatment may be reduced. For one thing, Internet-based resources—including smartphone applications—are becoming more accessible, useful, and comprehensive. Communication among physicians, counselors, psychologists, and other specialists may need to be promoted and encouraged. Group practices that include experts from several specialties might be one way to ensure this collaboration. Collaboration might also include greater communication with patients to ensure that they are aware of the issues associated with their medications, especially in regard to polypharmacy. Moreover, there have not been many truly new psychiatric drugs in recent years; most have been derived from the classic agents. Therefore, the side effects are generally similar to those of the first generation of psychiatric medications. These considerations help to alleviate concerns about the increasing complexity of current and developing pharmacological treatments of mental disorders.

STUDY QUESTIONS

1. For the past two decades, there have been few new pharmacological treatments for mental illnesses. What other therapies or approaches to the treatment of mental disorders have been reexamined as a result?

2. What are the major revisions of the *Diagnostic and Statistical Manual of Mental Disorders* (DSM-5)?

3. What are the Research Domain Criteria and why were they developed?

4. What are some of the major shortcomings of current pharmacological treatment for mental illness?

5. What are the main proposals of the 21st Century Cures Act?

6. Do you find any of the case studies particularly relevant and if so, why? What are the three most important factors in regard to patient compliance with drug therapy? Do you have any vignettes you might add?

REFERENCES

Bishop, T. F., et al. (2016). "Population of US Practicing Psychiatrists Declined, 2003–13, Which May Help Explain Poor Access To Mental Health Care." *Health Affairs (Millwood)* 35: 1271–1277. doi: 10.1377/hlthaff.2015.1643.

Boggs, W. (2014). "Pharmacotherapy or Psychotherapy? No Easy Answer." *PsychCongress Network*. May 8. http://www.psychcongress.com/article/pharmacotherapy-or-psychotherapy-no-easy-answer.

Center for Behavioral Health Statistics and Quality. (2016). *2015 National Survey on Drug Use and Health: Detailed Tables*. Rockville, MD: Substance Abuse and Mental Health Services Administration. https://www.samhsa.gov/data/sites/default/files/NSDUH-DetTabs-2016/NSDUH-DetTabs-2016.pdf.

Clay, R. A. (2013). "The Next DSM: A Look at the Major Revisions of the Diagnostic and Statistical Manual of Mental Disorders." *Monitor on Psychology* 44: 26.

Crump, C., et al. (2013). "Mental Disorders and Vulnerability to Homicidal Death: Swedish Nationwide Cohort Study." *BMJ* 346: f557. doi: 10.1136/bmj.f557.

Cuthbert, B. (2014). "Research Domain Criteria (RDoC)." *The Carlat Report Psychiatry* 12: 1, 4, 7.

Davey, G. C. L. (2014). "Overprescribing Drugs to Treat Mental Health Problems: 10 Reasons Why Drugs Shouldn't Be a Treatment of Choice for Mental Disorders." *Psychology Today*. January 30. https://www.psychologytoday.com/blog/why-we-worry/201401/overprescribing-drugs-treat-mental-health-problems.

Doellinger, O. V., et al. (2016). "Spontaneous Seizures After ECT in a Patient Medicated with Bupropion, Sertraline and Risperidone." *Trends Psychiatry and Psychotherapy* 38: 111–113. doi: S2237-60892016005012105.

Farrelly, S., et al. (2014). "Anticipated and Experienced Discrimination Amongst People with Schizophrenia, Bipolar Disorder and Major Depressive Disorder: A Cross Sectional Study." *BMC Psychiatry* 14: 157. doi: 10.1186/1471-244X-14-157.

Friedman, R. A. (2015). "Psychiatry's Identity Crisis." *New York Times*. July 19. https://www.nytimes.com/2015/07/19/opinion/psychiatrys-identity-crisis.html?_r=0.

Fuller, D. A., et al. (2016). *Going, Going, Gone: Trends and Consequences of Eliminating State Psychiatric Beds: A Report from the Office of Research and Public Affairs*. Arlington, VA: Virginia Treatment Advocacy Center. http://www.treatmentadvocacycenter.org/storage/documents/going-going-gone.pdf.

Huhn, M., et al. (2014). "Efficacy Of Pharmacotherapy and Psychotherapy For Adult Psychiatric Disorders: A Systematic Overview Of Meta-Analyses." *JAMA Psychiatry* 71: 706–715. doi: 10.1001/jamapsychiatry.2014.112.

Kinderman, P. (2014). "Why We Need to Abandon the Disease-Model of Mental Health Care." *Scientific American MIND Guest Blog*. November 17. https://blogs.scientificamerican.com/mind-guest-blog/why-we-need-to-abandon-the-disease-model-of-mental-health-care/.

Kupfer, D. J., et al. (2013). "DSM-5 – The Future Arrived." *JAMA* 309: 1691–1692. doi: 10.1001/jama.2013.2298

Luhrmann, T. M. (2015). "Redefining Mental Illness." *New York Times*. January 17. https://www.nytimes.com/2015/01/18/opinion/sunday/t-m-luhrmann-redefining-mental-illness.html?_r=0.

Makari, G. (2015). "Psychiatry's Mind-Brain Problem." *New York Times*. November 11. https://www.nytimes.com/2015/11/11/opinion/psychiatrys-mind-brain-problem.html?_r=0.

McHugh, R. K., et at. (2013) "Patient Preference for Psychological vs Pharmacologic Treatment of Psychiatric Disorders: A Meta-Analytic Review." *Journal of Clinical Psychiatry* 74: 595–602. doi: 10.4088/JCP.12r07757.

Ostermann, K., et al. (2013). "Possible Association of Severe Major Depression with Acute Cessation of Long-Term Excessive Triptan Use." *Journal of Clinical Pharmacy and Therapeutics* 38: 77–79. doi: 10.1111/jcpt.12009.

Pies, R. W. (2015). "The Bogus 'Epidemic' of Mental Illness in the US." *Psychiatric Times*. June 18. http://www.psychiatrictimes.com/couch-crisis/bogus-epidemic-mental-illness-us.

Pratt, L. A., and Brody, D. J. (2014). *Depression in the U.S. Household Population, 2009–2012*. *NCHS Data Brief, No. 172*. Hyattsville, MD: National Center for Health Statistics. https://www.cdc.gov/nchs/data/databriefs/db172.pdf.

Seeman, N., et al. (2016). "World Survey of Mental Illness Stigma." *Journal of Affective Disorders* 190: 115–121. doi: http://dx.doi.org/10.1016/j.jad.

Substance Abuse and Mental Health Services Administration. (2016). *Key Substance Use and Mental Health Indicators in the United States: Results from the 2015 National Survey on Drug Use and Health* (HHS Publication No. SMA 16-4984, NSDUH Series H-51). Rockville, MD. https://www.samhsa.gov/data/sites/default/files/NSDUH-FFR1-2015/NSDUH-FFR1-2015/NSDUH-FFR1-2015.pdf.

Thomas, S., et al. (2012). "Suicidal Ideation and Self-Harm Following K2 Use." *Journal of the Oklahoma State Medical Association* 105: 430–433.

Walker, E. R., et al. (2015). "Mortality in Mental Disorders and Global Disease Burden Implications." *JAMA* 72: 334–341. doi: 10.1001/jamapsychiatry.2014.2502.

World Health Organization. (2001). "World Health Report: Mental Disorders Affect One in Four People." http://www.who.int/whr/2001/media_centre/press_release/en/.

APPENDIX A

QUICK REFERENCE TO PSYCHOTROPIC MEDICATION

This appendix provides several quick-reference medication tables initially prepared by John Preston, Psy.D., ABPP, and reproduced and modified by the authors with his permission. Additional references included the Clinical Handbook of Psychotropic Drugs Online (hogrefe publishers 22nd edition) and Epocrates™ (online application). The tables present a list of recommended doses and side effects for psychotherapeutic drugs. To our knowledge, the information is accurate—but it is only intended for general reference, not as a guideline for prescribing for individual patients. These tables supplement the discussion of the pharmacology of these medicines presented in earlier chapters. The tables are designed to answer questions about the therapeutic doses of psychotherapeutic medicines encountered in clinical practice. They also detail the effects of therapeutic drugs on production of sedative side effects, potential for inducing weight gain, potential for producing cognitive impairments, and availability in generic (less expensive) formulations. Please check the manufacturer's product information sheet or the Physicians' Desk Reference (PDR) for any changes in dosage schedule or contraindications. (Brand names are registered trademarks.)

Antidepressants

| Names | | Therapeutic dose range | Sedation | Weight gain | Cognitive impairment | Generic available |
Generic	Brand					
Imipramine	Tofranil	75–300 mg	mid	mid	mid	yes
Desipramine	Norpramin	75–300 mg	low	0–low	mid	yes
Amitriptyline	Elavil	75–300 mg	high	0–low	mid	yes
Nortriptyline	Aventyl, Pamelor	50–150 mg	mid	0–low	low	yes
Protriptyline	Vivactil	5–60 mg	mid	0–low	mid	yes
Trimipramine	Surmontil	75–300 mg	high	0–low	mid	yes
Doxepin	Sinequan, Adapin	75–300 mg	high	0–low	mid	yes
Clomipramine	Anafranil	75–300 mg	high	0–low	mid	yes
Maprotiline	Ludiomil	75–225 mg	high	0–low	low	yes
Amoxapine	Asendin	100–600 mg	mid	0–low	low	yes
Trazodone-XR	Desyrel, Oleptro	50–600 mg	mid	0–low	low–mid	yes
Fluoxetine[a]	Prozac, Sarafem	20–80 mg	low	low	low	yes
Bupropion-ER	Wellbutrin-ER	150–450 mg	low	0	0	yes
Sertraline	Zoloft	50–200 mg	low	low	low	yes
Paroxetine	Paxil, Pexeva	20–50 mg	low	low	low	yes
Venlafaxine-XR	Effexor-XR	75–225 mg	low	low	0	yes
Desvenlafaxine	Pristiq, Khedezla	50 mg	mid	low	0	yes
Fluvoxamine	Luvox	50–300 mg	low	low	low	yes
Mirtazapine	Remeron	15–45 mg	mid	low–mid	low	yes
Citalopram	Celexa	10–40 mg	low	low	low	yes

Antidepressants (continued)

Generic	Brand	Therapeutic dose range	Sedation	Weight gain	Cognitive impairment	Generic available
Escitalopram	Lexapro	10–20 mg	low	low	low	yes
Duloxetine	Cymbalta	60–120 mg	low	low	0	yes
Atomoxetine (for ADHD)	Strattera	40–100 mg	low	0	0	yes
Vilazodone	Viibryd	20–40 mg	low	low	low	no
Vortioxetine	Trintellix	5–20 mg	low	low	0	no
Levomilnacipram	Fetzima	40–120 mg	0-low	0-low	0-low	no
MAO Inhibitors						
Phenelzine	Nardil	30–90 mg	low	0	0	yes
Tranylcypromine	Parnate	20–60 mg	low	0	0	yes
Selegiline	Emsam (patch)	6–12 mg	low	0	0	no

aProzac available in 90-milligram time-release/weekly formulation.

Bipolar disorder medications

Generic	Brand	Serum level[a]	Weight gain	Cognitive impairment	Generic available
Lithium salts	Eskalith, Lithonate	0.8–1.2* 0.6-1.0**	high	high	yes
Olanzapine/ Fluoxetine	Symbyax	—	high	high	no
Carbamazepine	Tegretol, Equetro	4–10[a]	low	low	yes
Oxcarbazepine	Trileptal	—[b]	low	low	yes
Valproic acid	Depakote	50–100[a]	mid	low	yes
Gabapentin	Neurontin	—[b]	low	low	yes
Lamotrigine	Lamictal	—[b]	0	0	yes
Topiramate	Topamax	—[b]	0	mid–high	yes
Tiagabine	Gabitril	—[b]	0	low–mid	yes

[a]Lithium levels are expressed in milliequivalents per liter; carbamazepine, valproic acid, and lamotrigine levels in micrograms per milliliter.
*Blood levels associated with acute treatment.
**Blood levels associated with maintenance treatment.
[b]Serum monitoring not necessary.

Psychostimulants

Generic	Brand	Therapeutic dose range[a]
Methylphenidate	Ritalin[b]	10–60 mg
	Concerta[c]	18–72 mg
	Metadate CD[c]	20–60 mg
	Daytrana[c] (patch)	10–30 mg
	Quillivant XR[c]	20–60 mg
	Quillichew ER[c]	
	Aptensio XR[c]	10–60 mg
Dexmethylphenidate	Focalin[b]	5–20 mg
Dextroamphetamine	Dexedrine[b]	5–40 mg
	ProCentra (liquid)	5–40 mg

Psychostimulants (continued)

Names		Therapeutic dose range[a]
Generic	**Brand**	
D- *and* L-*Amphetamine*	Adderall	
	IR	5–40 mg
	XR[c]	10–30 mg
	Mydayas ER[c]	12.5–50 mg
Amphetamine	Adzenys XR[c] ODT[d]	12.5 mg
	Dyanavel XR[c] (suspension)	2.5–20 mg
	Evekeo	5–40 mg
Lisdexamfetamine	Vyvanse	30–70 mg
Modafinil	Provigil, Sparlon	100–400 mg
Armodafinil	Nuvigil	150–250 mg

[a]Adult doses.
[b]Available in generic formulation.
[c]Sustained release.
[d]Orally disintegrating tablet.

Drugs used to treat obsessive-compulsive disorder

Names		Therapeutic dose range[a]
Generic	**Brand**	
Clomipramine	Anafranil	150–250 mg
Fluoxetine	Prozac	20–80 mg
Sertraline	Zoloft	50–200 mg
Paroxetine	Paxil	20–60 mg
Fluvoxamine	Luvox	50–300 mg
Citalopram	Celexa	20–60 mg
Escitalopram[b]	Lexapro	10–20 mg
Venlafaxine[b]	Effexor	75–375 mg
Duloxetine[b]	Cymbalta	60–120 mg

[a]Often higher doses are required to control obsessive-compulsive symptoms than the doses generally used to treat depression.
[b]Off-label.

Antipsychotics

Names		Therapeutic dose range	Weight gain	Cognitive impairment	Generic available
Generic	Brand				
Low Potency					
Chlorpromazine	Thorazine	250–1000 mg	high	mid	yes
Thioridazine	Mellaril	150–800 mg	high	mid	yes
Clozapine	Clozaril	300–900 mg	high	low	yes
Quetiapine	Seroquel (XR)	400–800 mg	mid	low	yes
High Potency					
Molindone	Moban	20–225 mg	low	low	yes
Perphenazine	Trilafon	8–64 mg	mid	low	yes
Loxapine	Loxitane	60–250 mg	0	low	yes
Trifluoperazine	Stelazine	4–40 mg	mid	low	yes
Fluphenazine	Prolixin[a]	2.5–40 mg	high	low	yes
Thiothixene	Navane	10–60 mg	mid	low	yes
Haloperidol	Haldol[a]	2–20 mg	mid	low	yes
Pimozide	Orap	2–10 mg	low	low	yes
Risperidone	Risperdal[a]	2–16 mg	mid	low	yes
Paliperidone	Invega[a]	6–12 mg	mid	low	yes
Olanzapine	Zyprexa[a]	5–20 mg	high	low	yes
Ziprasidone	Geodon	40–160 mg	low	0	yes
Aripiprazole	Abilify[a]	10–30 mg	low	0	yes
Iloperidone	Fanapt	4–24 mg	mid	low	no
Asenapine	Saphris	5–20 mg	mid	low	no
Lurasidone	Latuda	40–160 mg	0	low	no
Brexpiprazole	Rexulti	2–4 mg	low	low	no
Cariprazine	Vraylar	1.5–6 mg	0	low	no

[a]Available in a time-release intramuscular form.

Drugs Used to Treat Insomnia

Names		Therapeutic
Generic	Brand	dose range
Benzodiazepines[a, d]		
Flurazepam[b]	Dalmane	15–30 mg
Temazepam[b]	Restoril	7.5–30 mg
Triazolam[b]	Halcion	0.125–0.5 mg
Estazolam[b]	ProSom	1.0–2.0 mg
Quazepam[b]	Doral	7.5–15 mg
Z Drugs[a]		
Zolpidem[b]	Ambien	5–10 mg
	Ambien ER	6.25–12.5 mg
Zaleplon[b]	Sonata	5–10 mg
Eszopiclone[b]	Lunesta	1–3 mg
Others		
Ramelteon	Rozerem	8 mg
Tasimelteon	Hetlioz	20 mg
Diphenhydramine[a, b]	Benadryl	25–50 mg
Doxepin[b, c]	Silenor	10–50 mg
Trazodone[b, c]	Deseryl	25–50 mg
Hydroxyzine[b]	Vistaril	50–100 mg
Chlorohydrate[b]	Noctec	500–1000 mg
Suvorexant	Belsomra	10–20 mg

[a]These drugs can produce cognitive impairment.
[b]Available in generic formulation.
[c]Also marketed for the treatment of depression (Chapter 12).
[d]Other benzodiazepines (see next table) can also be used to treat insomnia.

Antianxiety (Anxiolytics)

Names		Therapeutic dose range
Generic	Brand	
Benzodiazepines[a]		
Diazepam	Valium	8–40 mg
Chlordiazepoxide	Librium	20–100 mg
Clorazepate	Tranxene	15–60 mg
Clonazepam	Klonopin	0.5–4.0 mg
Lorazepam	Ativan	2.0–10.0 mg
Alprazolam	Xanax,	0.25–4.0 mg
	Xanax ER	0.5–1.0 mg
Oxazepam	Serax	30–120 mg
Other Antianxiety Agents[b]		
Buspirone	BuSpar	10–60 mg
Propranolol[c]	Inderal	10–80 mg
Atenolol[c]	Tenormin	25–100 mg
Guanfacine[c]	Tenex	0.5–3 mg
Clonidine[c]	Catapres	0.1–0.3 mg

[a]All benzodiazepines produce cognitive impairment and are available in a generic form.
[b]All agents listed are available in a generic form.
[c]Antihypertensive drugs which are used off-label to treat certain anxiety disorders.

Common side effects

Anticholinergic Effects (block acetylcholine)	
Dry mouth	Blurred vision
Constipation	Memory impairment
Urinary retention	Confusional states
Extrapyramidal Effects (dopamine blockade in basal ganglia)	
Parkinsonlike effects: rigidity, shuffling gait, tremor, flat affect, lethargy	
Dystonias: spasms in neck and other muscle groups	
Akathisia: intense, uncomfortable sense of inner restlessness	
Tardive dyskinesia: often a persistent movement disorder (lip smacking, writhing movements, jerky movements)	

Note: These are common side effects. All medications can produce specific or unique side effects.

APPENDIX B

INTRODUCTION TO EPIGENETICS

Inside the nucleus of each cell in our bodies is our DNA, our genetic code. That DNA represents the blueprints, or instructions, that make us who we are. But this fact gives rise to an important question. If each cell in our body has the same DNA, how does a cell that is supposed to become a skin cell actually turn into a skin cell instead of some other type of cell, such as a neuron? In other words, during gestation, when the embryo develops into a fetus and eventually a complete human being, what is responsible for the process that ensures a liver cell does not turn into a blood cell? That question has led to the realization that the DNA sequence is only one part of the story, and that the answer involves the phenomenon of *epigenetics*, which literally means "over or above genetics." Although there is still debate about the specific meaning of this term, most sources agree that at its simplest, epigenetics is the study of changes in gene activity that do not involve changes in the genetic code itself (DNA or genome), but which still get passed down to at least one successive generation.

One way to conceive of this concept is to think of the DNA code as a musical score that cannot be heard without an orchestra (the cells of the body) or a conductor who controls the performance. Epigenetics represents the "conductor." Another common analogy is that the DNA, that is, the genome, is the "hardware," while the epigenome is the "software" of our genetic makeup. Regardless of the way it is expressed, it has become clear that epigenetics may help us to understand the answer to some scientific questions that are not explained by the genome alone. For example, if identical twins have the same DNA, how come only one might develop schizophrenia, bipolar disorder, or any other disorder, such as cancer? Although monozygotic twins have the same genes, we have come to realize that some genes might be active (or inactive) in one twin, but not the other. In other words, they are *genetically* identical but not *epigenetically* the same.

STRUCTURE OF THE GENOME

To begin to understand how this might work, it is helpful to know something about the structure of the *genome*. If all of the DNA in each of our cells were stretched out, it would be over 6 feet in length. The nucleus of the cell, however, is only 1/10,000th of an inch across. Obviously, our DNA has to be packaged very tightly to fit into such a small space. Furthermore, in spite of this cramped environment, there has to be some way for all the functions to be performed for normal development—some genes need to be activated and copied, and others turned off at appropriate times. For over a century, scientists have been studying how genes are compacted. Our current understanding of how this is accomplished is shown in Figure B.1.

As indicated in the figure, the strands of our DNA are wound around "spools" of protein, called *histones*, of which there are different versions. These histone proteins

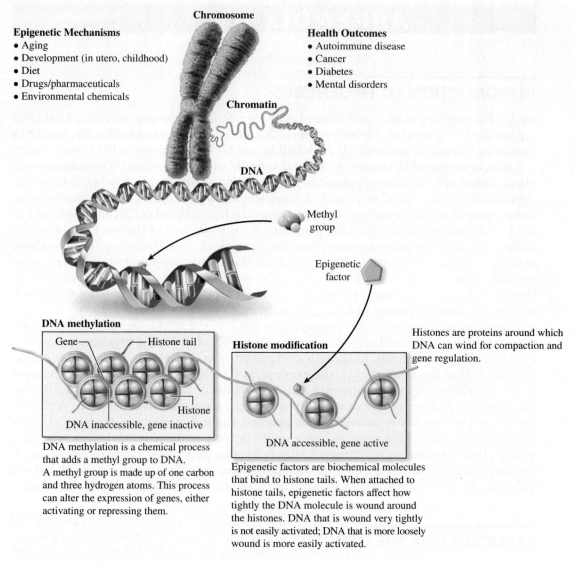

Epigenetic Mechanisms
- Aging
- Development (in utero, childhood)
- Diet
- Drugs/pharmaceuticals
- Environmental chemicals

Health Outcomes
- Autoimmune disease
- Cancer
- Diabetes
- Mental disorders

Chromosome

Chromatin

DNA

Methyl group

Epigenetic factor

Histones are proteins around which DNA can wind for compaction and gene regulation.

DNA methylation

Gene — Histone tail

Histone

DNA inaccessible, gene inactive

DNA methylation is a chemical process that adds a methyl group to DNA. A methyl group is made up of one carbon and three hydrogen atoms. This process can alter the expression of genes, either activating or repressing them.

Histone modification

DNA accessible, gene active

Epigenetic factors are biochemical molecules that bind to histone tails. When attached to histone tails, epigenetic factors affect how tightly the DNA molecule is wound around the histones. DNA that is wound very tightly is not easily activated; DNA that is more loosely wound is more easily activated.

FIGURE B.1   Schematic description of epigenetic processes.

are positively charged, which helps to attract the negatively charged DNA. There are also thin "tails" that extend from each histone. Together, the combination of histones and DNA is called *chromatin*. The basic repeating structural and functional unit of chromatin is the *nucleosome*, which consists of a group of eight histones plus about 166 base pairs (the components) of DNA. (In Figure B.1, we can see only one side of the nucleosomes, which shows four of the eight histones.)

Every chromosome in the nucleus of our cells contains hundreds of thousands of nucleosomes and the DNA that runs between them. In other words, the *chromosome* is made up of *chromatin*, which is a long chain of *nucleosomes*, composed of *histones*, which looks like a string of beads under an electron microscope. Many higher-order levels of chromatin folding are required for the incredible compaction necessary for the DNA to fit into the nucleus.

As indicated in the figure, under normal conditions, when histones are tightly compacted, genes on the DNA are "hidden" within the nucleosome and not exposed, which means that they cannot be activated and turned on. To turn genes on—"read" them or express them—and off—"not read" them or silence them—the structure of chromatin has to be altered. This is the job of epigenetic processes. The function of epigenetics is to control the activation and inactivation of appropriate genes, at the appropriate time.

Currently, there are several different types of epigenetic processes, which include the biochemical mechanisms of *methylation, acetylation, phosphorylation, ubiquitylation, sumoylation*, and more will likely be discovered. For this introduction, only the first two will be described to provide an overview of the importance of these phenomena.

EPIGENETIC FUNCTION

The best-known epigenetic process so far is DNA methylation. As seen in Figure B.1, certain sites on the DNA strands (associated with certain cytosine bases on the DNA) are "tagged" with a *methyl* group, a fundamental unit of organic chemistry. A methyl group consists of one carbon atom attached to three hydrogen atoms ($-CH_3$). Histones may also be methylated. Methyl groups, and other epigenetic factors associated with histones, are located on the small extensions of the histone tails. When DNA or histones are methylated, this compacts the chromatin, [which makes DNA inaccessible and means that] the gene(s) in this region is (are) 'silenced' (not expressed)" (Stahl, 2010, 221). (In some situations, histone methylation may activate a gene, depending on location.) Methyl groups are attached to the DNA by enzymes, often near the beginning of a gene— the same place where proteins attach to activate the gene. If the protein cannot attach due to a blocking methyl group, then the gene usually remains off. So, attaching a methyl group to a gene usually means it is turned off, because the protein that would activate the gene is blocked.

As explained by Stahl (2010), "Histones are methylated by enzymes called histone methyltransferases, [and enzymes called *histone demethylases* reverse this]. Methylation of DNA is regulated by DNA methyltransferase (DNMT) enzymes and demethylation of DNA by DNA demethylase enzymes. There are many forms of methyltransferase enzymes" (221).

Another epigenetic process is histone acetylation. This biochemical reaction removes positive charges, thereby reducing the affinity between histones and DNA. This makes it easier to access genes; therefore, in most cases, histone acetylation enhances gene activation, while histone deacetylation represses gene activation. Histone acetylation is catalyzed by histone acetyltransferases (HATs) and histone deacetylation is catalyzed by histone deacetylases (HDs or HDACs). Furthermore, the two processes of methylation and acetylation may affect each other. That is, "methylation of DNA can eventually lead to deacetylation of histones, by activating HDACs" (Stahl, 2010). These are not the only known interactions. There are substances that can expose DNA by sliding or even detaching histones.

In summary, methylation and deacetylation compress chromatin and silence genes. On the other hand, demethylation and acetylation do the opposite; they decompress chromatin and thus activate genes. Effects on chromatin will determine how accessible the chromosomes are to the molecules, such as RNA, that perform all the necessary functions of copying, synthesizing, and repairing our genetic machinery.

EPIGENETIC EFFECTS

It is epigenetic "marks" such as these that tell your genes to switch "on" or "off," and this is how environmental factors such as diet, stress, and toxins can have an effect on genes that may be passed on to other generations. For example, methyl groups are obtained from the diet; they cannot be produced by the body. Methyl groups are critical to the building blocks of RNA and DNA, and they are important in the synthesis of the biogenic amines: dopamine, norepinephrine, and serotonin. Further, they "are also involved in the synthesis of melatonin and epinephrine, and in the inactivation of dopamine and norepinephrine, the latter by the methyltransferase enzyme known as catechol-o-methyl transferase (COMT)" (Stahl, 2010, 223). The crucial involvement of methyl groups in the processes of genetics, epigenetics, and the transmitters suggests that the study of methyl groups, called *methylomics*, may be relevant to the etiology of mental illnesses.

While the psychiatric implications of epigenetics have yet to be determined, scientists have discovered that some diseases, such as Prader–Willi syndrome, Angelman syndrome, and Rett syndrome, have epigenetic etiologies. The most extensive amount of research has been in the area of cancer. Because some cancers are caused by deactivation of tumor-suppressing genes, researchers have worked to develop medications that reactivate them. The drug azacitidine, for example, treats leukemia in this manner. Unfortunately, it also produces serious side effects of nausea, anemia, vomiting, and fever, which might be expected for substances that have such a nonspecific action. Nevertheless, research continues on epigenetic mechanisms in immune disorders, aging-related changes, including Alzheimer's disease, and the possibility of abnormal methylation in schizophrenia. One of the most active areas of epigenetic research in psychiatry is that of addiction. More generally, the possibilities are being explored that "unfavorable epigenetic mechanisms may be triggered [when someone becomes] addicted to drugs [or acquires other] forms of "abnormal learning," [such as developing] an anxiety disorder or a chronic pain condition" (Stahl, 2010, 222).

CRISPR-Cas9

"Think about a film strip," said biochemist Jennifer Doudna. "You see a particular segment of the film that you want to replace. And if you had a film splicer, you would go in and literally cut it out and piece it back together—maybe with a new clip. Imagine being able to do that in the genetic code, the code of life" (CBS News, 2015).

CRISPR-Cas9 is one of the most significant developments in the field of genetics, perhaps since the discovery of the molecular makeup of DNA itself. CRISPR-Cas9 refers to a genetic editing tool that can modify the structure of DNA faster, cheaper, and more accurately than any previous method. With this technique, it is possible to go to a specific location on a strand of DNA, then remove, add, or alter a section of the DNA sequence. By using this procedure, scientists can, for example, remove or inactivate part of a (defective) gene, so that it will not be turned on, or insert a new set of DNA instructions, to perhaps correct for the genetic defect. It is a way to "cut and paste" the genetic code so that defective DNA may be eliminated, or replaced, with normal DNA.

Physically, CRISPR is a short strand of RNA. The CRISPR RNA is called a guide RNA (gRNA). The letters are an acronym for the term **C**lustered **R**egularly **I**nter-spaced **S**hort **P**alindromic **R**epeats. This refers to the fact that, in 1987, bacteria was discovered that had segments of DNA *repeated* multiple times along the strand. In between these repeated segments of DNA were nonrepetitive segments referred to as "spacers."

Later, it was realized that a second set of DNA sequences were always associated with the CRISPR sequences. These *Cas genes*, short for CRISPR-associated genes, are coded for enzymes often likened to a pair of molecular scissors, which can cut the DNA strands so that bits of DNA can be added or removed.

The CRISPR gRNA is located within a larger section of RNA, called a "scaffold." The scaffold part binds to DNA and the gRNA sequence guides Cas9 to the right location. This ensures that the Cas9 enzyme cuts at the right point in the genome. The gRNA is designed to locate and bind to a specific sequence in the DNA by "matching" the target DNA sequence. That is, the RNA nucleotide bases are complementary to the matched DNA section. This guarantees that the gRNA will only bind to the target sequence and no other regions of the genome. The Cas9 enzyme follows the gRNA to the same location in the DNA sequence and makes a cut across both strands of the DNA. At this stage, the cell recognizes that the DNA is damaged and tries to repair it.

CRISPR-Cas9 is not the only method available, but it has some advantages over previous methods of altering DNA. First, it can be used to add or remove more than one gene at a time. This means that the process can occur much faster than with other techniques, in a matter of weeks rather than years. Second, it is not restricted to any one species, but can be applied to organisms, both plants and animals, that could not be affected by earlier methods.

There are numerous applications for this process. In agriculture, it could result in new types of grains or fruits. In regard to health, it could lead to new treatments for rare metabolic and genetic disorders, such as hemophilia and Huntington's disease, or to corrections of some disorders, such as cystic fibrosis or Tay-Sachs disease.

In 2008, the Danisco department of DuPont first put the CRISPR-Cas9 system to practical use to improve bacterial culture immunity against viruses. Now the procedure is employed in the making of cheese and yogurt.

Jennifer Doudna and Emmanuelle Charpentier of the Massachusetts Institute of Technology (MIT) published a paper in 2012 showing how, by using the natural CRISPR-Cas9 system as a tool, any DNA strand could be cut in a test tube (Jinek et al., 2012). Soon after, in 2013, papers by Feng Zhang at MIT-Harvard Broad Institute [Ran et al., 2013], George Church at Harvard Medical School [Mali et al., 2013], as well as Doudna [Jinek et al., 2013] were published, showing that the genome of human cells could be edited by the CRISPR-Cas 9 system.

In 2015, researchers were able to use Crispr-Cas9 to restore muscle function in mice with muscular dystrophy. It has also been reported that this technique can cure a rare liver disease and make human cells immune to the AIDS virus. Finally, there are efforts to modify the genetics of mosquitoes to prevent them from transmitting malaria, and the possibility of eliminating ticks' ability to infect people with Lyme disease is being investigated.

The first reported application of CRISPR-Cas9 to (nonviable) human embryos was in April 2015 by a Chinese laboratory. But this breakthrough, while exciting, raised serious ethical issues. The first ethical question concerns the extent to which this process should be used to change the genes of the next generation. The potential benefit of curing diseases by altering defective DNA in the cells in the body might not be controversial. But the possibility of creating "designer babies" through genetic manipulation of sperm or eggs raised significant ethical issues. Some scientists, including some who were responsible for developing CRISPR-Cas9, have called for a moratorium on this application.

The second issue is one of safety. Because the technology is so new, a lot of work is still necessary to ensure that the changes are precise, and that altering one section of DNA does not produce unpredictable changes in another location. The possibility of unforeseen consequences is extremely worrisome. Ongoing research is intensely focused on reducing these so-called off-target effects. A related concern is that once a change is made in a plant or animal, they may not be distinguishable from the "normal" species and, after release into the environment, they could be a danger to other organisms.

There is much debate about what ethical and safety limitations of the technology might be necessary. The U.S. National Institutes of Health published a statement in April 2015 noting that any experiments using CRISPR or similar methods of gene editing in human embryos will not be funded (NIH, 2015). On the other hand, current restrictions in the United Kingdom are less severe.

Furthermore, the technology has become embroiled in several major patent disputes. DuPont, various biotechnology companies, and several universities have filed patents covering hundreds of claims; even if some of these patents are granted, they may be challenged. It will take a while for these disputes to be settled.

Meanwhile, research continues at a fast pace. On October 28, 2016, scientists at West China Hospital in Chengdu reported that they had given a patient stricken with lung cancer an injection of cells that had been altered by CRISPR-Cas9. They edited a gene that impairs the cell's ability to trigger an immune response. The hope is that these altered cells will be able to kill the cancerous cells. The first step in this long-term effort is to determine how safe the technology is. Initially, a small group of 10 patients will be examined during a 6-month period to assess whatever side effects might occur. A trial of the CRISPR-Cas 9 technique to be used against a variety of cancers will also be conducted in humans in the United States during 2017 (Dicker, 2016). Clearly, this phenomenon has the potential to revolutionize life in ways that have not yet even been conceived.

REFERENCES

Dicker, R. (2016). "Gene Editing Tool CRISPR-CAS9 Used in a Human for the First Time." *U.S. News & World Report*. November 17. https://www.usnews.com/news/national-news/articles/2016-11-17/gene-editing-tool-crispr-cas9-used-in-a-human-for-the-first-time.

Stahl, S. M. (2010). "Methylated Spirits: Epigenetics Hypotheses of Psychiatric Disorders." *CNS Spectrum* 15: 220–230.

CBS NEWS November 30, 2015, Could revolutionary gene-editing technology end cancer? https://www.cbsnews.com/news/crispr-jennifer-doudna-gene-editing-technology-diseases-dangers-ethics/

NIH, 2015. Statement on NIH funding of research using gene-editing technologies in human embryos. Accessed at: https://www.nih.gov/about-nih/who-we-are/nih-director/statements/statement-nih-funding-research-using-gene-editing-technologies-human-embryos.

Jinek, M., et al. (2012). "A programmable dual-RNA-guided DNA endonuclease in adaptive bacterial immunity." *Science* 337: 816–821. doi: 10.1126/science.1225829.

Jinek, M., et al. (2013). "RNA-programmed genome editing in human cells." *Elife* 2: e00471 PMCID: PMC3557905.

Mali, P., et al. (2013). "RNA-guided human genome engineering via Cas9." *Science* 339: 823–826. doi: 10.1126/science.1232033.

Ran, F. A., et al. (2013). "Genome engineering using the CRISPR-Cas9 system." *Nature Protocols* 8: 2281–2308.

GLOSSARY

Abstinence syndrome. State of altered behavior that follows cessation of drug administration. See also **Withdrawal syndrome**

Acamprosate. A structural analogue of glutamate, it is an anticraving drug used to maintain abstinence in alcohol-dependent patients.

Acetylcholine. Neurotransmitter in the central and peripheral nervous systems, which activates two types of receptors, muscarinic and nicotinic. See **Muscarine; Nicotine**

Additive effect. Effect that occurs when two drugs that have similar biological actions are administered. The net effect is the sum of the independent effects exerted by the drugs.

Adenosine. Chemical neuromodulator in the CNS, primarily at inhibitory synapses.

Adenylate cyclase. Intracellular enzyme that catalyzes the conversion of cyclic AMP to adenosine monophosphate.

Adrenaline (epinephrine). Hormone secreted by the adrenal gland that activates the sympathetic nervous system, as part of the "fight or flight" response.

Affective disorder. Type of mental disorder characterized by recurrent episodes of mania, depression, or both.

Affinity. Ability of a drug to bind to its receptor.

Agonist. Drug that attaches to a receptor and produces actions that mimic or potentiate those of an endogenous transmitter.

Akathisia. A movement disorder, characterized by a feeling of inner restlessness and an inability to sit still.

Aldehyde dehydrogenase. Enzyme that carries out a specific step in alcohol metabolism: the metabolism of acetaldehyde to acetate. This enzyme may be blocked by the drug disulfiram (Antabuse).

Allosteric. A substance that indirectly alters the effect of another molecule (such as an agonist or inverse agonist) at the receptor binding site.

Alzheimer's disease. Progressive neurological disease that occurs primarily in the elderly. It is characterized by a loss of short-term memory and intellectual functioning. It is associated with a loss of function of acetylcholine neurons.

Amyloid. A starch-like protein that is deposited in the liver, kidneys, spleen, or other tissues in certain diseases.

Amphetamine. Behavioral stimulant that acts by increasing the amount of biogenic amines in neuronal synapses.

Amygdala. A pair of almond-shaped neural structures in the cerebral hemispheres, which mediate emotional responses.

696

Anabolic steroid. Testosterone-like drug that acts to increase muscle mass and produces other masculinizing effects.

Anandamide. Endogenous chemical compound that attaches to cannabinoid receptors in the CNS and to specific components of the lymphatic system.

Anandamide receptor. Receptor to which anandamide and tetrahydrocannabinol bind.

Anesthetic. Sedative-hypnotic compound used primarily in doses capable of inducing a state of general anesthesia that involves both loss of sensation, amnesia, and loss of consciousness.

Antagonist. Drug that attaches to a receptor and blocks the action of either an endogenous transmitter or an agonistic drug.

Anticonvulsant. Drug that blocks or prevents epileptic convulsions. Some anticonvulsants (for example, carbamazepine and valproic acid) are also used to treat certain nonepileptic psychiatric disorders.

Antidepressant. Drug that is useful in treating mentally depressed patients but does not produce stimulant effects in nondepressed persons. Subdivided into several categories.

Antinociceptive. Decreasing sensitivity to painful (nociceptive) stimulation; analgesic.

Antipsychotic. Medication effective in the treatment of psychosis, particularly for reducing the positive symptoms of schizophrenia, such as hallucinations, delusions, and thought disorder.

Anxiolytic. Drug used to relieve the symptoms associated with defined states of anxiety. Classically, the term refers to the benzodiazepines and related drugs.

2-arachidonoyl glycerol (2-AG). One of the endogenous cannabislike substances.

Arrythymia. A condition in which the heart beats with an irregular or abnormal rhythm.

Ataxia. A lack of muscle coordination that may affect speech, eye movements, the ability to swallow, walking, picking up objects and other voluntary movements.

Attention deficit/hyperactivity disorder (ADHD). Learning and behavioral disorder characterized by reduced attention span, impulsivity, and/or hyperactivity.

Atypical antipsychotic. Drug that alleviates the positive symptoms of schizophrenia (hallucinations, delusions, and thought disorder) without necessarily causing the neurological side effect of abnormal motor movements. Also used in the treatment of mania.

Autonomic nervous system. Portion of the peripheral nervous system that controls, or regulates, the visceral, automatic, usually involuntary functions of the body, such as heart rate and blood pressure.

Autoreceptor. A receptor located on the presynaptic neuronal membrane, which is activated by the neurotransmitter released by that neuron (or by substances that interact with that receptor).

Ayahuasca (also called hoasca). A hallucinogenic beverage made from the bark and stems of a tropical South American vine.

Barbiturates. Class of chemically related sedative-hypnotic compounds that share a characteristic six-membered ring structure.

Basal ganglia. An anatomical system in the brain consisting of three primary nuclei (the caudate nucleus, the putamen, and the globus pallidus) located at the base of the brain that are primarily responsible for coordinating and organizing smooth voluntary motor functions. The basal ganglia are abnormal in a number of important neurological conditions, including Parkinson's disease and Huntington's disease. This system may also be referred to as the *extrapyramidal system* to distinguish it from the pyramidal component of the motor system, which is responsible for controlling fine motor responses.

"Bath Salts." The term refers to a group of drugs containing one or more synthetic chemicals related to cathinone, an amphetaminelike stimulant.

Benzodiazepines. Class of chemically related sedative-hypnotic agents, of which chlordiazepoxide (Librium) and diazepam (Valium) are examples. Primarily used in the treatment of anxiety and in alcohol withdrawal.

Bioavailability. The degree and rate at which a substance (such as a drug) is absorbed into a living system and has access to the site of physiological activity.

Biomarker. A measurable substance in an organism whose presence is indicative of some phenomenon such as disease, infection, or environmental exposure.

Bipolar disorder. Affective disorder characterized by alternating bouts of mania and either depression or euthymia (normal affective state). Also called *manic-depressive illness*.

Blackout. Period of time during which a person may be awake, but memory is not imprinted. It frequently occurs in people who have consumed excessive alcohol or to whom have been administered (or who have taken) large doses of sedative drugs.

Blood alcohol concentration (BAC). The weight of alcohol in a fixed volume of blood, used as a measure of the degree of intoxication in an individual. The BAC depends on body weight, the quantity and rate of alcohol ingestion, and the rates of alcohol absorption and metabolism.

Bradykinesia. Slowness and poverty of movement.

Brain syndrome, organic. Pattern of behavior induced when neurons are either reversibly depressed or irreversibly destroyed. Behavior is characterized by clouded sensorium, disorientation, shallow and labile affect, and impaired memory, intellectual function, insight, and judgment.

Brand name. Unique name licensed to one manufacturer of a drug. Contrasts with *generic name*, the name under which any manufacturer may sell a drug.

Bronchospasm. Abnormal contraction of the smooth muscle of the bronchi, resulting in an acute narrowing and obstruction of the respiratory airway.

Caffeine. Behavioral and general cellular stimulant found in coffee, tea, cola drinks, and chocolate. Acts by blocking an adenosine receptor.

Caffeinism. Habitual use of large amounts of caffeine.

Cannabis sativa. Hemp plant; contains marijuana.

Carbidopa. Drug that inhibits the enzyme dopa decarboxylase, allowing increased availability of dopa within the brain. Contained in the medication Sinemet.

Central nervous system (CNS). Brain and spinal cord.

Cerebellum. Structure located at the base of the brain, just above the brain stem, where the spinal cord meets the brain, whose function is to coordinate voluntary movements, posture, and balance.

Cerebral cortex. The outer layer of the cerebrum (cerebral hemispheres), composed of gray matter and responsible for mediating higher brain functions.

Cerebrum. The most dorsal, primary part of the brain, consisting of left and right hemispheres, separated by a fissure. It is responsible for the integration of complex sensory and neural functions and the initiation and coordination of voluntary activity in the body.

Chemoreceptor trigger zone. An area in the medulla oblongata that responds to bloodborne signals that cause nausea and vomiting.

Chromatin. Substance made up of DNA, RNA and proteins (histones), in the cell nucleus, which makes up chromosomes.

Chromosome. Composed of condensed chromatin fibers, it contains the genes.

Cirrhosis. Serious, usually irreversible liver disease. Usually associated with chronic excessive alcohol consumption.

Clonidine (Catapres). Antihypertensive drug useful in alleviating the symptoms of narcotic withdrawal.

Cocaine. Behavioral stimulant. Acts primarily by blocking reuptake of the transmitter dopamine into the neuron from which it was released.

Codeine. Sedative and pain-relieving agent found in opium. Structurally related to morphine but less potent; constitutes approximately 0.5 percent of the opium extract.

Comorbid disorder. Psychiatric disorder that coexists with another psychiatric disorder (for example, multisubstance abuse in a patient with major depressive disorder).

Compulsion. Repetitive or ritualistic behaviors or mental acts performed over and over in response to an obsessive thought, such as repeated hand washing.

Convulsant. Drug that produces convulsions (seizures) by blocking inhibitory neurotransmission.

Cotinine. The primary metabolite of nicotine.

COX inhibitors. Aspirin-like analgesic drugs that produce their actions by inhibiting the enzyme cyclooxygenase. Two variants of the enzyme occur: COX-1 and COX-2. Some drugs are specific for COX-2; others are nonspecific inhibitors.

Crack. Street name for a smokeable form of potent, concentrated cocaine.

Cross-dependence. Condition in which one drug can prevent the withdrawal symptoms associated with physical dependence on a different drug.

Cross-tolerance. Condition in which tolerance of one drug results in a lessened response to another drug.

Cytochrome P450 enzyme family. A large group of proteins, mostly (but not only) found in the liver, responsible for metabolizing a wide variety of endogenous and exogenous substances.

Delirium tremens (DTs). Syndrome of tremulousness with hallucinations, psychomotor agitation, confusion and disorientation, sleep disorders, and other associated discomforts, lasting several days after alcohol withdrawal.

Delta receptor. One of the 3 classes of opiate receptors (DOR), which is activated by the endogenous opiates and synthetic opioids.

Dementia. Loss of mental ability severe enough to interfere with normal activities of daily living, lasting more than six months, not present since birth, and not associated with a loss or alteration of consciousness.

Detoxification. Process of allowing time for the body to metabolize and/or excrete accumulations of drug. Usually a first step in drug abuse evaluation and treatment.

Diagnostic and Statistical Manual of Mental Disorders (DSM-5). A classification system of mental disorders, published by the American Psychiatric Association, that proposes objective criteria to be used in diagnosis.

Diencephalon. The posterior part of the forebrain, whose major components are the thalamus and hypothalamus.

Differential diagnosis. Listing of all possible causes that might explain a given set of symptoms.

Dimethyltryptamine (DMT). Psychedelic drug found in many South American plants.

Disulfiram (Antabuse). An antioxidant used in the treatment of chronic alcoholism that interferes with the normal metabolic degradation of alcohol in the body, producing an unpleasant reaction when a small quantity of alcohol is consumed.

Dopamine. One of the monoaminergic (catecholamine) neurotransmitters in the central nervous system, considered to be the primary reward neurotransmitter in the brain and important in mediating voluntary movement (loss of dopamine neurons produces Parkinson's disease). It is the precursor to norepinephrine.

Dopamine transporter. Presynaptic protein that binds synaptic dopamine and transports the neurotransmitter back into the presynaptic nerve terminal.

Dorsal root ganglia. A group of neurons on the dorsal roots of the spine that carry signals from sensory organs toward the appropriate part of the nervous system.

Dose-response relation. Relation between drug doses and the response elicited at each dose level.

Drug. Chemical substance used for its effects on bodily processes.

Drug absorption. Mechanism by which a drug reaches the bloodstream from the skin, lungs, stomach, intestinal tract, or muscle.

Drug administration. Procedures through which a drug enters the body (oral administration of tablets or liquids, inhalation of powders, injection of sterile liquids, and so on).

Drug dependence. State in which the use of a drug is necessary for either physical or psychological well-being.

Drug distribution. Movement of drug between the blood and various tissues of the body.

Drug interaction. Modification of the action of one drug by the concurrent or prior administration of another drug.

Drug misuse. Use of any drug (legal or illegal) for a medical or recreational purpose when other alternatives are available, practical, or warranted or when drug use endangers either the user or others with whom he or she may interact.

Drug receptor. Specific molecular substance in the body with which a given drug interacts to produce its effect.

Drug tolerance. State of progressively decreasing responsiveness to a drug.

Dual-action antidepressants. Antidepressant drugs that act by inhibiting the active presynaptic reuptake of more than one neurotransmitter, for example, norepinephrine and serotonin.

Dyskinesia. A movement disorder that consists of adverse effects, including diminished voluntary movements and the presence of involuntary movements, similar to tics or chorea.

Dystonia. A state of abnormal muscle tone producing muscular spasm and abnormal posture, typically due to neurological disease or a side effect of drug therapy.

Efficacy. The ability of a drug to produce its intended effect.

Electroconvulsive therapy (ECT). A procedure in which an electric current is passed through the brain to produce controlled convulsions (seizures) to treat patients with depression, particularly for those who cannot take or are not responding to antidepressants, have severe depression, or are at high risk for suicide.

Electronic (e) cigarette (EC). A cigarette-shaped device containing a nicotine-based liquid that is vaporized and inhaled, used to simulate the experience of smoking tobacco.

Endorphin. Naturally occurring protein that causes endogenous morphinelike activity.

Enkephalin. Naturally occurring protein that causes morphinelike activity.

Entactogens. A class of psychoactive drugs that presumably produce distinctive empathic, emotional, and social effects.

Enteral route. Anything involving the gastrointestinal tract, from the mouth to the rectum.

Environmental tobacco smoke (ETS). Secondhand smoke; passive smoke. Exhaled smoke from cigarette smokers, which is inhaled by persons other than the smoker.

Enzyme. Large organic molecule that mediates a specific biochemical reaction in the body.

Enzyme induction. Increased production of drug-metabolizing enzymes in the liver, stimulated by certain drugs (inducers). As a result of induction, drugs that are metabolized by the induced enzyme will be degraded more rapidly. It is one mechanism by which pharmacological tolerance is produced.

Epigenetics. The study of heritable changes in gene expression caused by mechanisms other than changes in the underlying DNA sequence.

Epilepsy. Neurological disorder characterized by an occasional, sudden, and uncontrolled discharge of neurons.

Epinephrine. See **Adrenaline**

Exocytosis. Secretion of the substances in synaptic vesicles, out of the neuron terminal.

Extrapyramidal symptoms (EPS). Motor symptoms, such as tremors, slurred speech, dystonia, and anxiety that are side effects to neuroleptic drugs caused by effects on the basal ganglia and associated structures within the brain.

Fasciculation. A brief, spontaneous, contraction affecting a small number of muscle fibers, often causing a flicker of movement under the skin.

Fetal alcohol syndrome (FAS). A congenital syndrome caused by excessive consumption of alcohol by the mother during pregnancy, characterized by retardation of mental development and of physical growth, particularly of the skull and face of the infant.

Fibromyalgia. A disorder of unknown etiology characterized by widespread pain, abnormal pain processing, sleep disturbance, fatigue, and often psychological distress.

First-order elimination. Elimination of a constant fraction of drug, per time unit, of the amount present in the organism. The elimination is proportional to the drug concentration.

First-pass metabolism (first-pass effect). The breakdown of drugs as they are transported through the liver before they reach the rest of the body through the circulatory system.

Flashback. See **Hallucinogen persisting perception disorder (HPPD)**

Forebrain. The anterior part of the brain, made up of the telencephalon and diencephalon, which includes the cerebrum, parts of the basal ganglia and limbic system, and the thalamus and hypothalamus.

G protein. Specific intraneuronal protein that links transmitter-induced receptor alterations with intracellular second-messenger proteins or with adjacent ion channels.

Gamma aminobutyric acid (GABA). Inhibitory amino acid neurotransmitter in the brain.

Generic name. Name that identifies a specific chemical entity (without describing the chemical). Often marketed under different brand names by different manufacturers.

Genetic Opioid Metabolic Defects (GOMD). Genetic variants of the enzymes responsible for the breakdown of opioids in the body, which may cause either an abnormal decrease (fast metabolizers) or increase (slow metabolizers) in levels of opiate medications.

Glutamic acid. Excitatory amino acid neurotransmitter. It is the precursor to GABA, the inhibitory neurotransmitter.

Half-life. Time it takes for half of the amount of drug in the circulation to be eliminated.

Hallucinogen. Psychedelic drug that produces profound distortions in perception.

Hallucinogen persisting perception disorder (HPPD). An unexpected recurrence of the effects of a hallucinogenic drug long after its initial use. See **Flashback**

Harmine. Psychedelic agent obtained from the seeds of *Peganum harmala*.

Hashish. Extract of the hemp plant (*Cannabis sativa*) that has a higher concentration of THC than does marijuana.

Herbal Marijuana Alternatives (HMAs). Classes of synthetic cannabinoid drugs.

Heroin. Semisynthetic opiate produced by a chemical modification of morphine.

Hindbrain. The lower part of the brainstem, consisting of the cerebellum, pons, and medulla oblongata.

Hippocampus. Part of the brain (limbic system) involved in learning and memory formation

Histones. Proteins found in the cell nucleus around which DNA is wound so that it is condensed into a smaller space.

Hookah. An oriental tobacco pipe with a long, flexible tube that draws the smoke through water contained in a bowl.

Hyperalgesia. Abnormally heightened sensitivity to pain.

Hypercortisolemia. Elevated levels of cortisol in the blood.

Hyperkinetic. An abnormal amount of uncontrolled muscular action; like a spasm or tic.

Hypocretin. See **Orexin**

Hypomania. A condition similar to mania, but less severe. The symptoms are similar, with elevated mood, increased activity, decreased need for sleep, grandiosity, racing thoughts, and the like. However, hypomanic episodes differ in that they do not cause significant distress or impair one's work, family, or social life in an obvious way while manic episodes do.

Hypothalamus. Brain structure located below the thalamus and above the pituitary gland that regulates bodily temperature, certain metabolic processes, and other autonomic activities.

Hypoxia. State of relative lack of oxygen in the tissues of the body and the brain.

Ice. Street name for a smokeable, freebase form of potent, concentrated methamphetamine.

Intramuscular injection. An injection into a muscle.

Intravenous injection. An injection into a vein.

Ionotropic receptor. A receptor that works by directly opening or closing ion channels that alter ionic movement across cell membranes.

Isomers. Each of two or more compounds with the same formula, but a different arrangement of atoms in the molecule and different properties.

Kappa receptor. One of several opiate receptor types.

Levodopa. Precursor substance to the transmitter dopamine; useful in alleviating the symptoms of Parkinson's disease.

Limbic system. Group of brain structures involved in emotional responses and emotional expression.

Lipid soluble. The ability of a chemical compound to dissolve in fats and oils.

Lithium. Alkali metal effective in the treatment of mania and depression.

Lysergic acid diethylamide (LSD). Semisynthetic psychedelic drug.

Major tranquilizer (archaic). See **Antipsychotic**

Mania. Mental disorder characterized by an expansive emotional state, elation, hyperirritability, excessive talkativeness, flights of ideas, and increased behavioral activity.

MAO. See **Monoamine oxidase**

Marijuana. Mixture of the crushed leaves, flowers, and small branches of both the male and female hemp plant (*Cannabis sativa*).

Medulla oblongata. The continuation of the spinal cord inside the skull, the lowest part of the brainstem, containing structures that control autonomic functions.

Mental Status Examination (MSE). An assessment of a patient's level of cognitive (knowledge-related) ability, appearance, emotional mood, and speech and thought patterns at the time of evaluation.

Mescaline. Psychedelic drug extracted from the peyote cactus.

Metabolic syndrome. The name for a group of risk factors that raises the risk for heart disease and other health problems, such as diabetes and stroke.

Metabotropic. A receptor type that is not linked directly to a membrane channel, but affects the channel indirectly through intermediate substances, such as second messengers.

Microtubule. Fibrous, hollow rods in the cells of body tissues, that function primarily to help support and shape the cell.

Midbrain. The short part of the brain, between the pons and the diencephalon.

Minor tranquilizer. Sedative-hypnotic drug promoted primarily for use in the treatment of anxiety.

Mixed agonist-antagonist. Drug that attaches to a receptor, producing weak agonistic effects but displacing more potent agonists, precipitating withdrawal in drug-dependent persons.

Monoamine oxidase (MAO). Enzyme capable of metabolizing norepinephrine, dopamine, and serotonin to inactive products.

Monoamine oxidase inhibitor (MAOI). Drug that inhibits the activity of the enzyme monoamine oxidase. Identifies one category of antidepressant medications.

Mood stabilizer. Drug used in the treatment of bipolar illness. Examples are lithium and any of the neuromodulator anticonvulsants.

Morphine. Major sedative and pain-relieving (analgesic) drug found in opium; makes up approximately 10 percent of the crude opium exudate.

Mu receptor. One of several types of opiate receptors, this type mediates the analgesic and rewarding effect of opiates.

Muscarine. Drug extracted from the mushroom *Amanita muscaria* that directly stimulates acetylcholine receptors.

Myelin sheath. A substance surrounding a nerve fiber which provides insulation and increases conduction speed.

Myristin. Psychedelic agent obtained from nutmeg and mace.

Neurodegenerative. Resulting in or characterized by degeneration of the nervous system, especially the neurons in the brain.

Neurofibrillary tangle. A pathological accumulation of paired helical filaments composed of abnormally formed tau protein that is found chiefly in the cytoplasm of nerve cells of the brain and especially the cerebral cortex and hippocampus and that occurs typically in Alzheimer's disease.

Neuroleptic malignant syndrome (NMS). The combination of hyperthermia, rigidity, and autonomic dysregulation that can occur as a serious complication of the use of antipsychotic drugs.

Neuromodulator. Antiepileptic drug used to treat bipolar illness, aggressive disorders, chronic pain, and a variety of other disorders.

Neuropathic pain. Pain caused by a primary lesion or dysfunction in the nervous system, that is, damage to nerves, to the brain, or the spinal cord.

Neurotransmitter. Endogenous chemical released by one neuron that alters the electrical activity of another neuron.

Neutrophil. Mature white blood cell.

Nicotine. Behavioral stimulant found in tobacco that directly stimulates acetylcholine receptors.

Nicotine replacement therapies (NRTS). Smoking cessation treatments that substitute another source of nicotine for the nicotine inhaled from smoking.

Nociceptive pain. Pain caused by damage to body tissue outside of the nervous system, usually described as a sharp, aching, or throbbing sensation.

Nociceptor. The sensory receptor for painful stimuli

Norepinephrine (also called *noradrenaline*). One of the monoaminergic (biogenic) excitatory neurotransmitters, a catecholamine in chemical structure, involved in alertness, concentration, aggression and motivation, among other actions.

Norepinephrine-specific reuptake inhibitor. See **Selective norepinephrine reuptake inhibitor**

Nucleosome. Any of the repeating subunits of chromatin occurring at intervals along a strand of DNA, consisting of DNA coiled around histone.

Obsession. Intrusive thoughts that produce anxiety and that lead to repetitive behaviors (compulsions) aimed at reducing anxiety.

Off-label. Term applied to the clinical use of a drug for an indication other than that for which the drug was approved by the U.S. Food and Drug Administration. Use is usually justified by medical literature, even though formal USDA approval for the use was not sought by the manufacturer of the drug. The manufacturer is not permitted to promote a drug for an off-label use.

Ololiuqui. Psychedelic drug obtained from the seeds of the morning glory plant.

Opioid. Natural or synthetic drug that exerts actions on the body similar to those induced by morphine, the major pain-relieving agent obtained from the opium poppy (*Papaver somniferum*).

Opium. Crude resinous exudate from the opium poppy. Contains morphine and codeine as active opioids.

Orexin. An excitatory neuropeptide hormone that stimulates appetite, wakefulness and energy use. See **Hypocretin**

Orthostatic hypotension (also called Postural hypotension). A drop in blood pressure that occurs when standing up from a sitting or lying position.

Parenteral. Located outside the gastrointestinal tract.

Parkinson's disease. Disorder of the motor system characterized by involuntary movements, tremor, and weakness, resulting from the loss of dopamine-producing neurons.

Partial agonist. Drug that binds to a receptor, contributing only part of the action exerted by the endogenous neurotransmitter or producing a submaximal receptor response. Buprenorphine (in Suboxone) is an example.

Peptide. Chemical composed of a chain-link sequence of amino acids.

Periaqueductal gray. The neural tissue surrounding the cerebral aqueduct within the tegmentum of the midbrain. It plays a role in the descending modulation of pain and in defensive behavior.

Peyote. Cactus that contains mescaline.

Pharmacodynamics. Study of the interactions of a drug and the receptors responsible for the action of the drug in the body.

Pharmacokinetics. Study of the factors that influence the absorption, distribution, metabolism, and excretion of a drug.

Pharmacology. Branch of science that deals with the study of drugs and their actions on living systems.

Phencyclidine (Sernyl, PCP). Psychedelic surgical anesthetic; acts by binding to and inhibiting ion transport through the NMDA-glutamate receptors.

Phenothiazine. Class of chemically related antipsychotic neuroleptic medications useful in the treatment of psychosis.

Physical dependence. State in which the use of a drug is required for a person to function normally. Physical dependence is revealed by withdrawing the drug and noting the occurrence of withdrawal symptoms (abstinence syndrome). Characteristically, withdrawal symptoms can be terminated by readministration of the drug.

Placebo. Pharmacologically inert substance that may elicit a significant reaction largely because of the mental set of the patient or the physical setting in which the drug is taken.

Plaque. A histopathologic lesion of brain tissue that is characteristic of Alzheimer's disease and consists of a dense proteinaceous core, composed primarily of beta-amyloid, that is often surrounded and infiltrated by a cluster of degenerating axons and dendrites.

Polypharmacy. The simultaneous use of multiple drugs to treat a single ailment or condition.

Pons. The part of the brainstem that links the medulla oblongata and the thalamus.

Postherpetic neuralgia. A painful condition that affects the nerve fibers and skin. Postherpetic neuralgia is a complication of shingles.

Potency. Measure of drug activity expressed in terms of the amount required to produce an effect of given intensity. Potency varies inversely with the amount of drug required to produce this effect—the more potent the drug, the lower the amount required to produce the effect.

Potentially reduced exposure products (PREPs). Cigarettes and smokeless tobacco products with purportedly lower levels of some toxins than conventional cigarettes and smokeless products.

Prodromal. Relating to or denoting the period between the appearance of initial symptoms and the full development of a disorder.

Prodrug. A biologically inactive compound that can be metabolized in the body to produce a drug.

Prolactin. A hormone released from the anterior pituitary gland that stimulates milk production after childbirth.

Psilocybin. Psychedelic drug obtained from the mushroom *Psilocybemexicana*.

Psoriasis. A skin disease marked by red, itchy, scaly patches.

Psychedelic. Drug that can alter sensory perception.

Psychoactive drug. Chemical substance that alters mood or behavior as a result of alterations in the functioning of the brain.

Psychological dependence. Compulsion to use a drug for its pleasurable effects. Dependence may lead to a compulsion to misuse a drug.

Psychopharmacology. Branch of pharmacology that deals with the effects of drugs on the nervous system and behavior.

Psychopharmacotherapy. Clinical treatment of psychiatric disorders with drugs.

Psychotherapy. Nonpharmacological treatment of psychiatric disorders utilizing a wide range of modalities from simple education and supportive counseling to insight-oriented, dynamically based therapy.

Racemate (racemic). Mixture of equal quantities of two enantiomers, substances whose molecular structures are mirror images of one another.

Rapid anesthesia-aided detoxification (RAAD). A procedure in which patients are placed under anesthesia while given treatment drugs, such as naltrexone, to avoid discomfort associated with drug detoxification.

Receptor. Location in the nervous system at which a neurotransmitter or drug binds to exert its characteristic effect. Most receptors are members of genetically encoded families of specialized proteins.

Receptor downregulation (desensitization). Decrease in a cellular response to a drug or transmitter due to a decrease in the number of receptors on the cell surface.

Receptor upregulation (supersensitivity). Increase in a cellular response to a drug or transmitter due to an increase in the number of receptors on the cell surface.

Reward circuit. Nerve pathways of the central nervous system connecting the neuronal structures that mediate feelings of pleasure and satisfaction.

Reye's syndrome. Rare CNS disorder that occurs in children; associated with aspirin ingestion.

Risk-to-benefit ratio. Arbitrary assessment of the risks and benefits that may accrue from administration of a drug.

Schizophrenia. Debilitating neuropsychiatric illness associated with disturbances in thought, perception, emotion, cognition, relationships, and psychomotor behavior.

Scopolamine. Anticholinergic drug that crosses the blood-brain barrier to produce sedation and amnesia; antagonist at the muscarinic receptor.

Second messenger. Intraneuronal protein that, when activated by a G protein, mediates the response that is initiated when neurotransmitter molecules bind to an extracellular receptor.

Sedative-hypnotic. Chemical substance that exerts a nonselective general depressant action on the nervous system.

Selective norepinephrine reuptake inhibitor (SNRI). Drug that blocks the active presynaptic transporter for norepinephrine. Used clinically to treat ADHD, depression, and other disorders, including seasonal affective disorder.

Selective serotonin reuptake inhibitor (SSRI). Second-generation antidepressant drug that blocks the reuptake transporter for serotonin.

Serotonin (5-hydroxytryptamine, 5-HT). Indoleamine neurotransmitter in both the brain and the peripheral nervous system (gut) that is involved in depression, appetite, sleep, and sexual responsiveness, among other functions.

Serotonin syndrome. Clinical syndrome resulting from excessive amounts of serotonin in the brain. The syndrome can follow use of excessive doses of SSRIs and is characterized by extreme anxiety, confusion, and disorientation.

Serotonin withdrawal syndrome. Clinical syndrome that can follow withdrawal or cessation of SSRI therapy. The syndrome is characterized by mental status alterations, severe flulike symptoms, and feelings of tingling or electrical shock in the extremities.

Side effect. Drug-induced effect that accompanies the primary effect for which the drug is administered.

Signal transduction. A basic process in molecular cell biology involving the conversion of a signal from outside the cell to a functional change within the cell.

Speedball. A mixture of cocaine and heroin.

"Spice." Street name for synthetic cannabinoids.

Spinal cord. The large group of nerves that runs through the center of the spine and carries messages between the brain and the rest of the body.

Steady state concentration. The concentration of drug at which the rate of administration and the rate of elimination are equal.

Subcutaneous. Under the skin.

Substance P. Protein neurotransmitter that regulates affective behavior, increasing the perception of pain. Substance P antagonists exhibit analgesic and antidepressant actions.

Substantia nigra. A layer of large pigmented nerve cells in the midbrain that produce dopamine and whose destruction is associated with Parkinson's disease.

Sudden sniffing death syndrome. Death that occurs very quickly in response to inhaled fumes, most commonly from butane, propane, and aerosol abuse.

Supersensitivity. See **Receptor**

Synapse. The junction between two nerve cells, consisting of a presynaptic neuronal membrane (which releases neurotransmitter), a postsynaptic neuronal membrane (which receives the transmitter signal) and a minute space between the two.

Synaptic cleft. The gap between the pre- and postsynaptic membranes of a synapse, across which neurotransmitter molecules diffuse.

Synaptic plasticity. Ability of synapses to strengthen or weaken over time, as a result of increases or decreases in their activity.

Tardive dyskinesia. Movement disorder that appears after months or years of treatment with neuroleptic (antipsychotic) drugs. It usually worsens with drug discontinuation. Symptoms are often masked by the drugs that cause the disorder.

Tectum. The uppermost part ("roof") of the midbrain.

Tegmentum. The base, or floor, of the midbrain.

Teratogen. Chemical substance that induces abnormalities of fetal development.

Testosterone. Hormone secreted from the testes that is responsible for the distinguishing characteristics of the male.

Tetrahydrocannabinol (THC). Major psychoactive agent in marijuana, hashish, and other preparations of hemp (*Cannabis sativa*).

Therapeutic drug monitoring (TDM). Process of correlating the plasma level of a drug with therapeutic response.

Therapeutic index. The ratio of the toxic dose and the therapeutic dose of a drug, which provides a measure of drug safety.

Therapeutic window. The range of drug dose, or blood concentration, that maintains a safe therapeutic effect.

Tobacco harm reduction (THR). Procedures or substances taken to lower the health risks associated with using nicotine.

Tolerance. Clinical state of reduced responsiveness to a drug; can be produced by a variety of mechanisms, all of which require increased doses of drug to produce an effect once achieved by lower doses.

Torsades de pointes. Variant of ventricular tachycardia that can be the result of lengthening the QT interval.

Toxic effect. Drug-induced effect either temporarily or permanently deleterious to any organ or system of an animal or person. Drug toxicity includes both the relatively minor side effects that invariably accompany drug administration and the more serious and unexpected manifestations that occur in only a small percentage of patients who take a drug.

Tumor necrosis factor. A protein produced by macrophages in the presence of an endotoxin and shown experimentally to be capable of attacking and destroying cancerous tumors.

Unipolar depression (also called clinical depression, major depression, and unipolar disorder). Mental disorder characterized by an all-encompassing low mood accompanied by low self-esteem and loss of interest or pleasure in normally enjoyable activities.

Ventral tegmental area (VTA). Group of neurons located on the floor of the midbrain (mesencephalon) that contain dopamine and serotonin; the VTA is a major component of the reward pathway in the brain.

Withdrawal syndrome. Onset of a predictable group of symptoms following the abrupt discontinuation or rapid decrease in dosage of a psychoactive substance on which the body has become dependent. May include anxiety, insomnia, delirium tremens, perspiration, hot flashes, nausea, dehydration, tremors, weakness, dizziness, convulsions, and psychotic behavior.

"Z drugs." Three drugs, the names of which all start with the letter "z," that are structurally not benzodiazepines, but which nevertheless bind to the same receptors to which benzodiazepines bind and exert the same agonist effects as the benzodiazepines.

Zero-order metabolism (kinetics). Condition in which the plasma concentration of a drug decreases (is metabolized) at a constant rate; the rate of metabolism does not depend on the amount (concentration) of the drug.

INDEX

Note: Page numbers followed by f indicate figures; those followed by t indicate tables; and those followed by n indicate footnotes.

Abilify. *See* Aripiprazole (Abilify)
Abnormal Involuntary Movement Scale (AIMS), 394
Abstinence syndrome, 35, 351
Abstral. *See* Fentanyl
ABT-126, 410
Acamprosate (Campral), 124, 143, 159–160, 162–163
Acetylation, histone, 691–692
Acetylcholine, 54–57, 55f, 56f, 192, 259f
Acetylcholine esterase, 80
Acetylcholine receptors, 55–56, 190–191
Acetylcholinesterase inhibitors, 55, 80, 644
N-Acetylcysteine (Mucomyst, NAC), 124, 244
    for cannabis dependence, 322
Acetylfentanyl, 372
Acomplia (rimonabant), 123, 306
Action potential, 49
Actiq. *See* Fentanyl
Active metabolites, 21n
Actos (pioglitazone), 651
Acurox (oxycodone/niacin), 355
Adapin (doxepin), 439t, 444
Adasuve (loxapine), 389t, 557
Adderall (amphetamine), 227, 602
Addiction. *See also* Drug abuse
    Brain Disease Model of Addiction and, 110, 117–120
    glutamatergic model of, 123–126
    neurobiology of, 109–119
    relapse in, 109–110, 114–115, 115f
    reward circuits and, 110–115
    stress and, 114–115

treatment of, 120–127. *See also* Drug abuse, treatment of
    vs. dependence, 35
Ademetionine (Strada), 477
Adenosine, 67, 185–186, 186f
S-Adenosylmethionine (SAM-e), 471
ADME, 3
Adolescents. *See also* Child and adolescent psychopharmacology
    psychological disorders in, 589–609
    substance abuse by, 582–588
        Adolescent Brain Cognitive Development Study for, 588
        alcohol, 148, 583
        inhalants, 164–166
        marijuana, 292, 584–586
        nicotine, 582–583
        prevention, diagnosis, and treatment of, 586–588
        screening for, 586–588
        stimulants, 228–229, 584
Adrenaline. *See* Epinephrine
Adrenergic antagonists, for cocaine abuse, 242–243
ADX-1149, 411
Adzenys, 603
Aero Shot Pure Energy, 177–178
Affective disorders, 435
Aggression
    alcohol and, 148
    antipsychotics for, 419
    in children and adolescents, 419, 597–598, 605–606, 674
    in elderly, 627–631
    varenicline and, 202, 203–205
Agitation
    antipsychotics for, 419
    in children and adolescents, 419
    in elderly, 627–631

Agomelatine (Thymanax, Valdoxan), 474, 507, 516
Agonist(s), 86–90, 87f, 89f
  biased, 370
  full, 335
  mixed agonist-antagonists, 335–337
  partial, 87f, 88, 121–122, 335
  vs. antagonists, 337
Agonist substitution treatment, 120–121
Agoraphobia, 490. *See also* Anxiety disorders
Agranulocytosis, 637
  clozapine-induced, 387, 402–403
Akathisia, 93n, 392, 393–394
Akineton (biperiden), 641
Alcohol
  caffeine and, 184–185
  concentration in beverages, 135–136, 138–139, 141f
  concentration in blood, 137–142, 141f
  distribution of, 136
  drink equivalents and, 138, 140, 175–176
  health risks and benefits of, 146
  memory impairment and, 149, 150f, 494
  metabolism of, 137–138, 138f, 139f
  pharmacodynamics of, 143–145
  pharmacokinetics of, 14, 31, 135–142, 138f, 139f, 141f
  pharmacological effects of, 145–147
  powdered, 142
  psychological and behavioral effects of, 147–148
  teratogenic effects of, 152–154
  toxicity of, 151–152
Alcohol breath, 136n
Alcohol dehydrogenase (ADH), 14, 136–137, 140–142
Alcohol dementia, 151
Alcohol myopia, 148
Alcohol use/abuse, 135–163
  addiction in. *See* Addiction
  by adolescents, 148, 583
  age at onset of, 154
  aggression and, 148
  binge drinking and, 146, 149, 154
  biomarkers of, 142
  blackouts and, 149, 150f, 494
  cannabis abuse and, 126–127, 144–145
  chronic care management for, 157
  clinical definition of, 154
  cocaine abuse and, 221
  cognitive effects of, 149
  comorbidity and, 108–109, 154–155
  criminal behavior and, 148
  cross-tolerance in, 140–142
  drug therapy for, 155–163

  for acute intoxication, 156
  combination therapy in, 158, 162–163
  for dependence, 155–156
  goals of, 156
  off-label drugs in, 157
  psychedelics in, 275–276
  for relapse prevention, 157–162
  for withdrawal, 156–157, 161–162
  drunk driving and, 145, 148, 307
  DSM classification of, 108–109
  early-onset, 162
  hangover prevention in, 140
  harm reduction approach to, 155
  intoxication in, 147–148, 147f
  long-term effects on brain, 148–149
  personality factors in, 148
  in pregnancy, 152–154, 575–576
  prevalence of, 135
  psychiatric disorders and, 108–109, 154–155
  self-medication in, 154–155
  sexual function and, 146–147
  side effects and toxicity in, 151–152
  stress and, 144, 154–155
  tolerance and dependence in, 140–142, 150–151
  varenicline and, 204
  withdrawal in, 150–151, 156–157, 161–162
Alcoholic liver disease, 151
Alcoholics Anonymous, 154
Alcohol-related neurodevelopmental disorder, 153
Alcosynth, 140
ALDH2i, for cocaine abuse, 244
Alfentanil (Alfenta), 357–358
ALKS-3831, 413
ALKS-5461, 474
ALKS-9072 (aripiprazole lauroxil), 413
Allergies, drug, 94, 349
Allosteric drugs, 71, 87
Alpha fentanyl, 358
Alpha-methylfentanyl, 372
Alpha-methyltryptamine (AMT), 267
Alprazolam (Xanax), 503–504
Alternative therapies. *See* Complementary and alternative therapies
Alvimopan (Entereg), 348
Alzheimer's disease, 642–654. *See also* Dementia
  amyloid deposition in, 644, 653–654
  benzodiazepines and, 505
  biomarkers in, 644, 653
  clinical example of, 674
  drug therapy for, 192–193, 644–654
    acetylcholinesterase inhibitors in, 646–648
    antidepressants in, 645
    antipsychotics in, 645

for behavioral disturbances, 645–646
cannabinoids in, 312
for depression and apathy, 645
limitations of, 653–654
memantine in, 644, 648–649
novel agents in, 650–654
principles of, 654
overview of, 642–644, 643f
unified theory of, 654
Amantadine (Symmetrel)
for cocaine abuse, 242
for Parkinson's disease, 641
Ambien (zolpidem), 508t, 510t, 511–513, 512f
Amidate (etomidate), 519
Amino acid neurotransmitters, 54t, 63–66
Amitifadine, 475
Amitiza (lubiprostone), 348
Amitriptyline (Elavil), 439t, 442, 443, 444, 517–518, 518t
Amnesia. *See* Anterograde amnesia
Amoxapine (Asendin), 447
AMPA receptors, 63, 64, 116, 125
Ampakines, 125
Amphetamine(s), 226–235
for attention-deficit/hyperactivity disorder, 600–601, 602–603, 605–606
for cocaine abuse, 242
for depression, 448–449
dosage of, 231
mechanism of action of, 229–230
medical uses of, 227–228
methamphetamine, 232–234. *See also* Methamphetamine
new formulations of, 602–603
pharmacokinetics of, 229
pharmacological effects of, 230–231
regulation of, 228
side effects and toxicity of, 231, 607–608
structure of, 226–227, 227f, 261f
Amphetamine abuse
drug therapy for, 126, 242–243
historical perspective on, 227–229
tolerance and dependence in, 234–235
withdrawal in, 235
AMT (alpha-methyltryptamine), 267
Amygdala, 44, 45f, 114, 114f
Amyl nitrite, 163
Anafrinal (clomipramine), 439t, 448
Analgesics. *See also* Opioid(s)
anticonvulsants as, 340
antidepressants as, 340–341
for children and adolescents, 553, 598–600
marijuana as, 310–311
mechanism of action of, 340–342
placebo effects of, 94–97

Anandamide, 145, 295f, 298–299, 300f
Anesthetics
for depression, 472–473
dissociative, 280–281
general, 518–519
inhalational, 163–167. *See also* Inhalant abuse
Anexate (flumazenil), 123, 506
Angel dust, 279–282
Anhedonia, 474
Ansofaxine, 475
Antabuse (disulfiram), 120–121, 158, 244
Antagonists, 87f, 88–90, 89f, 120–121, 337
mixed, 335–336, 365, 367–368
Anterior cingulate cortex, 44, 45f, 47
Anterograde amnesia
alcohol-induced, 494
benzodiazepine-induced, 503, 504
Antianxiety drugs. *See* Anxiety disorders, treatment of
Antibipolar drugs. *See* Mood stabilizers
Antibodies
for cocaine abuse, 246–247
for methamphetamine abuse, 248
Anticholinergic psychedelics, 258–260, 258t. *See also* Psychedelic drugs
Anticholinergics, 640–641
Anticonvulsants, 489, 519–524, 519t, 520f
for alcohol abuse, 157, 161–162
for anxiety, 504
for bipolar disorder, 519, 535–541, 535t, 549–555, 560
clinical uses of, 519, 549
for cocaine abuse, 124–125, 243–244
for disruptive behavior disorders, 598
for drug abuse, 124–125, 243–244
for insomnia, 518, 518t
for pain, 340
in pregnancy, 523–524, 549, 581–582
suicide risk and, 524
Antidepressant(s), 433–477, 682t–683t
for alcohol abuse, 144
for Alzheimer's disease, 645
with antipsychotics, 393–394, 468
for anxiety disorders, 504, 507
for attention-deficit/hyperactivity disorder, 604
atypical (second-generation), 439t, 440, 447–449
augmenting agents for, 468–469
for bipolar disorder, 533–534, 540–541
caffeine and, 179–180
classification of, 438–440, 439t, 441t
for cocaine abuse, 242
codeine and, 353
under development, 474–477
development of, 438–440

Antidepressant(s) *(Continued)*
    drug interactions with, 24
    dual-action, 452t
    effectiveness of, 434–435, 451, 464–466
    for elderly, 631–633
    first-generation, 391, 439t, 442–447
    indications for, 452t
    for insomnia, 510t, 518
    ketamine as, 279
    mechanism of action of, 436–438
    mixed serotonin-norepinephrine reuptake
        inhibitors, 441t, 448
    monoamine oxidase inhibitors, 57, 80,
        438–440, 445–447
    needed improvements in, 440
    neurogenesis and, 436–438
    for nicotine dependence, 202, 204
    nonresponse to, 433–434, 451
    noradrenergic/specific serotonergic, 441t,
        462–463
    norepinephrine-dopamine reuptake inhibitors,
        441t
    for pain, 340, 444
    for pediatric depression, 589–591
    poop-out effect and, 458–459
    in pregnancy, 443, 457, 577–579
    for premenstrual dysphoric disorder, 456
    sedative effects of, 439t, 442t, 443, 444, 510t
    selective norepinephrine reuptake inhibitors,
        441t
    selective serotonin reuptake inhibitors, 61,
        439t, 440, 449–459. *See also* Selective
        serotonin reuptake inhibitors (SSRIs)
    serotonin + norepinephrine reuptake
        inhibitors, 441t, 452t, 459–461
    serotonin syndrome and, 93, 358, 361, 453
    serotonin-2 antagonists/reuptake inhibitors,
        441t, 461–462
    for stimulant abuse, 242
    tramadol and, 361
    tricyclic, 438, 439t, 442–445
    withdrawal and, 35
Antidepressant tachyphylaxis, 459
Antidiabetic agents, for drug abuse, 127
Antiepileptics. *See* Anticonvulsants
Antihistamines, for insomnia, 518, 518t
Antimuscarinics, 258–260, 259f
Antipsychotics, 686t
    for aggression, 419
    for agitation, 419
    for Alzheimer's disease, 645
    with antidepressants, 393–394, 468
    atypical, 387–388
    for autism spectrum disorder, 419
    for bipolar disorder, 415–416, 555–559, 559t

    for borderline personality disorder, 420–421
    for children and adolescents, 592–593
    costs of, 409–411
    for dementia, 417–418, 629
    for depression, 415, 416–417, 468
    under development, 410–414
    for disruptive behavior disorders, 598
    dopamine receptor antagonists, 383f, 384
    effectiveness of, 408–410
    for elderly, 417–418, 627–631
    first-generation, 388–396, 389t
        indications for, 389t
        negative symptoms and, 390
        pharmacokinetics of, 388
        pharmacologic effects of, 390
        side effects and toxicity of, 391–396, 391t
        types of, 389t
    for hallucinogen persisting perception
        disorder, 272
    historical perspective on, 396–410
    for insomnia, 518, 518t
    for LSD flashbacks, 272
    for nonschizophrenic disorders, 415–421
    for obsessive-compulsive disorder, 420
    off-label uses of, 397, 398t
    for Parkinson's disease, 421
    for PCP/ketamine intoxication, 282
    for posttraumatic stress disorder, 419–420
    in pregnancy, 558, 579–580
    for schizophrenia, 386–415
    second-generation, 384, 386–422, 387–388, 397t
        development of, 387
        effectiveness of, 396–397
        mechanism of action of, 388
        side effects of, 400–408, 401t
    selection of, 396–397
    side effects of, 384, 387, 400–408, 401t, 402f
    third-generation, 397
    weight gain and, 400, 401t, 402f, 403, 404
Antiseizure agents. *See* Anticonvulsants
Anxiety disorders
    in adolescents, 589
    caffeine and, 184
    in children and adolescents, 594–596
    classification of, 490
    clinical examples of, 674, 675–676
    depression and, 435
    marijuana and, 306, 312–313
    treatment of, 489–524, 688t. *See also*
        Anxiolytics; Benzodiazepine(s);
        Sedative-hypnotics
    anticonvulsants for, 504
    antidepressants for, 435, 448, 504, 507, 597
    benzodiazepines for, 500–502
    new approaches for, 506–507

opioids for, 347, 500–502
psychedelics for, 275–278
sedative-hypnotics for, 489–524
Anxiolytics, 688t. *See also* Benzodiazepine(s)
for depression, 474
indications for, 489–490
overdoses of, 492
Apadz, 355
Apathy, in Alzheimer's disease, 645
Aplenzin. *See* Bupropion
Apolipoprotein E, 652
Apomorphine (Apokyn), 639
Appetite stimulation, by marijuana, 306
Aptiom (eslicarbazene), 523
AQW051, 410
2-Arachidonoyl glycerol (2-AG), 299
Arachidonoylethanolamine (anandamide, AEA),
145, 295f, 298–299, 300f
2-Arachidonoylglycerol (2-AG), 300f
2-Arachidonoylglycerylether (Noladin ether),
299, 300f
N-Arachidonyldopamine (NADA), 299, 300f
O-Arachidonylethanolamine (Vinodhamine), 298,
300f
Aricept (donepezil), 646–647
Aripiprazole (Abilify), 397, 397t, 399–400
akathisia and, 393–394
for autism spectrum disorder, 419
for bipolar disorder, 415, 535t, 555–558
for borderline personality disorder, 420–421
for cocaine addiction, 122
for dementia, 630
for depression, 416, 468, 633
for disruptive behavior disorders, 598
indications for, 398t
for obsessive-compulsive disorder, 420
for posttraumatic stress disorder, 419
for schizophrenia, 399–400, 409
side effects of, 401t, 407
for stimulant abuse, 242
Aripiprazole lauroxil (Aristada), 413
Armodafinil (Nuvigil), 240, 241–242, 469
Arrhythmias
antipsychotic-induced, 405, 406f, 407f
in inhalant abuse, 166–167
quetiapine-related, 405, 406f
Artane (trihexyphenidyl), 641
Arymo ER, 352
Asenapine (Saphris), 397t, 398t, 400, 401t, 402f,
407–408, 415, 535t, 555, 556
Asendin (amoxapine), 447
Ataxia, 41
Atherosclerosis, smoking and, 195
Ativan (lorazepam), 4–5, 5f, 158, 492t
Atomoxetine (Strattera), 452t, 604

Atropine, 258
Attention-deficit/hyperactivity disorder, 600–609
in adults, 607
alternative drugs for, 604–605
amphetamines for, 600–601, 602–603, 605–606
antidepressants for, 445
clinical trials for, 605–606
investigational drugs for, 609
methylphenidate for, 240, 240f, 601–602
in pregnancy, 576
prenatal methamphetamine exposure and, 234
stimulants for, 600–603, 605–608
Atypical antidepressants. *See* Antidepressant(s)
Austedo (deutetrabenazine), for tardive
dyskinesia, 394
Autism spectrum disorder, 419, 593, 597
antidepressants in pregnancy and, 579
Autonomic nervous system, 226
Autoreceptors, 51
AV-101, 475
Avandia (rosiglitazone), 651
Aventyl. *See* Nortriptyline (Aventyl, Pamelor)
AVL-3288, 410
AVN-211, 411
AVP-786, 475
Axons, 49, 50f
AXS-05, 476
Ayahuasca, 273, 277
AZD6423, 475
Azilect (rasagiline), 637, 640

Baclofen (Lioresal), 123, 160–161, 243
Bagging, 163–167. *See also* Inhalant abuse
BALANCE study, 548
Banzel (rufinamide), 522
Bapineuzumab, 650
Barbiturates, 491, 491f, 495–497, 520. *See also*
Sedative-hypnotics
sites and mechanism of action of, 493–494,
493f
Bariatric surgery, alcohol metabolism after, 136,
137
Barnes Akathisia Rating Scale, 394
Basal ganglia, 41, 43–44, 43f
Basimglurant, 476
"Bath salts," 236–238
Beers Criteria, 418, 626
Behavioral conditioning, 35
Behavioral disruptive disorders, 597–598,
605–606, 674
Belbuca, 362
Belladonna, 259
Belsomra (suvorexant), 508t, 517
Benadryl (diphenhydramine), 517, 518t, 641
Benzedrine, 228

Benzhydrocodone (KP201), 355
Benzodiazepine(s), 500–506, 688t
  abuse of, flumazenil for, 123
  for alcohol withdrawal, 156–157, 504
  alternatives to, 504
  classification of, 492t
  clinical uses of, 502–504
  complex sleep-related behaviors and, 509
  development of, 491–492
  in elderly, 501–502
  GABA receptors and, 493–494
  intermediate-acting, 492t
  limitations of, 502–504
  long-acting, 492t
  opioids and, 339–340
  overdoses of, 492
  for PCP/ketamine intoxication, 282
  pharmacokinetics of, 492t, 500–502, 501f
  pharmacological effects of, 502
  in pregnancy, 506
  short-acting, 492t
  side effects and toxicity of, 491–493, 504–505,
    510t
  sites and mechanism of action of, 493–494
  sleep-related activities and, 504, 509
  structure of, 491f
  tolerance and dependence and, 505
Benzodiazepine receptor agonists, 493–494,
    508–514, 510t, 512f
  full, 514
  nonbenzodiazepine, 511–514
  partial, 514
Benzoylecgonine, 221, 222f
Benzoylindoles, 315
Benztropine (Cogentin), 641
1-Benzylpiperazine (BZP), 266
Beta-blockers, 506
Beta-hydroxythiofentanyl, 372
Bexarotene (Targretin), 652
Bhang, 295
BI-409306, 413
Biased agonists, 370
Binge drinking, 146, 146n, 149, 154
  in pregnancy, 154
Bioavailability, 3
Biomarkers, in Alzheimer's disease, 644, 653
Biotransformation. *See* Drug metabolism
Biperiden (Akineton), 641
Bipolar disorder, 531–561
  brain changes in, 538
  in children and adolescents, 593, 595–597
  clinical examples of, 673–674, 676
  course and prognosis of, 533
  diagnosis of, 534
  drug therapy for, 684t

  antidepressants in, 533–534, 540–541
  antipsychotics in, 468, 555–558, 559t
  BALANCE study of, 548
  combination therapy in, 547
  fluoxetine/olanzapine in, 416, 456
  guidelines for, 536
  LiTMUS Study of, 480–481
  mood stabilizers in, 468, 519, 534, 535–555,
    580–582. *See also* Mood stabilizers
  nonadherence to, 547
  in pregnancy, 580–582
  STEP-BD study of, 539–541
  genetic factors in, 534
  monoamine (receptor) hypothesis of, 442
  nicotine and, 193
  omega-3 fatty acids for, 558–559
  in pregnancy, 546–547, 553, 579–582
  psychotherapeutic/psychosocial treatment for,
    560–561
  remission maintenance in, 557–559
  substance abuse and, 533
  subtypes of, 532
  suicide in, 533, 547
  symptoms of, 533
  vs. postpartum depression, 534
  vs. unipolar depression, 534
Birth defects, 152–154, 225–226
Bk-amphetamines, 236
Blackouts, 149, 150f
Bladder, ulcerative colitis of, ketamine-induced, 281
Blonanserine (Lonasen), 412
Blood alcohol concentration, 137–142, 141f
Blood-brain barrier, 16, 18–19, 18f, 574
Blue mystic, 264
Borderline personality disorder, 420–421
Botox, 476
Bowman's capsule, 27, 28f
Brain, organization and structures of, 39–47,
    40f–43f, 45f–48f
Brain Disease Model of Addiction, 110, 117–120.
    See also Addiction; Reward circuits
Brain injury, marijuana for, 311
Brain mapping, 47
Brain stem, 40–41, 41f
Brain-derived neurotrophic factor (BDNF), 117,
    436–438, 538
Breastfeeding, anticonvulsants and, 582
Breathalyzer test, 136n
Brevital (methohexital), 519
Brexpiprazole (Rexulti), 397, 397t, 398t, 399,
    401t, 402f, 408, 416
  with antidepressants, 468
Brief Intervention and Referral to Treatment,
    587–588
Brivaracetam (Briviact), 523

Bromo, 265
4-Bromo-2,5-dimethoxyphenethylamine (2C-B), 265
Bromocriptine (Parlodel), 225, 242, 269f, 395, 639
BTRX-246040, 477
Bufotenine, 268, 269f, 273
Bunavil, 362
Buphenyl (sodium phenylbutyrate), 653
Buprenex, 362
Buprenorphine (Subutex), 336t, 361–365, 599
    abuse of, 364
    for chronic pain, 362
    implanted, 362
    for opioid abuse, 121, 363–364
    as partial agonist, 335
    in pregnancy, 364–365
    for psychological disorders, 363
    side effects of, 363
    for stimulant abuse, 245
Buprenorphine-naloxone (Probuphine, Suboxone), 10, 362
Buprenorphine-samidorphan, 474
Bupropion, 449, 459
    for attention-deficit/hyperactivity disorder, 449
    for bipolar disorder, 556
    clinical uses of, 449, 452t
    dependence on, 449
    for depression, 449
    for nicotine dependence, 202, 204, 449
    side effects of, 449
    for stimulant abuse, 242
"Businessman's lunch," 272
Buspirone (BuSpar)
    absorption of, 7–8
    for alcohol abuse, 162
    for cocaine abuse, 243
Butalbital, 496
Butorphanol (Stadol), 336t, 365
Butrans patch, 362
Butyrlfentanyl, 372
Butyrophenones, 387. *See also* Antipsychotics
Butyrylcholinesterase, for cocaine abuse, 247
BZP (1-benzylpiperazine), 266

Caffeine, 177–187
    adenosine and, 185–186, 186f
    adverse effects of, 183–185
    alcohol interaction with, 184–185
    for alcohol intoxication, 156
    antidepressants and, 179–180
    beneficial effects of, 180–183
    dose-response curve for, 85–86, 85f
    nicotine and, 178t
    pharmacokinetics of, 179–180, 179f
        pharmacological effects of, 180–183
        in pregnancy, 186–187
        sources and amounts of, 177–178, 178t
        structure of, 179f
        tolerance and dependence and, 187
        withdrawal and, 187
Caffeine mist, 177–178
Caffeine powder, 185
Caffeine use disorder, 187
Caffeinism, 184
CAM2038, 363–364
cAMP response-element binding protein (CREB), 437
Campral (acamprosate), 124, 143, 159–160
Cancer
    alcohol and, 146, 152
    caffeine and, 181–182
    medical marijuana for, 311
    psilocybin therapy for, 277
    smoking and, 195
    testicular, marijuana and, 309
Cannabidiol (CBD), 295–298, 296f, 303–304
    for cannabis dependence, 322
Cannabinoid receptors, 295f, 296–298
    alcohol and, 144–145
Cannabinoids, opioids and, 126–127
Cannabis. *See also* Marijuana
    components of, 295, 295f
    dopamine and, 297
    forms of, 295
    THC content of, 295, 295f
Cannabis Use Disorder, 320
Carbamazepine (Equetro, Tegretol), 520f, 521
    for alcohol withdrawal, 157
    for bipolar disorder, 535t, 549–550
    in pregnancy, 581
    side effects of, 550
Carbidopa, 242, 635–636
4-Carbomethoxyfentanyl, 372–373
Cardiac arrhythmias
    antipsychotic-induced, 405, 406f, 407f
    in inhalant abuse, 166–167
    quetiapine-related, 405, 406f
Cardiovascular disorders
    alcohol and, 146
    antidepressants and, 455
    caffeine and, 181
    cocaine and, 224
    marijuana and, 305
    methamphetamine and, 232
Cardura (doxazosin), 123, 243, 507, 508t
Carfentanyl, 372–373
Cariprazine (Vraylar), 397, 399–400, 401t, 402f, 408, 417, 535t, 557
Carisoprodol (Soma), 491, 498

Carrier proteins, 77–80, 79f
Cataplexy, 499
Catecholaminelike psychedelics, 258, 258t
Catecholaminergic psychedelics, 261–268
Catecholamines, 54t, 57–60, 58f. *See also*
    Dopamine; Epinephrine; Norepinephrine
Catha edulis (khat), 235
Cathine, 235
Cathinones, 235, 236–238
CATIE study, 408–410
Caudate nucleus, 43, 43f
CB1/CB2 receptors, 296–298
CBD. *See* Cannabidiol (CBD)
CDP-choline, 246
Ceftriaxone, for drug abuse, 124
Celexa. *See* Citalopram (Celexa)
Cell membranes, drug distribution and, 16–17,
    16f
Cellular-adaptive tolerance, 35
Cenobamate, 560
Central Intelligence Agency, LSD experiments
    of, 276
Central nervous system, 39. *See also* Brain;
    Spinal cord
Centrax (prazepam), 492t
Century Cures Act, 672–673
CEP-26401 (Irdabisant), 412
CERC-301, 475–476
CERC-501, 474
Cerebellum, 41, 41f
Cerebral cortex, 44, 46f
Cerebrospinal fluid, 15–16, 15f
Cerebrum, 44, 46f
Cesamet (nabilone), 306, 308, 315, 321
Chantix. *See* Varenicline (Chantix)
Charas, 295
Chemoreceptor trigger zone, 347
Chiari type I malformation, 578
Child and adolescent psychopharmacology,
    582–609. *See also* Adolescents; Pregnancy
  for anxiety disorders, 594–596
  for attention-deficit/hyperactivity disorder,
    593, 600–608
  for autism spectrum disorder, 419, 593, 597
  for bipolar disorder, 593, 595–597
  for depression, 445, 589–591
  desipramine-related sudden death and, 445
  for disruptive behavior disorders, 597–598
  for pain, 353, 558–600
  for posttraumatic stress disorder, 595
  for psychotic disorders, 592–593
  substance abuse and, 582–589
"China white," 358
Chloral hydrate (Noctec), 497
Chlorazepate (Tranxene), 492t
Chlordiazepoxide (Librium), 157, 491, 492t

Chlorpromazine (Largactil, Thorazine), 386, 389t
Cholinergic receptors, 55–56
Cholinesterase inhibitors, for Alzheimer's
    disease, 644
Chromatin, 690
Chronic care management, for alcohol
    dependence, 157
Cigarettes. *See also* Nicotine; Smoking
  electronic, 199–202, 301, 582–583
  menthol, 191
Cingulate cortex, 44, 45f
Cinnamaldehyde, 653
Circadin, 516
Circulatory system
  anatomy of, 9f
  capillaries in, 17–18, 17f
  drug distribution in, 14
Cirrhosis, 151
Citalopram (Celexa), 441t, 450, 451t, 452t,
    457–458
Citoline, 246
Clinical examples, 673–678
Clobazam (Onfi), 492t, 522–523
Clomipramine (Anafranil), 439t, 448
Clonazepam (Klonopin), 492t
Clonidine, 604
Clozapine (Clozaril), 387, 397t, 398–399
  for bipolar disorder, 415
  drug interactions with, 24
  effectiveness of, 408–409
  for Parkinson's disease, 421
  side effects of, 400–403, 401t, 402f
  for tardive dyskinesia, 394
Club drugs
  GHB, 498–499
  ketamine, 279–282
  MDMA, 237, 260, 263–265
  MDMA-related, 265–267
  PCP, 279–282
Cocaethylene, 221, 222f
Cocaine, 217–226
  as anesthetic, 222
  crack, 219, 354
  forms of, 219
  freebase and, 219
  historical perspective on, 217–219, 228
  mechanism of action of, 222–223, 223f
  pharmacokinetics of, 220t, 221, 229
  pharmacological effects of, 224–225
  preparations of, 219, 220t
  as psychostimulant, 223
  regulation of, 219
  routes of administration of, 219, 220t, 224
  side effects and toxicity of, 224–225
  in speedballs, 225
  structure of, 222f

tolerance to, 224
as vasoconstrictor, 222
Cocaine abuse
alcohol abuse and, 221
comorbidity and, 225
drug therapy for
anticonvulsants in, 124–125, 243–244
antidepressants in, 242
disulfiram in, 121, 244
dopaminergic/adrenergic approaches in, 242–243
GABAergic/glutamatergic approaches in, 123–126, 243–244
metabolizing enzymes in, 246–247
heroin abuse and, 225, 354
in pregnancy, 221, 225–226
tolerance in, 224–225
vaccine for, 247–248
Codeine, 335, 336t, 353, 599. *See also* Opioid(s)
Coffee. *See* Caffeine
Cogentin (benztropine), 641
Cognex (tacrine), 646
Cognitive-behavioral therapy, 561
for insomnia, 509
for pediatric depression, 590
Cogwheel-type rigidity, antipsychotics and, 393
COMBINE study, 158, 162–163
Comorbidity, 109
in alcohol abuse, 108–109, 154–155
in bipolar disorder, 533
in cocaine abuse, 225
Compazine (prochlorperazine), 389t
Competitive antagonists, 88–89, 89f
Complementary and alternative therapies.
        See also Omega-3 fatty acids
for Alzheimer's disease, 645–646, 648
for depression, 470–471
drug interactions with, 25
for psychotic disorders, 422
Complex sleep-related behaviors, 509, 513
COMT gene, placebo effect and, 96
COMT inhibitors, 637–638
Comtan (entacapone), 636
Conditioning
addiction and, 117
behavioral, 35
relapse and, 115, 115f
Congenital heart disease, antidepressants in pregnancy and, 578
Conjugation, 21–22
Connectome, 47, 48f
Conotoxins, 511
Conscious sedation, 495
Constipation, opioid-induced, 348
Controlled substance schedules, 105, 106t
Corpus striatum, 43, 43f

Corydalis spp., 244
Cotinine, 190, 651
Cough suppression, opioids for, 347
CPP-115, 123
CR845 (difelikefalin), 368
Crack cocaine, 219, 354. *See also* Cocaine
CRAFFT screening too, 587
Crank, 232. *See also* Methamphetamine
Craving. *See also* Relapse
in alcohol abuse, 151
glutamate and, 117
neuroadaptation and, 109, 114–115
Crenezumab, 650
Criminal behavior, alcohol and, 148
CRISPR-Cas9, 692–694
Cross-tolerance, 24
Crystal meth, 232. *See also* Methamphetamine
Curcumin, 653
CUtLASS studies, 408–410
Cyclic AMP, 75–77, 78f
Cyclohexylphenols, 315
Cycloserine, 126
Cylert (pemoline), 240f, 260
Cymbalta (duloxetine), 441t, 452t, 461
CYP-3A4, 8
Cystine, for nicotine addiction, 121–122
Cystine-glutamate exchanger (xCT), 117, 123–124
Cystitis, ketamine-induced, 281
Cytidine diphosphate-choline, 246
Cytisine (Tabex), 202
Cytochrome P450 enzymes, 21–26, 23f

Dabbing, 301
Dalgan (dezocine), 365
Dalmane (flurazepam), 492t, 508t
Dantrolene, 263, 395
Darvon (propoxyphene), 357
Dasotraline, 609
Date rape drugs, 495, 499, 503. *See also* Club drugs
Datura spp., 259
Deadly nightshade, 259
Death receptor, 62
Decosahexaenoic acid (DHA), 645–646
Deep brain stimulation, 127
Default-mode network, 278
Delirium tremens, 151
Delta receptor, 67, 343, 343t
ΔFosB, 117
Dementia. *See also* Alzheimer's disease
alcohol-induced, 151
antipsychotics for, 417–418, 627–631
caffeine and, 182
clinical example of, 674
cognitive enhancers for, 192–193
drug-induced, 151, 494–495
hallucinations in, 418

Demerol (meperidine), 336t, 357
Dendrites, 49, 50f
Depacon/Depakene/Depakote. *See* Valproic
    acid (Depakene, Depakote, Depacon,
    Divalproex)
Dependence, 35
Depot administration, 12
Depression, 434–440
    in adolescents, 589
    anesthetics for, 472–473
    antidepressants for. *See* Antidepressant(s)
    antipsychotics for, 416–417, 468
    anxiety and, 435
    anxiolytics for, 474
    atypical, 445
    bipolar. *See* Bipolar disorder
    brain changes in, 538
    in cancer patients, 277
    in children and adolescents, 589–591
    clinical examples of, 674, 675–676, 677
    cocaine abuse and, 225
    complementary and alternative therapies for,
        470–471
    diet and, 470–471, 472
    genetic factors in, 437, 466–467
    monoamine (receptor) hypothesis of, 442
    neurogenic theory of, 436
    nicotine and, 193
    pathophysiology of, 435–438
    postpartum, 534
    in pregnancy, 443, 457, 577–579
    psychedelics for, 275–278
    psychostimulants for, 448–449, 468–469
    stress and, 436
    symptoms of, 435
    treatment-resistant, 433–434, 451
    unipolar vs. bipolar, 533
Designer drugs, 261f, 262, 267
Desipramine (Norpramin), 439t, 442, 445
Desmedetomidine (Precedex), 519
O-Desmethyltramadol, 372
Desmorphine, 371
Desoxyn (methamphetamine), 234
Desvenlafaxine (Pristiq, Khedezla), 441t, 452,
    460
Desyrel (trazodone), 447
Deutetrabenazine (Austedo), for tardive
    dyskinesia, 394
Devil's apple, 259
Dexamfetamine, 243
Dexanabinol, 311
Dexing, 282
Dextroamphetamine (Dexedrine, DextroStat),
    226–227, 227f, 231, 602
    in pregnancy, 577

Dextromethorphan, 282–283, 476
Dextrorotatory isomers, 80, 81f
Dezocine (Dalgan), 365
Diabetes, type 2
    antipsychotics and, 403
    caffeine and, 181
    smoking and, 195–196
Diacetylmorphine (heroin), 353–354. *See also*
    Heroin abuse
Diacomit (stiripentol), 523
*Diagnostic and Statistical Manual of Mental
    Disorders* (DSM), 108–109, 669–670
Dianicline, 203
Diarrhea, opioids for, 347–348
Diazepam (Valium), 157, 492t, 506
    half-life of, 30–31
Diencephalon, 40f, 42, 42f
Diet, depression and, 470–471, 472
Difelikefalin (CR845), 368
Diffusion, passive, 6
Dihexa, 652
Dihydrodesoxymorphine, 371
Dilantin (phenytoin), 520–521, 520f
Dilaudid (hydromorphone), 336t, 354, 356–357
Dimebon (latrepirdine), 650
2,5-Dimethoxy-4-propylthiophenethylamine, 265
Dimethoxymethamphetamine (DOM), 261f
Dimethoxymethylamphetamine (DMA), 261f,
    263, 267
1,3-Dimethylamylamine (DMAA), 239–240
Dimethylserotonin, 273
Dimethyltryptamine (DMT), 268, 269f, 273–274
Diphenhydramine (Benadryl), 517, 518t, 641
Diphenoxylate, 348
Diprovan (propofol), 519
Discontinuation syndrome, 36
Disruptive behavior disorders, 597–598, 605–606,
    674
Dissociation rate, 85
Dissociative anesthetics, 280–281
Disulfiram (Antabuse), 120–121, 137, 158, 244
Divalproex. *See* Valproic acid (Depakene,
    Depakote, Depacon, Divalproex)
Diviner's sage, 283–285
DMA (dimethoxymethylamphetamine), 261f,
    263, 267
DMAA (1,3-dimethylamylamine), 239–240
DMT (dimethyltryptamine), 260, 268, 269f,
    273–274
DNA, 689–691, 690f
Dolophine. *See* Methadone (Dolophine)
DOM (dimethoxymethamphetamine), 261f, 263,
    267
Donepezil (Aricept), 646–647
Donepezil-memantine (Namzaric), 649

Dopamine, 42, 57–60, 60f
  in addiction, 110–112, 113–114, 121, 122
  amphetamines and, 229–230
  biosynthesis of, 57, 58f
  cannabis and, 297
  cocaine and, 223, 223f
  nicotine and, 192
  in Parkinson's disease, 633–637, 636f
  in reward circuits, 110–114, 110f
  in schizophrenia, 382–384. *See also*
      Antipsychotics
  structure of, 227f
  synthetic cathinones and, 236–237
Dopamine agonists, for stimulant abuse, 121,
    242
Dopamine phosphoprotein modulator, 412
Dopamine receptor agonists, for Parkinson's
    disease, 639
Dopamine-acetylcholine balance theory, 640
Doriden (glutethimide), 491f, 498
Dormalin (quazepam), 492t
Dorsal horn, 340
Dorsal root ganglia, 340
  in pain, 340, 341f
Dorsal-lateral prefrontal cortex, 44–46, 46f
Dose
  ED$_{50}$, 91–92
  LD$_{50}$, 91–92
  reference tables for, 681–688
  therapeutic index and, 90–92
Dose-response curves, 84–90, 84f, 87f, 89f
Downregulation, 35
Doxazosin (Cardura), 123, 243, 507, 508t
Doxepin (Adapin, Silenor, Sinequan), 439t, 444,
    508t, 510t, 518
DRESS syndrome, 405, 406
Drink equivalents, 138, 140, 175–176
Driving, impaired
  by alcohol, 145, 148, 307
  by benzodiazepines, 504–505, 509
  by marijuana, 145, 307
  sleep driving and, 509
Dronabinol (Marinol), 306, 315, 321
  for cannabis dependence, 321
Drug absorption, 3, 6–8
Drug abuse. *See also specific drugs*
  addiction in. *See* Addiction
  alcohol abuse and, 149
  by children and adolescents, 582–589
  controlled substance schedules and, 105, 106t
  craving in, 109–110, 114–115, 117, 151
  dependence in, 35
  DSM classification of, 108–109, 669–670
  eating and, 127
  epidemiology of, 105–108

  nosology of, 108–109
  overview of, 105–108
  psychiatric disorders and. *See* Comorbidity
  rates of, 105–108, 107f
  relapse in, 109–110, 114–115, 115f
  societal impact of, 105–108
  therapeutic applications of abused drugs in,
      102–103
  tolerance in, 34–36, 82, 83f, 112
  treatment of. *See also specific agents*
    agonist substitution in, 120–121
    antagonists in, 120–121
    antidiabetic agents in, 127
    chronic care management in, 157
    deep brain stimulation in, 127
    GABAergic drugs in, 123
    glutamatergic drugs in, 123–126
    new directions in, 127–128
    partial agonists in, 121–122
    religion in, 128
    vaccines in, 127
  urine testing in. *See* Urine testing
  withdrawal in. *See* Withdrawal
Drug administration. *See* Routes of
    administration
Drug allergies, 94, 349
Drug concentration
  half-life and, 29–33, 30f, 31t, 32f
  steady-state, 31–33, 32f
  therapeutic drug monitoring and, 33, 34f, 443
Drug dependence, 35
Drug distribution, 3, 14–20
  blood-brain barrier and, 18–19, 18f
  cell membranes and, 16–17, 16f
  in circulatory system, 9f, 14
  half-life and, 29–33, 30f, 31t, 32f
  placental barrier and, 19–20
  redistribution and, 29
Drug elimination, 3, 26–28, 28f
Drug hangover, 30
Drug interactions, 23–24
  cross-tolerance and, 24
  with food, 6–8, 446
  with herbs and dietary supplements, 26
  metabolic tolerance and, 23–24
  pharmacodynamics and, 92–93
  pharmacokinetics and, 23–24, 92–93
Drug metabolism, 3, 20–31, 24t
  active metabolites in, 21n
  conjugation in, 21–22
  drug interactions and, 23–24
  first-order elimination and, 31
  first-pass, 7, 14
  glucuronidation in, 22
  half-life and, 29–33, 30f, 31t, 32f

Drug metabolism (*Continued*)
  kidneys in, 26–28, 28f
  liver in, 23f, 28–29
  non-CYP enzymatic, 26, 27t
  P450 enzymes in, 21–26, 23f
  phase I reactions in, 21
  phase II reactions in, 21–22
  time course of, 29–33
  zero-order elimination and, 31, 138n
Drug names, 5n
Drug sensitization, 35
Drug testing. *See* Urine testing
Drug toxicity, 93–94
  definition of, 14
  receptors and, 81–82
Drug-receptor binding, 69, 80–82, 81f, 86–90, 87f,
    89f. *See also* Pharmacodynamics; Receptors
Drunk driving, 145, 148, 307
DSM (*Diagnostic and Statistical Manual of
    Mental Disorders*), 108–109, 669–670
DSP-1053, 474
Dual diagnosis, 109. *See also* Comorbidity
Duloxetine (Cymbalta), 441t, 452t, 461
Durapatch. *See* Fentanyl
Dyanavel XR, 603
Dynorphins, 54t, 343
Dysthymia, 435
Dystonia, 393

Early-onset alcoholism, 162
Eating, drug abuse and, 127
E-cigarettes, 199–202, 301, 582–583, 585
Ecstasy (MDMA), 237, 260, 263–265
ED$_{50}$, 91–92
Edluar (zolpidem), 510t, 511–513, 512f
Effexor. *See* Venlafaxine (Effexor)
Efficacy, 85f, 86
Eicosahexaenoic acid (DHA), 645–646
Elavil (amitriptyline), 439t, 442, 443, 444,
    517–518, 518t
Eldepryl (selegiline), 439t, 446, 639–640
Elderly, 625–654
  antipsychotics for, 417–418, 627–631
  benzodiazepines for, 501–502
  dementia in, 417–418, 627–631, 642–654.
    See also Alzheimer's disease; Dementia
  depression in, 631–633
  drugs under development for, 641–642
  inappropriate drug use in, 626–627
  most commonly used drugs for, 628t
  neuroprotective agents for, 642
  Parkinson's disease in, 633–637
  sedative-hypnotics for, 495
Electronic nicotine devices, 199–202, 301, 582–583
Elemicin, 261f, 267–268
Embeda-ER (morphine/naltrexone), 367

Empathogenic reactions, MDMA-induced, 264
Emsam (selegiline), 439t, 446–447, 634–640
Enantiomers, 80, 81f
Endocannabinoids, 298–300, 300f
Endorphins, 54t, 67, 343
Energy drinks, 177–178, 178t, 183–184. *See also*
    Caffeine
  for alcohol intoxication, 156
Enerzer (isocarboxazid), 439t
Enkephalins, 54t, 67, 343
Entacapone (Comtan), 636
Entereg (alvimopan), 348
Environmental tobacco smoke, 196
Enzyme induction, 23, 35
Enzyme receptors, 80
Ephedrine, 227–228, 235
Epicatechin, 653
Epidural injections, 11, 11t, 13
Epigenetics, 689–694
  genome structure and, 689–691, 690f
  methylation and, 691
Epilepsy. *See* Seizures
Epinephrine, 57–60, 227f
Epinephrine receptors, 57
Equanil (meprobamate), 491, 491f, 498
Equetro. *See* Carbamazepine (Equetro, Tegretol)
Erlotinib (Tarceva), 652
Erowid, 278
Erythoxylon coca, 217–218
Escitalopram (Lexapro), 441t, 450, 451t, 452t,
    458–459
  for children and adolescents, 591
  for elderly, 632
Esketamine, 473
Eslicarbazene (Aptiom), 523
Estazolam (ProSom), 492t, 508t
Eszopiclone (Lunesta), 508t, 510t, 511, 512f, 514
Ethanol. *See* Alcohol
Ethchlorvynol (Placidyl), 491f, 498
Ethosuximide, 520f, 521
Ethyl alcohol. *See* Alcohol; Alcohol use/abuse
Etomidate (Amidate), 519
Euphoria, opioid-induced, 345
Evekeo, 602–603
Exalgo (hydromorphone), 336t, 356–357
Exelon (rivastigmine), 646, 647
Exenatide (Ex-4), for drug abuse, 127
Exocytosis, 49–50
Extrapyramidal side effects, 384, 387, 393–394
Ezogabine (Potiga), 523

FAAH inhibitor, 321
Family Smoking and Prevention and Tobacco
    Control Act, 188
Family-focused therapy, 561
Fanapt (iloperidone), 397t, 398t, 401t, 402f, 407

Fazaclo. *See* Risperidone
Fecal microbiota transplant, 26
Fefitinib (Iressa), 652
Felbamate (Felbatol), 520f
Females, blood alcohol concentration in, 137
Fentanyl, 10, 336t, 357–358
    synthetic derivatives of, 372–373
Fertility, marijuana and, 309
Fetal alcohol effects, 153
Fetal alcohol syndrome, 152–154, 576
Fetal solvent syndrome, 167
Fetzima (levomilnacipran), 441t, 461
First-order elimination (kinetics), 31
First-pass metabolism, 7, 14
Flakka (α-pyrrolidinovalerophenone), 238–240
Flashbacks, LSD, 272
Flumazenil (Anexate, Romazicon), 123, 245, 506
Flunitrazepam (Rohypnol), 503
Fluoxetine (Prozac, Sarafem), 441t, 450, 451t,
        452t, 455–456
    drug interactions with, 24
    for pediatric depression, 590–591
Fluphenazine (Prolixin), 389t
Flurazepam (Dalmane), 492t, 508t
Fluvoxamine (Luvox), 450, 451t, 452t, 457
Folate, for depression, 470–471
Food, caffeine in, 178t
Food-drug interactions, 6–8, 446
Forebrain, 39, 40f, 42, 42f, 44
Forfivo. *See* Bupropion
Formication, 224
49-methyl-α-propiophenone (4-MePP), 238
Fospropofol (Lusedra), 519
4-MEC (4-methyl-N-ethylcathinone, 238
Foxy (5-methoxy-diisopropyltryptamine), 267
Freebase cocaine, 219
Frontal lobe, 44, 46f, 113–114, 114f, 128
Full opioid agonists, 335
Furanyl-fentanyl, 372
Fycompa (perampanel), 125, 523

GABA, 63, 65–66, 66f
    nicotine and, 192
    in reward circuits, 111
GABA receptor(s), 493–494, 493f
    alcohol and, 143
    benzodiazepines and, 493–494
    type A, 65–66, 66f, 71–72, 72f, 111
    type B, 66, 66f, 123
GABA receptor agonists, 493, 502
GABA transaminase inhibitors, 243
GABAergic drugs, 123, 243–244
Gabapentin (Gralise, Neurontin), 520f, 521
    for alcohol abuse, 125, 157, 161
    for bipolar disorder, 535t, 554
    for cannabis dependence, 123, 322
    for insomnia, 518t
    for marijuana abuse, 322
    for stimulant abuse, 245
Gabitril (tiagabine), 244, 520f, 522
Galantamine (Razadyne), 646, 647–648
Gambling, pathological, 155, 367
Gamma aminobutyric acid. *See* GABA
Gamma hydroxybutyrate (GHB, Xyrem), 498–499
Gamma-vinyl-GABA (Sabril, vigabatrin), 123,
        243, 522
Ganja, 295
Gastric bypass surgery, alcohol metabolism after,
        136, 137
Gastritis
    alcohol-induced, 152
    alcohol-related, 152
Gastrointestinal bleeding, SSRI-induced, 455
Gastrointestinal disorders, marijuana-induced, 306
General anesthetics, 518–519
Generalized anxiety disorder, 490. *See also*
        Anxiety disorders
Generic drug names, 5n
Genetic factors
    in bipolar disorder, 534
    in depression, 437, 466–467
    in drug metabolism, 22–23, 24t
    in nicotine dependence, 194
    in placebo effect, 96
    in schizophrenia, 381–383, 385–386
Genetic opioid metabolic defects, 349–350
Genome, structure of, 689–691, 690f
Geodon. *See* Ziprasidone (Geodon)
GHB (gamma hydroxybutyrate), 498–499
Glaucoma, marijuana for, 311–312
Glia, 48
Glial cells
    in glutamate regulation, 117
    types of, 48–49
Glial sheath, 19
Glial-glutamate transporter (GLT-1), 117, 123–124
Globus pallidus, 43, 43f
Glomerulus, 27, 28f
GLP-1, 127
GLT-1 (glial-glutamate transporter), 117, 123–124
Glucophage (Metformin), 554, 651
Glucuronidation, 22
Glue sniffing, 163–167. *See also* Inhalant abuse
Glutamate, 63–65, 64f
    in addiction, 116–117, 116f, 123–126
    biosynthesis of, 63
    neuronal toxicity of, 65
    nicotine and, 192
    in schizophrenia, 382
Glutamate receptors, 63–65, 143
Glutamatergic drugs, for stimulant abuse,
        243–244

Glutamatergic model of addiction, 123–126
Glutaminergic NMDA receptor antagonists, 279–282, 279f, 472–473
Glutaminergic psychedelics, 258, 258t. *See also* Psychedelic drugs
Glutethimide (Doriden), 491f, 498
GLYX-13 (rapastinel), 473, 476
G-protein-coupled (metabotropic) receptors, 63, 71f–77f, 72–77, 87, 343–344, 344f
Gralise. *See* Gabapentin (Gralise, Neurontin)
Grapefruit, drug absorption and, 8
Guanfacine (Intuniv), 604
Gut microbiome, 25–26
    depression and, 472
Gut-brain peptides, 67

Halazepam (Paxipam), 492t
Halcion (triazolam), 4–5, 5f, 492t, 508t, 511
Half-life, 29–33, 30f, 31t, 32f
Hallucinations. *See also* Psychedelic drugs
    alcohol and, 151
    in dementia, 418
    DMT and, 273
    LSD and, 268–270, 271, 272
    MDMA and, 263
    MDMA substitutes and, 265–267
    in schizophrenia, 275
Hallucinogen persisting perception disorder, 272
Hallucinogens, 257. *See also* Psychedelic drugs
Haloperidol (Haldol), 389t
    for bipolar disorder, 535t, 555–558
    for schizophrenia, 409
Harm reduction, 155
Harmine, 273
Harrison Narcotic Act, 339
Hashish, 292. *See also* Marijuana
Head injury, marijuana for, 311
Heart disease. *See also* Cardiovascular disorders
    alcohol and, 146
    antipsychotic-induced, 405, 406f, 407f
    cocaine abuse and, 224
    in inhalant abuse, 166–167
    methamphetamine abuse and, 232
    quetiapine-related, 405, 406f
    smoking and, 195, 196
Hemp, 295
Hepatocytes, drug metabolism in, 28–29
Heroin abuse, 353–354. *See also* Opioid(s)
    cocaine abuse and, 225, 354
    drug therapy for
        LAAM in, 360
        methadone in, 120, 359–360, 369
        nalmefene in, 336t, 367
        naloxone in. *See* Naloxone (Narcan)
        naltrexone in, 122, 366–367, 370

immune system in, 370
outcome in, 369–370
reward system in, 370
TLR4 receptor in, 370
urine testing for, 353
vaccine for, 370
Heterocyclic antidepressants. *See* Antidepressant(s)
Heteromer, 186
Hindbrain, 39, 40f
Hippocampus, 44, 45f
    in addiction, 114, 114f, 117
    in depression, 436–437
Histones, 689–691, 690f
    acetylation of, 691–692
    methylation of, 691–692
Hoasca, 273
Hookahs, 198
HS665, 368
5-HT. *See* Serotonin
Huffing, 163–167. *See also* Inhalant abuse
Human Connectome Project, 47
Huperzine A, 648
Hydrocodone, 336t, 354–355. *See also* Opioid(s)
Hydrocodone/acetaminophen (Lortab, Vicodin), 336t, 354–355
Hydromorphone (Dilaudid, Palladone), 336t, 354, 356–357
Hydronephrosis, ketamine-induced, 281
5-Hydroxy DMT, 273
5-Hydroxytryptamine (5-HT). *See* Serotonin
Hydroxyzine, 245
Hyoscyamine, 258
Hyperglycemia, antipsychotic-induced, 403
Hyperthermia, malignant, 263
Hypofrontality, 113–114
Hyponatremia, SSRI-induced, 455
Hypothalamus, 42, 42f
Hypoxia, in inhalant abuse, 166
Hysingla, 355

Ibudilast, 245–246
"Ice," 228, 232. *See also* Methamphetamine
Idalopirdine, 652
Ifenprodil, 126
Iloperidone (Fanapt), 397t, 398t, 401t, 402f, 407
Imipramine (Tofranil), 439t, 442, 443, 590
Immovane (zoplicone), 514
Immunosuppression, marijuana-related, 305–306
Imodium (loperamide), 348
IMPACT model, 631–632
Inderal. *See* Propranolol (Inderal)
Indolamine neurotransmitters, 54t, 61f, 62, 62f.
        See also Serotonin
Infertility, marijuana and, 309
Ingrezza (valbenazine), for tardive dyskinesia, 394

Inhalant abuse, 163–167, 164t, 518
  acute effects of, 166
  by children and adolescents, 164–166
  chronic effects of, 166–167
  inhaled substances in, 163, 164t, 518
  long-term effects of, 166–167
  treatment of, 167
  withdrawal in, 167
Inhalation anesthetics, 518
Inhalational administration, 8–9, 9f
Injections
  epidural, 11, 11t, 13
  intramuscular, 11t, 12–13
  intrathecal, 11, 11t, 13
  intravenous, 11–12, 11t
  subcutaneous, 11t, 13
Inosine, 642
Insomnia, 687t
  anticonvulsants for, 518, 518t
  antidepressants for, 510t, 518
  antihistamines for, 518, 518t
  antipsychotics for, 518, 518t
  benzodiazepine receptor agonists for, 508–514,
    510t, 512f
  benzodiazepines for, 503, 508–510, 508t, 510t
  cognitive-behavioral therapy for, 509
  conotoxins for, 511
  melatonin receptor agonists for, 510t, 514–516
  nonbenzodiazepines for, 508t, 510t, 511–514
  off-label agents for, 517–518, 518t
  orexin antagonists for, 510t, 516–517
Insula (insular cortex), 46
  nicotine dependence and, 206
Insulin resistance, antipsychotic-induced, 403
Intermezzo (zolpidem), 510t, 511–513, 512f
International Classification of Diseases, 669–670
Interpersonal and social rhythm therapy, 561
Intramuscular administration, 11t, 12–13
Intrathecal injections, 11, 11t, 13
Intravenous administration, 11–12, 11t
Intravenous immunoglobulin, for Alzheimer's
    disease, 651
Intuniv (guanfacine), 604
Invega (paliperidone), 397t, 398t, 401t, 402f, 407
Inverse agonists, 87, 87f
Ion channel (ionotropic) receptors, 55–56, 63–65,
    65f, 70–72, 71f–73f
Ionsys. *See* Fentanyl
iQOS, 199
Irdabisant (CEP-26401), 412
Iressa (fefitinib), 652
Irreversible acetylcholine esterase inhibitors, 80
Irreversible antagonists, 89, 89f
Irritable bowel syndrome, placebo effects in, 95
Isocarboxazid (Enerzer, Marplan), 439t, 445–446

Isomers, 80–82, 81f
Isradipine (Prescal), 642
ITI-007 (lumateperone), 412

Jamestown weed, 259
Jimsonweed, 259
JNJ-42847922, 476

"K2" (synthetic marijuana), 315–318, 677
Kainate receptors, 63, 64
Kappa receptor, 67, 343, 343t
Kappa receptor agonists, 368
Kappa receptor antagonists, 474
Kapvay (clonidine), 604
Keppra (levetiracetam), 522, 523
Ketamine (Ketalar), 279–282, 279f, 385
  for alcohol dependence, 163
  for bipolar disorder, 472–473
  for depression, 472–473
Khat *(Catha edulis)*, 235
Khedezla (desvenlafaxine), 441t
Kidney
  in drug elimination, 26–28, 28f
  ketamine-induced injury of, 281
Kindling, alcohol withdrawal seizures and, 151
Klonopin (clonazepam), 492t
Korsakoff's syndrome, 151–152
KP201 (benzhydrocodone), 355
Kratom, 371
Krypton, 361

LAAM (levo-alpha acetylmethadol), 361
Lacosamide (Vimpat), 522
Lamotrigine (Lamictal), 520f, 522
  for alcohol abuse, 125, 157
  for bipolar disorder, 469, 535t, 540–541,
    552–553, 596
  for cocaine abuse, 244
  in pregnancy, 553, 581
Largactil (chlorpromazine), 386, 389t
Latrepirdine (Dimebon), 650
Latuda (lurasidone), 397t, 398t, 401t, 402f, 408,
    559t
Laudanum, 300, 338
LD$_{50}$, 91–92
L-dopa. *See* Levodopa
Leu-enkephalin, 343
Levetiracetam (Keppra), 162, 522, 523
Levo-alpha acetylmethadol (LAAM), 361
Levodexedrine, 227
Levodopa
  for cocaine abuse, 242
  new formulations of, 641
  "off-on" episodes with, 638, 641
  for Parkinson's disease, 635–639

Levodopa/carbidopa (Sinemet), 635
Levodopa/carbidopa/entacapone (Stalevo), 636, 638
Levomilnacipran (Fetzima), 441t, 461
Levorotatory isomers, 80, 81f
Levorphanol (Levo Dromoran), 336t
Levo-tetrahydropalmatine (l-THP), 245
Lexapro. See Escitalopram (Lexapro)
Liberation phase, 3n
Librium (chlordiazepoxide), 157, 491, 492t
Limbic system, 43–44, 45f
    in addiction, 116–117, 116f
    in reward circuits, 110f, 111
Lioresal (baclofen), 123, 160–161, 243
Lipid-soluble drugs, 6–7, 16–17
    distribution of, 16–17
    excretion of, 27–28
Lisdexamfetamine (Vyvanse), 6, 229, 608
Lithium, 474–548
    BALANCE study of, 548
    clinical example of, 673–674
    in combination therapy, 547
    for depression, 468–469
    for disruptive behavior disorders, 598
    drug interactions with, 26
    effectiveness of, 535t, 542–544, 543f, 543t
    LiTMUS study for, 547–548
    mechanism of action of, 539–541
    nonadherence to, 547
    for pediatric patients, 547
    pharmacodynamics of, 544–545
    pharmacokinetics of, 544
    in pregnancy, 546–547, 580–582
    side effects and toxicity of, 545–547
LiTMUS study, 547–548
Liver
    alcohol-induced injury of, 151
    in drug metabolism, 23f, 28–29
Locus coeruleus, 57, 59f
Lofexidine, for cannabis dependence, 321
Lomotil, 348
Lonasen (blonanserine), 412
Loperamide (Imodium), 348
Lophophora williamsii, 262
Lorazepam (Ativan), 4–5, 5f, 158, 492t
Lortab (hydrocodone/acetaminophen), 354–355
Loxapine (Adasuve, Loxitane), 389t, 557
LSD, 260, 268–272
    adverse effects and toxicity of, 272
    CIA's use of, 275, 276
    flashbacks and, 272
    historical perspective on, 268–270
    pharmacokinetics of, 270
    physiological effects of, 270
    psychological effects of, 270–271
    regulation of, 275, 276
    serotonin and, 61, 384
    therapeutic use of, 275–278
    tolerance and dependence and, 272
Lu AF35700, 410
Lubiprostone (Amitiza), 348
Ludiomil (maprotiline), 447
Lumateperone (ITI-007), 412
Lunch-hour drug, 272
Lunesta (eszopiclone), 508t, 510t, 511, 512f, 514
Lung
    drug absorption by, 9f, 16–17
    smoking-related diseases of, 195
Lurasidone (Latuda), 397t, 398t, 401t, 402f, 408, 535t, 559t
Lusedra (fospropofol), 519
Luvox (fluvoxamine), 450, 451t, 452t, 457
LY-2940094, 477
Lyrica (pregabalin), 157, 505, 507, 554
Lysergic acid amide, 274
Lysergic acid diethylamide. See LSD

Mace, 267–268
Magic mint, 283–285
Magic mushrooms (psilocybin), 260, 268, 273–274, 277
Ma-huang (ephedrine), 227, 235
Major depressive disorder. See Depression
Malathion, 55
Malignant hyperthermia, 263
Mandragora officinarum, 259
Mandrake, 259
Mania, monoamine (receptor) hypothesis of, 442
Manic-depressive disorder. See Bipolar disorder
MAOIs (monoamine oxidase inhibitors), 57, 80, 93, 438–440, 445–447, 683t. See also Antidepressant(s)
Maprotiline (Ludiomil), 447
Margin of safety, 91–92, 91f
Marijuana, 292–323. See also Cannabis
    cannabinoid receptors and, 295f, 296–298
    delivery methods for, 301–303
    edible, 302, 303
    endocannabinoids and, 298–300, 300f
    mechanism of action of, 296–298, 297f
    pharmacokinetics of, 301–304, 304f
    physiological effects of, 301–304
    psychoactive effects of, 306–310
    regulation of, 293–294
    rewarding effects of, 307
    synthetic, 108, 291, 315–318, 586, 676–677
    THC in, 295, 295f, 301–302
    therapeutic applications of, 293–294, 310–313
    urine testing for, 302
    vaping of, 301, 585

Marijuana use/abuse, 319–321
  by adolescents, 584–586
  alcohol abuse and, 126–127, 144–145
  dependence in, 319–320
  epidemiology of, 107–108, 292
  historical perspective on, 292–294
  legalization of, 320–321
  medical uses, 293–294, 310–313
    by adolescents, 584
    for Alzheimer's disease, 312
    for anxiety disorders, 312–313
    for appetite stimulation, 306
    for brain injury, 311
    for cancer, 311
    for epilepsy, 311
    for glaucoma, 311–312
    for multiple sclerosis, 306
    for neuroprotection, 311
    for pain and spasticity, 310–311
    for posttraumatic stress disorder, 312–313
    for schizophrenia, 313
  memory impairment and, 308
  in pregnancy, 309–310, 576
  psychological disorders, 315
  rates of, 107–108
  tolerance in, 319
  treatment of, 123, 321–322
  urine testing for, 302
  withdrawal in, 319
Marinol (dronabinol), 306, 315, 321
Marplan (isocarboxazid), 445–446
Mazindol, 609
mCPP (meta-chlorophenylpiperazine), 266
MDA (methylenedioxyamphetamine), 263, 267
MDAI (5,6-methylenedioxy-2-aminoindane), 265
MDE (methylenedioxyethylamphetamine), 261f, 263, 267
MDMA (Ecstasy), 237, 260, 263–265
MDMA-related drugs, 265–267
MDPV (3,4-methylenedioxypyrovalerone), 236f, 237–238
4-MEC (4-methyl-N-ethylcathinone, 238
Medial forebrain bundle, 44, 45f
Medical marijuana. *See* Marijuana use/abuse, medical uses
Medulla, 40, 40f, 41f
Melatonin, 514–515
Melatonin receptor agonists, 510t, 514–516
Mellaril (thioridazine), 389t
Memantine (Namenda)
  for alcohol abuse, 125
  for Alzheimer's disease, 644, 648–649
  for Parkinson's disease, 641
Memory
  alcohol and, 149

  antidepressants and, 444
  marijuana and, 308
  MDMA and, 264
Mental illness, epidemiology of, 668–669
Mental time travel, 278
Menthol cigarettes, 191
5-MeO-DIPT, 263
Meperidine (Demerol), 336t, 357
Mephedrone (methcathinone), 236–238, 236f, 265
Meprobamate (Equanil, Miltown), 491, 491f, 498
Mescaline, 260, 261f, 262
Mesocortical pathway, 60
Mesolimbic dopamine pathway, 60, 110–112, 110f
Metabolic syndrome, antipsychotic-related, 400, 401t, 403, 404
Metabolic tolerance, 23
Metabolism. *See* Drug metabolism
Metabolites, active, 21n
Metabotropic (G-protein-coupled) receptors, 55–56, 63, 71f–77f, 72–77, 87, 343–344, 344f
Meta-chlorophenylpiperazine (mCPP), 266
Met-enkephalin, 343
Metformin (Glucophage), 554, 651
Methadone (Dolophine), 336t, 359–360
  for chronic pain, 359
  for heroin abuse, 120, 359–360, 369
  in pregnancy, 364–365
Methamphetamine. *See also* Amphetamine(s)
  for cocaine abuse, 242–243
  dose-response curve for, 85–86, 85f
  historical perspective on, 227–229
  mechanism of action of, 229–230
  pharmacokinetics of, 229
  pharmacological effects of, 230–231
  preparations of, 232
  side effects and toxicity of, 231, 232–234, 607–608
  smokeable, 228, 232
  structure of, 226–227, 227f
Methamphetamine abuse
  by adolescents, 228–229, 584, 608
  in pregnancy, 234
  tolerance and dependence in, 234–235
  treatment of, 242–243
    dopaminergic/adrenergic approaches in, 242–243
    GABAergic/glutamatergic approaches in, 243–244
    vaccines in, 247–248
Methaqualone (Quaalude), 491f, 498
Methcathinone (Mephedrone), 236–238, 236f, 265

Methohexital (Brevital), 519
Methoxetamine, 282
5-Methoxy-diisopropyltryptamine (5-MeO-DIPT, Foxy), 267
49-Methyl-α-propiophenone (4-MePP), 238
Methylation, histone, 691–692
Methylene blue, 652
Methylenedioxyamphetamine (MDA), 261f, 263, 267
Methylenedioxyethylamphetamine (MDE), 261f, 263, 267
Methylenedioxymethamphetamine (MDMA, Ecstasy), 260, 263–265
3,4-Methylenedioxypyrovalerone (MDPV), 236f, 237–238
3-Methyl-fentanyl (TMF), 372
Methylhexaneamine (DMAA), 239–240
4-Methylmethcathinone (Mephedrone), 236, 237f, 265
Methylnaltrexone (Relistor), 348
4-Methyl-N-ethylcathinone (4-MEC), 238
Methylone, 237
Methylphenidate (Ritalin)
    for attention-deficit/hyperactivity disorder, 240, 240f, 600–602, 603, 605
    for cocaine abuse, 242
    for depression, 448–449
    for disruptive behavior disorders, 598
    in pregnancy, 577
    receptor effects and, 82
Methylprylon (Noludar), 491f
α-Methyltryptamine, 267
Metyrapone, 245
MH6, 248
Mickey Finn, 498
Microbiome, 25–26
    depression and, 472
Midazolam (Versed), 492t, 495
Midbrain, 39, 40, 40f, 41, 41f
Mifepristone (RU-486), 477
Milnacipran (Savella), 452t
Miltown (meprobamate), 491, 491f, 498
MIN-101, 411
MIN-117, 474
Minipress (prazosin), 507
Miosis, opioid-induced, 348
Mirapex (pramipexole), for Parkinson's disease, 639
Mirtazapine (Remeron)
    for akathisia, 393
    for depression, 441t, 452t, 462–463, 632
Mixed agonists-antagonists, 335–336, 365, 367–368
Mixed opioid agonist-antagonists, 335–337
Mixed serotonin-norepinephrine reuptake inhibitors, 448

Moban (molindone), 389t
Moclobemide, 446
Modafinil (Provigil), 240–241, 240f
    in agonist substitution treatment, 120–121
    with antidepressants, 468–469
    for drug abuse, 124
    for methamphetamine abuse, 246
    for stimulant abuse, 243
"Mojo" (synthetic marijuana), 315–318
Molindone (Moban), 389t
Monitoring the Future study, 108
Monoamine (receptor) hypothesis, for depression and mania, 442
Monoamine oxidase, 57, 80
Monoamine oxidase inhibitors (MAOIs), 57, 80, 93, 438–440, 445–447. *See also* Antidepressant(s)
Monoaminergic (serotonergic) hallucinogens, 268–278
Monoaminergic neuroreceptors, 57–67
Monoaminergic psychedelics, 260
Mood stabilizers, 535–555, 535t, 684t. *See also* Lithium
    for alcohol withdrawal, 157
    anticonvulsants as, 535t, 549–555
    for bipolar disorder, 535–538
    for children and adolescents, 547
    clinical example of, 673–674
    for disruptive behavior disorders, 598
    drug interactions with, 26
    mechanism of action of, 539–541
    in pregnancy, 546–547, 553, 579–582
    STEP-BD study of, 539–541
    types of, 535t
Moonflower, 259
Morning glory seeds, 274
Morphine (MS-Contin, Rylomine), 335, 336t, 337n, 338–339, 351–353. *See also* Opioid(s)
Morphine/naltrexone (Embeda-ER), 367
Movantik (naloxegol), 348
Movement disorders
    antipsychotic-induced, 384, 387, 394–396
    levodopa-induced, 637
MS-Contin (morphine), 336t, 338–339, 351. *See also* Opioid(s)
M-smack, 265
Mu (μ) receptor, 67, 126, 342–345, 343t
Mu (μ) receptor agonists/antagonists, 474
Mucomyst (*N*-acetylcysteine), 123–124, 244
Mucous membranes, drug absorption by, 10
Multiple sclerosis
    caffeine and, 182
    marijuana for, 310
    nicotine and, 195
Muscarinic receptor antagonists, 640–641

Muscarinic receptors, 55–56
Mushrooms, psilocybin in, 260, 268, 273–274, 274, 277
Myelin sheath, 49
Myristicin, 261f, 267–268

Nabilone (Cesamet), 306, 308, 315, 321
Nabiximols (Sativex), 310–311
Nalbuphine (Nubain), 365
Nalfurafine (Remitch), 368, 369
Nalmefene (Revex, Selincro), 159, 336t, 367
Naloxegol (Movantik), 348
Naloxone (Narcan), 122, 336t, 366, 370, 599
   with buprenorphine, 362
   for opioid-induced constipation, 348
   for respiratory depression, 346, 366
Naltrexone (ReVia, Trexan, Vivitrol), 336t, 366–367
   administration of, 12
   for alcohol abuse, 126, 144, 158–159, 160, 162–163, 367
   for amphetamine abuse, 126
   for cannabis dependence, 365
   for cocaine abuse, 245
   for heroin abuse, 122, 366–367, 368, 370
   implant for, 159
   with morphine, 367
   with oxycodone, 368
Namenda. See Memantine (Namenda)
Namzaric (memantine/donepizil), 649
Nanocolumns, 50
Narcan. See Naloxone (Narcan)
Narcolepsy
   GHB for, 498–499
   modafinil for, 240–241
Narcotics, 335. See also Opioid(s)
Nardil (phenelzine), 439t, 445–446
Narghiles, 198
National Drug Control Strategies, 105–106
National Survey on Drug Use and Health (NSDUH), 107
Nausea and vomiting
   marijuana-induced, 306
   opioid-induced, 347
Navane (thiothixene), 389t
Nefazodone (Serzone), 441t, 461–462
Nephron, 27, 28f
Nepicast, 244
Nervous system
   autonomic (visceral), 226
   central, 39. See also Brain; Spinal cord
   parasympathetic, 226n
   peripheral, 39
   sympathetic, 226n
Neupro (rotigotine), 639
Neurodevelopmental disorder, alcohol-related, 153

Neurogenesis, 49
   antidepressants and, 436–438
Neurogenic theory of depression, 436–438
Neuroleptic malignant syndrome, 395
Neuromodulators, 549–555
Neurons, 49, 50f
Neurontin. See Gabapentin (Gralise, Neurontin)
Neuroprotective agents, 642
   marijuana as, 311
Neurotoxicity
   of MDMA, 263–264
   of methamphetamine, 232–234
Neurotransmitters, 49–67
   acetylcholine, 54–57
   amino acid, 63–66
   catecholamine, 57–60
   classification of, 53, 54t
   co-release of, 67
   indolamine, 62
   monoaminergic, 57–67
   in pain transmission, 340–342
   peptide, 67
   processing of, 51–53
   release of, 49–51
   types of, 53–67
Neurotransporters, 19, 77–80, 79f
Neurotrophins, 437
New psychoactive substances, 102–103
Nexus, 265
NIC002 vaccine, 205
Nicotinamide adenine dinucleotide (NAD), 137
Nicotine, 187–206. See also Smoking
   absorption of, 189
   adolescent use of, 582–583
   bipolar disorder and, 193
   cancer and, 195, 196
   cardiovascular disease and, 195, 196
   cognitive effects of, 192–193
   delivery methods for, 188, 197–202
   depression and, 193
   mechanism of action of, 190–191, 191f
   menthol and, 191
   pharmacokinetics of, 189–190
   pharmacological effects of, 192–194
      acute, 193–194
      on brain, 192–193
   pulmonary disease and, 195, 196
   schizophrenia and, 193
   tolerance to, 194
   toxicity of, 194–196
   vapor products and, 199–202
Nicotine dependence, 194
   agonist substitution therapy for, 120
   behavioral approaches to, 197
   bupropion for, 202, 204

Nicotine dependence (*Continued*)
  cravings and, 194
  cytisine for, 198
  dianicline for, 202
  e-cigarettes for, 199–202
  genetic factors in, 194
  insular cortex and, 206
  nicotine replacement therapy for, 120, 202, 205
  nortriptyline for, 202
  partial agonist substitution therapy for, 121–122
  pharmacological approaches for, 197–206
  vaccines for, 205
  varenicline for, 121, 202
  withdrawal and, 194
Nicotinic receptors, 55–56, 190–191, 191f
NicQbeta, 205
NicVAX, 205
Nilotinib (Tasigna), 642
Nitrite inhalants, 163–164. *See also* Inhalant abuse
Nitrous oxide, 164t, 165–166, 518. *See also* Inhalant abuse
NKTR-181, 369
NMDA receptor(s), 64–65, 65f
  in addiction, 116, 125–126
  alcohol and, 143
  dextromethorphan and, 283
  ketamine and, 280
  methoxetamine and, 282
  PCP and, 280
  in schizophrenia, 280
NMDA receptor agonists/antagonists, 279–282, 279f, 475–476
Nocebo effects, 96
Nociceptin receptor, 343, 343t, 477
Noctec (chloral hydrate), 497
Noladin ether, 300f
Noludar (methylprylon), 491f, 498
Nonbenzodiazepines, for insomnia, 508t, 510t, 511–514
Noncompetitive antagonists, 89, 89f
Nonsteroidal antiinflammatory agents, lithium and, 26
Noradrenaline, synthetic cathinones and, 236–237
Noradrenergic/specific serotonergic antidepressants, 441t, 462–463. *See also* Antidepressant(s)
Norco, 354
Norepinephrine, 57–60
  amphetamines and, 229–230
  biosynthesis of, 57, 58f
  structure of, 227f, 261f
Norepinephrine pathways, 57–59, 59f
Norepinephrine receptors, 57

Norepinephrine-dopamine reuptake inhibitors, 441t. *See also* Antidepressant(s)
Norpramine (desipramine), 439t, 442, 445
Nortriptyline (Aventyl, Pamelor)
  for depression, 439t, 442, 443
  for nicotine dependence, 202
Novel psychoactive substances, 102–103
Novocaine (procaine), 218
NRX-1074, 476
NSAIDs (nonsteroidal antiinflammatory agents), lithium and, 26
NSI-189, 477
Nubain (nalbuphine), 365
Nucleosomes, 690–691
Nucleus accumbens, 44, 45f, 110–112, 110f, 116, 116f
  nicotine and, 192
  therapeutic stimulation of, 127
Nucleus basilis, 56
Nucynta (Tapentadol), 336t, 358–359
Numorphan (oxymorphone), 356–357
Nuplazid (pimavanserin), 384, 411–412, 417, 637, 645
Nutmeg, 267–268
Nuvigil (armodafinil), 240, 241–242, 469
NW-3509, 411

Obesity. *See also* Weight gain
  caffeine and, 181
Obsessive-compulsive disorder, 490, 685t. *See also* Anxiety disorders
  antidepressants for, 448
  antipsychotics for, 420
  brain abnormalities in, 494–495
  in children and adolescents, 594–595
Occipital lobe, 44, 46f
Olanzapine (Relprevv, Zydis, Zyprexa), 397t, 401t, 404–405, 408–410
  with antidepressants, 468–469
  for bipolar disorder, 415–416, 535t, 555–558, 559t
  for borderline personality disorder, 420–421
  for dementia, 629–630
  for disruptive behavior disorders, 598
  indications for, 398t
  for obsessive-compulsive disorder, 420
  for Parkinson's disease, 421
  for posttraumatic stress disorder, 419
  side effects of, 401t, 402f
Olanzapine/fluoxetine (Symbyax), 416, 456, 468, 556, 559t
N-Oleoylethanolamine (OEA), 300f
Oleptro (trazodone), 447
Oliceridine (Olinvo), 370
Ololiuqui, 274

Omega-3 fatty acids
    for Alzheimer's disease, 645–646
    for bipolar disorder, 558–559
    for depression, 421–422, 470
OMS 824, 413
Ondansetron (Zoftran), 162
Onfi (clobazam), 492t, 522–523
Onsolis. *See* Fentanyl
Opana (oxymorphone), 336t, 356–357
Opioid(s), 333–373
    adverse reactions to, 339–340
    allergic reactions to, 349
    analgesic effects of, 345
    benzodiazepines and, 339–340
    Boxed Warnings for, 340
    cannabinoids and, 126–127
    for children and adolescents, 553, 598–600
    classification of, 335–337, 336t
    constipation and, 348
    under development, 368–369
    for diarrhea, 347–348
    drug interactions with, 24, 339–340, 349–350
    euphoric, 345
    historical perspective on, 337–340
    mechanism of action of, 340–341, 340–342
    metabolism of, genetic defects in, 349–350
    overdose of
        genetic defects and, 349–350
        naloxone reversal for, 346
    overview of, 333–334
    pharmacological effects of, 345–349
    placebo effects of, 94–97
    regulation of, 339–340
    semisynthetic, 335
    synthetic, 335
    terminology of, 335–337
Opioid agonists
    biased, 370
    full, 351–360
    mixed agonist-antagonist, 335–336, 365,
        367–368
    partial, 361–365
    pure, 366–368
Opioid agonists-antagonists, 365, 367–368
Opioid antagonists, 122–123, 337
    for alcohol dependence, 158–159
    mixed, 365, 367–368
    pure, 366–368
Opioid misuse/abuse
    abstinence syndrome in, 351, 351t
    government policy and, 334–335
    illicit drugs in, 371–372
    immune system in, 370
    outcome in, 369–370
    overdose deaths in, 334–335, 335f

overview of, 333–335
    potential for, 345
    in pregnancy, 352
    rates of, 107–108
    reward system in, 370
    TLR4 receptor in, 370
    tolerance and dependence in, 350–351, 351t
    treatment of
        buprenorphine in, 121, 361–363
        future directions in, 369–370
        methadone in, 120, 336t, 359–360
        nalmefene in, 367
        naloxone in, 122, 336t, 366, 370
        naloxone/oxycodone in, 367–368
        naltrexone in, 122, 366–367
        naltrexone/morphine in, 367
        naltrexone/oxycodone in, 368
        office-based, 10
        vaccines in, 370
    withdrawal in, 350–351, 351t
Opioid peptides, 54t, 67
Opioid receptors, 67, 126, 144, 341–345, 343t, 344f
Opium, 337–339, 338f. *See also* Opioid(s)
Optogenetics, 53
Oral administration, 6–8
Orap (pimozide), 389t
Orbital prefrontal cortex, 44, 46f
Orcein, 651
Orexin antagonists, 476, 510t, 516–517
Organelles, 49, 50f
Orthosteric binding sites, 87
Oxazepam (Serax), 245, 492t
Oxcarbazepine (Trileptal), 520f, 522, 523, 535t
    for alcohol withdrawal, 157
    for bipolar disorder, 535t, 550–551
Oxycodone (OxyContin, Percodan, Xtampza-ER,
        Remoxy), 336t, 355–356, 599–600. *See also*
        Opioid(s)
Oxymorphone (Numorphan, Opana), 336t,
        356–357
Oxytocin, 246

P450 system, 21–26, 23f
Pain
    acute, 333
    alcohol and, 147
    antidepressants for, 444
    buprenorphine for, 361–362
    chronic, 333
    insensitivity to, 342
    marijuana for, 310–311
    methadone for, 359
    terminology of, 335–337
    transmission of, 340–341, 341f
Pain management. *See* Analgesics; Opioid(s)

Paliperidone (Invega, Sustenna, Maintena), 397t, 398t, 401t, 402f, 407, 535t
Palladone (hydromorphone), 336t, 356–357
N-Palmitoylethanolamine (PEA), 300f
Pamelor. *See* Nortriptyline (Aventyl, Pamelor)
Pancreatitis, alcohol-induced, 152
Panic disorder, 490. *See also* Anxiety disorders
Papaverine, 335
Paraldehyde, 497
Parasympathetic nervous system, 226n
Parathion, 55
Paraxanthine, 179, 179f
Parietal lobe, 44, 46f
Parkinsonism, 393
Parkinson's disease, 633–639
  antipsychotics for, 421
  caffeine and, 182
  levo-dopa for, 635–639
  nicotine and, 192–193
  placebo effects in, 96–97
Parlodel (bromocriptine), 225, 242, 269f, 395, 639
Parnate (tranylcypromine), 439t, 445–446
Paroxetine (Paxil), 441t, 450, 451t, 452t, 457
  for bipolar disorder, 556
  for children and adolescents, 590
  for elderly, 632
Partial agonist substitution treatment, 121–122
Partial agonists, 87f, 88, 121–122, 335
Partial nicotine receptor agonists, 203–205
Passive diffusion, 6
Passive smoking, 196
Patches, transdermal, 10–11
Pathological gambling, 155, 367
Paxil. *See* Paroxetine (Paxil)
Paxipam (halazepam), 492t
PBT2, 651
PCP. *See* Phencyclidine (PCP)
PDE9 inhibitors, 413
Pediatric psychopharmacology. *See* Child and adolescent psychopharmacology
Pemoline (Cylert), 240, 240f
Penicillin, 19
Pentazocine (Talwin), 336t, 365
Pentothal (thiopental), 519
Peptide neurotransmitters, 54t, 67
Perampanel (Fycompa), 125, 523
Percodan (oxycodone), 336t, 355–356, 367–368
Periaqueductal gray, 340
  in pain, 340, 341f
Peripheral nervous system, 39
Perphenazine (Trilafon), 389t
Persistent depressive disorder, 435
Personality disorders, 420–421

Peyote, 262
PF329, 369
PF-04457845, 120
PF-04958242, 411
P-glycoproteins, 19
Pharmacodynamic tolerance, 35
Pharmacodynamics, 1, 2, 69–97
  definition of, 69
  dose-response curves and, 84–90, 87f, 89f
  drug interactions and, 92–93
  drug-receptor interaction and, 69–84. *See also* Receptors
  drug-receptor specificity and, 80–82, 81f
  nocebo effects and, 96
  placebo effects and, 94–97
  second messengers and, 75–77, 78f
  side effects and, 81–82, 84
  therapeutic index and, 90–97
Pharmacokinetics, 1–2, 31–36
  absorption and, 3, 6–8
  bioavailability and, 3
  definition of, 3
  distribution and, 3, 14–20
  drug interactions and, 23–24, 92–93
  elimination and, 3, 26–31
    first-order, 31
    zero-order, 31, 138n
  half-life and, 29–33, 30f, 31t, 32f
  metabolism and, 3, 20–31
  overview of, 3, 4f
  steady-state concentration and, 31–33, 32f
  therapeutic drug monitoring and, 33, 34f, 443
Pharmacology, definition of, 1
Phencyclidine (PCP), 279–282, 279f
  glutamate and, 89–90, 385
Phenelzine (Nardil), 439t, 445–446
Phenobarbital, 490–491, 491f, 520
Phenothiazines, 386
Phenylisopropylamine, 227
Phenytoin (Dilantin), 520–521, 520f
Phobias, 490. *See also* Anxiety disorders
Phospholipids, 16
Pimavanserin (Nuplazid), 384, 411–412, 417, 421, 637, 645
Pimozide (Orap), 389t
Pioglitazone (Actos), 651
Piperazines, 266
Placebo effects, 94–97
Placental barrier, 19–20, 574
Placidyl (ethchlorvynol), 491f, 498
Plasticity, synaptic, 2
  NMDA receptor in, 64–65
Polycystic ovary syndrome, 540
Polypharmacy, 92. *See also* Drug interactions

Polyunsaturated fatty acids, for bipolar disorder, 558–559
Pons, 40, 40f, 41f
Poop-out effect, 458
Posterior cingulate cortex, 44, 45f
Postinjection delirium/sedation syndrome, 405
Postpartum depression, 534
Postsynaptic membrane, 49, 52f
Posttraumatic stress disorder, 490. *See also* Anxiety disorders
  antipsychotics for, 419–420
  in children and adolescents, 595
  clinical example of, 674
  marijuana for, 312
  MDMA for, 276
Potency, dose-response curves and, 84–86, 84f
Potentially reduced exposure products, for nicotine dependence, 197
Potiga (ezogabine), 522
Powdered alcohol, 142
Pramipexole (Mirapex), for Parkinson's disease, 639
Pravidoline, 315
Prazepam (Centrax), 492t
Prazosin (Minipress), 507
Precedex (desmedetomidine), 519
Prefrontal cortex, in addiction, 113–114, 114f, 128
Pregabalin (Lyrica), 157, 505, 507, 554
Pregnancy
  alcohol use in, 152–154, 575–576
  anticonvulsants in, 523–524, 549, 581–582
  antidepressants in, 443, 457, 577–579
  antipsychotics in, 579–580
  attention-deficit/hyperactivity disorder in, 576
  benzodiazepines in, 506
  buprenorphine in, 364–365
  caffeine in, 186–187
  cocaine in, 221, 225–226
  criminalization laws and, 577
  drug distribution in, 19–20
  drug therapy in, 573–582
  inhalants in, 167
  lithium in, 546–547
  marijuana in, 309–310, 576
  methadone in, 364–365
  mood stabilizers in, 546–547, 553, 579–582
  opioids in, 352
  placental barrier in, 19–20, 574
  psychostimulants in, 576–577
  smoking in, 196–197, 574–575
  teratogens in, 152–154, 225–226, 574, 575t
Premenstrual dysphoric disorder, 456
Prescal (isradipine), 642

Presynaptic carrier proteins, 78, 79f
Presynaptic membrane, 49, 52f
Priapism, 448
Primary afferents, 340
Primidone, 520f, 521
Pristiq (desvenlafaxine), 441t, 452t, 460
Probuphine (buprenorphine-naloxone), 10, 362
Procaine (Novocaine), 218
Prochlorperazine (Compazine), 389t
Prodrugs, 6
Prolixin (fluphenazine), 389t
Prometa, 245
Propofol (Diprovan), 519
Propoxyphene (Darvon), 357
Propranolol (Inderal)
  for akathisia, 393
  for anxiety, 393
ProSom (estrazolam), 492t, 508t
Protriptyline (Vivactil), 439t
Provigil. *See* Modafinil (Provigil)
Prozac. *See* Fluoxetine (Prozac, Sarafem)
Pseudoephedrine, 235
Psilocin, 268, 269f, 273–274
Psilocybin, 260, 268, 269f, 273–274, 277
Psychedelic drugs, 257–285
  anticholinergic, 258–260, 258t
  catecholaminergic, 258t, 261–268
  classification of, 258, 258t
  designer, 261f, 262, 267
  glutaminergic NMDA receptor antagonists, 279–282
  monoaminergic, 260
  overview of, 257–258
  serotonergic, 268–278, 269f
  serotonin syndrome and, 93
  terminology for, 257
  therapeutic uses of, 275–278
Psychedelic therapy, 275
Psychiatric disorders, substance abuse and. *See* Comorbidity
Psychoactive drugs, definition of, 39
Psycholytic therapy, 275
Psychopharmacology
  challenges facing, 667–678
  definition of, 1
  geriatric, 625–654
  overview of, 1–2
  pediatric. *See* Child and adolescent psychopharmacology
  psychotherapy and. *See* Psychotherapy
Psychosis. *See also* Schizophrenia
  antipsychotics for. *See* Antipsychotics
  ketamine/PCP-induced, 281–282
  methamphetamine-induced, 232
  THC-induced, 298

Psychostimulant(s), 217–248, 684t–685t
  amphetamines, 226–235
  for attention-deficit/hyperactivity disorder, 600–608
  cocaine, 217–226
  for depression, 448–449, 468–469
  for disruptive behavior disorders, 598
  nonamphetamine, 235–242
  in pregnancy, 576–577
  serotonin syndrome and, 93
  side effects of, 607–608
Psychostimulant abuse
  by adolescents, 228–229, 584
  drug therapy for
    dopaminergic/adrenergic approaches in, 242–243
    GABAergic/glutamatergic approaches in, 123–126, 243–244
    metabolizing enzymes in, 246–247
  vaccines for, 247–248
Psychotherapy, 671–672
  cognitive-behavioral therapy, 509, 561, 590
    for insomnia, 509
    for pediatric depression, 590
Psychotomimetics, 257. *See also* Psychedelic drugs
Pupillary constriction, opioid-induced, 348
Pure GABA agonists, 502
Putamen, 43, 43f
α-Pyrrolidinovalerophenone, 238–240

Qsymia (topiramate-phenteramine), 554
Quaalude (methaqualone), 491f, 498
Quazepam (Dormalin), 492t, 508t
Qudexy XR, 554
Quetiapine (Seroquel), 397t
  for bipolar disorder, 415, 535t, 555–558
  for dementia, 628t, 629–630
  for depression, 468
  effectiveness of, 408–410
  indications for, 398t
  for insomnia, 518, 518t
  for obsessive-compulsive disorder, 420
  for Parkinson's disease, 421
  for posttraumatic stress disorder, 419
  for schizophrenia, 405–406, 408–410
  side effects of, 401t, 405–406
QuilliChew ER, 603
Quillivant XR, 602. *See also* Methylphenidate

Racemic mixtures (racemates), 81
Ramelteon (Rozerem), 510t, 515
Rapastinel (GLYX-13), 473, 476
Raphe nuclei, 61
Rasagiline (Azilect), 637, 640
Raves, 263. *See also* Club drugs

Razadyne (galantamine), 646, 647–648
RBP-6000, 363
RBP-7000, 414
Receptors, 49, 50, 50f, 70–84. *See also*
    Pharmacodynamics *and specific types*
  acute vs. chronic effects of, 82–84, 83f
  affinity for, 70
  autoreceptors, 51
  carrier (transport) protein, 77–80, 79f
  cholinergic, 55–56
  definition of, 69
  dose-response curves and, 84–90, 87f, 89f
  downregulation (desensitization) of, 82–84, 83f, 350
  drug binding to, 69
  enzyme, 80
  G-protein-coupled (metabotropic), 55–56, 63, 71f–77f, 72–77, 343–344, 344f
  ion channel (ionotropic), 55–56, 63–65, 65f, 70–72, 71f–73f
  muscarinic, 55–56
  nicotinic, 55–56
  number of, 82n
  side effects and, 81–82
  specificity of, 80–82, 81f
  structure of, 70–80
  subtypes of, 70
  supersensitivity of, 82–84, 83f
  upregulation of, 82–84, 83f
Rectal administration, 8
Relapse, 108–109, 114–115, 115f
Releasing factors, 42
Religion, in drug abuse treatment, 128
Relistor (methylnatrexone), 348
Relprevv. *See* Olanzapine (Relprevv, Zydis, Zyprexa)
REM rebound, 496, 504
Remeron. *See* Mirtazapine (Remeron)
Remifentanyl (Ultiva), 357–358
Remitch (nalfurafine), 368, 369
Remoxy (oxycodone), 355–356
Renal drug elimination, 26–28
Reproductive function, marijuana and, 308–310
Requip (ropinirole), 639
Research Domain Criteria, 670–671
Residence time, 85
Respiratory depression, opioid-induced, 346–347
  naloxone reversal for, 346, 366
Respiratory disease, marijuana-related, 305
Restoril (temazepam), 492t, 508t
Reverse tolerance, 35
Revex (nalmefene), 336t
ReVia. *See* Naltrexone (ReVia, Trexan, Vivitrol)
Reward circuits, 41–42, 44, 45f, 110–115, 110f, 114f, 115f

Brain Disease Model of Addiction and, 110, 117–120

Rexulti (brexpiprazole), 397, 397t, 398t, 399, 401t, 402f, 408, 416, 468

Rimonabant (Acomplia), 123, 306

Risperdal Consta, 414

Risperidone (Risperdal, Fazaclo), 397t
  for autism spectrum disorder, 419
  for bipolar disorder, 415, 535t, 540–541, 555–558
  for borderline personality disorder, 420
  for dementia, 418, 629–630
  for disruptive behavior disorders, 598
  effectiveness of, 408–410
  indications for, 398t
  long-acting depot form, 414
  for obsessive-compulsive disorder, 420
  for Parkinson's disease, 421
  for posttraumatic stress disorder, 419
  side effects of, 404

Ritalin. *See* Methylphenidate (Ritalin)

Rivastigmine (Exelon), 646, 647

RO5545965, 413

Robo-tripping (roboing), 282

Rohypnol (flunitrazepam), 503

Romazicon (flumazenil), 123, 506

Ropinirole (Requip), 639

Rosiglitazone (Avandia), 651

Rostral ventral medulla, 340
  in pain, 340, 341f

Rotigotine (Neupro), 639

Routes of administration, 6–13
  inhalational, 8–9, 9f
  intramuscular, 11t, 12–13
  intravenous, 11–12, 11t
  mucosal, 10
  nasal, 10
  oral, 6–8
  rectal, 8
  spinal, 11t, 13, 13f
  subcutaneous, 11t, 13
  sublingual, 10
  transdermal, 10–11

Rozerem (ramelteon), 510t, 515

RP-5063 (RP-5000), 412, 560

RU-486 (mifepristone), 477

Rufinamide (Banzel), 522

Rylomine (morphine), 336t, 338–339, 352

Sabril (gamma-vinyl-GABA, vigabatrin), 243, 522

St. John's wort, 471

Sally-D, 283–285

Salsolinol, 137n

Salvinorin A, 283–285, 284f, 343n

SAM-e (*S*-adenosylmethionine), 471

Saphris (asenapine), 397t, 398t, 400, 401t, 402f, 407–408, 415, 535t, 555, 556, 559t

Sarafem (fluoxetine), 441t, 456

Sarin, 55

Sativex (nabiximols), 310–311

Savella (milnacipran), 452t

Sazetidine-A, for nicotine dependence, 122, 205

Schizophrenia, 381–386
  cannabis and, 298
  causes of, 381–382
  in children and adolescents, 592–593
  clinical example of, 676
  course and prognosis of, 381, 382
  dopamine in, 382–384
  genetic factors in, 381–382, 385–386
  glutamate in, 382, 385
  hallucinations in, 275
  ketamine and, 279
  marijuana and, 313–315
  neurochemistry of, 382–385
  nicotine and, 193
  NMDA receptors in, 280
  PCP and, 279
  prevention of, 421–422
  risk factors for, 382
  serotonin in, 384
  symptoms of, 381, 384, 390
  treatment of
    agents in, 383f
    antipsychotics in. *See* Antipsychotics
    early intervention in, 421–422
    experimental agents in, 422
    for first episode, 421–422
    future directions for, 421–422
    omega-3 fatty acids in, 421–422, 470
    recommendations for, 414–415

Scopolamine, 258–260, 259f

Screening, for adolescent substance abuse, 586–588

Second messengers, 75–77, 78f, 436

Sedation
  antidepressant-induced, 439t, 441t, 442, 444
  antipsychotic-induced, 401t, 402
  conscious, 495
  opioids for, 347

Sedative-hypnotics, 489–524, 687t
  amnestic effect of, 493–494
  barbiturates, 495–497
  benzodiazepines, 500–506. *See also* Benzodiazepine(s)
  brain dysfunction from, 493–494
  complex sleep-related behaviors and, 511
  conscious sedation and, 495
  for elderly, 495, 501–502
  historical perspective on, 490–493

Sedative-hypnotics (*Continued*)
  indications for, 489
  for insomnia, 508–509, 510t
  memory and, 493–494
  nonbarbiturate, 497–499
  nonbenzodiazepine, 511–514
  overview of, 490–493
  sites and mechanism of action of, 493–494, 493f
  sleep behaviors and, 493–496
  structure of, 491f
Seizures
  alcohol withdrawal, 151
  anticonvulsants for, 519–524, 520f
  benzodiazepines for, 504
  clozapine-induced, 402
  medical marijuana for, 311
Selective norepinephrine reuptake inhibitors
    (SNRIs), for depression, 441t
Selective serotonin reuptake inhibitors
    (SSRIs), 61, 439t, 449–459. *See also*
    Antidepressant(s)
  for alcohol abuse, 144, 162
  codeine and, 353
  drug interactions with, 24
  efficacy of, 433–434, 450, 451, 464–467
  indications for, 450–451, 451t, 452t
  mechanism of action of, 450, 451t
  for nicotine dependence, 202
  opioids and, 24
  pharmacokinetics of, 450, 451t
  serotonin syndrome and, 93, 358, 361, 450, 453
  side effects of, 454–455
  SSRI discontinuation syndrome and, 453–454
  for stimulant abuse, 242
  suicide and, 454, 455f
  withdrawal and, 35
Selective serotonin-norepinephrine reuptake
    inhibitors (SSNRIs), 452t
Selegiline (Eldepryl, Emsam, Zelapar), 439t,
    446–447, 639–640
Selincro (nalmefene), 159, 336t, 367
Septal nuclei, 56
Serax (oxazepam), 245, 492t
Seroquel. *See* Quetiapine (Seroquel)
Serotonergic psychedelics, 268–278, 269f
Serotonin, 61, 61f
  biosynthesis of, 61, 62f
  LSD and, 61, 384
  in schizophrenia, 384
Serotonin pathways, 61–62, 61f
Serotonin receptor antagonists
  for bipolar disorder, 559, 560
  for schizophrenia, 384, 388. *See also*
    Antipsychotics
Serotonin receptors, 61–62, 144

Serotonin syndrome, 93, 358, 361, 453
Serotonin-2 antagonists/reuptake inhibitors,
    441t, 461–462, 474–475. *See also*
    Antidepressant(s)
Serotoninlike psychedelics, 258, 258t. *See also*
    Psychedelic drugs
Serotonin-norepinephrine reuptake inhibitors,
    441t, 459–461
Serotonin-norepinephrine-dopamine reuptake
    inhibitors, 475
Sertindole, 409
Sertraline (Zoloft), 439, 441t, 450, 451t, 452t,
    456–457
  for alcohol abuse, 144, 162
  for bipolar disorder, 556
Serzone (nefazodone), 441t, 461–462
Sexual function
  alcohol and, 146–147
  antidepressants and, 454
  marijuana and, 308–310
  opioids and, 348–349
Shisas, 198
Side effects, 93–94
  definition of, 14
  receptors and, 81–82
Sigma-1 receptor, 273
Silenor (doxepin), 439t, 444
Sinemet (levodopa/carbidopa), 635
Sinequan (doxepin), 439t, 444
Sintocinon, 413
Skin, drug absorption by, 10–11
SKL-PSY/FZ-016, 560
Sleep disturbances
  barbiturates and, 494–495, 496
  benzodiazepines for, 503
  caffeine and, 184
  complex sleep-related activities and, 511
  complex sleep-related behaviors and, 514
  marijuana and, 305
  sedative-hypnotics and, 494–495, 496
  SSRIs and, 454
Sleep driving, 509
Sleep-related behaviors, benzodiazepines and, 509
Smoking. *See also* Nicotine
  age-related restrictions on, 188
  cancer and, 195, 196
  cardiovascular disease and, 195, 196
  cessation of, 189
    benefits of, 189
    craving and, 194
    difficulty of, 194
    mental illness and, 193
    nicotine replacement therapy for, 120, 202,
      205
    pharmacological approaches for, 197–206

vaccines for, 105
vapor products and, 200–202
weight gain after, 194
withdrawal and, 194
e-cigarettes and, 199–202, 301, 582–583
mental health and, 193
menthol cigarettes and, 191
passive smoke and, 196
in pregnancy, 196–197
prevention of, 188
public policy and, 187–189
pulmonary disease and, 195, 196
rates of, 188
regulation of, 188
social costs of, 188–189
Snail toxins, 511
Sniffing, 163–167. *See also* Inhalant abuse
Snus, 198
Social anxiety disorder, 490. *See also* Anxiety
    disorders
Sodium oxybate (Xrem), 499
Sodium phenylbutyrate (Buphenyl), 653
Solaneuzumab, 650
Soma (carisoprodol), 491, 498
Soma (cell body), 49, 50f
Soman, 55
Sonata (zaleplon), 508t, 512f, 513
Souvenaid, 652
Spasticity, marijuana for, 310–311
"Special K," 279–282
Spectrum, 265
Speed, 232. *See also* Amphetamine(s);
    Methamphetamine
Speedballs, 225
"Spice" (synthetic marijuana), 315–318
Spinal cord, 39–40
SSRIs. *See* Selective serotonin reuptake
    inhibitors (SSRIs)
Stablon (tianeptine), 473–474
Stadol (butorphanol), 336t, 365
Stalevo (levodopa/carbidopa/entacapone), 636, 638
Steady-state concentration, 31–33, 32f
Stelazine (trifluoperazine), 389t
STEP-BD study, 539–541
Stephania rotunda, 244
Stevens-Johnson syndrome, 405–406, 550
Stimulants. *See* Psychostimulant(s)
Stinkweed, 259
Stiripentol (Diacomit), 523
Strada (ademetionine), 477
Strattera (atomoxetine), 452t, 604
Stress
    addiction and, 114–115
    alcohol and, 144, 154–155
Striatum, 43

Stroke
    alcohol and, 146
    marijuana and, 305
    smoking cessation after, 206
Structural drug names, 5n
Subcutaneous administration, 11t, 13
Sublimaze. *See* Fentanyl
Sublingual administration, 10
Sublocade, 363
Suboxone (buprenorphine-naloxone), 10, 362
Substance abuse. *See* Alcohol use/abuse; Drug
    abuse; Smoking
Substance Abuse and Mental Health Services
    Administration (SAMHSA), 107
Substance P, 67
Substance Use Disorder, 109
Substantia nigra, 41, 43f, 44
Subsys. *See* Fentanyl
Subthalamic nucleus, 43f, 44
Subutex. *See* Buprenorphine (Subutex)
Succinyl norcocaine, 247
Sudden cardiac death, antipsychotic-induced,
    405, 407f
Sudden sniffing death syndrome, 166
Sufentanil (Sufenta), 357–358
Suicide
    in bipolar disorder, 533, 534, 547
    in pediatric depression, 591
    in schizophrenia, 398–399
    SSRIs and, 454, 455f
    varenicline and, 204
Surmontil (trimipramine), 439t
Sustenna (paliperidone), 397t, 398t
Suvorexant (Belsomra), 508t, 517
Symbyax (olanzapine/fluoxetine), 416, 456, 468,
    556, 559t
Symmetrel. *See* Amantadine (Symmetrel)
Sympathetic nervous system, 226n
Sympathomimetics, 217. *See also*
    Psychostimulant(s)
Synapses, 49–51, 52f
Synaptic cleft, 49, 52f
Synaptic plasticity, 2
    NMDA receptor in, 64–65
Synaptic transmission, 48–53. *See also*
    Neurotransmitters
Synaptic vesicles, 49, 52f
Synthetic fentanyl derivatives, 372–373
Synthetic marijuana, 108, 315–318, 316, 586
    clinical example of, 676–677
    current abuse, 316–317
    effects and toxicity of, 317, 318f
    forms of, 315, 316n
    treatment for, 316
    vaping and, 316

T7, 265
Tabex (cytosine), 202
TA-CD vaccine, 247–248
Tachyphylaxis, 35
Tacrine (Cognex), 646
TAK-063, 413
Talampanel, 125
Talwin (pentazocine), 336t, 365
Tapentadol (Nucynta), 336t, 358–359
Tarceva (erlotinib), 652
Tardive dyskinesia, 384, 387, 394–396
Tarenflurbil, 650
Targiniq-ER, 367–368
Targretin (bexarotene), 652
Tasigna (nilotinib), 642
Tasimelteon, 516
Tasmar (tolcapone), 638
Tau kinase inhibitors, 653
Tea. See Caffeine
Tectum, 41
Tedatioxetine, 475
Teenagers. See Adolescents
Tegmentum, 41
Tegretol. See Carbamazepine (Equetro, Tegretol)
Telencephalon, 40f, 43f, 44, 45f
Temazepam (Restoril), 492t, 508t
Temporal lobe, 44, 46f
Teratogens, 152–154, 225–226, 574, 575t
Testicular cancer, marijuana and, 309
Tetrabenazine (Xenazine), for tardive dyskinesia, 394
Tetrahydrocannabinol (THC), 295–298, 295f, 296f, 301–302
Tetrahydrocannabinolic acid (THCa), 295–296, 295f, 301–302
Tetrahydropalmatine, 244–245
Tezampanel, 125
TFMPP (1,(3-trifluoromethylphenyl) piperazine, 266
Thalamus, 42, 42f
THC (delta-9 tetrahydrocannabinol), 295–298, 295f, 296f, 301–302
THCa (tetrahydrocannabinolic acid), 295–296, 295f, 301–302
Thebaine, 335
Theobromine, 177, 179, 183
Theophylline, 177, 179
Therapeutic drug monitoring, 33, 34f, 443
Therapeutic index, 90–97
Therapeutic window, 33
Thiopental (Pentothal), 519
Thioridazine (Mellaril), 389t
Thiothixene (Navane), 389t
Thorazine (chlorpromazine), 386, 389t
Thorn apple, 259

Thrombotic thrombocytopenic purpura, 356
Thymanax (agomelatine), 474, 507, 516
Tiagabine (Gabitril), 244, 520f, 522
Tianeptine (Stablon), 473–474
TK-301, 516
TLR4 receptor, in opioid abuse, 370
TMA (trimethoxyamphetamine), 261f, 263, 267
TMF (3-methyl-fentanyl), 372
Tofranil (imipramine), 439t, 442, 443
Tolcapone (Tasmar), 638
Tolerance, 34–36, 82, 83f, 112
Toluene abuse, 164t, 167. See also Inhalant abuse
Toonies, 265
Topiramate (Topamax, Topiragen), 520f, 522
    for alcohol abuse, 157, 161–162
    for bipolar disorder, 535t, 554–555
    for cannabis dependence, 321
    for drug abuse, 124–125, 244, 321
    in pregnancy, 554–555, 581
Topiramate-phenteramine (Qsymia), 554
Torsade de pointes, antipsychotic-induced, 405, 406f, 407f
Toxic epidermal necrolysis, 550
Toxicity. See Side effects
Trade drug names, 5n
Tramadol (Ultram), 336t, 361, 593
Tramiprosate, 650
Tranquilizers, 498. See also Anxiolytics
Transcytosis, 19
Transdermal patches, 10–11
Transporters, 19, 77–80, 79f
Tranxene (chlorazepate), 492t
Tranylcypromine (Parnate), 439t, 445–446
Traumatic brain injury, cannabinoids for, 311
Trazodone (Desyrel, Oleptro), 439t, 447, 518t
Tremor, antipsychotics and, 393
Trexan. See Naltrexone (ReVia, Trexan, Vivitrol)
Triazolam (Halcion), 4–5, 5f, 492t, 508t, 511
Tricyclic antidepressants, 434f, 438–440, 439t, 442–445. See also Antidepressant(s)
Trifluoperazine (Stelazine), 389t
Trifluoromethylphenylpiperazine (TFMPP), 266
Trihexyphenidyl (Artane), 641
Trilafon (perphenazine), 389t
Trileptal. See Oxcarbazepine (Trileptal)
Trimethoxyamphetamine (TMA), 261f, 263, 267
Trimipramine (Surmontil), 439t
Trintellix (vortioxetine), 441t, 449
Trinza (paliperidone), 397t, 398t
Tripelennamine, 365
Triple reuptake inhibitors, 475
Tripstay, 265
Triptans, serotonin syndrome and, 93
Trokendi XR, 554
"Ts and blues," 365

Tweety-Bird Mescaline, 265
2C-B (4-bromo-2,5-dimethoxyphenethylamine), 263, 265, 266
2C-T-7, 265
2s, 265
Tyramine, MAOIs and, 446

U-47700, 373
Ulcerative colitis of bladder, ketamine-induced, 281
Ultiva (remifentanyl), 357–358
Ultram (tramadol), 336t, 361, 593
UMB-425, 369
Urine testing, 20n
  for heroin, 353
  for marijuana, 302

Vaccines, 127
  for cocaine abuse, 247–248
  for methamphetamine abuse, 247–248
  for nicotine dependence, 205
  for opioid abuse, 370
Valbenazine (Ingrezza), for tardive dyskinesia, 394
Valdoxan (agomelatine), 474, 507, 516
Valium. *See* Diazepam (Valium)
Valnoctamide, 552
Valproic acid (Depakene, Depakote, Depacon, Divalproex), 520f, 521, 524, 559t
  for alcohol withdrawal, 157
  for bipolar disorder, 535t, 536, 540, 551–552, 559t
  for cocaine abuse, 243
  for disruptive behavior disorders, 498
  polycystic ovary syndrome and, 540
  in pregnancy, 581
Vantrela, 355
Vaping
  of natural marijuana, 301, 585
  of synthetic marijuana, 316
  of tobacco, 199–202
Varenicline (Chantix)
  for alcohol addiction, 121
  for nicotine addiction, 121, 202
Venlafaxine (Effexor), 452t, 460
  for bipolar disorder, 556
  for depression, 441t, 590
Ventral tegmental area (VTA), 41, 44, 45f, 110–112, 110f, 116, 116f, 192
Venus, 265
Versed (midazolam), 492t, 495
Vicodin (hydrocodone/acetaminophen), 336t, 354–355
Vigabatrin (gamma-vinyl-GABA, Sabril), 123, 243, 522
Vilazodone (Viibryd), 441t, 449, 451t, 452t, 463
Vimpat (lacosamide), 522
Vinodhamine, 299, 300f

Virtioxetine (Trintellix), 449
Visceral (autonomic) nervous system, 226
Vivactil (protriptyline), 439t
Vivitrol. *See* Naltrexone (ReVia, Trexan, Vivitrol)
Voke, 199
Vomiting
  marijuana-induced, 306
  opioid-induced, 347
Von Economo neurons, 46–47
Vortioxetine (Trintellix), 441t, 463–464
Vraylar (cariprazine), 397, 399–400, 401t, 402f, 408, 417, 535t, 557
Vyvanse (lisdexamfetamine), 6, 229, 608

W-18, 373
Water pipes, 198
Weight gain
  after smoking cessation, 194
  antipsychotic-related, 400, 401, 401t, 402f, 403, 404
Weight loss, caffeine and, 181
Wellbutrin. *See* Bupropion
Whippets, 518
WIN-55212-2, 315
Withdrawal, 35, 109–110
  alcohol, 150–151, 156–157, 161–162
  amphetamine, 235
  antidepressant, 35
  caffeine, 187
  in cocaine-exposed infants, 226
  inhalant, 167
  marijuana, 319
  nicotine, 194
  opioid, 350–351, 351t
  stress and, 114–115
  synthetic marijuana, 317
Women, blood alcohol concentration in, 137, 141f

Xanax (alprazolam), 492t, 503–504
Xanthines, 177, 179–180, 179f
Xartemix-XR, 356
xCT (cystine-glutamate exchanger), 117, 123–124
Xenazine (tetrabenazine), for tardive dyskinesia, 394
Xrem (sodium oxybate), 499
Xtampza-ER (oxycodone), 355
Xyrem (gamma hydroxybutyrate), 498–499

YXP-3089, 560

Z drugs, 511, 512f
Zaleplon (Sonata), 508t, 512f, 513
Zelapar (selegiline), 439t, 639–640
Zero-order elimination (kinetics), 31, 138n
Zinc cysteine, for Alzheimer's disease, 651

Ziprasidone (Geodon), 6, 409
   for bipolar disorder, 535t, 555–558, 559t
   for depression, 468
   indications for, 398t
   for posttraumatic stress disorder, 419
   side effects of, 401t, 405–406
Zoftran (ondansetron), 162
Zohydro (hydrocodone), 355
Zoloft. *See* Sertraline (Zoloft)

Zolpidem (Ambien, Edluar, Intermezzo),
   511–513, 511t, 512f
Zonisamide (Zonegran), 162, 522, 535t
Zoplicone (Immovane), 514
Zotepine, 409
Zyban. *See* Bupropion
Zydis. *See* Olanzapine (Relprevv, Zydis, Zyprexa)
Zyprexa (olanzapine). *See* Olanzapine (Relprevv,
   Zydis, Zyprexa)